Operative Arthroscopy

Fourth Edition

Operative Arthroscopy

Fourth Edition

Editor-in-Chief

Donald H. Johnson, MD, FRCSC
Director
Sports Medicine Clinic
Carleton University
Assistant Professor
Orthopaedic Surgery
University of Ottawa
Ottawa, Canada

Annunziato Amendola, MD
Professor, Department of Orthopedic
Surgery and Rehabilitation
Kim and John Callaghan Chair
Director of Sports Medicine
University of Iowa
Iowa City, Iowa

F. Alan Barber, MD, FACS
Fellowship Director
Plano Orthopedics Sports Medicine
and Spine Center
Plano, Texas

Larry D. Field, MD
Director, Upper Extremity Service
Mississippi Sports Medicine &
Orthopaedic Center
Clinical Instructor
University of Mississippi School of Medicine
Jackson, Mississippi

John C. Richmond, MD
Chairman, Department of Orthopedic Surgery
New England Baptist Hospital
Professor, Orthopaedic Surgery
Tufts University School of Medicine
Boston, Massachusetts
Boston Sports and Shoulder Center
Chestnut Hill, Massachusetts

Nicholas A. Sgaglione, MD
Chairman, Department of
Orthopaedic Surgery
Professor of Orthopaedic Surgery
Hofstra North Shore-LIJ School of Medicine
North Shore Long Island Jewish
Medical Center

 Wolters Kluwer | Lippincott Williams & Wilkins
Health
Philadelphia • Baltimore • New York • London
Buenos Aires • Hong Kong • Sydney • Tokyo

Acquisitions Editor: Brian Brown
Product Manager: Dave Murphy
Marketing Manager: Lisa Lawrence
Design Manager: Doug Smock
Manufacturing Manager: Benjamin Rivera
Production Services: S4 Carlisle Publishing Services

© Copyright 2013

Printed in China

978-1-60547-860-9
1-60547-860-1

Library of Congress Cataloging-in-Publication Data

Operative arthroscopy.—4th ed. / editor-in-chief, Donald H. Johnson . . . [et al.].
    p. ; cm.
Rev. ed. of: Operative arthroscopy / editor-in-chief, John B. McGinty. 3rd ed. c2003.
Includes bibliographical references and index.
Summary: "Arthroscopy has become the major tool for orthopaedic surgeons fixing ligament problems in almost every anatomic joint in the human body. Chapter format to focus on how-to-do-it material. The anatomic areas now covered are those that the sports medicine specialist will typically handle" —Provided by publisher.
ISBN 978-1-60547-860-9 (alk. paper)
I. Johnson, Donald (Donald Hugh)
[DNLM: 1. Joints—surgery.   2. Arthroscopy—methods. WE 312]
LC classification not assigned
617.4'720597—dc23
                                 2012029433

DISCLAIMER

Dedication

To my wife Sherry and my children Shannon, Collin and Cameron for all their love and support.

—ALAN BARBER

To my wife Leslie whose magnificent love, exquisite beauty and deep strength of being have always been and always will be the source of my inspiration and purpose.

To my children Nicholas, Caroline, Jonathan and Matthew, whose bright futures and rich blessings abound. Your daily gifts are far greater than I could ever give back to each of you.

To my parents Jennie and Nick for your unconditional love and guidance.

—NICK SGAGLIONE

To my wonderful wife, Cindy, and our three children, Eric, Evelyn, and Adam. Thank you for your sacrifices and understanding. Your love and support make everything possible.

—LARRY D. FIELD

"To my wife Chris and my children Scott and Mike for all that they have given to me through the years."

—JOHN RICHMOND

I dedicate this book to my best friend and wife Alison, and four wonderful children Richie, Julie, Andy and Christine, who have made my life beautiful.

—ANNUNZIATO AMENDOLA

DEDICTATION – FOURTH EDITION OF OPERATIVE ARTHROSCOPY

The Fourth Edition of Operative Arthroscopy is dedicated to John B. McGinty, M.D. He is the retired Professor and Chairman of the Department of Orthopedic Surgery at the Medical University of South Carolina in Charleston, S.C. He was the Editor-in-Chief of the first three editions of this text, and has clearly left a lasting imprint in the field of arthroscopic surgery. Jack McGinty was the first President of the Arthroscopy Association of North America (AANA) from 1982 to 1983. AANA has thrived and remains committed to Dr. McGinty's love for education and arthroscopy. Dr. McGinty went on to be the President of the American Academy of Orthopedic Surgery in 1990.

We as arthroscopic surgeons all owe Dr. McGinty a debt of gratitude for his vision and his commitment to education. He has been our inspiration as we put together the Fourth Edition of Operative Arthroscopy. We thank him for his commitment to create the definitive textbook of operative arthroscopic surgery, and dedicate this Fourth Edition to him.

Contents

Contributors

Sami Abdulmassih, MD
Foot and Ankle Fellow
Department of Orthopedic Surgery
and Rehabilitation
University of Iowa, Iowa

Jeffrey S. Abrams, MD
Medical Director
Princeton Orthopaedic &
Rehabilitation Associates
Chief, Shoulder Surgery
Sports Medicine Princeton
Attending Surgeon
Department of Surgery
University Medical Center at
Princeton
Princeton, New Jersey

Olusanjo Adeoye, MD
Fellow, Sports Medicine
Sports Medicine, Department of
Orthopaedic Surgery
Stanford University
Redwood City, California

Robert Afra, MD
Assistant Clinical Professor
Department of Orthopaedic
Surgery
University of California, San Diego
San Diego, California

David W. Altchek, MD
Co-Chief Sports Medicine Service
Hospital for Special Surgery
New York, New York

Annunziato Amendola, MD
Professor
Department of Orthopaedics and
Rehabilitation
Director and Callaghan Chair
UI Sports Medicine
University of Iowa
Iowa City, Iowa

Richard L. Angelo, MD
Clinical Professor
Department of Orthopedics
University of Washington
Seattle, Washington
Evergreen Orthopedic Clinic
Kirkland, Washington

Evan Argintar, MD
Resident Physician
Georgetown University Hospital
Center for Hand and Elbow
Specialists
Washington, DC

Amar Arora, MD
Department of Orthopaedic
Surgery
Sharp Rees-Stealy Medical Group
San Diego, California

Champ L. Baker III, MD
Staff Physician
The Hughston Clinic
Columbus, Georgia

Champ L. Baker Jr., MD
Staff Physician
The Hughston Clinic
Columbus, Georgia
Clinical Assistant Professor
Department of Orthopaedics
Medical College of Georgia
Augusta, Georgia

F. Alan Barber, MD, FACS
Fellowship Director
Plano Orthopedics Sports Medicine
and Spine Center
Plano, Texas

William R. Beach, MD
Orthopaedics Research of Virginia
Tuckahoe Orthopaedic
Associates Ltd
Richmond, Virginia

Timothy C. Beals, MD
Associate Professor
Department of Orthopaedics
University of Utah
Salt Lake City, Utah

R. Cole Beavis, MD, FRCSC
Clinical Assistant Professor of
Surgery
University of Saskatchewan
Saskatoon, SK Canada

John D. Beck, MD
Resident
GHS Orthopaedics
Danville, Pennsylvania

Robert H. Bell, MD
Associate Professor
Department of Orthopaedics
Northeastern Ohio University
School of Medicine
Rootstown, Ohio
Chief of Shoulder and Elbow
Surgery
Department of Orthopaedics
Summa Health Systems
Akron, Ohio

Massimo Berruto, MD
Knee Surgery Department
Ist.Ort. G. Pini
Milan, Italy

Jack M. Bert, MD
Summit Orthopedics, Ltd
Adjunct Clinical Professor
University of Minnesota School of
Medicine
St. Paul, Minnesota

Patrick Birmingham, MD
Department of Orthopaedic
Surgery
Hospital for Special Surgery
New York, New York

Brad D. Blankenhorn, MD
Visiting Instructor
Department of Orthopaedic
    Surgery
University of Utah Health Care
Salt Lake City, Utah

Yaw Boachie-Adjei, MD
Department of Orthopaedics
University of Virginia School of
    Medicine
Charlottesville, Virginia

Davide Edoardo Bonasia, MD
University of Iowa Sports Medicine
    Fellow
University of Iowa
Iowa City, Iowa
University of Turin Medical School
Mauriziano "Umberto I" Hospital
Turin, Italy

Kevin F. Bonner, MD
Jordan-Young Institute
Virginia Beach, Virginia

Andrea L. Bowers, MD
Senior Clinical Instructor
Department of Orthopedic
    Surgery
Weill Cornell Medical College
Fellow
Sports Medicine & Shoulder
    Service
Hospital for Special Surgery
New York, New York

John H. Brady, MD, MPH
San Diego Sports Medicine &
    Orthopaedic Center
San Diego, California

Paul C. Brady, MD
Tennessee Orthopaedic Clinics
Orthopaedic Surgeon
Shoulder Specialist
Tennessee Orthopaedic Clinics
Knoxville, Tennessee

Karen K Briggs, MPH
Steadman Philippon Research
    Institute
Vail, Colorado

Peter U. Brucker, MD
Department of Orthopaedic Sports
    Medicine
Klinikum Rechts der Isar
Technische Universität München
Munich, Germany

Joseph P. Burns, MD
Southern California Orthopaedic
    Institute
Van Nuys, California

James A. Bynum, MD
Plano Orthopedic Sports Medicine
    and Spine Center
Plano, Texas

J. W. Thomas Byrd, M.D.
Nashville Sports Medicine
    Foundation
Nashville, Tennessee

Lawrence Camarda, MD
Department of Orthopaedic Surgery
University of Palermo
Palermo, Italy

Filippo Castoldi, MD
Assistant Professor in Orthopaedics
    and Traumatology,
University of Turin Medical School
Mauriziano "Umberto I" Hospital
Turin, Italy

Terence Y. P. Chin, MBBS, FRACS
Fellow
Dalhousie University Orthopedics
Halifax, Nova Scotia

James Campbell Chow, MD
Hip & Knee Specialist
Arizona Center for Bone & Joint
    Disorders
Phoenix, Arizona

James C. Y. Chow, MD
Orthopaedic Center of Southern
    Illinois
Mt Vernon, Illinois

Benjamin I. Chu, MD
Orthopaedic Research of Virginia
Richmond, Virginia

OrthopaediCare
Chalfont, Pennsylvania

Brian J. Cole, MD, MBA
Division of Sports Medicine
Department of Orthopaedic
    Surgery
Rush University Medical Center
Rush Medical College of Rush
    University
Chicago, Illinois

Andrew J. Cosgarea, MD
Professor
Department of Orthopaedic Surgery
Johns Hopkins University
Director
Division of Sports Medicine and
    Shoulder Surgery
Johns Hopkins Hospital
Baltimore, Maryland

Alan S. Curtis, MD
Assistant Clinical Professor
Tufts University School of
    Medicine
Orthopedic Surgeon
New England Baptist Hospital
Boston, Massachusetts
Boston Sports and Shoulder Center
Chestnut Hill, Massachusetts

Thomas DeBerardino, MD
Associate Professor
University of Connecticut Health
    Center
Farmington, Connecticut

Michael J. Defranco, MD
Shoulder Fellow
Department of Orthopaedic
    Surgery
Harvard Shoulder Service
Fellow
Department of Orthopaedics
Massachusetts General Hospital
Boston, Massachusetts

Peter A.J. de Leeuw, MD, PhD
Fellow
Academic Medical Centre
Department of Orthopedic Surgery
Amsterdam, The Netherlands

Matthew Denkers, MD, FRCSC
Arthroscopy Fellow
Department of Surgery
University of Calgary
Calgary, AB, Canada

Robert C. Dews, MD
Fellow
Mississippi Sports Medicine and
    Orthopaedic Center
Jackson, Mississippi

David B. Dickerson, MD
Fellow
Orthopaedic Foundation for Active
    Lifestyles
Plancher Orthopaedics & Sports
    Medicine
Cos Cob, Connecticut and
    New York, New York

Christopher C. Dodson, MD
Attending Orthopaedic Surgeon
Rothman Institute
Philadelphia, Pennsylvania

Jonathan A. Donigan, MD
Department of Orthopaedics and
    Rehabilitation
University of Iowa Hospitals and
    Clinics
Iowa City, Iowa

Ryan M. Dopirak, MD
Lakeshore Orthopaedics
Manitowoc, Wisconsin

Raymond R. Drabicki, MD
Fellow
Mississippi Sports Medicine &
    Orthopaedic Center
Jackson, Mississippi

Alex Dukas, MA
SUNY Downstate Medical Center
Brooklyn, New York

Cory Edgar, MD, PhD
Assistant Professor
Department of Orthopedic Surgery
Boston Medical Center Team
    Physician
Boston University
Boston, Massachusetts

Craig J. Edson, MS, PT, ATC
Fanelli Sports Injury Clinic
Geisinger Medical Center
Danville, Pennsylvania

Scott G. Edwards, MD
Associate Professor
Georgetown University Hospital
Center for Hand and Elbow Specialists
Washington, DC

Alberto N. Evia-Ramirez, MD
Clinical and Research Fellow at the
    Service of Adult Hip and Knee
    Reconstruction of the National
    Rehabilitation Institute of Mexico

Paul Fadale, MD
Department of Orthopaedic Surgery
Division of Sports Medicine
Rhode Island Hospital
Warren Alpert Medical School of
    Brown University
Providence, Rhode Island

Gregory C. Fanelli, MD
GHS Orthopaedics
Danville, Pennsylvania

Kevin W. Farmer, MD
Adjunct Clinical Postdoctoral
    Associate
Department of Orthopaedic Surgery
The University of Florida
Gainesville, Florida

John E. Femino, MD
Associate Clinical Professor
Department of Orthopaedics &
    Rehabilitation
University of Iowa
Iowa City, Iowa

Richard D. Ferkel, MD
Associate Clinical Professor
Department of Orthopaedic Surgery
University of California, Los Angeles
Los Angeles, California
Program Director
Sports Medicine Fellowship
Southern California Orthopedic
    Institute
Van Nuys, California

Larry D. Field, MD
Director
Upper Extremity Service
Mississippi Sports Medicine &
    Orthopaedic Center
Clinical Instructor
University of Mississippi School of
    Medicine
Jackson, Mississippi

Giuseppe Filardo, MD
Biomechanic's Lab IX Div.
Ist. Ort. Rizzoli
Bologna, Italy

Craig J. Finlayson, MD
Fellow
Children's Hospital Boston
Department of Orthopaedic
    Surgery
Division of Sports Medicine
Boston Massachusetts

Donald C. Fithian, MD
Department of Orthopedic Surgery
Southern California Permanente
    Medical Group
El Cajon, California

Nicole A. Friel, MS
Division of Sports Medicine
Department of Orthopaedic
    Surgery
Rush University Medical Center
Rush Medical College of Rush
    University
Chicago, Illinois

Freddie H. Fu, MD, DSci(Hon),
DPs(Hon)
David Silver Professor and Chairman
Department of Orthopaedic Surgery
University of Pittsburgh Medical
    Center
Pittsburgh, Pennsylvania

John P. Fulkerson, MD
Clinical Professor of Orthopedic
    Surgery
University of Connecticut
Orthopedic Associates of
    Hartford, PC
Farmington, Connecticut

Aaron Gardiner, MD
Assistant Clinical Professor
Tufts University School of Medicine
Orthopedic Surgeon
Newton-Wellesley Hospital
Newton Wellesley Orthopedic
    Associates
Newton, Massachusetts

William B. Geissler, MD
Professor and Chief
Division of Hand and Upper
    Extremity Surgery
Chief-Arthroscopic Surgery and
    Sports Medicine
Department of Orthopaedic
    Surgery and Rehabilitation
University of Mississippi Health
    Care
Jackson, Mississippi

Neil Ghodadra, MD
Department of Orthopaedic Surgery
Rush University
Chicago, Illinois

Steven A. Giuseffi, MD
Orthopedic Surgery Resident
Mayo Clinic
Rochester, Minnesota

Mark Glazebrook, MSc, PhD,
MD, FRCS(C), Dip Sports Med
Assistant Professor
Dalhousie University
    Orthopaedics
Director of Foot and Ankle
    Orthopaedics
The Department of Orthopaedic
    Surgery
New Halifax Infirmary, Queen
    Elizabeth II HSC
Halifax, Nova Scotia, Canada

Ronald E. Glousman, MD
Kerlan-Jobe Orthopaedic Clinic
Los Angeles, California

Alberto Gobbi, MD
Oasi Bioresearch Foundation
    Gobbi NPO
Milan, Italy

John, P. Goldblatt, MD
University of Rochester
Rochester, New York

Matthew J. Goldstein, MD
Resident
Department of Orthopaedic Surgery
North Shore-Long Island Jewish
    Health System
Great Neck, New York

Troy M. Gorman, MD
Orthopaedic Surgeon
Intermountain Healthcare—LDS
    Hospital
Salt Lake City, Utah

Robert C. Grumet, MD
Department of Orthopaedic Surgery
St Joseph Medical Center
Orthopaedic Specialty Institute
Orange, California

Carlos A. Guanche, MD
Southern California Orthopedic
    Institute
Van Nuys, California

James J. Guerra, MD, FACS
Collier Sports Medicine and
    Orthopaedic Center
Naples, Florida

Onur Hapa, MD
Plano Orthopedic Sports Medicine
    and Spine Center
Plano, Texas

David Hergan, MD
Department of Orthopaedic Surgery
NYU Medical Center
New York, New York

Laurence D. Higgins, MD
Associate Professor
Department of Orthopaedics
Harvard Medical School
Chief
Sports Medicine and Shoulder
    Service
Brigham and Women's Hospital
Boston, Massachusetts

Beat Hintemann, MD
Associate Professor
Department of Orthopaedic Surgery
University of Basel
Basel, Switzerland
Chairman
Clinic of Orthopaedic Surgery
Kantonsspital
Liestal, Switzerland

E. Rhett Hobgood, MD
Mississippi Sports Medicine and
    Orthopaedic Center
Jackson, Mississippi

Victor M. Ilizaliturri Jr., MD
Chief of Adult Hip and Knee
    Reconstruction
The National Rehabilitation
    Institute of Mexico
Professor of Hip and Knee Surgery
Universidad Nacional Autónoma
    de México
The National Rehabilitation
    Institute of Mexico
Mexico City, Mexico

Andreas M. Imhoff, MD
Department of Orthopaedic Sports
    Medicine
Klinikum Rechts der Isar
Technische Universität München
Munich, Germany

Darren L Johnson, MD
University of Kentucky
Department of Orthopaedic Surgery
    and Sports Medicine
Lexington, Kentucky

Donald H. Johnson,
MD, FRCSC
Director, Sports Medicine Clinic
Carleton University
Assistant Professor
Orthopaedic Surgery
University of Ottawa
Ottawa, Canada

Georgios Karnatziko, MD
O.A.S.I. Bioresearch Foundation
N.P.O. Milan, Italy

Ronald P. Karzel, MD
Attending Orthopedic Surgeon
Southern California Orthopedic
    Institute
Van Nuys, California

Bryan T. Kelly, MD
Hospital for Special Surgery
New York, New York

Gino M. M. J. Kerkhoffs,
MD, PhD
Orthopaedic Surgeon
Academic Medical Centre
Department of Orthopedic Surgery
Amsterdam, The Netherlands

Elizabeth A. Kern, BA
Orthopaedic Foundation for Active
    Lifestyles
Plancher Orthopaedics & Sports
    Medicine
Cos Cob, Connecticut and
    New York, New York

Graham J. W. King, MD, MSc,
FRCSC
Professor
Department of Surgery
University of Western Ontario
Chief
Orthopaedic Surgery
St. Joseph's Health Centre
Hand and Upper Limb Centre
London, Ontario, Canada

Chlodwig Kirchhoff, MD
Department of Orthopedic Sports
    Surgery
Klinikum Rechts der Isar
Technische Universitaet Muenchen
Munich, Germany

Mininder S. Kocher, MD, MPH
Associate Professor
Department of Orthopaedic Surgery
Harvard Medical School
Associate Director
Orthopaedics—Division of Sports
    Medicine
Children's Hospital Boston
Boston, Massachusetts

Jason Koh, MD
NorthShore University
    HealthSystem
A Teaching Affiliate of the
    University of Chicago Pritzker
    School of Medicine
Department of Orthopaedic Surgery
Evanston, Illinois

Elizaveta Kon, MD
Biomechanic's Lab IX Division
Ist. Ort. Rizzoli
Bologna, Italy

Sumant G. "Butch" Krishnan, MD
Director, Shoulder Fellowship
Baylor University Medical Center
Attending Orthopaedic Surgeon
Shoulder Service
The Carrell Clinic
Dallas, Texas

Peter R. Kurzweil, MD
Memorial Orthopaedic Surgical
    Group
Long Beach, California

Marc R. Labbé, MD
Clinical Assistant Professor
Department of Orthopaedic
    Surgery
Baylor College of Medicine
Houston, Texas
Clinical Assistant Professor
Department of Orthopaedic
    Surgery
University of Texas Medical
    Center
Galveston, Texas

Robert F. LaPrade, MD, PhD
Sports Medicine and Complex Knee
    Surgery
The Steadman Clinic
Chief Medical Research Officer
Steadman Philippon Research
    Institute
Adjunct Professor
Department of Orthopaedic
    Surgery
University of Minnesota
Vail, Colorado

Christopher M. Larson, MD
Director of Education
Minnesota Sports Medicine
    Fellowship Program
Minnesota Orthopaedic and Sports
    Medicine Institute
Twin Cities Orthopaedics
Eden Prairie, Minnesota

Johnny Tak-Choy Lau, MSc, MD,
FRCS(C)
Assistant Professor
University of Toronto Orthopaedics
Toronto, Ontario

Matthew R. Lavery, MD
OrthoIndy
Sports Medicine
Indianapolis, Indiana

Sheryl L. Lipnick, DO
Fellow
Orthopaedic Foundation for Active
    Lifestyles
Plancher Orthopaedics & Sports
    Medicine
Cos Cob, Connecticut and
    New York, New York

Ian K.Y. Lo, MD, FRCSC
Assistant Professor
McCaig Junior Professor of
    Orthopedics
Department of Surgery
University of Calgary
Calgary, AB, Canada

Emilio Lopez-Vidriero, MD, PhD
Fellow in Sports Medicine and
    Arthroscopy
Department of Orthopaedics,
    Ottawa Hospital
Ottawa, Ontario, Canada

James H. Lubowitz, MD
Director
Taos Orthopaedic Institute Research
    Foundation and Orthopaedic
    Sports Medicine Fellowship
Active Staff
Department of Surgery
Holy Cross Hospital
Taos, New Mexico

Robert M. Lucas, MD
Department of Orthopaedic
    Surgery
University of California, San
    Francisco
San Francisco, California

Milford H. Marchant Jr., MD
Kerlan-Jobe Orthopaedic
    Clinic
Los Angeles, California

Craig S. Mauro, MD
University of Pittsburgh Medical
    Center
Burke and Bradley Orthopedics
Pittsburgh, Pennsylvania

Augustus D. Mazzocca, MS, MD
Associate Professor of Orthopaedic
    Surgery
University of Connecticut
Orthopaedic Team Physician
University of Connecticut
    Athletics
Director of the Human Soft Tissue
    Research Laboratory
Director of Orthopaedic Resident
    Education
Shoulder and Elbow Surgery
Farmington, Connecticut

Mark McCarthy, MD
Department of Orthopaedic
    Surgery
University of Iowa
Iowa City, Iowa

Mark E. McKenna, MD
Resident
GHS Orthopaedics
Danville, Pennsylvania

Mark D. Miller, MD
S. Ward Casscells Professor of
    Orthopaedic Surgery
University of Virginia Team
    Physician
James Madison University
JBJS Deputy Editor for Sports
    Medicine
Director, Miller Review Course
Charlottesville, Virginia

Suzanne L. Miller, MD
Assistant Clinical Professor
Tufts University School of
    Medicine
Orthopedic Surgeon
New England Baptist Hospital
Boston, Massachusetts
Boston Sports and Shoulder
    Center
Chestnut Hill, Massachusetts

Bryan Mitchell, MD
University of Rochester
Rochester, New York

Keith O. Monchik, MD
Foundry Orthopedics & Sports
    Medicine
Clinical Assistant Professor
Brown Alpert Medical School
Providence, Rhode Island

Jill Monson, PT, CSCS
University Orthopaedics Therapy
    Center
Minneapolis, Minnesota

Mark Morishige, MD
Fellow
Mississippi Sports Medicine and
    Orthopaedic Center
Jackson, Mississippi

Steven Mussett, MBChB, FRCS(C)
Fellow
University of Toronto
    Orthopaedics
Toronto, Ontario

Adam Nasreddine, BS
Research Coordinator
Children's Hospital Boston
Department of Orthopaedic
    Surgery
Graduate Students
Boston University, School of
    Medicine
Boston, Massachusetts

Florian Nickisch, MD
Associate Professor
Department of Orthopaedic Surgery
University of Utah Health Care
Salt Lake City, Utah

Curtis R. Noel, MD
Instructor
Department of Orthopaedics
Summa Health Systems
Akron, Ohio

Keith D. Nord, MD, MS
Sports, Orthopedics & Spine, PC
Shoulder Arthroscopy & Sports
    Medicine Fellowship Director
Sports, Orthopedics & Spine
    Educational Foundation
Sports, Orthopedics & Spine
Jackson, Tennessee

Frank Noyes, MD
Chairman and Medical Director
Cincinnati Sports Medicine and
    Orthopaedic Center
President
Cincinnati Sports Medicine
    Research and Education
    Foundation
Volunteer Professor
Department of Orthopaedic
    Surgery
University of Cincinnati
Cincinnati, Ohio

Michael J. O'Brien, MD
Assistant Professor
Tulane University
Department of Orthopaedics
New Orleans, Louisiana

Athanasios A. Papachristos, MD
Fellow
Orthopaedic Research Foundation
    of Southern Illinois
Mt. Vernon, Illinois

Derek F. Papp, MD
Resident
Department of Orthopaedic Surgery
Johns Hopkins University
Baltimore, Maryland

Robert A. Pedowitz, MD, PhD
Professor of Orthopaedic
    Surgery
David Geffen School of Medicine at
    UCLA
Los Angeles, California

Fernando Pena, MD
Assistant Professor
Department of Orthopaedics
University of Minnesota
Minneapolis, Minnesota

Michael Pensak, MD
University of Connecticut Health
Center
Farmington, Connecticut

Marc J. Philippon, MD
Steadman Philippon Research
Institute
Vail, Colorado

Phinit Phisitkul, MD
Assistant Clinical Professor
Department of Orthopaedic Surgery
University of Iowa
Iowa City, Iowa

Kevin D. Plancher, MD
Associate Clinical Professor
Albert Einstein College of Medicine
New York, New York
Fellowship Director
Plancher Orthopaedics &
Sports Medicine/Orthopaedic
Foundation for Active Lifestyles
Cos Cob, Connecticut and
New York, New York

Chris Pokabla, MD
Memphis Orthopaedics Group
Memphis, Tennesee

Matthew T. Provencher, MD,
CDR, MC, USN
Department of Orthopaedic Surgery
Naval Medical Center San Diego
San Diego, California

Jay H. Rapley, MD
Rockhill Orthopedics
Lee's Summit Missouri

Jesus Rey II, MD
Attending Orthopaedic Surgeon
Charlton Methodist Medical Center
Southwest Orthopedics & Sports
Medicine, PA
Dallas, Texas

John T. Riehl, MD
Resident
GHS Orthopaedics
Danville, Pennsylvania

Daniel T. Richards, DO
Granger Medical Riverton Clinic &
Associates
Riverton, Utah

Samuel P. Robinson, MD
Jordan-Young Institute
Virginia Beach, Virginia

James R. Romanowski, MD
Fellow
Orthopaedic Sports Medicine
University of Pittsburgh School of
Medicine
UPMC Center for Sports Medicine
Pittsburgh, Pennsylvania

Anthony A. Romeo, MD
Department of Orthopaedic
Surgery
Rush University
Chicago, Illinois

Roberto Rossi, MD
Assistant Professor in Orthopaedics
and Traumatology
University of Turin Medical
School
Mauriziano "Umberto I" Hospital
Turin, Italy

J.R. Rudzki, MD
Clinical Assistant Professor of
Orthopaedic Surgery
The George Washington University
School of Medicine
Orthopaedic Surgery, Shoulder
Surgery, & Sports Medicine
Washington Orthopaedics & Sports
Medicine
Washington, DC

Michell Ruiz-Suárez, MD, MSc
Attending Physician
Shoulder and Elbow Reconstruction
Department
Instituto Nacional de
Rehabilitación
Mexico City, Mexico

David S. Ryan, MD
Orthopaedic Research of Virginia
Richmond, Virginia

Richard K. N. Ryu, MD
Ryu Hurvitz Orthopedic Clinic
Santa Barbara, California

Marc R. Safran, MD
Professor
Orthopaedic Surgery, Sports
Medicine
Department of Orthopaedic Surgery
Stanford University
Redwood City, California

Charles L. Saltzman, MD
Chairman,
Department of Orthopaedics
Louis S Peery MD Presidential
Endowed Professor
University of Utah

Thomas G. Sampson, MD
Medical Director of Hip Arthroscopy
Post Street Surgery Center
Post Street Orthopaedics and Sports
Medicine
San Francisco, California

Benjamin Sanofsky, BA
Research Assistant
Department of Orthopaedics
Harvard Shoulder Service
Research Assistant
Brigham and Women's
Hospital
Boston, Massachusetts

Felix H. Savoie III, MD
Lee C. Schlesinger Professor and
Chief
Tulane Institute of Sports Medicine
Tulane University
Department of Orthopaedics
New Orleans, Louisiana

Verena M. Schreiber, MD
Resident
Department of Orthopaedic
Surgery
University of Pittsburgh
Pittsburgh, Pennsylvania

Bruno G. Schroder e Souza, MD
Steadman Philippon Research
    Institute
2009/2010 Visiting Scholar in Hip
    Arthroscopy and Biomechanics
    at Steadman Philippon Research
    Institute
Scholarship provided with grants
    from the Instituto Brasil de
    Tecnologias da Saude.
Steadman Philippon Research
    Institute
Vail. Colorado

Jon K. Sekiya, MD
Associate Professor
Department of Orthopaedic
    Surgery
University of Michigan
Team Physician
Medsport
University of Michigan Medical
    Center
Ann Arbor, Michigan

Nicholas A. Sgaglione, MD
Chairman
Department of Orthopaedic
    Surgery
Professor of Orthopaedic
    Surgery
Hofstra North Shore-LIJ School of
    Medicine
North Shore Long Island Jewish
    Medical Center

Benjamin Shaffer, MD
Washington Orthopaedics and
    Sports Medicine
Washington, DC

Orrin Sherman, MD
Associate Professor
Department of Orthopaedic
    Surgery
NYU Medical Center
New York, New York

Matthew V. Smith, MD
Assistant Professor
Orthopedic Surgery
Washington University
St. Louis, Missouri

Patrick A. Smith, MD
Department of Orthopaedic Surgery
University of Missouri
Columbia Orthopaedic Group
Columbia, Missouri

Stephen J. Snyder, MD
Southern California Orthopedic
    Institute
Van Nuys, California

Mark E. Steiner, MD
Clinical Instructor
Harvard Medical School
Clinical Instructor
Tufts University School
    of Medicine
Orthopedic Surgeon
New England Baptist Hospital
Boston, MA
Sports Medicine Associates
Brookline, Massachusetts

Scott P. Steinmann, MD
Professor of Orthopedic Surgery
    and Consultant
Mayo Clinic
Rochester, Minnesota

William B. Stetson, MD
Associate Clinical Professor
USC Keck School of Medicine
Stetson Powell Orthopaedics
    and Sports Medicine
Burbank, California

Daniel R Stephenson, MD
Beach Cities Orthopedics
    and Sports Medicine
Manhattan Beach, California

James Stone, MD
The Orthopedic Institute of
    Wisconsin
Franklin, Wisconsin

Christian Sybrowsky, MD
UI Sports Medicine Center
Department of Orthopaedics and
    Rehabilitation
University of Iowa Hospitals and
    Clinics
Iowa City, Iowa

James P. Tasto, MD
San Diego Sports Medicine &
    Orthopaedic Center
Clinical Professor
University of California –
    San Diego
Department of Orthopaedics
San Diego, California

Ettore Taverna, MD
Department of Shoulder Surgery
IRCCS Istituto Ortopedico
    Galeazzi
Milan, Italy

Robert A. Teitge, MD
Professor of Orthopaedics
Residency Program Director
Research Co-Director
Department of Orthopaedic
    Surgery
Wayne State University
Detroit, Michigan

David Thut, MD
Department of Orthopaedic
    Surgery
NYU Medical Center
New York, New York

John W. Uribe, MD
Professor and Chairman
Department of Orthopaedic
    Surgery
Florida International University
    School of Medicine
Miami, Florida
Chief
Department of Orthopaedics Sports
    Medicine
Doctor's Hospital
Coral Gables, Florida

C. Niek van Dijk, MD, PhD
Professor
Department of Orthopaedic
    Surgery
University of Amsterdam
Chief of Service
Department of Orthopaedic
    Surgery
Academic Medical Centre
Amsterdam, The Netherlands

Maayke N. van Sterkenburg,
MD, PhD
Fellow
Academic Medical Centre
Department of Orthopedic Surgery
Amsterdam, The Netherlands

Tanawat Vaseenon, MD
Department of Orthopaedics and
    Rehabilitations
University of Iowa Hospitals and
    Clinics
Iowa City, Iowa

James E. Voos, M.D.
Orthopaedic and Sports Medicine
    Clinic of Kansas City
Leawood, Kansas

Bradford A. Wall, MD
Georgia Bone and Joint
    Surgeons
Orthopaedic Surgeon
Cartersville, Georgia

David W. Wang, MD
Sports Medicine Fellow
Southern California Orthopedic
    Institute
Van Nuys, California
Sacramento Knee & Sports
    Medicine
Sacramento, California

Samuel Ward, PT, PhD
Departments of Radiology,
    Orthopaedic Surgery, and
    Bioengineering
University of California, San Diego
San Diego, California

Thomas L. Wickiewicz, MD
Professor
Department of Orthopedic Surgery
Weill Cornell Medical College
Attending Orthopaedic Surgeon
Sports Medicine & Shoulder Service
Hospital for Special Surgery
New York, New York

Richard Woodworth, MD
Orthopaedic Institute of Henderson
Henderson, Nevada

Brian R. Wolf, MD, MS
Assistant Professor
University of Iowa Hospitals and
    Clinics
Team Physician University of Iowa
Iowa City, Iowa

Corey A. Wulf, MD
Fellow
Orthopaedic Sports Medicine
Minnesota Sports Medicine
Twin Cities Orthopaedics
Eden Prairie, Minnesota

Gautam P. Yagnik, MD
Attending Physician
Department of Orthopaedic Surgery
DRMC Sports Medicine
Dubois, Pennsylvania

Darryl K. Young, MD, FRCSC
Orthopaedic Surgeon
Queensway Carleton Hospital
Ottawa, Ontario, Canada

Scot A. Youngblood, MD, CDR,
MC, USN
Department of Orthopaedic
    Surgery
Naval Medical Center San Diego
San Diego, California

Bashir A. Zikria, MD
Assistant Professor
Orthopedic Surgery
Johns Hopkins University
Baltimore, Maryland

Preface

Arthroscopy was one of the major orthopaedic advances of the 20th century, along with total joint replacement, and open reduction and internal fixation of fractures.

In the 21st century arthroscopy has continued to evolve with some minimally invasive procedures that we couldn't even envisage in the past, such as arthroscopic repair of gluteus medius tears, release of the ligament to decompress the suprascapular nerve, and all inside ACL and PCL reconstruction.

It is an exciting time to watch the progress of arthroscopy, and to try and imagine what the future holds.

In this textbook the most recent procedures are described in detail. This is an advanced text on the procedures, and hands-on training is suggested at cadaver labs such as the Orthopaedic Learning Center in Chicago.

I would like to thank all the authors, their staff, and the associate editors for all their many hours of hard work to bring this book to fruition.

A special thanks to Dr. Jack McGinty whose early vision inspired many of us to pursue arthroscopic training and practice.

A further thank you to WoltersKluwer for making the 4th edition possible.

Don Johnson MD FRCS C
Editor in Chief

The Shoulder

Arthroscopic Setup: Approaches and Tips for Success

Richard L. Angelo

PATIENT POSITIONING

The safety and ease with which an arthroscopic shoulder procedure is accomplished frequently relates to how the patient is positioned and how accurate and utilitarian are the portals that have been established. Although minor variations exist, most surgeons employ either the lateral decubitus or the beach chair positions, and each has its proponents. The choice is largely influenced by the familiarity gained while the surgeon was learning shoulder arthroscopy, the ease and anticipated likelihood of converting to a mini-open procedure, and the availability of surgical assistants and supportive devices for arm positioning. Equipment is readily available to facilitate the use of either position.

Lateral Decubitus Orientation

The supine position is used during the induction of general anesthesia. The patient is then repositioned in the lateral decubitus orientation on a vacuum bag (Fig. 1.1A, B). A gel pad can be layered on top of the bean bag, particularly if there is the anticipation that the procedure may be prolonged. A soft axillary roll is placed beneath the upper thorax to minimize direct pressure on the axilla, and the head is supported in a neutral orientation. The patient is allowed to roll back approximately 15° orienting the glenoid parallel with the floor. The vacuum bag is then evacuated to maintain support. All bony prominences must be appropriately padded, in particular the fibular head to protect the peroneal nerve. The operating table is then rotated to position the anesthesiologist and necessary equipment in an area near the middle of the operating table near the patient's abdomen. The surgeon is thus provided with unrestricted access to the involved shoulder. Monitors are located for easy viewing.

If the primary procedures are to be performed in the subacromial region, that is, rotator cuff repair, the primary monitor is positioned superior and anterior to the patient's head. A secondary monitor for use by the surgical assistant may be located in front of and above the patient's abdomen. When the work to be completed is primarily in the

glenohumeral joint, that is, a Bankart or SLAP repair, the monitor is set across from the surgeon near the patient's abdomen as the general viewing direction for glenohumeral procedures is anterior. The arm is supported in 30° to 40° of abduction and 15° of forward flexion using 10 lb (4.5 kg) to suspend rather than place significant traction on the arm. This shoulder position is varied during the case depending on the access necessary to specific locations. Numerous sterile sleeves and gauntlet devices are commercially available to support the arm.

Arthroscopic Bankart repairs may be facilitated by directing 10 lb (4.5 kg) of accessory traction laterally (perpendicular to the humerus) to distract the shoulder and improve access to the anterior aspect of the glenohumeral joint. Alternatively, a similar manual maneuver can be accomplished by an assistant. A routine sterile prep and drape are then performed. The lateral decubitus method eliminates the need for an assistant or mechanical device to support the arm. Internal and external rotation of the suspended arm affords acceptable access to the entire rotator cuff. If range of motion is to be assessed, that is, at the completion of a Bankart repair, the arm is removed from suspension for the motion exam while maintaining sterility of the sleeve suspension loop.

While working in the glenohumeral joint, the monitor view of the glenoid is typically oriented parallel with the floor. When working in the subacromial space, however, the surgeon may elect to either maintain this orientation (the acromion is vertical) or rotate the camera head to view the acromion in a position parallel with the floor (as it would appear with the patient standing).

If converting to an open procedure through a standard deltopectoral approach for the glenohumeral joint, subscapularis, or biceps tendon, the unsterile portion of the suspension apparatus is removed and the patient's arm is allowed to rest on the ipsilateral hip. The vacuum bag is at least partially inflated (softened) and the patient allowed to roll back into a more supine position. A draw sheet is used to center the patient on the operating table. The table is then configured to a gentle beach chair orientation with acceptable position and support for the head and neck

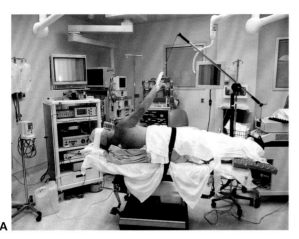 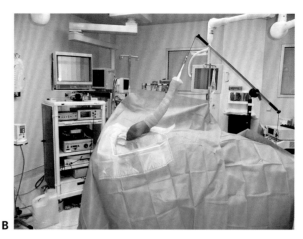

FIGURE 1.1. A: Patient positioned in the lateral decubitus orientation; anesthesia setup is near the chest. Dual monitors are helpful, particularly for the viewing of an assistant. **B:** Once draping is complete, easy access to the entire shoulder is afforded; the arm is "suspended" with 10 lb through a disposable arm sleeve.

verified. Although it is unnecessary to completely reprep and redrape, it is prudent to replace the clean, sterile barrier sheet anterior to the shoulder to shield the anesthesiologist and related equipment.

If the surgeon elects to convert to a mini-open approach to the subacromial region, repositioning is unnecessary although some prefer to tilt the table posteriorly toward the surgeon to improve access to the anterior shoulder. An approach to the supraspinatus and infraspinatus is readily obtained by extending the lateral subacromial (LSA) portal proximally. An absorbable suture is introduced transversely through the deltoid at the inferior extent of the portal defect to prevent inadvertent distal extension and iatrogenic injury to the axillary nerve. The deltoid is then divided proximally along its fibers to the level of the acromion.

Beach Chair Orientation

Some surgeons prefer the beach chair position due to its more anatomic orientation, which conforms to the familiar open approach (1). The patient's thorax is positioned to permit the involved shoulder to overhang the side of the table. Once the hips are flexed 70° to 80° and the legs 30°, the back is then elevated approximately 70°. After padding bony prominences, a vacuum pack supports the hips and thorax, but is displaced from the ipsilateral periscapular region.

Alternatively, a specially designed table with a removable wing for exposure of the operative shoulder may be employed (Fig. 1.2A, B). A relatively more vertical orientation for the back will minimize the dependent position of the camera when the scope is in the posterior portal and also minimize lens fogging. However, a more upright position for the thorax increases the hydrostatic pressure gradient between the head and the brachium. The anesthesiologist sets up near the patient's uninvolved shoulder, and the viewing monitor is placed opposite the surgeon near the foot of the table. A surgical assistant or a sterile, maneuverable mechanical arm holder adjusts the position of the shoulder during the procedure, depending on the access necessary. Somewhat greater mobility of the arm exists when compared with the lateral decubitus position.

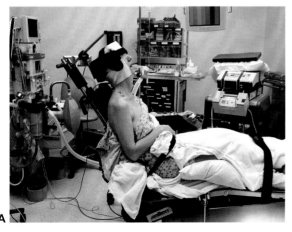 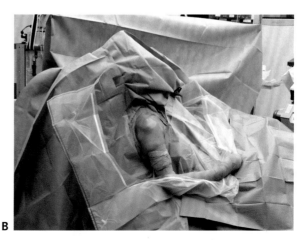

FIGURE 1.2. A: Patient positioned in the beach chair orientation; anesthesia setup is near the contralateral shoulder; a table with a removable wing affords easy access to the entire shoulder. **B:** The anterior and posterior aspects of the shoulder are readily accessed; a sterile arm positioner can be added if desired.

The upright (anatomic) orientation for the arthroscope and monitor view is maintained while working in both the glenohumeral and the subacromial regions. Conversion to an open procedure for all regions of the shoulder is relatively simple and only requires reducing the degree of thorax elevation. The vacuum pack must be at least partially inflated in order to safely change the patient's position without creating pressure points. Alternatively, a relatively more supine position for the thorax can often be accomplished by tilting the entire table into greater Trendelenberg.

A recent case report identified four patients who underwent shoulder surgery in the sitting position, which resulted in one death and three patients with severe brain damage (2). Cerebral hypoperfusion, rather than cardiovascular risk factors, was believed to be the cause and may be attributable to differences in blood pressure reference points. A blood pressure difference as great as 90 mm Hg between the head and the calf may exist in the sitting position based on hydrostatic factors alone. Potentially catastrophic cerebral hypoperfusion may be avoided by precautions including placing the blood pressure cuff on the brachium rather than the calf (3), maintaining perioperative blood pressure values at a minimum of 80% of preoperative resting values, and ensuring that the intraoperative blood pressure is at a minimum of 100 mm Hg at the level of the head. Loss of vision and ophthalmoplegia have also been reported following general anesthesia with the patient in the beach chair position, but the exact mechanisms for this pathology are unclear (3). Thromboembolic events are also possible with the patient in the sitting position and make the use of cyclical pneumatic compression cuffs around the calves prudent.

ANESTHESIA CHOICES

General Anesthesia

Both endotracheal intubation and a laryngeal mask airway (LMA) provide safe, reliable options for maintaining the airway during general anesthesia. No durable analgesia is afforded once the patient awakens, and nausea/vomiting can sometimes be difficult to manage in the perioperative period.

Interscalene Regional Block

Interscalene blocks (ISBs) provide anesthesia, muscle relaxation, and postoperative analgesia although supportive parenteral pain medication may be necessary during the immediate postoperative period (4). An ISB can be used as the primary means of anesthesia or as an adjunct to general anesthesia. As with any invasive procedure, the risk/benefit ratio determines its use. Proponents note its effectiveness despite the frequent need for some additional narcotic support during the immediate postoperative period and its relatively low risk of serious complications. Dedicated anesthesia teams committed to regional anesthesia and that perform a large number of blocks will be helpful to minimize untoward events (5). Potential serious complications have been reported including cardiac arrest, grand mal seizures, hematoma, and pneumothorax. Possible neurologic injuries include damage to the recurrent laryngeal, vagal, and axillary nerves. Phrenic nerve dysfunction is common and can give rise to significant respiratory distress. Brachial plexus pathology may include transient paresthesias (which have been reported to be as high as 9% at 24 hours and 3% at 2 weeks post-op) (6), or a brachial plexus palsy, which may be transient, require prolonged recovery or be permanent in a very small number of cases.

It is essential that the block be performed in the awake patient who is able to provide critical feedback during administration of the block. More recently, the use of ultrasound to guide placement of the needles has added a measure of safety. Even with a successful block, the duration of pain relief averages only 9 to 10 hours following surgery, which may make pain management challenging in an outpatient setting (4). A thorough disclosure of the potential risks should be discussed with the patient, preferably beforehand in an office setting during the preoperative visit.

Adjunctive Pain Management

The suprascapular nerve supplies 70% of the sensation to the shoulder joint. Instillation of 20 cc of 0.25% bupivacaine adjacent to the suprascapular nerve may result in up to a 30% reduction in postoperative narcotic usage and a five-fold reduction of nausea (7, 8). This block carries a low risk when performed with a blunt-tipped needle, and may be repeated as necessary, even in an office setting on the first postoperative day (9). In addition, local infiltration of the portal sites with 0.5% bupivacaine leads to further reduction in pain. Pain pumps remain controversial, but have been consistently used in the subacromial space with safety provided that the glenohumeral joint is not exposed to the catheter and infiltrate. Cooling jackets using circulating ice water may also substantially improve patient comfort.

PORTALS

When arthroscopic portals are properly placed, they will provide the necessary field of view and instrument access to desired locations within the glenohumeral joint, acromioclavicular joint, and subacromial space (10–14). A thorough knowledge of the regional anatomy, particularly the palpable bony landmarks, will improve safety and ensure accuracy in establishing the desired portals. There is a greater margin of safety in creating access to the subacromial space where the use of various accessory portals is routine.

General Technique

Bony landmarks are identified by careful palpation and mapped at the beginning of the case prior to soft tissue distortion from fluid extravasation. Anticipated portal sites are referenced from the landmarks and identified using a surgical marker. All anatomical references and diagrams provided here are for a right shoulder with the patient in the lateral decubitus position. Minor adjustments to the recommended distances from anatomic landmarks may be necessary if the patient is supported in the beach chair orientation or for particularly large or small patients. As experience is gained, surgeon preference may also lead to subtle adjustments in the skin entry site for various portals. The posterior glenohumeral portal is typically established first. It is recommended that all subsequent portals be made in an outside-in manner under direct vision after first establishing the desired tract with a spinal needle. A small skin incision is made at the chosen entry site and a trocar and cannula directed along the path identical to the spinal needle and into the glenohumeral joint or subacromial space.

Glenohumeral Portals (Fig. 1.3)

Posterior (P) serves as the primary intra-articular viewing portal and provides instrument access to the posterior glenoid labrum and rim, posterior capsule, and articular surface of the infraspinatus. The field of view includes the glenoid, posterosuperior humeral head, anterior capsule, biceps, superior subscapularis, glenohumeral ligaments, and articular surface of the supraspinatus and superior subscapularis tendons (Fig. 1.4A, B). The entry site is 1.0 to 1.5 cm inferior and 1.0 cm medial to the posterolateral (PL) corner of the acromion.

After creating a small skin incision, the cannula is introduced and directed toward the coracoid tip. If it is anticipated that this portal will be employed to drill or insert anchors along the posterior glenoid rim, the entry

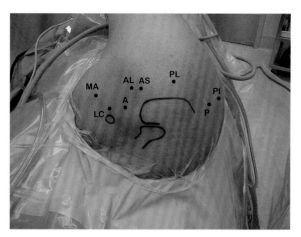

FIGURE 1.3. Right shoulder in the lateral decubitus orientation viewed from superior (anterior is to the left); bony landmarks are mapped out and the common glenohumeral portals are identified; P, posterior; A, anterior; PI, posteroinferior; PL, posterolateral ("Port of Wilmington"); AS, anterosuperior; AL, anterolateral; MA, midanterior; LC, lateral coracoid.

site must be adjusted 1 cm further lateral to account for the anterior glenoid version. This modification will enable the approach to be approximately 45° to the glenoid in the transverse plane. If this lateral modification is not made, the portal will be too "shallow" and create a risk that instruments will either skive off the articular cartilage or be directed too far medial along the glenoid neck.

Anterior (A) enters through the middle of the rotator interval and provides instrument access to the biceps, anterior labrum, glenoid rim, anterior and superior capsule, articular surfaces of the supraspinatus, infraspinatus, and the superior aspect of the subscapularis tendons. The field of view includes the posterior glenoid and labrum,

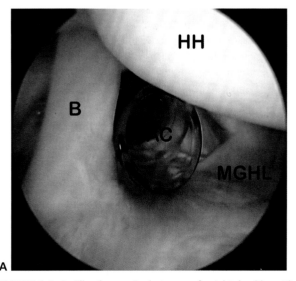

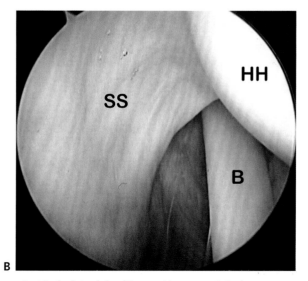

FIGURE 1.4. A: All arthroscopic photos are of a right shoulder with the patient in the lateral decubitus position; scope is in the posterior portal viewing anteriorly; HH, humeral head; B, biceps; MGHL, middle glenohumeral ligament; AC, anterior cannula. **B:** Scope is in the posterior portal viewing anteriorly; HH, humeral head; B, biceps; SS, capsule overlying the articular surface of the supraspinatus just posterior to the biceps.

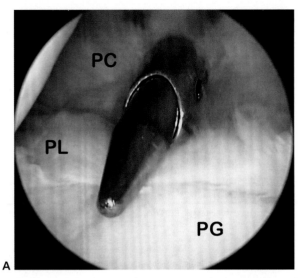
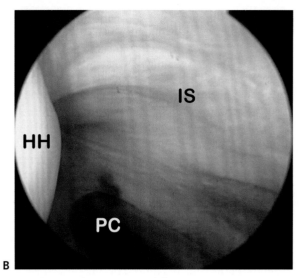

FIGURE 1.5. A: Scope is in the anterior portal viewing posteriorly; PC, posterior capsule; PL, posterior labrum; PG, posterior glenoid. **B:** Scope is in the anterior portal viewing posterosuperiorly; HH, humeral head; IS, capsule underlying the infraspinatus tendon; PC, posterior cannula.

anterosuperior (AS) humeral head, articular surface of the infraspinatus, posterior capsule, and the biceps origin (Fig. 1.5A, B). The entry site is midway between the coracoid tip and the anterolateral (AL) corner of the acromion. The cannula is directed toward the center of the glenohumeral joint while viewing from the posterior portal.

Midanterior (MA) is the preferred portal to instrument the anterior glenoid rim with drills and anchors in preparing the neck for a Bankart repair. In addition, it affords access to the anterior and inferior capsule for suture-passing instruments. The entry site is 1.5 cm lateral and 1.5 cm inferior to the coracoid tip. A spinal needle identifies the appropriate track, which, after penetrating the skin, is

directed somewhat superiorly over the superior border of the subscapularis. A small superficial skin incision is made, and an obturator and cannula are initially directed superiorly, then over the top of the subscapularis, and finally inferiorly to enable ready access to the inferior glenoid. Instruments passing through this portal should be able to approach the glenoid at a 45° angle in the transverse plane.

AS provides a tangential view to the anterior glenoid rim and neck (for Bankart repairs), the superior insertion of the subscapularis onto the lesser tuberosity, the superior and posterior capsule, labrum, and glenoid rim (Fig. 1.6A, B). The entry site is 1.0 cm directly lateral to

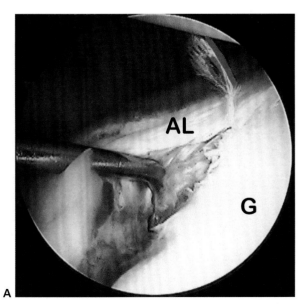
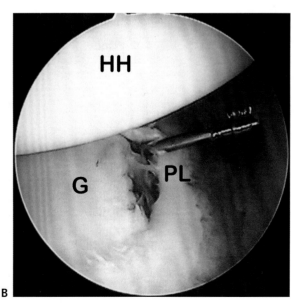

FIGURE 1.6. A: Scope is in the AS portal viewing anteroinferiorly; probe is demonstrating a Bankart lesion; G, glenoid; AL, anterior labrum. **B:** Scope is in the AS portal viewing posteroinferiorly; probe is inside a posterior labral tear; HH, humeral head; G, glenoid; PL, posterior labrum.

I. The Shoulder

the AL corner of the acromion, and the cannula is directed immediately anterior to the anterior border of the supraspinatus and then either anterior or posterior to the biceps tendon, depending on the intended primary use.

AL serves to enable instrument access to the posterior aspect of the coracoid, the anterior, superior, and posterior aspects of the subscapularis for release, and to the lateral border of the subscapularis (e.g., for use with antegrade suture-passing instruments). The entry site is 1.0 cm anterior and 1.0 to 1.5 cm lateral to the AL corner of the acromion. The cannula or instrument is directed toward the posterior aspect of the tip of the coracoid or somewhat more inferiorly toward the biceps groove.

Lateral coracoid (LC) enables instrument access to the lesser tuberosity for subscapularis repair from an intra-articular view. The entry site is 1.0 to 1.5 cm directly lateral to the middle of the coracoid tip and the instrument is then directed somewhat laterally toward the lesser tuberosity.

PL (or Port of Wilmington) facilitates placement of anchors at the posterosuperior glenoid rim for labral repair. The portal may penetrate the infraspinatus tendon. Concern has been raised regarding the defect in the tendinous portion of the rotator cuff and it is advisable to limit this portal to the smallest diameter practical for a given anchor and its preparation. The entry site is 1.5 cm anterior and 1.5 cm lateral to the PL corner of the acromion. Viewing from an anterior portal, a spinal needle is directed approximately 45° from lateral to medial to establish the proper track.

Posteroinferior (PI) provides instrument access to the posterior capsule and axillary recess for capsular excoriation and suture plication. The entry site is 2.0 cm inferior and 1 cm lateral to the posterior portal. A spinal needle is used to establish the proper track while viewing from the AS portal. Care must be taken not to err too far inferior and risk injury to the axillary nerve.

Subacromial Portals (Fig. 1.7)

Posterior subacromial (PSA) is a primary viewing portal and offers instrument access to the posterior bursa, cuff, the acromion, and the greater tuberosity. The field of view includes the entire subacromial space, acromioclavicular joint, extra-articular biceps and sheath, the coracoclavicular ligaments, and suprascapular notch (Fig. 1.8A, B). The entry site is the same as the posterior glenohumeral portal. The trocar is directed anterosuperiorly, immediately inferior to the inferior surface of the acromion.

LSA provides a "50-yd line" view of the supraspinatus–infraspinatus insertion onto the greater tuberosity and a lateral view of the acromioclavicular joint, the anterior

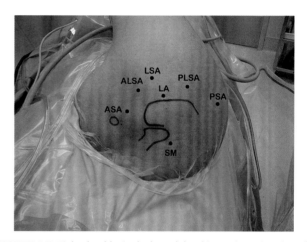

FIGURE 1.7. Right shoulder in the lateral decubitus orientation viewed from superior (anterior is to the left); bony landmarks are mapped out and the common glenohumeral portals are identified; PSA, posterior subacromial; PLSA, posterolateral subacromial; LSA, lateral subacromial; LA, lateral acromial; ALSA, anterolateral subacromial; ASA, anterior subacromial; SM, Superomedial

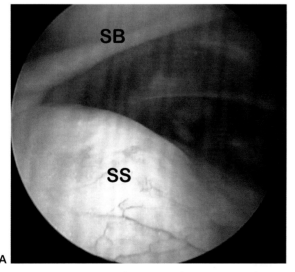

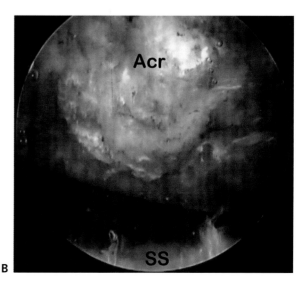

FIGURE 1.8. A: Scope is in the PSA portal viewing anteriorly; normal subacromial bursal region; SS, normal supraspinatus with vascular pattern; SB, ASA bursal fold. **B:** Scope is in the PSA portal viewing anteriorly; SS, bursal surface of supraspinatus; Acr, large anterior acromial spur.

acromion, and the posterior bursal curtain. Instruments are able to approach the rotator cuff, greater tuberosity, and acromion. The entry site is 2.5 to 3.0 cm lateral and 0 to 1.0 cm posterior to the AL corner of the acromion. Instruments roughly parallel the inferior surface of the acromion.

Anterolateral subacromial (ALSA) portal is the same as AL glenohumeral portal, but is placed into the subacromial space. When in the anterior subacromial (ASA) space, it provides a view of the extra-articular biceps, the intertubercular groove, the bursal surface of the subscapularis, and the lesser tuberosity (once the clavipectoral fascia has been excised). Instruments can approach the subscapularis tendon for release and suture passage as well as to perform a coracoplasty. The entry site is 1.0 cm anterior and 1.0 to 1.5 cm lateral to the AL corner of the acromion.

ASA is the same as the anterior glenohumeral portal, but enters the subacromial space. It offers a view of most of the subacromial space, but is commonly used for suture management. Instruments can be introduced into the anterior aspect of the rotator cuff for a side-to-side repair. Once through the skin, the trocar is directed immediately beneath the anterior margin of the acromion. When instrument access to the biceps groove is intended, the optimal portal entry site is identified with a spinal needle. While viewing from the AL portal, the needle is directed toward the biceps groove with the humerus internally rotated approximately 20°.

Posterolateral subacromial (PLSA) serves as a primary viewing portal to address rotator cuff pathology. Once established, a 30° scope offers a "50-yd line" view of the rotator cuff and subacromial space (Fig. 1.9). The entry site is approximately 1.0 cm anterior and 1.0 cm lateral to the PL corner of the acromion. An arthroscope in the PL

portal may interfere with instruments introduced through the LSA portal if a minimum of 3 cm is not maintained between the two sites.

Lateral acromial (LA) is primarily used for instrument approach to the greater tuberosity (e.g., drill, tap, and anchor insertion for rotator cuff repair). The entry site is immediately lateral to the lateral border of the acromion. The optimal anteroposterior location is identified using a spinal needle. Access to the entire greater tuberosity is possible with internal and external rotation of the humerus. When attempting to place anchors into the medial aspect of the greater tuberosity adjacent to the articular cartilage, it is essential to nearly completely adduct the humerus to avoid approaching the tuberosity at too shallow an angle and potentially violating the articular surface of the humeral head.

Superomedial (SM—Neviaser) is employed to introduce suture-passing and retrieving instruments toward the rotator cuff. The entry site is 1.0 cm medial to the posterior aspect of the acromioclavicular joint. With the arthroscope in the subacromial space and the arm abducted <45°, a spinal needle is directed from medial to lateral at approximately 60° in the frontal plane. If the portal is introduced too close to the acromioclavicular joint, the mobility of the instrument is significantly restricted.

Anterior acromioclavicular (AAC) affords an anterior approach for resection of the distal clavicle. The entry site is 2.0 cm anteroinferior to and in line with the acromioclavicular joint. The optimal path is identified with a spinal needle. Alternatively, when approaching the acromioclavicular joint in a direct fashion, two small portals can be established. One is directly AS and a second posterosuperior to the AC joint. A small-diameter arthroscope and shaver are used initially until a greater space can be established.

SUTURE MANAGEMENT

Suture management is one of the most challenging aspects of accurately completing an effective arthroscopic shoulder procedure. By employing a systematic routine, suture can be passed, manipulated, and tied in an efficient manner. Simplifying the steps involved results in time saved and frustration avoided. Suture must be handled carefully to avoid fraying and nicking with the possibility of eventual breakage. Loop rather than jaw-type graspers help maintain this suture integrity. It is optimal to isolate the suture being manipulated whenever possible by placing all other nonworking sutures in a separate portal. Tangling and mistaking various limbs and suture mates can thus be avoided. Once all sutures from a given anchor have been passed, the working cannula is withdrawn and then reinserted placing the sutures outside the cannula, which can then be used to manage a new set of sutures.

In order for sutures to securely reapproximate tissue, they must be optimally placed. When manipulating tissues and suture-passing instruments, efficiency can be gained

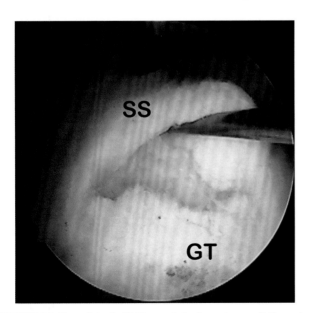

FIGURE 1.9. Scope is in the PLSA portal viewing anteromedially; probe demonstrates a bursal-sided rotator cuff tear; SS, supraspinatus; GT, greater tuberosity.

by having an assistant hold the arthroscope to maintain an acceptable field of view. The surgeon is then able to secure the tissue with graspers in one hand while controlling the suture-passing device with the other, similar to using forceps and a needle driver in an open technique. Antegrade devices, which often simplify suture passage by minimizing the number of steps involved, can be made more efficient by using a counterforce traction suture to control the tissue and prevent it from being pushed away during instrument delivery. When using a penetrating device in retrograde fashion, its mobility can be restricted significantly once it has passed through the tissue. Rather than attempt to "chase" the desired suture with the open jaw, deliver the selected anchor suture to the penetrator with a loop grasper or knot pusher. Various cannulated instruments, with or without an attached suture retrieval loop, do not require the use of a cannula and are able to be introduced through a very small skin nick such as the SM (Neviaser) portal.

Entanglements are avoided by managing sutures in an orderly fashion. When passing sutures through the rotator cuff, it is helpful to pass them from "far to near." Those sutures that are to be passed furthest from the viewing arthroscope are introduced first (Fig. 1.10). Consequently, as subsequent sutures are delivered closer to the arthroscope, the field of view remains unobstructed by previously passed sutures. The suture pairs are then progressively tied in the opposite sequence, that is, those closest to the scope tied first and those furthest tied last. This method permits adherence to the principle of working with sutures in isolation as much as possible.

When working with sutures that pass through anchors, care must be taken to avoid "offloading" the suture from the anchor. The location of the involved anchor should be kept in view while a limb is being retrieved to verify that the suture is being pulled through the anchor. Stop, reorient yourself, and select the proper limb if the suture is moving through the anchor.

Many methods exist for tying knots. When using a sliding knot, the post limb must pass through the tissue being repaired so that the knot is delivered toward the tissue and away from the anchor. Otherwise, as the knot is introduced, it can become "bound up" at the entry site for the anchor and fail to slide further, compromising loop security. In addition, prominent knots near articular surfaces may generate significant chondral scuffing and abrasion. As half hitches are introduced to secure the knot, the post should be alternated, the throw reversed, and each half hitch seen to "lay down" without inappropriate twists.

PEARLS AND PITFALLS

Accurate portal placement is essential. If the initial portal placement is malpositioned or misdirected, time, frustration, and potential complications can be avoided by establishing a new portal in the optimal location. Using sharp trocars or excessive force to penetrate the capsule can lead to inadvertent damage to the articular cartilage. Once established, screw-in or lock-in cannulas are more secure, particularly when instruments are passed through them frequently. A relatively tight portal of entry through the skin will also help prevent inadvertent withdrawal of the cannula. Clear cannulas improve the visibility of instruments and sutures that are within the tip of the cannula.

It is essential to obtain a clear field of view. Relative hypotensive anesthesia, a hydrodynamic balance of inflow and outflow pressures, irrigation containing epinephrine, and selective radiofrequency cauterization can lead to improved visibility. Repositioning of the joint often improves the view, especially in relatively tight regions (e.g., posterior displacement of the humeral head to improve access to the anterior glenoid or improve working space when addressing subscapularis lesions; adducting the shoulder to safely approach the medial aspect of the lesser tuberosity). Anatomic relationships should be verified prior to resecting or altering any tissue. Motorized instruments and sharp tools must be kept in view to prevent iatrogenic tissue damage.

If a suture is inadvertently offloaded from an anchor with a suture loop eyelet, a new suture can be reintroduced into the anchor (Fig. 1.11A–E). Reposition the suture remaining in the anchor to create asymmetric limbs. Load a free suture in a small atraumatic needle and then pass that needle through the braids of the longer limb of the remaining anchor suture where it exits the working cannula. By placing traction on the short limb of the

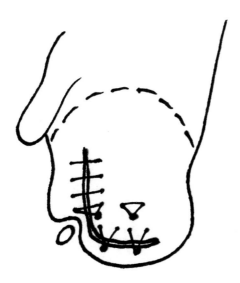

FIGURE 1.10. Diagram of a right shoulder viewed from superiorly depicting a large "L"-shaped rotator cuff tear; consider placing most medial (farthest from scope) sutures first and working progressively laterally (closest to scope); consider tying most lateral sutures first and then progressing medial with suture pairs.

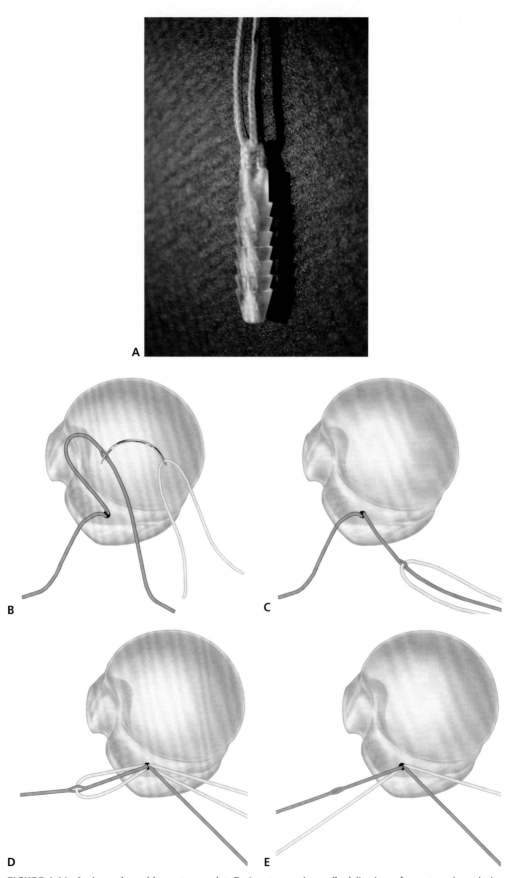

FIGURE 1.11. A: An anchor with a suture eyelet. **B:** An atraumatic needle delivering a free suture through the braids of the suture, which remains in the anchor. **C:** A completed pass of the free suture through the anchor suture. **D:** By pulling on the short limb of the anchor suture, it acts as a shuttle to deliver the free limb through the suture eyelet. **E:** Both suture limbs are now through the anchor eyelet in a normal fashion.

remaining anchor suture, the free suture can be "shuttled" through the anchor eyelet. Once the two sutures are disengaged, both pass through the suture eyelet.

When a suture is accidently offloaded from an anchor with a rigid eyelet and multiple sutures, a new suture can be secured to the anchor (Fig. 1.12A–C). A simple overhand throw is created outside the cannula with the suture, which still passes through the anchor. A second free suture is passed beneath the loop that has been created. As the half hitch is delivered down the cannula, it draws the second (free) suture to the anchor head. A second and third alternating half hitch are introduced to secure the free strand. Once all limbs are passed through the tissue, the suture passing through the anchor eyelet is tied first, which helps further secure the free strand. Nonsliding knots must be used for both pairs of sutures.

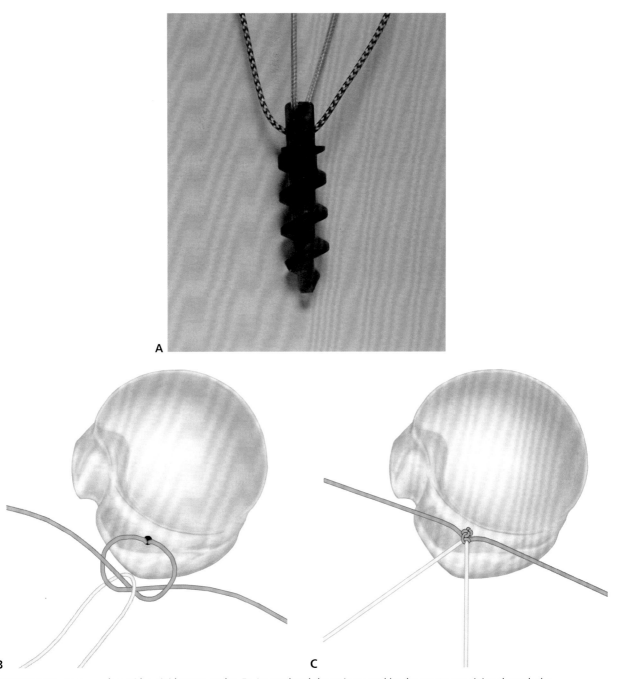

FIGURE 1.12. A: An anchor with a rigid suture eyelet. **B:** An overhand throw is created by the suture remaining through the eyelet and a separate free suture is passed through the loop that is created. **C:** The anchor suture is tied to the anchor head and backed up with two half hitches. Both sutures are now secured to the anchor, but require nonsliding knots to be employed once the sutures are passed through the tissue.

CONCLUSIONS

Either the beach chair or lateral decubitus positions can be used to position patients safely for shoulder arthroscopy. Adequate cerebral blood flow must be maintained when the head and thorax are significantly elevated. General anesthesia is routinely performed and permits greater blood pressure management compared with an ISB. ISBs should be performed by experienced anesthesiologists with a detailed knowledge of the regional anatomy and an opportunity to perform blocks on a routine basis to maintain their skills. The use of ultrasound guidance is recommended.

Accurate portal placement can either greatly facilitate and inaccurate portal placement can hinder the performance of any arthroscopic procedure. An 18G spinal needle will aid in identifying the optimal entry site and path for specific portals. The choice of camera and view orientation is largely surgeon preference, particularly when working in the subacromial space. Manipulating the position and displacement of the shoulder will aid in optimizing the view and working space. A systematic routine for handling sutures will prevent tangling, suture damage, and insecure knots with poor loop security.

REFERENCES

1. Correa MC, Concalves LB, Andrade RP, et al. Beach chair position with instrumental distraction for arthroscopic and open shoulder surgeries. *J Shoulder Elbow Surg.* 2008;17:226–230.
2. Pohl A, Cullen DJ. Cerebral ischemia during shoulder surgery in the upright position: a case series. *J Clin Anesth.* 2005;17:463–469.
3. Papadonikolakis A, Wiesler ER, Olympio MA, et al. Avoiding catastrophic complications of stroke and death related to shoulder surgery in the sitting position. *Arthroscopy.* 2008;24:481–482.
4. Weber S, Jain R. Scalene regional anesthesia for shoulder surgery in a community setting: an assessment of risk. *J Bone Joint Surg Am.* 2002;84:775–779.
5. Bishop JY, Sprague M, Gelber J, et al. Interscalene regional anesthesia for shoulder surgery. *J Bone Joint Surg Am.* 2005;87:974–979.
6. Urban MK, Urquhart B. Evaluation of brachial plexus anesthesia for upper extremity surgery. *Reg Anesth.* 1994;19:175–182.
7. Ritchie ED, Tong D, Chung F, Norris AM, Miniaci A, Vairavanathan SD. Suprascapular nerve block for postoperative pain relief in arthroscopic shoulder surgery: a new modality? *Anesth Analg.* 1997;84:1306–12.
8. Matsumoto D, Suenaga N, Oizumi N, et al. A new nerve block procedure for the suprascapular nerve base on a cadaveric study. *J Shoulder Elbow Surg.* 2009;18:607–611.
9. Barber FA. Suprascapular nerve block for shoulder arthroscopy. *Arthroscopy.* 2005;21:1015.
10. Nottage WM. Arthroscopic portals: anatomy as risk. *Orthop Clin North Am.* 1993;24:19–26.
11. Stanish WD, Peterson DC. Shoulder arthroscopy and nerve injury: pitfalls and prevention. *Arthroscopy.* 1995;11:458–466.
12. Lo IK, Lind CC, Burkhart SS. Glenohumeral arthroscopy portals established using an outside-in technique: neurovascular anatomy at risk. *Arthroscopy.* 2004;20:596–602.
13. Meyer M, Graveleau N, Hardy P, et al. Anatomic risks of shoulder arthroscopy portals: anatomic cadaveric study of 12 portals. *Arthroscopy.* 2007;23:529–536.
14. Woolf SK, Buttmann D, Karch MM, et al. The superior-medial shoulder arthroscopy portal is safe. *Arthroscopy.* 2007;23:247–250.

I. The Shoulder

Arthroscopic Shoulder Evaluation: Normal Anatomy and How to Thoroughly Evaluate It

Joseph P. Burns • David W. Wang

Although initial arthroscopies were quite primitive, Burman described using an arthroscope to evaluate a cadaver shoulder in 1931. Few further advances in shoulder arthroscopy were made until 1959 when Watanabe introduced an illuminated arthroscope with an offset tungsten bulb at the tip, the No. 21 arthroscope (1). Innovations in the 1970s included improved arthroscopic illumination and magnification, and it was during this period that the rapid expansion of arthroscopic applications occurred. In 1978, Watanabe described the anterior and posterior shoulder portals and the next year reported his arthroscopic findings of shoulder pathology. In 1979, Conti used an anterior arthroscopic cannula to perform a capsular release on 18 patients with adhesive capsulitis, but it appears he did this without joint visualization (2).

Johnson (3) is one of the pioneers of shoulder arthroscopy. He authored the classic textbook on the subject *Diagnostic and Surgical Arthroscopy of the Shoulder*. Perhaps his greatest contribution was the introduction of the motorized shaver in 1980. Many subsequent advances in knowledge and techniques have expanded the field of shoulder arthroscopy and helped revolutionize the diagnosis and management of shoulder pathology that was previously difficult or impossible to treat.

In contrast to open surgery, arthroscopy allows the direct, magnified visualization of the structures of the shoulder without the morbidity of a muscle or tendon splitting dissection, resulting in decreased postoperative pain and a more rapid rehabilitation. Because of the advances in recent years, shoulder arthroscopy has become a popular and common procedure for the examination and treatment of shoulder problems. This chapter reviews the equipment required, the setup and positioning of the patient, basic technique for diagnostic arthroscopy, and review of normal shoulder anatomy.

EQUIPMENT NEEDED

Personnel

The first requirement for shoulder arthroscopy is an effective team that will assist the surgeon. Attention to detail from all members of the team is necessary to make the procedure run smoothly without unnecessary problems. The anesthesiologist must have a basic understanding of the technical procedure to be performed in order to plan for a regional nerve blockade and/or general anesthesia. He must also be comfortable with maintaining the blood pressure at a lower level, ideally around 90 mm Hg systolic or mean arterial pressure of 50 mm Hg in order to diminish bleeding from the synovium and subacromial bursa (4). The scrub technician should be familiar with all of the arthroscopic equipment, utilize an efficient instrument setup and be able to troubleshoot any problems that may arise with the equipment. A good circulating nurse will be able to assist in positioning the patient correctly. They must know how to set up the equipment and maintain the arthroscopy fluid and pump, as well as be familiar with any medication needed for the irrigation bags (e.g., epinephrine or glycine). It may be prudent to perform a "dry run" or hold an in-service with the entire team before undertaking your first shoulder arthroscopy.

Operating Room

The optimal operating room should be at least 30 × 30 ft (9.1 × 9.1 m) in size, with adequate overhead lighting for the scrub table, nurse, and anesthesiologist (Fig. 2.1). If additional light sources, that is, windows or light boxes, cause glare on the video monitor, they should be covered or turned off. The operating table should be placed in the center of the room, and the video tower placed directly across from the primary surgeon. A Mayo stand should be placed anterior to the patient with the equipment most commonly used, such as the motorized

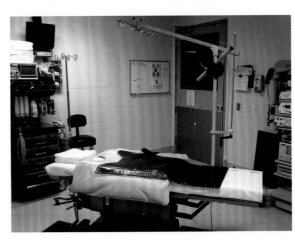

FIGURE 2.1. The operating room should have adequate overhead lighting and space.

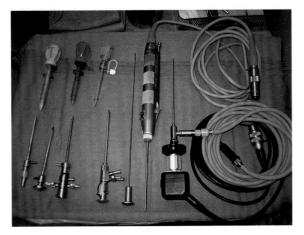

FIGURE 2.2. The Mayo stand should contain the equipment most commonly used.

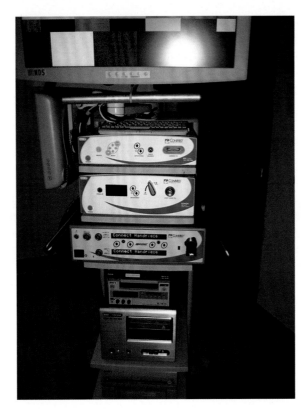

FIGURE 2.3. The equipment tower allows a convenient way to store and move needed equipment.

shaver, electrosurgical pencil or radiofrequency ablator, the remote control to the pump, and the various cannulas, sheaths, and guide rods that will be used (Fig. 2.2). Another Mayo stand will be placed behind the surgeons that will hold the instruments needed to begin the procedure and introduce the arthroscope camera into the joint.

Tower Equipment

Most of the important electronic equipment will be placed onto a tower, which allows a more convenient way to connect the equipment and move it around the room as one unit. This includes the video monitor, camera box, light source, shaver/burr power unit, printer, and CD/DVD burner with a USB type connection. (Fig. 2.3). Several commercially available products are on the market. In recent years, high-definition cameras and monitors have become available, as have digital recordings of intraoperative pictures and videos. The arthroscopic pump system is placed next to the video tower. It is an essential part of shoulder arthroscopy. Many systems allow the surgeon to control the inflow rate, the pressure maintained in the joint, as well as

the outflow rate. The surgeon should be familiar with the nuances of the system. Because of the propensity for fluid under pressure to be forced into the surrounding soft tissue, an accurate and sensitive pressure reading from inside of the joint or bursa is necessary.

Hand Equipment

Various cannulas exist for use in shoulder arthroscopy. Depending on the arthroscopic system chosen, interchangeable metal cannulas may be available, which can make switching portals easier. Some surgeons prefer to use slightly larger plastic cannulas, which allow fluid outflow through the cannula instead of exclusively through the shaver or burr. A shaver or burr can provide inconsistent outflow if it clogs during heavy use. Larger cannulas must be used when larger, more intricate instruments are used to pass or shuttle sutures through tissue. Electrosurgical probes can be used to cauterize small bleeders and to perform precise soft tissue releases. Radiofrequency ablators are commonly used to ablate tissue and achieve hemostasis, which in turn helps shorten procedure times. They can also cauterize bleeders using the coagulation setting. Many different arthroscopic instruments exist including probes, graspers, scissors, rasps, hooks, suture passers, and shuttling devices of all shapes and sizes. We prefer to use a simple grasper, crochet hook, switching sticks, and a curved shuttling device for most of our procedures. In addition, suture anchors of differing materials and sizes exist for rotator cuff, labrum, instability, and biceps tendon procedures. It is important for the surgeon to intimately know the equipment before using it on a patient. This requires lots of practice either in a dry lab on a shoulder model or on cadavers.

Exam Under Anesthesia

A good time to perform a thorough examination under anesthesia is after induction of the general anesthesia while the patient is lying supine on the operating table. Shoulder ranges of motion along with laxity or stiffness can be assessed and compared with the preoperative exam findings. Many times the office examination can be complicated by significant pain or the patient's body habitus. Important physical exam findings consistent with adhesive capsulitis or instability can be clarified during an exam under anesthesia. A comparison with the normal nonoperative shoulder can be helpful.

Beach-Chair Position

The beach-chair position is often preferred for shoulder arthroscopy. The patient is first aligned so that the operative shoulder is slightly off the table while the remaining torso, hips, and lower extremities remain on the table (Fig. 2.4). The hips should be placed at the break in the table to make positioning easier once the patient is moved upright. The head is placed into a cushioned rest. The upper body is then flexed at the hips to about 45°. The knees are then flexed approximately 20° to prevent the patient from sliding down the table. Make sure the knees and heels are well padded with pillows or other cushioning devices to avoid pressure points. The upper table and torso are then flexed completely into a sitting position, which typically positions the acromion 60° relative to the floor. A padded side post is placed against the patient's pelvis to prevent sideways sliding. The neck and endotracheal tube positioning is checked by the anesthesiologist. Standard prepping and draping protocols are then followed. The operative arm can be left free and placed across the patient's lap at rest. Any positioning in abduction, internal,

or external rotation must be done by an assistant during the procedure. Various commercially available arm-holding devices exist, which can facilitate arm positioning without an assistant.

Advantages of the beach-chair position include the upright position which allows the surgeon to operate "right side up." This is particularly helpful when working in the subacromial space so that the camera does not have to be rotated to make the image appear correct. The weight of the arm also provides some traction to open up the subacromial space to make instrumentation somewhat easier. The beach-chair position may be a disadvantage when working in the glenohumeral joint. It can be quite cumbersome to achieve and hold lateral traction to the arm while working in the joint. Access to some anterior and inferior locations is difficult to achieve without an assistant. Newer devices such as the Spider limb positioner (Tenet Medical, Calgary, Canada) have helped offset this limitation. The Spider is a pneumatically powered unit that allows the surgeon to place the arm in the desired position and hold it without assistance.

Lateral Decubitus Position

The lateral decubitus position for shoulder arthroscopy is another common position (Fig. 2.5). A 3-ft (0.91 m) vacuum beanbag is placed with the U side at the level of the patient's scapula. An axillary roll is prepared prior to moving the patient. It can be a gel roll or simply a liter bag of intravenous saline solution wrapped with a cotton cloth. Four people are needed to safely position the patient. While the anesthesiologist controls the head and neck, the surgeon and assistant stand anterior and posterior to the trunk with a nurse holding the legs. After induction of general anesthesia and securing of the endotracheal tube, a draw sheet is used to lift the patient and move him laterally several inches to the posterior side of the operative table before tilting him to the lateral decubitus position. Next, the axillary roll is placed in the U portion of the beanbag to support the chest and prevent pressure on the dependent shoulder and axillary structures. Adequate

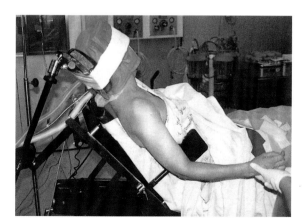

FIGURE 2.4. Beach-chair position.

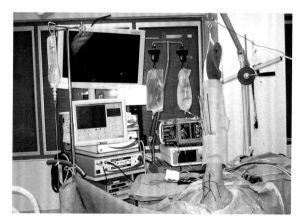

FIGURE 2.5. Patient in lateral position fully prepped and draped.

foam padding is placed at the dependent elbow, knee, and ankle, and pillows are placed between the legs. The hips and knees are flexed into a balanced position; usually around 30° is adequate. Finally, the beanbag is molded around the patient with the torso slightly tilted posteriorly about 20°, and the nurse applies the suction to deflate the bag. The table is then unlocked and rotated 45° posteriorly to allow the surgeon to step around the head and access the superior shoulder. The primary surgeon stands behind the patient closer to the axilla, whereas the assistant stands at the head. The patient's arm is then prepped and draped in the preferred manner.

In the lateral decubitus position, the arm is placed into a commercially available arm holder, usually a foam or silicone sleeve that is then connected by an S-hook to the cable system of a 3-point traction system. Approximately 10 lb (4.5 kg) attached to the upper cable (pulley at the end of the boom) is needed to suspend the average-sized arm in 70° of abduction and 15° of forward flexion.

The advantage of the lateral decubitus position is that it allows for slight traction to be placed onto the arm to open up the joint for instruments. This is achieved by placing the correct amount of weight on the cable establishing a balanced suspension. This allows the surgeon to gain better access to the entire glenohumeral joint without the need of an assistant. The abduction of the arm is also easily changed by moving the pulley down the boom (partially adducting) or by simply moving the weights to the inferior cable to completely adduct the arm down to the patient's side (the so-called bursal position). If external or internal rotation is needed, an assistant or scrub tech can hold the arm in a satisfactory position while the surgeon works. In the lateral position, the glenohumeral joint is viewed with the glenoid being the floor of the screen and the humeral head being the roof. This view, in combination with the extra room from the distraction, allows one to easily work on the glenoid and capsule and lends itself to instability repair. One potential disadvantage of this position is working in the subacromial space. In order for the acromion to appear as the "roof" on the monitor, the camera-arthroscope must be rotated approximately 90°. Without some practice, this can be disorienting for the surgeon.

ARTHROSCOPIC EVALUATION OF NORMAL ANATOMY

Surface Anatomy

The first part of any successful shoulder arthroscopy is accurately marking out the bony landmarks of the shoulder (Fig. 2.6). It is important to first identify the posterolateral edge of the acromion. It is necessary to mark the inferior edge of the bone because that is the portion that will interfere with the instruments. Next, the remaining acromion is marked posteriorly and

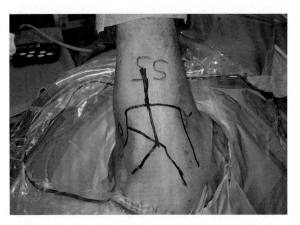

FIGURE 2.6. Mark the bony landmarks of the shoulder before starting the arthroscopy.

laterally. The anterior edge of the clavicle is then found and marked. Then the junction between the posterior clavicle and the acromion is marked along with the posterior clavicle and the anterior scapular spine. The posterior aspect of the AC joint is located anterior to this V-shaped mark and is usually palpable in line with the coracoid process. Finally, an orientation line is marked starting at the posterior clavicle and extending laterally in line with the humerus and continuing 4 cm lateral to the acromion. This line represents the posterior aspect of the subacromial bursa and is the limit of safe incision extension laterally to avoid iatrogenic injury to the axillary nerve.

Posterior Portal

Most standard shoulder arthroscopy procedures start with the creation of the posterior portal. It is where the camera and inflow cannula are placed to begin glenohumeral arthroscopy. It is also often used for subacromial arthroscopy. Traditionally, it has been described as 2 cm inferior and 1 cm medial to the posterolateral edge of the acromion. However, patients come in all shapes and sizes and this often does not correlate well to the actual anatomy. All additional appropriate information regarding bony and muscular anatomy must be used to determine the location of this portal. Since this portal is created without the benefit of the camera, it is supremely important to get it right. If it is inaccurately placed, the rest of the procedure may become much more difficult than anticipated.

Palpation of the "soft spot," which is the interval between the infraspinatus and teres minor muscles, is the most reproducible method for correct posterior portal placement (Fig. 2.7). In patients who are obese, the soft spot may not be palpable. Another method to confirm correct placement is by translating the humeral head anteriorly and posteriorly to locate the interface between the glenoid and the humeral head. A 1-cm incision is made with a no. 11 blade only through the dermis. A blunt

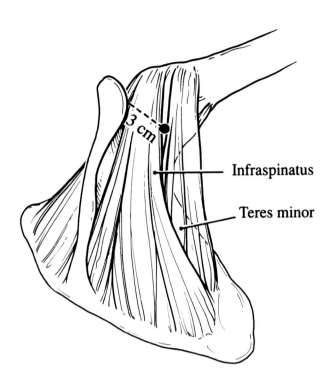

3 cm

Infraspinatus

Teres minor

FIGURE 2.7. Palpation of the "soft spot" at the interval between the infraspinatus and teres minor muscles identifies the correct site for posterior portal placement.

trocar tip is advanced carefully with steady, constant pressure through the deltoid and then the infraspinatus and teres minor interval to the posterior capsule. Running the tip of the trocar back and forth lightly over the posterior humeral head and glenoid will confirm the correct placement. Rotating or translating the humeral head will also give the surgeon tactile feedback. Lateral traction/abduction is placed on the humerus and the trocar is advanced into the joint. A palpable pop is usually felt and the trocar should move freely superiorly and inferiorly along the glenohumeral interface. Ideally, the posterior portal is introduced near the equator of the humeral head to allow easy access both superiorly and inferiorly.

Some surgeons distend the joint with saline before placing a cannula in the joint. Theoretically, the advantage of this distention is that the glenoid and humeral head are distracted and separated by the fluid and are less likely to be damaged by the insertion of the trocar. However, because the insertion into the joint is "blind," the likelihood of damaging articular cartilage by the needle is relatively high. In addition, if the needle is placed outside the joint in the subacromial space or soft tissue, unnecessary iatrogenic trauma and swelling may change the orientation of the markings and make the subsequent introduction of the trocar and cannula more difficult. We do not distend the joint and have found that relying on tactile feedback and an anatomic appreciation makes joint access reproducible, quick, and safe.

Anterior Portal

Once the arthroscope is inside the glenohumeral joint, the surgeon should establish the anterior portal. The location and method will depend on the type of procedure planned. The simplest method is inside out. When no significant anterior glenohumeral pathology such as a superior labral, anterior to posterior labral lesion (SLAP), Bankart, or subscapularis tendon lesion is observed, this method is quite satisfactory. Simply place the tip of the arthroscope into the anterior rotator cuff interval between the biceps and the subscapularis tendons. The tip is angled slightly superiorly and laterally. The camera is removed from the cannula and either a long sharp trocar or a taper-tipped guide rod is advanced into the cannula to gently puncture the anterior capsule and tent the skin. A 1-cm stab incision is created at the guide rod. To double-check the location, it should be approximately 2 cm inferior and 1 cm medial to the anterolateral edge of the acromion. The rod is advanced through the stab wound and another cannula placed over the guide rod and into the glenohumeral joint, thus creating the anterior portal. The guide rod is removed from the posterior cannula and the camera reinserted to confirm the satisfactory anterior portal placement.

If a SLAP, Bankart, or other anterior lesion is expected, the surgeon should utilize the outside-in technique. Position the anterior portal superiorly in the rotator interval. Place a spinal needle into the skin approximately 1 cm off the anterior acromion and follow it into the joint just underneath the biceps tendon under direct vision. Make a skin incision and then place a cannula with a blunt trocar into the joint in the same angle and location as the spinal needle. A second, more inferior anterior midglenoid portal is placed in a similar manner just above the subscapularis tendon, usually approximately 2 cm distal and 1 cm medial to the first anterior-superior portal. It is important to maximize the distance between these two cannulas in order to optimize the working area. Once the anterior cannula or cannulas are placed, the outflow drainage tubing is connected and the diagnostic glenohumeral arthroscopy performed.

GLENOHUMERAL JOINT EVALUATION: 15-POINT ANATOMY REVIEW

This 15-point review was developed by Snyder (5) for use in the lateral decubitus position so that the examination flows naturally from one anatomic point to the next. However, it can easily be used in the beach-chair position as well. For the purposes of this description, it is assumed that the video image is always oriented such that the glenoid surface is horizontal, comprising the "floor" of the monitor. This allows the entire surgical team to immediately understand and orient themselves during the procedure. The first 10 points are visualized from the posterior portal.

Position 1 visualizes the biceps tendon and its insertion onto the superior labral anchor (Fig. 2.8). Carefully

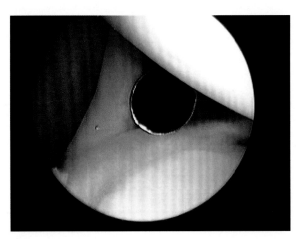

FIGURE 2.8. Position 1—long head of biceps and its insertion onto the superior labral anchor.

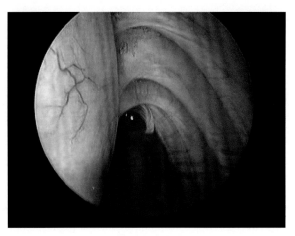

FIGURE 2.9. Position 3—inferior axillary recess.

examine the intra-articular biceps tendon on both of its sides. Angle the arthroscope toward the entry of the biceps into the intertubercular groove, and use an arthroscopic angled probe or looped grasper to pull as much of the tendon as possible into the joint for evaluation. This maneuver can reveal pathologic tendon that cannot be seen within the joint. Normal biceps tendon is white and glossy in texture. Next, inspect the biceps anchor on the superior labrum. It should be well attached to the underlying glenoid.

Several normal variants exist for the superior labrum, which can be quite confusing for the novice. The superior labrum is loosely attached and meniscoid in appearance in approximately 15% of patients. This is often incorrectly mistaken for a SLAP tear. Upon closer examination, the articular cartilage underneath the superior labrum extends on top of the glenoid to the point of the labral attachment. Traction upon the labrum flap does not pull it away from bone nor does it transfer any tension to the middle glenohumeral ligament.

Another unusual variant is the bifid biceps tendon. One portion attaches onto the supraglenoid tubercle, and the other attaches to the rotator cuff tendon. Very rarely does the entire biceps tendon attach onto the rotator cuff ridge without any attachment to the glenoid.

Position 2 includes the posterior labrum and posterior recess. In order to visualize this area, retract the camera without coming out of the posterior capsule and rotate the angle back toward the surgeon. This area is often difficult to visualize, particularly if the posterior portal is placed suboptimally. One technique to improve the view is to lift the arthroscope off the posterior labrum several millimeters to allow some room between the camera and the glenoid. The labrum should be attached tightly to the posterior glenoid rim but often has redundant synovium.

Position 3 is the inferior axillary recess (Fig. 2.9). The camera is rotated from along the posterior glenoid rim around and up toward the capsular attachments onto the humeral head. There should be a smooth capsule present

with normal synovium and a smooth attachment onto the head. The axillary recess may be difficult to access when adhesive capsulitis is present. Conversely, with chronic, repetitive subluxations or dislocations, the capsule may be patulous and the pouch quite large. Rarely, the capsular attachment may be disrupted in association with a traumatic dislocation.

Position 4 is situated over the inferior labrum and glenoid articular surface. The inferior labrum is first evaluated as the camera is aimed at the inferior glenoid. Again, the labrum should be smooth and white and fused to the articular cartilage. The capsular edge should be elevated off the glenoid cartilage a few millimeters. Attention is then turned to the glenoid surface. It has a shallow concavity with an area in the center with thinned-out cartilage, which is a normal finding. The anterior glenoid often has a notch or indentation that demarcates the inferior and superior portions of the glenoid.

Position 5 is the insertion of the supraspinatus and infraspinatus tendons onto the greater tuberosity (Fig. 2.10). The camera is brought around the humeral head superiorly and the tip angled up toward the insertion of these rotator cuff tendons. The tendons should be smooth and

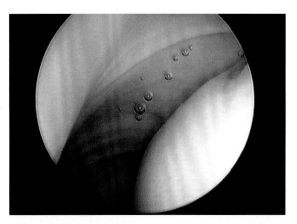

FIGURE 2.10. Position 5—attachment of supraspinatus and infraspinatus to greater tuberosity.

firmly attached to the bone. The probe and cannula can be brought through the anterior portal above the biceps tendon to provide easier access to the cuff. Attention should be paid to any fibrillation or patulousness of the tissue. This is usually indicative of a partial tear or intratendonous delamination that often cannot be fully appreciated from the intra-articular side. To aid in localizing the same area of the cuff on the bursal side, a spinal needle is introduced into the joint through any abnormal tissue and a no. 1 PDS "marker" suture is passed into the joint and cut off with a tail extending out of the skin.

Position 6 is the posterior aspect of the rotator cuff at its attachment near the "bare area" of the humeral head. The camera is slowly pulled back posteriorly and the bevel angled to approximately 10 or 2 o'clock. There is not much space in this area to view the bare area, so small movements should be used to prevent the arthroscope slipping back out of the joint. The bare area can be normally fenestrated and appear somewhat irregular. It can be quite extensive in size covering up to several centimeters in diameter. However, do not confuse this with a Hill-Sachs lesion. A Hill-Sachs lesion is more medial in location and surrounded by normal articular cartilage.

Position 7 is the portion of the humeral head that can be visualized from the posterior portal (Fig. 2.11). Position the arthroscope medially from the bare area to obtain the "equator" view and rotate the arm back and forth as well as moving the camera from 9 to 3 o'clock. Typically, glenohumeral osteoarthritis begins posteriorly, so this is a particularly important area to examine for early fibrillations or softening of the cartilage.

Position 8 is the area around the rotator interval bounded by the biceps and subscapularis tendons and the anterior-superior labrum (Fig. 2.12). This triangle includes the superior and middle glenohumeral ligaments. Because of the high degree of normal anatomic variation, this area can be quite confusing. Begin by examining the anterior-superior labrum just below the biceps anchor. In approximately 80% of cases, the labrum is firmly attached to the glenoid. However, in 14% of

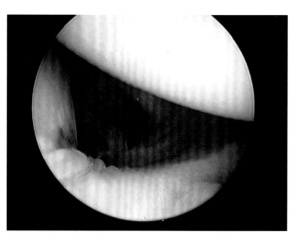

FIGURE 2.12. Position 8—rotator interval bounded by biceps tendon, subscapularis tendon, MGHL, and anterior-superior labrum.

patients a sublabral foramen exists (Fig. 2.13). This hole under the labrum can vary in size from a few millimeters to involve the entire anterior-superior labrum. It is of utmost importance to probe the tissue and differentiate this from a SLAP or Bankart tear. In these pathologic conditions, the detachment obviously extends into the biceps anchor or anterior-inferior labrum (inferior to the anterior glenoid notch).

Another variation is the so-called Buford complex, which occurs in approximately 6% of shoulders. In this interesting anatomic variant, the anterior-superior labrum is replaced with a cord-like middle glenohumeral ligament. This tissue crosses the subscapularis tendon at a 45° angle and attaches to the superior labrum just anterior to the base of the biceps anchor. The Buford complex appears quite striking and a novice surgeon can easily mistake it for a significant tear of the labrum and middle glenohumeral ligament. On closer inspection, however, the tissue is usually smooth and without fraying.

The superior glenohumeral ligament crosses between the biceps and subscapularis tendons. It courses from the labrum at the superior glenoid tubercle to the upper portion of the lesser tuberosity. It frequently appears frayed without significant consequence. The subscapularis

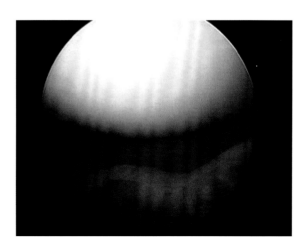

FIGURE 2.11. Position 7—posterior humeral head.

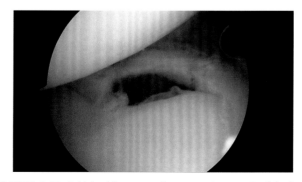

FIGURE 2.13. Sublabral foramen—loose anterior-superior labral attachment, with normal superior and inferior labral attachments.

tendon passes vertically from its attachment onto the lesser tuberosity to disappear down below the glenoid rim. Normally, the middle glenohumeral ligament drapes across the tendon at a 45° angle, although there are several variations as will be discussed below. Rarely, the leading edge of the tendon will have a bifid appearance without fraying or surrounding synovial irritation. This occurs in approximately 3% of patients.

The middle glenohumeral ligament has the most variable appearance of all the anterior structures. As mentioned, it normally crosses the subscapularis tendon to insert on the anterior-superior neck of the glenoid. In this case, the only opening to the subscapularis recess is above the leading edge of the ligament. Also, the cord-like ligament mentioned above is the most common variant and occurs in approximately 20% of shoulders. The cord can attach in its normal position on the glenoid neck or can insert onto the anterior-superior labrum. In either of these cases, the subscapularis recess can be accessed from both above or below the ligament. The final variation is simply a thin veil or complete absence of the middle glenohumeral ligament, which occurs in 10% of shoulders. Usually, the anterior band of the inferior glenohumeral ligament is hypertrophied, presumably as compensation.

Position 9 is the anterior-inferior labrum. Angle the arthroscope inferiorly to visualize the attachment of the labrum to the glenoid (Fig. 2.14). Often, the humeral head will need to be pushed posteriorly to obtain an unobstructed view. The labrum should attach firmly onto the neck of the glenoid and fuse with the edge of the cartilage. In about 5% of shoulders, a meniscoid attachment occurs in which the base of the labrum is still well attached to the glenoid, but the edge of the labrum is separated from the glenoid. Traction to the labrum does not allow it to pull away.

Position 10 includes the inferior glenohumeral ligament and anterior-inferior capsule. The anterior band of the inferior ligament usually inserts onto the anterior labrum. The remaining capsule should be smooth and covered by thin synovium. If the patient has adhesive capsulitis, it is usually impossible to view these structures from this angle. On the other hand, if the ligaments are overly lax, such as with recurrent instability or multidirectional instability,

then the arthroscope passes down with no difficulty at all, demonstrating the so-called drive-through sign.

This completes the portion of the arthroscopic glenohumeral examination viewed from the posterior portal. The final five steps require switching the arthroscope to the anterior portal and moving the outflow cannula to the posterior portal. This is accomplished with "switching sticks," which are metal rods that allow the removal and placement of the cannulas in and out of the joint without having to reintroduce a trocar.

Position 11 is the posterior labrum and capsule. The camera in the anterior portal is pointed inferiorly. The posterior labrum is attached directly to the glenoid rim. In about 5% of cases, the posterior labrum has a meniscoid attachment. Upon probing, normal labrum does not pull away and beneath the edge of the labrum the articular cartilage extends to the labral attachment. Occasionally, the posterior band of the inferior glenohumeral ligament can be seen running at a 45° angle from the midposterior labrum to the humeral head. Rarely, the ligament and posterior capsular attachment can be avulsed off the humerus in what is called a reverse humeral avulsion of the glenohumeral ligament, or RHAGL lesion.

Position 12 includes the posterior-superior capsule and the posterior insertion of the rotator cuff. The camera is angled superiorly to obtain this view (Fig. 2.15). The arthroscope can be retracted and replaced superior to the biceps tendon. The rotator ridge is the posterior attachment of the capsular thickening where it arches across the cuff to attach to the humeral head. Next, rotate the bevel of the arthroscope posteriorly to the 6 o'clock position to visualize the superior glenoid recess. Then move around the biceps tendon back into the glenohumeral joint.

Position 13 is the anterior labrum and anterior-inferior glenohumeral ligament. Rotate the arthroscope inferiorly and lift the humeral head away from the glenoid. Palpate the labrum, ligament, and capsule to confirm normal attachments. This is the most important view when evaluating for anterior instability. A probe should be brought

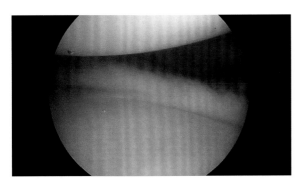

FIGURE 2.14. Position 9—anterior-inferior labrum.

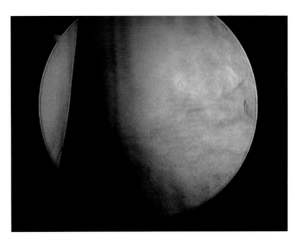

FIGURE 2.15. Position 12—posterior rotator cuff attachment.

from the posterior portal. If in fact there is an abnormality, then the anterior midglenoid portal should be created as described earlier. This more inferior portal will become the main "working portal" during the repair of the Bankart lesion. Next, rotate the arthroscope laterally to examine the attachments of the capsule anteriorly. This is important to rule out the presence of the HAGL lesion, or humeral avulsion of the glenohumeral ligament.

Position 14 is the anterior attachment of the middle glenohumeral ligament and the subscapularis recess. As mentioned before, the MGHL crosses over the subscapularis tendon to insert onto the labrum or glenoid neck. Follow the leading edge of the tendon medially down into the subscapularis recess. Loose bodies may be lodged in this area.

Position 15 is the attachment of the subscapularis to the humeral head and the anterior surface of the humeral head (Fig. 2.16). Look up laterally at the insertion of the subscapularis tendon onto the lesser tuberosity. This is the most common location of tears. The superior glenohumeral ligament also attaches to the humeral head in this area, which is often associated with some irregularity of the synovium. Rotate the arthroscope toward the anterior humeral head. Occasionally, there is a normal bare area or at least an area of thinned cartilage located superior to the attachment of the subscapularis tendon. This should not be confused with a defect caused by the impact of the glenoid rim in posterior dislocations.

DIAGNOSTIC BURSOSCOPY

Once all intra-articular procedures have been completed, a diagnostic bursoscopy may be performed. The most common indications for a bursoscopy include suspected subacromial impingement, acromioclavicular joint pathology, rotator cuff tears, and calcific tendinitis. The anatomy of the subacromial bursa is less complicated than the glenohumeral joint but is often more difficult for the surgeon to navigate in because of the lack of easily identifiable landmarks. It does not have a sturdy ligamentous capsule and the fascicle attachments are usually quite thin. This often leads to problems with fluid extravasation into the muscle

and subcutaneous envelope of the shoulder. Therefore, every effort to minimize surgical time, fluid pump pressure, and flow are of the utmost importance.

The first step is to reposition the arm for optimal visualization of the bursa. Reposition the arm from 70° of abduction to 20° of abduction and 5° forward flexion. A few more pounds may be placed on the cable for the bursal position but >15 lb (6.8 kg) are seldom needed. This position opens up the subacromial space by moving the greater tuberosity inferiorly and laterally out of the way.

Place the arthroscopic cannula into the posterior portal aiming for the posterolateral border of the acromion. Advance the cannula to the posterior acromial edge. Push the cannula underneath the acromion staying in a plane parallel to that of the acromion. Do not scrape the trocar directly under the acromion because you are apt to end up above the bursa. Conversely, aiming the trocar inferiorly may penetrate the infraspinatus and miss the bursa inferiorly. Make sure the cannula is aimed toward the anterior and middle (medial to lateral) third of the acromion because the subacromial bursa is located in the anterior half of the subacromial space in front of the orientation line drawn at the beginning of the case (Fig. 2.17).

Once in position, insert a long guide rod and use it to palpate the coracoacromial ligament. Push the rod underneath the ligament and out through the anterior-superior portal made earlier. In a retrograde manner, place an outflow cannula over the guide rod back into the bursa. Insert the arthroscope and camera and turn on the pump. The distended bursal space should immediately open up into "a room with a view" (Fig. 2.18). If you see muscle or fatty tissue, remove the instruments and repeat these steps until a bursal view is achieved. If you continue to have difficulty, place your shaver into the anterior portal and carefully remove the bursa, aiming the blades superiorly toward the acromion and away from the rotator cuff tendons. Now, you are ready for the 8-point bursal anatomy examination.

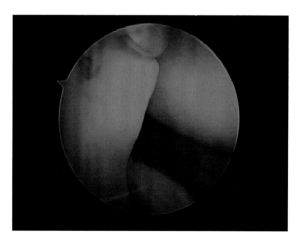

FIGURE 2.16. Position 15—subscapularis tendon insertion.

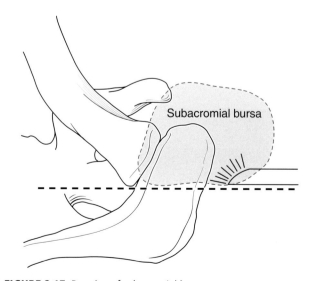

FIGURE 2.17. Drawing of subacromial bursa.

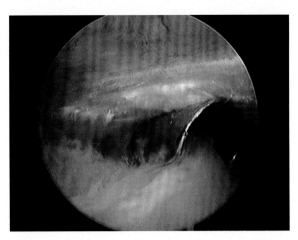

FIGURE 2.18. The distended bursal space opens up into "a room with a view."

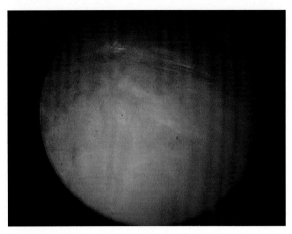

FIGURE 2.19. Bursal side of rotator cuff.

Subacromial Bursal Exam: 8-Point Anatomy Review

Position 1 is the inferior acromion and the CA ligament. The convention is to hold the camera such that the acromion is superior and the cuff is inferior. Angle the arthroscope superiorly toward the "roof" of this "room." The CA ligament usually attaches onto the anterolateral edge of the acromion and has various extensions. It can extend under the entire anterior half of the acromion, attach solely to the central portion, or extend laterally under the deltoid attachment. The ligament then dives anteromedially to attach to the coracoid. The normal appearance of the ligament is smooth and glistening. Any fraying or reactive bursitis should raise the suspicion of impingement.

Position 2 is the lateral edge of the acromion and any lateral bursal shelf. Aim the camera laterally to find the anterolateral edge of the acromion. A plica-like shelf of bursal tissue often lies there and is quite variable in appearance. It must be differentiated from the underlying rotator cuff.

Position 3 is the greater tuberosity and the insertion of the supraspinatus and infraspinatus tendons (Fig. 2.19). Angle the arthroscope inferolaterally to observe the cuff insertion. If the lateral bursal shelf obstructs this view, it may be necessary to carefully remove it with the mechanical shaver, making sure to protect the cuff from injury. Slowly rotate the arm internally and externally to completely view the entire footprint. The tendon should appear smooth without any fraying or roughness. Any fraying is suggestive of impingement.

Position 4 is the rotator cuff located just medial to the tendon–bone interface. Rotate the camera inferiorly and move the tip of the arthroscope medially to observe this location. This is a critical portion of the cuff as it is very poorly vascularized and tends to be the first area to fail. Also, calcific tendinitis seems to be localized to this area of the rotator cuff.

Position 5 includes the medial wall of the subacromial bursa. Aim the camera medially. This tissue separates the

subacromial bursal cavity from the subclavicular region. Normal bursa is smooth and vascular. When inflamed, the tissue can be quite hypertrophic with significant vascular fatty tissue. This tissue needs to be removed in order to gain access to the acromioclavicular joint. If this area is not exposed, large osteophytes can be easily overlooked in the area of the medial facet of the acromion and lateral clavicle. The AC joint should not be violated unless a Mumford procedure (distal clavicle resection) will be performed. The spine of the scapula that divides the supraspinatus and infraspinatus muscle bellies is visualized more posteriorly. Do not instrument medially to the spine because the suprascapular nerve lies within this region as it curves around the spinoglenoid notch to innervate the infraspinatus muscle. The remaining three positions are viewed from the anterior portal with the outflow cannula located posteriorly.

Position 6 is the posterior bursal curtain (Fig. 2.20). It extends from the posterior border of the AC joint to the lateral border of the acromion. This curtain separates the bursa from the posterior subacromial space and is the reason the camera must be inserted into the anterior half of the space to visualize the "room with a view." With

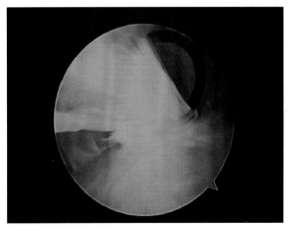

FIGURE 2.20. The posterior bursal curtain.

I. The Shoulder

significant bursitis, the curtain may become hypertrophic and obstruct the view. If this is the case, the instruments need to be switched and the curtain debrided at the beginning of the bursoscopy before proceeding to position 1.

Position 7 is the posterior aspect of the infraspinatus tendon attachment on the greater tuberosity. Move the tip of the arthroscope laterally and aim the camera inferomedially to observe the infraspinatus tendon attachment. Rotate the arm internally to fully view the posterior segment.

Position 8 includes the anterior portion of the rotator cuff, the rotator interval, and the anterior bursal recess. From the anterior portal, withdraw the arthroscope maintaining the bevel angled inferiorly to visualize this area. Small cuff tears are often located anteriorly near the rotator interval and can be missed from the posterior view. Continue down anteriorly to find the interval and then the recess.

These steps result in a comprehensive arthroscopic examination of the shoulder and permit the surgeon to evaluate all the visible anatomy of the shoulder. It is important to develop a rigid protocol for evaluating both the

glenohumeral joint and the subacromial space in order to minimize overlooking any pathology. It may make sense to perform surgical procedures at different points in this comprehensive examination, but once the procedure is complete, the comprehensive evaluation should be reinitiated. Following this rigorous examination will instill confidence in your diagnostic abilities and ultimately benefit your patients, which is most important of all.

REFERENCES

1. Bigony L. Arthroscopic Surgery: a historical perspective. *Orthop Nurs.* 2008;27;349–354.
2. Strafford BB, Del Pizzo W. A historical review of shoulder arthroscopy. *Orthop Clin North Am.* 1993;24;1–4.
3. Johnson LL. *Diagnostic and Surgical Arthroscopy of the Shoulder.* New York, NY: Elsevier; 1993.
4. Morrison DS, Schaefer RK, Friedman RL. The relationship between subacromial space pressure, blood pressure, and visual clarity during arthroscopic subacromial decompression. *Arthroscopy.* 1995;11:557–560.
5. Snyder SJ. *Shoulder Arthroscopy.* Philadelphia, PA: Lippincott Williams & Williams; 2002.

Acromioclavicular Separations: Soft Tissue (Weaver–Dunn or Allograft) Techniques

Robert F. LaPrade and Corey A. Wulf

Injuries to the acromioclavicular joint (AC) are common. AC separations, subluxations, and dislocations represent 9% of all injuries to the shoulder girdle. They more commonly occur in males during the second and third decades (1). There is a high incidence among collision athletes. It is the third most common injury in Division I hockey (2) players. The reported incidence in American collegiate football players and National Football League quarterbacks is 41% and 40%, respectively (3).

Despite the commonality of AC separations, very little was known in regard to its kinematics and biomechanics until recently. This lack of fundamental understanding has resulted in the development of surgical procedures that failed to stabilize the AC joint and restore more normal kinematics and function of the joint. It is the goal of this chapter to review the anatomy, biomechanics, and kinematics of the AC joint while incorporating these principles into the selection of a surgical technique for reconstruction of the AC joint.

BASIC SCIENCE

The shoulder girdle is capable of complex movements through multiple articulations involving the chest wall, scapula, proximal humerus, and clavicle. Movements through the aforementioned articulations are powered by the 20 muscle/tendon units that originate or insert on it (4). The clavicle functions as a strut to maintain the lateral positioning of the glenohumeral joint relative to the thorax. The clavicle also provides the origin of the coracoclavicular (CC) ligaments, the conoid, and the trapezoid, which suspend the scapula and contribute to the stability of the AC joint. Bony prominences on the undersurface of the clavicle mark the origins of each ligament. The trapezoidal ridge marks the lateral extent of the trapezoid, whereas the conoid tubercle marks the posterior extent of the conoid. These landmarks can be useful when determining the correct placement for graft fixation while reconstructing the AC joint.

The AC joint is the point of articulation between the scapula and the clavicle. The AC joint is a diarthrodial joint composed of the distal, or lateral, end of the clavicle and the medial aspect of the acromial process of the scapula. Hyaline cartilage is present on the articulating surfaces of the acromion and clavicle. There is a meniscal homologue interposed within the articular space. The meniscal homologue is composed of fibrocartilage and is quite variable in size and shape. The function of the meniscal homologue is unknown and thought to be negligible because it undergoes degeneration in the second and third decades. The articular surfaces are surrounded by the joint capsule and capsular ligaments. The capsule and joint are dually innervated by both the suprascapular and the lateral pectoral nerves.

The AC joint is stabilized both statically and dynamically. The static stabilizers are composed of the joint capsule/ligaments (acromioclavicular or AC ligaments) and the CC ligaments. The fascia of the trapezius and deltoid are the predominant dynamic stabilizers of the AC joint. The AC ligaments are the primary stabilizers of the AC joint at low forces, with the superior ligaments being the strongest and thickest. The CC ligaments are the primary stabilizers at greater forces. They work in concert to stabilize the AC joint as well as to link movement between the clavicle and the scapula. The trapezoid ligament is the broader of the two. It originates on the undersurface of the clavicle, medial to the trapezoidal ridge, and inserts broadly on the posterior, dorsal half of the coracoid. The trapezoid ligament's main function is to resist AC joint compression and posterior displacement of the clavicle during loading of the glenohumeral joint. The conoid ligament has an oval footprint as it originates anterior to the conoid tubercle on the undersurface of the clavicle. It narrows while passing inferiorly to insert on the posterior and dorsal most portion of the coracoid, including the angle.

Historically, the clavicle and AC joint together were thought to be relatively immobile and simple in regard to their kinematics. This has changed over the years as biomechanical evaluation has demonstrated the intricate role that the clavicle and its articulation with the scapula play in movements of the upper extremity. The clavicle is not stationary in its relation to the acromion. Motion about the clavicle occurs in three axes: anterior–posterior, superior–inferior, and axial rotation around the anatomic axis of the clavicle. The clavicle hinges on the sternoclavicular joint, allowing up to 35° of motion in the anterior, posterior, and superior directions (4). The axial rotation of the clavicle is greater in relation to the sternum than it is to the acromion, 45° to 50° and 5° to 8°, respectively (4). Despite the multitude of stabilizing constraints, the clavicle may show moderate amounts of displacement in all planes. Debski et al. (5) demonstrated that the clavicle may translate up to 5 mm in the anterior, posterior, and superior directions during application of a 70-N force.

Most historic procedures failed to account for the normal kinematics of the AC joint and led to high rates of failure. Rigid constructs that inhibited AC motion and translation, such as CC screws, failed due to fatigue or pull out. Kirshner (K)-wire fixation tended to migrate. Soft tissue reconstructions restore more normal kinematics while maintaining the reduction of the AC joint.

CLINICAL EVALUATION

Injuries and separations of the AC joint do not typically present a diagnostic dilemma to the evaluating clinician. The mechanism of injury, deformity, and location of pain are reliable findings that lead the clinician to the correct diagnosis. The most common mechanism of injury is through direct trauma with an impact onto the acromion while the arm is in an adducted position. However, it may also occur with a fall onto a hand or elbow that drives the humerus into the undersurface of the acromion. The proposed mechanism for the rare, inferiorly displaced clavicle involves a force applied axially to the upper extremity while the arm is in hyperabduction and external rotation with the scapula in a retracted position. Patients often complain of pain over the superior aspect of the shoulder in the region of the AC joint, but may note pain that radiates into the anterior portion of the neck. Deformity about the AC joint is also a common finding in both the acute and the chronic settings. Prominence of the distal clavicle in the superior, or cranial, direction in relation to the acromion is the most common finding, but displacement in the anterior–posterior planes may be found in association with superior displacement. Less commonly, patients may sustain an AC joint separation with inferior displacement of the clavicle in relation to the acromion.

Evaluation of the patient starts with a detailed history. The key elements include the mechanism, previous injuries, and identification of any unrecognized or masked injuries. A detailed history is followed with a thorough physical examination. Inspection often identifies the deformity about the AC joint. Palpation elicits pain over the AC joint, but one should palpate the entire length of the clavicle and sternoclavicular joint, as concomitant injuries have been reported. Range of motion (ROM) is often limited by pain, especially when the arm is placed in adduction and forward elevation. The cross-body adduction test is performed with the arm in 90° of forward elevation and passively adducting the arm. A positive test is present when pain is reproduced superiorly at the AC joint. The O'Brien's test is helpful in differentiating patients with Superior Labrum Anterior and Posterior (SLAP) lesions from those with AC joint injuries. However, approximately 18% of patients with type V AC joint injuries had concomitant SLAP lesions (6). It is also important to palpate around the coracoid to evaluate for avulsion fractures of the coracoid. Neurovascular documentation is important, especially in the setting of an inferiorly displaced clavicle.

Imaging

Radiographic evaluation is directed by the clinician's physical exam findings. Standard shoulder series including AP, scapular Y, and axillary views are routinely ordered. Historically, visualization of the AC joint on a standard shoulder series has been difficult due to the overpenetration that can occur with more superficial structures. We have found this to be less of an issue with the introduction of digital X-rays, which allow the user to adjust the contrast and brightness for better visualization. A Zanca view can be added to allow for optimal visualization of the AC joint. It is performed with the X-ray beam centered over the AC joint and angled 10° to 15° cephalad while using half the penetration strength of a standard AP. CT scans more accurately define bony abnormalities or fracture patterns, both of which are uncommonly encountered in the authors' practice. As such, a CT scan is rarely obtained since it adds very little information to the plain radiographs that would affect treatment. MRI may be considered if there is concern for associated or concomitant glenohumeral joint pathology. We do not routinely obtain MRIs as a part of the initial evaluation or index procedures, but it may be of benefit in the setting of failed treatment due to persistent or recurrent pain in the absence of ongoing AC instability.

Classification

AC joint separations are commonly classified using the Tossy/Rockwood system. There are six types based on the amount and direction of displacement. The types correlate with the structures injured. Type I represents a sprain of the AC ligaments without appreciable displacement of the clavicle in relation to the acromion. Type II injuries involve complete disruption of the AC ligaments while the CC ligaments remain intact. The clavicle is usually subluxated superiorly in relation to the acromion. The clavicle is unstable upon direct stress. Type III injuries present as a dislocation of the AC joint with 100% subluxation displacement of the clavicle relative to the acromion. Type III injuries represent tears of the AC and CC ligaments, whereas the trapezial and deltoid fascias remain intact. The clavicle is unstable in the horizontal and vertical planes. Type IV injuries are characterized by complete dislocation of the AC joint as a result of the disruption of the AC and CC ligaments and posterior displacement of the clavicle through the trapezial fascia. The posterior displacement of the clavicle is best visualized on the axillary radiograph. Type V separations result in displacement of the clavicle between 100% and 300% of the width of the clavicle in relation to the acromion due to failure of the AC ligaments, CC ligaments, and deltotrapezial fascia. Finally, type VI injuries are rare injuries with complete inferior displacement of the clavicle into a subacromial or subcoracoid position.

TREATMENT

Nonoperative

Conservative treatment remains the mainstay for type I, II, and III injuries. However, the treatment of type III injuries remains controversial and an area of intense debate. In a systematic review, Spencer (7) performed an analysis of the English-language literature to determine whether grade III AC joint separations were best treated operatively or nonoperatively. The author concluded that nonoperative treatment was deemed more appropriate than traditional operative treatments because the results of the latter were not clearly better and were associated with higher complication rates, longer convalescence, and longer time away from work and sports. This conclusion was based upon a relatively low level of evidence with the most data coming from level IV studies with very few level I and II studies reported. We prefer to initially treat patients with type III injuries nonoperatively, especially if the patient is in an athletic season, and reserve surgical management for those who fail conservative treatment.

Generally nonathletic patients are treated with a regimen that includes a period of sling immobilization for up to 7 days, analgesics, and progressive activity as tolerated. Gladstone et al. (8) described a nonoperative regimen for athletes with AC separations. It consists of four phases: (1) pain control with immediate protected ROM and isometric exercises; (2) strengthening exercises using isotonic contractions and proprioceptive neuromuscular facilitation (PNF) exercises; (3) unrestricted functional participation with the goal of increasing strength, power, endurance, and neuromuscular control; and (4) return to activity with sports-specific functional drills. The authors allowed the patients to progress through the phases as symptoms abated, noting that patients with type III injuries progressed slower than those with type I and II injuries. Gladstone et al. (8) recommended return to play when the following criteria are met: full ROM, no pain

or tenderness, satisfactory clinical exam, and demonstration of adequate strength on isokinetic testing. More commonly, athletes are allowed to return to play when they can demonstrate full ROM, minimal symptoms on exam, and protective strength. Additional padding, vests, and foam cutouts may provide additional comfort and cushioning for contact athletes. The author is unaware of any study that confirms that additional padding or cushioning will prevent or lessen additional trauma after return to play.

Operative

There have been numerous surgical procedures described for instability about the AC joint. Techniques are quite variable and range widely from rigid fixation to anatomic soft tissue reconstruction. Although some techniques have fallen out of favor, there continue to be various techniques employed by surgeons for the treatment of AC joint dislocations. The focus of this chapter will be on soft tissue reconstruction. However, we will briefly explore the different described methods.

Surgical management is usually reserved for type III, IV, V, and VI separations that have failed nonoperative management. Ongoing instability, pain, and inability to effectively participate in sports or difficulty performing daily activities are indications for surgery. Cosmesis tends to be a common complaint, but is a relatively weak indication for surgical treatment. Deformity at the AC joint may cause discomfort for female patients from overlying undergarment straps. Contraindications are relative and include in season athletes and acute injuries.

Rigid fixation includes differing techniques such as screws, plates, and threaded K-wires. Screw and K-wire fixation are plagued by relatively low failure loads and concerns for fatigue failure with retained implants, whereas plates may involve intra-articular placement with associated arthrosis or prominent and painful hardware. These techniques have been abandoned for more biologic and anatomic reconstructions.

Soft tissue reconstructions of the AC joint also have many variations in methods that range from anatomic to nonanatomic repairs with variable tissue sources. Tissue sources include the CA ligament, the short head of the biceps, conjoined tendon, and hamstring tendon autograft or allograft. Augmentation of soft tissue reconstructions has also been described with nonbiologic materials such as suture, screws, and K-wires. The modified Weaver–Dunn (9) and semitendinosus tendon graft reconstruction of the CC ligaments are the most popular of the various soft tissue techniques. The variations in descriptions in the literature of the modified Weaver–Dunn and especially allograft reconstructions are overwhelming and outside the scope of this chapter. However, the principles for successful reconstruction among the various descriptions are relatively constant and include strength of the tissue used in the reconstruction and the ability of the reconstruction to allow for relatively normal kinematics, thus reducing the stress placed on the reconstruction.

The modified Weaver–Dunn procedure is the most popular of the nonanatomic soft tissue reconstructions. The CA ligament is transferred to the distal aspect of the clavicle after resection of the articular portion of the clavicle. LaPrade et al. (10) noted the modified Weaver–Dunn reconstruction was found to restore motion of the AC to near-intact values, but created a more anterior and inferior position of the clavicle with respect to the acromion. Total translatory motion of the AC in the cut state was significantly greater than both the intact and the reconstructed states in the medial/lateral (intact, 4.3 mm; cut, 7.9 mm; reconstructed, 2.6 mm), anterior/posterior (intact, 4.8 mm; cut, 6.1 mm; reconstructed, 4.9 mm), and superior/inferior (intact, 4.1 mm; cut, 8.0 mm; reconstructed, 4.8 mm) directions. Clinically, this is born out in the literature with numerous reports of successful reconstructions using this technique. However, the load to failure of the CA ligament is approximately one-fifth that of the CC ligaments (11), and may be partially responsible for reported failures with recurrent deformity and pain. The modified Weaver–Dunn procedure also disrupts the CA arch with loss of a secondary static stabilizer to superior translation of the humeral head in relation to the glenoid.

Reconstruction of the CC ligaments with the use of allograft or autograft tendon provides the benefits of a similar load to failure profile to the CC ligaments (11), less elongation under loading than reconstruction with the CA ligament (11), restores both superior/inferior and anterior/posterior stability (12), and maintains the integrity of the CA arch. CC ligament reconstruction, as previously mentioned, has numerous variations. Allograft semitendinosus tendon is the most common graft type used. Described variations include a cerclage technique with the graft looped around the coracoid and clavicle, holes drilled in both the clavicle and the coracoid with the graft traversing the bony tunnels, tunnels in the clavicle only, and any of the aforementioned techniques augmented with nonbiologic materials such as braided suture or Dacron tape. Graft fixation also varies with suture fixation and interference screws being the most commonly reported techniques. Bone tunnels allow for anatomic placement of the graft but also produce stress risers that can be of concern in collision athletes. Care should be taken to minimize the size of the bone tunnels while maintaining an adequate bone bridge between multiple tunnels.

Mazzocca et al. (12) compared a CA ligament transfer with an anatomic double-bundle reconstruction of the CC ligaments with bone tunnels and interference screw fixation in a cadaveric model. There were no significant differences with load to failure, superior migration over 3,000 cycles, or superior displacement. The anatomical CC reconstruction had significantly less (*P* < .05) anterior and posterior translation than the modified Weaver–Dunn procedure. Failure of the modified Weaver-Dunn to control anterior and posterior displacement may allow for impingement and pain

when the clavicle displaces posteriorly into the acromion and scapular spine.

Finally, Tauber et al. (13) performed a prospective study comparing the surgical treatment with a modified Weaver–Dunn procedure to an autologous semitendinosus tendon reconstruction with drill holes in the clavicle and secured by suturing the tendon to itself. There were 24 patients, 12 in each reconstruction group, with a mean follow-up of 37 months. The mean American Shoulder and Elbow Surgeons shoulder score improved from 74 ± 7 points preoperatively to 86 ± 8 points postoperatively in the Weaver–Dunn group and from 74 ± 4 points to 96 ± 5 points in the semitendinosus tendon group (*P* < .001 for both techniques). The mean constant score improved from 70 ± 8 points to 81 ± 8 points in the Weaver–Dunn group and from 71 ± 5 points to 93 ± 7 points in the semitendinosus tendon group (*P* < .001). The results in the semitendinosus tendon group were significantly better than those in the Weaver–Dunn group (*P* < .001). The radiologic measurements showed a mean CC distance of 12.3 ± 4 mm in the Weaver–Dunn group increasing to 14.9 ± 6 mm under stress loading, compared with 11.4 ± 3 mm increasing to 11.8 ± 3 mm under stress in the semitendinosus tendon group. The difference during stress loading was statistically significant (*P* = .027). The authors concluded that the semitendinosus tendon graft for CC ligament reconstruction resulted in significantly superior clinical and radiologic outcomes compared with the modified Weaver–Dunn procedure. We prefer reconstruction with allograft semitendinosus (14) based on the presented biomechanical and clinical data. Allograft does carry the small risk of disease transmission, but does not have the associated comorbidities of graft harvesting.

AUTHORS' PREFERRED TECHNIQUE

Patients are placed in the beach chair position. A standard deltopectoral incision with extension more proximally is made. The incision allows for visualization of the distal clavicle and coracoid. The deltopectoral groove is identified and the cephalic vein is retracted medially. The coracoid is identified as well as the conjoined tendon and pectoralis minor attachments on the coracoid. The superior aspect of the distal clavicle is exposed over its borders by subperiosteal dissection to allow for complete visualization from its lateral aspect to the level of the normal CC ligament attachment medially on the clavicle, leaving the anterior deltoid attachment on the clavicle intact. We then prepare for placement of the semitendinosus graft by first drilling a 6 mm hole, superior to inferior, at approximately the anterior third of the distal clavicle at the region of the normal CC ligament attachment (Fig. 3.1). An 8- to 10-mm bone bridge from the anterior aspect of the clavicle is preserved. A Chandler retractor is then placed inferiorly, to protect against overpenetration by the drill when reaming superior to inferior through the distal clavicle.

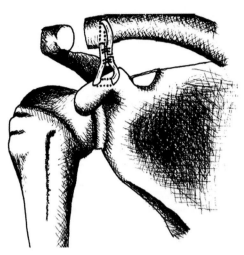

FIGURE 3.1. Schematic demonstrating the location of drill holes in both the coracoid and the clavicle and orientation of the graft.

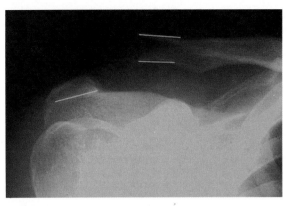

FIGURE 3.2. Anteroposterior radiographic view, right shoulder, shows proximal migration of the distal clavicle after a failed modified Weaver–Dunn reconstruction (white lines drawn to supplement visualization under acromion and superior/inferior surfaces of distal clavicle).

The coracoid is then identified with an attempt to minimally detach the deltoid attachments on the clavicle. A coracoid tunnel is then drilled slightly proximal and medial to the conjoined tendon from lateral to medial. A Chandler retractor is placed posterior to the coracoid for protection of the neurovascular structures. Two incomplete 6-mm holes are drilled, one along the medial and one along the lateral edges of the coracoid. The tunnels are then connected using a 90°-angled hemostat by placing the hemostat into each tunnel and gently twisting. The graft is prepared on the back table by tubularizing each end of the semitendinosus allograft with No. 2 sutures to allow it to be easily passed through the bony tunnels. A No. 2 suture is then placed through the coracoid tunnel and tied to the passing stitches within the hamstring allograft, and the sutures are pulled through the coracoid tunnel. The graft is pulled through the tunnel, routed under the deltoid, and positioned under the distal clavicle. The graft is passed from inferior to superior through the distal clavicle tunnel.

The two arms of the graft are pulled under the deltoid by axial traction until the distal clavicle elevation is completely reduced. Multiple No. 2 nonabsorbable sutures are stitched in a horizontal mattress fashion to fix both ends of the graft together while the clavicle is held in a reduced position. The clavicle is then tested in the newly reduced position to confirm that there is no slack of the graft in situ, and stiff graft resistance occurs while attempting to elevate the clavicle superiorly away from the coracoid. Motion is tested to observe the tension on the repair. If >90° of forward elevation can be achieved with no obvious tension on the hamstring/CC reconstruction suture repair, the tail ends of the newly sutured graft loop are excised and the wound is closed. After skin closure, 30 mL of 0.25% bupivacaine without epinephrine is injected to aid in postoperative analgesia, and patients are placed in a cold compression device, a shoulder sling, and taken to the recovery room (Figs. 3.2 and 3.3).

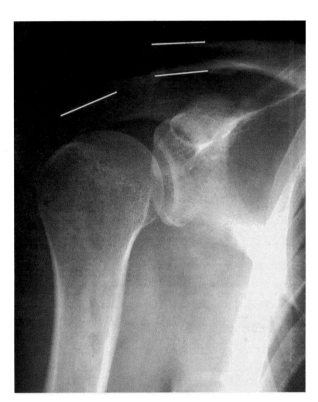

FIGURE 3.3. Anteroposterior radiographic view, right shoulder, shows the appearance after reconstruction of the CC ligament with a semitendinosus graft for a failed right modified Weaver–Dunn reconstruction (white lines drawn to supplement visualization under acromion and superior/inferior surfaces of distal clavicle).

COMPLICATIONS

To date we have not experienced any complications or failures related to allograft reconstruction of the CC ligaments for treatment of AC joint injuries. However, we have a relatively short period of follow-up and although the biomechanical data support allograft reconstructions, only long-term results will provide the evidence needed to support the described technique. Although there are no reported cases, potential stress risers in both the clavicle and the coracoid pose a theoretical risk of fracture, especially in contact athletes.

PEARLS

1. A standard deltopectoral approach provides excellent visualization of the pertinent anatomic structures for safe and accurate placement of tunnels in both the coracoid and the clavicle.
2. Protection of the neurovascular structures while working about the coracoid, especially posterior and medial, will reduce the risk for iatrogenic injury.
3. Adequate bone bridges should be preserved to reduce the risk of fracture.
4. Reduction of the AC joint is best performed with downward pressure on the distal clavicle using an instrument, such as a Picador ball spike, while the surgical assistant forces the humerus upward by placing a hand under the elbow.

PITFALLS

1. Care is taken to close the wound in layers to minimize any prominence of the graft as it passes over the clavicle.
2. Strict postoperative therapy regimen and return to play criteria reduce the risk of recurrence.

REHABILITATION

Initial physical activities for the operative shoulder included pendulum exercises four times daily and passive elevation four times daily to a maximum of 90° for 6 weeks. Patients are allowed to initiate active motion at 6 weeks postoperatively and rotator cuff and scapular stabilizer exercises are started at 8 weeks. Full activities are allowed once full strength has been restored after 4 months postoperatively.

CONCLUSIONS AND FUTURE DIRECTIONS

Acromioclavicular separations are common injuries to a joint of which we are only beginning to understand its contributions to upper extremity function. The majority of injuries may be treated nonoperatively with most experiencing good outcomes. For patients who fail nonoperative therapy or sustain a more severe separation of the AC joint, anatomic reconstruction of the CC ligaments with a tendon graft appears to be a good treatment with promising short-term results. The biomechanical evidence would suggest that CC ligament reconstruction as described may produce fewer failures and better outcomes than more historic procedures and the modified Weaver–Dunn. Only mid- and long-term follow-up will provide definitive information on the true safety and efficacy of a CC ligament reconstruction.

REFERENCES

1. Rockwood CJ, Williams G, Young D. Disorders of the AC joint. In: Rockwood CJ, Matsen F, eds. *The Shoulder*. Vol 1. Philadelphia, PA: WB Saunders; 1998:483–553.
2. Flik K, Lyman S, Marx RG. American collegiate men's ice hockey: an analysis of injuries. *Am J Sports Med.* 2005;33:183–187.
3. Kaplan LD, Flannigan DC, Norwig J, et al. Prevalence and variance of shoulder injuries in elite collegiate football players. *Am J Sports Med.* 2005;33:1142–1146.
4. Buckwalter JA, Einhorn TA, Simon SR. *Orthopedic Basic Science, Biology and Biomechanics of the Musculoskeletal System*, 2nd ed. Rosemont, IL: AAOS;2000:741.
5. Debski RE, Parsons IM 3rd, Fenwick J, et al. Ligament mechanics during three degree-of-freedom motion at the acromioclavicular joint. *Ann Biomed Eng.* 2000;28:612–618.
6. Tischer T, Salzmann GM, El-Azab H, et al. Incidence of associated injuries with acute acromioclavicular joint dislocations types III through V. *Am J Sports Med.* 2009;37:136–139.
7. Spencer EE Jr. Treatment of grade III acromioclavicular joint injuries: a systematic review. *Clin Orthop Relat Res.* 2007;455:38–44.
8. Gladstone J, Wilk K, Andrews J. Nonoperative treatment of acromioclavicular injuries. *Oper Tech Sports Med.* 1997;5:78–87.
9. Ponce BP, Millett PJ, Warner JP. Acromioclavicular joint instability: reconstruction indications and techniques. *Oper Tech Sports Med.* 2004;12:35–42.
10. LaPrade RF, Wickum DJ, Griffith CJ, et al. Kinematic evaluation of the modified Weaver-Dunn acromioclavicular joint reconstruction. *Am J Sports Med.* 2008;36:2216–2221.
11. Lee SJ, Nicholas SJ, Akizuki KH, et al. Reconstruction of the coracoclavicular ligament with tendon grafts: a comparative biomechanical study. *Am J Sports Med.* 2003;31:648–654.
12. Mazzocca AD, Santangelo SA, Johnson ST, et al. A biomechanical evaluation of an anatomical coracoclavicular ligament reconstruction. *Am J Sports Med.* 2006;34:236–246.
13. Tauber M, Gordon K, Koller H, et al. Semitendinosus tendon graft versus a modified Weaver-Dunn procedure for acromioclavicular joint reconstruction in chronic cases: a prospective comparative study. *Am J Sports Med.* 2009;37:181–190.
14. LaPrade RF, Hilger B. Coracoclavicular ligament reconstruction using a semitendinosus graft for failed acromioclavicular separation surgery. *Arthroscopy.* 2005;21:1279.e1–1279.e5

Acromioclavicular Separations: Arthroscopic Reconstruction of the Acromioclavicular Joint

Daniel T. Richards • James J. Guerra

Acromioclavicular (AC) joint dislocations are common injuries encountered in orthopedic medicine. Treatment strategies vary greatly ranging from nonsurgical to complete reconstruction. Despite a recent resurgence of interest in the orthopedic literature about AC joint injuries, treatment recommendations remain controversial. For lesser grade injuries, current literature has reaffirmed the success of nonoperative treatment for many AC joint separations. However, for injuries with significant displacement, surgical management is recommended to restore the normal kinematics of the shoulder. Modern biomechanical testing and recent anatomical dissection have demonstrated inconsistencies related to the more traditionally recommended surgical techniques while providing insight into improving the surgical management of both acute and chronic injuries. Much of this research has focused on the combined use of ultrastrong synthetic materials in combination with biologic grafts.

This chapter presents the most current anatomical, biomechanical, and surgical considerations relating to the treatment of AC joint injuries with a particular focus on arthroscopic surgical techniques.

CLINICAL EVALUATION

History and Physical Exam Findings

As with any acute injury, a complete history and physical exam should be performed for any patient suspected of having an injured AC joint. The history will help determine treatment options for the patient and should focus on the injury mechanism, treatment timing, and the potential for postinjury morbidity. Age, desired sport, and occupational demands warrant special consideration should operative intervention be contemplated. On physical exam, concomitant traction injuries should be noted and a careful examination of the affected shoulder be completed.

Incomplete injuries to the AC joint will likely result in pain localized to the upper shoulder. At times, this pain

can be poorly localized. The AC joint has dual innervation from the suprascapular nerve as well as the lateral pectoral nerve, and pain can be referred to their respective dermatomal distributions. Isolation of the AC joint as the location of injury can be accomplished by eliciting pain with direct palpation or provocative maneuvers such as the cross-chest adduction test. Relief of pain with injection of a local anesthetic confirms the diagnosis. With complete injuries, there is almost always pain, swelling, and deformity of the AC joint. Subtle deformities can be confirmed with radiographs.

Diagnostic Imaging

Radiographs are usually sufficient for evaluating potential AC joint injuries. Specific views for optimal assessment have been described. In general, three orthogonal views are adequate to initially evaluate the shoulder for a traumatic injury. These views include an AP, a scapular-Y, and an axillary. If an AC joint injury is further suspected, additional views may be indicated.

Although the AP and scapular-Y views of the shoulder can indicate an AC joint injury, more specific views can reveal additional, more subtle findings. The Zanca view angles the X-ray beam 10° to 15° cephalad in a true AP orientation to eliminate the overlap of the scapular spine (1). The X-ray power should be reduced to 30% to 50% of normal to avoid overpenetration of the less dense AC joint. The Zanca view will reveal any relative displacement of the clavicle. Bilateral Zanca views on the same X-ray cassette allow for comparison with the contralateral side (Fig. 4.1). Bearden et al. (2) demonstrated in their study

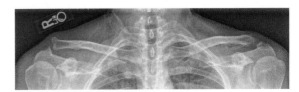

FIGURE 4.1. Bilateral Zanca view: allows for comparison with unaffected shoulder.

that the mean distance between the superior border of the coracoid and the inferior border of the clavicle was 1.1 to 1.3 cm. As this distance will vary between patients and radiographic techniques, it is necessary to compare side-to-side differences. Distances of >25% to 50% compared with the unaffected side have been shown to be diagnostic for a complete CC ligament disruption (3).

The axillary view, although not specific, can be helpful in type IV injuries in which the clavicle is posteriorly displaced. In addition, the cross-arm view can illuminate the degree of injury by accentuating the displacement of the clavicle (4) (Fig. 4.2). Although classically described and often cited in the evaluation of AC joint injuries, weighted stress radiographs are no longer thought to be the gold standard and have been largely superseded by bilateral Zanca views.

Classification of AC Joint Injury

Most AC joint injuries are the consequence of a force directed inferiorly at the acromion with the arm adducted. This motion forces the entire shoulder girdle down. During the initial motion, the AC joint remains congruent. However, the clavicle eventually impacts the first rib, inhibiting further inferior translation. The clavicle will

either fracture, with the first rib acting as a fulcrum, or the AC ligament complex will sequentially fail.

Although first recognized by Hippocrates (5), it was not until 1917 when the first description of the sequential failure of the AC joint complex was published by Cadenat (6). Tossy (7) later proposed a classification scheme including three degrees of injury ranging from type I injuries, which represent a sprain of the AC ligaments, to type III with complete disruption and separation of the clavicle and scapula. Rockwood et al. (3) expanded Tossy's classification, adding three additional injury grades for a total of six.

Rockwood's classification (Fig. 4.3) begins with a minimal injury to the AC joint proper. This injury pattern, type I, represents a sprain of the joint capsule and surrounding ligaments without displacement. In a type II injury, the AC joint capsule and surrounding ligaments are disrupted but without significant elevation of the clavicle, usually <50%. The coracoclavicular (CC) ligaments are intact preventing superior displacement but increased anterior–posterior translation will often be apparent. With further significant force a type III injury occurs. The AC ligament complex as well as the CC ligament complex rupture resulting in up to 100% displacement of the clavicle relative to the scapula. Type IV injuries, best visualized on axillary radiographs, occur when the clavicle is forced posteriorly through the trapezius and are generally irreducible

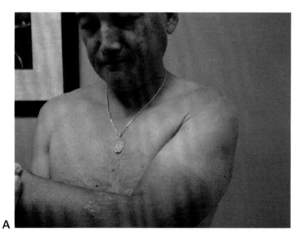
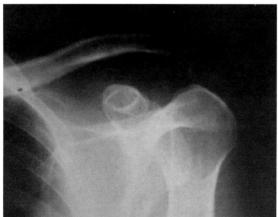

FIGURE 4.2. A: Clinical photograph of a cross-chest adduction view. **B:** Radiograph demonstrating the accentuated displacement of the clavicle.

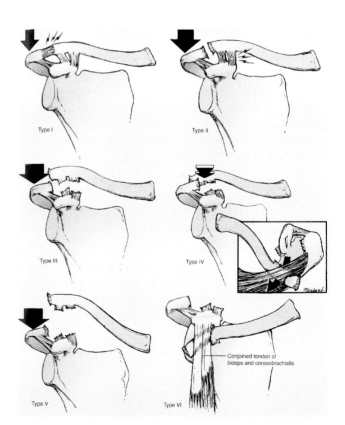

FIGURE 4.3. Rockwood classification AC injuries. (From Johnson D, Pedowitz RA, *Practical Orthopaedic Sports Medicine*. Philadelphia, PA: Lippincott William and Wilkins; 2006 with permission.)

on physical exam due to soft-tissue interposition. Type V injuries are secondary to violent force and represent complete soft-tissue disruption of the clavicle from the scapula with up to 300% displacement of the clavicle. This displacement occurs because of the disruption of the deltotrapezial fascia. Finally, the extremely rare type VI injury occurs when the clavicle becomes displaced and entrapped beneath the coracoid or acromion.

TREATMENT

Nonoperative Treatment Considerations

Lesser grade AC joint injuries, types I and II, can be treated successfully nonoperatively and conservative care is the mainstay of management. Various regimes have been used effectively. Initial immobilization with a sling for comfort followed by unrestricted use and symptomatic pain relief usually affords excellent results. Use of a corticosteroid and anesthetic preparation for high demand patients or athletes may speed recovery. If symptoms persist despite extensive conservative care, an arthroscopic distal clavicle resection of no more than 8 to 10 mm is appropriate. Conversely, treatment strategies for types IV, V, and VI almost always include surgical intervention. Patients with these injury types will often suffer significant morbidity if left untreated, and an AC stabilization procedure is generally indicated.

The controversy lies in the treatment for type III injuries. At the onset, these injuries can be debilitating and painful with a cosmetic deformity that may be unacceptable to patients. However, many patients will do well with conservative care and return to near normal function despite persistent deformity. The general consensus currently is to treat most type III injuries initially conservatively and surgery is reserved for recalcitrant cases that remain persistently symptomatic beyond 3 months (8–10).

Operative Indications for Surgical Reconstruction

Hundreds of techniques have been proposed to stabilize or reconstruct the AC joint. Many have proven inadequate or physiologically unsound. AC joint separations that are considered for surgery are usually divided into acute and chronic categories, with approximately 6 weeks defining the two. As our understanding of the biomechanics and surgical techniques has improved, that distinction has become increasingly less defined. For the purpose of simplicity, however, we will maintain that division between acute and chronic injuries.

If an acute injury is determined to be best managed surgically, the use of an AC joint stabilization technique such as a Bosworth screw, suture or wire cerclage, K-wire fixation or ultrastrong suture pulley system is favored (11). For chronic cases, it is necessary to utilize a soft-tissue graft, preferably a free graft, along with a synthetic backup to reconstruct the AC joint complex. Although

the Weaver–Dunn procedure has been traditionally recommended to reconstruct chronic AC joint separations, recent studies have demonstrated that the transferred coracoacromial ligament has a quarter of the strength of the native CC complex. Moreover, even with modern surgical techniques, failures with the Weaver–Dunn procedure have been reported in up to 50% of patients (12, 13).

Special Anatomic and Motion Considerations

The AC joint is more than just a link between two bones. It provides for a complex articulation and multiplanar motion between the axial and appendicular skeleton. Appreciating the complex anatomy and motion of the joint is the key to a satisfactory reconstruction.

The AC joint is usually described as an arthrodial joint linking the distal clavicle to the medial border of the acromion of the scapula. The components of this joint consist of the AC capsular ligaments (anterior, posterior, superior, and inferior), the articular disk and the synovial membrane. The CC ligaments as detailed in Grey's Anatomy are usually described in conjunction with the AC joint since "they form a most efficient means of retaining the clavicle in contact with the acromion." The CC ligaments consist of two fasciculi, named for their particular geometric shapes: the conoid and the trapezoid. The term AC joint complex is used when referring to both the AC joint proper and the CC ligaments.

Each end of the AC joint is surfaced with hyaline cartilage surrounded by a synovial membrane. Interposed is a meniscal type of fibrocartilage disk. The size, shape, and presence of the meniscus are highly variable and often absent. Its particular function is not clear as it seems to degenerate with age (14–16).

The capsular ligaments of the AC joint proper consist of the anterior, posterior, superior, and inferior capsular thickenings and are the primary horizontal stabilizers of the AC joint. Serial sectioning of the AC joint ligaments have shown that the superior and posterior ligaments contribute 56% and 25% of the resistance to posterior translation, respectively (17). Therefore, when performing an arthroscopic distal clavicle resection, care should be taken to maintain the superior and posterior capsule of the AC joint to avoid the painful complication of the posterior clavicle impinging on the spine of the scapula.

Although not part of the AC joint proper, the CC ligament complex with its two bundles contributes greatly to the inherent stability of the articulation (18). Historically, and despite its importance in AC joint stability, the CC ligament has received little in the way of an anatomic description. Improved surgical interventions may be realized through a better understanding of that particular anatomy.

Each ligament bundle assumes the shape of its namesake (Fig. 4.4). Both originate from the coracoid process and insert on the clavicle. The trapezoid ligament is a thin, quadrilateral ribbon-like structure that has a linear origin and insertion both on the coracoid and the clavicle.

I. The Shoulder

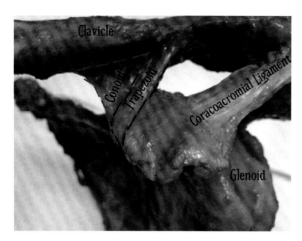

FIGURE 4.4. Cadaver dissection of the coracoclavicular ligaments. Note that the conoid lies in the coronal plane, whereas the trapezoid lies in the sagittal plane

The coracoid attachment is along the medial border of the "tubercle of Naples," sometimes referred to as the coracoid "knuckle." The tubercle lies just lateral to the scapular notch. The broad width of the trapezoid then wraps over the superior surface of the coracoid in a 45° angle to insert laterally on the clavicle. The clavicular insertion is oriented obliquely in the sagittal plane with its anterior border free and posterior border joining the conoid ligament in an orthogonal orientation, analogous to two contiguous walls of a box.

The conoid ligament is noted to be more vertical in orientation. It originates posteriorly on the Naples tubercle or "knuckle" and fans out into a cone to insert linearly along the very posterior aspect of the clavicle in the coronal plane. The conoid tubercle of the clavicle is where most of the conoid fibers attach. The conoid's most posterior and medial fibers of the coracoid attachment are confluent with the superior transverse ligament of the scapula.

For purposes of surgical reconstruction, it is helpful to note the average distance of insertion on the clavicle from its lateral edge. The trapezoid insertion was found to be 26 mm from its lateral edge, whereas the conoid was 46 mm (19). The ligament span between the coracoid and the clavicle is reported as 1.1 to 1.3 cm (2).

AC Joint Motion

The motion of the AC joint is complex and perhaps incompletely understood. This lack of appreciation of its complexity is perhaps partially to blame for the legion of surgical interventions that ultimately fail. It is generally accepted that the AC joint translates as well as rotates about three axes. These motions are guided by the AC joint complex, which includes the CC ligament. The distal clavicle is able to glide in a vertical and horizontal fashion. The scapula, at the acromion, also rotates forward and backward. Simply put, the clavicle glides up and down and the scapula pivots in an anterior–posterior direction. It is important to understand that the connection

of the clavicle and scapula, while strong, is not rigid. Fukuda (17) concluded that maximal horizontal translation in the posterior direction was restricted by the superior and posterior AC ligaments. Loss of these structures can lead to excessive posterior motion and impingement of the distal clavicle on the spine of the scapula.

Vertical translation of the joint is mediated primarily by the CC ligament. The scapula is suspended from the clavicle mainly by the CC ligament. Both inferior and superior motion is possible. Inferior motion is restricted in part by the AC joint but mainly by the proximity of the clavicle to the coracoid and the interposed mass of CC ligament. Superior translation is check-reined by the conoid and trapezoid like two portions of a rope. The vertical orientation of the conoid places it as the primary restraint to superior displacement. In biomechanical testing, the conoid consistently fails first followed by the trapezoid. The angled orientation of the trapezoid provides a relatively longer length, allowing it to "unwind" with superior displacement of the clavicle, hence, a secondary check-rein.

The third axis of rotation is the forward and backward pivoting of the scapula on the distal clavicle. The extent of this motion is restricted by the CC ligament complex. The complex orientation of the CC ligament suspends the scapula from the clavicle while allowing for the compound motions of the scapula in relation to the chest wall. The trapezoid limits backward rotation, whereas the conoid limits forward rotation of the suspended scapula.

Biomechanical Testing of the AC Joint Complex

Extensive research continues to evaluate the biomechanical properties of both the native AC joint complex and the diverse group of stabilization and reconstruction techniques. Various studies have shown the native CC complex to have an ultimate load to failure of 500 to 725 N. Evaluation of the popular Weaver–Dunn reconstruction has shown it to be biomechanically insufficient in the laboratory. The load to failure of the transferred coracoacromial ligament has been reported to be 145 N (12, 20). The high number of reported failures with the Weaver–Dunn may be attributed to its inability to restore physiologic restraints (21, 22).

TECHNIQUE—ARTHROSCOPIC STABILIZATION AND RECONSTRUCTION OF THE AC JOINT

Traditionally, AC joint reconstructions have been performed as an open procedure. With the ever-increasing use of the arthroscope, AC stabilization and reconstruction can now be performed as an arthroscopically assisted procedure with the ability to minimize soft-tissue trauma and incision length. There are two main objectives involved in any attempt at AC reconstruction. The first is access to the clavicle, and the second is access to the coracoid. The relatively superficial clavicle is easily accessed by incising the skin and delto-trapezial fascia in the area of interest. The size of the incision is determined by the procedure being performed.

The coracoid is the second area of interest as this holds the key to a strong, lasting construct. The coracoid is not as superficial, not readily accessible, and in open procedures requires extensive dissection to access the inferior border. What is fundamental to any arthroscopic AC joint surgery is the approach and exposure of the coracoid base regardless of the construct being placed. Use of the arthroscope has provided a safe and reproducible way to gain access and exposure of the coracoid, especially its inferior surface.

AUTHORS' PREFERRED TREATMENT

The authors' preferred technique for AC joint reconstruction is to use the GraftRope (Arthrex, Naples, FL) (Fig. 4.5). It is a second generation AC fixation device intended for use in both acute and chronic AC joint separations. It utilizes the strength of the double pulley system while incorporating a biologic soft-tissue graft that together is placed through bone tunnels in the coracoid and clavicle. After adequate reduction of the AC joint, the joint is maintained by the double pulley/button system consisting of four strands of the ultrastrong No. 5 braided suture. The biologic graft tails are then appropriately tensioned and secured with an interference screw in the clavicle. The combination of synthetic and biologic

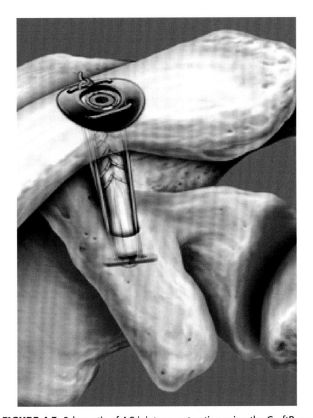

FIGURE 4.5. Schematic of AC joint reconstruction using the GraftRope.

fixation allows for treatment of both acute and chronic AC joint disruptions.

Graft Preparation

The procedure begins with preparation of the construct, which consists of a soft-tissue graft and a commercially available pulley system. Graft options vary and include either autogenous or allograft tissue, usually a semitendinosus or gracilis tendon. These grafts folded have been shown to be biomechanically comparable to the native CC ligament complex (16, 17). The selected graft is then prepared to a length of 13 cm (6.5 cm folded) and then trimmed as needed longitudinally such that the folded diameter should pass easily through a 5-mm spacer. Next, a No. 2 braided whipstitch approximately 1.5 cm in length is placed on each respective end of the graft.

The graft is then placed within the pulley system. The folded end is secured to the coracoid button by tying it with No. 2 braided ultrastrong suture. The whip-stitched free ends of the graft are then brought through the center of the clavicle washer (Fig. 4.6). Confirm that the entire construct (the graft and pulley system) now pass through a 6-mm in diameter spacer since this represents the future tunnel diameter in the clavicle and coracoid.

Create Unicortical Pilot Hole in the Clavicle

Prior to starting the arthroscopic portion of the procedure, a unicortical hole is made in the clavicle, which will serve as a rest for the superior sleeve of the C-ring drill guide. Selecting the starter hole in the clavicle at the outset greatly reduces the technical difficulty of placing the guide in the correct location under the coracoid while at the same time making certain the superior drill sleeve is in the correct location on the top of the clavicle.

After visual inspection, the topographical anatomy of the shoulder is marked. A 2-cm transverse skin incision is centered 3.5 cm from the distal aspect of the clavicle. After splitting the superior delto-trapezial fascia, the clavicle is exposed subperiosteally. At this point, the AC joint can be inspected for reduction and the need for a distal clavicle resection determined. It is the authors' preference to err on the side of preserving the distal clavicle so as to avoid further destabilization of the AC joint. However, occasionally in chronic cases, a distal clavicle resection may be necessary to achieve a satisfactory reduction and to minimize any cosmetic deformity.

Measuring 3.5 cm from the distal tip of the clavicle, a 2.4-mm guide pin is centered and drilled through both cortices of the clavicle. The location of the starter hole 3.5 cm from the distal tip of the clavicle is based upon anatomic studies of the attachment of the CC ligaments on the undersurface of the clavicle and splits the distance between the conoid and trapezoid attachments. The pin is then overdrilled through only the superior cortex of the clavicle with a 6-mm cannulated reamer (Fig. 4.7). The pin and reamer are then removed and attention is next directed to the arthroscopic aspect of the procedure.

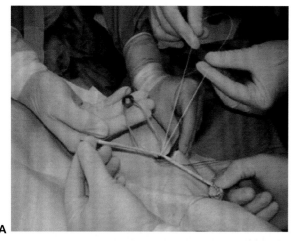

A

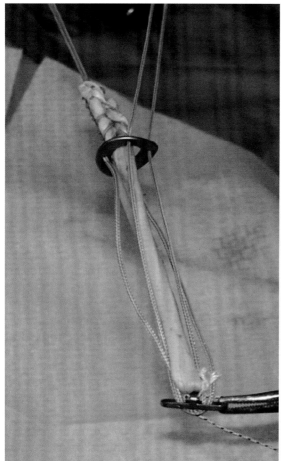

B

FIGURE 4.6. A: Intraoperative preparation of the graft and pulley device. **B:** Graft and pulley prepared.

Arthroscopic Exposure of the Undersurface of the Coracoid

The procedure can be performed readily in either the beach chair or the lateral decubitus position, and the coracoid may be approached either from the subacromial space or from the glenohumeral joint through the rotator interval. It is the authors' preferred technique to perform the procedure in the lateral decubitus position approaching the coracoid through the rotator interval.

A standard posterior portal is established and a general inspection of the glenohumeral joint is performed. Next, an anterosuperior portal is established similar in location to one for an arthroscopic Bankart procedure. Identify the borders of the rotator interval by visualizing the superior glenohumeral ligament and the superior border of the subscapularis. Use a motorized shaver to create a rent in the rotator interval just superior to the subscapularis tendon. Upon opening of the interval, the tip and lateral border of the coracoid should be apparent (Fig. 4.8). Ascending obliquely from the coracoid tip will be the coracoacromial ligament while the subscapularis will appear to dive posteriorly and medially. The inferior border of the coracoid is exposed using a combination of motorized shaver and electrocautery. The inferior border will begin to broaden as it transitions to its projection off the scapula. Anatomic studies have shown the average width of the coracoid at its base to be 2.5 cm. It is imperative to have adequate visualization of the inferior surface of the coracoid. A 70° arthroscope can greatly enhance visualization of the desired area as can an additional anteroinferior viewing portal.

The C-ring guide is then assembled and the aiming arm is placed beneath the coracoid through the anterosuperior portal. Proper placement of the aiming arm is paramount. It should lie centered in the width of the coracoid and placed as close as possible to the inferior base of the coracoid where it is widest projecting off the scapula. This places the hole in the widest part of the coracoid allowing for the greatest margin of safety to avoid tunnel blowout. An excellent reference landmark is the subscapularis tendon. The subscapularis tendon can be traced medially as it crosses the coracoid process. The aiming guide should be placed on the undersurface of the coracoid at the level or medial to where the subscapularis crosses the coracoid. Ideally, place the side of the aiming guide up against the body of the scapula (Fig. 4.9).

Tunnel Creation in the Clavicle and Coracoid

Having arthroscopically exposed and selected the correct location for the aiming guide on the undersurface of the coracoid, the bullet-nosed drill sleeve of the C-ring guide is placed in the unicortical hole on the superior surface of the clavicle (Fig. 4.10). It is not necessary to have the AC joint anatomically reduced at this point. With the guide in place, and under direct arthroscopic visualization, drill a 2.4-mm guide pin from superior to inferior through the clavicle and coracoid until it hits the drill stop. Remove the aiming device and verify proper placement of the guide pin. Overream the guide pin with the 6-mm cannulated reamer to create a hole in both the clavicle and the coracoid. To avoid errant advancement of the guide pin while reaming, secure the end of the guide pin with a curette or open-faced shaver. Leave the reamer in place and remove the guide pin.

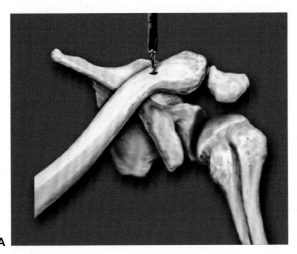

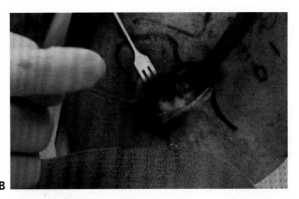

FIGURE 4.7. A: Preparation of a 6-mm unicortical hole in the clavicle. **B:** Unicortical drill hole established.

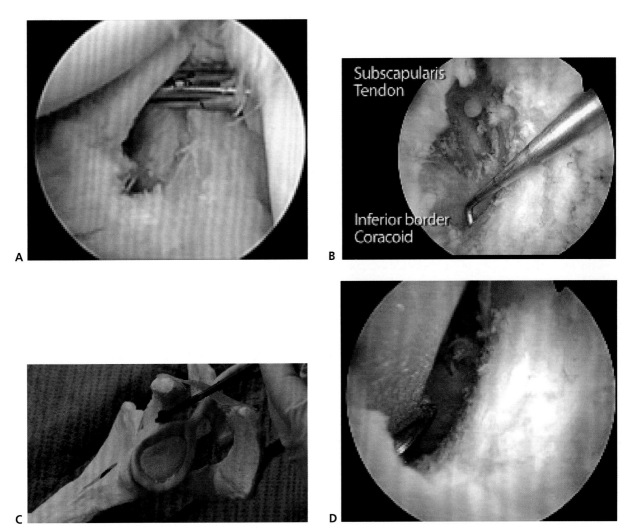

FIGURE 4.8. Arthroscopic exposure of the coracoid. **A:** Create a rent in the interval between the subscapularis tendon and the superior glenohumeral ligament. **B:** Skeletonize the inferior surface of the coracoid. **C:** Sawbones depiction of guide placement on the inferior surface of the coracoid. **D:** Arthroscopic photograph of guide arm placed on inferior surface of the coracoid at its confluence with the scapular body.

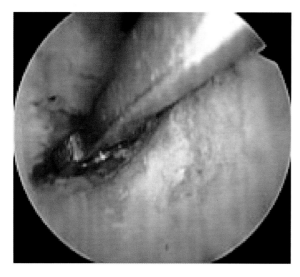

FIGURE 4.9. Arthroscopic photo demonstrating position of the guide on the coracoid relative to the subscapularis tendon.

Graft Passage

A wire loop is then passed through the cannulated reamer, which will shuttle the prepared graft, sutures, and coracoid button. The wire loop is grasped below the coracoid as it exits the cannulated reamer and brought out the anterior portal. After removing the reamer, place the pull suture that is attached to the coracoid button of the graft construct through the wire loop and shuttle the pull suture through the clavicle and coracoid. Pull the graft construct through the clavicle and coracoid until the entire length of the button is visible arthroscopically below the coracoid. Often a forked probe or knot pusher must be used to assist the force vector while pulling. This will also prevent the suture cutting through the coracoid (Fig. 4.11). Seat the button on the inferior cortex of the coracoid by pulling back on the sutures. The button can easily be repositioned to a satisfactory position using a simple probe.

Reduce the AC Joint and Secure the Construct

Next, reduce the clavicle. This is best accomplished by stabilizing the clavicle while bringing the arm and shoulder into a superior position, thus placing the clavicle in an anatomic position. While an assistant holds the clavicle reduced, cinch the suture pulley system tight and place 5 to 6 alternating half hitches in the No. 5 ultrastrong braided suture (Fig. 4.12). Adequate reduction can be confirmed by several methods. The simplest way is to palpate the AC joint itself. The distal clavicle can also be visualized from the subacromial space. An image intensifier can ultimately confirm an acceptable reduction of the AC joint.

The last step is securing the free ends of the graft into the clavicle. While gently pulling on the grafts tails, place a flexible 1.1-mm guide wire through both cortices of the clavicle. Tension the graft tails to remove any undesired slack and insert a 5.5-mm × 12-mm cannulated interference screw (Fig. 4.13). The remaining graft can be removed or used to augment reconstruction of the AC joint proper.

SPECIAL CONSIDERATIONS AND CONTROVERSIES

Type III AC Injuries: Surgical Versus Conservative Treatment

Although the treatment for type III injuries remains controversial, the scientific literature has historically supported conservative treatment for the initial management. Surgical intervention is typically reserved for those who fail conservative measures. In a review, Bradley and Elkousy (8) concluded that no perfect study existed that demonstrated the clear superiority of surgical versus non-surgical treatment. Although they concede that multiple factors must be considered in the decision to perform surgery, it is their opinion that all type III injuries should be treated with conservative care initially and only those who fail appropriate conservative care undergo surgery (8). More recently, Spencer (9) reviewed the literature regarding type III injuries and concluded that nonoperative treatment was superior to surgical intervention. The operative patients' results were not clearly better than those treated conservatively and were associated with more complications and a longer recovery.

Schlegel (23) performed a prospective study to determine the natural history of untreated type III AC separations. The bench press was the only strength test that showed a significant difference, with the injured extremity being on average 17% weaker at short-term follow-up. However, 20% of the patients thought their results were suboptimal.

Despite the lack of an overwhelming advantage for conservative initial treatment for type III injuries, it is the authors' opinion, like Bradley and Elkousy (8) and others (10), that patients should be treated conservatively for up to 12 weeks with an emphasis on rehabilitation. Those who are unsatisfied or otherwise considered to have failed conservative treatment can be considered for surgical intervention.

PEARLS AND PITFALLS

Arthroscopic Access to the Coracoid is the Key

Exposure of the coracoid can be accomplished either directly through the glenohumeral joint or by way of a subacromial approach. Both approaches use standard posterior, lateral, and anterosuperior portals. When approaching from the glenohumeral joint, a 30° arthroscope is placed through a posterior portal for initial visualization and dissection. A standard anterosuperior portal similar in location to that used for an arthroscopic stabilization

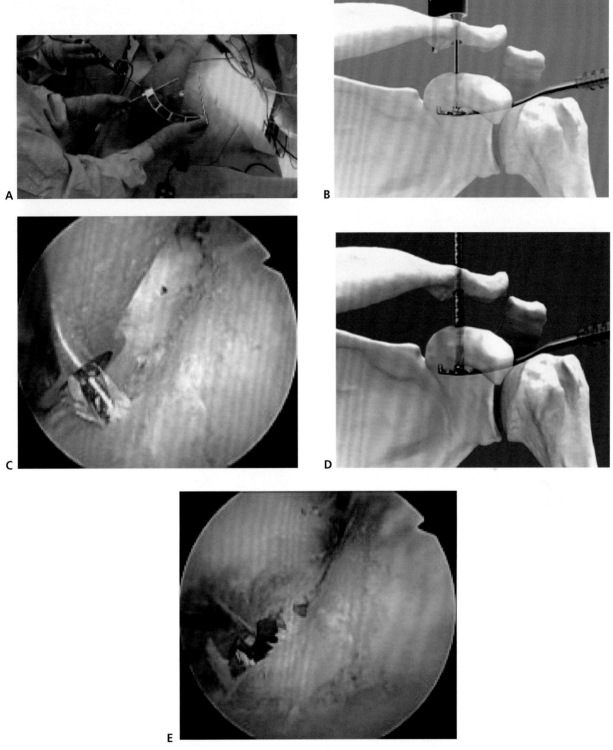

FIGURE 4.10. A: C-ring guide demonstrated prior to insertion through the anterior portal. **B:** Schematic showing placement of the aiming guide beneath the coracoid. The drill sleeve rests superiorly in the unicortical hole already established in the clavicle. **C:** A 2.4-mm guide pin is drilled through the clavicle and coracoid until it hits the drill stop. **D:** The guide wire is then overreamed to 6 mm. **E:** The drill is left in place and the guide wire removed and a passing wire loop is placed through the cannulated reamer and pulled out the anterior portal.

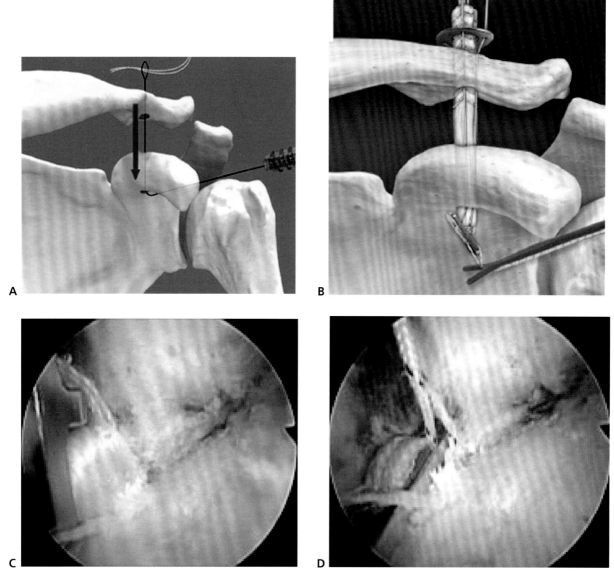

FIGURE 4.11. A: After removal of the drill, the wire loop is used to shuttle the passing suture from the graft/pulley construct. **B:** The graft and coracoid button are pulled through both clavicle and coracoid. Use of a forked probe facilitates passage. **C:** Arthroscopic view of the button emerging from the inferior coracoid hole. **D:** Button is flipped and positioned.

procedure is then established. The coracoid lies out of the arthroscopic field of view just anterior to the rotator interval. The subscapularis is identified and a small rent is made with a motorized shaver in the rotator interval just superior to the subscapularis tendon. The coracoid is immediately encountered and easily dissected with a combination of motorized shaver and electrocautery. The coracoid is widest (2.5 cm) near its projection off the scapula and tapers dramatically to 1 cm near the coracoid tip. It is therefore imperative to expose the most medial aspect of the inferior base of the coracoid for proper coracoid tunnel placement. This is greatly facilitated by a 70° arthroscope. The subscapularis tendon is an excellent landmark for appropriate tunnel placement in the coracoid. The subscapularis can be followed medially toward the scapula to where the tendon crosses the coracoid. The tunnel in the coracoid should exit at the location where the subscapularis crosses the coracoid or medial to it, never lateral (Fig. 4.14).

Although the authors prefer to approach the coracoid through the glenohumeral joint through the rotator interval, the coracoid can also be readily approached from subacromial space with only slight modification of the technique. The arthroscope is placed posteriorly into the subacromial space and a thorough bursectomy is performed from a lateral portal. The coracoacromial ligament is identified and followed inferomedially to its attachment on the coracoid. The arthroscope is then placed through the lateral portal and an anterior working portal established. The scope is positioned to best visualize the inferior

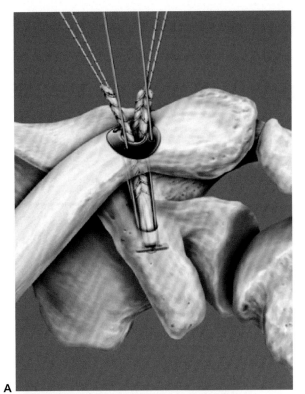

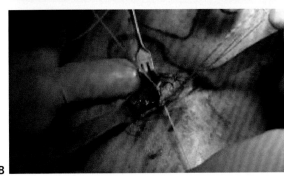

FIGURE 4.12. A: Schematic of the graft and buttons placed prior to joint reduction and suture fixation. **B:** Surgical photograph of joint reduction and tying of No. 5 suture.

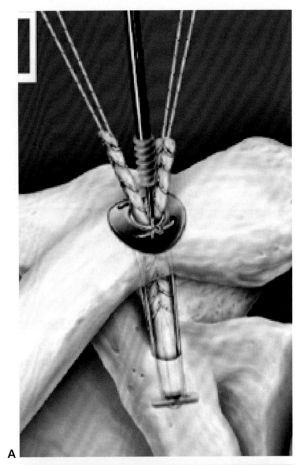

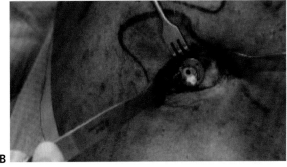

FIGURE 4.13. A: Schematic of interference screw being placed bicortically while the graft limbs are tensioned. **B:** The excess graft may be removed or used to augment the AC joint proper.

surface of the coracoid and the inferomedial aspect of the coracoid is exposed in an analogous fashion to what has been described above. As before, a 70° arthroscopic greatly facilitates the exposure.

REHABILITATION AND POSTOPERATIVE CARE

With the recent improved appreciation of the complex anatomy and biomechanical demands of the AC joint, advancements in the reconstructive techniques have resulted in superior outcomes. Despite the supraphysiologic biomechanical strength of current reconstructions, rehabilitation should be approached with prudence.

Immediately following the procedure and before the patient is awakened, the arm is placed into a well-supported sling. The arm should be so positioned as to prevent the weight of the arm from causing excessive strain on the AC joint. At the first postoperative visit, radiographs are taken to confirm the reduction (Fig. 4.15). Gentle range of motion of the hand, wrist, and elbow are encouraged, whereas motion at the shoulder is only permitted in the supine position.

The sling is discontinued at 6 weeks at which point the patient can initiate free range of motion and gentle strengthening. Isometric and isotonic exercises dominate the second 6 weeks with slow advancement to weight training at 4 months. Return to contact sports is permitted at 6 months.

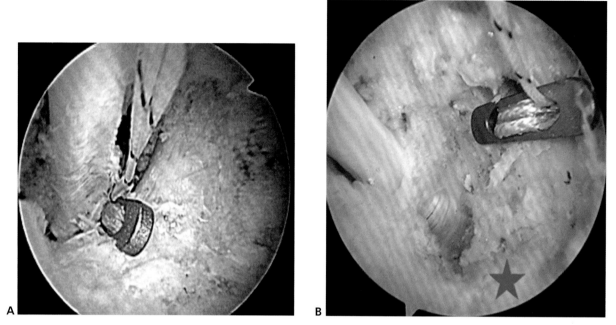

FIGURE 4.14. Correct position of the coracoid button and graft. **A:** Relative to the subscapularis tendon, the coracoid should be drilled so that the graft and button lie in the same plane. **B:** Incorrect location of the coracoid tunnel. The star marks the correct location for the graft superior to the subscapularis tendon.

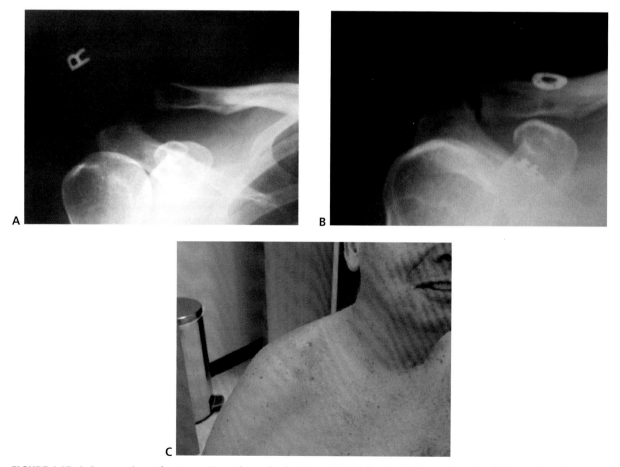

FIGURE 4.15. A: Preoperative and postoperative radiographs showing original deformity. **B:** Correct location of the tunnels and buttons with the clavicle reduced. **C:** Postoperative clinical photo of a right arthroscopic AC joint reconstruction.

CONCLUSIONS AND FUTURE DIRECTIONS

The AC joint is a complex joint. In reality, it is only part of a complex biologic mechanism that regulates the intricate motion that occurs between the axillary and appendicular skeleton. Owing to its complex nature, reconstruction of the injured AC joint can be challenging and perhaps explains the inability of surgeons to achieve a consensus on the ideal treatment for such injuries. Renewed interest and research suggest that the use of a biologic soft-tissue graft in conjunction with a synthetic, stable fixation mechanism holds the promise of lasting results. Ultimately, the use of these so-called hybrid reconstructions may dominate not only in chronic AC joint injuries but in acute cases as well.

It is beyond the scope of this chapter to review all of the reported arthroscopic techniques for AC joint reconstruction. Common to almost all is the visualization of the coracoid through the arthroscope while utilizing a small incision to access the clavicle. Presented is an arthroscopic technique that utilizes a free graft and a suture pulley system to achieve a physiologically sound construct. The ultrastrong No. 5 sutures are placed through a specially designed "washer" and "button" that create a pulley-like mechanism, thus bridging the coracoid and the clavicle. Interposed within the pulley mechanism is a load sharing, free biologic graft that is suspended within bone tunnels of the coracoid and clavicle. The suture pulley maintains the provisional reduction of the AC joint, whereas the biologic graft is incorporated for long-term stability. This can be utilized for both acute and chronic AC joint injuries and is easily modified for unique cases or revision surgery.

Arthroscopic AC reconstruction represents an evolving technique and is clearly in its infancy. Although a specific procedure has been presented in this chapter, alternative methods abound. However, the concept of arthroscopically passing a biologic graft through or around the coracoid combined with synthetic support seems to be consistent throughout most techniques. Ultimately, it is probably the combination of a free graft with a synthetic support that will prove to be the strongest and have lasting results.

REFERENCES

1. Zanca P. Shoulder pain: involvement of the acromioclavicular joint (analysis of 1,000 cases). *Am J Roentgenol Radium Ther Nucl Med.* 1971;112:493–506.
2. Bearden JM, Hughston JC, Whatley GS. Acromioclavicular dislocation: method of treatment. *J Sports Med.* 1973;1:5–17.
3. Rockwood CJ, Williams G, Young D. Disorders of the acromioclavicular joint. In: Rockwood CJ, Matsen FA III, eds. *The Shoulder.* 2nd ed. Philadelphia, PA: WB Saunders; 1998:483–553.
4. Trainer G, Arciero RA, Mazzocca AD. Practical management of grade III acromioclavicular separations. *Clin J Sport Med.* 2003;18:162–166.
5. Adams FL. *The Genuine Works of Hippocrates.* Vols. 1 and 2. New York, NY: William Wood; 1886.
6. Cadenat F. The treatment of dislocations and fractures of the outer end of the clavicle. *Int Clin.* 1917;1:145–169.
7. Tossy J, Mead N, Sigmond H. Acromioclavicular separations: useful and practical classification for treatment. *Clin Orthop Relat Res.* 1963; 28:111–119.
8. Bradley JP, Elkousy H. Decision making: operative versus nonoperative treatment of acromioclavicular joint injuries. *Clin Sports Med.* 2003; 22:277–290.
9. Spencer EE Jr. Treatment of grade III acromioclavicular joint injuries: a systematic review. *Clin Orthop Relat Res.* 2007; 455:38–44.
10. Trainer G, Arciero RA, Mazzocca AD. Practical management of grade III acromioclavicular separations. *Clin J Sports Med.* 2008; 18:162–166.
11. Bosworth BM. Acromioclavicular dislocation: end-results of screw suspension treatment. *Ann Surg.* 1948; 127:98–111.
12. Harris RI, Wallace AL, Harper GD, et al. Structural properties of the intact and the reconstructed coracoclavicular ligament complex. *Am J Sports Med.* 2000; 28:103–108.
13. Lee SJ, Nicholas SJ, Akizuki KH, et al. Reconstruction of the coracoclavicular ligaments with tendon grafts: a comparative biomechanical study. *Am J Sports Med.* 2003; 31:648–654.
14. Petersson C. Degeneration of the acromioclavicular joint: a morphological study. *Acta Orthop Scand.* 1983; 54:434–438.
15. DePalma A, Callery G, Bennett G. Variational anatomy and degenerative lesions of the shoulder joint. *Instr Course Lect.* 1949; 6:255–281.
16. Salter EG Jr, Nasca RJ, Shelley BS. Anatomical observations on the acromioclavicular joint and supporting ligaments. *Am J Sports Med.* 1987; 15:199–206.
17. Fukuda K, Craig EV, An KN, et al. Biomechanical study of the ligamentous system of the acromioclavicular joint. *J Bone Joint Surg Am.* 1986; 68:434–440.
18. Harris RI, Vu DH, Sonnabend DH, et al. Anatomic variance of the coracoclavicular ligaments. *J Shoulder Elbow Surg.* 2001; 10:585–588.
19. Rios CG, Arciero RA, Mazzocca AD. Anatomy of the clavicle and coracoid process for reconstruction of the coracoclavicular ligaments. *Am J Sports Med.* 2007; 35:811–817.
20. Motamedi AR, Blevins FT, Willis MC, et al. Biomechanics of the coracoclavicular ligament complex and augmentations used in its repair and reconstruction. *Am J Sports Med.* 2000; 28:380–384.
21. Weaver JK, Dunn HK. Treatment of acromioclavicular injuries, especially complete acromioclavicular separation. *J Bone Joint Surg Am.* 1972; 54:1187–1194.
22. Weinstein DM, McCann PD, McIlveen SJ, et al. Surgical treatment of complete acromioclavicular dislocations. *Am J Sports Med.* 1995; 23:324–331.
23. Schlegel TF, Burks RT, Marcus RL, et al. A prospective evaluation of untreated acute grade III acromioclavicular separations. *Am J Sports Med.* 2001; 29:699–703.

Arthroscopy of the AC Joint: Two and Three Portal Approaches

James P. Tasto • Amar Arora

KEY POINTS

- The acromioclavicular (AC) joint has a complex anatomic structure that needs to be understood prior to attempting open or arthroscopic procedures.
- Arthroscopic resection of the AC joint appears to be an improvement over traditional open procedures as it results in enhanced ligament preservation, reduced infection rate, improved cosmesis, and accelerated rehabilitation.
- Differential diagnosis of AC joint pain can include AC joint arthritis, osteolysis, microinstability, symptomatic meniscal derangement, rheumatoid arthritis, infection, and gout and polymyalgia rheumatica.
- Nonoperative management including nonsteroidal anti-inflammatory drugs (NSAIDs), rest, local intra-articular injections is usually successful.
- Three portal and two portal techniques can be used to treat AC joint pathology arthroscopically.
- The three portal technique is useful for all sources of AC joint pathology and can be combined with rotator cuff surgery or isolated subacromial decompression.
- The two portal (direct) superior approach is somewhat more difficult because of the limited access to the AC joint but is useful in patients not requiring subacromial surgery.
- The two portal (direct) arthroscopic technique is useful in competitive athletes with isolated AC joint pathology (e.g., osteolysis) who do not require a subacromial decompression and wish to return quickly to sports.

Pain derived from the AC joint is a prevalent complaint and can be the result of various specific disorders. Since first being described by Mumford and Gurd in 1941, methods for excision of the distal clavicle have evolved to incorporate both open and arthroscopic techniques. After attempts of nonsurgical pain management have been unsuccessful, surgical resection of the joint can be employed to address AC joint pathology and effectively relieve pain. Current arthroscopic techniques have evolved over the past 20 to 25 years and can lead to reproducible favorable outcomes.

However, if not done correctly, arthroscopic AC joint resection can lead to increased morbidity over traditional open procedures. It is therefore important to have a good understanding of the anatomy prior to undertaking surgical correction of AC joint pathology.

ANATOMY

The AC joint is a diarthrodial joint with fibrocartilaginous articular surfaces, allowing for dynamic movement. A fibrocartilaginous meniscal homolog is usually present. In the sagittal view, the joint slopes superior lateral to inferior medial, whereas in the coronal plane, it slopes anterior lateral to posterior medial. The AC joint lies directly over the supraspinatus muscle and musculotendinous junction. The AC and coracoclavicular ligaments contribute to the stability of the AC joint and are the chief restraints to motion. The conoid ligament primarily restricts anterior and superior displacement of the clavicle. The trapezoid ligament is the chief constraint against compression of the distal clavicle into the acromion. The AC joint has been shown to allow for up to 3 mm of laxity with stress and allow for 5° to 8° of rotation. There appears to be little motion between the clavicle and the scapula. Synchronous motion is usually obtained as the clavicle rotates upward allowing the scapula to rotate downward. Preservation of the AC ligaments that make up the posterior superior capsule is critical when performing surgery. If performed correctly with recognition and protection of distinct anatomical structures, arthroscopic resection appears to be an improvement over traditional open procedures as it results in enhanced ligament preservation, reduced infection rate, improved cosmesis, and accelerated rehabilitation.

CLINICAL EVALUATION

History

It is important to determine the contribution of the AC joint in a patient who presents with shoulder pain. Obtaining a detailed history is an essential component used to design an appropriate treatment plan. It is necessary to ascertain a history of joint separation, a posttraumatic event, generalized osteoarthritis, and/or conditions isolated to sports-specific injuries such as osteolysis in weight lifters. Ascertaining a history of instability or previous separation of the AC joint is paramount and cannot be overemphasized.

Physical Exam

It is imperative to clinically evaluate the AC joint. Differentiation between classical impingement, subcoracoid impingement, early frozen shoulder, and AC joint pathology is critical. Most patients may initially complain of global shoulder pain. Patients may present with tenderness to direct palpation of the AC joint and may have swelling as well as a clinical deformity in the region. Physical tests have been used to identify AC pathology and include the following: (1) Pain may be elicited by passive and active horizontal adduction and internal rotation; (2) a positive O'Brien's test with the arm adducted and forward elevated to 90° producing greater pain localized to the AC joint with a thumbs down position when compared with a thumbs up position; (3) AC joint tenderness with attempts at AP translation; (4) localized pain at the AC joint during conventional impingement testing. In addition, patients often respond positively to an injection of lidocaine with or without additional steroid into the AC joint. Proper injection technique into the joint should take into account the normal superolateral to inferomedial sagittal inclination and is commonly limited to approximately 1 to 2 cc of fluid.

Imaging

X-ray analysis is critical before any type of shoulder surgery to define acromial morphology, the presence of any AC joint involvement, presence or absence of an os acromiale, any calcification in the area, and to help rule out a diagnosis of neoplasia. A radiographic shoulder series should include an anteroposterior view taken in the scapular plane with humeral internal and external rotation, an outlet, and an axillary view. In addition, the following studies can be helpful: (1) 15° cephalic coned-down view with a comparative view of the contralateral AC joint, (2) 30° tangential glenoid view, (3) a bone scan, and (4) magnetic resonance imaging, which can be used to evaluate the pathology of the rotator cuff, detect AC synovitis and localize osteophytes. A bone scan may be helpful if a history of osteolysis is suspected.

Differential Diagnosis

- The most common cause of symptomatic AC joint pain remains degenerative AC arthritis in the setting of rotator cuff disease. In this particular setting, pain can be caused by the AC joint itself, from the degenerative tear of the rotator cuff, or from impingement of inferior osteophytes from the acromion or the AC joint compressing the rotator cuff.
- Posttraumatic arthritis of the AC joint is also a very common diagnosis. In this setting, a careful history usually reveals an episode of AC joint separation. With this diagnosis, a careful physical examination is mandatory to evaluate the presence or absence of AC joint instability.

- Osteolysis of the clavicle is a less common cause of AC joint pathology but should be thought of with a history of trauma, active weight lifting, or with certain metabolic disorders especially hyperparathyroidism. Radiographs may show massive bony resorption of the distal clavicle and bone scans usually show increased activity in that same area.
- Other causes of AC joint pathology include symptomatic meniscal derangement, rheumatoid arthritis, infection, gout, and polymyalgia rheumatica.

Decision-Making Algorithms/Indications for Resection

- There are several indications for arthroscopic resection of the distal clavicle including arthritis, osteolysis, and meniscal derangement. The role of the AC joint in the impingement syndrome remains somewhat controversial. Some surgeons resect a large percentage of AC joints associated with a subacromial decompression, whereas others are quite selective and resect only a small percentage of AC joints. The contribution of inferior osteophytes in the production of pain is contested. Each surgeon needs to determine whether the inferior osteophytes play any role in the creation of symptoms or are simply a reaction to the patient's degenerative process.
- Patients who present with prior second degree, third degree, or fourth degree AC joint separations with obvious displacement of the distal clavicle may be poorer candidates for isolated AC joint resection. A significant component of this pain syndrome is often due to ligamentous instability and a reconstruction or reinforcement of the distal clavicle following AC joint resection is often necessary.

NONOPERATIVE TREATMENT

Most patients are improved with an initial course of rest, nonsteroidal anti-inflammatory medication, or local steroid/lidocaine injection. If symptoms do not improve with such measures, surgical treatment should be considered.

SURGICAL TREATMENT

Arthroscopic techniques produce reliably good outcomes in the appropriately selected patients. There are several arthroscopic techniques that have been described over the past few decades. This chapter will focus on three techniques: (1) the three portal technique, (2) two portal (direct) technique, and (3) co-planing in the setting of subacromial decompression.

Equipment Setup

Various commercial radiofrequency (RF) devices are available, which may assist the surgeon in debridement and visualization of the morphology of the acromion and

AC joint. These RF devices are both monopolar and bipolar and are chosen at the surgeon's discretion. Conventional electrocautery has largely been supplanted by these devices because of the ease of use, rapid vaporization of tissue, better delineation of the bony landmarks, and a quicker and more precise soft tissue ablation mode. Conventional shavers and burr devices (3.5 and 4.5 mm) can be employed. Plum and spinal curettes with narrow shafts are also recommended. In addition to the standard arthroscopic equipment, a 4.0-mm 30° arthroscope and arthroscopic pump are utilized. Epinephrine can be used in the fluid bags to help with managing hemostasis.

Patient and Equipment Position

Patient positioning can be either in the beach chair or in the lateral decubitus position with approximately 12 lb (5.44 kg) of balanced suspension. The arm is placed in 20° to 30° of abduction and 20° of forward flexion for all subacromial and AC work. After the patient is positioned, the arm is prepped and draped. If deemed medically appropriate, the systolic blood pressure should be maintained between 90 to 95 mm Hg. In addition, hemostasis can also be adequately obtained by keeping the difference between the systolic blood pressure and the subacromial pressure through the pump to around 40 mm Hg.

THREE PORTAL TECHNIQUE

Indications

The three portal technique can be used for all diagnosed sources of AC joint pathology. It is most convenient to use this technique in combination with rotator cuff surgery or isolated subacromial decompression.

Operative Technique

This technique utilizes the conventional posterior viewing portal and an anterior portal directly aligned with the AC

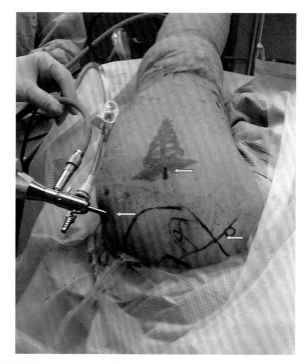

FIGURE 5.1. Location of portal placement for the three portal technique. The arthroscope is located in the posterior portal.

joint, as well as a lateral portal. Initial subacromial injection of marcaine with epinephrine can help with hemostasis. The posterior viewing portal can be used throughout the entire case and the arthroscope generally does not have to be moved (Fig. 5.1). Next, commonly from the lateral portal, conventional burrs, shavers, and RF are used to delineate the AC joint. A portion of the acromial facet is removed for better visualization. This is referred to as the "window to the AC joint." A small predetermined portion of the inferior distal clavicle is resected from the lateral portal (Figs. 5.2 to 5.4). Once this inferior component

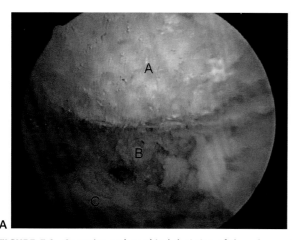

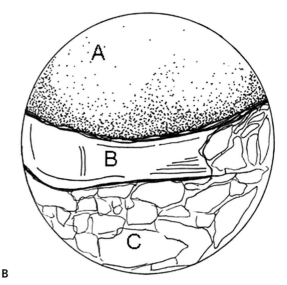

FIGURE 5.2. Operative and graphical depiction of the subacromial space prior to acromioplasty viewed from the posterior portal. A, acromion; B, distal clavicle; C, soft tissue.

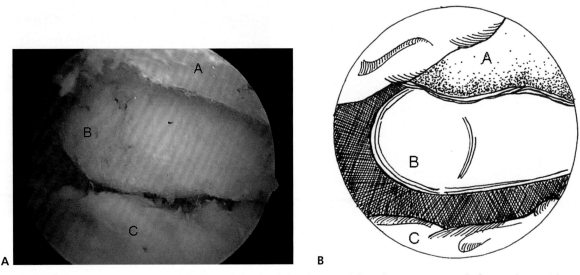

FIGURE 5.3. Operative and graphical depiction of the distal clavicle viewed from the posterior portal after a subacromial decompression. A, acromion; B, distal clavicle.

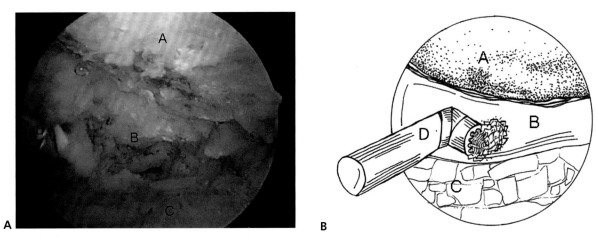

FIGURE 5.4. Operative and graphical depiction of a RF device initiating soft tissue resection, viewed from the posterior portal. A, acromion; B, distal clavicle; C, soft tissue; D, RF device.

has been removed, the outflow is changed to the lateral portal and the working portal becomes the anterior portal. At this time, the remaining component of the distal clavicle and/or a portion on the acromion is resected to a predetermined distance. The general recommendation for distal clavicle resection is between 5 and 10 mm.

Usually the burr or shaver can be used to quantitate that distance. Periscoping the arthroscope allows full visualization of the AC joint from superior to inferior and anterior to posterior. Judicious use of conventional RF will help delineate the osseous margins so that no residual osteophytes or spurs are left. Most work done on the distal clavicle is through the anterior portal. Care must be taken to remove the entire circumference of the distal clavicle to avoid residual osteophytes and to preserve the integrity of the superior acromial clavicular joint capsule and ligamentous structures. This provides for some residual stability following this operative procedure.

A surgical tool can be used to ensure that the predetermined amount of bone has been resected. If difficulty is encountered while evening out the distal clavicle from the anterior portal a two handed technique can be used on the shaver and burr while an assistant holds the camera in position in the lateral or posterior portal. This can help stabilize the instrument and allow for the proper placement of the instrument in the AC joint. Because the entire inferior capsule and a portion of the anterior and posterior ligamentous and capsular structures have been violated during this procedure, the maintenance of the superior components is critical to avoid long-term instability and symptoms. Further evaluation of the resection can be accomplished by placing the arthroscope in the anterior portal (Figs. 5.5 and 5.6). The portal sites are then closed using the surgeon's preferred technique followed by injection into the subacromial space of a local anesthetic.

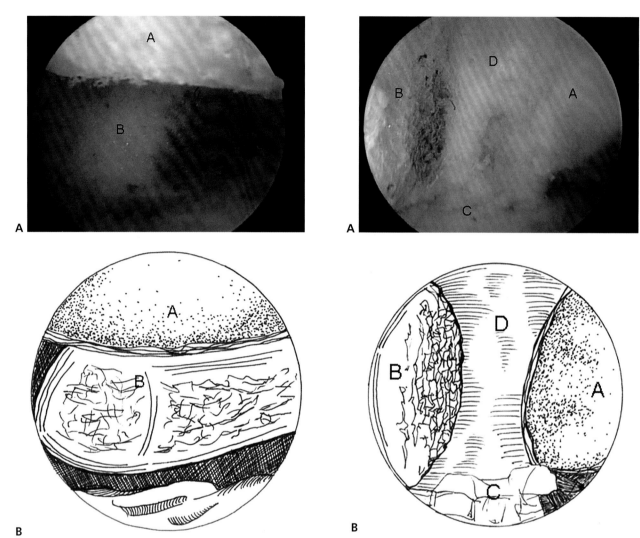

FIGURE 5.5. Operative and graphical depiction of the distal clavicle after resection has been completed viewed from the posterior portal. A, acromion; B, distal clavicle.

FIGURE 5.6. Operative and graphical depiction of the acromioclavicular (AC) joint resection viewed from the anterior portal. A, acromion; B, distal clavicle; C, soft tissue; D remaining superior joint capsule.

TWO PORTAL (DIRECT) TECHNIQUE

Indications

The direct superior approach is more difficult because of the limited access to the AC joint but is certainly useful in those patients who do not require subacromial surgery. Although the two portal technique can be used for all the above mentioned sources of AC joint pathology, it certainly has its greatest benefit with isolated AC joint pathology. Competitive athletes who present with isolated AC joint pathology such as osteolysis, with no indication for a subacromial decompression, and who wish to return to sports quickly may be the best candidates for this technique. An added advantage of this approach is the almost complete preservation of the circumferential stabilizing ligaments and capsule of the AC joint, thereby reducing the potential for iatrogenic creation of microinstability.

Operative Technique

Precise location of the AC joint is achieved with the placement of two or three 22-gauge spinal needles positioned anterosuperiorly, posterosuperiorly, and in the joint center. The joint is then insufflated and the portals are injected using a local anesthetic with epinephrine to obtain capsular hemostasis. The anterosuperior portal is established 0.75 cm anterior to the AC joint and the posterosuperior portal is made 0.75 cm posterior to the AC joint (Fig. 5.7). An 11-blade scalpel is used to incise the skin and the capsule of the AC joint both anterior and posteriorly. At this point, if the AC joint is narrow, a 2.7-mm arthroscope is placed in the anterosuperior portal otherwise a standard 4.0-mm 30° arthroscope can be used.

A small shaver placed in the posterosuperior portal is used to begin the resection of the meniscal remnant and joint debris. A small burr is employed to start the bony resection. A panoramic view of the area is then attained

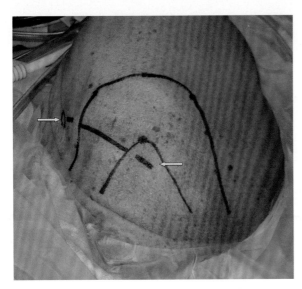

FIGURE 5.7. Portal placement for two portal technique. Arrows point to the suggested placement of the portals. The circle represents location of the coracoid process.

with insertion of a 4-mm arthroscope. Electrocautery using an RF probe is used to subperiosteally "shell out" the distal clavicle while cautiously preserving the superior AC ligaments. This "shelling out" process helps avoid uneven resection of the distal clavicle that may leave bone peripherally and result in continued pain. A burr is then used to complete the resection of the distal clavicle. The arthroscope is switched to the posterosuperior portal to allow the burr access to the most anterior portion of the clavicle. Final beveling of the bone surface can be performed manually with an arthroscopic rasp followed by a shaver. The AC joint is insufflated with an anesthetic and closure of the portals is performed using the surgeon's desired technique.

COPLANNING THE AC JOINT

Some surgeons prefer to remove inferiorly based bone spurs of the AC joint while performing a subacromial decompression. Arthroscopic subacromial decompression specifically is an accepted procedure. One must be careful in assessing the value of coplanning of the AC joint in the absence of clinical findings supporting AC joint pathology. By removing the inferior osteophytes of the distal clavicle and acromion, a significant increase in motion at the AC joint can be iatrogenically created by the removal of the inferior capsular and bony architecture of this joint. This may lead to increased superior translation and rotational motions that may lead to persistent symptoms and poor clinical results.

REHABILITATION

Initially a sling is used for comfort following surgery regardless of the type of technique used. Simple pendulum exercises can be initiated the day of surgery followed by passive and active range of motion exercises as tolerated. If isolated AC resection has been performed, strengthening exercises can be initiated when tolerated but usually is around the 2- and 3-week mark. Full activity and contact sports may resume around 6 weeks. If an AC resection has been performed in addition to a subacromial decompression, full activity can be resumed between 10 and 12 weeks.

SUGGESTED READINGS

Branch TP, Burdette HL, Shahriari AS, et al. The role of the AC ligaments and the effect of distal clavicle resection. *Am J Sports Med.* 1996;24:293–297.

Charron KM, Schepsis AA, Woloshin I. Arthroscopic distal clavicle resection in athletes: a perspective comparison of the direct and indirect approach. *Am J Sports Med.* 2007;35:53–58.

Deshmukh AV, Perlmutter GS, Zilberfarb JL, Wilson DR., et al. Effect of subacromial decompression on laxity of the acromioclavicular joint: biomechanical testing in a cadaveric model. *J Shoulder Elbow Surg.* 2004;13:338–343.

Edwards SL, Wilson NA, Flores SE, et al. Arthroscopic distal clavicle resection: a biomechanical analysis of resection length and joint compliance in a cadaveric model. *Arthroscopy.* 2007;23:1278–1287.

Flatow EL, Bigliani LU. Arthroscopic acromioclavicular joint debridement and distal clavicle resection. *Oper Tech Orthop.* 1991;1:240–247.

Flatow EL, Cordasco FA, Bigliani LU. Arthroscopic resection of the outer end of the clavicle from a superior approach: a critical, quantitative, radiographic assessment of bone removal. *Arthroscopy.* 1992;8:55–64.

Levine WN, Barron OA, Yamaguchi K, et al. Arthroscopic distal clavicle resection from a bursal approach. *Arthroscopy.* 1998;14:52–56.

I. The Shoulder

Subacromial Decompression: Lateral and Posterior (Cutting Block) Approach

Kevin D. Plancher • David B. Dickerson • Elizabeth A. Kern

Arthroscopic subacromial decompression is a safe and effective technique to treat impingement syndrome refractory to conservative management. Two techniques have been described to resect the anteriorinferior acromion, subacromial bursa, and release the coracoacromial ligament and thus increase the volume of the subacromial space. The lateral approach was initially described by Ellman in 1988. Sampson subsequently described a posterior approach commonly referred to as the "cutting block" technique. Good to excellent outcomes of refractory impingement syndrome treated with arthroscopic subacromial decompression have been reported in up to 88% of patients.

CLINICAL EVALUATION

Introduction

Impingement syndrome is a common cause of shoulder pain, which often leads to a decreased ability to perform athletic and daily activities. Subacromial decompression has been used to treat impingement syndrome refractory to conservative treatment since Neer's description of an open procedure in 1972. Neer (1) described a procedure to increase the volume of the subacromial space and relieve external compression of the rotator cuff by combining debridement of the subacromial bursa with resection of the coracoacromial ligament and the anteriorinferior acromion (acromioplasty). A 25-year follow-up study reported 88% positive patient satisfaction after open acromioplasty (2). However, there has been a general trend to perform procedures using minimally invasive techniques and return patients to their normal activities sooner. Since Ellman's description of an arthroscopic technique in 1985, the arthroscopic skills of many surgeons and technology have improved leading many surgeons to transition from an open to an arthroscopic approach to accomplish the same goals with comparable results (3–10).

Although equipment needs are greater, arthroscopic subacromial decompression offers several important advantages to the open procedure. Arthroscopy allows for the evaluation of underlying intra-articular and extra-articular pathology that can be treated concurrently. The smaller incisions needed for arthroscopic portals cause minimal disruption to the deltoid muscle insertion, allowing for a quicker rehabilitation, less postoperative pain, improved cosmesis, and most importantly, allowing patients an earlier return to activities and sports.

Two arthroscopic techniques have been popularized that resect the anteriorinferior acromion. The lateral technique described by Ellman (6) and the "cutting block" technique described by Sampson (11). There is no clear benefit to either technique and different patient outcomes have never been reported. Techniques used are based on surgeon preference. We advocate the use of the lateral technique, but recommend learning both techniques.

Anatomy/Pathoanatomy

Understanding the relationship between the bony anatomy and the interposed subacromial bursa is essential for the diagnosis of an impingement syndrome and avoiding complications during surgical intervention. The relevant bony structures include the acromion, coracoid process, distal clavicle, acromioclavicular joint, and the greater tuberosity of the humerus. The shape of the anterior acromion has been attributed to the symptoms caused by external impingement. Bigliani (12) described three acromial shapes: type I (flat), type II (curved), and type III (hooked) (Fig. 6.1). A type III acromion decreases the subacromial space and is associated with underlying rotator cuff tears. The acromial type is best evaluated with a supraspinatus outlet view radiograph and aids in planning the amount of the undersurface of the acromion that is surgically resected to establish a flat acromion.

Abnormalities in soft tissues structures around the shoulder are associated with external impingement. The important soft tissue structures relevant are the coracoacromial ligament and the subacromial bursa. The

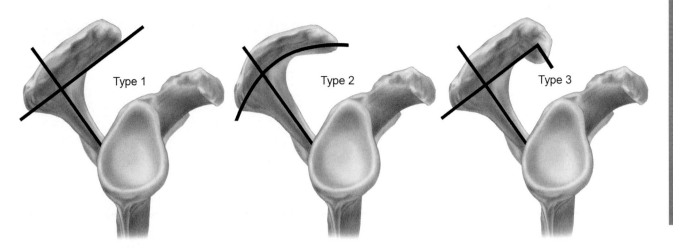

FIGURE 6.1. Acromial shapes as described by Bigliani: type I (flat), type II (curved), and type III (hooked).

subacromial bursa lies between the undersurface of the acromion and the superior surface of the rotator cuff. Inflammation of the subacromial bursa leads to a decrease in the subacromial space due to hypertrophy and pain with overhead movements. The coracoacromial ligament extends from the coracoid process to the anterior aspect of the acromion. Hypertrophy of the coracoacromial ligament also causes a decrease in the subacromial space and subsequent impingement. We believe the release of the coracoacromial ligament and a thorough subacromial bursectomy are essential for an arthroscopic subacromial decompression.

History and Physical Examination

Patients often relate a history of a gradual and progressive onset of symptoms located in their shoulder noted while performing overhead activities or when placing an arm in their coat. Frequently, patients will also complain of weakness and limitations of shoulder movement as a result of this shoulder pain. Many individuals cannot reach to put on their seatbelt or reach items in the back seat of their car. Some patients complain of sudden pain after a traumatic event or when pursuing a new sport. Pain due to impingement is most commonly localized to the anterolateral aspect of the acromion. Patients will often wake at night due to this pain or have difficulty sleeping on the affected shoulder. Although anterolateral shoulder pain is not specific for impingement syndrome, it guides the examiner to a spectrum of disorders of the rotator cuff and the subacromial space.

An insidious onset of symptoms due to extrinsic impingement is more commonly seen in athletes and workers that perform activities with repeated overhead motion. The traumatic onset of an impingement syndrome can be seen after a direct blow to the superolateral aspect of the shoulder or an axial load on the upper extremity, compressing the humeral head into the inferior aspect of the acromion (snow skiing fall, a football or hockey player

poorly fitted shoulder pads). The resultant inflammation of the subacromial bursa or contusion of the underlying rotator cuff causes the discomfort noted with overhead motion.

The physical examination is the key to making the diagnosis of an impingement syndrome. In order to perform an adequate examination, the patient must wear a shirt that allows for inspection of the neck, shoulder, and periscapular musculature. The exam should begin with an evaluation of the cervical spine and shoulder girdle. Limitations in neck range of motion, pain reproduced with provocative testing of the cervical spine, and pain radiating from the neck into the shoulder may indicate underlying cervical pathology and should not be confused with an impingement syndrome. The shoulder contours and musculature should be compared with the contralateral shoulder observing any muscle atrophy or squaring of the shoulder girdle. Changes in the resting position, contours, or atrophy of shoulder musculature indicate a possible neurological cause for abnormal shoulder motion resulting in secondary impingement. Tenderness localized to the subacromial bursa and rotator cuff, anterior or anterolateral to the acromion, and along the coracoacromial ligament is a common finding noted in patients who have extrinsic impingement syndrome.

Active forward flexion and abduction of the shoulder is frequently limited secondary to pain. However, passive range of motion must be tested to adequately assess terminal pain in forward flexion and/or abduction to ensure that the diagnosis of adhesive capsulitis is not made in error. Strength testing may also be limited due to pain and may suggest rotator cuff dysfunction, specifically with supraspinatus and infraspinatus testing differentiated with a lidocaine test. Subtle dynamic scapular winging of the shoulder during range of motion may be present. This denotes scapular dyskinesis, although it will not distinguish impingement as a primary or secondary condition.

Several tests have been described to aid in the diagnosis of an impingement syndrome. The "impingement sign" initially described by Neer, along with the Hawkins–Kennedy test, the painful arc sign, and the infraspinatus muscle test, offer the high sensitivity and specificity needed to distinguish this disease. The Neer sign is positive when pain at the anterior or lateral edge of the acromion is produced when the examiner stabilizes the scapula and passively forward flexes the arm with the humerus internally rotated. Hawkins and Kennedy described an alternative impingement test. This test is positive when pain is reproduced with forward flexion of the humerus to 90° and gentle internal rotation of the shoulder. These tests place the greater tuberosity, rotator cuff, or biceps tendon against the undersurface of the acromion or coracoacromial ligament causing aggravation of an inflamed subacromial bursa. The Neer sign has a sensitivity and specificity of 68.0% and 68.7%, respectively. The Hawkins–Kennedy sign has a slightly higher sensitivity (71.5%) and slightly lower specificity (66.3%). The sensitivities increase when patients without underlying rotator cuff disease are excluded.

A third test, the painful arc sign, has a sensitivity of 73.5% and specificity of 81.1%. This test is positive when a patient has pain or painful catching between 60° and 120° of elevation when actively elevating the arm in the plane of the scapula. The infraspinatus muscle test also has diagnostic value with a sensitivity of 41.6% and a specificity of 90.1%. This test is performed with the arm adducted to the side and the elbow flexed to 90°. The patient is then asked to resist an internal rotation force. A test is considered positive if the patient gives way due to pain or weakness, or has an external rotation lag sign. The likelihood of an impingement syndrome is >95% if the Hawkins–Kennedy impingement sign, painful arc sign, and infraspinatus muscle test are all positive. If these three tests are all negative, the likelihood of an impingement syndrome is <24% (13). Confidence in the diagnosis can be improved with the lidocaine test. Injection of 10 mL of lidocaine into the subacromial space through an anterior approach (as this is where the pathology lies) often alleviates the patient's symptoms. The alleviation of symptoms during provocative testing after injection confirms the diagnosis of an impingement syndrome.

Diagnostic Imaging

Radiographic evaluation of the shoulder is essential to evaluate the shape of the acromion and rule out concomitant pathology. A true anterior–posterior radiograph of the shoulder allows assessment of the glenohumeral joint. To obtain this view, the body is rotated 35° toward the side of the involved shoulder, and the scapula is placed flat against the film. This position places the glenoid perpendicular to the X-ray beam and allows for the assessment of the glenohumeral joint to note any arthritic

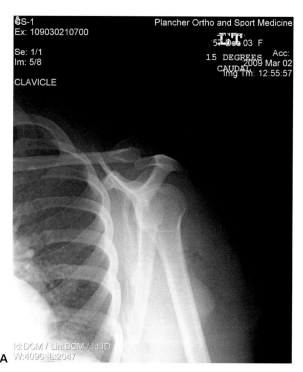

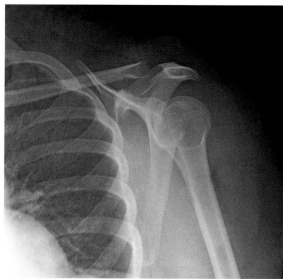

FIGURE 6.2. A: Supraspinatus outlet view radiograph showing a type III acromion. **B:** Supraspinatus outlet view radiograph after acromioplasty now showing a type I acromion.

changes. A second view, the supraspinatus outlet view, allows for the assessment of acromial morphology and is essential for preoperative planning. We advocate a repeat supraspinatus outlet view postoperatively to evaluate the acromial shape after arthroscopic acromioplasty (Fig. 6.2A and B). This view is obtained by positioning the patient for a scapular lateral view and tilting the X-ray beam caudally 10° to 15°. Additional routine radiographs of the shoulder that may be helpful include the axillary view and Zanca view. The axillary view further evaluates the glenohumeral joint and acromion and more importantly, may reveal an os acromiale. The Zanca view is best to evaluate the acromioclavicular joint for arthrosis or any incongruity.

Further evaluation of the painful shoulder with ultrasound, CT, and MRI is not necessary to make the diagnosis of an impingement syndrome. If the diagnosis of impingement is uncertain, the lidocaine test is equivocal, and there is suspicion of concomitant pathology involving the glenohumeral joint or other soft tissues around the shoulder (i.e., rotator cuff, SLAP lesions, etc.) an MRI should be obtained. The MRI may show increased signal intensity in the subacromial bursa due to subacromial bursitis, or underlying rotator cuff pathology may be revealed.

TREATMENT

Preoperative Considerations

Operative intervention is suggested for patients that do not respond to a prolonged course of conservative treatment or have a recurrence of symptoms after initial improvement. The indications for subacromial decompression are

1. Structural abnormalities causing extrinsic impingement (type II or III acromion, hypertrophic coracoacromial ligament, inferior spur from the acromioclavicular joint, or hypertrophic subacromial bursa)
2. Patients that fail nonoperative management but have previously responded to subacromial injections
3. Patients undergoing debridement of a bursal-sided partial rotator cuff tears
4. Patients having a rotator cuff repair

Acromioplasty and release of the coracoacromial ligament is contraindicated in patients with massive or irreparable rotator cuff tears. Patients with instability and resultant secondary impingement should also not have an acromioplasty and release of the coracoacromial ligament. A cautious approach with further diagnostic workup is recommended for patients with impingement symptoms who fail to receive any symptomatic relief after a subacromial injection. Performing an acromioplasty as an adjunct to subacromial bursal debridement in patients with adhesive capsulitis is controversial and beyond the scope of this chapter.

Operative Considerations

A conservative approach is the preferred initial treatment for patients with an isolated impingement syndrome. The goal is to limit inflammation while preserving range of motion. The offending overhead movement should be identified and limited to help symptoms resolve. Nonsteroidal anti-inflammatory medications and modalities such as ice, heat, iontophoresis, and ultrasound are beneficial in reducing inflammation and should be started early in the course of treatment. Physical therapy that includes range of motion, scapular stabilization, and strengthening exercises should be implemented once symptoms begin improving. An anesthetic injection with a corticosteroid can be therapeutic and will often help reduce bursal inflammation. This form of nonoperative treatment is successful in most cases. Those patients who have recurrent symptoms after responding to the subacromial injections may need operative intervention. In contrast, patients who have concomitant pathology and secondarily develop impingement syndrome will be unlikely to respond to conservative treatment.

SURGICAL TECHNIQUE

Lateral Approach

Patient positioning, anesthesia, and draping are identical for the lateral acromioplasty technique and the posterior "cutting block" technique. An interscalene block with or without general anesthesia is used in most patients. If possible, hypotensive anesthesia with the systolic blood pressure in the range of 95 to 105 mm Hg is preferred. Maintenance of a systolic blood pressure <100 mm Hg will limit the need for higher arthroscopic pump pressures and will allow for perfect visualization and minimize fluid extravasation. A pump pressure of 40 to 50 mmHg is often sufficient. We prefer the beach chair position for isolated acromioplasty and subacromial decompression. This is also the preferred position if a concomitant procedure such as a rotator cuff repair is being performed. The key in either method is sterility with multiple layers of drapes. Drapes are placed to the middle of the sternum anteriorly and to the medial border of the scapula posteriorly.

Once the patient is properly positioned, all palpable shoulder landmarks are marked with a skin marker. The arm is placed in full adduction and parallel with the trunk prior to marking the skin. If the arm is forward flexed or extended, the posterior viewing portal may be improperly placed. Also, the arm should be allowed to hang freely at that patient's side. The standard posterior portal is placed 1 to 2 cm medial and 2 cm inferior to the posterolateral corner of the acromion. This position is variable based on the patient size and body habitus and may be adjusted to the "soft spot." An alternative posterior portal is marked 1 cm superior and 0.5 to 1 cm lateral to the standard posterior viewing portal in the case of use of the "cutting block" technique. The lateral working portal is marked 2 cm lateral to the lateral border of the acromion and in line with the midportion of the clavicle. This portal can be "cheated" slightly anterior or posterior if this position is advantageous to access associated pathology (Fig. 6.3).

A 30° arthroscope is placed through the posterior portal into the glenohumeral joint. Standard glenohumeral arthroscopy is performed prior to performing

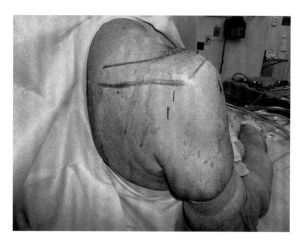

FIGURE 6.3. Portal placement for subacromial decompression. We mark the standard posterior portal 1 to 2 cm medial and 2 cm inferior to the posterolateral corner of the acromion, an alternative posterior portal is marked 1 cm superior and 0.5 to 1 cm lateral to the standard posterior viewing portal, and the lateral working portal is marked 2 cm lateral to the lateral border of the acromion and in line with the midportion of the clavicle.

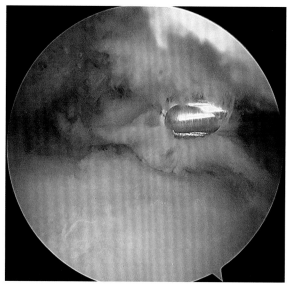

FIGURE 6.4. Arthroscopic view using an arthroscopic shaver to completely debride the subacromial bursa.

acromioplasty and subacromial decompression. The technique for glenohumeral arthroscopy is discussed elsewhere in this text. All associated pathology is treated at this time. The arthroscope is removed from the cannula and the trocar is inserted. The trocar and cannula are withdrawn together from the glenohumeral joint, but not past the posterior deltoid. These instruments are then redirected superiorly into the subacromial space and advanced until the undersurface of the acromion is identified. A medial to lateral "sweep" is performed from the medial border of the acromion to the level of the lateral portal. This "sweep" will break up bursal adhesions and creates the "room with a view." A lateral portal is made and a 5.5-mm cannula is placed through the deltoid into the subacromial space. With the arthroscope's trocar in the posterior portal, the tip of the arthroscope's trocar and the tip of the cannula trocar should meet. With the arthroscopic sheath held in position, the 30° arthroscope is inserted into the subacromial space and directed to the tip of the cannula. A radiofrequency device may be used to ablate and debride the bursal adhesions and the posterior bursal curtain (posterior "veil of tears"). Without debridement of this posterior bursal curtain, visualization can be hindered throughout the procedure. Creating a "room with a view" (adequate space) allows for excellent visualization and helps make the procedure more efficient. The anterolateral corner of the acromion is localized and marked with a spinal needle. In order to delineate the subacromial space and widen it, the anterior and lateral borders of the acromion should be delineated and the undersurface of the acromion debrided using the radiofrequency device. The remaining bursa

overlying the rotator cuff is debrided using a full-radius motorized shaver (Fig. 6.4). It is our preference to debride the entire bursa until the blood vessels overlying the superior rotator cuff can be clearly seen (Fig. 6.5). Bleeding is commonly encountered when using the motorized shaver medial to the supraspinatus myotendinous junction and this should be avoided. The medial edge of the acromion should be visualized, but the acromioclavicular joint capsule should not be violated unless a clavicular coplaning or distal clavicle resection is planned. Release of the hypertrophic coracoacromial ligament is performed in all cases except in patients with massive or unrepairable rotator cuff tears. Bleeding from the acromial branch of the thoracoacromial artery is commonly encountered when releasing the coracoacromial ligament and should be ablated with the radiofrequency device. When performed, the release should be performed at the

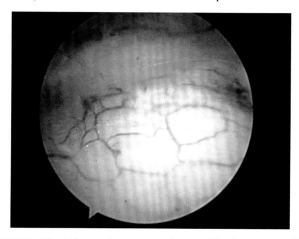

FIGURE 6.5. Arthroscopic view showing the blood vessels on the superior aspect of the rotator cuff signifying a complete bursectomy.

most lateral extend to avoid this vessel. The extent of the acromial hook may be difficult to appreciate from the posterior viewing portal and moving the camera to the lateral portal provides an understanding of the acromial morphology from another angle (Fig. 6.6).

A 6.0-mm oval hooded burr is placed through the lateral portal and oriented along the anterior border of the acromion (Fig. 6.7). For smaller individuals, a 4.0 mm

burr is utilized. The depth of the acromial resection is established by burying the burr to the diameter of the burr (Fig. 6.8). This resection should start just medial to the acromioclavicular joint to avoid violation of the acromioclavicular joint capsule. Once the extent of the most anterior resection is established, the remaining hook of the acromion is resected until the acromion is flat (Fig. 6.9). Using the burr in reverse for most acromioplasty procedures is suggested, especially when the surgeon is converting from an open to an arthroscopic technique. Using a burr in reverse is also prudent in patients with soft bone. More control can be achieved which limits the creation of an uneven surface or overzealous resection. A narrow ENT nasal rasp inserted through the lateral portal can be used to smooth any remaining rough edges.

When first transitioning to an arthroscopic technique, palpation with a digit through the lateral portal

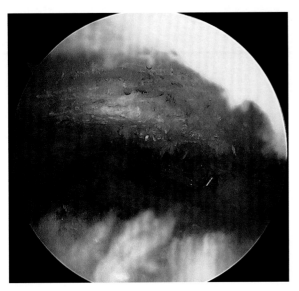

FIGURE 6.6. Arthroscopic view from the lateral portal of a type III acromion after complete bursectomy and debridement of the undersurface of the acromion with a radiofrequency device.

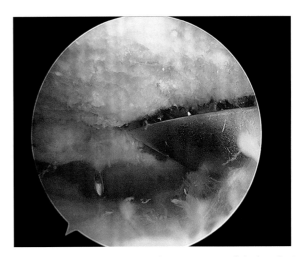

FIGURE 6.8. Lateral technique. Arthroscopic view of the burr buried the diameter of the burr. The remainder of the acromioplasty will be based off the depth set during this step.

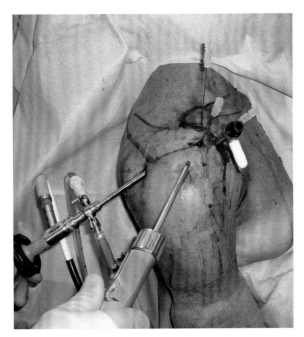

FIGURE 6.7. Lateral technique. The arthroscope is in the posterior portal and the burr is placed through the lateral portal. The burr is parallel to the front of the acromion when burying burr to begin the acromioplasty.

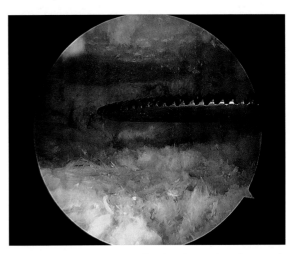

FIGURE 6.9. Arthroscopic view of coplaned acromion after completed acromioplasty.

can provide a better assessment of the finished resection. This technique is helpful to insure that the acromioplasty is smooth and the lateral border has been adequately resected. The arthroscope should always be placed through the lateral portal to check for any remaining acromial spurs and to insure that a complete resection has been accomplished. (Note: The most common missed bony spurs are medial near the acromioclavicular joint.) Prior to withdrawing the arthroscope, a spinal needle is once again placed in the subacromial space. The remaining fluid in the subacromial space is then suctioned out and the arthroscope is withdrawn. All portal sites are closed with subcutaneous and subcuticular sutures. Any anesthetic or other medications can then be placed through the spinal needle. A sterile dressing is placed over the wounds and a sling is fitted for patient comfort.

Posterior (Cutting Block) Approach

The "cutting block" technique is an alternative method for a subacromial decompression. The setup for this technique is identical to the lateral approach. The posterior portal created for glenohumeral arthroscopy is commonly too low to perform a true "cutting block" coplaning of the acromion. If this portal is too low, the posterior acromion cannot be used as a guide and the risk of overresection of the anterior aspect of the acromion increases (Figs. 6.10 and 6.11). Therefore, we prefer to create an additional portal 1 to 2 cm superior and slightly lateral to the usual posterior portal (Figs. 6.12 and 6.13). The 6.0-mm oval burr is placed through this new posterior portal and the arthroscope

is placed in the lateral portal. It is helpful as previously stated to use the burr in reverse for most acromioplasty procedures.

Coplaning of the acromion is begun at the posterior border of the clavicle and advanced forward

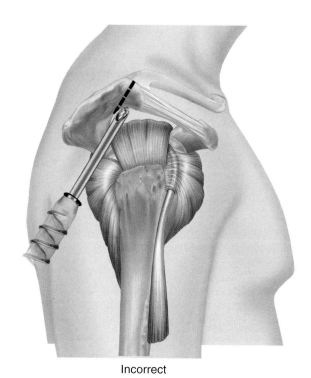

Incorrect

FIGURE 6.11. Cutting block technique. A posterior portal placed too inferiorly results in a vertically oriented angle of the burr. This vertically oriented angle of the burr will likely result in overresection of the anterior acromion.

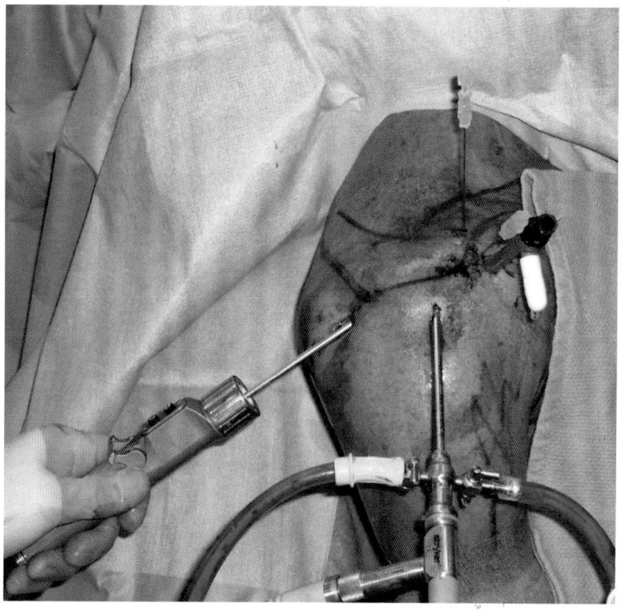

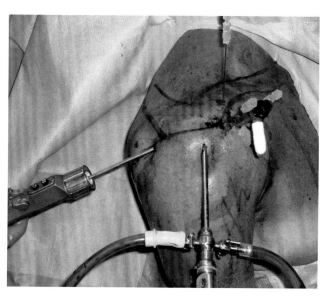

FIGURE 6.10. Cutting block technique. This position of the burr in the posterior portal is too vertical and likely will result in overresection of the anterior acromion.

FIGURE 6.12. Cutting block technique. By using the alternate posterior portal, the burr can be oriented parallel to the posterior acromion. This allows proper use of the posterior acromion as a cutting block.

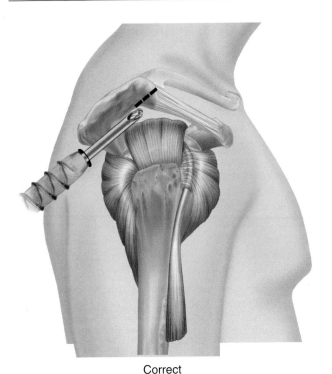

Correct

FIGURE 6.13. Cutting block technique. By using the alternate posterior portal, the burr can be oriented parallel to the posterior acromion. This allows proper use of the posterior acromion as a cutting block.

to the anterior border of the acromion using the undersurface of the posterior acromion as the "cutting block." Each pass of the burr will serve as the guide for the next pass (Fig. 6.14). The resection should begin at the medial acromion and move toward the lateral

border with each successive pass of the burr. A change in pitch of the burr will occur as it transitions from bone to soft tissue at the lateral border. Noting this will limit the need for placing the burr in the lateral portal to complete the acromioplasty. Commonly, the medial-most border of the acromion at the AC joint is missed during resection and may cause recurrence of symptoms. The capsule of the AC joint should never be violated unless preoperative X-rays show a corresponding infraclavicular spur that will be resected based on preoperative planning.

Once coplaning of the acromion is complete, the hooded portion of the burr can be used to check the "flatness" of the acromioplasty (Fig. 6.15). The arthroscope is placed in the posterior portal to check the lateral edge of the acromion for any remaining spurs. A narrow nasal rasp inserted through the lateral portal can be used to smooth any rough edges. Prior to withdrawing the arthroscope, a spinal needle is placed in the subacromial space. The remaining fluid in the subacromial space is then suctioned out and the arthroscope is withdrawn. All portal sites are closed with subcutaneous and subcuticular sutures. Any anesthetic or other medications can then be placed through the spinal needle. A sterile dressing is placed over the wounds and a sling is fitted for patient comfort.

COMPLICATIONS

Complications from an arthroscopic subacromial decompression can be limited by proper patient selection and diligent preoperative planning. Performing an isolated subacromial decompression in patients with concomitant

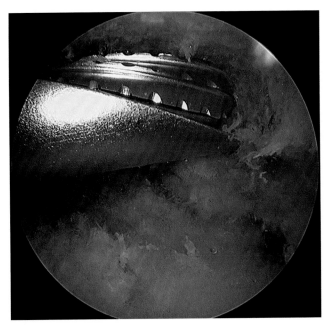

FIGURE 6.14. Cutting block technique. The posterior acromion is used as the cutting block guide. Each successive pass from medial to lateral is used as the guide for the next pass.

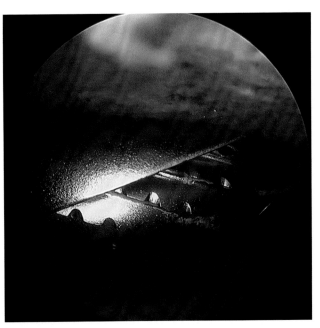

FIGURE 6.15. Cutting block technique. The hooded portion of the burr can be used to assess the flatness of the acromioplasty.

glenohumeral pathology or shoulder instability will more often than not fail and result in persistent symptoms. Failures can be limited by a meticulous history and thorough physical exam, proper diagnosis, and can be confirmed by performing a lidocaine test. Preoperative evaluation of the radiographs is essential to understand the topography of the acromion and any osteophytic spurs that should be resected. Proper posterior portal placement is imperative to avoid under- or overresection of the acromion when using the cutting block technique. The placement of a posterior portal 1 to 2 cm superior and slightly lateral to the standard posterior portal can minimize this complication. Other complications include deltoid detachment from an overzealous anterior or lateral resection, infection, postoperative stiffness, and failure to identify a symptomatic os acromiale.

PEARLS

1. Careful preoperative planning and critical evaluation of the radiographs help to avoid under or overresection of the acromion.
2. Safe hypotensive anesthesia limits intraoperative bleeding and maintains visualization.
3. Proper portal placement is crucial, especially with the cutting block technique. It is better to create an additional portal than to attempt the acromioplasty with an improperly placed portal.
4. Thorough bursal debridement is crucial for visualization, and an inflamed bursa may irritate the rotator cuff.
5. Outlining the anterior and lateral borders of the acromion with a radiofrequency device allows for excellent visualization, helps maintain your orientation, and often prevents overresection of the acromion.
6. Use the arthroscopic burr in reverse when first learning the arthroscopic technique as well as when the patient has soft bone. The creation of divots will be avoided with this technique.

PITFALLS

1. Failure to resect the posterior bursal curtain ("vale of tears") will impede visualization throughout the procedure and make completion of the subacromial decompression more difficult. Unresected bursa will also swell with the influx of fluid and further impede visualization.
2. Failure to sweep the cuff with the scope to break up bursal adhesions and create a "room with a view" will make the procedure more difficult and lengthy.
3. When using the cutting block technique, poor posterior portal placement can lead to under or overresection of the acromion.
4. Avoid overdetachment of the deltoid insertion at the anterior and lateral border of the acromion.

POSTOPERATIVE REHABILITATION PROTOCOL

All patients are placed in a sling immediately postoperatively. For isolated subacromial decompression, early motion and physical therapy are encouraged. On the first postoperative day, all dressings are changed and patients are encouraged to begin Codman exercises and gentle active and passive range of motion. By the end of the first week, patients are weaned from the sling and encouraged to return to daily activities as tolerated. During the subsequent weeks, progressive strengthening of the shoulder girdle and scapular stabilization is encouraged. A return to full activities is allowed once the patient is pain free and has regained strength equal to 90% of the contralateral shoulder. For patients who undergo a procedure for concomitant pathology, the postoperative rehabilitation protocol is based on the protocol for that procedure.

CONCLUSION

Satisfactory results have been reported in 67% to 88% of arthroscopic subacromial decompression for impingement (3,6,9,10). These results are comparable to the results reported by Neer using an open technique. Both the lateral and "cutting block" techniques for arthroscopic subacromial decompression are safe and efficacious methods of treating an impingement syndrome with results equivalent to open surgical techniques. Although there is no difference in outcomes with the two arthroscopic techniques, we prefer the lateral technique because it is less dependent on portal placement. We recommend having both techniques at your disposal and believe with proper patient selection, careful preoperative planning, and meticulous surgical technique, impingement syndrome can be safely treated arthroscopically with low morbidity and rapid return to activities.

REFERENCES

1. Neer CS. Anterior acromioplasty for the chronic impingement syndrome in the shoulder: a preliminary report. *J Bone Joint Surg Am.* 1972;54:41–50.
2. Chin PYK, Sperling JW, Cofield RH, et al. Anterior acromioplasty for the shoulder impingement syndrome: long-term outcome. *J Shoulder Elbow Surg.* 2007;16:697–700.
3. Altchek DW, Warren RF, Wickiewicz TL, et al. Arthroscopic acromioplasty: technique and results. *J Bone Joint Surg Am.* 1990;72:1198–1207.
4. Altchek DW, Carson EW. Arthroscopic acromioplasty: current status. *Orthop Clin North Am.* 1997;28:157–168.
5. Barfield LC, Kuhn JE. Arthroscopic versus open acromioplasty: a systematic review. *Clin Orthop Relat Res.* 2007;455:64–71.

6. Ellman H. Arthroscopic subacromial decompression: a preliminary report. *Orthop Trans.* 1985;9:49.

7. Ellman H. Arthroscopic subacromial decompression: analysis of one to three year results. *Arthroscopy.* 1987;3:173–181.

8. Hawkins RH, Plancher KD, Saddemi SR, et al. Arthroscopic subacromial decompression. *J Shoulder Elbow Surg.* 2001; 10:225–230.

9. Spangehl MJ, Hawkins RH, McCormack RG, et al. Arthroscopic versus open acromioplasty: a prospective, randomized, blinded study. *J Shoulder Elbow Surg.* 2002;11:101–107.

10. Stephens SR, Warren RF, Payne LZ, et al. Arthroscopic acromioplasty: a 6- to 10-year follow-up. *Arthroscopy.* 1998;14:382-388.

11. Sampson TG, Nisbet JK, Glick JM. Precision acromioplasty in arthroscopic subacromial decompression of the shoulder. *Arthroscopy.* 1991;7:301–307.

12. Bigliani LU, Morrision D, April EW. The morphology of the acromion and its relationship to rotator cuff tears. *Orthop Trans.* 1986;10:228.

13. Park HB, Yokota A, Gill HS, et al. Diagnostic accuracy of clinical tests for the different degrees of subacromial impingement syndrome. *J Bone Joint Surg Am.* 2005;87:1446–1455.

I. The Shoulder

The Treatment of the Symptomatic Os Acromiale

Richard K.N. Ryu • Ryan M. Dopirak

The acromion develops from four different centers of ossification: the preacromion, mesoacromion, meta-acromion, and basiacromion. These ossification centers appear between the ages of 14 to 18, with complete fusion typically evident by age 18 to 25.

An os acromiale is an anatomic variant that represents the failure of the acromial apophysis to fuse. It occurs in approximately 6% to 8% of the population and is bilateral in 33% to 41% of individuals. It has been observed to be more frequent in males than in females and is also more common in blacks than in whites. The most common site of an os acromiale is between the mesoacromion and the meta-acromion and is called a mesoacromiale.

Although often an incidental radiographic finding, an os acromiale may be pathologic in some patients. An unstable os acromiale may cause pain directly due to motion at the non-union site. Additionally, it may be a source of symptoms due to external impingement with resultant rotator cuff pathology.

The initial treatment of a symptomatic os acromiale is typically nonoperative consisting of rest, activity modification, nonsteroidal anti-inflammatory drugs (NSAIDs), and physical therapy. Subacromial corticosteroid injections may also play a role in selected individuals although this may not be indicated in younger patients with significant rotator cuff pathology. When nonoperative measures fail to provide lasting symptomatic relief, surgery is often considered. Surgical options for an os acromiale include standard acromioplasty, complete fragment excision, or open reduction and internal fixation (ORIF).

There are currently no controlled studies comparing these various treatment options. Therefore, several factors should be considered during the decision-making process, including patient age and functional demands, location of the os acromiale, radiographic findings on MRI and bone scan, and intraoperative stability of the anterior fragment (1,2).

CLINICAL EVALUATION

Pertinent History

A careful history is important in evaluating the patient with an os acromiale, as this may simply be an incidental finding unrelated to their true source of pain or dysfunction. However, when an os acromiale is symptomatic, it may cause symptoms by two different mechanisms. Motion between the fragments may be a direct cause of pain similar to that of a painful nonunion elsewhere in the body. In this scenario, patients typically report pain in the superior aspect of the shoulder, which may be exacerbated by overhead activity, heavy lifting, or repetitive use of the involved extremity.

Alternatively, an unstable os may cause a dynamic impingement syndrome where the mobile anterior fragment impinges upon the anterior aspect of the rotator cuff during deltoid contraction. In these patients, symptoms are those of a classic impingement syndrome. There may be pain in the anterolateral shoulder that is exacerbated by overhead activity and repetitive use of the extremity. Night pain and weakness are often present, especially in patients with concomitant rotator cuff pathology.

In some patients, the onset of symptoms may occur after a significant trauma to the shoulder with disruption of a previously stable fibrous union. However, in most patients the onset of symptoms is insidious without a significant traumatic event.

Physical Examination

A standard comprehensive physical examination is performed when evaluating the patient with an os acromiale. An unstable os may be painful due to motion at the nonunion site. In this situation, the examiner may elicit tenderness with palpation directly at the site of the os. Ballotment of the anterior mobile fragment can create motion at the nonunion site and reproduce the patient's symptoms. It is sometimes possible for the examiner to appreciate motion of the anterior fragment although this is typically only possible in slender patients with a grossly unstable anterior fragment.

When the os acromiale causes symptoms due to a dynamic impingement upon the rotator cuff, physical findings are similar to those of a classic impingement syndrome. Patients demonstrate a painful arc of motion as well as positive impingement signs. Active forward elevation in the scapular plane may be limited secondary to pain. Significant weakness of the rotator cuff may be present if concomitant rotator cuff pathology is present. Subacromial injection of local anesthetic is sometimes helpful in differentiating between weakness that is pain induced and weakness that is due to actual rotator cuff pathology.

Imaging

Standard shoulder radiographs are obtained when evaluating the patient with an os acromiale. A standard anteroposterior (AP) view can sometimes suggest the diagnosis of an os acromiale, as one may notice an apparent double density of the acromion. The scapular Y view can clearly demonstrate the os in most cases although in some patients this can be a subtle finding that may be overlooked. In a small number of patients, the Y view will reveal osteophytes on the superior aspect of the acromion. This is secondary to motion at the nonunion site and would be analogous to a hypertrophic nonunion elsewhere in the body. The axillary lateral is the view that is most essential in the diagnosis of the os acromiale. It will reliably demonstrate the presence of the os and will allow the surgeon to classify it according to its location (Fig. 7.1).

Although plain radiographs are a reliable and cost-effective method of diagnosing an os acromiale, a shoulder MRI is also be obtained in many patients to rule out associated shoulder pathology. The os can be demonstrated on both the axial and the sagittal oblique MR images (Fig. 7.2). One must ensure that the axial cuts begin above the superior margin of the acromion or the diagnosis may be missed. On sagittal oblique views, it is important to recognize that the os can be mistaken for the acromioclavicular (AC) joint and may be overlooked.

When evaluating an os acromiale on MRI, an increased signal on the T2 sequences signifies the presence of fluid within the nonunion site and/or adjacent bone marrow edema within the fragment and is presumably due to repetitive motion and microtrauma. When present, many surgeons consider this finding to be diagnostic of instability of the anterior fragment.

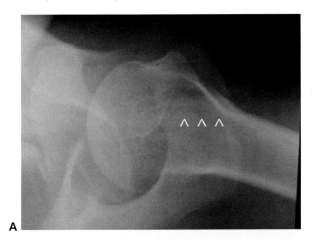

A

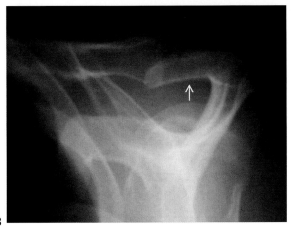

B

FIGURE 7.1. Radiographic examination of a mesoacromiale. **A:** Axillary view, white arrowheads indicate site of the mesoacromiale. **B:** Outlet view, white arrow indicates site of the mesoacromiale.

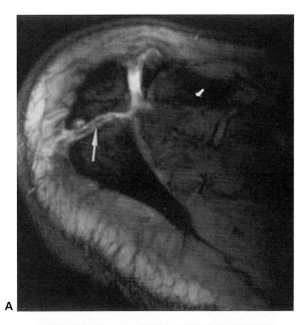

A

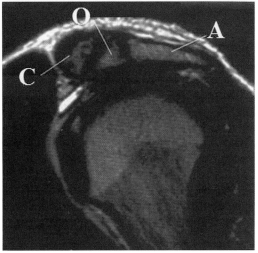

B

FIGURE 7.2. MRI evaluation of an os acromiale. **A:** Axial image, white arrow indicates site of the os acromiale. **B:** Sagittal oblique image; A, acromion; O, os acromiale; C, clavicle.

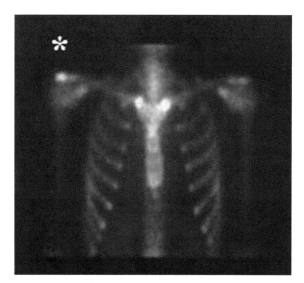

FIGURE 7.3. Tc 99 bone scan showing increased asymmetric uptake at site of os acromiale. Asterisk indicates site of os acromiale.

Technetium (Tc 99) bone scanning is often utilized in the evaluation of an os acromiale. Significant asymmetric uptake in the acromion signifies instability of the anterior fragment with resultant motion and microtrauma at the nonunion site (Fig. 7.3). This test is an important part of the decision-making algorithm for the treatment of the os acromiale.

Classification

The acromion develops from four different centers of ossification: the preacromion, mesoacromion, meta-acromion, and basiacromion. When the diagnosis of os acromiale is made, it is commonly classified according to the anatomic location of the nonunion site. The ossification center directly anterior to the nonunion site is the fragment that is clinically unstable and thus the source of clinical symptoms; therefore, the os acromiale will derive its name from this fragment (Fig. 7.4).

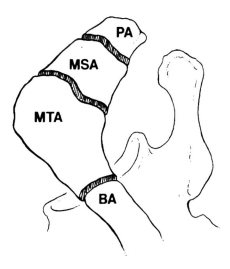

FIGURE 7.4. Classification of os acromiale. PA, preacromion; MSA, mesoacromion; MTA, meta-acromion; BA, basiacromion.

The most common type of os acromiale is a mesoacromiale, which represents a failure of fusion between the mesoacromion and the meta-acromion. Preacromial fragments occur less frequently than the mesoacromiale, but are not uncommon. In some patients, the preacromial fragment is small and may be overlooked on radiographic studies. The meta-acromiale is relatively uncommon.

When considering the diagnosis of os acromiale, it is important to remember that complete fusion of the acromial ossification centers does not typically occur until age 18 to 25. Therefore, in patients under age 25 an unfused acromial apophysis may represent nothing more than a normal developmental finding.

TREATMENT

Nonoperative

The initial treatment for an isolated os acromiale should be nonoperative consisting of rest, activity modification, NSAIDs, and formal physical therapy. Subacromial corticosteroid injections may also play a role in selected individuals although this may not be indicated in younger patients with significant rotator cuff pathology.

Nonoperative management has empirically been recommended for a minimum of 6 months. In the current medical environment, however, it is becoming increasingly difficult to get physical therapy authorized for an extended period of time. Despite this fact, all conservative measures should be exhausted prior to consideration of surgical intervention.

In patients with a symptomatic os acromiale and a concomitant full thickness rotator cuff tear, extended nonoperative management may not be appropriate for all patients. In this situation, the decision-making process should be guided by standard protocols for the treatment of rotator cuff tears.

Operative Indications

When patients fail to improve with conservative measures as outlined above, surgical intervention may be considered. Several surgical options exist, including arthroscopic subacromial decompression (ASAD), complete fragment excision, and ORIF. There are currently no prospective controlled studies comparing these various treatment options. Therefore, several factors should be considered during the decision-making process, including patient age and functional demands, location of the os acromiale, radiographic findings on MRI and bone scan, and intraoperative stability of the anterior fragment.

TECHNIQUE

Arthroscopic Subacromial Decompression

The primary advantage of ASAD for an os acromiale is that it avoids the potential complications associated with ORIF and complete fragment excision, including nonunion and symptomatic hardware, and deltoid dysfunction, respectively. However, if the os acromiale is unstable, resulting in painful motion at the nonunion site, simple ASAD is not likely to provide meaningful symptomatic relief as the underlying source of pathology has not been addressed.

Hutchinson and Veenstra (3) performed ASAD in three patients with impingement syndrome and an associated os acromiale. After 1 year, all three patients had a recurrence of their symptoms. The authors concluded that simple ASAD was not appropriate for the treatment of os acromiale.

Aboud et al. (4) also evaluated outcomes after SAD for an os acromiale in 11 patients and found satisfactory results in only 64%. However, the SAD was arthroscopic in five patients and open in the remaining six patients. Furthermore, 5 of the 11 patients underwent concomitant rotator cuff repair. The diverse study group makes it difficult to draw conclusions from this study on the efficacy of ASAD for os acromiale.

Armengol et al. (5) performed modified acromioplasty in 23 patients with an os acromiale; seven of the surgeries were arthroscopic. In their technique, the undersurface was burred relatively aggressively so that only a thin cortical shell remained superiorly. Satisfactory results were achieved in 87% of patients.

Wright et al. (6) treated 12 patients (13 shoulders) with a mesoacromiale with extended arthroscopic acromioplasty. None of these patients had pain or tenderness at the nonunion site preoperatively. Their technique was similar to that of Armengol et al. (5) and consisted of more bone resection than the typical arthroscopic acromioplasty. The goal was to resect the mobile anterior lip to the point that it would be unable to impinge upon the rotator cuff while minimizing disruption to the deltoid and AC joint capsule. Satisfactory results were achieved in 85% of patients (6).

Based on the available literature, we believe ASAD may be indicated in selected patients with an os acromiale. The most critical factor in evaluating the patient with an os acromiale is determining whether the os is stable or unstable. ASAD should be performed only for an os acromiale that is determined to be relatively stable. This can be evaluated in three different ways. First, during the physical examination, assess tenderness to palpation directly at the site of the nonunion. Second, obtain a bone scan preoperatively to assess any asymmetric increased uptake at the site of the os acromiale. Third, evaluate the stability of the anterior fragment intraoperatively (Fig. 7.5). Through direct pressure on the superior aspect of the anterior fragment, significant motion may be appreciated if the fragment is grossly unstable (Fig. 7.6). In patients with no preoperative tenderness over the site of the os, a negative bone scan, and no evidence of instability intraoperatively, ASAD is the most appropriate treatment option for impingement of the anterior fragment upon the rotator cuff.

The technique is similar to that of a standard ASAD, but may at times involve more bone resection than the

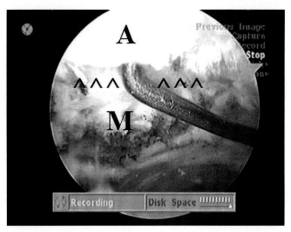

FIGURE 7.5. Arthroscopic view of a mesoacromiale with arthroscope in posterior subacromial portal. Tip of probe in the site of the nonunion. A, acromion; M, mesoacromial fragment; arrowheads, site of nonunion.

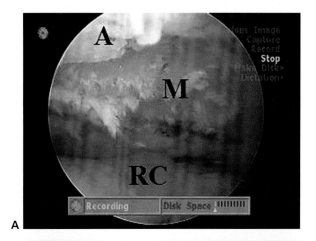

A

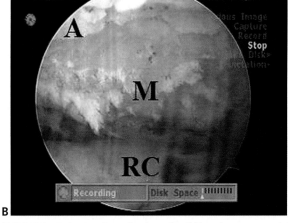

B

FIGURE 7.6. Arthroscopic evaluation of stability of a mesocromiale, arthroscope in posterior subacromial portal. **A:** Photo taken without external manual pressure. **B:** Photo taken during application of external downward pressure on anterior fragment. Anterior fragment is depressed inferiorly, indicating fragment is mobile and unstable. A, acromion; M, mesoacromial fragment; RC, rotator cuff.

typical acromioplasty. The goal should be to remove an adequate amount of bone so that the anterior acromial undersurface does not impinge upon the rotator cuff. All efforts should be made to preserve the integrity of the coracoacromial ligament (CAL). The CAL will need to be released from the anterior aspect of the acromion in order to obtain adequate visualization. However, the ligament should remain in continuity and its attachment to the lateral margin of the acromion should be preserved. An overly aggressive release of the ligament may actually destabilize a previously stable os acromiale. Disruption of the acromioclavicular joint capsule should also be minimized, if possible. Performing a complete distal clavicle excision, or even an aggressive coplaning, may compromise the stability of the os acromiale.

Rehabilitation

Postoperative care will be similar to that after standard ASAD without an os acromiale. Patients remain in a sling for comfort as needed for up to 1 to 2 weeks after surgery. Formal physical therapy is initiated after the first post-op visit, which is approximately 10 days after surgery. Physical therapy initially focuses on regaining full range of motion (ROM), as well as maintenance of proper scapulothoracic mechanics. Strengthening typically begins at 6 weeks post-op. If ASAD is performed in conjunction with rotator cuff repair, then standard postoperative rotator cuff repair protocols are utilized.

Complete Fragment Excision

The primary advantage of complete fragment excision is that the source of clinical symptoms is definitively addressed. The disadvantage of this procedure is that it involves alteration of the deltoid insertion, which may result in unsatisfactory outcomes due to significant pain and weakness. Several authors have reported outcomes after open excision of the anterior fragment. Although these were generally small case series, a significant percentage of patients experienced unsatisfactory outcomes in all these studies (5,7,8).

In contrast, Pagnani et al. (9) reported relatively favorable results after arthroscopic fragment excision in nine patients (11 shoulders) with an unstable mesoacromiale. All patients were competitive male athletes between the ages of 18 to 25. All patients were able to return to full athletic participation postoperatively. Isokinetic strength testing was performed in seven patients and revealed no strength deficits in the operative shoulder as compared with the contralateral shoulder. The authors felt that their results were superior to those after open excision because arthroscopic fragment excision did not violate the insertion of the deltoid fascia into the acromion.

Complete fragment excision may be indicated in certain individuals with an os acromiale. Open excision is rarely recommended as a primary procedure, but may be performed as a salvage procedure for failed ORIF with persistent nonunion if concomitant hardware removal is necessary. In most circumstances when fragment excision is considered, an arthroscopic approach is preferable to an open approach. For preacromial fragments, arthroscopic resection has little morbidity and is typically the procedure of choice. For a mesoacromiale that is deemed to be significantly unstable, as determined by tenderness at the nonunion site, increased uptake on the bone scan, and intraoperative instability of the anterior fragment, surgical options include either complete fragment excision or ORIF. Arthroscopic fragment excision is preferable in older, sedentary patients. In younger, high-demand patients, either ORIF or fragment excision may be considered. Based on the findings of Pagnani et al. (9), arthroscopic fragment excision appears to be both safe and effective in younger athletic patients. However, there are no controlled studies comparing these two treatment options, so it is unknown at this time which procedure is superior. It is important to discuss the risks and benefits of both procedures with each patient and allow them to participate in the decision-making process.

The principles of arthroscopic excision of an os acromiale are similar to those of standard ASAD. One must be comfortable with arthroscopic visualization as well as manipulation of instruments through all three portals. It is essential to visualize the final resection from the posterior, lateral, and anterior portals prior to concluding the case, in order to ensure that residual bony fragments have not been overlooked. A common area to leave residual bone is superiorly at the posterior margin of the anterior fragment. This area is difficult to visualize from the posterior portal and must also be evaluated from either the lateral or the anterior portal.

The primary advantage of the arthroscopic approach is the preservation of the deltoid insertion. Use of a standard burr has the potential to damage the deltoid fascia when resecting the final portion of the acromion superiorly. Pagnani et al. (9) recommended use of a bone-cutting shaver to avoid this complication. Alternatively, one may use a standard arthroscopic burr on the reverse setting.

Rehabilitation

The postoperative regimen is similar to that described by Pagnani et al. (9) Patients remain in a sling for 3 to 4 weeks. During this time, the patients may remove the sling to perform elbow, wrist, and hand motion, as well as gentle pendulum exercises. Passive and active-assisted ROM begins at 3 to 4 weeks post-op and active ROM begins at 6 weeks. Strengthening begins at 10 weeks. The postoperative protocol is intentionally more conservative than that of a standard ASAD in order to minimize the risk of postoperative deltoid detachment. If concomitant rotator cuff repair is performed, standard postoperative protocols for rotator cuff repair are utilized.

Open Reduction and Internal Fixation

The primary advantage of ORIF is the potential to preserve the normal anatomy and biomechanics of the acromion and deltoid. However, nonunion occurs in a significant number of patients and symptomatic hardware is a common occurrence postoperatively. Outcomes after ORIF for os acromiale have been reported by numerous authors and have been somewhat inconsistent.

Warner et al. (8) performed ORIF and bone grafting in 11 patients (12 shoulders) with an os acromiale. Radiographic union was achieved in only 58% of shoulders. However, ORIF with cannulated screws appeared to be superior to simple tension banding with pins and wires. The rate of union after ORIF with cannulated screws and tension banding was 86% (6/7 shoulders); radiographic union after tension banding with pins and wires alone was only 20% (1/5 shoulders).

Hertel et al. (10) performed ORIF with tension band wiring in 12 patients (15 shoulders) with a symptomatic mesoacromiale. Two different surgical approaches were utilized: an anterior approach and a transacromial approach. When an anterior approach was used union was achieved in 43% (3/7 shoulders). In contrast, when a transacromial approach was used the rate of union was 88% (7/8 shoulders). The authors noted that an anterior approach may potentially devascularize the anterior fragment, as exposure of the anterior acromion entails detachment of the anterior deltoid and thus disruption of the acromial branch of the thoracoacromial artery. They concluded that a transacromial approach was superior to an anterior deltoid-detaching approach, presumably because it preserves the vascularity of the anterior acromion.

Peckett et al. (11) performed ORIF and bone grafting in 26 patients with an os acromiale. Radiographic union occurred in 96% of patients at an average of 4 months postoperatively. Satisfactory outcomes were achieved in 92% of patients. Hardware removal was required in 31% of patients.

Abboud et al. (4) performed ORIF in eight patients with a mesoacromiale. Radiographic union occurred in all eight patients. However, satisfactory clinical results were achieved in only 38% of patients. Ryu et al. (12) reported on four patients undergoing ORIF with cannulated screws and local bone graft. Union was achieved in all four patients.

We believe that ORIF is indicated in certain patients with an os acromiale. In all patients with a meta-acromiale, ORIF should be the standard of care. Excision of the fragment would compromise the anterior and lateral portions of the deltoid and may lead to significant postoperative morbidity. In patients with an unstable mesoacromiale, treatment options include either complete fragment excision or ORIF. In younger patients and those with higher functional demands, ORIF may be preferable. Assuming union is achieved, the normal anatomy and biomechanics of the acromion and deltoid will be preserved. This is attractive for patients who desire to maintain normal strength at and above shoulder level.

When performing ORIF, one may use either an anterior approach as described by Ryu et al. (12,13) or a transacromial approach as described by Hertel et al. (10). The nonunion site is identified and curetted until healthy

bleeding bone is encountered on both sides. Reduction is performed and provisional fixation is achieved with two parallel guide wires. Bone graft is then harvested from the greater tuberosity using a Craig needle and packed into the nonunion site. The two cannulated screws are inserted over the guide wires using a standard AO technique. Final screw tightening is performed only after packing the bone graft is complete. The stability of the construct is assessed after insertion of the cannulated screws. Although typically unnecessary, a figure-of-eight tension band wire may be passed through the cannulated screws if additional stability is desired.

Rehabilitation

Postoperatively patients are maintained in an external rotation brace for 6 weeks. During this time they may come out of the sling to work on elbow, wrist, and hand motion, as well as gentle pendulum exercises. Early passive ROM is initiated under the supervision of a physical therapist. Active ROM begins at 6 weeks post-op. Radiographs are obtained at the first post-op visit to assess reduction and fixation and then on a serial basis to assess the progression of radiographic healing (Fig. 7.7). The strengthening phase of physical therapy is not permitted until

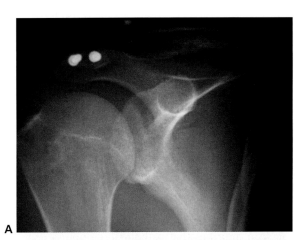

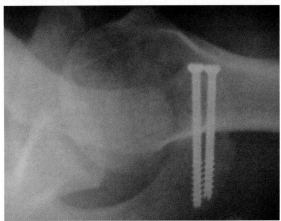

FIGURE 7.7. Postoperative radiographs after ORIF of an unstable mesoacromiale. **A:** AP view. **B:** Axillary view.

radiographic union is achieved, which typically occurs by 10 to 12 weeks.

AUTHORS' PREFERRED TREATMENT

Surgical treatment of an os acromiale is indicated when an appropriate course of conservative management has been attempted and has failed to provide significant symptomatic relief. For preacromial fragments, excision is usually the most appropriate procedure. It has little associated morbidity and will completely eliminate the pathologic lesion. One may consider ORIF for larger preacromial fragments, but this is rarely necessary. For a symptomatic meta-acromion, the fragment is too large to excise without causing significant dysfunction of the deltoid. Therefore, in lesions that are unstable, ORIF is the preferred treatment.

The mesoacromion is the most commonly encountered type of os acromiale. Although numerous authors have published outcomes after surgical treatment of mesoacromiale, most of these studies are case series. Currently, there are no controlled studies comparing these various treatment options. We believe that in order to determine which surgical option is most appropriate for each patient, it is first necessary to determine if the os is stable or unstable. This is based on the findings of the clinical examination and preoperative bone scan, as well as the intraoperative assessment of the stability of the fragment.

During the physical examination, assess tenderness to palpation directly at the site of the nonunion. Significant tenderness at the nonunion site signifies an unstable nonunion, resulting in painful motion between the anterior fragment and the remainder of the acromion. If significant tenderness is present, one may assume the nonunion is symptomatic and a bone scan may not be necessary. In patients without appreciable tenderness, we typically obtain a bone scan to assess any asymmetric increased uptake at the site of the os acromiale. Increased uptake on the bone scan indicates that pathologic motion is occurring at the nonunion site and the os is unstable. Finally, evaluate the stability of the anterior fragment intraoperatively. Through direct manual pressure on the superior aspect of the anterior fragment, significant motion may be appreciated if the fragment is grossly unstable. In larger patients, it may be difficult to assess stability in this manner. In this situation, one may also assess stability of the fragment by probing it with an arthroscopic instrument in the subacromial space.

Preferred Treatment Algorithm

Our preferred algorithm for the treatment of the symptomatic mesoacromiale is based on multiple factors, including the stability of the os acromiale (as defined above), presence of concomitant rotator cuff pathology, as well as patient age and activity level. As with any procedure, it is important to discuss the risks and benefits of each procedure with each patient and allow them to participate in the decision-making process.

Isolated Os Acromiale Without Rotator Cuff Tear

1. Os stable
   • Preferred treatment: arthroscopic acromioplasty

2. Os unstable
   a. Young patient or high-demand patient
      • Preferred treatment: ORIF with bone graft
   b. Older patient or sedentary patient
      • Preferred treatment: arthroscopic fragment excision

Os Acromiale in Patient Undergoing Concomitant Rotator Cuff Repair

1. Os stable
   a. Type 1 acromion
      • Preferred treatment: treat rotator cuff only; no treatment of os acromiale indicated
   b. Type 2 or type 3 acromion
      • Preferred treatment: arthroscopic acromioplasty

2. Os unstable
   c. Young patient or high-demand patient
      • Preferred treatment: ORIF with bone graft
   d. Older patient or sedentary patient
      • Preferred treatment: arthroscopic fragment excision

COMPLICATIONS

Complications after ASAD for an os acromiale are similar to those after standard ASAD. In addition to the standard risks of ASAD, one must also realize it is possible for an os that was stable preoperatively to become unstable and symptomatic postoperatively. Although the cause for this is not known with certainty, it may be due to the destabilizing effect of release of the CAL and/or AC joint capsule. The initial treatment for this should be conservative, consisting of NSAIDs, activity modification, and formal physical therapy. If conservative measures fail to provide symptomatic relief, revision surgery may be considered. If sufficient bone is present, ORIF may be attempted. However, in a patient who has had a prior acromioplasty, ORIF may not be a viable option if significant bone was resected. In this scenario, the procedure of choice would be complete arthroscopic fragment excision.

One of the potential complications of complete fragment excision is alteration of the deltoid insertion and lever arm. In some patients, this may result in clinical weakness with activities at and above shoulder level. Patients should be counseled on this risk as a part of the informed consent process, as there is not a good salvage procedure for this problem.

Potential complications after ORIF for an os acromiale include symptomatic hardware, loss of fixation, or persistent nonunion. For symptomatic hardware, removal of hardware is usually successful in providing symptomatic relief. This is only performed after radiographic union is achieved. For loss of fixation or persistent nonunion, the salvage procedure is fragment excision.

PEARLS AND PITFALLS

ASAD: The technique for ASAD for an os acromiale is similar to that of a standard ASAD, but may at times involve more bone resection than the typical acromioplasty. As with a standard ASAD, the goal is to remove an adequate amount of bone so that the anterior acromial undersurface does not impinge upon the rotator cuff.

During the exposure of the anterior acromion, all efforts should be made to preserve the integrity of the CAL. The ligament will need to be released from the undersurface of the anterior acromion in order to obtain adequate visualization. However, the ligament should remain in continuity and its attachment to the lateral margin of the acromion should be preserved if possible. An overly aggressive release of the CAL has the potential to compromise the stability of the anterior fragment. Disruption of the acromioclavicular joint should also be minimized if possible, as the distal clavicle and ligaments of the AC joint may impart some stability to the anterior fragment. Performing a complete distal clavicle excision, or even an aggressive coplaning, may potentially compromise the stability of the os acromiale.

During the preoperative visit, it is important to inform each patient that the arthroscopic assessment of the stability of the os will play a significant role in the final decision-making process. What was thought to be a stable os preoperatively may be found to be unstable intraoperatively after release of the CAL and/or AC joint capsule. In this situation, the surgeon should be prepared to convert from standard ASAD to complete fragment excision or ORIF intraoperatively, based on your preoperative discussions with the patient.

Complete fragment excision: The basic principles of arthroscopic excision of an os acromiale are similar to those of standard ASAD. The surgeon must be comfortable with arthroscopic visualization as well as manipulation of instruments from all three portals. It is essential to visualize the final resection from the posterior, lateral, and anterior portals, in order to ensure that the resection is complete. It is especially important to confirm that superior margin of the posterior aspect of the anterior fragment has been completely resected, as residual bone in this location may predispose to persistent symptoms postoperatively. It is difficult to assess this area from the posterior portal with a 30° arthroscope. Therefore, one must ensure that the resection is complete by directly visualizing this area with the arthroscope in the lateral or anterior portal (Figs. 7.8 and 7.9).

As compared with open fragment excision, the primary advantage of the arthroscopic approach is that disruption of the deltoid fascia is minimized. During the procedure, one should exercise caution when the resection reaches the level of the superior cortical plate. Excessive upward force has the potential to cause the burr to plunge through the bone, causing iatrogenic damage to the deltoid fascia. When resecting the superior cortex, using the burr on the reverse setting may help to minimize this risk. Another option is to use a bone-cutting shaver instead of a standard burr, as recommended by Pagnani et al. (9).

During the final portion of the case, it is not uncommon to notice small fragments of bone superiorly that appear to be embedded in the deltoid fascia. Ideally, all bone debris should be removed. However, aggressive attempts to remove these small final remnants of bone may have the potential to damage the deltoid fascia unnecessarily. There is probably minimal morbidity associated with leaving these minute fragments of bone behind if they cannot be safely resected.

Some patients may have symptomatic AC joint arthritis in addition to an unstable os acromiale. A mesoacromiale is typically located at the posterior margin of the AC joint. In these patients, excision of the os alone should be sufficient to treat both the symptoms caused by the os as well as the AC joint pathology. Distal clavicle excision is typically unnecessary, unless the location of the mesoacromiale is more anterior than usual.

ORIF with bone grafting: If a significant inferior spur is present in a patient with a thin acromion, it may be desirable to avoid formal acromioplasty in order to preserve enough bone to ensure the fixation will be adequate. During debridement of the nonunion site, resecting slightly more bone on the superior surface of the acromion will enable you to perform a dorsally based closing wedge osteotomy. This will make it possible to tilt the mobile fragment superiorly and effectively decompresses the subacromial space without formal acromioplasty.

From a biomechanical perspective, fixation with cannulated screws is a superior to tension banding with pins and wires alone. However, in some patients the acromion may be extremely thin and fixation with cannulated screws may not be possible. In this situation, simple tension band wiring may be the only available option. When tension band wiring is used as the sole method of fixation, we typically utilize a transacromial approach, as Hertel et al. (10) demonstrated that this resulted in superior rates of radiographic union as compared with a standard anterior deltoid detaching approach.

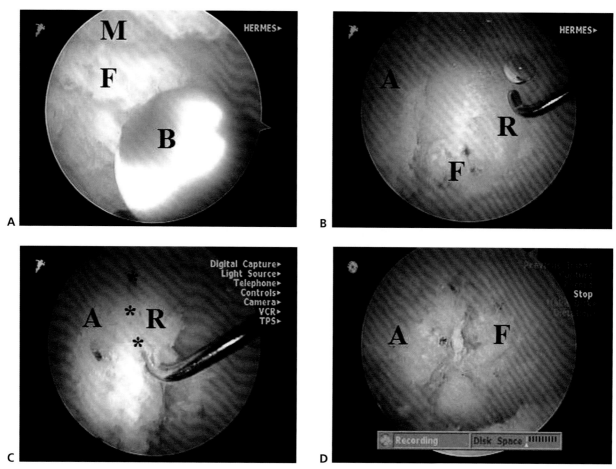

FIGURE 7.8. Arthroscopic excision of an os acromiale. **A:** Os being resected, arthroscope in posterior portal. **B:** View from lateral portal demonstrating residual superior bone. **C:** View from lateral portal demonstrating residual bone adjacent to site of nonunion. Probe is palpating residual mesoacromial bone. **D:** View from lateral portal showing final resection. Superior fascia is completely intact. A, acromion; B, burr; F, deltoid fascia; M, mesoacromion being resected; R, residual mesoacromial bone; *, site of nonunion.

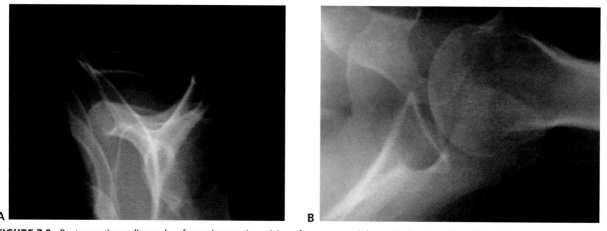

FIGURE 7.9. Postoperative radiographs after arthroscopic excision of an os acromiale. **A:** Outlet view. **B:** Axillary view.

CONCLUSIONS AND FUTURE DIRECTIONS

Os acromiale is an anatomic variant that will be commonly encountered by orthopedic surgeons, as it is present in approximately 6% to 8% of the population. Although it is probably an incidental radiographic finding in most patients, an os acromiale may be pathologic in some patients.

The initial treatment of a symptomatic os acromiale is typically nonoperative. When conservative measures fail to provide lasting symptomatic relief, surgery is often considered. Surgical options for a symptomatic os acromiale include standard acromioplasty, complete fragment excision, or ORIF.

Although numerous authors have reported outcomes after the surgical treatment of os acromiale, most of these studies are small case series. There are currently no controlled studies comparing these various treatment options. Further comparative studies with larger patient populations are needed in order to determine which surgical options provide the best long-term outcomes.

REFERENCES

1. Kurtz CA, Humble BJ, Rodosky MW, et al. Symptomatic os acromiale. *J Am Acad Orthop Surg.* 2006;14(1):12–19.
2. Ortiguera CJ, Buss DD. Surgical management of the symptomatic os acromiale. *J Shoulder Elbow Surg.* 2002;11(5):521–528.
3. Hutchinson MR, Veenstra MA. Arthroscopic decompression of shoulder impingement secondary to os acromiale. *Arthroscopy.* 1993;9(1):28–32.
4. Aboud JA, Silverberg D, Pepe M, et al. Surgical treatment of os acromiale with and without associated rotator cuff tears. *J Shoulder Elbow Surg.* 2006;15(3):265–270.
5. Armengol J, Brittis D, Pollock RG, et al. The association of an unfused acromial epiphysis with tears of the rotator cuff: a review of 42 cases. *Orthop Trans.* 1994;17:975–976.
6. Wright RW, Heller MA, Quick DC, et al. Arthroscopic decompression for impingement syndrome secondary to an unstable os acromiale. *Arthroscopy.* 2000;16(6):595–599.
7. Mudge MK, Wood VE, Frykman GK. Rotator cuff tears associated with os acromiale. *J Bone Joint Surg Am.* 1984;66(3):427–429.
8. Warner JJ, Beim GM, Higgins L. The treatment of symptomatic os acromiale. *J Bone Joint Surg Am.* 1998;80(9):1320–1326.
9. Pagnani MJ, Mathis CE, Solman CG. Painful os acromiale (or unfused acromial apophysis) in athletes. *J Shoulder Elbow Surg.* 2006;15(4):432–435.
10. Hertel R, Windisch W, Schuster A, et al. Transacromial approach to obtain fusion of unstable os acromiale. *J Shoulder Elbow Surg.* 1998;7(6):606–609.
11. Peckett WR, Gunther SB, Harper GD, et al. Internal fixation of symptomatic os acromiale: a series of twenty-six cases. *J Shoulder Elbow Surg.* 2004;13(4):381–385.
12. Ryu RK, Fan RS, Dunbar WH 5th. The treatment of symptomatic os acromiale. *Orthopedics.* 1999;22(3):325–328.
13. Ryu RK. Operative treatment of symptomatic os acromiale. In: Barber FA, Fischer SP, eds. *Surgical Techniques for the Shoulder and Elbow.* New York, NY: Thieme; 2003:42–45.

I. The Shoulder

Partial Rotator Cuff Tears: Treatment Options

William B. Stetson

Partial thickness tears of the rotator cuff may involve either the articular surface, bursal surface or both sides of the rotator cuff or can be intratendinous. They may be asymptomatic or a potential source of shoulder dysfunction. With the advent of magnetic resonance imaging (MRI) and shoulder arthroscopy, more tears are being recognized. However, the optimal clinical approach to these tears has not been completely defined (1). To gain a better understanding of these tears, we must first understand the anatomy, pathogenesis, and natural history of these tears and then agree on a classification system to develop a rational approach to their treatment.

ANATOMY

The suprascapular artery is the primary vascular supply to the supraspinatus tendon. The vascular studies of Rathbun and McNab have demonstrated the articular side of the rotator cuff is hypovascular as compared to the bursal side. This finding has been suggested as a factor in the tendency for partial tears to occur on the articular surface of the cuff (Fig. 8.1). Perfusion of the rotator cuff is a dynamic phenomenon with markedly reduced perfusion when the arm is in full adduction. Collagen bundles located near the articular surface of the cuff are thinner and

less uniform than the thick parallel bundles found closer to the bursal surface (Fig. 8.2). The articular surface of the cuff has an ultimate failing stress only half as high as the bursal surface. This lack of uniformity of the collagen bundles along with the hypovascularity of the articular surface of the cuff are contributing factors for partial tears to occur more commonly on the articular surface (1).

The anatomic footprint of the rotator cuff has been proposed as an important landmark for the insertional point of the supraspinatus tendon and for recognizing the degree of partial tearing of the articular surface of the rotator cuff. In a cadaveric study, Curtis studied the anatomic insertions of the rotator cuff musculature. He found the supraspinatus had a rectangular insertion from approximately the 11:30 position to the 1 o'clock position with an average length of 23 mm (range 18 to 33 mm) and a width of 16 mm (range 12 to 21 mm) (Fig. 8.3A, B). The infraspinatus wraps and interdigitates with the supraspinatus tendon. The infraspinatus frames the bare spot of

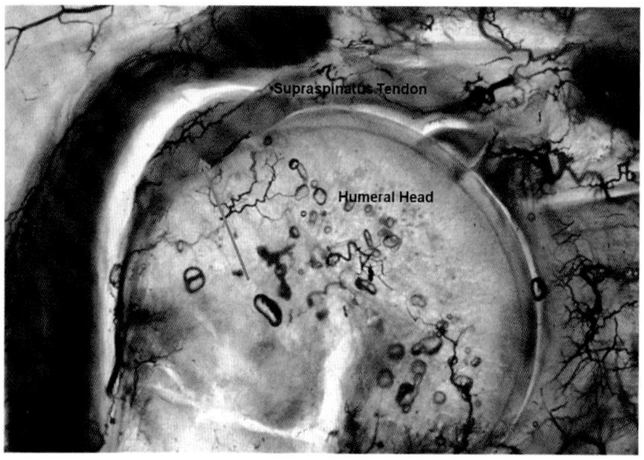

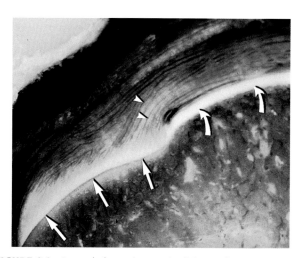

FIGURE 8.2. Coronal photomicrograph of the tendinous insertion of the supraspinatus tendon. The small arrowheads point to the thinner, less uniform collagen bundles of the articular side of the supraspinatus tendon. (From Seibold CJ, Mallisee TA, MD, Erickson SJ, et al. Rotator Cuff: Evaluation with US and MR Imaging. RadioGraphics May 1999, 19, 685-705. With permission)

FIGURE 8.1. Coronal photomicrograph of the zone of diminished vascularity of the supraspinatus tendon. The arrow points to the critical zone of hypovascularity of the articular side of the tendon.

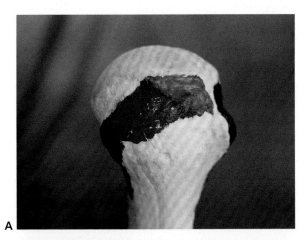

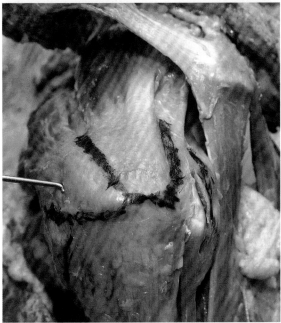

FIGURE 8.3. The insertional footprint of the supraspinatus *(green)* tendon is depicted in this model **(A)** and cadaver specimen **(B)**. It inserts approximately from the 11:30 position to 1:00 with an average length of 23 mm (range 18 to 33 mm) and a width of 17 mm (range 12 to 24 mm). (Reprinted with permission from the author, Alan Curtis.)

the humeral head, has an average length of 28 mm (range 20 to 45 mm) and a width of 18 mm (range 12 to 24 mm) (2). Nottage and his colleagues found the mean anteroposterior dimension of the supraspinatus tendon was 25 mm. The mean superior to inferior tendon thickness at the rotator interval was 11.6 mm, 12.1 mm at mid-tendon, and 12 mm at the posterior edge (3). Mochizuki and colleagues studied the humeral insertions of the supraspinatus and infraspinatus tendons in 113 cadaver shoulders. The footprint of the supraspinatus was triangular in shape with an average medial to lateral length of the tendon to be 6.9 mm (±1.4 mm). The average anterior to posterior width was 12.6 mm (±2.0 mm) on the medial margin and 1.3 mm (±1.4 mm) on the lateral margin. The infraspinatus had a long tendinous portion in the superior half of the

muscle, which curved anteriorly and extended to the anterolateral area of the highest impression of the greater tuberosity. The footprint of the infraspinatus was trapezoidal in shape with an average medial to lateral length of 10.2 mm and an average anterior–posterior width of 32.7 mm. They found that the footprint of the supraspinatus on the greater tuberosity was smaller than previously believed and that this area of the greater tuberosity is actually occupied by a substantial amount of the infraspinatus. The normal cuff is 9 to 12 mm thick but ranges from 9 to 22 mm of thickness.

PATHOGENESIS

The pathogenesis of partial rotator cuff tears are multifactorial and may be classified as intrinsic, extrinsic, traumatic or a combination of all of these. Intrinsic changes in the cuff are related to intrinsic tendinopathy with failure of collagen fibers within the cuff. This may be due to a lack of uniformity of the collagen bundles especially on the articular side causing partial tearing on the articular side. The lack of cuff vascularity also contributes to weakness of the cuff on the articular side leading to degenerative tears associated with the aging process. These degenerative tears are often associated with extensive delamination or can remain entirely intratendinous.

Histologic evidence supporting an intrinsic, degenerative cause of rotator cuff tears with aging by some researchers has shown a loss of cellularity, loss of vascularity, and loss of fibrocartilage mass at the site of the cuff insertion. Hashimoto and colleagues found seven characteristic features of age-related degeneration in tissue specimens which included thinning and disorientation of the collagen fibers, myxoid degeneration, and hyaline degeneration. Other degenerative changes included vascular proliferation, fatty infiltration, chondroid metaplasia and calcification. The authors felt that vascular proliferation was part of the reparative process. Histologic evidence from surgical specimens does not support a significant reparative process nor any significant inflammatory process. Although inflammation may play a role in the initiation of rotator cuff pathology, it appears not to play a role in the propagation and progression of the disease process. These specimens typically showed hypercellularity, a loss of tightly bundled collagen appearance, an increase in proteoglycan content, and neovascualization. This is felt to be a failed healing response. Therefore, the term tendinopathy may be more appropriate than tendonitis or tendinosis as a generic descriptor of the clinical condition seen in the shoulder.

Smooth muscle actin (SMA) has been found within the nonvascular connective tissue cells immediately surrounding torn rotator cuff edges. SMA in vitro leads to contraction of collagen-glysosaminoglycan compounds, substances found in considerable concentrations in the rotator cuff. In vivo, this may translate into SMA cells

I. The Shoulder

causing the damaged cuff to retract with the increasing distances at the repair margin, which results in an inhibition of healing.

The role of altered collagen fiber quality has also been proposed as an intrinsic mediator of cuff degeneration. The healthy central zone of the supraspinatus tendon is primarily composed of type I collagen with smaller amounts of type III collagen. The fibrocartilaginous zone of the tendon insertion against the humerus is primarily composed of type II collagen, a collagen subtype associated with withstanding compressive loads. In diseased rotator cuff there is an increase in the levels of type III collagen within the fibrocartilaginous zone, a collagen subtype associated with tendon healing and a decrease in type II collagen. The change in collagen composition could reduce the tendon's ability to withstand the compressive loads traditionally associated with type II collagen.

Extrinsic impingement due to narrowing of the supraspinatus outlet caused by coracoacromial arch abnormalities can result in cuff irritation and may play a major role in many partial cuff tears (1). Histologic changes have been found on the undersurface of cadaveric acromion specimens with bursal surface tears but not in those with articular surface tears. This suggests that bursal-surface tears may be more likely to be related to abrasion of the cuff by the acromion (1). Gartsman and Milne (4) believe that extrinsic impingement due to coracoacromial arch narrowing can lead to partial tears on the articular side as well as the bursal surface of the cuff. A differential shear stress affecting the layered anatomy of the cuff has been proposed as another mechanism involved in the production of articular surface tears (1).

Walch et al. (5) and Jobe have described a subset of partial articular-sided rotator cuff tears that develop secondary to "internal impingement." Glenohumeral instability and traction stress on the rotator cuff in the throwing athlete can lead to undersurface tears in the absence of extrinsic impingement. In addition, throwers and other overhand athletes may experience posterior shoulder pain when repetitive contact occurs between the undersurface of the supraspinatus and the posterosuperior glenoid during the late cocking phase of the throwing motion. Fatigue of the dynamic stabilizers and excessive external rotation secondary to overstretching of the anterior capsule may predispose individuals to development of internal impingement (1). A subset of these patients may develop a glenohumeral internal rotation deficit (GIRD) with a significant loss of internal rotation on the affected side.

Trauma is more often associated with articular surface tears than with bursal surface tears (6). This may be due to a direct fall on the shoulder or to repetitive microtrauma seen in laborers or athletes with repetitive overhead activities. Repetitive stresses may lead to small injuries within the tendon that are given an insufficient time to heal before further trauma. The combination of weaker cuffs with

a single traumatic insult, or progressive microtrauma can then lead to cuff tearing. This is consistent with the early studies of Codman that demonstrated that partial cuff tears typically began on the articular side of the tendon, because the load capacity of the bursal side is higher than that of the articular side, making the articular side more prone to damage. Typically, after the deep fibers tear, they retract because they remain under tension even with the arm at rest. This results in an increased load on the remaining fibers that increases the likelihood of further rupture.

Repetitive trauma and chronic overuse have been studied in the rat model and angiogenic and inflammatory markers have been identified and support the hypothesis that both of these play an important role in tendon degeneration. Substance P, a proinflammatory mediator, has been found to be increased in rotator cuff tendinopathy. Acute increases in angiogenic messenger ribonucleic acid (mRNA) markers for vascular endothelial growth factor (VEGF) have been found in the cuff of rats undergoing repetitive microtrauma injuries. Overuse also leads to a progressive down regulation of transforming growth factor beta-1 (TGF-β1), altering the normal collagen constituents within the rat supraspinatus tendon and leading to a lower load to failure with respect to controls. Overload not only affects the collagen and proteoglycans but also elicits an essential response in tenocytes that appears designed to adapt the collagen matrix to increased load. Matrix load is transmitted into the cell and alters protein and enzyme production and can actually cause nucleus deformation. Clearly, this is one of the most intriguing and dynamic fields of research.

The current human in vivo evidence base for a strong inflammatory component remains relatively weak as histologic studies have failed to find a significant chronic inflammatory environment in rotator cuff tears and other tendinopathies in cadaveric and postsurgical specimens.

In summary, degeneration and partial tearing of the rotator cuff tendon is multifaceted. A combination of growth factors and neurotransmitters affects the tenocytes, their nuclei and the collagen infrastructure of the rotator cuff tendon. On a histologic level, degeneration is characterized by loss of cellularity, vascularity, tissue architecture, and fibrocartilaginous mass within the cuff tendon resulting in a mechanically inferior tendon. This is then compounded by repetitive microtrauma—mechanical loading of a degenerative tendon leading to several small tears that only partially heal until the tendon is so weakened that a full-thickness tear develops.

NATURAL HISTORY

The natural history and progression of these partial rotator cuff tears is a controversial topic. Codman first described changes in the musculotendinous cuff as a rim rent (partial tear) in the undersurface of the supraspinatus tendon at the point of attachment near the articular surface of the humeral head (7). We do know that partial tears of the articular surface are two to three times more common than bursal surface tears (8, 9). Most tears involve the supraspinatus tendon with the infraspinatus, subscapularis, and teres minor tendons much less commonly involved (4). Intratendinous tears are intrasubstance and therefore have no communication with either surface (10). As anticipated, cadaveric studies have demonstrated a higher incidence of intratendinous tears than that reported in clinical studies since inspection is limited to the tendon surfaces (11). MRI techniques have improved our ability to detect intrasubstance tears and tendon degeneration.

Fukuda et al. (11) reported a 13% incidence of partial rotator cuff tears in a cadaveric study of 249 anatomic specimens. The prevalence of these partial thickness tears increases with age. DePalma studied 96 shoulders of patients aged 18 to 74 years without a history of shoulder dysfunction and found partial ruptures of the supraspinatus tendon in 37%.

Sher and colleagues (12) in an MRI study of 96 asymptomatic individuals, found a high incidence of partial rotator cuff tears. They were increasingly frequent with advancing age and were compatible with normal, painless, functional activity.

In 1934, Codman (7) described four categories of incomplete rupture of the rotator cuff. He suggested that spontaneous healing of partial thickness rotator cuff tears might occur. In 1996, Fukuda et al. (10) examined histologic sections of partial thickness rotator cuff tears and found no evidence of active tissue repair. The question of whether or not these partial tears heal or progress is controversial. However, second look arthroscopies of patients with documented partial rotator cuff tears have demonstrated no evidence of healing (4, 9). Yamanaka studied 40 patients with symptomatic articular-sided partial rotator cuff tears treated nonoperatively with serial arthrography. At a mean follow-up of 13.5 months, repeat arthrography showed that four tears (10%) had disappeared and were presumed to have healed, reduction of the size of the tear occurred in 4 patients (10%), but enlargement of tear size occurred in 79% with 21(51%) of the partial tears increasing in size, and 11 (28%) progressed to a full thickness tear. Mazoue and Andrews followed 11 baseball pitchers who had arthroscopic debridement of partial rotator cuff tears but were unable to return to pitching. At the time of repeat arthroscopy, 9 progressed to a full thickness tear. With repetitive microtrauma seen in overhead athletes such as pitchers, the risk of progression to a full thickness tear can be as high as 81% (13).

The prognosis of articular-sided tears appears to be worse with increasing age, a larger initial tear size, and the absence of a traumatic episode. The patients in Yamanaka's study in whom follow-up arthrography showed a disappearance of the tear often had a history of trauma. Conversely, a history of trauma was seldom noted in those with progressive tear enlargement, resulting in a full thickness tear. Therefore, the risk of progression of partial thickness tears to a full thickness tear is significant and ranges from 28% to 81% (13).

A recent MRI study published in 2009 of partial thickness rotator cuff tears treated nonoperatively showed a progression of the tear in only 17%. However, this may be explained by the use of different diagnostic techniques of arthrography in Yamanaka's study compared with MRI in this recent study by Maman. Future studies using magnetic resonance arthrography (MRA) may be helpful in explaining this discrepancy as MRA has been found more sensitive in detecting partial articular-sided rotator cuff tears (14).

The role of operative treatment in modifying the natural history of partial thickness rotator cuff tears is poorly defined (1). Although Codman felt debridement of partial tears stimulated a healing response (7), there is no evidence that debridement of a partially torn cuff stimulates a healing response (4,9) in second look arthroscopies. The role of subacromial decompression and its ability to reduce narrowing of the subacromial outlet in those with external impingement has been proposed to delay the progression of cuff pathology but has never been proven in prospective, clinical studies.

The question of which partial tears may progress and why still needs to be clearly defined. At this point, it appears prudent to follow patients clinically and monitor their symptoms. If their symptoms progress or do not resolve after being treated with proper nonoperative means, the partial tear may be a cause of their symptoms or the tear may be progressing in size and may need to be addressed surgically. Overhead athletes may be more prone to progression of their partial thickness tears to complete tears because of the repetitive stresses placed on the rotator cuff (13).

CLINICAL EVALUATION

Pertinent History and Physical Examination

The prevalence of partial tears of the rotator cuff in asymptomatic individuals was studied by Sher et al. in 1995 (12). Magnetic resonance images of the shoulders of 96 asymptomatic individuals found 19 partial thickness tears (20%). It is evident from this study that partial tears may be asymptomatic and must be evaluated on a case-by-case basis to determine if the partial tear is truly causing symptoms.

It is important to take a detailed history of the patient starting with the duration of symptoms and the mechanism of injury. Patients may present with an insidious onset of shoulder pain without any discrete injury or accident. They may also have a history of trauma or repetitive stress to the shoulder as seen with overhead athletes. Pain is the predominant symptom, often most troubling at night and with overhead activities (11). Their symptoms may be nonspecific and may overlap with impingement, rotator cuff tendonitis or tendinopathy, and small, full thickness rotator cuff tears (15). Most patients have a painful arc of motion between 60° and 120° of elevation (6). They may also have loss of motion (10) with posterior capsular tightness and a resultant restriction of internal rotation (4). This may cause anterosuperior translation of the humeral head from a posterior capsular contracture and may potentiate impingement-like symptoms (1).

The impingement signs described by Neer (pain with forced passive forward elevation) and Hawkins (pain with passive internal rotation of the arm placed in 90° of abduction) are positive in nearly all patients with symptomatic partial thickness rotator cuff tears (4). Differentiating between impingement alone and impingement with a partial rotator cuff tear can be very difficult. It is at times difficult to determine what is causing the pain. Is it more the impingement or is the pain caused more by the partial rotator cuff tear? The lidocaine test, an injection of 10 cc of 1% lidocaine into the subacromial space, can be helpful. After the injection, the maneuvers may be repeated and diminution of pain on repeat testing may be indicative of pure impingement (1).

Strength is usually preserved on clinical examination. However, pain inhibition may result in an apparent loss of strength and a decrease in active range of motion in these patients with a partially torn rotator cuff (1). Patients may also have pain with active resistance to shoulder abduction with the shoulder positioned in 90° of abduction in the scapular plane (Jobe test).

Throwing athletes with partial thickness rotator cuff tears may also have nonspecific posterior shoulder pain, indicative of "internal impingement." They may develop a GIRD or contracture with an obligate increase in external rotation (5). Impingement of the deep surface of the supraspinatus tendon may occur as the cuff abrades against the posterosuperior glenoid rim (5). It is a matter of debate whether or not rotator cuff injuries observed in individuals with internal impingement develop as a result of pathologic anterior glenohumeral subluxation or repetitive cuff abrasion in an otherwise stable shoulder (1). Posterosuperior labral lesions (SLAP variants) may also be present in throwing athletes and predispose to articular surface partial thickness rotator cuff tears (5).

The clinical course of patients with partial thickness rotator cuff tears is often indistinguishable from that of patients with impingement syndrome, tendonitis or tendinopathy, or small, full thickness rotator cuff tears. Symptoms may also be difficult to differentiate from bicipital tendonitis, labral or SLAP lesions, and mild cases of adhesive capsulitis (1). These associated conditions may also be present in addition to rotator cuff pathology creating a confusing clinical presentation.

Imaging

Imaging techniques to detect partial thickness rotator cuff tears have improved over the last 10 years. With the advent of MRA and newer fat suppression techniques, sensitivity has increased in detecting partial tears.

Radiographic evaluation is the first imaging tool used when evaluating shoulder pathology. Initial X-rays include an anteroposterior view of the glenohumeral joint, an axillary view, and a supraspinatus outlet view. The supraspinatus outlet view is especially important because it not only demonstrates acromial morphology (types I to III), but it also ascertains the thickness of the acromion which is important in preoperative planning for an arthroscopic subacromial decompression. In general, radiographic findings are nonspecific for partial thickness tears but may be helpful in ruling out other causes of shoulder pain (1).

Arthrography of the glenohumeral joint is limited for detecting partial tears. Although proponents have reported an accuracy of >80% (6), other authors have been unable to duplicate these results (4, 5).

Bursography may be performed as an adjunct to arthrography to aid in the detection of partial thickness tears involving the bursal surface. However, subacromial inflammation and adhesive capsulitis may limit the value of this technique (1). The accuracy of bursography has been reported to range from 25% to 67% (6, 10, 11). However, a negative arthrogram or bursogram cannot reliably rule out the presence of a partial thickness rotator cuff tear (15).

Ultrasound may be of limited value in detecting partial thickness tears. Weiner and Seitz reported a sensitivity of 94% and a specificity of 93% in a series of 69 partial thickness rotator cuff tears. However, its clinical use is limited by the availability of personnel experienced in the performance and interpretation of the study and its limitations in diagnosing other concomitant pathology. In comparing preoperative ultrasound to MRI in arthroscopically confirmed partial-thickness rotator cuff tears, Teefey found that 13 of 19 tears were correctly identified by ultrasound, whereas 12 of 19 tears were correctly identified by MRI. Iannotti found the preoperative diagnostic accuracy of ultrasound to be 70% and MRI to be 73%.

MRI, although a useful and established technique for detecting full thickness rotator cuff tears, has been found to be less reliable in detecting partial tears. Newer techniques have been developed to increase sensitivity. Using a T1-weighted image, a diagnosis of a partial tear is suggested by increased signal in the rotator cuff without evidence of tendon discontinuity. Further increase in signal changes on a T2-weighted with a focal defect can suggest an intratendinous tear (Fig. 8.4A, B, C). Signal changes on the bursal side can be indicative of a bursal-sided tear, which can be accentuated by fluid within the subacromial space (Fig. 8.5). Signal changes on a T2-weighted image can also show an articular surface tear (Fig. 8.6). Rotator cuff tendonitis or tendinopathy may be distinguished from partial thickness tears by an increased signal on T1 images but a decreased signal on T2 (Fig. 8.7A, B). However, many cases of tendinopathy may actually be partial thickness rotator cuff tears (15).

Standard magnetic resonance techniques are relatively insensitive in the detection of partial thickness

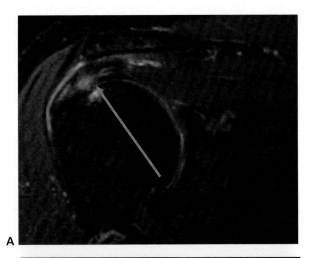

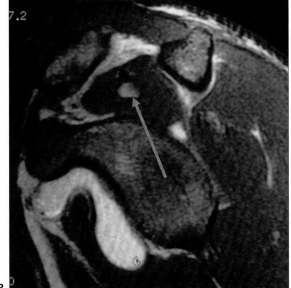

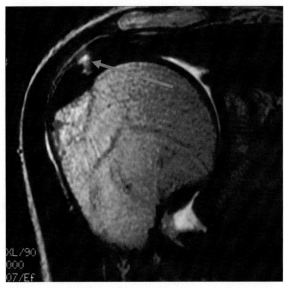

FIGURE 8.5. Coronal oblique T1 image of a partial, bursal-sided supraspinatus tendon tear. Note the signal changes within the supraspinatus tendon near its insertion *(blue arrow).*

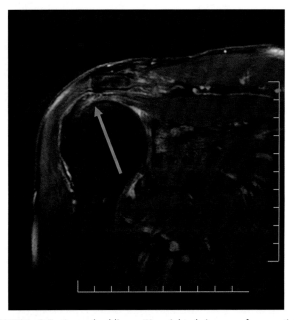

FIGURE 8.6. Coronal oblique T2-weighted image of a partial, articular-sided tear of the supraspinatus tendon *(blue arrow).*

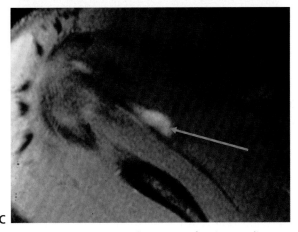

FIGURE 8.4. A: Oblique coronal MRI view of an intratendinous tear of the supraspinatus tendon *(blue arrow).* **B:** Sagittal view of an intratendinous tear of the supraspinatus *(blue arrow).* **C:** Axillary view of an intratendinous tear of the supraspinatus *(blue arrow).*

tears. In 1992, Traughber and Goodwin reported a sensitivity of 56% to 72% and a specificity of 83% to 85% for arthroscopically proven partial thickness cuff tears.

Other studies such as that by Hodler and Snyder in 1992 have reported an 83% rate of false negative results with arthroscopically proven partial tears. Wright and Cofield found only six definite partial tears on preoperative MRI studies in 18 patients with arthroscopically proven partial tears.

Fat suppression techniques accentuate fluid signal contrast on T2-weighted images and have been suggested as a means of increasing detection of partial thickness tears. Clinical results have varied using this technique (Fig. 8.8A, B). Quinn et al. found a sensitivity of 82% and a specificity of 99% in 11 arthroscopically proven partial

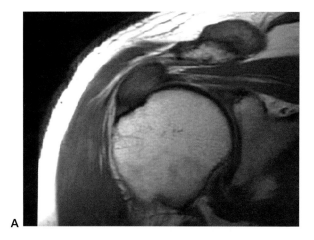

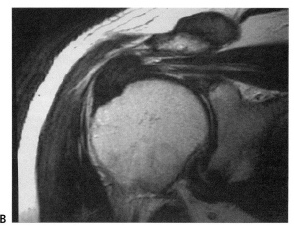

FIGURE 8.7. A and B: Coronal oblique MR images of signal changes within the supraspinatus tendon characteristic of rotator cuff tendonitis or tendinopathy.

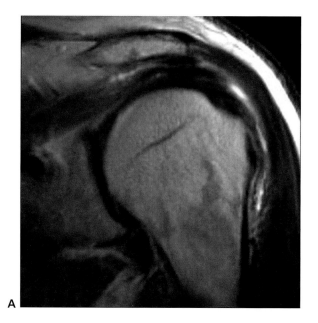

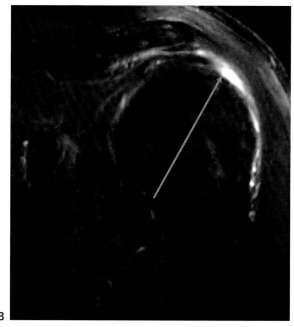

FIGURE 8.8. A: Coronal oblique view using a T1 technique. **B:** Fat suppression T2 technique accentuates fluid signal contrasts in partial thickness tears *(blue arrow)*.

tears using fat suppression techniques. Reimus and colleagues, however, increased the sensitivity only from 15% to 35% using this technique.

MRA improves sensitivity in detecting partial thickness cuff tears but early studies found a high false-negative rate. In 1992, Hodler and Snyder found that intraarticular gadolinium improved sensitivity, but that 5 of 13 tears found at the time of arthroscopy were missed by MR arthrogram. Lee et al. examined MR arthrograms in a retrospective study of 16 patients who underwent shoulder arthroscopy. Standard MR arthrogram oblique coronal images detected only 5 partial tears (21%). Using the ABER (abduction and external rotation) view increased the accuracy to 100% for detecting partial articular-sided tears.

In a recent prospective study of 50 patients, we found that MRA had 91% sensitivity with only a 9% false negative rate for partial articular-sided rotator cuff tear, which were verified arthroscopically (14). At this time, it seems prudent to use intraarticular gadolinium if the diagnosis is uncertain or one is suspicious of a partial thickness rotator cuff tear (Fig. 8.9A, B). The ABER position is not routinely used and has not been necessary when intra-articular gadolinium is used.

The occurrence of abnormal MRI signal changes in asymptomatic individuals makes it important to fully evaluate the patient including a thorough history and physical examination before concluding that the MRI findings are the cause of the patient's complaints. In a prospective, randomized study of 96 asymptomatic individuals, magnetic resonance images of the shoulder were evaluated to determine the prevalence of findings consistent with a tear of the rotator cuff. There were 14 full thickness tears (15%) and 19 partial thickness tears (20%). The frequency of each type of tear increased with age. In those >60 years of age, 26% had a partial thickness tear, all of which were

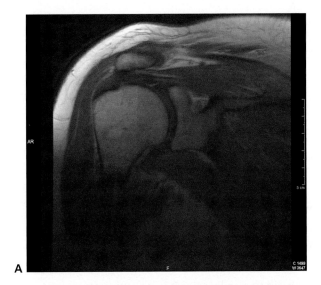

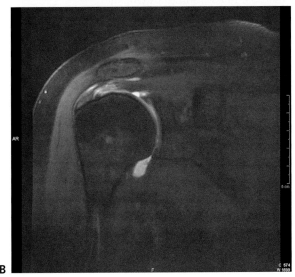

FIGURE 8.9. A: Coronal oblique T1 image showing a normal rotator cuff. **B:** T2 image with intraarticular gadolinium showing a partial, undersurface tear of the supraspinatus tendon.

asymptomatic. The results of the study emphasize the potential hazards of the use of MRI scans alone as a basis for the determination of operative intervention in the absence of associated clinical findings (12).

Classification

At present, there is no widely accepted classification system for partial thickness rotator cuff tears. This makes it difficult to compare studies because partial tears can vary widely in size and involve the articular, bursal or both sides of the rotator cuff tendon (14). Neer first described three stages of rotator cuff disease looking at histologic specimens of the rotator cuff. Stage I is characterized by hemorrhage and cuff edema, stage II by cuff fibrosis, and stage III by a cuff tear. However, this system has significant limitations clinically and does not address partial thickness tears.

Ellman recognized the difficulty in using Neer's classification system and proposed a classification for partial thickness rotator cuff tears. For partial thickness tears, grade I is <3 mm deep, grade II is 3 to 6 mm deep, and grade III tears are >6 mm deep. He also recognized that partial tears could occur on the articular side, bursal side, or be interstitial. He felt that grade III tears involving >50% of the tendon should be repaired (assuming an average cuff thickness of 9 to 12 mm) (8).

Many authors have recommended a simple system of grading tears based on whether or not the tear depth exceeds 50% of the cuff thickness (2, 3, 16). If one assumes that the average cuff is approximately 12 mm in size, it is possible to grade the percentage of tearing. Using the supraspinatus footprint as a guide, if >6 mm of the footprint is exposed, a >50% tear of the supraspinatus insertion (2, 3) has occurred (Fig. 8.10A, B). However, the cuff may range from 9 to 22 mm in thickness (2), which makes this classification system not always reliable. At a recent international shoulder conference, three case presentations with arthroscopic video clips were presented and the audience of over 400 participants was asked

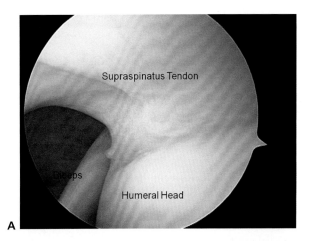

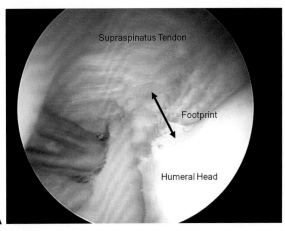

FIGURE 8.10. A: The normal footprint of the supraspinatus tendon. **B:** A partial tear of the supraspinatus footprint. The tear can be graded from the distance of the intact supraspinatus fibers to the articular surface. (Reprinted by permission from Alan Curtis.)

Table 8.1

Snyder classification of partial rotator cuff tears (17)

Location of Tears

A   Articular surface
B   Bursal surface

Severity of Tear

0   Normal cuff, with smooth coverings of synovium and bursa
I   Minimal, superficial bursal or synovial irritation or slight capsular fraying in a small, localized area; usually <1 cm
II   Actually fraying and failure of some rotator cuff fibers in addition to synovial, bursal, or capsular injury; usually <2 cm
III   More severe rotator cuff injury, including fraying and fragmentation of tendon fibers, often involving the whole surface of a cuff tendon (most often the supraspinatus); usually <3 cm
IV   Very severe partial rotator tear that usually contains, in addition to fraying and fragmentation of tendon tissue, a sizable flap tear, and often encompasses more than a single tendon

whether the tears involved greater or less than 50% of the tendon. In each case, there was only 67% agreement as to the degree of tearing. Clearly, a better classification system is needed.

Snyder and coworkers proposed a comprehensive classification system for both partial and complete tears (17). At the time of a complete 15-point glenohumeral diagnostic shoulder arthroscopy, the articular side of the rotator cuff is fully evaluated. The degree of tearing is graded from 0 to IV with 0 being normal and IV being a significant partial tear >3 cm in size (Table 8.1). A designation of IV implies that the partial tear is very severe, having tendon damage over a large area, with fragmentation and often flap formation. For all practical purposes, a grade IV tear is tantamount to a full thickness lesion even though there are a few remaining fibers (Fig. 8.11) (17).

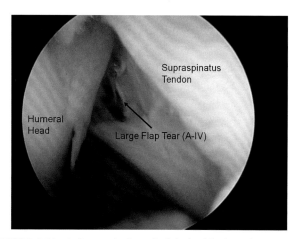

FIGURE 8.11. Arthroscopic view of a left shoulder from the posterior portal looking anteriorly of a partial articular-sided rotator cuff tear with fraying and a large flap component (Snyder grade A-IV).

Localizing and classifying both the articular and bursal sides of the partial rotator cuff tear is important not only for decision making in determining treatment but also in describing partial tears with a system that can be reproduced. Viewing from the posterior portal and looking anteriorly within the glenohumeral joint, a marker suture is placed using the technique described by Snyder and co-workers (17). An 18-gauge spinal needle is placed percutaneously through the partial articular-sided tear. An absorbable suture (no. 1 PDS) is then placed via the spinal needle into the glenohumeral joint (Fig. 8.12A). The spinal needle is then removed leaving the suture through the partial rotator cuff tear. The bursal side of the tear can be easily located during the bursal exam by locating the marker suture (Fig. 8.12B). The bursal side of the cuff is then inspected and is graded in a similar fashion as the articular side. For example, an A-IV, B-I type of partial tear has partial tearing >3 cm on the articular side of the cuff (Fig. 8.13A) and tearing on the bursal side of <1 cm (Fig. 8.13B). An A-I, B-III partial tear has mild fraying <1 cm on the articular side with <3 cm of partial tearing on the bursal side.

We performed a prospective, randomized study of 27 orthopedic surgeons at the AAOS annual meeting in Chicago in 2006 to test the reproducibility of the Snyder classification system. They were shown 10 case studies of arthroscopic shoulder video clips and then asked to classify the partial rotator cuff tears using the Snyder classification system. The interobserver reliability demonstrated a Kappa coefficient of 0.512 making the reliability of this classification system for partial rotator cuff tears to be strongly statistically significant.

To date, other clinical studies validating any classification system are lacking. In the meantime, one must be careful when interpreting studies that fail to quantify

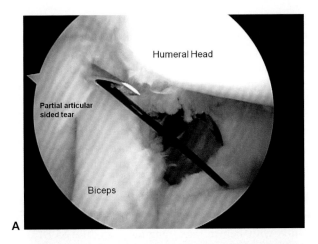

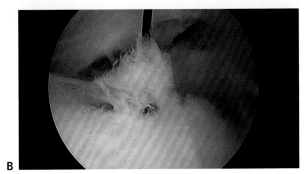

FIGURE 8.12. A: Viewing from the posterior portal anteriorly in a right shoulder, a marker suture is placed through a partial articular-sided rotator cuff tear using an 18-gauge spinal needle. **B:** The bursal side of the tear is easily located with the aid of the marker suture.

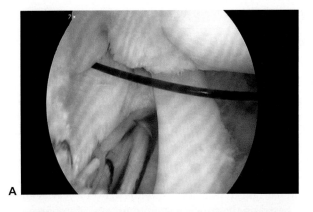

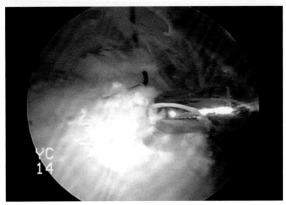

FIGURE 8.13. A: Viewing from the posterior portal anteriorly, a spinal needle is placed in an A-IV partial tear of the articluar side. **B:** On the bursal side, the maker suture is localized, a B-I type of partial tear on the bursal side of <1 cm is seen.

partial rotator cuff tears and also fail to mention whether or not the tears occurred on the articular side, bursal side, or both.

NONOPERATIVE TREATMENT

There is no simple treatment algorithm for partial thickness rotator cuff tears (1). Treatment of the symptomatic shoulder with a partial tear is directed toward correcting the primary diagnosis, such as impingement, or treating underlying instability which is secondarily producing the partial tear. As we know from the work of Sher and colleagues, not all partial tears are symptomatic (12). Therefore, it is reasonable to direct the initial nonoperative treatment toward the primary diagnosis.

Individuals with a suspected partial tear due to extrinsic impingement or intrinsic tendinopathy are treated in a similar fashion as those with an impingement syndrome. Subacromial bursal inflammation is controlled with activity modification, nonsteroidal anti-inflammatory medication, and the judicious use of injectable corticosteroids. Although recent reports by Alvarez published in 2005 have questioned the efficacy of corticosteroid injections, it is still considered a useful tool in reducing pain and inflammation in the

subacromial space. Rehabilitation to restore normal joint mechanics and strengthen the rotator cuff and parascapular musculature has been proposed to reduce the progression of rotator cuff disease in those with both external and internal impingement. The role of the external rotators that act as humeral head depressors may play a role in reducing external impingement thus reducing further mechanical impingement of the cuff from the coracoacromial arch. Rehabilitation of the parascapular musculature may serve to restore normal scapulothoracic mechanics and minimize impingement secondary to scapulothoracic dyskinesis (1). In those with "internal impingement" and those with underlying instability, restoring normal range of motion, stretching the posterior capsule, and reducing internal rotation contractures (so-called GIRD), may prevent pathologic contact between the supraspinatus and the superior labrum, especially in the overhead athlete.

There are very few studies that analyze the clinical outcome of the conservative treatment of partial rotator cuff tears. Although there is no hard and fast rule as to how long conservative measures should be used before surgical intervention is performed, it is reasonable to continue nonoperative treatment for a minimum of 3 months or until symptoms do not improve.

OPERATIVE TREATMENT

Operative Indications

The timing of surgical intervention when conservative treatment fails is controversial. Surgical intervention is considered for patients whose symptoms do not improve with conservative management and are of sufficient duration and intensity. A minimum of 3 months to as long as 6 months of nonoperative treatment has been recommended before considering surgical intervention. However, the literature is unclear as to the timing of surgery and has ranged from a few months to over a year. It should be based on the patient's symptoms, rate of improvement, as well as the goals of each individual patient.

The underlying cause of the tear must be clarified. For example, debridement of a partial articular-sided tear in an overhead athlete with instability has been associated with a high-failure rate. Jobe and Kvitne recommended treatment of the underlying shoulder instability at the time of surgery, particularly in overhead athletes.

The surgical treatment of partial thickness rotator cuff tears is also controversial. The lack of uniformity in describing rotator cuff tears and an acceptable classification system has made it difficult to compare study results. Surgical treatment options include tear debridement, acromioplasty with tear debridement, and arthroscopic or mini-open rotator cuff repair with or without acromioplasty. Surgery may be performed open, arthroscopically assisted, or entirely as an arthroscopic procedure.

Diagnostic Arthroscopy

A complete 15-point arthroscopic diagnostic examination of the glenohumeral joint should be done initially not only to evaluate the articular side of the rotator cuff but also to diagnose and to treat labral lesions and other glenohumeral pathology (17). The diagnosis of partial thickness tears is often not made with certainty until the rotator cuff is examined arthroscopically (1). Partial tears have been found unexpectedly in as many as 15% to 35% of patients undergoing arthroscopic treatment for impingement syndrome (11). A marker suture (no. 1 PDS, an absorbable monofilament) may be placed through an 18-gauge spinal needle laterally off the edge of the acromion into the partial tear as previously described. The needle is then removed leaving the suture in place. The subacromial space is then entered, the marker suture localized, and the extent of any bursal tearing determined. After debridement of hypertrophic bursal tissue, the area surrounding the marker suture is carefully inspected. Complete visualization of the cuff is done by internally and externally rotating the arm. After debridement of any damaged bursal rotator cuff fibers with a full radius shaver, the extent of the tear can be better assessed.

Arthroscopy affords no substantial advantage in the evaluation and treatment of intratendinous tears as these typically cannot be identified arthroscopically (1).

Preoperative tests such as MRI most often show significant signal changes within the supraspinatus tendon, but at the time of diagnostic arthroscopy, no tear can be identified. Tissue appearance and palpation with the tip of the shaver may help to identify these lesions. In 2002, Lo, Gonzalez, and Burkhart described "The Bubble Sign" as an arthroscopic indicator of an intratendinous rotator cuff tear. This is a bulging expansion of the rotator cuff tendon following injection of saline into the suspected lesion. This is an interesting technique, which requires further investigation.

Arthroscopic Debridement

Arthroscopic debridement of partial tears has led to mixed results with failure rates ranging from 14% to 81% (5). Many of the studies are limited by their description of the tears and the length of follow-up. In 1985, Andrews, Broussard, and Carson reported that debridement alone in 34 patients led to 85% satisfactory results with an average of only 13 months of follow-up. The average age was 22 years old and most were competitive overhead athletes. However, the question of whether these patients actually had underlying instability, the degree of tearing and whether the partial tear was really the cause of the patient's symptoms is a matter of debate. This study was published in 1985 and our understanding of glenohumeral instability has improved considerably.

In 1991, Snyder proposed arthroscopic debridement of partial rotator cuff tears and reported 84% satisfactory results in a mixed series of articular and bursal-sided tears with an average follow-up of 23 months. However, over one half of the patients had a subacromial decompression performed at the same time. In 9 of 31 cases, the bursal side of the cuff was not inspected. This paper was one of the first to describe a classification system reflecting the size of both articular and bursal-sided tears and found no correlation between the grade of the tear and the result.

In 2005, Budoff and colleagues reported 79% good or excellent results in a retrospective review of 62 shoulders in 60 patients treated with debridement with an average follow-up of 9.5 years. However, only 39% were available for physical examination, and the remainder were interviewed by telephone. Only 58% were able to return to recreational activities without difficulty. Fifty-eight percent had no pain while the remainder had mild (19%), moderate (8%), or severe pain (15%).

Other authors have reported less satisfactory results with debridement alone. In 1986, Ogilvie-Harris and Wiley reported on 57 patients treated with arthroscopic debridement without subacromial decompression who had a 50% failure rate. The average follow-up was only 1 year and no exact description of the tears was given making it hard to compare this study with others. In 1992, Walch (5) also reported poor results with arthroscopic debridement of partial tears secondary to "internal impingement," emphasizing the importance of treating the underlying cause of the tear.

In 2006, Mazoué and Andrews reported on 11 over-head athletes (baseball pitchers) who had arthroscopic debridement of partial thickness rotator cuff tears. Nine of 11 progressed to full thickness rotator cuff tears over 20.6 months (range of follow-up 9 to 69 months) (13). Although the size and classification of these partial thickness rotator cuff tears is hard to determine from the manuscript, it raises the question of whether debriding partial tears especially in overhead athletes is effective treatment.

Arthroscopic Debridement with Subacromial Decompression

Arthroscopic subacromial decompression with arthroscopic debridement of partial tears has also led to mixed results with failure rates ranging from 15% to 35%. (9) The studies are again limited by the tear description and length of follow-up. In 1990, Ellman reported on 20 patients with partial tears involving the articular surface (12 patients), the bursal surface (7 patients), or both sides of the tendon (1 patient). With a short follow-up period, which was not documented, he reported a 20% failure rate (5 patients) (8). Esch reported on 34 patients with a partial rotator cuff tear treated with debridement and subacromial decompression and had a 24% failure rate with an average follow-up of 19 months. No mention is made of bursal or articular-sided tears.

In 1992, Ryu reported on 35 patients treated with an arthroscopic subacromial decompression and debridement with a follow-up of 23 months and had 86% good results. Bursal-sided tears had more favorable results while only one of four articular-sided tears had a good result.

In 1990, Gartsman reported on 40 patients with partial rotator cuff tears treated with arthroscopic debridement and arthroscopic subacromial decompression. There were 32 tears of the supraspinatus tendon on the articular side, four on the bursal side, four tears of the infraspinatus, all but one on the articular side. The tears ranged from 0.3 to 3 cm in size averaging 1.1 by 1.6 cm in size. There was no mention of whether any of the tears had both articular and bursal side involvement. With an average follow-up of 28.9 months, 33 of 40 patients had marked improvement.

Stephens, Warren, and colleagues reported on 11 patients with a long-term follow-up of 8 years with partial tears treated with debridement with arthroscopic subacromial decompression. Three patients (27%) required further surgery and 2 of 3 had progressed to a full thickness tear. Cordasco found an overall failure rate of 32% (4 of 14 patients with bursal-sided tears and 2 of 63 with articular-sided tears) treated with debridement and subacromial decompression. Weber reported a failure rate of 29% of 31 patients with a follow-up of 2 to 7 years. Six of the 9 patients with poor results underwent reoperation and 3 had progressed to a full thickness tear and the other 3 showed no evidence of healing (9).

Adequate acromioplasty alone does prevent rotator cuff progression (9) and long-term follow-up studies have shown a high-failure rate. It is clear from reviewing the literature, especially the histologic sections performed by Fukuda (which showed no evidence of active repair) (10) and the second look arthroscopies performed by Gartsman and Weber (4, 9), that debridement does not stimulate a healing response as originally theorized nor does it prevent tear progression. Debridement of high-grade partial rotator cuff tears with or without subacromial decompression without surgical repair has led to unacceptable failure rates in long-term studies. Many of the studies in the current literature are retrospective in nature with short follow-up and combine patients with articular-sided and bursal-sided tears with a variable amount of tearing. Future prospective, long-term studies using an acceptable and reproducible classification system is needed before definitive treatment guidelines can be agreed upon.

Arthroscopic Debridement with Completion of the Tear

Repair of extensive partial rotator cuff tears has been recommended because of concerns about cuff integrity and tear progression (4, 8, 9, 11, 16, 18). Ellman was one of the first to recommend arthroscopic subacromial decompression along with open repair of significant, partial tears of the rotator cuff. He recommended open repair when more than one half of the cuff thickness was involved. Empirically, grading and treating tears in this manner appears reasonable but it is often difficult to estimate the thickness of the tear clinically (8).

Fukuda and colleagues (11) reported on 66 patients with partial tears treated with open acromioplasty and repair. Satisfactory results were obtained in 94% with an average follow-up of 32 months. Location and size of the tears were meticulously recorded. Few if any other studies have been as thorough and as complete. Itoi and Tabata (6) had 82% satisfactory results in 38 patients treated in a similar fashion with a follow-up averaging 4.9 years. With newer arthroscopic techniques, these studies may be the gold standard to which others are compared.

Weber has been at the forefront of the controversy surrounding arthroscopic debridement versus mini-open repair versus arthroscopic repair of partial rotator cuff tears. In a retrospective review of 65 patients with partial cuff tears, 32 were treated with arthroscopic subacromial decompression with arthroscopic debridement and 33 with arthroscopic subacromial decompression with mini-open repair. Treatment was not randomized and follow-up ranged from 2 to 7 years. The groups were similar in age and types of tear with the majority being articular-sided tears (29/32 in the arthroscopic group and 28/33 in the mini-open group). Statistically significant differences in long-term outcomes were noted with a UCLA score of 22.7 in the arthroscopic debridement group versus a 31.6 in the mini-open group. There were 9 poor results in the arthroscopic debridement group versus only one in the mini-open group. In the debridement group, a second look arthroscopy showed 3 of 6 patients had tear progression to a full thickness tear and 3 showed no evidence of healing (9).

In a follow-up study, Weber (19) compared another group of 29 mini-open repair patients to a group of 33 patients with partial articular-sided tears who underwent an arthroscopic repair. Arthroscopically completing the articular-sided tear from the bursal side, debriding the damaged tissue, and then advancing the healthy tendon back to its attachment site with suture anchors resulted in outcomes similar for both groups (UCLA scores 30.67 for the arthroscopic group and 29.84 for the mini-open group).

Deutsch reported on 41 patients with >50% partial thickness rotator cuff tears which were treated with debridement, conversion to full thickness tears, and repaired with suture anchors. Thirty-three (80%) were articular-sided tears and with a follow-up of 38 months, 98% were satisfied with their results (17). Another study by Porat and Nottage using a similar technique reported 83% good or excellent results and 17% fair scores with no poor results (18). Determining when a tear's thickness is greater or less than 50% is challenging and difficult, but both of these studies along with the study by Weber show that completing the tear and repairing it leads to good or excellent results in most patients.

Arthroscopic PASTA Repair

The arthroscopic trans-tendon technique for treating significant partial articular-sided rotator cuff tears, the so-called PASTA (partial articular-sided tendon avulsion) lesion has been described by Snyder. This method seeks to reattach the torn surface to its native "footprint" area on the tuberosity while preserving the remaining fiber attachment (17). It is an alternative to arthroscopic debridement and completion of the tear as described by Weber. Using the Snyder classification system for grading partial rotator cuff tears, the ideal tear is an A-3 or an A-4 PASTA tear. At least 30% of the native tendon must remain intact. This is a technically demanding procedure and many authors have written about their specific technique, but few have reported on their long-term results.

Only one long-term study has been published using this technique. In 2005, Ide and colleagues published their results on 17 patients with a follow-up of 39 months. They used a calibrated probe and repaired PASTA tears having >6 mm of exposed footprint. They reported 16 good to excellent results, but only 2 of 6 overhead athletes were able to return to their previous level of competition (20).

Arthroscopic Intraarticular Side-to-Side Repair

Other arthroscopic repair techniques have been proposed for partial rotator cuff tears. In 2005, Lyons, Savoie, and Field described arthroscopic debridement of articular-sided tears to evaluate tear depth as well as to attempt to promote a healing response. Following tear debridement, the arthroscopic shaver is used to lightly abrade the greater tuberosity adjacent to the tear while avoiding the articular surface. An arthroscopic side-to-side suture pulled the debrided tendon end in contact with the abraded humeral surface. This inhibited further progression of the tear in patients with Ellman grade I or grade II partial tears and selected grade III tears. They reported on 28 patients with a short follow-up of 8 months with good preliminary results. In 2008, Brockmeier and colleagues reported a similar technique using multiple side-to-side mattress sutures used in 8 patients with a 5-month follow-up. Further long-term studies are needed but this could be a promising technique.

Arthroscopic Repair of a Partial Bursal-Sided Tear (Monk's Hood)

Similar to the articular side PASTA lesion of the supraspinatus tendon, a partial bursal-sided tear can be seen with intact fibers on the articular side. This is the so-called Monk's Hood lesion as described by Snyder (17) (Fig. 8.14A). While the articular side of the cuff is intact, the bursal-sided fibers are often retracted but mobile. This bursal tissue can be advanced laterally and repaired to the lateral footprint with the use of suture anchors (Fig. 14B, C).

Arthroscopic Repair of an Intratendinous Tear

Arthroscopy provides no substantial advantage in the evaluation and treatment of intratendinous tears since these typically cannot be identified arthroscopically (1). Although a preoperative MRI may show significant signal changes within the supraspinatus tendon, at the time of diagnostic arthroscopy, no tear can be identified. Tissue appearance and palpation with the tip of the shaver may help to identify these lesions. Lo, Gonzalez, and Burkhart described the "Bubble Sign" as an arthroscopic indicator of an intratendinous rotator cuff tear. This is a bulging expansion of the rotator cuff tendon following injection of saline into the suspected lesion. This is an interesting technique, which requires further investigation. If an intratendinous tear is suspected, debridement with a full radius shaver will allow removal of damaged tissue and then subsequent arthroscopic repair can be performed depending on how much tissue is removed.

DECISION-MAKING ALGORITHM

At this time, there is no accepted management algorithm for the treatment of partial rotator cuff tears. Critical decision-making factors include the patient's age, occupation and/or sport, location of the tear (bursal vs. articular vs. intratendinous), etiology including acute trauma, repetitive overhead trauma, and possible underlying instability. Clinical symptoms include pain, motion loss and associated weakness. Nonsurgical management should be the mainstay of treatment. When the patient fails to progress, surgical intervention is discussed and may be

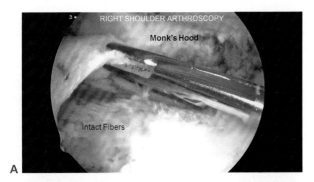

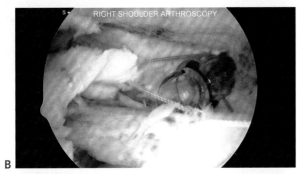

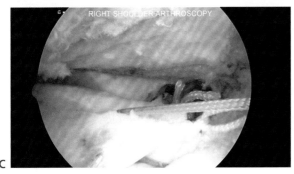

FIGURE 8.14. A: A bursal-sided tear can be seen with intact fibers on the articular side, the so-called Monk's Hood. The articular side of the cuff is usually intact but the bursal-sided fibers are retracted but mobile. **B:** With the use of a suture anchor, the bursal side of the tendon can be brought out laterally. **C:** Multiple sutures are often necessary and the tendon is repaired back into the area of the footprint.

entertained. Depending on the patient's expectations and desires, surgical intervention can be discussed as early as 3 months, but in most cases, 6 to 12 months of conservative treatment should be tried.

The simplistic view of repairing tears with >50% involvement of the tendon and debriding those with <50% involvement is appealing. But, sometimes it is difficult to determine the amount of involvement at the time of diagnostic shoulder arthroscopy. Using the footprint as a marker to determine whether a tear involves greater or less than 50% of the tendon has been proposed (2, 3). Since tendon thickness and tendon cross-sectional area vary widely from 26.4 ± 11.3 mm^2 of the anterior belly and 31.2 ± 10.1 mm^2 in the posterior belly of the supraspinatus tendon, further clinical studies are needed before this promising technique can be recommended.

Separating younger, overhead athletes, those with so-called internal impingement, and those with underlying instability from older patients with external impingement, can simplify the complex treatment algorithm. Young overhead athletes rarely need decompression but require treatment for their underlying instability.

In those patients in whom instability has been ruled out as an underlying cause of the partial rotator cuff tear, the size and thickness of the tear dictates the appropriate treatment. In those patients with impingement like symptoms and good strength on clinical examination and only partial fraying of the articular or bursal side of the cuff (Snyder grade A-I, A-II or B-I, B-II; Ellman grade I or II; <50% of the tendon involved), it is reasonable to debride the rotator cuff and perform an arthroscopic subacromial decompression (Fig. 8.15).

For an older individual with a significant partial articular-sided tear (Snyder grade A-III, A-IV; Ellman grade III type of tear: >50% of the tendon involved) with a normal bursal surface, simple debridement with an arthroscopic subacromial decompression in may provide significant pain relief. However, in a younger, more active individual, this treatment may be inadequate and lead to tear progression with residual pain and weakness. Repairing the high-grade articular-sided partial tear, the so-called PASTA lesion, using the technique of completing the tear and repairing it with suture anchors has led to good to excellent clinical results (9, 16, 19). These significant partial articular-sided tears may be amenable to the trans-tendon technique described previously in order to reproduce the anatomic footprint (Fig. 8.16A, B). Further long-term studies are needed using this promising technique. However, postoperative stiffness is a potential problem.

In those patients with a normal articular surface (Snyder grade A-0) but with significant fraying on the bursal surface (Snyder grade B-III or BIV) (Fig. 17A, B), arthroscopic subacromial decompression is recommended.

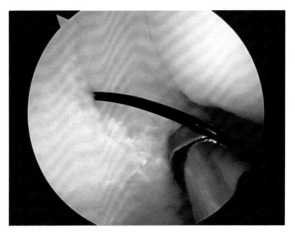

FIGURE 8.15. A partial articular-sided rotator cuff tear with a marker suture in place measuring <2 cm in size consistent with an A-2 tear.

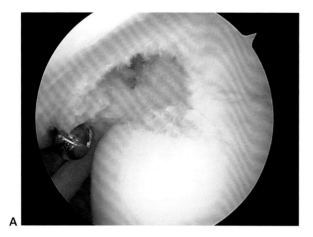

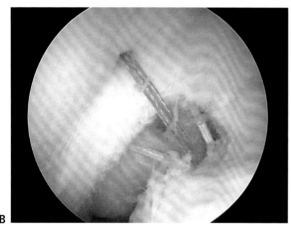

FIGURE 8.16. A: Partial tear of the supraspinatus tendon of a right shoulder with exposed footprint and the degree of tearing is measured from the edge of the articular surface to the intact tendon. **B:** An anchor has been placed into the greater tuberosity with two nonabsorbable sutures. These are woven through the rotator cuff, retrieved in the subacromial space and then tied. (Reprinted by permission of Alan Curtis.)

The surgeon then faces the dilemma of deciding between debridement and repair. Higher demand and younger patients may benefit from an aggressive approach focusing on restoring fiber integrity by a repair. Even older patients may benefit from a repair. Which technique to use for these partial bursal-sided tears is controversial and hopefully further studies will answer this question. If there is mobility in the bursal-sided tear, the so-called Monk's Hood, the remaining articular-sided fibers can be left intact and the bursal fibers repaired with suture anchors. It also is reasonable to complete the tear and repair it if the bursal-sided fibers are not amenable to repair. A side-to-side soft tissue technique or a suture anchor technique can be used.

When both sides of the cuff are involved, the risk of tear progression is more likely and more aggressive repair measures must be considered. For example, a partial articular-sided tear (Snyder grade A-II or A-III) and a partial tear of the bursal side (Snyder grade B-II, B-III, or

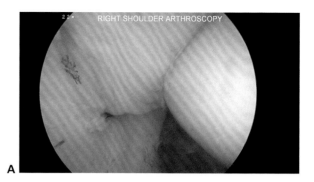

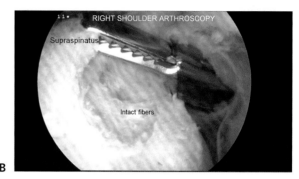

FIGURE 8.17. A: A normal articular surface of the supraspinatus (A-0). **B:** Viewing from the posterior portal, a partial tear of the bursal surface of the supraspinatus (B-3).

B-IV) treated with only debridement may lead to residual pain and weakness. A reasonable approach would be to debride the damaged tissue, complete the tear, and repair the healthy tissue with suture anchors along with a subacromial decompression (Fig. 18A–E).

AUTHOR'S PREFERRED TREATMENT AND TECHNIQUE

Each partial rotator cuff tear must be individually evaluated to determine if indeed the tear is actually the source of the clinical symptoms. Before proceeding with surgery, it is important to discuss with the patient the possibility of a high-grade partial rotator cuff tear and to discuss the decision-making process and expectations of the patient.

A complete diagnostic arthroscopy with a 15-point glenohumeral examination is critical in order to assess other intraarticular pathology such as a SLAP tear or chondral injuries, which may not have been diagnosed with a preoperative MRI. This pathology should be addressed before the rotator cuff.

A marking suture technique is invaluable in localizing the articular side of the tear and the bursal side of the tear in the subacromial space. In the glenohumeral joint, viewing from the posterior portal looking anteriorly and superiorly at the supraspinatus just off the edge of the humeral head, a marker suture (no. 1 absorbable monofilament PDS suture) is placed through an 18-gauge spinal

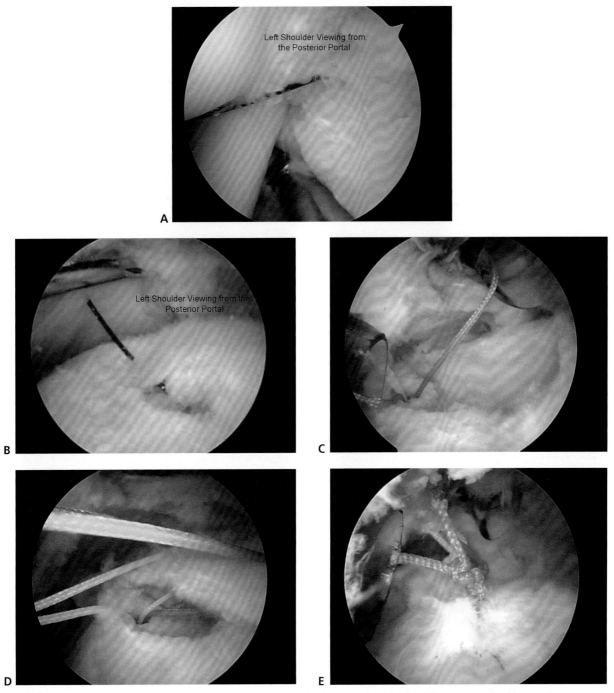

FIGURE 8.18. A: Partial articular-sided tear with a marker suture (A-II). **B:** The bursal side of the rotator cuff with a marker suture (B-III). This would be considered an A-II, B-III type of tear using the Snyder classification system. **C:** After debridement of the damaged tissue and converting it to a complete tear, an anchor is placed at the edge of the articular surface into the greater tuberosity loaded with two nonabsorbable sutures. **D:** The sutures are woven through the leading edge of the cuff in a mattress type of stitch. **E:** The sutures are tied arthroscopically repairing the cuff to its anatomic position.

needle laterally off the edge of the acromion through the partial tear. The needle is then removed leaving the suture in place. The subacromial space is then entered, the marker suture localized, and the extent of any bursal tearing determined. If a subacromial decompression is to be performed, it is easier to do this first and then to look for the marker suture. After debridement of hypertrophic

bursal tissue, the area surrounding the marker suture is carefully inspected. Complete visualization of the cuff is facilitated by internally and externally rotating the arm.

After debridement with a full radius shaver of any damaged bursal rotator cuff fibers, the extent of the tear can be better assessed. If the partial tear is limited in size (A-I or A-II with a normal bursal side, B-0; normal articular side A-0, with mild tearing on the bursal side, B-I or B-II) and associated with impingement, a simple decompression may solve the problem.

The high-grade partial tear continues to be the clinical challenge. In the case of a significant partial articular-sided tear in patients over 40 (A-III, A-IV even with a normal bursal surface), completing the tear and repairing it with suture anchors along with an arthroscopic subacromial decompression provides significant pain relief and return to function. I continue to use a single row with triple-loaded suture anchors because the current studies using double-row fixation have not shown any clinical difference. My early treatment of these partial rotator cuff tears with debridement only and subacromial decompression led to failures and patient dissatisfaction. This led me to a more aggressive treatment regimen of completing the tear and repairing it.

The high-grade partial tear involving the bursal surface (Snyder grade B-III or B-IV) with a normal articular surface (A-0), the so-called Monk's Hood, can usually be repaired by leaving the articular fibers intact and repairing the bursal fibers with side-to-side sutures or often with suture anchors placed laterally near the footprint combined with an arthroscopic subacromial decompression. These patients often go through postoperative rehabilitation quickly and the surgeon must monitor their postoperative course carefully to make sure they do no return to sports or activities too soon.

The risk of tear progression may be more likely when both sides of the tendon are involved. This is usually seen in patients older than 50 years and debridement with an arthroscopic subacromial decompression may give adequate pain relief but usually does not allow patients to return to overhead activities or even lifting without residual pain. Therefore, more aggressive repair measures must be considered in this patient population as patients expect not only pain relief but also a return to function without residual pain or weakness. In these patients over 50 years old, I use Snyder's classification system and call it the "Rule of 4's." When there is damage to both the articular side, for example, a partial articular-sided tear (Snyder grade A-I, A-II or A-III) and a partial tear of the bursal side (Snyder grade B-I, B-II, B-III), if these add up to "4" or greater, then I am more aggressive in treating the tear by debriding it, completing the tear, and repairing it with suture anchors.

For patients younger than 40 and in overhead athletes, the high-grade PASTA lesion continues to be a challenging problem. Our reluctance to complete the tear has led to the technique of keeping the remaining fibers intact and restoring the footprint with suture anchors placed percutaneously through the intact cuff and tying the sutures in the subacromial space. Determining how much of the cuff remains (greater or less than 50%) can be challenging even if one measures from the exposed footprint. These patients are often young, active, and wish to return

to overhead sporting activities. Once we have ruled out instability and GIRD as underlying causes, we are faced with a significant partial rotator cuff tear that needs to be addressed. This type of patient is the ideal candidate for a PASTA repair (Fig. 19A–G). This is a technically demanding procedure and can be made more difficult if not impossible if the edge of the acromion overhangs too far laterally and does not allow a suture anchor placement at an appropriate angle. It is also important to note that the only long-term study in the literature using this PASTA technique resulted in only two of six overhead throwing athletes returning to their previous level of competition (20). The surgeon may feel more comfortable completing the tear and repairing it with suture anchors, which is a reasonable alternative.

COMPLICATIONS, CONTROVERSIES, AND SPECIAL CONSIDERATIONS

Mechanical failure is one of the most common complications with any arthroscopic procedure. It is the responsibility of the surgeon and his operative team to make sure that all equipment is functioning properly before beginning a procedure. With that said, some things are out of the control of the surgeon and mechanical failure of the arthroscope, pump system, shaver system, and other specialized equipment can occur at any time. It is important to have back up equipment readily available before beginning any procedure. With more procedures being done in outpatient surgery centers, some centers are reluctant to purchase back up equipment but this can compromise patient care. It is up to the surgeon to make sure that these backup systems are available.

When performing arthroscopic shoulder surgery, it is also very important to be prepared to address any shoulder pathology. Preoperative MRIs do not always detect partial rotator cuff tears or SLAP lesions. Partial rotator cuff tears are found in over 35% of patients undergoing routine arthroscopic subacromial decompression. Any surgeon performing arthroscopic shoulder surgery should always be prepared to repair SLAP lesions, partial rotator cuff tears or other pathology, which may not have been diagnosed preoperatively. The surgeon should make sure that he always has a full set of cannulas, anchors, and other instrumentation to address any unforeseen pathology before beginning an arthroscopic shoulder procedure.

The optimal clinical approach for partial rotator cuff tears is still controversial. Subacromial decompression offers predictable pain relief and the ability to reduce subacromial outlet narrowing in those with external impingement. However, it has never been proven to delay the progression of cuff pathology. Therefore, significant partial rotator cuff tears should be treated aggressively using the technique the surgeon is most comfortable

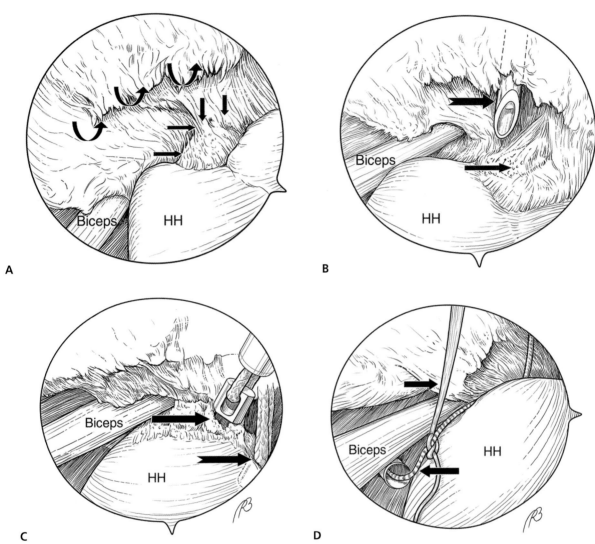

FIGURE 8.19. A: Identify and quantitate the tear utilizing the anatomic "footprint" as the reference point. Prepare the exposed footprint with a motorized shaver utilizing a standard anterior portal. Debride the partial articular-sided tear. **B:** Pass a percutaneous spinal needle lateral to the edge of the acromion. This needle will traverse through the substance of the remaining attached rotator cuff into the exposed footprint. This will serve as a guide for anchor insertion. **C:** A narrow diameter sleeve or instrument-specific cannula is then passed percutaneously through the rotator cuff (trans-tendon) and the appropriate instrumentation is used to place one or two anchors, each double-loaded, depending on the size of the tear. **D:** For each anchor in sequence, one suture limb of the anchor is grasped through the anterior portal. A spinal needle loaded with a passing suture (no. 1 absorbable suture, PDS) is then passed through the bursal side of the cuff, aiming for the edge of the partial tear. Some manipulation of the shoulder may be necessary, for example, abduction and/or rotation in order to pass the loaded needle accurately. The suture is introduced into the joint and grasped through the anterior portal and will serve as a suture shuttle. A simple loop is tied in the absorbable suture and one of the limbs from the anchor, which has been bought through the anterior portal is loaded on the shuttle outside the joint by tightening the loop. The shuttle and accompanying anchor suture is then pulled retrograde, in order, through the cannula, the tear edge, into the subacromial space and out through the skin.

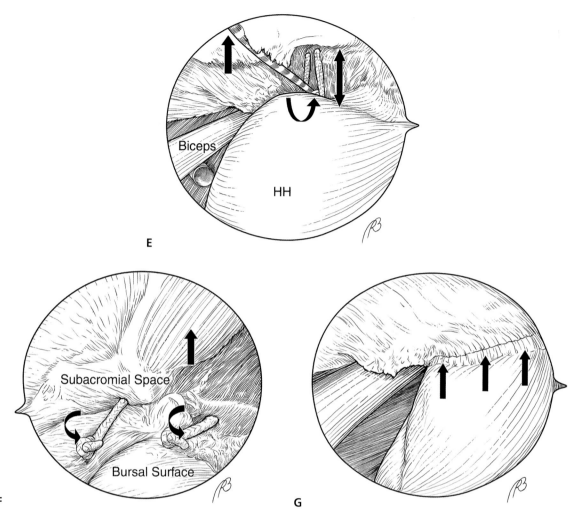

FIGURE 8.19. (Continued) **E:** After the shuttle is brought through the cuff *(left arrow)*, the remaining sutures are passed in a similar manner and eventually tied to reproduce the anatomic footprint *(right arrow)* to the humeral head (HH). **F:** The arthroscope is then introduced into the subacromial space. Color-coded sutures facilitate identification of matched sutures. The appropriate suture pairs are separated and then tied through a lateral or anterior cannula. **G:** The arthroscope is reintroduced into the glenohumeral space and the edge of the partial tear should be contiguous with the articular margin, completely effacing the previously exposed footprint. The shoulder is then taken through a range of motion to evaluate the quality of the repair, to make sure undue tension is not present, and to make sure a near anatomic repair has been performed.

performing. The literature is also unclear as to which patients require subacromial decompression at the time of arthroscopic rotator cuff repair. At present, it is reasonable to recommend arthroscopic subacromial decompression in patients over 40 or in patients with a history and physical examination consistent with an impingement syndrome.

Because there is no widely accepted classification system for partial thickness rotator cuff tears, it is important that the surgeon try to describe the type of tear found. We believe that the Snyder classification system is the best one for describing partial rotator cuff tears as it addresses both articular and bursal-sided tears. However, this is a controversial point. Grading the partial tears with greater or less than 50% is appealing, but not always reproducible.

The literature is unclear and controversial as to the timing of surgery, and recommendations have ranged from a few months to over a year. Surgery should be based on the patient's symptoms, rate of improvement, as well as the goals of each individual patient.

The treatment of intratendinous tears remains problematic. As discussed, arthroscopy affords no substantial advantage in the evaluation and treatment of intratendinous tears as these typically cannot be identified arthroscopically (1). Preoperative tests such as MRI often show significant signal changes within the supraspinatus tendon, but at the time of diagnostic arthroscopy no tear can be identified. Depending on the patient's age, symptoms, and activity level, aggressive debridement and repair may be necessary. Tissue appearance and palpation with the shaver tip may help to identify these lesions and if suspected, debridement and repair should be performed.

The arthroscopic treatment of partial rotator cuff tears in overhead athletes is also controversial as there has been a high-failure rate in treating these types of tears with debridement only. If internal impingement and multidirectional instability is ruled out, completion of the tear with arthroscopic repair with suture anchors has led to good results in a few selected studies. A PASTA repair technique is also possible and may be the best alternative in this select group of patients. However, there is only one long-term study in the literature, which reported mixed results in this difficult subgroup of patients.

PEARLS AND PITFALLS

1. **Pearl:** With the advent of MRI and shoulder arthroscopy, more tears are being recognized.
   Pitfall: Not all partial tears are symptomatic and they can be present in over 20% of the shoulders of asymptomatic patients. Partial tears increase with age and may not be the cause of the patient's symptoms.

2. **Pearl:** Pain, often most troubling at night, along with pain with overhead activities is the predominant symptom.
   Pitfall: The symptoms are nonspecific and may overlap with an impingement syndrome and often are treated nonoperatively for an extended period without improvement.

3. **Pearl:** Glenohumeral instability and traction stress on the rotator cuff in the throwing athlete can lead to undersurface tears in the absence of extrinsic impingement.
   Pitfall: Misdiagnosing this patient population, treating them with a subacromial decompression and not addressing the underlying disorder can lead to a poor result.

4. **Pearl:** The histologic examination and second look arthroscopies of partial thickness rotator cuff tears have confirmed that no active tissue repair occurs after debridement.
   Pitfall: Symptoms can persist after arthroscopic debridement of a partial rotator cuff tear and more aggressive treatment may be necessary.

5. **Pearl:** MRI can have a high false-negative rate for detecting partial rotator cuff tears.
   Pitfall: Ignoring this high false-negative rate can lead to misdiagnosis of patients with chronic shoulder pain.

6. **Pearl:** Rotator cuff tendonitis or tendinopathy may be distinguished from partial thickness tears by an increased signal on T1 images but a decreased signal on T2 images.
   Pitfall: A diagnosis of tendonitis or tendinopathy on MRI does not preclude a partial rotator cuff tear. Many cases of rotator cuff tendonitis or tendinopathy may actually be partial thickness rotator cuff tears.

7. **Pearl:** The use of intraarticular gadolinium with MRA can increase the sensitivity of detecting partial articular-sided rotator cuff tears.
   Pitfall: This technique does not help in the detection of partial bursal-sided tears.

8. **Pearl:** Using MRA is prudent if the diagnosis is uncertain, especially in a younger patient population where the history and physical examination can be confusing.
   Pitfall: The presence of a partial rotator cuff tear, even in a young, overhead athlete, does not mean that surgery is necessary. The initial treatment should be nonoperative before surgery is considered.

9. **Pearl:** The lidocaine injection test, an injection of 10 ml of 1% lidocaine into the subacromial space, can be helpful in differentiating impingement from a symptomatic partial rotator cuff tear.
   Pitfall: A posterior injection does not always reach the subacromial space because of posterior bursal curtain thickness and the posterior musculature.

10. **Pearl:** The diagnosis of partial thickness rotator cuff tears is often not made with certainty until the rotator cuff is examined arthroscopically.
    Pitfall: Failure to do a complete arthroscopic and bursal examination can lead to failure to adequately diagnose and treat these partial rotator cuff tears.

11. **Pearl:** With repetitive microtrauma such as seen in overhead athletes, the risk of progression to a full thickness rotator cuff tear can be as high as 81%.
    Pitfall: Arthroscopic debridement only in these patients may not give adequate pain relief and may not allow them to return to competitive activities. However, the optimal clinical approach is still controversial.

12. **Pearl:** The use of a marker suture technique in the glenohumeral joint for partial articular-sided tears is helpful in localizing the bursal side of the tear.
    Pitfall: Without the use of a marker suture, it can be very difficult and sometimes impossible to localize the bursal side of the tear, which can lead to misdiagnosis and improper treatment.

REHABILITATION

After arthroscopic debridement and subacromial decompression, an early aggressive range of motion program is instituted with early strengthening. The postoperative protocol for those patients with either with a PASTA repair or a completed and repaired partial thickness tear is similar to the program for a full thickness rotator cuff repair.

Early passive range of motion is instituted. However, many patients have little pain following an arthroscopic repair and may want to do more actively than appropriate. Typically, 4- to 6-week time is needed to allow these repairs to heal before any active motion is allowed. It is been the author's experience that many patients do more than they are instructed to do during this time. We may learn from our experience with anterior cruciate ligament reconstruction rehabilitation that patients may be able to accelerate their rehabilitation.

CONCLUSIONS AND FUTURE DIRECTIONS

The treatment of partial rotator cuff tears remains a controversial topic. Some of the controversy stems from our current lack of knowledge regarding the natural history of partial tears as well as from the abundance of confusing clinical studies. Partial tears may be asymptomatic or may be a significant cause of pain and disability in any age group. Treatment must be based on the patient's age, occupation or sport, etiology, and depth of tear. Suffice it to say that each partial rotator cuff tear must be individually evaluated to determine if indeed the tear is actually the source of clinical symptoms. If a partial tear is deemed to need treatment, ascertaining any associated pathology is critical. If the partial tear is a secondary phenomenon resulting from labral or ligamentous insufficiency, treatment should be directed toward the primary problem initially before rotator cuff surgery is discussed. Arthroscopic debridement of partial tears (Snyder A-I, A-II) along with treating the underlying labral tear or ligamentous insufficiency is often all that is necessary. The role of acromioplasty in these patients should be individualized but is usually not necessary in a younger population.

If the partial tear is of limited size and associated with impingement (Snyder A-I, A-II or B-I, B-II), a simple decompression may solve the problem entirely. The high-grade partial tear continues to be the clinical dilemma. The challenge remains choosing debridement versus arthroscopic repair and how to repair the cuff tear. Recent studies have shown that completing the tear and repairing it with suture anchors gives very good results. Using newer techniques such as a PASTA repair or side-to-side sutures for partial articular-sided tears may provide acceptable results especially in overhead athletes. However, long-term studies are needed to determine if these techniques are better than completing the tear and repairing it.

With our increasing understanding of rotator cuff anatomy and with the ability to grossly measure tear depth arthroscopically, the goal of restoring the integrity to the rotator cuff in the younger, higher demand patient becomes more compelling. Future long-term studies evaluating the treatment of partial rotator cuff tears utilizing a standardized classification system that is reproducible and using the techniques described are clearly needed before any treatment algorithm can be fully validated. As for rehabilitation, further prospective studies comparing different rehabilitation protocols are also needed to determine if rehabilitation may be safely accelerated in patients whose tears are repaired using these newer arthroscopic techniques.

REFERENCES

1. McConville OR, Iannotti JP. Partial thickness tears of the rotator cuff: evaluation and management. *J Am Acad Orthop Surg.* 1999;7:32–43.
2. Curtis AS, Burbank KM, Tierney JJ, et al. The insertional footprint of the rotator cuff: an anatomic study. *Arthroscopy.* 2006;22:603–609.
3. Ruotolo C, Fow JE, Nottage WM. The supraspinatus footprint: an anatomic study of the supraspinatus insertion. *Arthroscopy.* 2004;20:246–249.
4. Gartsman GM, Milne JC. Articular surface partial-thickness rotator cuff tears. *J Shoulder Elbow Surg.* 1995;4:409–415.
5. Walch G, Boileau P, Noel E, et al. Impingement of the deep surface of the supraspinatus tendon on the posterosuperior glenoid rim: an arthroscopic study. *J Shoulder Elbow Surg.* 1992;1:238–245.
6. Itoi E, Tabata S. Incomplete rotator cuff tears: results of operative treatment. *Clin Orthop Relat Res.* 1992;284:128–135.
7. Codman EA. *The Shoulder.* Boston, MA: Thomas Todd; 1934.
8. Ellman H. Diagnosis and treatment of incomplete rotator cuff tears. *Clin Orthop Relat Res.* 1990;254:64–74.
9. Weber SC. Arthroscopic debridement and acromioplasty versus mini-open repair in the management of significant partial-thickness tears of the rotator cuff. *Orthop Clin North Am.* 1997; 28:79–82.
10. Fukuda H, Craig EV, Yamanaka K, et al. Partial-thickness cuff tears. In: Burkhead WZ Jr, ed. *Rotator Cuff Disorders.* Baltimore, MD: Williams and Wilkins; 1996:174–181.
11. Fukuda H, Mikasa M, Yamanaka K. Incomplete thickness rotator cuff tears diagnosed by bursography. *Clin Orthop Relat Res.* 1987;223:51–58.
12. Sher JS, Uribe JW, Posada A, et al. Abnormal findings on magnetic resonance images of asymptomatic shoulders. *J Bone Joint Surg Am.* 1995;77:10–15.
13. Mazoué CG, Andrews JR. Repair of full-thickness rotator cuff tears in professional baseball players. *Am J Sports Med.* 2006;34:182–189.
14. Stetson WB, Phillips T, Deutsch A. Magnetic resonance arthrogram for detecting partial rotator cuff tears. *J Bone Joint Surg Am.* 2005;87(suppl 2):81–88.
15. Stetson WB, Ryu RKN, Bittar ES. Arthroscopic treatment of partial rotator cuff tears. *Op Tech Sports Med.* 2004;6: 135–148.
16. Deutsch A. Arthroscopic repair of partial thickness tears of the rotator cuff. *J Shoulder Elbow Surg.* 2007;16:193–201.
17. Snyder SJ. *Shoulder Arthroscopy.* 2nd ed. Philadelphia, PA: Lippincott Williams and Wilkins; 2003.
18. Porat S, Nottage W, Fouse MN. Repair of partial thickness rotator cuff tears: a retrospective review with minimum of two year follow-up. *J Shoulder Elbow Surg.* 2008;17:729–731.
19. Weber SC. Arthroscopic repair of partial thickness rotator cuff tears: the safety of completing the tear. Presented at the 22nd Annual Meeting of the Arthroscopy Association of North America; 2003; Phoenix, Arizona.
20. Ide J, Maeda S, Tabagi K. Arthroscopic transtendon repair of partial-thickness articular-side tears of the rotator cuff: anatomical and clinical study. *Am J Sports Med.* 2005;33:1672–1679.

Arthroscopic Cuff Repair: Single-Row Options

Matthew R. Lavery • Joseph P. Burns • Stephen J. Snyder

The origins of rotator cuff surgery date back to Codman's 1911 description of the first supraspinatus repair to its insertion on the greater tuberosity and the subsequent publication of his treatise on the shoulder in 1934. The succeeding decades produced refinement in the description of anatomy, terminology, and surgical treatment of rotator cuff tears. Neer provided us with a definition of "impingement" in 1972 and elucidated many of the important concepts in the etiology and treatment of rotator cuff disease followed today. The development of arthroscopy in the 1970s may have paved the way for modern shoulder surgery, but the past decade has provided even more rapid advancement in the techniques and implants available to surgeons treating rotator cuff disease.

Arthroscopic rotator cuff repair techniques offer significant advantages to both the surgeon and the patient. Some of these advantages include better visualization of the pathoanatomy, deltoid preservation, greater versatility in treatment, and less postoperative pain and scarring. As an increasing number of surgeons develop the skills necessary to perform these operations, we have amassed sufficient experience to document the success of arthroscopic rotator cuff repair.

In recent years, the sports medicine and arthroscopy literature has demonstrated the short- and long-term success of these techniques. Morse et al. published a meta-analysis in 2008 in the *American Journal of Sports Medicine* comparing outcomes between all-arthroscopic and mini-open repairs. The study found no difference in outcomes between the two techniques (1). Successful outcomes and a satisfied patient population validate the incorporation of arthroscopic rotator cuff repair into the armamentarium of any surgeon with the appropriate skill set.

Today, there is little debate over the safety and efficacy of arthroscopic cuff repair techniques although controversy remains regarding the appropriate method of fixation. Both single-row and double-row options are being extensively studied. We advocate a single-row, minimally tensioned repair that emphasizes the need for biologic healing in conjunction with an adherence to the biomechanical principles of adequate tendon to bone fixation.

CLINICAL EVALUATION

Pertinent History

The clinical history of patients with rotator cuff disease can be stratified based upon patient age. Young patients with rotator cuff problems are usually involved in aggressive overhead athletics, sustain a high-impact injury, or engage in heavy overhead manual labor. Pain typically occurs during the overhead phase of the activity and seems to diminish with rest. When pain persists after the offending activity ceases or intensifies at night, a partial thickness cuff tear should be suspected.

As patients progress toward middle age, their history often reveals a pattern of chronic overuse, especially when they routinely perform overhead work. Full-thickness cuff tears may be present, particularly in cases with shoulder trauma. Patients will report a chronically aching shoulder with radiating pain into the lateral deltoid area. This pain may be associated with weakness or catching. Often the patient has recently increased upper extremity activity secondary to a new exercise routine or job. Other patients may report more chronic impingement syndrome-type symptoms in which the rotator cuff and biceps tendon are insidiously eroded by a subacromial spur. Symptoms are often more pronounced at night and may result in the patient sleeping in a semi-sitting position or using sleeping medications to achieve some degree of rest. In severe cases, active shoulder elevation and external rotation may be weak or nearly impossible to perform.

As patients age beyond 65 years, rotator cuff pathology is extremely common, possibly affecting more than 40% of the population (2). Symptoms may be less pronounced in this age group as activity levels decline, and the chronic nature of the disease results in more compensatory movements. Weakness and chronic aching are the most pronounced complaints in this age group.

Physical Examination

Patients undergoing surgery should undergo a comprehensive physical examination. However, the evaluation of rotator cuff pathology should involve a specific and standardized subset of tests. It is useful to inspect both shoulders for symmetry of the bony and muscular anatomy. Scars, incisions from previous surgery, and visible irregularities may give clues regarding previous trauma or treatments.

Palpation and Range of Motion

After a general inspection, assess the patient's active and passive range of motion. Observe the patient for signs of pain during this portion of the exam. A painful arc in which the patient displays pain between 60° and 140° of flexion is a classic finding. This often indicates that the rotator cuff has been disrupted and is being pinched between the anterior edge of the greater tuberosity and the acromion. Palpate the entire shoulder including the sternoclavicular joint. Assess ligamentous integrity when there is any suspicion of instability (e.g., younger patient).

Neuromuscular Testing

Strength and function of the intrinsic and extrinsic shoulder muscles should be assessed and graded from zero to five. Resisted internal and external rotation with the arm adducted to the side allows for grading of subscapularis and infraspinatus strength, respectively. To test supraspinatus strength, the arm should be positioned in 60° of abduction and 45° of forward flexion with the shoulder in internal rotation and the thumb pointing toward the ground as resistance is applied. This maneuver is often quite painful in patients with rotator cuff pathology and should be performed with care.

Because there are several neurologically mediated conditions that can mimic the pain of rotator cuff disease, careful neurologic testing should be performed. Two of the more common conditions affecting shoulder pain and function are cervical radiculitis and suprascapular nerve dysfunction. These conditions may result in profound atrophy of the rotator cuff musculature. Patients with suprascapular nerve dysfunction often report pain that is deep in the joint and has a more constant presence as opposed to the activity-related pain of cuff pathology. Cervical nerve root pathology may produce pain that radiates down the arm and is associated with burning or numbness; deep tendon reflexes may be altered. The performance of a Spurling's maneuver (extension, rotation, and axial compression of the neck) may reproduce these symptoms in patients with cervical nerve root irritation. An electromyogram may help more clearly define the location of a neurologic lesion.

Impingement Tests

Impingement signs are often positive in patients with rotator cuff pathology. While no impingement test is completely reliable, they are a valuable component of the routine shoulder examination. We utilize the Neer test (impingement test 1) and the Hawkins test (impingement test 2) (Fig. 9.1A, B). These maneuvers are performed with the patient in the supine position to stabilize the scapula

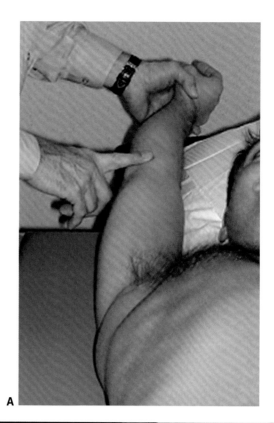

A

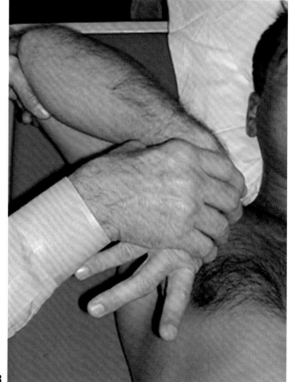

B

FIGURE 9.1. **A**: Neer test. **B**: Hawkins test.

against the exam table. To perform the Neer test (impingement test 1), position the internally rotated arm into a forward-flexed overhead position. This causes the greater tuberosity to compress under the anterior acromion and against any spur that may be present. The Hawkins test (impingement test 2) requires that the elbow be position in flexion and the shoulder in 90° of abduction. The arm is then maneuvered into an arc of adduction, elevation, and internal rotation. This maneuver results in a similar compression of the rotator cuff structures beneath the lateral and anterior acromial arch, resulting in pain when pathology is present. In addition to rotator cuff injury, biceps disease, labral pathology, and bursal inflammation may also result in positive impingement signs (3).

Imaging

Radiography

Four radiographic shoulder views: a true anterior–posterior (AP perpendicular to the plane of the scapula), an axillary lateral, a lateral supraspinatus outlet view, and a Zanca (acromioclavicular joint) view are obtained on patients presenting with shoulder complaints. Taken together, these four radiographs generally provide adequate information for preoperative planning in conjunction with a good quality MRI scan.

Part of that preoperative plan involves assessing the need for subacromial decompression. The supraspinatus outlet view aids in this determination as do the intraoperative findings. Based upon the supraspinatus outlet view, we apply the Bigliani and Morrison classification to the acromion: type I, flat acromion; type II, gently curved acromion; type III, acromion with a sharp inferior "beak" (4). Because acromial thickness can vary significantly, we also classify the thickness of the acromion: type A, less than 8 mm; type B, 8 to 12 mm; type C, greater than 12 mm (5). This measurement is made on the supraspinatus outlet view in an area that corresponds to the posterior aspect of the AC joint for consistency (Fig. 9.2). This information is extremely useful in the preoperative planning of a subacromial decompression.

Magnetic Resonance Imaging

Most of our patients have obtained an MRI scan prior to rotator cuff repair. A high-quality, noncontrast MRI scan provides a multitude of information regarding the status of the rotator cuff tendons and their muscle bellies, the

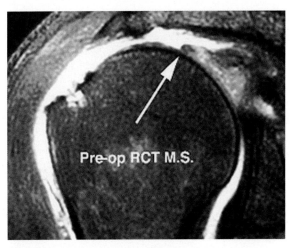

FIGURE 9.3. This coronal oblique MRI documents a large, retracted somewhat degenerative rotator cuff tear.

subscapularis, the biceps, as well as the AC and glenohumeral joints. Our protocol is to obtain sagittal oblique (perpendicular to the scapula), coronal oblique (parallel to the scapula) (Fig. 9.3), and axial sequences. The coronal images provide the most immediate assessment of the supraspinatus tendon. The most lateral cuts in the sagittal sequence can provide information regarding the amount of footprint involved in a tear, whereas the medial cuts help to assess fatty infiltration in the muscle bellies of the rotator cuff. Significant fatty infiltration of the muscle may portend a poorer prognosis following repair, and patients should be counseled accordingly preoperatively (Fig. 9.4A, B). Axial images provide a clear look at the subscapularis and posterior rotator cuff tendons. In cases where a recurrent tear or a PASTA (partial articular supraspinatus tendon avulsion) lesion is suspected, we utilize a gadolinium arthrogram in conjunction with the MRI to more clearly define the pathoanatomy.

Decision Making

Indications for arthroscopic rotator cuff repair hinge on both the patient and the surgeon. The nature of the tear (i.e., chronicity, size, and quality of the cuff musculature) has an impact on its suitability for repair. Other patient factors include age and the physical demands placed on the shoulder. Full-thickness tears do not heal or reattach to the bone without intervention and are likely to progress in size (6). Essentially all young, active patients should be considered for early repair of a torn rotator cuff tendon. In middle-aged and older patients, pain, loss of strength, and range of motion are also generally indications for operative repair, assuming a repairable tendon and adequate bone stock for secure anchor purchase.

Contraindications to rotator cuff repair are relatively few. Inadequate bone stock or large subchondral cysts may prevent adequate bone purchase and holding strength of the suture anchor. Other contraindications include advanced degenerative joint disease, overriding medical comorbidities, or activity demands low enough to tolerate

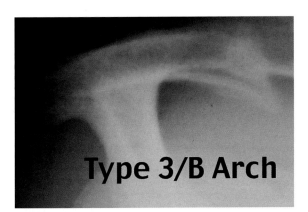

FIGURE 9.2. Supraspinatus outlet view.

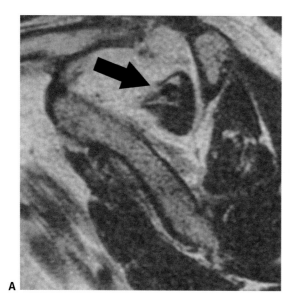

A

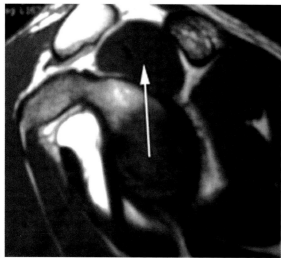

B

FIGURE 9.4. A. the sagittal oblique MRI demonstrates moderate atrophy of the supraspinatus muscle belly with surrounding fat (arrow). **B.** The normal muscle fills the entire supraspinatus fossa often bulging up between the clavicle and acromial spine.

cuff deficiency. Patients with large, retracted, chronic, or recurrent tears and significant fatty infiltration should be counseled that outcomes are less predictable than with more standard tears. A capsular release and manipulation are performed at the time of repair for patients with concomitant adhesive capsulitis. We counsel the patient that they are likely to have a protracted postoperative course requiring more physical therapy to restore motion and possibly another manipulation or release to regain motion. Delaying the operation risks more atrophy and a more difficult repair.

Classification

The ability to precisely evaluate and classify rotator cuff pathology facilitates recording, studying, and communicating treatment strategies with others. This should be done routinely as a component of the permanent operative record. The Southern California Orthopedic Institute (SCOI) rotator cuff classification system is a simple descriptive scheme that uses letters and numbers to designate the pathologic conditions of the tendon. The capital letter indicates the side of the cuff where the tear is located: "A" for articular side partial tears, "B" for bursal side partial tears, and "C" for complete thickness or transtendon damage. The degree of tendon damage is classified using a numeric designation of 0 to 5 (Table 9.1).

When recording the information, all three areas are represented even if they are normal. As an example, a tear designated A2/B4/C0 would indicate a small area of fraying on the articular surface with minimal cuff fiber damage. The bursal surface would have a significant injury with tendon fragmentation and a flap formation. Despite the severe nature of the damage, there is still no full-thickness component, hence C0. Larger, full-thickness tears can be further described by their morphology, such as crescent, U-shaped, L-shaped, reverse L-shaped, and massive degenerative tear patterns.

TREATMENT

Nonoperative Versus Operative Treatment

As previously alluded to, we recommend repairing rotator cuff tears in the majority of patients. Individuals with significant medical comorbidities, those with massive tears that may require grafting, or those who are reluctant or unwilling to undergo an operation should be counseled regarding nonoperative options for treatment of their pain. In addition, scapular strengthening exercises and biofeedback training can be employed to allow compensatory shoulder musculature to function more effectively. Patients should be appropriately counseled that although this will not cause a torn tendon to heal back to bone, it may reduce their painful symptoms.

Timing

The quality of the rotator cuff tendon tissue and amount of retraction are important factors in the decision-making process and in appropriately timing surgery. Because chronic tears have the propensity to increase in size and degree of fatty muscle infiltration, we generally recommend earlier repair in suitable candidates. When neglected for an extended period, reparable rotator cuff tears having a good prognosis can become irreparable with a poor prognosis. Our experience has shown that a full-thickness tear that includes two or three cuff tendons and is retracted medial to the level of the glenoid, especially when coupled with significant muscle atrophy, is often untreatable by direct surgical repair. However, a partial rotator cuff repair may be helpful in some of these patients if they qualify for surgery. Additionally, several methods of biologic augmentation have shown promise in bridging previously irreparable gaps (7).

Table 9.1
Tear classification

Location of Tear

A. Articular surface
B. Bursal surface
C. Complete tear

Severity of Tear

0. Normal cuff with smooth coverings of synovium and bursa
1. Minimal superficial bursal or synovial irritation or capsular fraying in localized area (<1 cm)
2. Actual fraying or failure of rotator cuff fibers in addition to synovial, bursal, or capsular injury (<2 cm)
3. More severe cuff injury, including fraying and fragmentation of tendon fibers, often involving the entire surface of a tendon (usually the supraspinatus and <3 cm)
4. Very severe partial rotator cuff tear that usually contains, in addition to fraying and fragmentation of the tendon, a sizable flap tear, usually larger in size than previous classifications, involving more than a single tendon
5. Large, irreparable tear with significant retraction of the tendon end

TECHNIQUE

We perform shoulder arthroscopy in the lateral position. As with all arthroscopic shoulder procedures, the evaluation begins with a 15-point glenohumeral examination. To completely evaluate articular-sided involvement, the surgeon must carefully visualize the rotator cuff tendon from both the posterior and the anterior portals. When a lesion is encountered on the underside of the cuff, its frayed edges should be carefully debrided from both the anterior and the posterior portals as this anatomy can be difficult or impossible to see and/or access from the bursal side.

When a partial thickness undersurface rotator cuff tear is encountered during the diagnostic glenohumeral examination, it can be difficult to determine the full extent of the lesion. To answer this question, the authors utilize a suture marker. An 18G spinal needle is inserted through the skin adjacent to the lateral border of the acromion, passing into the joint directly through the articular side cuff defect. Ten centimeters of no. 1 PDS suture is passed through the needle and into the joint. The needle is removed, leaving the suture in place (Fig. 9.5A, B). When evaluating the subacromial space the surgeon can therefore locate the suture and readily evaluate the area of the cuff corresponding to the articular side defect.

Following the diagnostic glenohumeral exam, the arm position is changed from 70° to 15° of abduction to evaluate the subacromial bursa. In this bursoscopy position, the greater tuberosity is situated more laterally, thereby opening the subacromial space and improving access to the cuff.

The arthroscopic cannula is inserted into the posterior superior portal (PSP). The transarticular guide rod is passed through the cannula and directed below the coracoacromial ligament and out anteriorly. An outflow cannula is placed over the anterior end and worked into the bursa. The bursal-sided anatomy is visualized systematically from both portals. The marker suture also should be identified at this time to prevent accidental removal. With the arthroscope in the anterior portal, carefully debride the posterior bursal curtain to improve visualization and clear the working area.

Reinsert the scope into the PSP to create the lateral acromial portal (LAP). Pass a spinal needle percutaneously to identify the "50-yd line," a position that is directly in line with the center of the cuff tear and at least 2.5 cm lateral from the acromial edge. Insert a smooth clear cannula with a tapered obturator.

Perform a selective subacromial decompression and mini or complete distal clavicle resection as needed, based upon the evaluation of the preoperative radiograph, the patient's symptoms, and the arthroscopic findings. Remove any thickened bursa from around the anterior and lateral portals to ensure an unobstructed view of the rotator cuff. Shave and, if necessary, lightly burr the cortical bone on the humerus adjacent to the cartilage edge, continuing laterally over the adjacent greater tuberosity. This area will be covered with neotendon as the healing cuff edge spreads out to regenerate the footprint of attachment (8).

AUTHOR'S PREFERRED TREATMENT

With the scope in the LAP, complete the preparation of the cuff. Remove the thin, dysvascular, feathered edge of tendon using a suction punch and shaver. Assess the pattern and mobility of the tear using a soft tissue grasper by way of the anterior and posterior cannulae. Plan the repair pattern to minimize tension and restore anatomy.

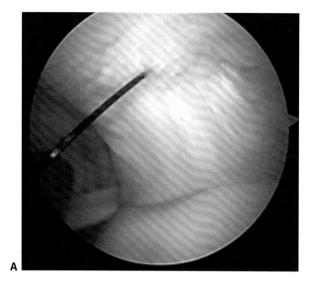

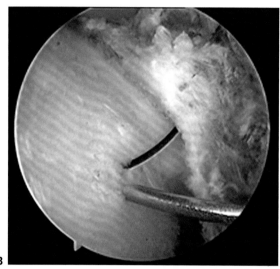

FIGURE 9.5. (A) A marker suture of PDS is placed into the articular side defect using a percutaneous spinal needle. **(B)** The PDS suture is located on the bursal side of the cuff and will mark the location of the underside cuff tear.

Side-to-Side Rotator Cuff Sutures

Placing side-to-side sutures to close the vertical component of an L-shaped tear has been an important advancement in the ability to repair larger lesions. The side-to-side sutures are important for two reasons: (1) they may help to realign the torn tendon ends with their insertion site on the humerus and (2) they relieve significant stress from the junction between the bone and the suture anchor.

To perform the stitch, use a suture hook loaded with a suture shuttling device. Insert the suture hook through the cannula that provides the most direct approach to the tear. Align the stitcher by laying it over the top of the tear in the direction of the desired stitch. If the tear is a V-shaped or an L-shaped tear, the first stitch should be medial near the apex.

At a point 1 cm from the edge, carefully pass the stitcher through the tendon, using a grasper for counter tension. Visualize the tip under the tendon, and pass it through the opposite side of the tear if possible. The shuttling device can then be advanced, grasped, and brought out the opposite portal. If the stitcher cannot reach through both sides of the tear a penetrating "bird beak"-type grasper can be used to retrieve the shuttle (or use a two-step suturing technique). Once outside the cannula, the shuttle is loaded with a strand of no. 2 braided suture and used to pass that suture across the tear (Fig. 9.6A–D).

Collect both braided suture limbs out the anterior or posterior cannula (whichever gives the best access to the tear) with a crochet hook, and tie them using a sliding/locking knot. The authors prefer the Samsung Medical Center (SMC) knot for braided sutures. Repeat the side-to-side stitches as often as needed to close the defect. It is debatable whether side-to-side sutures result in any healing of the rotator cuff, but there is good evidence that they result in a reduction in tear volume and in tension at the bone–anchor interface (9).

Suture Anchor Fixation of Rotator Cuff Tears to Bone

Modern implants offer multiple sutures per anchor. This advance provides the surgeon with the option of maximizing the number of effective sutures holding the tendon from each point of anchor fixation in the available greater tuberosity. Coons et al. (10) have shown biomechanical advantages of constructs with three simple sutures, thus lending support to the use of triple-loaded suture anchors. More recently, the use of triple-loaded anchors and three simple stitches has been further validated in comparison with various double-row configurations (11).

Viewing from the LAP, insert a spinal needle percutaneously next to the acromion to determine the proper position and angle for placement of the suture anchors. With careful positioning of the needle at the center of the tear, it may be possible to use one 3-mm stab incision for two or three anchors (Fig. 9.7). For larger tears, additional stab incisions may be required. The goal should be to direct the tip of the anchor slightly medially to achieve purchase in the denser subchondral bone as opposed the softer bone of the tuberosity. After identifying the best location, make a small stab incision with a no. 11 blade scalpel. The posterior anchor is inserted first unless an arthroscopic biceps tenodesis is planned, in which case the anterior anchor is implanted initially and used for the biceps and the first anterior cuff stitch.

The normal medial extent of the rotator cuff footprint is approximately 2 mm from the edge of the articular cartilage of the humeral head. Beginning posteriorly and working anteriorly, we prefer to create pilot holes for each anchor approximately 1 cm apart in the prepared bone, approximately 3 mm lateral from the articular edge

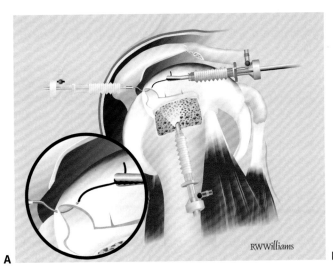

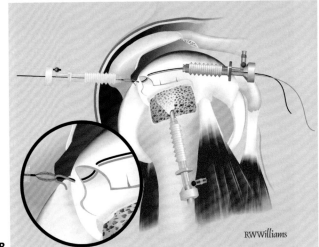

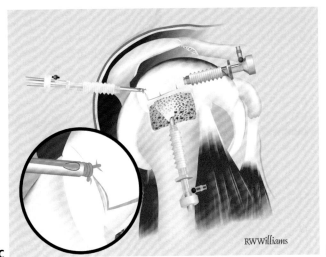

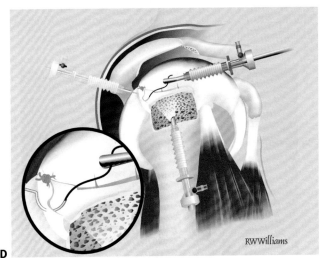

FIGURE 9.6. (**A**) A crescent shaped suture hook is passed the through the side to side cuff tear and a shuttle is retrieved out the opposite cannula. (**B**) A strand of braided suture is loaded in the shuttle and carried across the tear. (**C**) The sutures are tied using a sliding-locking knot. (**D**) Additional sutures are added using either the single pass technique or the "two-step" shuttle method to complete the repair.

(Fig. 9.8). The pilot holes serve as guides to the location and direction of anchor placement. Placing anchors medially instead of laterally minimizes tension on the repair while reestablishing a strong medial footprint. Insert the bone punch through the previously localized stab incision. For repairs requiring multiple anchors, direct each punch vector parallel or divergent to ensure that each anchor has a solid wall of surrounding bone. We utilize a 1-mm punch that is significantly smaller than the diameter of our self-tapping anchor as the pilot hole functions as a guide, but is not a necessity with this type of implant.

At this stage, insert the working cannula. We prefer to use a "docking cannula," or 7-mm Dry-Doc (ConMed/Linvatec, Largo, FL) for the anterior and posterior portals. A docking cannula is able to maintain the portal while minimizing fluid extravasation and permitting passage of all common stitching tools, affording easy removal and reinsertion without the need to screw the cannula through the tissues.

The ThRevo (ConMed Linvatec, Largo, FL) triple-loaded suture anchor is loaded with high-strength braided sutures in three different colors. Other brands of anchors may come triple loaded or may accommodate the addition of a third suture through the eyelet. The insertion handle for the ThRevo anchor has a vertical guide mark on the shaft positioned perpendicular to the eyelet opening. This mark allows the surgeon to identify the alignment of the sutures in relation to the rotator cuff. The alignment of the sutures becomes important later during knot tying in maintaining the ability of all three sutures to slide within the eyelet.

Insert the first anchor through the same small skin incision used for the punch. Screw it through the muscle and seat the tip in the pilot hole. Align the screw so that it follows the medial direction of the pilot hole, seating the anchor in the strong subchondral bone. The sutures are unloaded from the driver handle and the handle is removed. Pull with gentle tension on the suture ends to confirm that the anchor is well seated. Note the orientation

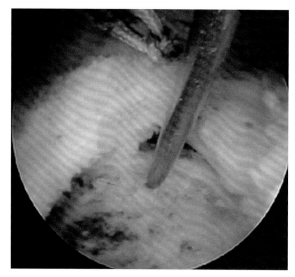

FIGURE 9.7. A spinal needle is used as a guide to select the appropriate position for the skin puncture for inserting the suture anchor.

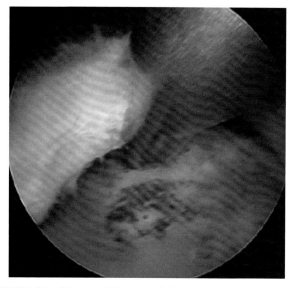

FIGURE 9.8. 9.8 A small bone punch is used to create a pilot hole for each suture anchor 4-5mm lateral from the edge of the articular cartilage.

of the sutures within the eyelet. Define the anterior, posterior, and middle sutures as well as which suture limbs exit the eyelet along the medial (cuff) side and which exit on the lateral (tuberosity) side. Retrieve the most posterior cuff-side suture out the anterior cannula using a crochet hook or suture grasper, taking care to stay medial to the remaining suture strands (Fig. 9.9A, B). This suture limb will be relayed through the cuff as the most posterior stitch in a posterior to anterior progression.

The suture hook that provides the best angle for stitching through the posterior portal should be chosen. A crescent-shaped hook is usually best for the most posterior stitch. Pass the hook through the cuff from top to bottom 8 mm posterior to the anchor and approximately 1 cm medial to the free edge. Visualize the needle tip exiting the

undersurface of the cuff end and feed the shuttle or relay suture into sight, taking care to include all undersurface lamina in the stitch.

Pass an arthroscopic grasper medial to the remaining sutures in the anchor through the anterior cannula. Grasp the shuttle near the tip of the needle. Feed the shuttle relay or PDS suture through the stitcher while carrying it out the anterior cannula with the grasper (Fig. 9.9C). It is imperative that the grasper, suture shuttle, and suture strand all follow the same medial path to avoid entanglement with the remaining unused strands.

Load the shuttle with the previously retrieved suture outside the anterior cannula and carry it back through the cuff from bottom to top and out the posterior portal. Retrieve the partner limb (tuberosity side) of this suture out the posterior cannula with the crochet hook (Fig. 9.9D, E). Because tying sutures at this point would restrict cuff mobility, we utilize Suture Savers (ConMed Linvatec, Largo, FL) to save the limbs outside the posterior cannula for later tying.

Placing multiple anchors in the shoulder can result in a somewhat crowded bursal space, making it critical to avoid inadvertent tangling of suture limbs and to keep partner sutures together. This task is simplified by placing paired limbs inside separate Suture Savers in a sequential manner as stitches are passed through the rotator cuff. This technique allows any number of sutures to be easily managed within the shoulder. Also, by leaving the initial sutures untied, it is much easier to pass the suturing devices under the edge of the tendon.

With the first suture pair in the posterior cannula, place a switching stick through the cannula into the bursa. Back the cannula out over the switching stick and retrieve the suture pair outside of the cannula. The paired limbs are then placed inside the first Suture Saver as it is advanced into the shoulder and the end is clamped to keep the Saver abutted against the cuff. Slide the cannula back into the shoulder over the switching stick. This completes the first stitch and demonstrates the cycle that will be repeated with the remaining sutures.

The cuff-side limb of the middle suture is then retrieved out the anterior cannula medial to the remaining unused sutures as previously described. Insert a suture hook again and pass it through the cuff from top to bottom in line with the middle of the anchor and 1 cm medial to the cuff edge. Depending on the tear configuration, a right- or left-curved suturing device is often better for passing this stitch. Advance the shuttle through the needle, carry it out the front, load the previously retrieved suture, and carry it back through the cuff (Fig. 9.10). This process is repeated for the anterior suture in the anchor, passing the suturing device through the cuff approximately 8 mm anterior to the anchor. Place these sutures in a Saver if additional anchors/sutures are to be placed.

Repeat the anchor, suture, and Saver steps for the remaining anchors as needed until the repair is complete (Fig. 9.11). By convention, we utilize the colored Suture Savers in the same order for all rotator cuff repairs

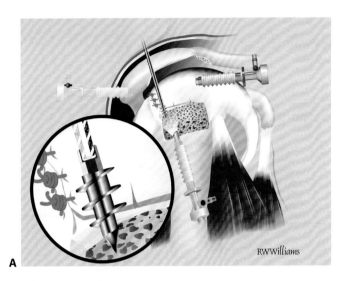

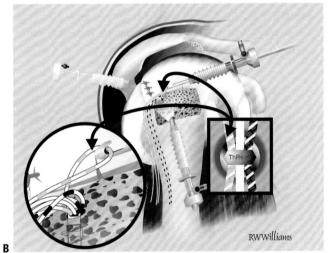

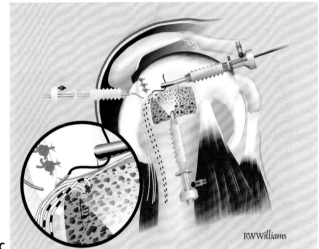

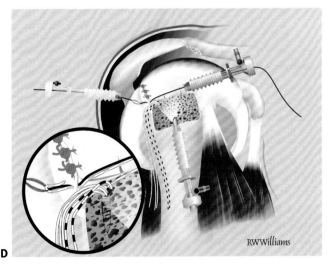

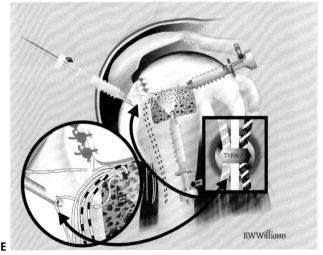

FIGURE 9.9. (**A**) The first anchor loaded with three sutures is inserted into the most poster pilot hole with eyelet aligned in the medial to lateral direction. (**B**) The medial limb of the posterior most suture is retrieved into the anterior cannula with a crochet hook. (**C**) A curved suture hook is passed through the most posterior free edge of the cuff tear about 5-6mm medial to the edge and a shuttle is passed and retrieved with a grasping clamp from the anterior cannula. (**D**) The shuttle is loaded with the suture in the anterior cannula and carried through the cuff and into the posterior cannula. (**E**) The partner of the first stitch is retrieved with a crochet hook into the posterior cannula taking care not to cross any of the sutures.

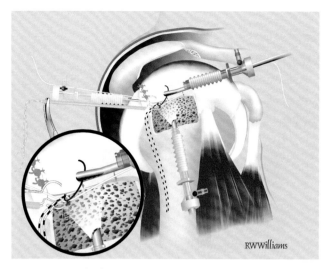

FIGURE 9.10. The first set of sutures is stored outside the posterior cannula using a small plastic straw which is clamped to keep it tight on the top of the cuff.

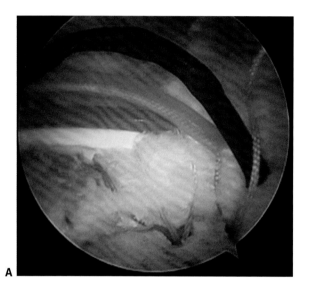

A

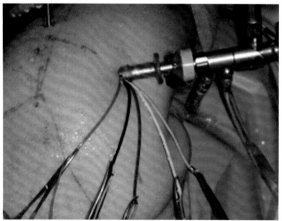

B

FIGURE 9.11. (A) The multicolored plastic suture straws hold the suture pairs together insuring that subsequent sutures are not entangled. (B) The multiple plastic suture straws are clamped outside the posterior cannula thereby holding the cuff is a reduced position.

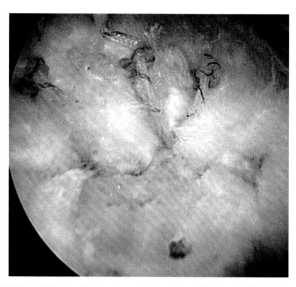

FIGURE 9.12. The finished repair has the cuff edge held firmly to the prepared bone with multiple simple sutures emanating from each anchor in a fan-like pattern.

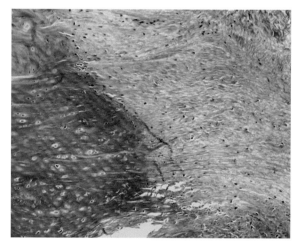

FIGURE 9.13. A biopsy of the regenerated footprint demonstrates the typical pattern of the multilayered enthesis of the rotator cuff tendon. The calcified cartilage stratum is not as wide as a normal tendon attachment but Sharpy's fibers are seen attaching into the bone.

to simplify the order of tying at the end of the case (Fig.9.12A, B). When tying the sutures, view from the posterior or anterior portal and retrieve the pairs with a crochet hook by way of the lateral portal. Discard the Saver and tie the sutures with a sliding locking knot (e.g., SMC knot) until the repair is complete (Fig. 9.12). (8, 12)

Crimson Duvet

Successful rotator cuff repair requires the reestablishment of the normal bone to tendon transition. This transition exists through an intermediate fibrocartilage zone that becomes progressively mineralized (Fig. 9.13). Uthoff and Himori noted that rotator cuff repairs would be subject to mechanical failure without this normal transition. Rodeo

(13) have clearly elucidated the progression toward collagen fiber continuity between tendon and bone during rotator cuff healing. Uthoff et al. (14) have demonstrated that the source of healing cells is from the bursa and proximal humerus, and that the tendinous stump has no intrinsic healing capacity.

Uthoff noted that establishing access through the subchondral bone permitted recruitment of marrow cells, thus allowing their participation in healing. A similar process is seen in the production of fibrocartilage through microfracture techniques commonly used in the knee and ankle. The access to marrow cells created results in a blanketing effect on the cuff footprint (Fig. 9.14A–C). This marrow blanket, or Crimson Duvet, provides the stem cells, platelets, and cytokines that result in formation of the normal bone tendon transition. Providing the appropriate biologic environment for healing of the rotator cuff tendon is every bit as important as creating secure biomechanical fixation of the tendon to bone.

COMPLICATIONS, CONTROVERSIES, AND SPECIAL CONSIDERATIONS

Avoidance of complications during arthroscopic rotator cuff repair requires attention to detail throughout the procedure. Anchor placement, stitching technique, and knot tying all present avenues for mistakes. Suboptimal surgical technique invites errors, which may affect outcomes. However, excellent technique will result in optimal tendon to bone fixation and lead to excellent surgical results (15–17).

Complications of rotator cuff repairs have been reported by various authors. Overall, reported complications are limited and include hardware failure as well as postoperative infections and stiffness. In well over 1,400 rotator cuff repairs performed by the senior author only three infections have been encountered. In two cases, anchors have become prominent and required removal. In these early cases, the anchors were placed too vertical in the footprint. Three patients required manipulation to restore motion caused by postoperative stiffness.

PEARLS

1. The technique should be practiced outside the operating room on models, at laboratories, or at courses. The surgeon who is comfortable with a mini-open approach can progress with the arthroscopic approach as far as possible and then convert to mini-open approach (possibly after a predetermined period of time) to critique the progress and technique.
2. Translucent cannulas should be used to maximize visualization. To accept most curved stitchers, flexible cannulas must be greater than 6.5 mm in diameter, whereas stiff cannulas must be greater than 8.0 mm. Two smooth metal switching sticks are invaluable when moving cannulas around the shoulder.

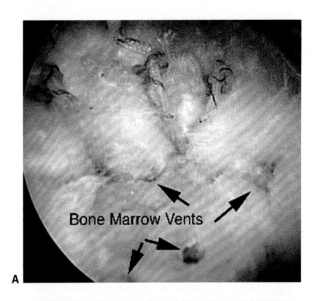

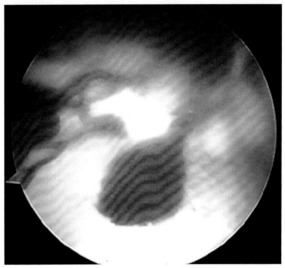

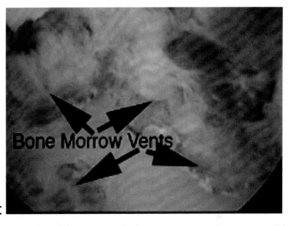

FIGURE 9.14. (A) Five to eight bone marrow vents are created by perforating the cortex of the tuberosity with a bone punch lateral to the rotator cuff attachment site. (B) When the fluid flow is turned off the bone marrow bubbles out of the vents and forms a rich velvety "super clot" bridging between the tuberosity and the cuff: the crimson duvet. (C) A plethora of vascular channels emanates from the bone marrow vents as seen in this second look evaluation.

3. Runoff bags should be carefully positioned to keep the patient dry.
4. Fluid pressure should be monitored and adjusted as needed to maximize visualization and minimize shoulder swelling.
5. Complete bursectomy, especially posteriorly and laterally, should be done early in the procedure because the bursa can swell over time and become a problem.
6. When grasping and shuttling sutures in and out of the shoulder, the surgeon must take care to watch the suture in the anchor eyelet so as to not unload it (i.e., pull it entirely out of the eyelet).

REHABILITATION

Appropriate rehabilitation following rotator cuff surgery is of great importance to successful operative outcomes. Many surgeons are concerned that patients will be non-compliant with their rehabilitation protocol. However, therapy that is too aggressive may be equally harmful to the patient. We advocate a phased rehabilitation that advances the patient based upon clinical symptomatology and the normal progression of rotator cuff tendon to bone healing.

The first phase of rehabilitation should emphasize preventing stiffness and decreasing pain and inflammation in the first 6 weeks after surgery. Patients are taught a set of gentle elbow, wrist, and hand range of motion exercises at the preoperative appointment and then reemphasize these exercises at their first post-op visit. Particular emphasis is placed on scapular mobilization and strengthening (e.g., shoulder shrugs), as well as gentle pendulum exercises and passive range of motion up to 90° of flexion. Patients are provided a printed copy of this simple protocol that includes diagrams. An abduction arm sling is used throughout the first phase of rehabilitation, but patients are encouraged to come out of their sling in the controlled environment of their own home to type on the computer, to feed themselves, and to perform waist to shoulder level activities of daily living.

During the second phase of rehabilitation, the patient builds upon the exercises from phase I by adding more active assist range of motion exercises. We also move patients toward their full-functional passive range of motion. During this phase, from weeks 6 through 12, we progressively increase strengthening activities starting with isometric cuff exercises and advancing to very gentle resistance band exercises near week 12. One of the primary goals of the second phase of therapy is to return the patient to the performance of all basic activities of daily living (ADL) with the operative extremity.

Phase III takes place from 12 to 24 weeks postoperatively and has the goal of returning the patient to pain-free overhead activities as well as progression to some activity-specific exercises. Patients who are clinically advancing at an appropriate pace are started on machine strengthening exercises as well as some basic coordination exercises (e.g., ball toss). The fourth phase of postoperative rehabilitation generally takes place after 24 weeks and has the goal of returning the patient to regular sporting activities with full strength in the operative shoulder.

CONCLUSIONS

Arthroscopic rotator cuff repair can be both challenging and rewarding to perform. Our technique was developed over many years, but is not the only one capable of achieving excellent results. We advocate a single-row repair due to the following advantages:

1. Minimizes tension
2. Utilizes the best bone for anchor purchase
3. Emphasizes biologic healing
4. Restores the anatomic footprint
5. Strength of triple-loaded suture anchors
6. Potential cost savings from a reduced number of anchors
7. No clinical difference versus double-row repairs in the literature

We encourage practicing these, and all arthroscopic shoulder techniques, on models or cadaveric specimens outside the operating room. With practice and experience, the numerous, seemingly complex steps can be mastered, enhancing the operative experience for both the surgeon and the patient.

REFERENCES

1. Morse K, Davis AD, Afra R, et al. Arthroscopic versus mini-open rotator cuff repair: a comprehensive review and meta-analysis. *Am J Sports Med.* 2008;36:1824–1828.
2. Kim HM, Teefey SA, Zelig A, et al. Shoulder strength in asymptomatic individuals with intact compared with torn rotator cuffs. *J Bone Joint Surg Am.* 2009;91:289–296.
3. Snyder SJ. Rotator cuff: introduction, evaluation, and imaging. In: *Shoulder Arthroscopy.* Philadelphia, PA: Lippincott Williams & Wilkins; 2003:189–200.
4. Bigliani LU, April EW. The morphology of the acromion and its relationship to rotator cuff tears. *Orthop Trans.* 1986;10:216.
5. Snyder SJ. A modified classification of the supraspinatus outlet view based on the configuration and the anatomic thickness of the acromion. In: *American Shoulder and Elbow Surgeons Annual Closed Meeting*; October 14, 1991; Seattle, WA.
6. Yamaguchi K, Tetro AM, Blam O, et al. Natural history of asymptomatic rotator cuff tears: a longitudinal analysis of asymptomatic tears detected sonographically. *J Shoulder Elbow Surg.* 2001;10:199–203.
7. Bond JL, Dopirak RM, Higgins J, et al. Arthroscopic replacement of massive, irreparable rotator cuff tears using a GraftJacket allograft: technique and preliminary results. *Arthroscopy.* 2008;24:403–409e1.

8. Burns JP, Snyder SJ, Albritton M. Arthroscopic rotator cuff repair using triple-loaded anchors, suture shuttles, and suture savers. *J Am Acad Orthop Surg.* 2007; 15:432–444.

9. Halder AM, O'Driscoll SW, Heers G, et al. Biomechanical comparison of effects of supraspinatus tendon detachments, tendon defects, and muscle retractions. *J Bone Joint Surg Am.* 2002;84:780–785.

10. Coons DA, Barber FA, Herbert MA. Triple-loaded single-anchor stitch configurations: an analysis of cyclically loaded suture-tendon interface security. *Arthroscopy.* 2006;22:1154–1158.

11. Barber FA, Schroeder FA, Aziz-Jacobo J, et al. Biomechanical advantages of triple loaded suture anchors compared with double row cuff repairs. *Arthroscopy.* 2010;26:316–323.

12. Kim SH, Ha KI. The SMC knot—a new slip knot with locking mechanism. *Arthroscopy.* 2000;16:563–565.

13. Rodeo SA. Biologic augmentation of rotator cuff tendon repair. *J Shoulder Elbow Surg.* 2007;16:S191–S197.

14. Uhthoff HK, Trudel G, Himori K. Relevance of pathology and basic research to the surgeon treating rotator cuff disease. *J Orthop Sci.* 2003;8 449–456.

15. Watson EM, Sonnabend DH. Outcome of rotator cuff repair. *J Shoulder Elbow Surg.* 2002;11:201–211.

16. Burns JP, Snyder SJ. Arthroscopic rotator cuff repair in patients younger than fifty years of age. *J Shoulder Elbow Surg.* 2008;17:90–96.

17. Murray TF Jr, Lajtai G, Mileski RM, et al. Arthroscopic repair of medium to large full-thickness rotator cuff tears: outcome at 2- to 6-year follow-up. *J Shoulder Elbow Surg.* 2002;11:19–24.

I. The Shoulder

Arthroscopic Cuff Repair: Double-Row Options

Robert A. Pedowitz

The purpose of rotator cuff repair is to restore a biomechanically sound, anatomically accurate, and durable connection between the torn cuff tendons and the humeral head. The surgeon has limited abilities to achieve these objectives due to various factors, many of which are out of his/her direct control. These factors include the preexisting state of the muscle–tendon unit (including tendon retraction and muscle atrophy, fatty infiltration, and connective tissue changes), the biomechanical stability of the repair construct, the healing potential of the bone–tendon interface, and the rehabilitation protocol and postoperative activities/compliance of the patient. The complex interplay between these factors makes objective interpretation of surgical repair strategies very difficult and probably explains the confusing discrepancies between laboratory biomechanical experiments and clinical outcome studies when we consider double-row rotator cuff repair.

Normal tendons rarely tear in the first place. Therefore, it seems logical that unraveling the underlying cause(s) of tendonopathy will provide important clues about possible solutions to this ubiquitous and challenging clinical problem. The biology of tendonopathy is germane to tendon disorders throughout the body. However, we should be very careful not to directly extrapolate findings from one tendon site to another because there may be subtle differences in cellular composition, gene expression, and local factors (such as blood supply or biomechanical factors) that would make therapeutic interventions highly variable in terms of regional efficacy. It is likely that in the future we will be better able to manipulate the biologic elements of the healing process, with a higher degree of clinical success. Nonetheless, a fundamental requirement will continue to be creation of a repair construct that is stable throughout the healing interval (even if that interval becomes shorter), so we will continue to strive for surgical strategies that are reproducible, reliable, and durable.

Arthroscopic rotator cuff repair has evolved to the point where patients can expect clinical outcomes that are similar to open or mini-open methods, and these results have been reviewed previously within this book. Arthroscopic outcomes are in part related to the surgical skill and experience of the operating surgeon, and there is a significant learning curve associated with these techniques. This field is rapidly advancing in terms of the surgical tools and implants at our disposal. We have almost reached a point where reports of clinical results are outdated by the time articles achieve publication because the surgical techniques are evolving so rapidly.

Advances in surgical technique, implants, and equipment have substantially improved our ability to tackle larger and more complex tears while simultaneously extending the general capabilities of surgeons to achieve good clinical outcomes (in other words, arthroscopic rotator cuff repair is no longer limited to the domain of "master arthroscopists"). It is critical to understand that the clinical outcome of rotator cuff repair depends upon surgical creation of a stable tendon–bone construct: regardless of whether that is achieved through arthroscopic or open methods (these principles are presented in Table 10.1). The surgical approach should therefore be dictated by the skill and preference of the operating surgeon in concert with informed consent regarding the pros and cons of the specific approach with the patient. At the current time, there is no clear evidence that long-term clinical outcome is markedly affected by the surgical approach with rotator cuff repair. However, patients clearly appreciate the advantages of less early postoperative pain and improved cosmetics associated with minimally invasive techniques, so it is likely that the indications for arthroscopic cuff repair will continue to expand (assuming at least long-term clinical equivalence).

HISTORY AND RATIONALE FOR THE DEVELOPMENT OF DOUBLE-ROW REPAIR

It is fascinating and humbling to look back at the history of surgery and to appreciate the amazing intuition of the early pioneers of orthopedic surgery. Early methods of rotator cuff repair involved wide open exposure of the rotator cuff, which was achieved by deltoid takedown and subsequent repair. Before the advent of suture anchors, the cuff was repaired to the bone with sutures that were

---

Table 10.1

Basic principles of rotator cuff repair, regardless of surgical approach

- Identification of tear pattern and extent, which usually requires bursectomy
- Removal of offending bone and soft tissue impingement (smoothing)
- Mental visualization of the repair strategy
- Mobilization of the tendon
- Stimulation of a biologic healing response
- Stable fixation of rotator cuff to bone
- Solid repair of structures violated by the approach, particularly the deltoid

---

passed through small holes in the greater tuberosity, the so-called transosseous repair. When the sutures were tied circumferentially around the tendon and the bone, the surgeon essentially achieved a footprint repair, with a point of medial fixation adjacent to the articular surface and a zone of more lateral compression of the tendon toward the tuberosity. Early strategies focused upon lateralizing the torn cuff to achieve a water tight repair if possible, and it is likely that the various patterns of cuff tearing and reduction were under-appreciated (with associated tension mismatch as attempts were made to overlateralize the cuff). The era of arthroscopy has clearly augmented our understanding of tear pattern (e.g., U-shaped vs L-shaped tears). Proper tendon reduction leads to better soft tissue balance, decreased tension overload, and a lower propensity for retear during the rehabilitation period.

The advent of suture anchors and early arthroscopic methods led to new surgical alternatives, including arthroscopic subacromial decompression and mini-open cuff repair. This method decreased the morbidity associated with deltoid takedown and repair. Deltoid splitting methods could also utilize transosseous cuff repair with sutures if desired; however, exposure of the greater tuberosity was somewhat limited by the acceptable extent of distal deltoid split (due to risk to the axillary nerve).

As arthroscopic skill and experience advanced, rotator cuff repair focused upon our surgical ability to place suture anchors in bone, pass sutures through cuff, manage multiple subacromial sutures, and tie reliable arthroscopic knots. In the 1990s, various tools and obturated cannulas were developed to assist with arthroscopic suture passage, and these tools continue to evolve today. Antegrade methods, retrograde methods, and shuttling techniques allowed for accurate passage of sutures through the tendon, which was further facilitated by various safe portals in the region to create the proper trajectories for arthroscopic instruments. Subsequently, so-called super-sutures were introduced that markedly decreased the tendency for suture breakage during knot tying. These sutures increase the

durability of the repair construct, assuming the suture anchors remain in their original position and solid knots that reliably resist suture slippage are created.

In the first decade of the new millennium, appreciation of the anatomy of the rotator cuff "footprint" reemerged. Although the medial–lateral extent of anatomic cuff attachment has been understood for many decades, arthroscopic application of this information became a topic of strong interest upon the presentation of compelling visual examples of normal footprint anatomy (Fig. 10.1). The theoretical and practical pros and cons of arthroscopic footprint repair are presented in Table 10.2. The rest of this chapter essentially deals with our current knowledge regarding these advantages and disadvantages. Suffice it to say, the jury is still out when it comes to double-row repair, and it is likely that our knowledge, experience, and clinical algorithms will mature substantially over the next 5 to 10 years.

FOOTPRINT RESTORATION AND BIOMECHANICAL STABILITY

The published data in regard to the biomechanics of double-row rotator cuff repair are relatively confusing (Table 10.3). To date, laboratory data are relatively compelling in terms of improved contact area and contact force between tendon and tuberosity, when comparing single-row against double-row constructs. It should be

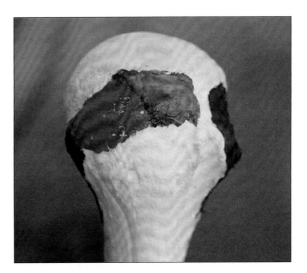

FIGURE 10.1. The rotator cuff has a broad medial–lateral insertional footprint. The supraspinatus (shown in *green*) extends from the articular surface of the humerus laterally approximately 15 mm. Note the oblique anterior extension of the infraspinatus (shown in *red*) whose fibers sweep forward and blend with the posterior fibers of the supraspinatus tendon. This architecture correlates with common L-shaped tears that propagate medially between the supraspinatus and the infraspinatus muscles and tend to have horizontal split components as well. (Reproduced with permission from Curtis AS, Burbank KM, Tierney JJ, et al. The insertional footprint of the rotator cuff: an anatomic study. *Arthroscopy* 2006;22(6):603–609.e1.)

Table 10.2	
Theoretical and practical pros and cons of arthroscopic footprint repair	
Pros	**Cons**
Increased contact area between tuberosity and cuff should augment bone–tendon healing	Overtension of a chronically retracted cuff could lead to tension overload/mismatch and early construct failure
Greater cuff apposition and more anchors and sutures should improve biomechanical stability	More suture anchors and longer surgical time may increase cost compared with simpler arthroscopic repair methods
Anatomic restoration of the footprint should lead to better long-term rotator cuff function and durability	Increased technical complexity may lead to an unacceptably long learning curve for the typical arthroscopist
Some double-row methods avoid arthroscopic knot tying, which should simplify the surgical technique	More implants and sutures could interfere with revascularization of the cuff, with a negative impact on healing

emphasized that most laboratory experiments use animal or human cadaveric tissue and involve creation of cuff defects that are repaired immediately, thus these models minimize the adverse but clinically relevant impact of excessive cuff tension (due to chronic retraction and/or tension mismatch). Nonetheless, laboratory data do support the notion that the area of tendon–bone apposition is augmented by double row and therefore it is logical to attempt footprint restoration if possible (assuming this theoretical advantage leads to better clinical results and the method is not outweighed by the "cons" noted in Table 10.2).

In contrast to the relatively consistent data regarding footprint restoration, laboratory studies of biomechanical stability/durability with double-row repair are more inconsistent and harder to interpret (Table 10.3). This is probably due to the wide variety of experimental paradigms and loading protocols that are applied in these studies. A thoughtful review by Reardon and Maffulli (6) provides a good overview of the background and scientific basis for double-row repair. This literature review suggests that there is good evidence for increased footprint coverage with double-row techniques and more inconsistent but generally positive biomechanical rationale. The authors conclude that we do not yet have strong clinical evidence of a difference in clinical outcome between single and double-row techniques.

Most experimental studies utilize a static position of the glenohumeral joint with direct medial pull of the supraspinatus to analyze cuff repair construct stability. However, recent evidence strongly suggests that the tendon–bone interface is asymmetrically loaded as a function of humeral rotation and abduction (13). Although this is a completely intuitive concept, relatively a few data are currently available in regard to the stability of various cuff repair constructs under these more physiologic

conditions. A critical implication of this concept is that it may be advantageous to avoid some rotational positions during the early postoperative period to minimize extremes of cuff tension: in other words, it may be better to limit passive motion until moderate healing and bone–tendon stability are achieved after rotator cuff repair. Solid clinical outcome data are not available to answer this important question, and a potentially adverse impact upon long-term shoulder range of motion must be considered as well.

Some of the footprint restoration constructs involve passage of sutures from medial, periarticular suture anchors, superiorly through the cuff, with lateral fixation of the sutures either by a direct lateral transfer or by a crossing configuration (see below). These methods are convenient because they do not require arthroscopic suture tying. However, from a biomechanical perspective, these techniques probably transfer a large part of the suture load to the lateral anchors when medial tension is applied to the construct. Unfortunately, bone quality is sometimes poor in the greater tuberosity (especially in the setting of a chronic cuff tear) and many of the current surgical methods involve a lateral "punch-in" anchor in order to fix the sutures in position. Punch-in anchors tend to be biomechanically weaker than similarly sized screw in anchors, especially in osteoporotic bone. In addition, simple passage of the sutures through the tendon (without a knot) is likely to increase the propensity of the sutures to cut through the tendon itself (compared with mattress sutures with bursal-sided knots or some kind of tendon augmentation with a suture loop just lateral to the point of suture egress). Unfortunately these methods require operative time and arthroscopic dexterity. Nonetheless, it is probably mechanically advantageous to stabilize the medial points of fixation prior to lateral suture

Table 10.3

Biomechanical studies of double-row rotator cuff repair

Better	No Difference
Double-row vs single-row	Double-row vs single-row
Footprint Restoration	
Mazzocca [AJSM] (2005) (15)	
Footprint area	
Tuoheti [AJSM] (2005) (16)	
Contact area, contact force (1)	
Meier and Meier [JSES] (2006)	
Footprint area	
Nelson (Arthroscopy) [2008] (17)	
Contact area	
Biomechanical Stability	
Waltrip [AJSM] (2003) (18)	
Tested with cyclic load	
Meier [ORS] (2005) (19)	Mazzocca [AJSM] (2005)
Cycles to 10-mm gap formation	Displacement or load to failure
Meier [AANA] (2005) (20)	
Displacement with internal/external rotation	
Kim [AJSM] (2006) (21)	
Gap formation, stiffness	
Ma [JBJS] (2006) (22)	Ma [JBJS] (2006)
Stronger vs single and Mason-Allen	Same as massive cuff stitch
Smith [JBJS] (2006) (23)	Mahar et al. [Arthroscopy] (2007)
Gap less, failure load higher	No difference single vs double row (2)
Baums [Knee Surg ST Arth] (2008) (27)	Nelson [Arthroscopy] (2008)
Compared with Mason-Allen sutures	No difference single vs double row
Hepp [Arch Orthop Trauma Surg] (2008) (25)	
Better double-layer, double-row repair	
Ahmad et al. [AJSM] (2008)	
Better when tested with rotational loads (3)	
Lorbach et al. [AJSM] (2008)	Zheng et al. [JBJS] (2008)
Different: various double-row methods (4)	Little difference: double-row methods (5)

bridging. In a recent study, Busfield and coworkers et al. (7) demonstrated the biomechanical advantage of medial knots in a double-row repair in human cadaveric shoulders, as opposed to simple transtendon sutures that were "bridged" laterally. We demonstrated very similar findings in our laboratory using a bovine cuff repair model utilizing suture anchors Leek et al. (26).

These biomechanical studies emphasize two very important points when critically assessing the laboratory literature in application to clinical practice: (1) cuff tears and "double-row repairs" are not created equal and therefore clinical results are expected to be quite variable (especially when we add the substantial clinical variables of tissue condition, technical performance, and postoperative rehabilitation) and (2) surgeons must spend sufficient time attending to the technical details of double-row repair in order to achieve biomechanically superior results (in other words, shortcuts such as avoidance of arthroscopic knot tying may not lead to improved clinical outcomes).

SURGICAL METHODS OF DOUBLE-ROW REPAIR

It is critical to understand cuff tear pattern and retraction before initiating repair. This is probably the single most important step in arthroscopic rotator cuff surgery. Anatomic understanding is augmented by reduction maneuvers that involve diagonal and lateral translation in various directions. Usually it becomes obvious where the tendons seem to "fit," if sufficient time is spent with the exercise. Occasionally traction sutures can be quite helpful, in order to minimize the crushing effect of powerful grasping tools. These traction sutures can also assist with subsequent suture passage maneuvers.

Tendon releases may be needed prior to determination of the ideal reduction position, freeing up the cuff from bursa, coracocohumeral ligament (anterior interval slide), labrum and capsule (internal release), and even through sectioning between the supraspinatus and the infraspinatus (posterior interval slide) or mobilization of the suprascapular nerve. These methods are described elsewhere in this text. Suffice it to say, when heroic tendon releases become necessary, there is a good chance that the rotator cuff repair will fail, regardless of the footprint repair strategy. In my opinion, the most important priority is creation of a stable construct that does not cause tension overload or tension mismatch, and in some cases, partial cuff repair with restoration of the anteroposterior force couple may be prudent, compared with heroic measures that are bound to be associated with a mechanical/biologic failure at the bone–tendon interface.

It is useful to carefully evaluate preoperative imaging studies because medial tear retraction and muscle atrophy/fatty infiltration are associated with greater difficulty in achieving anatomic footprint restoration. In addition, cuff tears that originally occurred medial to the enthesis will lead to relative difficulty when we try to pull the residual edge of the cuff to the normal lateral footprint margin, due to associated lack of tendon tissue for repair. In this situation, it might be prudent to create a periarticular repair configuration to avoid tension overload.

In our zeal to cover the anatomic footprint, it is easy to overtension the cuff or create a nonanatomic configuration, particularly when the cuff is fixed with the arm in a position of significant abduction. Overtension is a particular pitfall for L-shaped tears that, with time, start to look like U-shaped tears. L-shaped tears should first be managed with side-to-side sutures that not only help to reduce the tear (thereby facilitating anatomic footprint restoration) but also help to stress relieve the tendon–bone interface. It is not known whether side-to-side sutures result in side-to-side healing of the cuff defect. Even if such healing does not occur, these sutures are still advantageous for stress relief of the suture anchors. Logically it is therefore not entirely clear whether absorbable or nonabsorbable sutures should be used for side-to-side repair. Surgeons should be thoughtful about the amount of permanent suture material in the subacromial space because large suture knots can occasionally rub against the undersurface of the acromion, and the associated clicking or squeaking can be irritating for the patient.

The footprint area should be gently "stimulated" in order to create a bleeding response since the bone appears to be critical for access to blood supply and possibly stem cells and growth factors that contribute to healing. Punctuate bleeding can be achieved by minimal decortication, which is clearly advantageous because cortical bone purchase is much better than cancellous bone purchase by suture anchors (especially in elderly, osteoporotic bone). Care should be taken if a burr is used for surface debridement, and in many cases, a shaver or small curette is a safer way to stimulate the bone without excess cortical removal. Some surgeons advocate deliberate access to marrow elements, essentially through a microfracture or drilling method to encourage creation of a local fibrin clot. If holes are created in the tuberosity, it is important not to violate the bone to the degree that mechanical stability of suture anchors becomes jeopardized. A positive clinical impact of tuberosity microfracture compared with superficial bone preparation has not been demonstrated, to date.

Early arthroscopic methods of cuff repair recapitulated traditional open methods of preliminary subacromial decompression. It has become clear in recent years that a large amount of acromial resection is not needed for successful clinical outcome. However, a basic biologic principle is that soft tissues do not "like" focal areas of compression, as compared with application of uniform tissue compression, which is actually tolerated quite well (a somewhat obtuse example is the deep sea diver who withstands enormous degrees of *uniform* tissue compression, without adverse effect). The point here is that biologic tissues do not thrive upon *points* of compression. The logical extension of this principle is that the acromion and coracoclavicular ligament should be sculpted in order to create a smooth and uniform undersurface. In my opinion, sufficient bursectomy and acromial exposure are required in order to evaluate and obviate spurs and points of compression that could compromise the cuff repair. Wide bone excision is not required.

Rotator cuff repair to bone should be performed upon completion of tissue mobilization, analysis of reduction, and tuberosity/subacromial preparation. Some surgeons choose to complete the acromial bone work after completion of the cuff repair in order to minimize bone bleeding that might interfere with visualization. The order of business is essentially "dealer's choice," but I have not found bone bleeding to be a major problem (given the combination of appropriate management of systemic blood pressure by the anesthesiologist, an arthroscopic pump, careful outflow and turbulence control, and radiofrequency ablation and coagulation). I personally like the idea of completion of bone work arthroscopically first, so that in the rare event of a need for "bail out" from arthroscopy, the cuff repair can be performed by extension of the lateral portal into a mini-open approach (without needing to do any more acromial work, which can be relatively difficult without taking down the deltoid).

The surgeon must now decide if a double-row repair/footprint restoration is feasible, and if so, various surgical methods can be utilized to achieve the goals of increased contact area and stable fixation. Early descriptions of arthroscopic double-row cuff repair involved placement of medial, periarticular anchors as well as laterally positioned anchors. The medial anchors were used for placement of medial mattress sutures, whereas the lateral anchors typically utilized simple sutures around the lateral margin of the cuff (Fig. 10.2). With this method, care must be taken to create a tight suture loop and a solid knot at the medial row, in order to position the medial repair margin against the tuberosity. The undersurface of the cuff is obviously impossible to see from the bursal surface, and it is educational to look at the undersurface of the cuff after completion of the repair (particularly watching this interface with gentle rotation of the arm).

The "second generation" of double-row repairs involves insertion of medial periarticular anchors, with superior transfer of sutures through the cuff and lateral capture of the sutures in a laterally based anchor. The lateral anchor is often a punch-in design although some methods involve a screw-in anchor that is designed to capture the suture. This construct has been coined the "transosseous equivalent" because it mimics the points of fixation achieved by open methods whereby sutures are passed through the tuberosity and circumferentially

around the cuff (Fig. 10.3). A variation on this theme involves a suture crossing strategy, whereby some sutures are passed obliquely from medial to lateral. The objective of this repair is to augment the compressed area of cuff against bone and to increase frictional purchase on the tendon itself (Fig. 10.4).

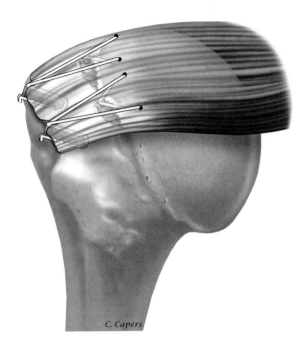

FIGURE 10.3. A double-row rotator cuff repair strategy utilizing medial "puncture" sutures that are bridged laterally to two additional points of fixation. This is a so-called transosseous equivalent repair.

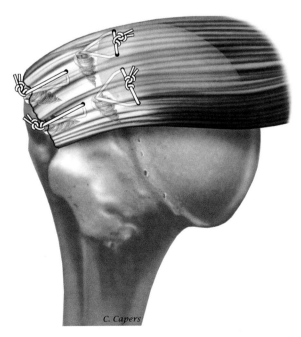

FIGURE 10.2. A double-row rotator cuff repair strategy utilizing two medial mattress sutures and two lateral simple sutures.

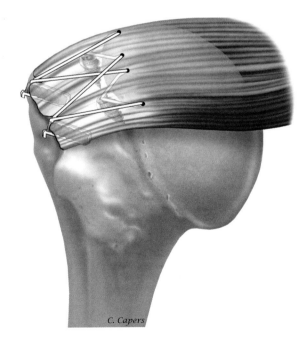

FIGURE 10.4. A double-row rotator cuff repair strategy utilizing medial "puncture" sutures, whereby some sutures are "crossed" laterally before being captured at the lateral points of fixation.

If simple lateral transfer of the sutures is selected, a nice alternative is creation of a small anteroposterior suture loop within the tendon (which still requires knot tying) just lateral to the point of egress of the sutures from the medial suture anchor, so that with lateral suture fixation/medial muscle tension, the transferred suture can load against the suture loop (instead of cutting through the tendon itself). However, this method does not solve the problem of stress transfer to the lateral punch-in anchor with potential anchor displacement, which is still a real concern in soft bone.

As noted previously, although it is relatively quick for the surgeon, there are some potential biomechanical disadvantages of simple transfer of the medial sutures through the tendon (without medial, bursal-sided knots), in terms of lateral anchor load and the potential for medial suture cut-through within the tendon itself. Therefore, some surgeons recommend medial mattress sutures and bursal-sided knots, prior to lateral suture transfer and stabilization, using a crossing technique for the laterally directed sutures (Fig. 10.5). This is my current preferred surgical method of footprint restoration even though it takes a bit of time to pass the medial sutures and create good arthroscopic knots.

PEARLS AND PITFALLS

The most important steps of arthroscopic cuff repair happen between the surgeon's ears, in terms of mental preparation, planning, and understanding of cuff reduction. In my opinion, the biggest pitfall is excessive emphasis upon

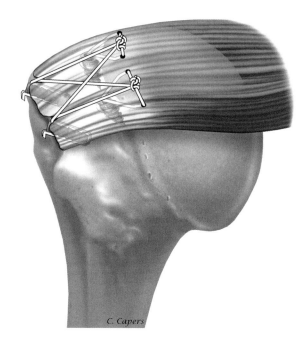

C. Capers

FIGURE 10.5. A double-row rotator cuff repair strategy utilizing medial mattress sutures, which are tied and then either crossed or passed directly for capture at the lateral points of fixation.

speed, which can lead to technical errors, significant frustration, and compromised outcomes. For example, sutures can tangle, anchors can unload, and knots can be inadequate, but these pitfalls are usually avoided by planning, practice, and patience.

Cuff visualization is a critical element of successful cuff repair. In my opinion, even though the bursa does contain some blood supply that might help with cuff healing, this biologic impact will be irrelevant if the cuff is not fixed securely and anatomically. For that reason, I recommend a wide and thorough bursectomy, taking care to control all small bleeders along the way. The bursa always seems to swell as the procedure goes along, particularly in the posterior part of the subacromial space, and it is better to be more thorough in the early part of the case. I like to take the bursa back posteriorly just anterior to the subdeltoid fascia. It is helpful to release the bursa down into the lateral gutter (taking care to protect the axillary nerve) and anteriorly as well. This can sometimes be accomplished using the blunt introducer from the scope, in a sweeping fashion down the gutters. This seems to allow deltoid to float away from the cuff and creates a useful working space. Sometimes a small "slit" can be created in the subdeltoid fascia to simplify instrument passage in and out of portals, but care should be taken not to be too aggressive because excessive fluid leakage from large portals will make hemostasis more difficult.

If a cuff repair is anticipated, it is very helpful to make the posterior scope portal somewhat lateral, just medial to the posterolateral margin of the acromion. This position is not ideal for intra-articular work (a more medial portal is better for labral and instability surgery), but usually the clinical indications for the arthroscopy make this decision easy preoperatively. However, having the scope a bit more lateral makes visualization of the cuff tear much easier. Placement of the scope in the lateral portal itself is also an important part of the case, and it is surprising how much different the cuff tear looks from this vantage point. If this so-called 50-yd line view is utilized, it helps to avoid pistoning in and out of the subacromial space with the scope. A good assistant is therefore a significant advantage for these kinds of procedures because the assistant will either need to hold the scope or pick up sutures during the case. It is much more difficult to perform a double-row cuff repair without a skilled and experienced surgical assistant.

Arthroscopic cannulas are essential for arthroscopic rotator cuff repair. These instruments are critical for passing sutures with antegrade suture passers (otherwise sutures will get caught up in the subcutaneous tissues), and they are absolutely required for arthroscopic knot tying. An important pearl is to always tie sutures alone within the cannula. It is much better to shuttle other sutures out of the way (and it just takes a moment to do this); otherwise sutures will become tangled within the cannula, with significant associated frustration. Usually there are several alterative locations to move sutures around. It is also generally better to make an extra portal for visualization or suture management than it is to struggle with poorly placed portals. There is little morbidity, and most patients do not find the cosmetic impact of an extra portal disturbing.

Placement of suture anchors should be performed using the appropriate trajectory, which is generally perpendicular to the cortical bone surface. For the medial anchors especially, the trajectory is rarely ideal through the lateral portal that was utilized for subacromial decompression. Use of this portal risks slipping of the anchor off the surface of the bone, with potential damage to the articular surface itself. The correct trajectory for the periarticular anchors usually involves creation of a small stab incision just off the anterolateral acromial margin. Skin markings that were placed at the beginning of the case always seem to migrate as the shoulder swells, so it is important to accurately localize this position using a spinal needle. This portal can be quite small—just large enough to pass the suture anchor insertion device and does not require a cannula (but the portal can be widened by the blunt introducer from the scope sheath, which makes passage of the anchor a bit easier). This can also be a useful portal for shuttling sutures around during knot tying (to get sutures out of the way), but it is not a good idea to tie sutures through this stab incision, as noted above.

It is usually possible to move around the humeral head under the acromion by internal/external rotation and abduction/adduction to achieve proper anchor trajectories. However, if needed, addition stab incisions can be created around the margin of the acromion. This may be particularly useful for anchors that are required for repair of far posterior cuff tears.

In terms of suture passage and order of knot tying, there are a couple of pearls worth mentioning. It is

generally better to place side-to-side sutures first, with knot tying, in order to help with cuff reduction and subsequent anatomic positioning. However, it is usually better to pass most or all the anchor-related sutures prior to knot tying because once the cuff is opposed to tuberosity, it can become difficult or impossible to pass instruments beneath the cuff for subsequent suture passage. Be careful with sharp suture passers and cuff "stabbers" because of the potential for articular cartilage damage and the risk of suture "nicking." This can significantly weaken the suture and lead to breakage during knot tying. A useful trick is to move posterior to anterior during suture placement and then anterior to posterior during suture tying. This approach tends to minimize risks of suture tangling and inadvertent snaring of previously placed sutures. Finally, it is important for the surgeon to be facile with both sliding and nonsliding knots. Sometimes a mattress suture or the second suture in a double-loaded suture anchors would not slide, and therefore a non sliding knot must be used for the repair. If that is needed, a nice trick is to have an assistant use a tool to oppose the cuff against the tuberosity while the surgeon passes hitches to create and lock the knot. This maneuver decreases the tendency for the tissue to spring away from the bone during knot tying.

CLINICAL OUTCOME OF DOUBLE-ROW ROTATOR CUFF REPAIR

Despite the theoretical advantages of footprint restoration, at this time there is no strongly compelling clinical evidence to support superiority of double-row repair compared with single-row repair (Table 10.4). An excellent critical review of clinical outcome data was presented by Reardon and Mafulli in 2007 (6), and there are some

Table 10.4

In vivo and clinical studies of double-row rotator cuff repair

Better	No Difference
Double-row vs Single-row	Double-row vs Single-row
Sugaya [Arthroscopy] (2005) (27)	Sugaya [Arthroscopy] (2005) (11)
Better MR appearance, double row	Clinical outcome same as single row
Charousset et al. [AJSM] (2007)	Charousset et al. [AJSM] (2007) (8)
Better "anatomy" by CT arthrography (8)	No clinical outcome difference
Ozbaydar [JBJS (Br)] (2008) (28)	Franceschi et al. [AJSM] (2007)
Better healing in rabbit tendon repairs	Randomized prospective study (9)
	Reardon and Mafulli [Arthroscopy] (2007)
	No evidence, critical literature review (6)
	Grasso et al. [Arthroscopy] (2009)
	Randomized prospective study (10)

important recent studies that further emphasize the point. It is likely that in the next few years, even in the interval between writing and publishing this chapter, more clinical information will become available to better clarify the best indications and methods of footprint restoration. Suffice it to say that, at the moment, this topic is still controversial and it is ultimately up to the judgment, skill, experience, and discretion of the treating surgeon to select a patient-specific course of action.

Charousset et al. (8) reported on a prospective, non-randomized clinical comparison of single- versus double-row repair. Although these authors noted a better healing rate with double-row repair by CT arthrography, there was no difference in observed clinical outcome measured by the constant score. Around the same time, Sugaya et al. (11) described their clinical results with double-row cuff repair. These authors noted general improvement with double-row repair, and an increased retear rate was noted on MRI with large and massive tears; however, there was no control or comparison group to assess a difference from single-row techniques. Lafosse and coworkers (2007) (29) described very good clinical outcomes with double-row methods, compared with historical outcomes, and observed better clinical results in patients with a healed cuff compared with patients with a residual or recurrent cuff defect. Huijsmans et al. (12) also noted good clinical outcomes after double-row repair in a large patient cohort. Park et al. (14) observed better clinical results in massive tears repaired with a dual-row method compared with single-row repair, whereas no clinical outcome differences were observed with small- to medium-sized tears according to repair method.

It should be emphasized that the articles noted in the prior paragraph are limited by the lack of randomized control groups (in terms of comparison with single-row repair methods), so strong clinical conclusions regarding superiority of double-row methods cannot be established by these reports. It is very important to understand that historical controls are not sufficient for strong evidence-based conclusions, especially in this setting, because surgical skills, instruments, and overall clinical experience have been in rapid evolution over the last decade or so (therefore any change in clinical outcomes might have nothing to do with the exact technical method of cuff repair and could have more to do with overall clinical experience in this field).

Franceschi et al. (9) published an excellent clinical investigation of double-row repair. This well-designed randomized prospective study found no significant difference in 2-year clinical outcome between single and double-row repairs although the number of patients in the two groups was relatively small (30 per group). Grasso et al. (10) also performed a randomized, prospective study of single-row versus double-row rotator cuff repair (medial mattress and lateral simple sutures). At 2-year follow-up, there was no difference in clinical outcome between the two groups.

AUTHOR'S RECOMMENDED TREATMENT ALGORITHM AND FUTURE DIRECTIONS

Given the clinical evidence provided above, it would be tempting to condemn double-row/footprint restoration and to rely upon single-row repair for arthroscopic cuff repair. However, the lack of strong clinical evidence is probably due to the complexity of this condition, the variability of surgical repair, and the challenges of postoperative rehabilitation. A more compelling question might be, Why not do a footprint restoration, if it is technically possible? This question is best answered by a look at the theoretical disadvantages of double-row repair, presented earlier in Table 10.2.

It is true that the cost of additional suture anchors is a real factor, and this must be a consideration in the "big picture" of healthcare costs and our local surgical environments (i.e., for hospitals and surgery centers). However, this should not be the driving factor for a specific patient who depends on our best efforts to create the ideal clinical outcome. Technical advances have made double-row repairs feasible for most surgeons, assuming they are willing to practice and rehearse on models and at appropriate courses prior to patient application. One unresolved question involves the potential adverse biologic impact of excessive implants or sutures, but this is probably a fairly minor issue. So it seems as if the major downside of double-row repair boils down to cost, time, and technical challenge, *assuming the method does not overtension the cuff and thereby cause a mechanical/biologic failure.*

It is likely that some of the conflicting clinical data are caused by the selection process employed for patient enrollment into the specific clinical study. For example, very small cuff tears that are inherently stable are likely to heal well (regardless of repair method), so a study based entirely upon small tears would be unlikely to demonstrate a substantial difference related to repair technique. Similarly, massive and chronically retracted tears are very unlikely to heal, regardless of repair method, due to their inherent biologic disadvantages. This group of patients is probably better managed by a low tension, medialized repair or by partial cuff repair in order to restore the A–P force couples, if possible. It seems like the most important subgroup of patients to prospectively study (in order to ultimately answer this question) will be those with a moderately sized cuff tear that can be repaired by footprint restoration without undue cuff tension. In my opinion, this is the best current indication for double-row repair and footprint restoration (Fig. 10.6). It will be exciting to watch this field continue to evolve, as we optimize our surgical methods and selection criteria for arthroscopic rotator cuff repair. The ultimate solutions will combine solid mechanical solutions with biologic augmentations to facilitate solid healing and recovery of relatively disadvantaged rotator cuff tendon and muscle.

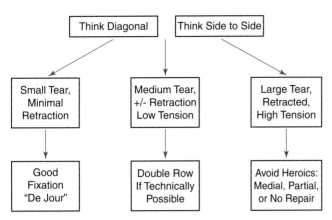

FIGURE 10.6. The author's current rotator cuff repair algorithm.

REFERENCES

1. Meier SW, Meier JD. Rotator cuff repair: the effect of double-row fixation on three-dimensional repair site. *J Shoulder Elbow Surg*. 2006;15(6):691–696.

2. Mahar A, Tamborlane J, Oka R, et al. Single-row suture anchor repair of the rotator cuff is biomechanically equivalent to double-row repair in a bovine model. *Arthroscopy*. 2007;23:1265–1270.

3. Ahmad CS, Kleweno C, Jacir AM, et al. Biomechanical performance of rotator cuff repairs with humeral rotation: a new rotator cuff repair failure model. *Am J Sports Med*. 2008;36(5):888–892.

4. Lorbach O, Bachelier F, Vees J, et al. Cyclic loading of rotator cuff reconstructions: single-row repair with modified suture configurations versus double-row repair. *Am J Sports Med*. 2008;36(8):1504–1510.

5. Zheng N, Harris HW, Andrews JR. Failure analysis of rotator cuff repair: a comparison of three double-row techniques. *J Bone Joint Surg (Am)*. 2008;90(5):1034–1042.

6. Reardon DJ, Mafulli N. Clinical evidence shows no difference between single- and double-row repair for rotator cuff tears. *Arthroscopy*. 2007;23(6):670–673.

7. Busfield BT, Glousman RE, McGarry MH, et al. A biomechanical comparison of 2 technical variations of double-row rotator cuff fixation: the importance of medial row knots. *Am J Sports Med*. 2008;36(5):901–906.

8. Charousset C, Grimberg J, Duranthon LD, et al. Can a double-row anchorage technique improve tendon healing in arthroscopic rotator cuff repair? A prospective, nonrandomized, comparative study of double-row and single-row anchorage techniques with CT arthrography tendon healing assessment. *Am J Sports Med*. 2007;35(8):1247–1253.

9. Franceschi F, Ruzzini L, Longo UG, et al. Equivalent clinical results of arthroscopic single-row and double-row suture anchor repair for rotator cuff tears: a randomized controlled trial. *Am J Sports Med*. 2007;35(8):1254–1260.

10. Grasso A, Milano G, Salvatore M, et al. Single-row versus double-row arthroscopic rotator cuff repair: a prospective randomized clinical study. *Arthroscopy*. 2009;25(1):4–12.

11. Sugaya H, Maeda K, Matsuki K, et al. Repair integrity and functional outcome after arthroscopic double-row rotator cuff repair. A prospective outcome study. *J Bone Joint Surg (Am)*. 2007;89(5):953–960.

12. Huijsmans PE, Pritchard MP, Berghs BM, et al. Arthroscopic rotator cuff repair with double-row fixation. *J Bone Joint Surg (Am)*. 2007;89(6):1248–1257.

13. Park MC, Idjadi JA, Elattrache NS, et al. The effect of dynamic external rotation comparing 2 footprint-restoring rotator cuff repair techniques. *Am J Sports Med*. 2008;36(5):893–900.

14. Park JY, Lhee SH, Choi JH, et al. Comparison of the clinical outcomes of single- and double-row repairs in rotator cuff tears. *Am J Sports Med*. 2008;36(7):1310–1316.

15. Mazzocca AD, Millett PJ, Guanche CA, Santangelo SA, Arciero RA. Arthroscopic single-row versus double-row suture anchor rotator cuff repair. Am J Sports Med. 2005; 33:1861–8.

16. Tuoheti Y, Itoi E, Yamamoto N, Seki N, Abe H, Minagawa H, Okada K, Shimada Y. Contact area, contact pressure, and pressure patterns of the tendon-bone interface after rotator cuff repair. Am J Sports Med. 2005; 33:1869–74.

17. Nelson CO, Sileo MJ, Grossman MG, Serra-Hsu F. Single-row modified mason-allen versus double-row arthroscopic rotator cuff repair: a biomechanical and surface area comparison. Arthroscopy. 2008; 24:941–8.

18. Waltrip RL, Zheng N, Dugas JR, Andrews JR. Rotator cuff repair. A biomechanical comparison of three techniques. Am J Sports Med. 2003; 31:493–7.

19. Meier SW, Meier JD. Rotator cuff repair: the effect of double-row fixation on three-dimensional repair site. J Shoulder Elbow Surg. 2006; 15:691–6.

20. Meier SW, Meier JD. The effect of double-row fixation on initial repair strength in rotator cuff repair: a biomechanical study. Arthroscopy. 2006; 22:1168–73.

21. Kim DH, Elattrache NS, Tibone JE, Jun BJ, DeLaMora SN, Kvitne RS, Lee TQ. Biomechanical comparison of a single-row versus double-row suture anchor technique for rotator cuff repair. Am J Sports Med. 2006; 34:407–14

22. Ma CB, Comerford L, Wilson J, Puttlitz CM. Biomechanical evaluation of arthroscopic rotator cuff repairs: double-row compared with single-row fixation. J Bone Joint Surg Am. 2006; 88:403–10.

23. Smith CD, Alexander S, Hill AM, Huijsmans PE, Bull AM, Amis AA, De Beer JF, Wallace AL. A biomechanical comparison of single and double-row fixation in arthroscopic rotator cuff repair. J Bone Joint Surg Am. 2006; 88:2425–31.

24. Baums MH, Buchhorn GH, Spahn G, Poppendieck B, Schultz W, Klinger HM. Biomechanical characteristics of single-row repair in comparison to double-row repair with consideration of the suture configuration and suture material. Knee Surg Sports Traumatol Arthrosc. 2008; 16:1052–60.

25. Hepp P, Engel T, Osterhoff G, Marquass B, Josten C. Knotless anatomic double-layer double-row rotator cuff repair: a novel technique re-establishing footprint and shape of full-thickness tears. Arch Orthop Trauma Surg. 2009; 129:1031–6.

26. Leek BT, Robertson C, Mahar A, Pedowitz RA. Comparison of mechanical stability in double-row rotator cuff repairs between a knotless transtendon construct versus the addition of medial knots. Arthroscopy. 2010; 26(9 Suppl):S127–33.

27. Sugaya H, Maeda K, Matsuki K, Moriishi J. Functional and structural outcome after arthroscopic full-thickness rotator cuff repair: single-row versus dual-row fixation. Arthroscopy. 2005; 21:1307–16.

28. Ozbaydar M, Elhassan B, Esenyel C, Atalar A, Bozdag E, Sunbuloglu E, Kopuz N, Demirhan M. A comparison of single-versus double-row suture anchor techniques in a simulated repair of the rotator cuff: an experimental study in rabbits. J Bone Joint Surg Br. 2008; 90:1386–91.

29. Lafosse L, Brzoska R, Toussaint B, Gobezie R. The outcome and structural integrity of arthroscopic rotator cuff repair with use of the double-row suture anchor technique. Surgical technique. J Bone Joint Surg Am. 2008; 90 Suppl 2 Pt 2:275–86.

Massive Cuff Repairs: A Rational Approach to Repairs

Jeffrey S. Abrams

KEY POINTS

- Massive rotator cuff tears include three or more of the rotator cuff tendons.
- Pathology anteriorly, superiorly, and posteriorly can be visualized by placing the arthroscope in multiple portals.
- Biceps tendon pathology is a common source of pain in shoulders with large and massive rotator cuff tears. Biceps tenotomy or tenodesis may be helpful in reducing the pain.
- Patient selection is a combination of factors including age, chronicity of the tear, radiographic imaging, and medical and physical comorbidities. Surgeons need to consider not only shoulders to be repaired but also shoulders that will heal.
- Surgical tear patterns are either based anteriorly surrounding the subscapularis–supraspinatus interval or posteriorly at the supraspinatus–infraspinatus interval. Recognition of patterns is helpful in creating a low-tension repair.
- Articular and bursal releases may include capsulotomy, coracohumeral releases, bursectomy, modified decompression, coracoid arch releases, and interval releases.
- After diagnostic arthroscopy, repairs begin anteriorly due to spatial limitations. Following subscapularis repair, anterior releases from a bursal perspective can be performed.
- Delaminations and mid-tendon tears need to be recognized to complete full-thickness repairs. Since the tendency is to create convergence of the cuff from multiple directions, anchor spreading is a preferred construct to stabilize the repair.

The massive rotator cuff tear includes at least three tendons. Many surgeons have incorrectly referred to the massive tear as one that is irreparable. Today, the massive rotator cuff tear has many surgical options, including arthroscopic repair (1–3). It is critical that the treating physician carefully evaluate the characteristics of the muscle, tear pattern, patient's comorbidities, and degree of disability to determine the best method of management.

The etiology of a massive tear may be trauma or an extension of an existing medium-sized tear following a specific event. These tears may be found at times in an older population with chronic changes noted on imaging studies. With improved imaging studies, rotator cuff tears are being diagnosed prior to significant muscular changes following trauma. This may present an opportunity to treat and repair symptomatic shoulders prior to permanent changes developing within the muscles and tendons. The possibility of successful healing and a "watertight" closure is best in the younger individual with minor changes to the detached cuff tendons. Delays in treatment may lead to tear extension and retraction, muscular atrophy, fatty changes within the muscles, superior migration of the humeral head, decreased tendon vascularity, and tuberosity osteopenia—all of which can impact the ability of healing.

Tear pattern recognition is important to understand how some small and medium tears can extend into a massive tear. Most rotator cuff tears begin along the anterior edge of the supraspinatus tendon. Tear extension is most common in a posterior direction, which eventually causes disruption of the entire supraspinatus and extends through the overlapping infraspinatus insertion. Some tears will also extend anteriorly across the rotator cuff interval to include the subscapularis. The massive cuff tear pattern is most often a crescent-shaped tear. The medial extension along the intervals, either anteriorly into the subscapularis or posteriorly into the infraspinatus, may create delaminations and a multilayered tear. In order to consider a repair that has minimal tension, these complex tear patterns need to be recognized and anatomically addressed when possible. The rotator interval may be included in this tear pattern, and disruption of the biceps pulley system is common (4). Treatment of biceps tears or instability may need to be included in the treatment of the massive rotator cuff tear.

Patients with a massive rotator cuff tear may exhibit a number of complaints ranging from resting pain to complete loss of function (Fig. 11.1). One role of the rotator cuff is to stabilize the glenohumeral articulation during functional elevation created by the deltoid. As the tear extends, certain shoulders are unable to compress the humeral head into the glenoid. This is rarely found with a

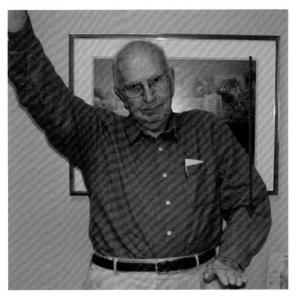

FIGURE 11.1. Patient with a massive rotator cuff tear attempts to elevate left arm.

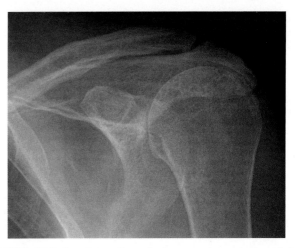

FIGURE 11.2. Standing radiograph demonstrating reduction of the acromiohumeral interval and chronic changes to the greater tuberosity and acromion.

single tendon tear and is more likely attributed to tears that include the superior portion of the subscapularis and the majority of the infraspinatus (5). This condition has been compared with a boutonniere deficiency seen with extensor capsule disruption of a finger. The remaining tendons sublux inferior to the axis of the joint creating an adductor force during an attempt of arm abduction. This results in a shrug sign. Over time, this dynamic loss may evolve into a fixed deformity reducing the humeral head acromion interval on a sitting or standing radiograph (Fig. 11.2).

An arthroscopic evaluation of a massive rotator cuff tear allows a thorough examination without deltoid detachment or retraction. There have been studies that recommend an open approach to a large and massive tear; however, these have been challenged by newer arthroscopic techniques, which mobilize tears and create secure repairs to the tuberosities (6,7). Advantages of arthroscopy include (1) reduced risk of infection, (2) reduced risk of postoperative stiffness, (3) reduced risk of deltoid injury, and (4) reduced morbidity during the early postoperative period.

CLINICAL EVALUATION

History

The key features obtained in a history include the patient's symptomatic problems and whether there was a traumatic onset. Treatment for pain has the best chance of successful results. Trauma suggests a recent onset. Patients who have had prior treatment including cortisone injections and therapy may have had a chronic cuff tear that was exacerbated with trauma. The development of chronic muscle and tendon changes include decreased vascularity to the damaged structures.

Select patients may present with the acute onset of weakness following a minor traumatic event. These patients may have had a well-compensated tear that was injured further. Details regarding the change in shoulder function are important to clarify. Although surgery for weakness has met with mixed results, acute repair of tear extensions and release of neurologic entrapment may return a patient's ability to elevate their arm (8,9).

Physical Exam

Observe the shoulder in a gown that does not cover the scapula and the deltoid. Look for significant degrees of atrophy in the supraspinatus, the infraspinatus, and the generalized shoulder musculature. Ask the patient to lift both arms to make comparisons with ranges of motion and whether movement is initiated by the glenohumeral joint or by raising the scapula. Measure flexion, external rotation with the elbow at the side, and internal rotation behind the back. Gentle strength testing can be performed by using the belly-press sign (subscapularis) and resistance against external rotation (infraspinatus and teres minor). The distal neurovascular examination may indicate whether a cervical problem may play a role in creating the shoulder symptoms.

Local tenderness can be elicited by direct pressure over the tuberosities and bicipital groove. Many patients will complain of tenderness along the margins of the tear posteriorly and anteriorly. Identify any associated symptoms including biceps pathology.

Imaging

In order to optimize patient selection, accurate imaging studies are important. Plain radiographs include three views. The anteroposterior view of the glenohumeral joint should be performed in an upright patient to identify "fixed" superior migration. A measurement of the acromiohumeral distance can be made. The literature suggests that 11 mm is normal and that less than 6 mm may suggest an irreparable tear and is suggestive of the need for surgical repair (10). Degenerative joint changes can be appreciated if this view is obtained tangentially to the glenoid surface. The Y view will best illustrate the acromial arch morphology, and the axillary view can demonstrate concentric reduction and further illustrate joint asymmetry.

Muscles and tendons are best illustrated with MRI. Europeans have popularized contrast CT to accomplish this goal. An MRI study does not require contrast for an initial exam, but may enhance the evaluation of shoulders previously repaired. The dimensions of the tear can be determined by coronal and sagittal cuts (Fig. 11.3). Transverse cuts will further identify subscapularis and posterior cuff tears.

A finding associated with torn muscle physiology is the development of atrophy and fat infiltration. Medial muscle cuts on sagittal MRI studies can demonstrate muscular deterioration with fatty substitution (Fig. 11.4). Since Goutallier's et al. original description of the infraspinatus on CT scans, there have been many opinions on

the reparability of chronic rotator cuff tears (11). An important question is whether repaired rotator cuff tendons actually heal if advanced stages of fatty infiltration exist. Most would agree that atrophy and fat infiltration are permanent and not reversible. These findings result in muscular weakness that does not improve with surgical repair. Although weakness may be permanent, pain relief has not necessarily been negatively impacted by these changes. For this reason, many patients continue to choose surgical repair as a viable option for a painful rotator cuff tear with moderate muscular changes (12).

Ultrasound has evolved into a dynamic assessment of the rotator cuff (13). The symptomatic shoulder can be easily compared with the opposite extremity and placed through a range of motion. Postoperative repair integrity can also be evaluated and metallic anchors and surgical debris seen on MRI exams can be evaluated with fewer artifacts.

Tear Patterns

Massive rotator cuff tears have two basic patterns—the anterosuperior and posterosuperior tears (14). The

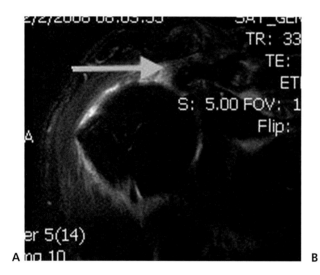
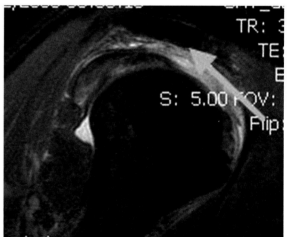
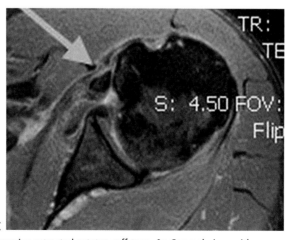

FIGURE 11.3. MRI views of a massive retracted rotator cuff tear. **A:** Coronal view with arrow pointing to supraspinatus tendon retracted to glenoid rim. **B:** Sagittal view with arrow pointing to posterior retraction away from greater tuberosity. **C:** Axial view with arrow pointing to a subscapularis retracted tear and the long head of the biceps dislocated out of the groove.

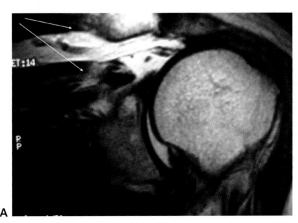

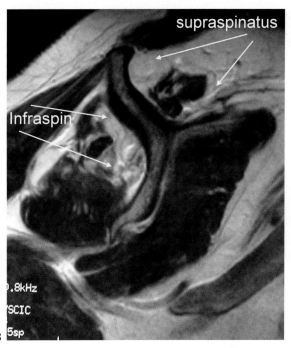

FIGURE 11.4. A: MRI of a massive tear with early fatty infiltration in the supraspinatus muscle. **B:** MRI medial sagittal view demonstrating advanced fatty infiltration into the supraspinatus and infraspinatus muscles.

anterosuperior tear centers along the rotator interval and extends through most of the subscapularis and supraspinatus insertions (Fig. 11.5). This is often a large crescent tear with medial retraction of the subscapularis creating a "comma sign" described by Burkhart and Tehrany (15) (Fig. 11.5). Anterior releases adjacent to the coracoid may assist in tendon repair to the lesser tuberosity. The superior and posterior extensions do not usually have significant retraction, and medial tear extension is uncommon.

The posterosuperior tear pattern involves the superior portion of the subscapularis and extends posteriorly exposing the majority of the greater tuberosity (Fig. 11.6).

This tear pattern often extends medially into the muscular tendinous junction as the tear margins enlarge. This pattern may require releases about the scapular spine allowing for tendon mobilization and margin convergence (Fig. 11.7). The posterior aspects of the tear are usually more mobile, and large defects can often be reduced with minimal tension (16).

Decision-Making Options

The optimal shoulder for repair is a middle-aged patient with a painful massive tear, trauma-precipitating symptoms, radiographs with the humeral head centered in the

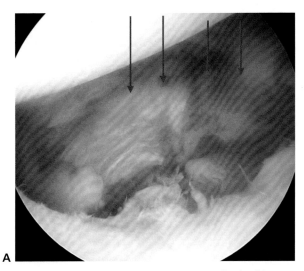

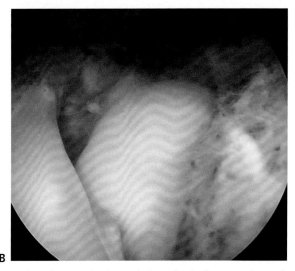

FIGURE 11.5. Massive anterosuperior tear, right shoulder. **A:** Comma sign of retracted subscapularis tendon in the rotator interval. **B:** Posterior tear extension through supraspinatus into the infraspinatus.

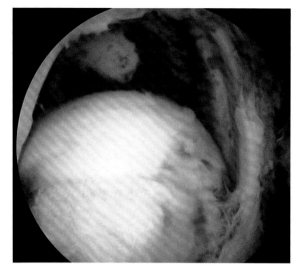

FIGURE 11.6. Massive posterosuperior tear viewed from lateral portal.

glenoid, and an MRI showing less than 50% fat changes within the muscles. The chances of healing a repaired cuff tear are less predictable when the humeral head has migrated superiorly (acromiohumeral interval less than 6 mm), there is muscular atrophy and fat infiltration of 50% to 75%, the patient is over 70 years, and vascular and medical comorbidities are present.

A biceps tenotomy may be considered as an option in patients with a compromised profile and painful shoulder limitations. Walch et al. (17) has shown symptomatic benefit without functional compromise in these patients. If a more favorable healing profile exists, patients can be considered for an arthroscopic repair if nonoperative treatment fails. This repair may include a complete or partial repair and a biceps tenodesis.

As patients approach the age of 67 and degenerative arthritis findings are present, a reverse prosthesis may be a more predictable operation to relieve pain and restore function. A number of patients may be considered too young for this prosthesis, but have an irreparable tear or failure of previous surgical attempts. Covering and augmenting the compromised tendons with either the biceps tendon or the use of an allograft may improve pain and humeral stability during overhead activities.

TREATMENT

Nonoperative

A number of elderly patients that present following an episode of trauma are unable to elevate their arm due to pain and weakness. After making a diagnosis, a conservative approach may be a very acceptable option. Indications for this conservative treatment include medical issues that may impact a decision of having elective surgery, social reasons limiting the ability to allow for immobilization postoperatively, transfer gait problems requiring the use of both upper extremities, and radiographic indicators that surgical repair is unlikely to make a measurable improvement. Acromiohumeral space on upright radiography less than 6 mm, excessive atrophy and fat infiltration on sagittal MRI view over 75%, patients over 70 years of age, and early arthritic glenohumeral findings are poor prognostic indicators. However, each of these factors has been challenged and successful pain relief can be achieved in selected patients.

Nonoperative treatment begins with the management of pain and maintaining a mobile glenohumeral joint. Simple exercises include pendulum rotations, supine-assistive flexion, actively assisted cross-chest stretches, and scapular shrugs. A cortisone shot in the subacromial space

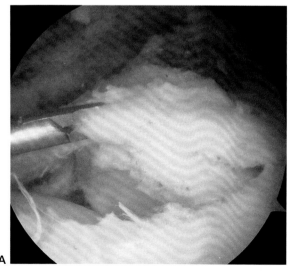
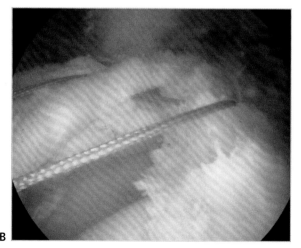

FIGURE 11.7. Techniques to repair. **A:** Tissue mobilization from the supraspinatus fossa to identify the tear pattern. **B:** Margin convergence sutures placed to medially reduce the massive tear extension.

may be helpful in reducing the initial discomfort. As the discomfort decreases and motion improves, upright exercises or semi-inclined exercises may be started. The goals of treatment include pain relief, use of the arm for hygiene and self-care, and useful strength when the arm is close to the side. Progression to overhead activities is based on the patient's needs and level of disability.

Biceps Tenotomy, Modified Decompression

There are a number of elderly patients who continue to have a painful shoulder in spite of nonoperative treatment. Many of these patients are active and are unable to either restrict movement or use their extremity. An option for these patients is to consider a modified decompression, debridement, and biceps tenotomy. The biceps tenotomy can be performed arthroscopically adjacent to the superior labrum. An ace bandage loosely applied to the upper arm postoperatively may limit the distal migration of the divided tendon. The sling can be discarded as comfort allows.

The subacromial decompression is performed as a "smoothing" surgery, removing any osteophytes directed inferiorly at the exposed humeral head (Fig. 11.8). The most inferior aspects of the coracohumeral ligament are gently elevated to expose the anterior acromial margin. The coracoacromial ligament is not removed or released from the superficial aspects of the acromion to preserve the coracoacromial arch. It is important to preserve this canopy to avoid the difficult complication of anterior superior escape of the humeral head.

Arthroscopic Rotator Cuff Repair

The diagnostic evaluation begins with the arthroscope in the posterior portal, 2 cm inferior to the junction of the spine of the scapula with the acromion. Determining the articular pattern of the tear begins with visualizing

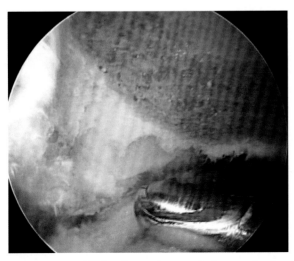

FIGURE 11.8. Modified arthroscopic acromioplasty maintains the coracoacromial ligament and removes the inferior osteophytes.

the long head of the biceps and its relationship with the inferior pulley and superior border of the subscapularis (Fig. 11.9). The middle glenohumeral ligament may be divided to visualize the inferior and medial extent of the tear. The arthroscope is then directed toward the greater tuberosity to visualize the posterior aspect of the tear. Replacing the arthroscope in the subacromial bursa allows for creation of a lateral portal 3 cm lateral to the anterior third of the acromion. Following a superficial bursectomy, the cuff margins can be visualized and cuff mobility evaluated.

The arthroscope is replaced in the posterior articular portal to repair the subscapularis. If the long head of the biceps is displaced from the groove or has tears, a suture can be placed through the biceps and a tenotomy completed adjacent to the superior labrum. The tear pattern of the subscapularis needs to be identified. This tear may vary from a superior border tear (Fig. 11.9) to a complete tendon detachment with medial retraction (Fig. 11.5). Start with articular releases consisting of a capsulotomy beginning at the interval and extending inferiorly. A window can be created in the rotator interval, and the arthroscope can be advanced allowing for the bursal perspective without removing the arthroscope. Coracoid releases including partial lateral bone resection can be performed in patients with adhesions and narrowing of the anterior space. The use of a 70° arthroscope allows for an improved angle of visualization as the subscapularis repair is being performed.

After preparation of the lesser tuberosity by removal of devitalized tissue, a series of suture anchors can be placed along the footprint of the lesser tuberosity. This is best performed adjacent to a percutaneous spinal needle directed lateral to the coracoid and with external rotation of the humerus. The superior subscapularis tears can often be repaired with a single anchor, whereas larger tears will likely need an additional more inferior anchor. Placing the subscapularis under lateral tension, the sutures can be passed through the tendon to create mattress sutures. It is beneficial to internally rotate the humerus during suture tying. Portions of the "comma sign" that are lateral to the subscapularis repair should be preserved for further reinforcement while visualizing from the bursa.

The arthroscope is switched to the anterior portal to visualize the posterior aspects of the tear. A capsulotomy can release the tendons and improve the multilayered appearance of the infraspinatus and its junction with the teres minor (Fig. 11.10). This capsulotomy should continue inferiorly through the posterior band of the inferior glenohumeral ligament.

The arthroscope can be replaced in the posterior subacromial portal. Tendon mobilization begins beneath the acromion, and a modified decompression can be performed to improve visualization and instrumentation. Releases should proceed anteriorly and medially to the spine of the scapula. The bursectomy continues laterally and posteriorly to define the posterior margins of the tear. If

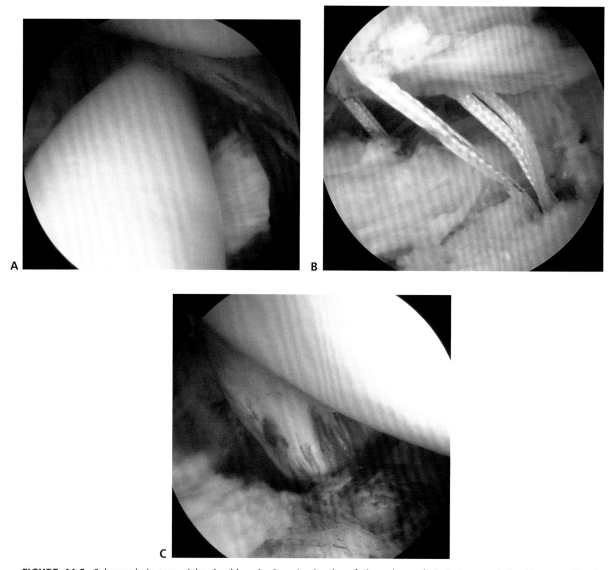

FIGURE 11.9. Subscapularis tear, right shoulder. **A:** Superior border of the subscapularis is torn and the biceps tendon is subluxed into the tear. **B:** Bursal view of a subscapularis repair with the scope posterior and a window created in the rotator interval. **C:** Articular view of the repair from a posterior portal with 30° arthroscope.

the tear extends into the tendinous structure posteriorly, margin convergence can be helpful to create closure with reduced tension in the repair (Fig. 11.7). If there is a split in the anterior interval (L-shaped tear), absorbable converging sutures placed between the supraspinatus and the interval may reposition the tendon.

Use a spinal needle to direct suture anchor placement along the posterior aspect of the greater tuberosity beginning posteriorly. In order to maximize the chances of improving external rotation strength, sutures will need to be passed through both deep and superficial aspects of the infraspinatus tendon. A common configuration uses a combination of mattress sutures and simple sutures from anchors that have multiple sutures (Fig. 11.10). If this anchor is not placed early in the repair, the posterior delaminated tendons are not well visualized and the tuberosity

is hidden, limiting spreading apart of the anchors. Sutures may be tied and placed away from the working cannula. These posterior sutures may later be used to incorporate the long head of the biceps to create a tenodesis.

The arthroscope can be placed in a posterior, posterolateral, or lateral portal to better visualize the remaining repair. An anchor is placed percutaneously along the anterior half of the medial footprint of the greater tuberosity. Mattress sutures are passed through the supraspinatus to maximize footprint coverage when possible. An anterior anchor is used to repair the important anterior margin of the supraspinatus. The single- versus double-row suture anchor controversy is often determined by tissue mobility and chronic tendon retraction. It is more important to spread anchors apart to improve soft tissue fixation while minimizing tension of the repair (Fig. 11.11).

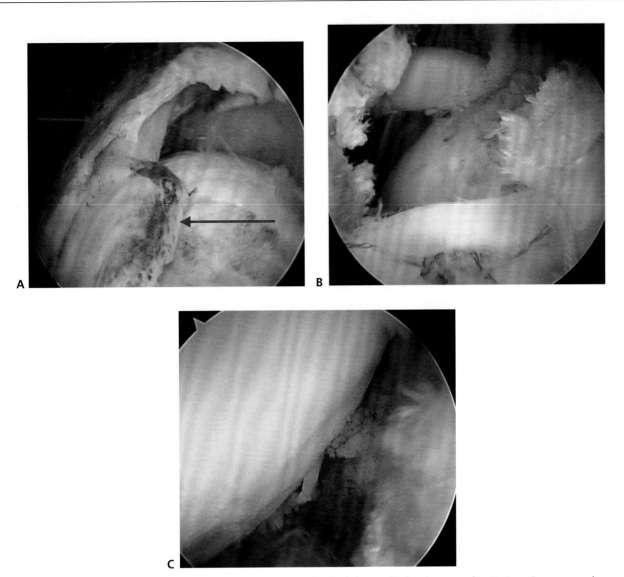

FIGURE 11.10. Infraspinatus tear techniques. **A:** Lateral view of multiple layers of infraspinatus tendon. **B:** Posterior suture anchor repairing both layers of infraspinatus. **C:** Articular view of repair from anterior portal.

Tissue from the comma sign composed of coracohumeral ligament and pulley can be attached to the anterosuperior anchor or lateral anchor to maximize cuff stability. If a biceps tenodesis is considered, pass the posterior infraspinatus sutures through the biceps to augment the repair and avoid the disrupting forces of tension.

Partial Repairs and Grafts

Certain shoulders may be improved with an attempt at repair, but tissue retraction will not allow complete tuberosity reattachment in spite of multiple releases and maximum tissue mobilization. Rather than risking tendon avulsion due to overtensioning the shoulder repair, a partial repair can be considered. This often consists of margin convergence sutures at the apex of the tear. Anchors are placed along the margins of the repair, leaving a defect exposing part of the tuberosity and articular surface

not completely covered by the rotator cuff. Depending on the size and quality of repaired tendons, there are several options to cover this area and reinforce the repair. Small defects can be covered with the tenotomized long head of the biceps and incorporated into the suture anchors bridging the defect (Fig. 11.12) (16). If the defect is considered too large or in patients with deficient tendons, an allograft may be considered to reinforce the repair.

A dermal matrix allograft (GraftJacket, Wright Medical Technology, Arlington, TN) has been used to repair complex rotator cuff tears when tendon-to-tuberosity repair is considered impossible (18). The graft is secured with medial mattress sutures placed at the muscular boundaries and laterally to anchors covering the defect and reinforcing tendon margins. Graft tension is beneficial to biologic in growth factors from the soft tissue margins. Biopsy-proven healing has occurred at both the native

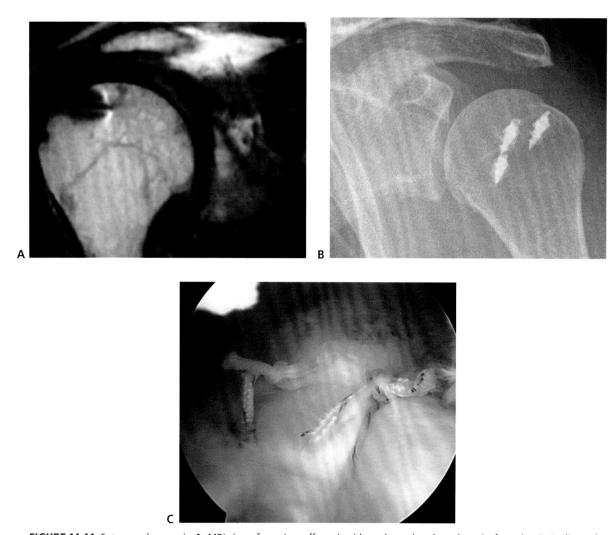

FIGURE 11.11. Suture anchor repair. **A:** MRI view of massive cuff repair with tendon reduced to tuberosity footprint. **B:** Radiographs of suture anchors spread apart to improve fixation. **C:** Suture anchors spread combining medial and lateral fixation to create footprint coverage. (Prior publication: US Musculoskeletal Review, 2007.)

soft tissue margins and the bone. Techniques to incorporate a graft have advanced, and both arthroscopic and arthroscopic-assisted mini-open approaches have been used to complete the repair (19).

Arthroplasty

The shoulder with a massive cuff tear, degenerative changes, and failed prior surgical attempts may be a candidate for a reverse shoulder arthroplasty. Currently this procedure is felt to be most appropriate in elderly patients over 67 years old. There are concerns that the longevity of this prosthesis may limit options for potential revision surgery that may become necessary during a patient's lifetime.

Benefits of a reverse shoulder arthroplasty include displacing the center of rotation inferiorly and laterally. The deltoid becomes the primary elevator and flexor of the shoulder. Rotation may be improved if partial repairs

of the cuff are completed or posterior tendon transfer may produce a tenodesis effect during arm elevation. Conventional arthroplasty may be considered if a cuff repair is possible. In patients with poor rotator cuff tendons, resurfacing the humeral head or a hemiarthroplasty is combined with a partial repair. Conventional glenoid components are not used due to concerns with loosening.

Postoperative Management

The postoperative management of an arthroscopic repair of a massive rotator cuff tear begins with sling immobilization in a neutral position. Patients are started on pendulum exercises, shoulder shrugs, and grip strength, and continue for 6 weeks.

Supine passive flexion will begin after 6 weeks. A gradual weaning from the sling will begin at 5 weeks and continue for 2 weeks. As passive flexion improves, semi-inclined and upright exercises may be started. Active

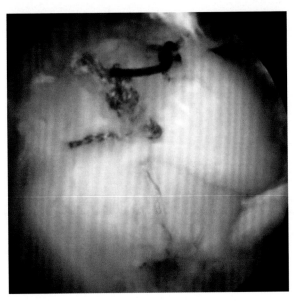

FIGURE 11.12. Biceps tenodesis. The long head of the biceps is sutured to a posterior anchor.

exercises are delayed until 8 to 10 weeks. Cross-chest stretches may begin at 8 to 10 weeks. Resistive exercises to strengthen flexion and external and internal rotation may begin at 12 weeks.

Consideration of the return to physical activities is dependent on repair integrity, pain relief, active motion, and strength demands. This may begin as early as 5 months for golf and 9 months for jobs requiring physical lifting above the shoulder level.

RESULTS

There have been studies that demonstrate the reparability of massive cuff tears. (1–3,7,12,14). There has been a direct correlation between patient age, medical comorbidities, and the successful healing of large repairs. Patient satisfaction has been rewarding, particularly if pain is the primary reason for surgical repair. Partial repairs and grafting have also shown a positive impact on pain relief and the return to functional activities (5,18).

From a personal series of 80 massive repairs, pain relief was achieved in 88%, active arm elevation gains were obtained in 75%, and a return of function observed in 75% (Fig. 11.11). Despite a chronic tear and muscular deterioration, pain relief may still be achieved but permanent weakness is likely. Most surgeons have suggested early surgical intervention in young, active individuals to limit the potential for irreversible muscle and tendon change.

In patients with a poor prognosis for healing a repair, biceps tenotomy, arthroscopic debridement, and a modified decompression will often improve patients' pain. Functional gains are equally dependent on the postoperative therapy when surgery is used to reduce painful changes.

The arthroscope has become a common technique to evaluate and repair a patient with a massive rotator cuff tear. Patient selection begins with an office evaluation, special imaging of the shoulder, and may proceed to arthroscopic treatment in select patients. Multiple options are available arthroscopically due to improved visualization and avoiding deltoid detachment. The advantages of the arthroscopic approach to the massive tear include a reduced risk of complications including stiffness, infections, and deltoid dehiscence.

REFERENCES

1. Burkhart SS, Danaceau SM, Pearce CE. Arthroscopic rotator cuff repair: analysis of results by tear, size, and by repair technique: margin convergence versus direct tendon-to-bone repair. *Arthroscopy.* 2001;17:905–912.
2. Jones CK, Savoie FH. Arthroscopic repair of large and massive rotator cuff tears. *Arthroscopy.* 2003;19:564–571.
3. Abrams JS. Arthroscopic approach to massive rotator cuff tears. *Inst Course Lect.* 2006;55:59–66.
4. Abrams JS. Repair of large anterosuperior cuff tears. In: Abrams JS, Bell RH, eds. *Arthroscopic Rotator Cuff Surgery: A Practical Approach to Management.* New York, NY: Springer, 2008:278–245.
5. Burkhart SS, Nottage WM, Ogilive-Harris DJ, et al. Partial repair of irreparable rotator cuff tears. *Arthroscopy.* 1994; 10:363–370.
6. Bishop J, Klepps S, Lo IK, et al. Cuff integrity after arthroscopic versus open rotator cuff repair: a prospective study. *J Shoulder Elbow Surg.* 2006;15:290–299.
7. Lafosse L, Brozska R, Toussaint B, et al. The outcome and structural integrity of arthroscopic rotator cuff repair with use of the double-row suture anchor technique. *J Bone Joint Surg Am.* 2007;89:1533–1541.
8. Warner JP, Krushell RJ, Masquelet A, et al. Anatomy and relationships of the suprascapular nerve: anatomical constraints to mobilization of the supraspinatus and infraspinatus muscles in the management of massive rotator cuff tears. *J Bone Joint Surg Am.* 1992;74:36–45.
9. Lafosse L, Tomasi A. Techniques for endoscopic release of suprascapular nerve entrapment at the suprascapular notch. *Tech Shoulder Elbow Surg.* 2006;7:1–6.
10. Hamada K, Fukuda H, Mikasa M, et al. Roentgenographic findings in massive rotator cuff tears. a long-term observation. *Clin Orthop Relat Res.* 1990;254:92–96.
11. Goutallier D, Postel JM, Bernageau J, et al. Fatty muscle degeneration in cuff ruptures: pre- and postoperative evaluation by CT scan. *Clin Orthop Relat Res.* 1994;304:78–83.
12. Galatz LM, Ball CM, Teefey SA, et al. The outcome and repair integrity of completely arthroscopically repaired large and massive rotator cuff tears. *J Bone Joint Surg Am.* 2004;86:219–224.
13. Teefey SA, Hasan SA, Middleton WD, et al. Ultrasonography of the rotator cuff: a comparison of ultrasonographic and arthroscopic findings in one hundred consecutive cases. *J Bone Joint Surg Am.* 2000;82:498–504.
14. Gerber C, Fuchs B, Hodler J. The results of repair of massive tears of the rotator cuff. *J Bone Joint Surg Am.* 2000;82:505–515.

15. Burkhart SS, Tehrany AM. Arthroscopic subscapularis tendon repair: techniques and preliminary results. *Arthroscopy.* 2002;18:454–463.

16. Abrams JS. Arthroscopic technique for massive rotator cuff repairs. *Tech in Shoulder Elbow Surg.* 2007;8:126–134.

17. Walch G, Edwards TB, Boulahaia A, et al. Arthroscopic tenotomy of the long head of the biceps in the treatment of rotator cuff tears: clinical and radiographic results in 307 cases. *J Shoulder Elbow Surg.* 2005;14:238–246.

18. Snyder SJ, Bond JL. Technique for arthroscopic replacement of severely-damaged rotator cuff using "GraftJacket" allograft. *Oper Tech Sports Med.* 2007;15:86–94.

19. Burkhead WZ, Schiffern SC, Krishnan SG. Use of GraftJacket as an augmentation for massive rotator cuff tears. *Semin Arthrop.* 2007;18:11–18.

Anthroscopic Cuff Repair: Tissue Graft Applications

Marc Labbé

The use of biologic grafts in rotator cuff repair and reconstruction is an area of burgeoning interest and focused research. The main problem is that rotator cuff repair is a challenging task. Our understanding of the problems involved, surgical tools available, and techniques has changed radically since Dr. Codman's first description of a repair in 1911. Despite these advances, we have come to learn that actually getting a complete repair in all cases remains a lofty goal. A recent multicenter study reported on the results of 576 arthroscopic repairs and noted a 25% rate of retear by MR or CT arthrogram. Functional results improved across the board although having an intact tendon was associated with even greater gains in activity level, motion, and especially strength. Pain, although significantly improved, was not statistically different in both healed and retear groups. Larger and more chronic tears were at greater risk of structural failure (1). Other studies have corroborated their finding that patients who are able to obtain a complete repair do better than those who do not.

For those cases where a repair is impossible, options are limited, especially for younger and more active patients. Where are we failing? Biologically! Technically, we now recognize tear patterns better and are able to mobilize the tissues as needed. The anchors and the sutures available have amazing strength and holding ability. Almost any tear is now repairable. There is just not enough healing ability within the time constraints of the rehabilitative process. Metaphorically, it is a race. The race begins once the brace is applied in the operating room. Will the cuff heal before the forces applied to it in rehabilitation pull it apart?

Several factors contribute to a bad biologic environment, which creates poor healing ability. Numerous studies describe the poor blood flow at the insertion of diseased rotator cuff tendons and the various forces applied there during activity. The surgeon must first deal with the possibility of tendon loss in addition to tissue stiffness in larger more chronic tears. Although surgeons try to avoid doing

so, the tendon is often placed under tension. The greater tuberosity with chronic tears also goes through degenerative changes resulting in osteopenia and cyst formation. The osteoblasts in the tuberosity show diminished ability to respond to mechanical stress, implying that they may not respond well to a repair process. Patient age and tear chronicity also play large roles with high recurrence rates reported in those older than 70 years who have significant fatty infiltration. Medications such as NSAIDs and other immune-modifying agents can also contribute to a surgical failure and should be stopped if possible. Surgeons are therefore often left trying to fix bad tissue to bad bone in a person with limited ability to heal: a daunting prospect.

Conceptually, grafting the rotator cuff would improve the strength of the primary fixation and add collagen at the repair site. Neviaser reported the use of grafts for massive tears. He used freeze-dried allograft rotator cuff tissue and reported good or excellent result in 14 of 16 patients (2). Ten years later, Nasca used a similar graft but reported functional improvement in only 2 of 7 patients, although all had pain relief (3). Almost 20 years later, Moore described his experience with allograft reconstruction. All of the patients who were imaged failed structurally, and outcomes were essentially the same as debridement(4). Despite the relatively poor early outcomes, grafting remains an area of significant interest and study today, thanks to the development of several novel grafts.

GRAFTS

The "modern" era of rotator cuff grafts began in 1999 with the introduction of the Restore (DePuy) xenograft. Since then, there has been a veritable explosion of graft development. There are properties inherent to each graft, which must be considered during selection. The source material, tissue preparation techniques, thickness, pliability, elasticity, and suture retention strength are all factors that can affect graft performance. Graft sources include allograft human cadaveric skin or tendon, xenograft skin

The author would like to recognize Dr. Toribio Natividad for his efforts in accumulating and organizing the data in the table.

or pericardium, porcine small intestine submucosa, and synthetic grafts made of polyurethane urea or poly-L-lactide/glycolide polymer. The tissue grafts are acellular and sterilized using various proprietary techniques. Some companies then choose to cross-link the collagen in order to limit or slow the natural process of enzymatic degradation after implantation. Controversy exists over whether or not cross-linking is beneficial or detrimental (5).

Ideally, any graft is slowly replaced with host tissue at such a pace that the structural integrity of the cuff repair is supported long enough to facilitate healing of the native cuff. This healing process may be on the order of months. In contrast, if the collagen fibers are too resistant to the enzymes, encapsulation and scar formation may occur around the graft. In addition, if the material elicits a large immunologic response, local soft tissue swelling and other signs of possible infection can occur. From a practical standpoint, trying to determine which patient is or is not infected could add unnecessary cost and delay recovery.

Grafts that are thinner tend to have less suture retention ability (6). Tissue pliability is also important in considering grafts for arthroscopic applications. Typically, a graft applied arthroscopically is passed through a cannula. Therefore, the graft must be able to fold and resist tearing while being pushed and/or pulled through the cannula. Cross-linked grafts tend to have more stiffness. Currently, there are no randomized trials comparing graft materials in humans. Perhaps there is no best choice. At the time of this writing, the GraftJacket material has the most published data, demonstrating its effectiveness and safety. The landscape in this area of orthopedics is constantly shifting, and the individual surgeon is wise to review the most current literature and decide for themselves which graft to choose. Currently, marketed grafts and their various properties are listed in Table 12.1 (7–8).

CLINICAL EVALUATION

As always, start with a good history and physical examination. The questions and exam maneuvers are those typically employed in evaluating someone with shoulder pain, although there are areas of specific focus. The chronicity of the tear is an important factor as well as the ability of the cuff to heal and regain function. Technically, an acute traumatic tear, even a large one, is easier to repair and more likely to heal than a chronic one. The tendons and muscle fibers are usually not so degenerative, although acute-on-chronic tears can create an acute large tear with relatively poor tissue. Visual inspection can reveal significant atrophy of the supraspinatus and infraspinatus in chronic cases.

Physical Examination

Both passive and active range of motion are important to measure. A shoulder that has become mechanically stiff associated with a chronic cuff tear will need either a capsular release or an alternative treatment considered before any

significant functional gains will be realized with a repair. The function of the cuff muscles must also be assessed to identify which are dysfunctional. The supraspinatus can be tested at 90° of forward flexion, or in scaption with the thumb up to avoid inadvertent pain from impingement that can occur with the thumb down. The infraspinatus is tested with the shoulder in 30° of abduction. The subscapularis can be tested with the belly press test, although care should be taken to keep the forearm parallel to the abdomen. The bear hug test is another option for testing subscapularis tendon integrity.

Imaging Tests

Imaging is of significant help in determining whether or not a graft may be beneficial. Plain X-rays can reveal elevation of the humeral head and acetabularization of the acromion found in chronic severe cases of cuff arthropathy. An MRI gives an understanding of the size and pattern of the tear. Early changes of glenohumeral arthritis can also be seen. Fatty infiltration of the muscle bellies can be identified and quantified.

Once the diagnosis of a rotator cuff tear has been established, a treatment plan must be created. A full thickness tear is a surgical problem if cuff repair is the ultimate goal. The natural history of full thickness tears is that they persist and most likely get larger over time. Steroid injections can offer pain relief, but this must be tempered with the possibility of further tissue degradation. Patients can maintain a high level of shoulder function as long as the shoulder maintains a balance with the anterior and posterior muscle forces equalized. The decision to surgically intervene is based upon the patient's goals and their health status.

Indications

The appropriate indications for the use of these graft materials are under development. It is important to know that these materials are FDA approved for the augmentation of soft tissue repairs. Specifically for the rotator cuff, the tendon edge must be repairable to within 1 cm of the greater tuberosity to fall within these guidelines. The current recommendations include the primary repair of large and massive tears in the setting of a bad biologic environment and any revision repair. A graft can also be used in cases of irreparable tears. While rotator cuff replacement or "bridging" of a defect falls outside the FDA guidelines, the procedure holds some promise for a very challenging patient population.

The main contraindication is severe cuff arthropathy. Other relative contraindications include early cuff arthropathy, shoulder stiffness, and a history of infection. The stiff shoulder should be assessed preoperatively and treated intraoperatively so that the humeral head can be appropriately reduced back into the glenoid before cuff repair. Efforts must be made to ensure complete resolution of any infection. The author recommends a period of at least 1 to 2 weeks off of any antibiotics followed by blood tests including a white blood cell count, erythrocyte

Table 12.1

List of currently available grafts

Grafts	Company	Material Source	Tissue Type	Cross-Link	Approved Use	Sterilization	Chemical Wash	Sterility Assurance Level (SAL) 10-6	Size	Rotator Cuff Clinical Reports
BioTape XM	Wright Medical	Porcine	Dermis	N		Ethylene Oxide				
Conexa	Tornier/ LifeCell	Porcine	Dermis	N	Rotator cuff reinforce/ augment soft tissue	Low-dose electron beam	Yes	Yes	1.3–1.4 mm thick 2 × 4 cm, 4 × 4 cm, 6 × 6 cm, 5 × 10 cm 1.7–1.8 mm thick 3 × 3 cm, 5 × 5 cm, 5 × 10 cm	
CuffPatch	Biomet and Organo- genesis	Porcine	SIS	Y	Rotator cuff reinforce/ augment soft tissue	Gamma irradiation		Yes	6.5 × 9 cm	
Gore-Tex soft tissue patch	W. L. Gore & Assoc	Synthetic	PTFE	Y	Soft tissue recon- struction	Yes				Hirooka et al.
GraftJacket	Wright Medical	Human	Dermis	N	Rotator cuff reinforce/ augment soft tissue	Yes. Asep- tically pro- cessed		No	0.5–2.29 mm thickness 5 × 5 cm 5 × 10 cm 5 × 30 cm 4 × 7 cm 2 × 4 cm	Burkhead et al. Dopirak et al. Labbe, Synder and Bond

I. The Shoulder

Product	Manufacturer	Species	Material	Crosslinked	Indication	Resorbable	Sterilization	Sterile	Dimensions	References
Matrix HD	RTI Biologics	Human	Dermis		Reinforce/augment soft tissue	Yes	Low-dose gamma	Yes		Audenaert et al.
Mersilene Mesh	Ethicon	Synthetic	Polyester	Y	Reinforce soft tissue		Yes			
OrthADAPT Bioimplant	Synovis Life Technologies, Inc.	Equine	Pericardium	Y EDC+ (carbodiimide)	Rotator cuff reinforce/augment soft tissue	Unknown	Ulti STER	No	0.5–0.8 mm thickness	
Restore	DePuy/J & J	Porcine	SIS	N	Augment soft tissue	Yes	Electron beam	No	0.5-mm thickness; 3 × 4 cm; 4 × 6 cm; 5 × 7 cm; 5 cm diameter	Dejardin et al.; Malcarney et al.; Schlamber et al.; Iannotti et al.; Walton et al.
SportMesh	Biomet	Synthetic	Polycaprolactone-based poly(urethane urea)	N	Reinforce/augment soft tissue	NA	Electron beam		0.9 mm thick	
TissueMend	Stryker/TEI Biosciences	Bovine	Dermis	N	Rotator Cuff Reinforce/augment soft tissue	Yes	Ethylene oxide gas	Yes	4 × 6 cm; 6 × 9 cm; 1-mm thickness	Seldes & Abramchayev

Table 12.1

List of currently available grafts (continued)

Grafts	Company	Material Source	Tissue Type	Cross-Link	Approved Use	Sterilization	Chemical Wash	Sterility Assurance Level (SAL) 10-6	Size	Rotator Cuff Clinical Reports
									3 × 3 cm	
									5 × 6 cm	
									6 × 10 cm	
ZCR Patch	Zimmer	Porcine	Dermis	Y	Rotator Cuff	Gamma	Yes	Yes	1.5-mm thickness	Badhe et al.
				HMDIC (hexamethylene diisoyanate)	Reinforce/augment soft tissue				5 × 5 cm	Soler et al.

Data was obtained from the available literature, promotional materials, and direct contact with the manufacturer/distributor.

From Dejardin LM, Arnoczky SP, Ewers BJ, et al. Tissue-engineered rotator cuff tendon using porcine small intestine submucosa: histologic and mechanical evaluation in dogs. *Am J Sports Med.* 2001;29:175–184; Burkhead W, Schiffern S, Krishnan S. Use of Graft Jacket as an augmentation for massive rotator cuff tears. *Semin Arthro plasty.* 2007;18:11–18; Hirroka A, Yoneda M, Wakaitani S, et al. Augmentation with gore-tex patch for repair of large rotator cuff tears that cannot be sutured. *J Orthop Sci.* 2002;7(4):451–456; Dopirak R, Bond J, Synder S. Arthroscopic total rotator cuff replacement with an acellular human dermal allograft matrix. *Int J shoulder Surg.* 2007;18:11–18; Labbe MR. Arthroscopic technique for patch augmentation of rotator cuff repairs. *Arthroscopy.* 2006;22(10): 113e1–1136e6; Synder S, Bond J. Technique for arthroscopic replacement of severely damaged rotator cuff using "Graftjacket" allograft. *Oper Tech Sports Med.* 2007;15:86–94; Audenaert E, Van Nuffel J, Schepens A, et al. Reconstruction of massive rotator cuff lesions with a synthetic interposition graft: prospective study of 41 patients. *Knee Surg Sports Tramatol Arthrosc.* 2006;14(4):360–364; Malcarney HL, Bonar F, Murrell GA. Early inflammatory reaction after rotator cuff repair with a porcine small intestine submucosal implant: a report of 4 cases. *Am J Sports Med.* 2005;33(6):907–911; Sclamberg SG, Tibone JE, Itamura JM, et al. Six-month magnetic resonance imaging follow-up of large and massive rotator cuff repairs reinforced with porcine small intestinal submucosa. *J Shoulder Elbow Surg.* 2004;13(5):538–541; Iannotti J, Codsi M, Kwon Y, et al. Porcine small intestinal submucosa (restore orthobiologic implant) augmentation of chronic two-tendon rotator cuff tears treated with open surgical repair: a randomized controlled trial. *J Shoulder Elbow Surg.* 16(2):e25–e26; Walton JR, Bowman NK, Khatib Y, et al. Restore orthobiologic implant not recommended for augmentation of rotator cuff repairs. *J Bone Joint Surg Am.* 2007;89(4): 786–791; Seldes RM, Abramchayev I. Arthroscopic insertion of a biologic rotator cuff tissue augmentation after rotator cuff repair. *Arthroscopy.* 2006;22(1):113–116; Badhe SP, Lawrence TM, Smith FD, et al. An assessment of porcine dermal xenograft as an augmentation graft in the treatment of extensive rotator cuff tears. *J Shoulder Elbow Surg.* 2008;17(1) (suppl 9):35S–39S; and Soler JA, Gidwani S, Curtis MJ. Early complications from the use of porcine dermal collagen implants (permacol) as bridging constructs in the repair of massive rotator cuff tears. A report of 4 cases. *Acta Orthp Belg.* 2007;73(4):432–436.

I. The Shoulder

sedimentation rate, C-reactive protein, and a joint aspiration with culture. In short, physiologically younger and more active patients with a mobile shoulder who can complete a rehabilitation program will benefit from an augmentation or replacement while older more sedentary patients with a stiff shoulder often will not.

TREATMENT

Rotator cuff repair should be performed as soon as is reasonable after that diagnosis is made for those patients who fit the indications. There is no absolute time frame within which a repair must be performed, but fatty muscle infiltration has been demonstrated in an animal model to occur in as little as 6 weeks. Those patients with glenohumeral stiffness should try to regain passive motion prior to surgery if possible.

Open Technique

The use of a graft through an open technique has been reported by Burkhead, Schiffern, and Krishnan. They performed the procedure for primary and recurrent massive tears and noted a close to 30% rate of retears although the tears were smaller than the original ones. The retear rate compares favorably to the nearly 100% rate seen in some studies for similar tears. No complications were observed.

A standard open approach is used and a minimal acromioplasty performed. The coracoacromial ligament is preserved and stitched for later repair. The tissue is mobilized and any side-to-side repairs needed are performed with Dacron (Deknatel, Teleflex Medical, Research Park, NC). The bone is prepared with a shallow but broad trough, and the edge of the articular cartilage is smoothed creating a level transition for the tendon. Metallic double-loaded anchors are used with a unique Transosseous Anchor Double Knot (TOAK) pattern. The suture ends are not cut, so they can be used for the graft. The graft is then prepared and attached to the cuff laterally with the sutures from the anchors. Extra anchoring sutures are then circumferentially placed around the graft. The deltotrapezial fascia and coracoacromial ligament are then repaired and wound closure performed (Figs. 12.1 to 12.4) (9).

Arthroscopic Augmentation

Successful arthroscopic augmentation of cuff tears has been reported by this author as well as Snyder and Bone and Barber et al. While there are some technical differences in these surgical techniques, the concept of suturing a graft to an intra-articular structure is the same. The author prefers to use a technique called the "4-corner augmentation." The idea is to arthroscopically place sutures in the four corners of the area where the graft is going to lie. An initial report of the technique showed satisfactory results in six patients using two different grafts. A recent prospective multicenter trial demonstrated a significant improvement in healing rates (85% v. 40%) in augmented repairs of tears greater than 3 cm. The initial results of the arthroscopic arm of the study were reported by Barber et al.

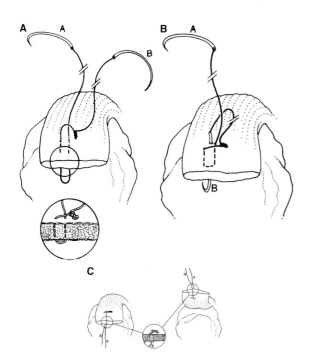

FIGURE 12.1. A: One suture limb (Limb A) from each pair of sutures is passed in a mattress fashion through the distal portion of the tendon. **B:** The second limb (Limb B) from each pair is now passed medial to the mattress suture from Limb A—completing the modified Mason–Allen stitch. **C:** Completed appearance of each pair of sutures after passing through distal portion of tendon. (From Nowinski RJ, Schiffern SC, Burkhead Jr WZ, et al. Biologic resurfacing of the glenoid: longer term results and newer innovations. *Semin Arthroplasty.* 2005;16(4);274 -280, with permission.)

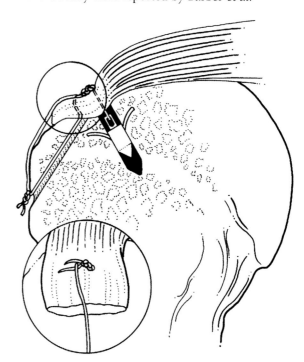

FIGURE 12.2. Inferior limb (Limb B) is now passed in a transosseous fashion. Knot is tied on lateral portion of greater tuberosity completing the TOAK technique. (From Nowinski RJ, Schiffern SC, Burkhead Jr WZ, et al. Biologic resurfacing of the glenoid: longer term results and newer innovations. *Semin Arthroplasty.* 2005;16(4);274 -280, with permission.)

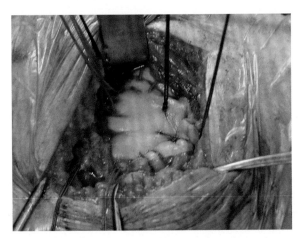

FIGURE 12.3. GraftJacket augmentation securely sutured over the previous rotator cuff repair, creating a watertight surface. (From Nowinski RJ, Schiffern SC, Burkhead Jr WZ, et al. Biologic resurfacing of the glenoid: longer term results and newer innovations. *Semin Arthroplasty.* 2005;16(4);274 -280, with permission.)

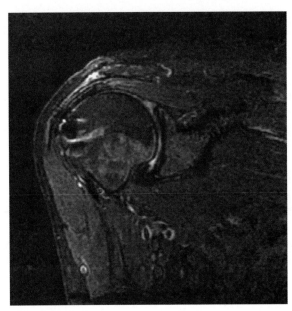

FIGURE 12.4. Postoperative MRI scan at 1-year follow-up. T2 coronal image shows an intact rotator cuff repair with tissue present all the way over the humeral head to the tuberosity. (From Nowinski RJ, Schiffern SC, Burkhead Jr WZ, et al. Biologic resurfacing of the glenoid: longer term results and newer innovations. *Semin Arthroplasty.* 2005;16(4);274 -280, with permission.)

AUTHOR'S PREFERRED TECHNIQUE: 4-CORNER AUGMENTATION

Step One

The first step is to perform a standard cuff repair arthroscopically. Repair the cuff laterally as far as it will go without threatening to slip out of the grasper. Single row, double row, suture-bridge, and other suture passing configurations are all reasonable options based on the tear pattern and tissue quality. For larger tears, consider more points of fixation and more complex suture patterns. Maximize the number of suture passes through tendon, distribute the stresses of the repair over the anchors, and provide as secure a fixation as possible. Too many anchors can cause problems by destabilizing the bone around them resulting in anchor pullout, which makes any necessary revision very difficult. The author prefers anchors that allow for bone marrow egress. Rehydrate the chosen graft if indicated so that it is ready when needed.

Step Two

Medially, at the muscle tendon junction, place two mattress sutures, one anteriorly and one posteriorly. They should be wide enough apart to span the width of your repair and should be placed medial in the tendon to the sutures used to repair the cuff. Use a penetrating retriever to go in and out of the cuff and hand yourself a suture through the opposite portal. Take both ends of the suture out of the opposite portal so that when completed the anterior mattress limbs exit the back of the shoulder and vice versa. Crossing the sutures facilitates management and retrieval later. Laterally place two anchors either in the lateral tuberosity or "over-the-edge" beyond the lateral margin of the cuff repair. The anchors should span the width of the repair. Using a device (e.g., probe with lines, knotted suture, Endobutton ruler), measure the width and

length of the area to be covered with the graft. Mark the graft on the back table and cut it to fit the application area. Most grafts have some innate elasticity. Cut the graft the same size as the graft area. When the sutures are placed 5 to 10 mm from the edge of the tendon to secure it, a natural tensioning of the graft will occur.

Step Three

Move the scope to the posterior portal if it is not there already. Place a large 8.5-mm (or larger) cannula in the lateral portal. Retrieve one of the four corner suture pairs and lay it outside the cannula in the corresponding direction. As the other sutures are retrieved, be sure to apply tension to the sutures already outside of the cannula and keep the retriever on the opposite side of the cannula to avoid crossing the sutures. Hold the graft in each corner with a small hemostat and place the sutures in their respective corners in a mattress pattern. For the medial sutures, identify which limb is most anterior and which is most posterior so that each is in its corresponding position in the graft. Grasp the medial end of the graft and slide it down the cannula into the subacromial space and do not let go. Do not apply tension to the sutures externally when sliding the graft. Once the graft is completely in the subacromial space pull tension on the external sutures in-line with the cannula as the graft is held in the space with the grasper. The slack is now out of the sutures, and the graft should be flat over the cuff.

Step Four

Retrieve one pair of sutures above the graft through a separate portal and tie them with standard arthroscopic knots. Tying the medial sutures first facilitates complete entry and deployment of the graft. Extra sutures can be placed along the margins of the graft to further secure it to the cuff as needed with the same technique used to pass the medial corner sutures (Figs. 12.5 to 12.13B).

The graft should completely cover the repair site in all directions. In addition, the repair site is "bridged" with fixation medial to the repair on the cuff and lateral to the repair on the tuberosity. The material can now load share with the repair, and add collagen to the site (10,11).

ARTHROSCOPIC ROTATOR CUFF REPLACEMENT

The bridging technique has been described and reported by Snyder and Bond. This technique offers the possibility of returning to an acceptable degree of function physiologically young and active patients with irreparable tears. Typically, these patients have massive tears involving both the supraspinatus and infraspinatus. The humeral head then subluxates superiorly resulting in significant pain and weakness. Over time cuff arthropathy develops. Treatment options in the past have included arthroscopic debridement, humeral hemiarthroplasty, and reverse arthroplasty. While each of these techniques has shown some benefit, none attempt to return the patient to a normal or near-normal state. A bridging graft has the potential to reconnect the cuff muscle to the tuberosity, restore the anterior/posterior muscle balance, and reduce the humeral head back into the glenoid. Snyder's original series showed complete incorporation of the graft in 12 of 13 patients with only one failure with a 2-year follow-up. No complications were noted.

The technique conceptually is the same as an augmentation. The cuff and tuberosity are prepared by placing sutures anteriorly and posteriorly in the cuff tendon and triple-loaded anchors in the bone at the articular margin. The anterior sutures can include the biceps tendon if the rotator interval tissue is deficient. Care is taken to abrade the tuberosity and create "bone marrow vents" with a small punch to allow the efflux of marrow elements.

The graft that has been measured and cut to fit the defect is prepared with short-tailed interference knot (STIK) sutures in the medial margin. The interference knots allow the graft to be pulled into the subacromial space and provide a grasping point for suture retrieval during the knot-tying phase. The medial sutures are first passed through the medial edge of the cuff from anterior to posterior followed by one suture from each anchor. The position of the sutures through the graft always matches the locations in the subacromial space.

Suture management is of key concern. When multiple sutures are passing in the cannula at the same time, the sutures must remain under tension and the retriever should pass laterally through the cannula to avoid suture entanglement. Snyder prefers to use suture savers (ConMed Linvatec, Largo, FL) to help manage the sutures throughout the procedure. Once the initial sutures are passed, the graft is pulled into the subacromial space. The STIK sutures are then retrieved in order and tied. The graft is now fixed medially and laterally with one suture from each anchor. The remaining sutures in the anterior and posterior

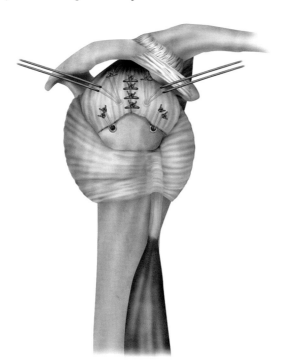

FIGURE 12.5. Repaired rotator cuff with medial mattress sutures in position.

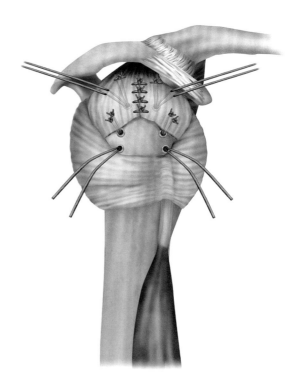

FIGURE 12.6. Lateral anchors are placed either on the lateral tuberosity or on the "over-the-edge" as indicated by the cuff repair forming a 4-corner framework.

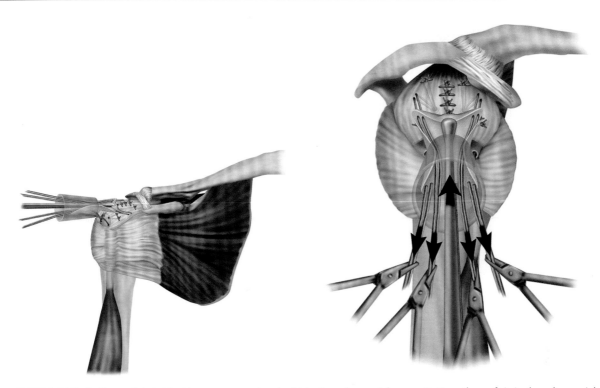

FIGURE 12.7. A: The graft is held with a grasper and pushed into the subacromial space. **B:** Once the graft is in the subacromial space, pull tension on the suture pairs in-line with the cannula to take out the slack.

margins of the cuff are then passed with a suture shuttle and tied. The anchors still have two sutures each remaining. One suture is passed through the lateral edge of the graft and the other through the closest edge of the native cuff. A third lateral anchor can be used if needed to secure the full width of the graft (Figs. 12.14 to 12.21) (12).

The author's preferred bridging technique is to place all of the sutures along the edge of the cuff medially, anteriorly, and posteriorly first along with two or three anchors as necessary into the tuberosity. The sutures are then exteriorized through a large lateral cannula and passed through the graft. The graft is then reduced into the subacromial space, and the sutures are retrieved and tied through a separate

cannula. In reality, these techniques are very similar. The difference lies in the order and location of suture passage. The techniques described can be modified to fit individual preferences so long as the basic concepts are maintained.

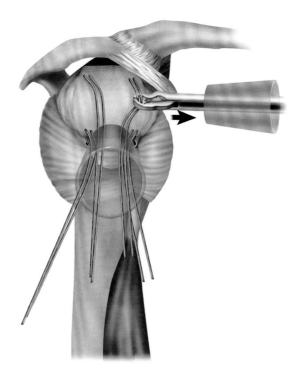

FIGURE 12.9. Retrieve suture pairs through a separate cannula and tie arthroscopically.

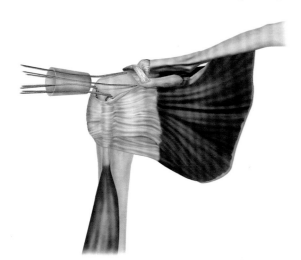

FIGURE 12.8. Graft in the subacromial space.

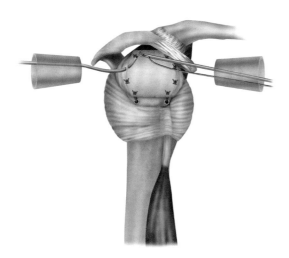

FIGURE 12.10. Add extra sutures as needed to secure the sides of the graft using a side-to-side suture passing technique.

POSTOPERATIVE CARE

The postoperative regime for each of the authors mentioned is very similar. The patients are placed into an abduction pillow and a 3- to 4-week period of rest follows. Depending upon the quality of the tissue and perceived strength of the repair, pendulum exercises can be performed. At 4 to 6 weeks, formal therapy begins for passive motion followed by active-assisted and then active motion at 6 to 8 weeks. Rotator cuff strengthening exercise starts no sooner than 12 weeks, although periscapular exercises may begin earlier.

COMPLICATIONS AND TECHNICAL CHALLENGES

The most common reported complication of grafting is an inflammatory reaction. To date, only the small intestine submucosa (Restore) graft has been reported to have a high

incidence of inflammatory reaction when used for rotator cuff augmentation (13). Recommendations have been made not to use this graft for rotator cuff augmentation.

Postoperative shoulder stiffness is a potential complication. The incidence of shoulder stiffness has not been reported but has been occasionally encountered by the author and others. The general sense is that the humeral head is freer to subluxate with the cuff torn and thus can be "captured" with an intact repair. There is also a normal incidence of adhesive capsulitis, which can develop after an arthroscopic repair. Care should be taken to preoperatively evaluate the shoulder prior to surgery to assess the "reducibility" of the shoulder into the glenoid. Those shoulders that demonstrate a resistance to being reduced should get concomitant capsular releases at the time of repair and grafting.

Postoperatively, treat the shoulder like a standard cuff repair. Various treatment algorithms have been proposed. Patients should have nearly full passive range of motion in forward flexion and abduction by 3.5 to 4.5 months. External and internal rotation can take longer to completely return. Treatments can include steroid injections, regional anesthesia with an indwelling catheter and aggressive therapy, dynamic bracing, surgical manipulation, and arthroscopic release.

Disease transmission is also a risk with allograft and xenograft tissues, although this has not been reported as a complication related to any specific graft. In the studies available, infection rates for either open or arthroscopic procedures are no greater than normal.

PEARLS AND PITFALLS

Technically, there are several challenges to the arthroscopic use of the graft. The first challenge is the cuff itself. Surgeons need advanced skills with the ability to perform various techniques of tissue mobilization, suture passage, and knot tying. The next challenge is the suture management

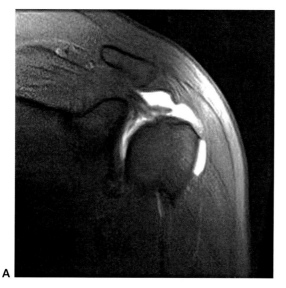
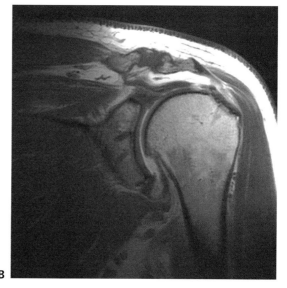

A   B

FIGURE 12.11. Before (**A**) and after (**B**) of an arthroscopic repair without augmentation examined with an MRI arthrogram 52 months out.

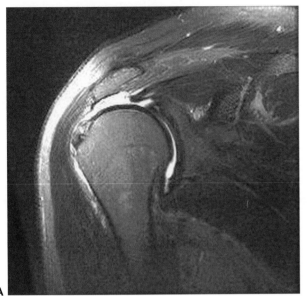
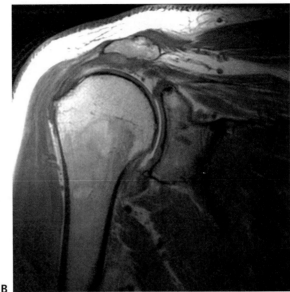

A   B

FIGURE 12.12. Before (**A**) and after (**B**) an arthroscopic repair augmented with GraftJacket studied by MRI arthrogram 11 months post surgery. This is the contralateral arm of the patient in Figures 12.11 (**A**) and (**B**). Note that this augmented side is completely healed and did not leak contrast into the subacromial space during the arthrogram.

required for successful graft placement. The arthroscopic techniques require that multiple sutures reside in the subacromial space and then pass through a single cannula. Using sutures of various colors greatly facilitates this process. In addition, the procedure must be performed in an orderly fashion with all participants focused on suture management in order to avoid entanglement. After a suture or suture pair is brought out the main cannula, it must be tensioned and pulled to one side of the cannula and the retriever brought down the opposite side so that it does not cross a suture as the next one is captured.

The surgical techniques described in this chapter provide a method of suture management in order to achieve this. There are many variations of these techniques that are possible. Each physician needs to master the techniques needed then practice the procedure either on a plastic model or on a cadaver specimen. Observing the procedure

first offers a better understanding of what the assistants can do to facilitate the operation. Once the suture management is mastered, the procedure breaks down to a series of simple steps, which can be accomplished relatively quickly.

CURRENT AND FUTURE DEVELOPMENTS

The future for the use of these materials is just starting to come into focus. As more procedures are performed, the evidence mounts that these grafts are useful tools in the treatment of difficult soft tissue problems and specifically the rotator cuff. The GraftJacket is currently being evaluated in a prospective, multicenter, single-blinded study although it is too early for any data to be released. As yet there is no consensus "best graft" although a few materials have been shown to be inferior for cuff repair. As the technique becomes more utilized, the grafts types will most

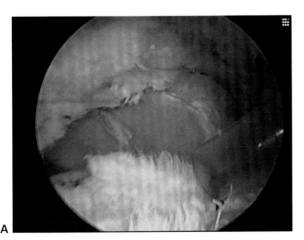
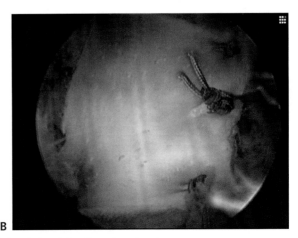

A   B

FIGURE 12.13. Arthroscopic view from the lateral portal before (**A**) and after (**B**) cuff repair and graft.

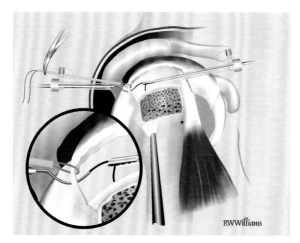

FIGURE 12.14. The irreparable tear is prepared by placing posterior and anterior "endzone" sutures across the tear and saving them in colored straws for later passage through the graft. Reprinted with permission from WoltersKluwer

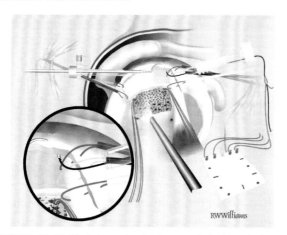

FIGURE 12.15. Medial suturing begins anteriorly through the posterior cannula. An anteromedial shuttle suture is used to pass the corresponding STIK suture from the graft across the tissue and out the posterior cannula. Reprinted with permission from WoltersKluwer

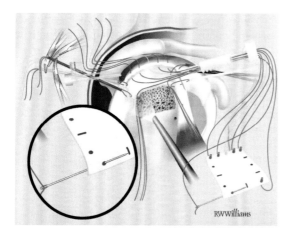

FIGURE 12.16. After careful passage and shuttling of all five medial STIK sutures in parallel, stabilization of the graft's anterior and posterior corners is achieved by passing a limb from each of the suture anchors up through the graft and tying a STIK on top. Reprinted with permission from WoltersKluwer

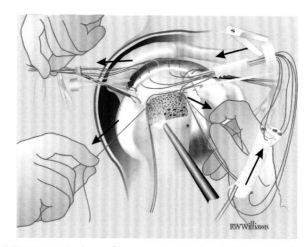

FIGURE 12.17. The graft can now be "push-pulled" into the shoulder through the anterior cannula, pulling on the free ends of all STIK sutures stabilizing the graft. Every suture has been carefully passed in parallel so that any entanglement can be avoided. Reprinted with permission from WoltersKluwer

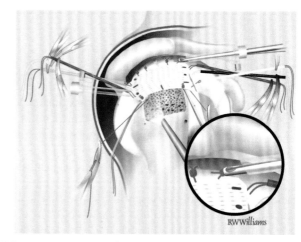

FIGURE 12.18. Once inside the shoulder, the medial STIK sutures are tied, stabilizing this side of the graft. Reprinted with permission from WoltersKluwer

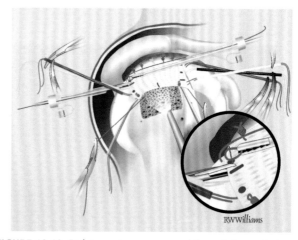

FIGURE 12.19. Endzone sutures are passed through the posterior and anterior sides of the graft and sequentially tied, stabilizing these sides of the graft. Reprinted with permission from WoltersKluwer

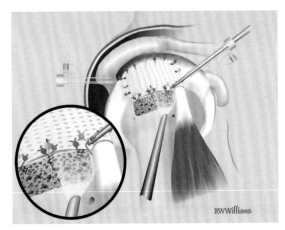

FIGURE 12.20. Finally, the lateral side of the graft is fixed to bone with suture anchors using standard rotator cuff repair technique. Reprinted with permission from WoltersKluwer

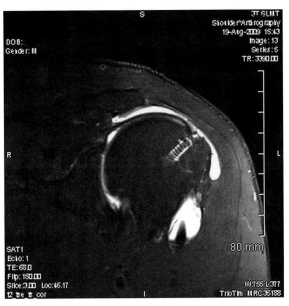

FIGURE 12.21. Ten months out from arthroscopic cuff replacement by the author. Graft is seen attached to cuff edge medially and the tuberosity laterally at the anchor site.

likely narrow because of the factors such as the supply of materials, price, and reimbursements assuming equal patient outcomes. Furthermore, advances will be made in instrumentation and techniques facilitating the procedure.

Conceptually, the graft addresses the issues of mechanical strength at the repair site and collagen deficiency. More can be done to induce the body to heal and the graft may act as a delivery mechanism. Even if grafting does not add much mechanically, the technique may prove worthy in this aspect. Already, many physicians use platelet-rich plasma at the time of repair. The plasma can be injected at the site or incorporated in the sutures at the bone–tendon or graft–tendon interface. In addition, growth factors such as transforming growth factor, fibroblast growth factor, cartilage-derived morphogenic protein, and bone morphogenic protein may separately or in combination have a strong effect on healing and can be delivered through

a graft (14). Stem cells are another area of interest. Cells could be injected at the time of surgery and/or infused. Alternatively or additionally, a graft may be preseeded with the cells prior to implantation. Some of this work had already started. The future looks very bright for this emerging technology. There is much work to be done evaluating the various factors, which can contribute to the success or failure of using a graft. As often is the case, the results can possibly be translated to other problems including wound care and ligament reconstruction. In short, biologic grafting of rotator cuff tears is a potentially powerful and emerging technology. What is emerging now is most likely the tip of the iceberg. Since only about 1/10th of an iceberg is above water, we need to explore for the rest.

REFERENCES

1. Flurin P-H, Landreau P, Gregory T, et al. Cuff integrity after arthroscopic rotator cuff repair: correlation with clinical results in 576 cases. *Arthroscopy*. 2007;7:340–376.
2. Nevaiser, JS, Nevaiser RJ, Nevaiser, TJ. The repair of chronic massive ruptures of the rotator cuff of the shoulder by use of a freeze-dried rotator cuff. *J Bone and Joint Surg Am*. 1978;60(5):681–4.
3. Nasca RJ. The use of freeze-dried allografts in the management of global rotator cuff tears. *Clin Orthop Relat Res*. 1988 March;(228):218–26.
4. Moore Dr, Cain EL, Schwartz ML, Clancy W. Allograft Reconstruction for Massive, Irreparable Rotator Cuff Tears *Am J Sports Med*. 2006;34(3):392–96.
5. Aurora A, McCarron J, Iannotti, JP, et al. Commercially available extracellular matrix materials for rotator cuff tears: state of the art and future trends. *J Shoulder Elbow Surg*. 2007;16:171S–178S.
6. Barber FA, Herbert MA, Coons DA. Tendon augmentation grafts: biomechanical failure loads and failure patterns. *Arthroscopy*. 2006;22:534–538.
7. Chen J, Xu J, Wang A, et al. Scaffolds for tendon and ligament repair: review of the efficacy of commercial products. *Expert Rev Med Devices*. 2009;6:61–73.
8. Walton JR, Bowman NK, Khatib Y, et al. Restore orthobiologic implant: not recommended for augmentation of rotator cuff repairs. *J Bone Joint Surg Am*. 2007;89:786–791.
9. Burkhead WZ, Schiffern SC, Krishnan SG. Use of graft jacket as an augmentation for massive rotator cuff tears. *Semin Arthro*. 2007;18:11–18.
10. Labbé M. Arthroscopic technique for patch augmentation of rotator cuff repairs. *Arthroscopy*. 2006;22:1136.e1–1136.e6.
11. Barber FA, Burns JP, Deutsch, Labbé MR, Litchfield RB. A Prospective, Randomized Evaluation of Acellular Human Dermal Matrix Augmentation for Arthroscopic Rotator Cuff Repair. *Arthroscopy*. 2012;28(1):8–15.
12. Burns JP, Snyder SJ. Biological patches for management of irreparable rotator cuff tears. *Tech Shoulder Surg*. 2009;10:11–21.
13. Sclamberg SG, Tibone JE, Itamura JM, Kasraeian S. Six-month magnetic resonance imaging follow-up of large and massive rotator cuff repairs reinforced with porcine small intestinal submucosa. *J Shoulder Elbow Surg*. 2004;13(5):538-41.
14. Rodeo SA. Biological augmentation of rotator cuff repair. *J Shoulder Elbow Surg*. 2007;16:191S–197S.

Arthroscopic Subscapularis Tendon Repair

Ian K.Y. Lo • Matthew Denkers

Due to their unique anatomy and pathoanatomy, subscapularis tears are commonly missed, particularly partial tears and full-thickness tears of upper subscapularis tendon. Although their incidence has been reported as high as 27%, many subscapularis tears occur in combination with other disorders particularly supraspinatus tendon tears. Importantly, the subscapularis tendon functions as a dynamic stabilizer, providing the anterior moment of the transverse force plane couple. Therefore, repair of subscapularis tendon tears is critical in balancing the force couples to provide a stable fulcrum for glenohumeral motion (1).

CLINICAL EVALUATION

Pertinent History

Patients with subscapularis tears usually present with pain as their predominant complaint. Although the reported mechanisms of injury are a forced external rotation or hyperextension load, many patients may not recall a traumatic episode, particularly in degenerative or combined tears of the subscapularis.

Physical Examination

Physical findings associated with subscapularis tendon tears are a painful arc of motion, a decrease in internal rotation strength, and an increase in passive external rotation. However, various special tests have been described to evaluate the integrity of the subscapularis tendon.

The lift-off test evaluates the patient's ability to lift the back of the hand posteriorly off the lumbar region using terminal internal rotation (i.e., subscapularis function). However, this classic test can be normal in patients with upper subscapularis tendon tears and may not be positive until greater than 50% to 75% of the subscapularis tendon is torn. Furthermore, some patients cannot bring the affected arm into the starting position because of pain or restricted range of motion. In this scenario, the belly-press test or Napoleon test may be used.

When performing the belly-press test (2,3), the patient presses on the abdomen with the palm of the hand and brings the elbow anterior to the mid-coronal plane of the body using internal rotation. The result of the test is considered positive (i.e., a subscapularis tear) when the patient's elbow drops posteriorly behind the mid-coronal plane and pressure on the abdomen is provided instead by extension of the shoulder. The Napoleon test (4) is similarly performed, but also considers the position of the wrist. In patients with a subscapularis tear, when the elbow drops posteriorly the wrist also correspondingly flexes against the abdomen (the position in which Napoleon commonly held his hand against his stomach during portraits). The amount of subscapularis tearing has been correlated with the degree of wrist flexion. Tears of less than 50% of the subscapularis tendon can have negative Napoleon signs (i.e., wrist fully extended), tears involving greater than 50% but not the entire tendon have an intermediate result (i.e., wrist flexed 30° to 60°), and tears involving the entire subscapularis tendon have a positive Napoleon test (i.e., wrist flexed 90°) (4) (Fig. 13.1).

The bear-hug test has been recently described and may be more sensitive than the previous tests for small upper subscapularis tendon tears (5). In the bear-hug test, the patient first positions the hand of the affected side on the contralateral shoulder with the elbow in a forward flexed position (5) (Fig. 13.2A). As the examiner pulls the patient's hand off the shoulder using an external rotational load, the patient resists using internal rotation. The result of the test is considered positive if the examiner is able to lift the patient's hand off the shoulder and is suggestive of at least a partially torn subscapularis (Fig. 13.2B).

In addition to subscapularis tendon insufficiency, patients should also be evaluated for subcoracoid impingement. Although controversial, subcoracoid impingement has been associated with subscapularis tears and may be an etiologic factor and a cause of persistent shoulder pain (6). Presumably, the origin of this pain is secondary to impingement between the subscapularis tendon/lesser

I. The Shoulder

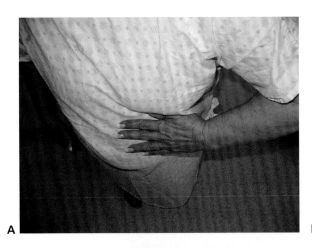
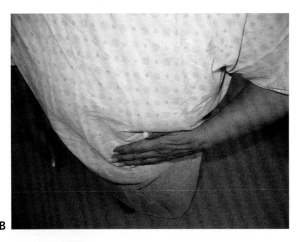
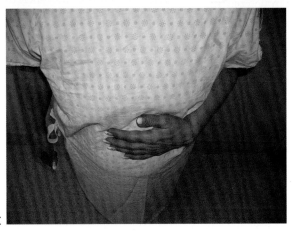

FIGURE 13.1. Napoleon test. **A:** Negative Napoleon test, the patient can press on the belly with the wrist at 0°, indicating normal subscapularis function. **B:** Intermediate Napoleon test, as the patient presses on the belly the wrist flexes 30° to 60°, indicating partial function of the subscapularis. **C:** Positive Napoleon test, indicating a nonfunctional subscapularis, in which the patient can press on the belly only by flexing the wrist 90°, using the posterior deltoid rather than subscapularis function.

tuberosity against the coracoid process. Most patients clinically will demonstrate pain and tenderness about the coracoid and subcoracoid region with a positive coracoid impingement test. This test result is considered positive when pain and/or clicking are elicited by passive forward flexion, adduction, and internal rotation (7,8).

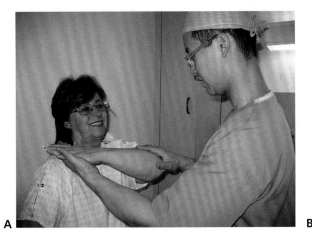
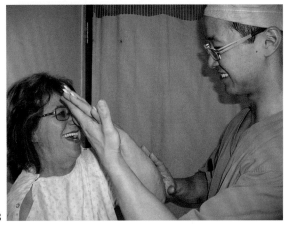

FIGURE 13.2. The bear-hug test. **A:** The patient tries to hold the starting position by means of resisted internal rotation as the examiner tries to pull the patient's hand from the shoulder with an external rotation force applied perpendicular to the forearm. **B:** A positive bear-hug test results when the patient cannot hold the hand against the shoulder as the examiner applies an external rotation force.

Diagnostic Imaging

A few studies have specifically evaluated the use of diagnostic imaging in the evaluation of the subscapularis tendon. Plain radiographs are usually nonspecific, but may demonstrate static anterior subluxation of the humeral head on axillary radiographs in patients with chronic subscapularis tendon insufficiency. In addition, proximal humeral head migration on anterior–posterior radiographs is highly suggestive of a massive, rotator cuff tear that may include the subscapularis tendon.

Ultrasound can provide an inexpensive, noninvasive, dynamic assessment of the rotator cuff, but is highly observer dependent. Ultrasound has been reported to be approximately 85% accurate in detecting full-thickness subscapularis tears, but is not as accurate in demonstrating partial thickness tears, particularly small upper subscapularis tendon tears.

MRI is considered the modality of choice for evaluating rotator cuff pathology. The addition of contrast enables better delineation of rotator cuff pathology and may improve diagnostic accuracy, particularly of upper subscapularis tears. Subscapularis tears can be demonstrated as areas of disorganization or disruption of normal tendon morphology and high signal intensity on T2-weighted images. In addition, adjacent pathology may be suggestive of subscapularis tearing. Medial dislocation of the long head of the biceps tendon is highly suggestive of a subscapularis tear since subscapularis tears commonly disrupt the medial sling of the biceps tendon resulting in biceps instability (Fig. 13.3A).

Although MRI arthrography has been reported to be 91% sensitive and 86% specific for detecting subscapularis tears (9), others have reported less promising results. Full-thickness, upper subscapularis tears and partial thickness tears are commonly missed on MRI. In one study, surgically confirmed subscapularis tears were identified in only 31% (5/16) of patients on MRI (10).

MRI may also be used to estimate the chronicity of the tear. Patients with severe atrophy and fatty degeneration on MRI or CT generally have poor tendon quality and limited tendon excursion, potentially indicating an irreparable subscapularis tear (11,12). However, other authors have argued that despite atrophy and fatty degeneration, many subscapularis tears are commonly reparable and may postoperatively function as a tenodesis to provide a stable fulcrum of motion (13).

In addition to subscapularis pathology, imaging studies should be evaluated for evidence of subcoracoid impingement. The subcoracoid space (i.e., between the lesser tuberosity and the coracoid) can be reduced by a number of potential causes including lesser tuberosity fracture, calcific tendinosis, postoperative changes (e.g., glenoid version alterations and coracoid osteotomy), or prominence of the coracoid. Importantly, it should be remembered when interpreting imaging that proximal humeral migration and anterior subluxation of the glenohumeral joint can exacerbate narrowing of the subcoracoid space, particularly when imaging studies are obtained supine (e.g., MRI).

One measurement technique, the coracoid index, measures the length of the coracoid tip, which projects lateral to a line drawn tangential to the glenoid face on axial CT scans. The normal projection of the coracoid lateral to this line was 8.2 mm (range: −2.5 to 25 mm) in 67 patients (14). Although not clearly defined, abnormal or excessive projection or angulation of the coracoid beyond this tangential line may predispose to subcoracoid impingement.

The more accepted method of measurement is to use the coracohumeral distance (i.e., the distance between the coracoid tip and the humerus/lesser tuberosity) as measured on axial CT or MRI images. In normal shoulders, the coracohumeral distance is 8.7 to 11.0 mm (7,8). In contrast, a narrowed coracohumeral distance is commonly associated with subscapularis tears (Fig. 13.3B). In one study of

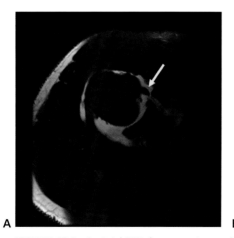 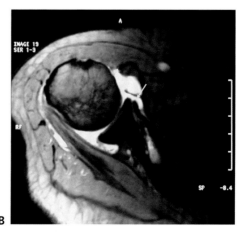

A   B

FIGURE 13.3. A: Axial MRI demonstrating medial dislocation of the long head of the biceps tendon *(arrow).* **B:** Axial T2-weighted MRI demonstrating a complete subscapularis tendon tear *(arrow)* with a narrowed coracohumeral distance *(yellow line).*

patients requiring a subscapularis repair, the coracohumeral distance was 5.0 ± 1.7 mm, compared with 10.0 ± 1.3 mm in a control group that had no rotator cuff, subscapularis, or subcoracoid pathology (15). Therefore, many authors consider a coracohumeral distance of less than 6 mm as evidence of narrowing although its exact role in the pathogenesis of subscapularis tendon tearing remains unclear.

TREATMENT

Nonoperative

Nonoperative treatment of subscapularis tears is similar to nonoperative treatment for standard posterosuperior rotator cuff tears. A few protocols have been specifically designed to address the subscapularis tendon. However, general conservative management may include cold/heat therapy, pain medications, nonsteroidal anti-inflammatories, injections (e.g., subacromial or glenohumeral), or physical therapy.

Operative Indications and Timing

The indications for arthroscopic subscapularis repair are essentially the same as indications for arthroscopic rotator cuff repair. Patients with significant pain and disability despite conservative management for 3 to 6 months are candidates for arthroscopic repair. Similar to acute tears of the posterosuperior rotator cuff, acute subscapularis tears should be treated urgently to prevent further retraction and atrophy. In patients with chronic tears, particularly those with significant tendon retraction and fatty infiltration of the subscapularis tendon, arthroscopic repair may still be attempted but may be unsuccessful. Alternative treatments including allograft or tendon transfer (e.g., split pectoralis major transfer) may be considered.

Although arthroscopic repair of full-thickness subscapularis tears is generally accepted following failure of nonoperative treatment, debridement alone may be considered in carefully selected patients. In contrast to younger patients, older patients can present with issues that complicate treatment and outcome including larger tear sizes, concomitant disease, and delayed presentation that can lead to tendon retraction, muscle atrophy, and fatty infiltration. Furthermore, some older patients may be unwilling to participate in the rehabilitation program required following repair. In one study, 9 of 11 such patients had good or excellent results following arthroscopic debridement of the subscapularis tear and release of the long head of the biceps (16).

OPERATIVE TECHNIQUE

Arthroscopic subscapularis repair is a relatively new technique. Due to its relative complexity, arthroscopic subscapularis repair should only be attempted when the arthroscopist is comfortable with standard rotator cuff repair. Two approaches may be generally used for arthroscopic subscapularis repair—bursal or articular approaches. The bursal approach repairs the subscapularis tendon while viewing through a lateral subacromial portal with instruments introduced through a separate anterolateral portal. This method provides improved visualization of the bursal surface of the subscapularis tendon and allows dissection of the axillary nerve. However, in our experience visualization and instrument spacing can be problems. Furthermore, axillary nerve dissection is rarely required. We prefer the articular approach, which maximizes instrument spacing, allows easy visualization and identification of the subscapularis tendon, and simplifies arthroscopic coracoplasty and subscapularis repair.

AUTHORS' PREFERRED TREATMENT

We perform all-shoulder arthroscopy in the lateral decubitus position, which maximizes surgical access circumferentially around the shoulder. The patient's arm is positioned in a Tenet Spider limb positioner with lateral arm attachment (Tenet Medical, Calgary, AB) and provides longitudinal traction. Although repair in the beach chair position is possible, limb positioning (in abduction, internal rotation, and posterior translation) is easier in the lateral position.

Standard anterior and posterior glenohumeral portals are established and a diagnostic arthroscopy performed. However, the critical portal is the anterosuperolateral portal created approximately 2 cm off the anterolateral corner of the acromion, anterior to the supraspinatus tendon but posterior to the long head of the biceps tendon. Importantly, the portal is created parallel to the lesser tuberosity and is the workhorse portal for releases, bone bed debridement, suture passage, and knot tying (Fig. 13.4).

Clear visualization during any arthroscopic procedure is essential. This can be particularly demanding during arthroscopic subscapularis repair. To visualize the

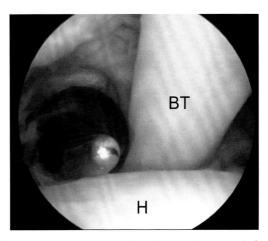

FIGURE 13.4. Arthroscopic view through a posterior portal of a left shoulder demonstrating the anterosuperolateral portal, adjacent to the biceps tendon, and parallel to the lesser tuberosity. BT, biceps tendon; H, humeral head.

procedure, we almost exclusively view through a posterior glenohumeral portal (Fig. 13.5A). However, manipulating the arm into abduction, internal rotation, and posterior translation can maximize visualization. This draws the fibers of the subscapularis away from the humeral head increasing the anterior working space and revealing the tendon insertion (Fig. 13.5B). A 70° arthroscope is used routinely in combination with arm positioning to maximize visualization (Fig. 13.5C). By using a combination of arm positioning and a 70° arthroscope, a top-down view of the subscapularis tendon and the entire footprint may be obtained and their relationship with adjacent structures assessed (e.g., medial sling and biceps tendon).

Once a subscapularis tear has been recognized (Fig. 13.6), the next step is to delineate the margins of the subscapularis tendon. This is particularly relevant in chronic complete, full-thickness tears of the subscapularis tendon. In this situation, the tendon stump commonly retracts medially scarring to the inner deltoid fascia. This obscures both the lateral and the superior borders of the subscapularis stump and can make the tendon stump difficult to locate.

The key to identifying the subscapularis tendon is to locate the pathoanatomic finding called the "comma sign." The comma sign is a comma-shaped arc of soft tissue located above the superolateral border of the torn subscapularis tendon (17) (Fig. 13.7A). This tissue is composed of the medial biceps sling (i.e., medial coracohumeral ligament and superior glenohumeral ligament) and interdigitates with the superior fibers of the subscapularis tendon at its humeral insertion. When the subscapularis tendon tears, the medial biceps sling tears along with it and stays attached to the superolateral corner of the subscapularis tendon forming this comma-shaped soft tissue. Applying traction along the "crook" of the comma, this draws out the subscapularis tendon from behind the glenoid and the superior and lateral borders of the subscapularis tendon may be identified (Fig. 13.7B).

A traction stitch is then passed through the superolateral corner of the subscapularis tendon to aid in tendon releases and reduction. An antegrade suture-passing

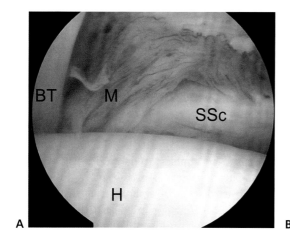

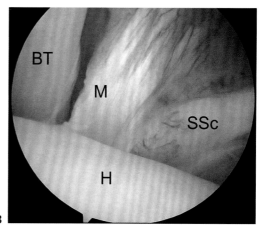

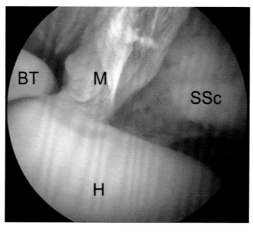

FIGURE 13.5. Arthroscopic views through a posterior portal of a left shoulder demonstrating the anterior structures in different arm positions. **A:** Normal. **B:** Internal rotation with posterior translation. **C:** Seventy-degree arthroscope. H, humeral head; BT, biceps tendon; SSc, subscapularis tendon; M, medial sling.

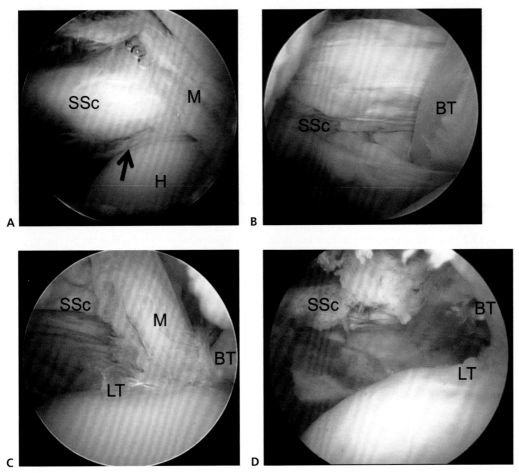

FIGURE 13.6. Arthroscopic views through a posterior portal of different right shoulders demonstrating various subscapularis tendon tears. **A:** A partial undersurface tear *(arrow)* of the upper subscapularis tendon. **B:** An upper subscapularis tendon tear with the biceps tendon subluxed through a split subscapularis tendon. **C:** A full-thickness, partial width upper subscapularis tendon tear involving the upper 33% of the footprint. **D:** A complete subscapularis tendon tear. SSc, subscapularis tendon; BT, biceps tendon; LT, lesser tuberosity; H, humeral head; M, medial sling.

instrument (e.g., Scorpion, Arthrex, Inc., Naples, FL) is introduced through the anterosuperolateral portal and a traction stitch placed. The traction stitch may be retrieved out a separate puncture wound or the anterosuperolateral portal.

During subscapularis repair, the long head of the biceps tendon usually must be addressed. Concomitant involvement of the long head of the biceps tendon occurs in the majority of cases and may include subluxation, dislocation, or rupture. Biceps instability is usually encountered since subscapularis tears are associated with disruption of the medial sling. Even in cases where the biceps tendon is not subluxed, some authors have recommended routine tenotomy or tenodesis, which is associated with improved subjective and objective results, independent of the preoperative condition of the biceps tendon (18). In general, we perform biceps tenodesis in the majority of cases except in elderly lower demand patients, in whom a simple biceps tenotomy is sufficient. The key principle is to tag and

release the biceps tendon early in the procedure, maximizing visualization for subsequent anterior shoulder work (i.e., releases and bone bed preparation). Tenodesis is performed low in the bicipital groove, after releases but prior to definitive tendon fixation to bone.

The next step is to mobilize the subscapularis tendon (1,4,13). Most complete subscapularis tears must be mobilized to allow a tension-free repair to bone. In general, releases begin superior and proceed anterior and posterior. A lateral release is sometimes required in chronically adhesed cases. Importantly, an inferior release is rarely required and avoids compromising the axillary nerve.

The superior release is performed first and essentially creates a window through the rotator interval (19). Pulling on the traction stitch draws the superior border of the subscapularis tendon out from behind the glenoid, and instruments (e.g., cautery and shaver) are introduced through the anterosuperolateral portal. Soft tissue resection begins superior to the subscapularis, keeping the lateral rotator

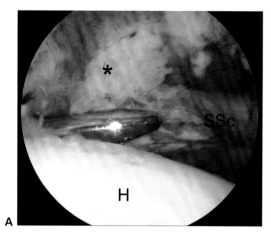
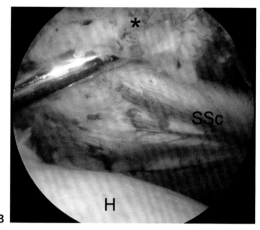

FIGURE 13.7. The comma sign. Arthroscopic views through a posterior portal of a left shoulder. **A:** The comma sign (*) is a comma-shaped arc of tissue above the superolateral border of the subscapularis tendon. The probe points to the superolateral corner of the subscapularis tendon. **B:** Traction along the "crook" of the comma sign draws out the superior and lateral borders of the subscapularis tendon. SSc, subscapularis.

interval tissue (i.e., the comma sign) intact (Fig. 13.8A). As the resection progresses, the underlying coracoid can be felt as a bony prominence and the coracoid is then exposed (Fig. 13.8B). It is important to stay on the posterolateral aspect of the coracoid, which prevents catastrophic neurovascular injury. Viewing with a 70° arthroscope can assist in visualizing the medial aspect of the superior border of the subscapularis tendon behind the glenoid and any superior adhesions may be released.

Once the rotator interval window has been created, the 70° arthroscope is advanced through the window and provides a top-down view of the structures anterior to the subscapularis tendon. The coracoid is identified and the anterior release is performed next. Instruments (e.g., shaver and cautery) are introduced through the anterosuperolateral portal directed anterior to the subscapularis

tendon. Fibrofatty tissue is removed from the subcoracoid space (Fig. 13.9A) and the posterolateral aspect of the coracoid is skeletonized essentially releasing the coracohumeral ligament (Fig. 13.9B).

The subcoracoid space is then assessed comparing the space with an instrument of known size (Fig. 13.10A). When indicated (subcoracoid space less than 6 mm), a coracoplasty is performed using a burr through the anterosuperolateral portal (20,21). The goal of the coracoplasty is to create a 7- to 10-mm space between the posterolateral tip of the coracoid and the anterior plane of the subscapularis tendon (Fig. 13.10B). Care is taken to protect the inferior conjoint tendon and the superolateral coracoacromial ligament. Subcoracoid decompression increases the anterior working space, facilitating repair and may protect the repaired subscapularis from any abrasive effect.

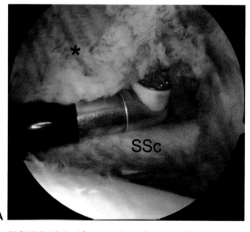
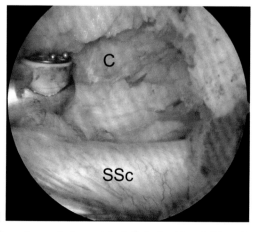

FIGURE 13.8. The superior release. Arthroscopic views through a posterior portal of a left shoulder. **A:** The soft tissue resection begins just above the subscapularis tendon, keeping the lateral comma sign intact. **B:** The rotator interval is resected exposing the coracoid and allowing visualization of structures anterior to the subscapularis tendon. C, coracoid; SSc, subscapularis tendon; *, comma sign.

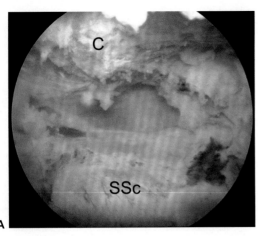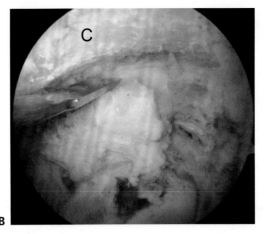

FIGURE 13.9. The anterior release. Arthroscopic views of a left shoulder through a posterior portal using a 70° arthroscope. **A:** The arthroscope is "driven" through the rotator interval window, providing a top-down view of the subscapularis tendon and coracoid. Fibrofatty tissue is removed from the subcoracoid space. **B:** The posterolateral arch of the coracoid is cleared releasing the coracohumeral ligament. C, coracoid; SSc, subscapularis tendon.

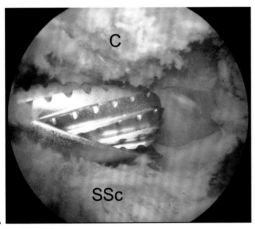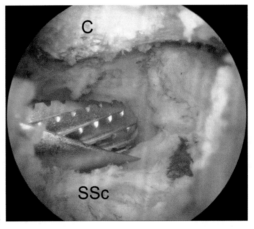

FIGURE 13.10. The coracoplasty. Arthroscopic view of a left shoulder through a posterior portal using a 70° arthroscope. **A:** The subcoracoid space is then assessed and appears slightly narrowed in this case. **B:** A burr is introduced through the anterosuperolateral portal anterior to the subscapularis tendon. A coracoplasty is then performed in line with the subscapularis tendon creating a space of approximately 7 to 8 mm. C, coracoid; SSc, subscapularis tendon.

The posterior release is performed next and the arthroscope is withdrawn out the rotator interval window. Using cautery and an elevator, the subscapularis tendon is released from the middle glenohumeral ligament and anterior capsule (Fig. 13.11). With a completed three-sided release (i.e., superior, anterior, and posterior), sufficient mobility is usually obtained for tendon repair to bone (Fig. 13.12).

In some chronically adhesed cases, a lateral release may also be necessary when the lateral margin of the subscapularis tendon is scarred to the inner deltoid fascia, coracoid, and conjoint tendon. In this case, the lateral margin must be defined and delineated (using the comma sign as a guide), and the soft tissue bursal leader lateral to the tendon is debrided (Fig. 13.13A). The dissection continues inferior until the subscapularis tendon is released

from the anterior structures (Fig. 13.13B,C), and the subcoracoid space is reconstituted.

Once the subscapularis has been released, the bone bed is prepared using a burr through the anterosuperolateral portal. The amount of bone bed exposed may be compared with cadaveric data (see above) to estimate the percentage of tendon torn. The average footprint measures 25.8 ± 3.2 mm in superior-to-inferior height, and the width measures 18.1 ± 1.6 mm (22,23). Occasionally the bone bed may be medialized by 5 mm to minimize repair tension and maximize tendon contact to bone.

Standard suture anchor-based techniques are used for definitive tendon fixation to bone. Starting inferiorly suture anchors (e.g., Bio-Corkscrew FT, Arthrex, Inc., Naples, FL) are percutaneously inserted in the lesser tuberosity using needle localization at a "Deadman's" angle.

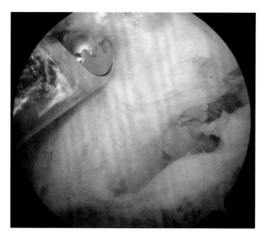

FIGURE 13.11. The posterior release. Arthroscopic views through a posterior portal of a left shoulder. Instruments are then introduced through the anterosuperolateral portal posterior to the subscapularis tendon releasing the capsule and middle glenohumeral ligament.

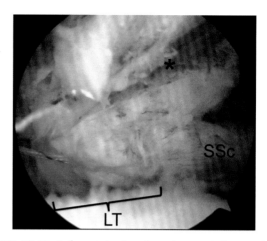

FIGURE 13.12. Arthroscopic view through a posterior portal of a left shoulder demonstrating reduction of the subscapularis tendon to the lesser tuberosity following release. SSc, subscapularis tendon; LT, lesser tuberosity; *, comma sign.

Antegrade suture passage through the anterosuperolateral portal is utilized (Fig. 13.14A) using the percutaneous anchor portal for suture management. To facilitate suture management and maximize visualization, tying as you go is the preferable technique (Fig. 13.14B). The repair proceeds superiorly with subsequent anchor insertion, suture passage, and knot tying. Usually two or three double-loaded anchors are required for a complete subscapularis tendon tear (Fig. 13.15). Double-row repair is possible when tendon excursion allows. However, only a single-row repair may be achievable and it has generally led to good clinical results.

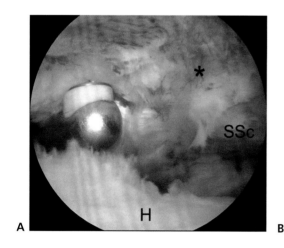

A

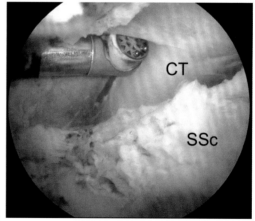

B

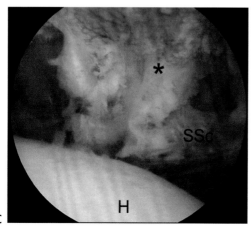

C

FIGURE 13.13. Arthroscopic view through a posterior portal of a left shoulder demonstrating an adhesed subscapularis tendon. A: The lateral margin of the subscapularis tendon is identified using the comma sign and released. B: The release continues inferior usually including release from the conjoint tendon. C: Completed release demonstrating reconstitution of the lateral border. SSc, subscapularis tendon; *, comma sign; CT, conjoint tendon, H, humeral head.

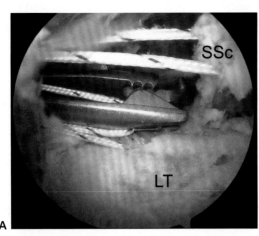 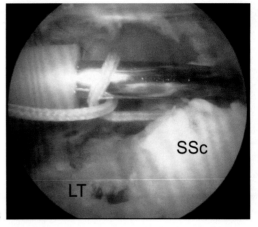

FIGURE 13.14. Suture anchor fixation. Arthroscope view through a posterior portal of a left shoulder. **A:** Following percutaneous anchor insertion, antegrade suture passer using a Scorpion suture passer (Arthrex, Inc., Naples, FL) is performed usually passing simple stitches. **B:** Knots are tied through the anterosuperolateral portal. LT, lesser tuberosity; SSc, subscapularis tendon.

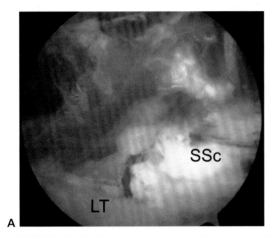 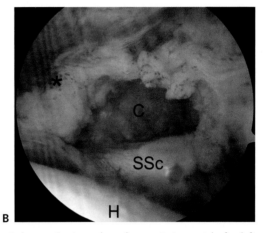

FIGURE 13.15. Completed subscapularis tendon repair. Arthroscopic views through a posterior portal of a left shoulder. **A:** View of the repair on the lesser tuberosity. **B:** Standard posterior arthroscopic view. The coracoid is visible through the rotator window. C, coracoid; SSc, subscapularis tendon; LT, lesser tuberosity; H, humerus; *, comma sign.

Once subscapularis repair is achieved, repair of the posterosuperior rotator cuff may proceed. If the lateral comma sign has been left intact, this tissue may be incorporated during posterosuperior rotator cuff repair (Fig. 13.16).

PEARLS AND PITFALLS

1. Maximize visualization of the subscapularis tendon by utilizing arm position (i.e., abduction, internal rotation, and posterior translation) and a 70° arthroscope.
2. Address biceps pathology by tagging and releasing the tendon early in the procedure to maximize visualization and facilitate repair.
3. Utilize the comma sign to identify the superior and lateral borders of the subscapularis tendon.
4. Place a traction stitch in the superolateral corner of the subscapularis tendon drawing the retracted

subscapularis tendon from behind the glenoid neck and into view.
5. Perform releases of the subscapularis tendon starting superiorly and progressing anterior and posterior. A lateral release may also be necessary in adhesed cases.
6. Standard suture anchor-based repair techniques utilizing antegrade suture passage are easiest for tendon fixation to bone.
7. Keep the lateral rotator interval tissue (i.e., the comma sign) intact, which can be useful in the repair of the posterosuperior rotator cuff.

REHABILITATION

Postoperatively, sling immobilization is recommended for 6 weeks during ambulation and sleep. Hand, wrist, and elbow motions are performed immediately, with active motion of the elbow restricted for 6 weeks if a biceps

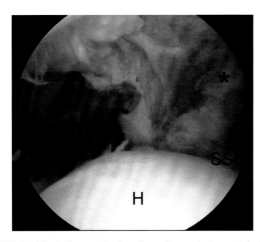

FIGURE 13.16. Arthroscopic view through a posterior portal of a left shoulder. The subscapularis tendon repair is complete with the residual posterosuperior rotator cuff tear still present. It is important to keep the comma sign intact, which may assist in the repair of the posterosuperior rotator cuff. SSc, subscapularis tendon; *, comma sign; H, humeral head; RCT, posterosuperior rotator cuff tear.

tenodesis was performed. Passive external rotation is also performed immediately limited to 0° or as assessed intraoperatively. Forward elevation is begun 6 weeks postoperatively progressing from active assisted to active range of motion. Rotator cuff and deltoid strengthening may begin at 12 weeks postoperatively.

CONCLUSIONS AND FUTURE DIRECTIONS

Arthroscopic subscapularis repair is a relatively difficult procedure and should not be attempted unless the surgeon is already familiar with standard arthroscopic rotator cuff repair. However, by adherence to the principles of maximizing visualization, delineating the margins of the subscapularis, and releasing and mobilizing the subscapularis, standard suture anchor-based techniques may be utilized for arthroscopic subscapularis tendon repair to bone.

Although arthroscopic techniques have developed considerably to allow routine arthroscopic subscapularis repair, the basic questions related to etiology and treatment remain unclear. In particular, its relationship between subcoracoid impingement and other factors (e.g., degeneration) requires further investigation. Future trials are necessary to define the indications for debridement versus repair for all lesions (i.e., partial thickness, partial width full thickness, and complete full thickness) and the treatment of concomitant pathology.

REFERENCES

1. Burkhart SS, Lo IK. Arthroscopic rotator cuff repair. *J Am Acad Orthop Surg.* 2006;14:333–346.
2. Gerber C, Krushell RJ. Isolated rupture of the tendon of the subscapularis muscle. Clinical features in 16 cases. *J Bone Joint Surg Br.* 1991;73:389–394.
3. Gerber C, Hersche O, Farron A. Isolated rupture of the subscapularis tendon. *J Bone Joint Surg Am.* 1996;78:1015–1023.
4. Burkhart SS, Tehrany AM. Arthroscopic subscapularis tendon repair: technique and preliminary results. *Arthroscopy.* 2002;18:454–463.
5. Barth JRH, Burkhart SS, De Beer JF. The bear-hug test: a new and sensitive test for diagnosing a subscapularis tear. *Arthroscopy.* 2006;22:1076–1084.
6. Lo IK, Burkhart SS. The etiology and assessment of subscapularis tendon tears: a case for subcoracoid impingement, the roller-wringer effect, and TUFF lesions of the subscapularis. *Arthroscopy.* 2003;19:1142–1150.
7. Gerber C, Terrier F, Sehnder R, et al. The subcoracoid space. An anatomic study. *Clin Orthop Relat Res.* 1987;215:132–138.
8. Friedman RJ, Bonutti PM, Genez B. Cine magnetic resonance imaging of the subcoracoid region. *Orthopedics.* 1998;21:545–548.
9. Pfirrmann CW, Zanetti M, Weishaupt D, et al. Subscapularis tendon tears: detection and grading at MR arthrography. *Radiology.* 1999;213:709–714.
10. Tung GA, Yoo DC, Levine SM, et al. Subscapularis tendon tear: primary and associated signs on MRI. *J Comput Assist Tomogr.* 2001;25:417–424.
11. Goutallier D, Postel JM, Bernageau J, et al. Fatty muscle degeneration in cuff ruptures. Pre- and post-operative evaluation by CT scan. *Clin Orthop Relat Res.* 1994;304:78–83.
12. Goutallier D, Postel JM, Bernageau J, et al. Fatty infiltration of disrupted rotator cuff muscles. *Rev Rheum Engl Ed.* 1995;63:415–422.
13. Burkhart SS, Brady PC. Arthroscopic subscapularis repair: surgical tips and pearls from A to Z. *Arthroscopy.* 2006;22:1014–1027.
14. Dines DM, Warren RF, Inglis AE, et al. The coracoid impingement syndrome. *J Bone Joint Surg Br.* 1990;72-B:314–316.
15. Richards DP, Burkhart SS, Campbell SE. Relation between narrowed coracohumeral distance and subscapularis tears. *Arthroscopy.* 2005;21:1223–1228.
16. Edwards TB, Walch G, Nové-Josserand L, et al. Arthroscopic debridement in the treatment of patients with isolated tears of the subscapularis. *Arthroscopy.* 2006;22:942–946.
17. Lo IK, Burkhart SS. The comma sign: arthroscopic guide to the torn subscapularis tendon. *Arthroscopy.* 2003;19:334–337.
18. Edwards TB, Walch G, Sirveaux F, et al. Repair of tears of the subscapularis. *J Bone Joint Surg Am.* 2005;87A:725–730.
19. Lo IK, Burkhart SS. The interval slide in continuity: a method of mobilizing the anterosuperior rotator cuff without disrupting the tear margins. *Arthroscopy.* 2004;20:435–441.
20. Lo IK, Burkhart SS. Arthroscopic coracoplasty through the rotator interval. *Arthroscopy.* 2003;19:667–671.
21. Lo IK, Parten PM, Burkhart SS. Combined subcoracoid and subacromial impingement in association with anterosuperior rotator cuff tears: an arthroscopic approach. *Arthroscopy.* 2003;19:1068–1078.
22. D'Addesi LL, Anbari A, Reish MW, et al. The subscapularis footprint: an anatomic study of the subscapularis tendon insertion. *Arthroscopy.* 2006;22:937–940.
23. Curtis AS, Burbank KM, Tierney JJ, et al. The insertional footprint of the rotator cuff: an anatomic study. *Arthroscopy.* 2006;22:603–609.

Labral (Including SLAP) Lesions: Classification and Repair Techniques

Jay H. Rapley • F. Alan Barber

KEY POINTS

- Superior labral injuries can be confused with normal variations or degenerative changes.
- Clinically significant superior labrum anterior and posterior (SLAP) lesions are most commonly found in throwing athletes or after shoulder dislocations.
- Glenohumeral arthritis and full thickness rotator cuff tears do not accompany true type II SLAP injuries.
- Described physical examination maneuvers and provocative tests provide inconsistent results and are not consistently accurate.
- An MRI with gadolinium can define labral anatomy and is a commonly chosen diagnostic imaging study.
- Posterior type II SLAP injuries commonly demonstrate a "peel back sign" during which the posterior superior labrum "peels back" off the glenoid rim when the arm is abducted to 90° and externally rotated.
- Three specific findings associated with significant superior labral pathology include sublabral fraying, superior glenoid chondromalacia, and injury to the superior glenohumeral ligament (SGHL).

Injuries to the biceps tendon attachment to the superior glenoid labrum can be chronic and can often present subtle findings. This type of injury was originally described in throwing athletes by Andrews et al. in 1985 (1). The initial classification system of what has come to be called SLAP lesions was defined in 1990 by Snyder et al. (2) and has been expanded by others over time (3, 4). Although these classifications present an organized approach to the defining SLAP pathology, the challenge is to diagnose these lesions preoperatively and to differentiate significant superior labral pathology from the many normal anatomic variations which exist. Compounding this challenge are the normal changes that occur to the labrum with increasing age. Reflecting this variability, the accepted mechanisms of injury are as varied as the different types of SLAP pathology. This chapter presents the current SLAP tear

classifications and an organized approach to their diagnosis and treatment. Clinical pearls are included to enhance an understanding of SLAP pathology and identification.

CLINICAL EVALUATION

Pertinent History

Clinically significant SLAP lesions are most commonly found in throwing athletes or after a specific traumatic event. These athletes often describe a long overhead throwing history starting as a child and may demonstrate significant humeral retroversion. The most prevalent complaints include anterior shoulder pain, clicking and popping in the shoulder, and reduced function (including decreased speed and power). Not uncommonly, patients will present because of pain with attempted overhead activities, decreased velocity in throwers (sometimes referred to as the "dead arm syndrome"), or increasing lap time in swimmers. In overhead throwing athletes, the symptoms may appear suddenly or over time.

SLAP lesions have various mechanisms of injury with no one specific mechanism predominating. These include falling on the outstretched arm creating shearing forces on the superior biceps labral complex, a tight posterior capsule, a sudden forced abduction and external rotation of the shoulder as might happen when a baseball runner slides head first into base, acceleration of the arm during the late cocking phase, a biceps traction overload caused by the long head of the biceps acting as a decelerator of the arm during the follow through phase of throwing, and the forces applied during a motor vehicle accident by a shoulder-lap belt restraining the ipsilateral chest wall causing the shoulder to roll around the seat belt on impact (5, 6).

The main difficulty for the clinician is differentiating a clinically significant superior labral injury (a real SLAP) from degenerative changes or normal variations. The patient's history is a key element during the decision-making process. In addition, the physical exam and mechanism of injury should be consistent with a SLAP lesion. Preoperative imaging studies are also helpful but can provide false-positive results and should not be the sole basis for the diagnosis.

Patient selection is the most important factor. It is important to understand which patients are likely to develop a true SLAP injury and those who are not. Age is an important consideration when determining whether a superior labral abnormality is actually symptomatic. Patients older than 40 years often have naturally occurring degenerative changes, which can be confused with pathologic injury (Fig. 14.1). This "senescence pattern" is seen in the superior labrum and can include labral separation as well as fraying. This can be a normal aging pattern and these changes are unlikely to cause symptoms. Pfahler et al. showed that there is a natural evolution of labral degeneration over time (7). A microscopic and macroscopic analysis of normal shoulders stratified by age demonstrated age-dependent changes at the labral attachment. Three stages were described: those younger than 10 years had a circumferential attachment; those between 30 and 50 years of age demonstrated fissuring and the development of sublabral recesses; and those older than 60 years demonstrated circumferential tearing, fissuring, and labral detachment.

The identification of a pathologic SLAP lesion is seldom an unexpected or incidental finding at the time of arthroscopy. Glenohumeral arthritis or full thickness rotator cuff tears do not accompany symptomatic true type II SLAP injuries. If these degenerative conditions are present, then the superior labral variation is most likely also part of the degenerative process and a surgical procedure to attach the labrum to the superior glenoid is unlikely to provide any clinical benefit.

SLAP injuries are most commonly found in the dominant arm of male patients younger than 40 years who have participated for many years in high-performance overhead or throwing activities. Another subgroup includes patients with previous shoulder trauma or instability. A history of a shoulder dislocation, a fall on an outstretched hand, or a motor vehicle accident during which the patient was wearing a shoulder lap belt over the involved shoulder are also suggestive of a SLAP injury (8).

Physical Examination

Several physical examination tests have been described to assist in diagnosing significant SLAP lesions. These tests usually apply stress during shoulder manipulation to the biceps anchor using torsion or tensile loads to recreate pain.

The O'Brien's test (9) positions the arm in 10° to 15° adduction and 90° of forward flexion. With the patient's thumb pointing toward the floor (full forearm pronation), the patient resists the examiner's downward pressure on the wrist of the outstretched arm (Fig. 14.2). Following this maneuver, the hand is fully supinated with the palm facing up and the examiner again applies pressure on the wrist while the patient resists. Pain in the shoulder with forearm pronation that is relieved in supination is considered a positive test and suggestive of a SLAP lesion. Tenderness at the acromioclavicular joint combined with local tenderness to palpation indicates AC joint pathology.

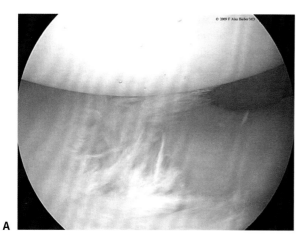

A

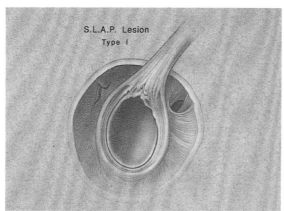

B

FIGURE 14.1. Patients older than 40 years often have naturally occurring degenerative changes classified as a type I SLAP lesion (photo **A**), which can be confused with pathologic injury (drawing **B**). (Photograph Figure 1A © F. Alan Barber MD.)

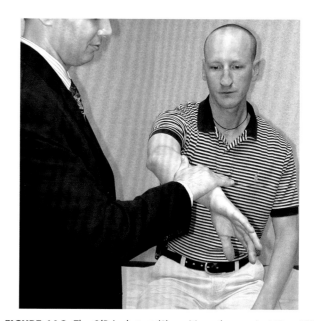

FIGURE 14.2. The O'Brien's test (9) positions the arm in 10° to 15° adduction and 90° of forward flexion. With the patient's thumb pointing toward the floor (full forearm pronation), the patient resists the examiner's downward pressure on the wrist of the outstretched arm. (Photograph © F. Alan Barber MD.)

In both instances, a positive test consists of less pain with the palm up position than the thumb down position.

When bicipital tendonitis is present, a positive Speed's test is elicited when pain is produced at the anterior bicipital groove by resisted forward flexion with the shoulder flexed at 90° and the forearm fully supinated.

A reduction in internal rotation when compared with the opposite shoulder is suggestive of a tight posterior capsule (Fig. 14.3). This reduction in internal rotation is suggestive of a SLAP injury especially if it is not resolved by a course of physical therapy. An accurate determination of internal rotation can be made with the patient supine and the examiner stabilizing the scapula by pressure on the anterior shoulder. The arm motion measured with a goniometer should be 180°. Long-term throwing athletes may develop humeral retroversion in which case, the dominant arm will demonstrate increased external rotation with a resultant decrease in internal rotation.

The previously mentioned provocative tests and others often provide inconsistent results and are often not independently diagnostic. The modified O'Brien's test, crank test, and anterior slide test have not been widely supported as solely diagnostic (10–12). The relocation test of Jobe was shown to be accurate in the hands of some individuals but not others. The biceps load test and the pain provocative test can be helpful in addition to other tests, but have not been validated independently. Despite the concerns about reliability of these tests (10–12), they do play a role in the physical examination of the shoulder.

Imaging

Diagnostic imaging may not be consistent for the identification of SLAP tears. Plain radiographs should be a mainstay to determine if there is any associated bony pathology. MRI with the addition of gadolinium enhances the anatomy of the superior labrum (Fig. 14.4), and interpretation by a musculoskeletal radiologist improves its accuracy. Community read scans were reported to have an accuracy of only 51%, but they were significantly more sensitive if an arthrogram was done in addition with the MRI (13). When reading the same studies, two fellowship-trained musculoskeletal radiologists increased the accuracy by 10% to 20%, but were still limited in their accuracy, sensitivity, and specificity (13).

Variations within the anatomy of the superior labrum have been identified which confound the diagnostic accuracy of this test. A normal sublabral separation from the glenoid surface is common and this may vary from a slight crease to a sulcus measuring 1 to 2 mm or more. These are not pathologic but may be filled in magnetic resonance arthrography. The presence of such a sulcus does not define a pathologic SLAP lesion. In contrast, the presence of a ganglion or sublabral cyst, often associated suprascapular nerve (SSN) compression, is very suggestive of a SLAP lesion (14, 15). Again, MRI should be used as an adjunct for diagnosis of a SLAP lesion and not relied upon independently.

Even among the "experts," there is a lack of consensus on making a SLAP diagnosis. The intraobserver and interobserver reliability for the diagnosis and treatment of various SLAP tears was greater than 50% among 70 experienced shoulder arthroscopic surgeons (16). Yet arthroscopy is considered one of the principal diagnostic tools for this condition.

Classification System

With the advancement of arthroscopy equipment and improved techniques, SLAP lesions have been better delineated from normal anatomy. The classification of SLAP

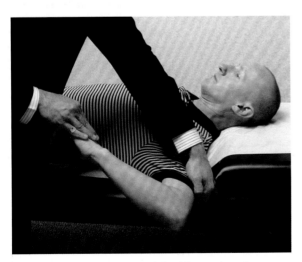

FIGURE 14.3. A decrease in internal shoulder rotation when compared with the opposite shoulder is suggestive of a tight posterior capsule. (Photograph © F. Alan Barber MD.)

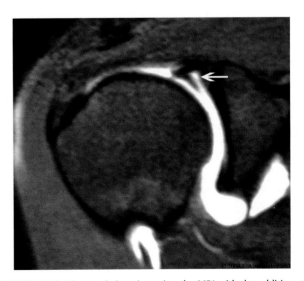

FIGURE 14.4. Diagnostic imaging using the MRI with the addition of gadolinium enhances the identification of the superior labral anatomy and interpretation by a musculoskeletal radiologist improves the accuracy. (Photograph © F. Alan Barber MD.)

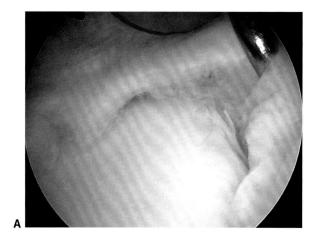

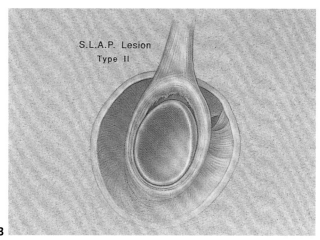

FIGURE 14.5. The type II SLAP (photo **A**) occurs when the superior labrum at the attachment of the biceps tendon pulls off the superior glenoid tubercle (drawing **B**). (Photograph A © F. Alan Barber MD.)

lesions has undergone expansion over the last 20 years by other authors beyond the initial description (2–4). A type I SLAP is considered by some to represent normal degenerative changes and the retreat of blood supply from the superior labrum that comes with increasing age and consists of fraying on the inner margin of the superior labrum (Fig. 14.1). Sometimes a larger meniscus-like superior labrum (meniscoid labrum—a normal variant) displays similar degenerative fraying of the inner rim and can also be considered a type I SLAP.

Although the degenerative type I SLAP is the most frequently observed abnormality, the most common clinically significant SLAP is the type II (Fig. 14.5). This occurs when the superior labrum at the attachment of the biceps tendon pulls off the superior glenoid tubercle. The type II SLAP can be further defined by the anatomic location of this elevation relative to the biceps tendon. The three subtypes described by Burkhart and Morgan are the anterior, posterior, and combined anterior and posterior (17).

In throwing athletes, the anterior type is the most common subtype of type II SLAP. This is observed to be

a labral avulsion from the anterosuperior quadrant of the glenoid. The posterior type II SLAP lesion is a labral avulsion in the posterosuperior quadrant of the glenoid. This subtype is most commonly seen in the throwing athletes (5, 6, 17, 18). A combined avulsion of both anterosuperior and posterosuperior quadrants of the glenoid is the least common subtype.

Applying traction to the biceps tendon of a posterosuperior quadrant labral lesion shifts the force of the tendon from an anterior-horizontal to a posterior-vertical position. The labrum detaches and slides back medially or peels off the posterior superior glenoid due to the force transmission of the biceps tendon base. This is the "peel back" phenomenon and was described by Morgan and Burkhart (6).

A type III SLAP lesion is a bucket handle tear of the superior labrum (Fig. 14.6) and usually extends from anterior to posterior at the biceps insertion. Unlike the

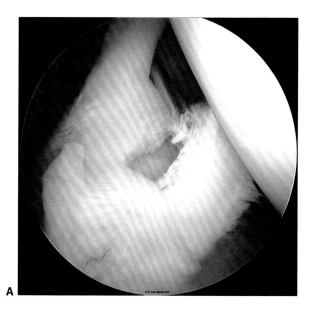

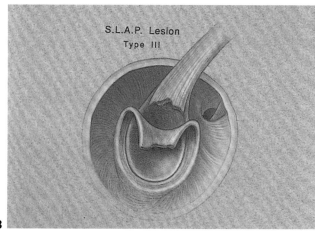

FIGURE 14.6. A type III SLAP lesion is a bucket handle tear of the superior labrum (photo **A**) and usually extends from anterior to posterior at the biceps insertion (drawing **B**). (Photograph A © F. Alan Barber MD.)

type II SLAP, the type III does not have any elevation of the biceps-labral attachment from the glenoid. The type IV SLAP is a bucket handle labral tear that extends into the biceps tendon resulting in a split in the tendon attachment (Fig. 14.7). Weber has further characterized the type IV SLAP (AAOS meeting 2009) into the type IV A, which has a white-on-red bucket handle portion best treated with excision of the bucket and repair of the remaining biceps anchor to the bone and a type IV B, which splits vertically into the biceps in a red-on-red pattern and can be repaired with side-to-side suturing.

This classification system was later expanded to include SLAP injuries associated with shoulder instability (3). In this expanded classification system, a type V SLAP is a Bankart lesion that extends superiorly to the biceps attachment (Fig. 14.8). A type VI SLAP is an anterior or posterior labral flap with a type II biceps elevation (Fig. 14.9). A type VII SLAP is a biceps attachment separation that extends into the middle glenohumeral ligament.

Additional classifications (4) added include a type VIII SLAP, which consists of a type II SLAP with posterior labral extension (Fig. 14.10), a type IX SLAP, which is a type II with circumferential labral tearing (Fig. 14.11), and a type X SLAP, which is a type II SLAP with a posterior inferior labral separation (19). With greater awareness of labral pathology, additional variations of labral pathology are to be expected. These include a type II SLAP injury with articular cartilage avulsions and loose bodies (Fig. 14.12).

A classification system is judged on the ability to provide an organized method of evaluating an injury

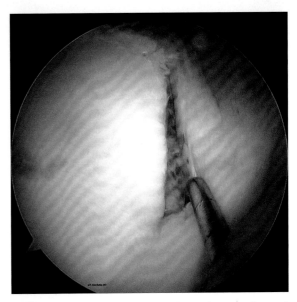

FIGURE 14.8. A type V SLAP is a Bankart lesion that extends superiorly to the biceps attachment. (Photograph © F. Alan Barber MD.)

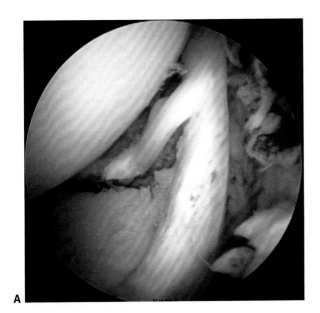

A

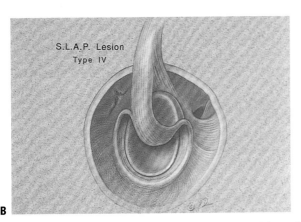

B

FIGURE 14.7. The type IV SLAP is a bucket handle labral tear (photo **A**) that extends into the biceps tendon, resulting in a split in the tendon attachment (drawing **B**). (Photograph A © F. Alan Barber MD.)

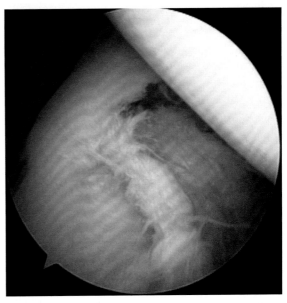

FIGURE 14.9. A type VI SLAP is an anterior or posterior labral flap with a type II biceps elevation. (Photoograph © F. Alan Barber MD.)

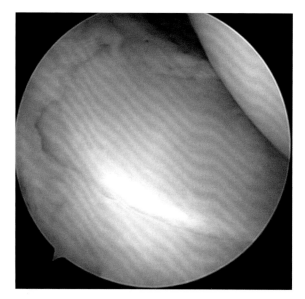

FIGURE 14.10. A type VIII SLAP consists of a type II SLAP with posterior labral extension. (Photograph © F. Alan Barber MD.)

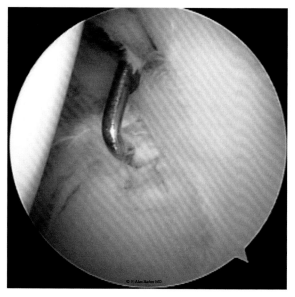

FIGURE 14.12. Additional variations of labral pathology include a type II SLAP injury with articular cartilage avulsions and loose bodies. (Photograph © F. Alan Barber MD.)

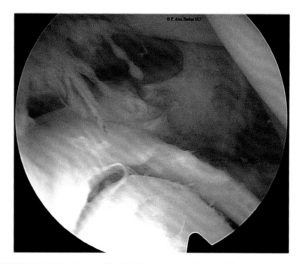

FIGURE 14.11. A type IX SLAP is a type II SLAP with circumferential labral tearing. (Photograph © F. Alan Barber MD.)

that can positively affect the treatment algorithm. One major point is that except for series dealing principally with shoulder instability, the overall incidence of SLAP tears is very low. A review of the frequency of these different SLAP types indicates that other than the type I SLAP, which is considered by most to be an incidental degenerative change, by far the most frequently observed SLAP lesion is the type II. Type II lesions represent 50% or more of SLAP pathology, but only 4% to 6% of all intra-articular pathology at time of arthroscopy (2, 3, 20, 21). The most frequent associated lesion for the group most likely to have a clinically significant type II lesion (those younger than 40 years) was shoulder instability. In contrast, those older than 40 diagnosed with a type II

lesion were frequently found to have either rotator cuff pathology or glenohumeral arthritis.

TREATMENT

Nonoperative Treatment

The initial treatment for SLAP injuries should be nonoperative and start with rest and include anti-inflammatory medication, stretching, and strengthening of specific muscular imbalances. Throwing and overhead athletes may have decreased internal rotation with a reduction in the arc of shoulder motion to be less than 180° indicating a tight posterior capsule. Physical therapy directed at posterior capsular stretching is the mainstay for initial treatment. Weakness of the scapular stabilizers and scapular dyskinesis may result in scapular winging and asymmetrical motion of the arm. A stretching program to attain full motion (especially internal rotation) should be undertaken before any surgical intervention. If symptoms persist after a period of 3 months of nonoperative treatment, surgery is indicated.

Surgical Treatment

Before directly assessing the superior labrum for pathological changes, the presence of a "drive through sign" during the initial arthroscopic examination of the glenohumeral joint can demonstrate the presence of laxity suggestive of a superior labral injury. Probing of the posterior superior labrum or taking the arm out of traction, abducting to 90°, and applying external rotation may demonstrate a "peel back sign" during which the posterior superior labrum "peels back" off the glenoid rim.

A careful review of the intra-articular structures should be performed to identify any other problems. Findings associated with a true SLAP lesion and helpful in confirming this diagnosis include SGHL laxity, sublabral chondromalacia, sublabral fraying, and associated biceps injury.

Anterior type II SLAP lesions are best approached through the normal anterior superior portal. Posterior or combined anterior and posterior type II SLAP lesions are best secured by placing an anchor posterior to the biceps tendon origin. This area can be accessed using a more posterior trans-cuff portal (Port of Wilmington) (17) placed 1 cm lateral and 2 cm anterior to the posterior lateral acromion corner.

The labrum should be elevated and mobilized in preparation for repairing the superior labrum to the glenoid neck (Fig. 14.13). Care must be taken during the elevation because inadvertent laceration of the labrum may occur. Debridement and abrasion of the superior surface of the glenoid is performed next. The site for biceps-labral complex reattachment is prepared by "dusting" the bone at the biceps attachment to create a bleeding bony bed. An aggressive decortication should be avoided because it can result in excessive superior glenoid bone loss or even labral damage.

Anchor insertion is the next step. If needed, a spinal needle can be used to identify the best position and trajectory for an accessory instrumentation portal. Regardless of the portal used, the anchor should be placed on the superior edge of the glenoid at a 45° angle. This may require some adjustment to accommodate the different thicknesses of the glenoid at different locations. The goal is to insert the anchor without cutting out medially or laterally into the articular cartilage. A single anchor immediately

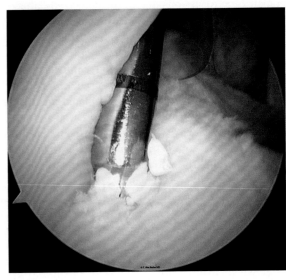

FIGURE 14.14. A single anchor immediately posterior to the biceps attachment is sufficient for most SLAP lesions. (Photograph © F. Alan Barber MD.)

posterior to the biceps attachment should be sufficient for most SLAP lesions (Fig. 14.14). After anchor insertion, the sutures are passed through the tissue using the methods deemed most appropriate by the surgeon. Arthroscopic knots are then tied and the repair is complete. A simple stitch will grasp and hold the labral tissue more strongly than a mattress suture and biomechanical testing suggests that a single anchor placed immediately posterior to the biceps is as effective as two stitches bracketing the biceps tendon (Fig. 14.15).

Recently, the use of a trans-rotator cuff portal has been brought into question (22). Placement is controversial for

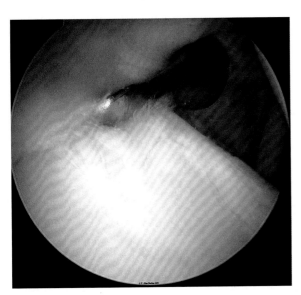

FIGURE 14.13. The labrum should be elevated and mobilized in preparation for repairing the superior labrum to the glenoid neck. (Photograph © F. Alan Barber MD.)

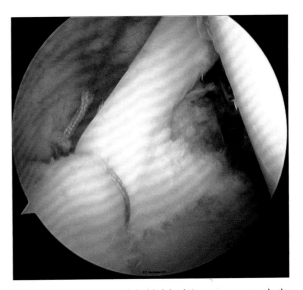

FIGURE 14.15. A simple stitch holds labral tissue more strongly than a mattress suture, and biomechanical testing suggests that a single anchor placed immediately posterior to the biceps is as effective as two stitches bracketing the biceps tendon. (Photograph © F. Alan Barber MD.)

the repair of SLAP lesions due to the perceived damage to the rotator cuff and later rotator cuff sequelae. The surgeon should objectively examine the portal placement technique and equipment used. The trans-rotator cuff portal may be innocuous if only a small hole is used for the placement of the suture anchor. When a cannula is used, its size and the resultant defect created should be evaluated arthroscopically. Smaller cannulas may not create a large enough defect for concern, but larger sizes (i.e., 8.0 and 8.5 mm) may necessitate a closure of the trans-cuff portal. Recent reports have demonstrated that a trans-cuff portal placement was efficient and safe for SLAP repairs (23).

The final outcome of surgical repair is reattachment of the biceps-labral complex to the superior glenoid and elimination of peel-back and drive-through signs. As postoperative problems associated with trans-labral tacks have become widely recognized, the use of suture anchors has become the fixation standard. The anterior type II SLAP can be secured by one suture anchor placed either beneath or slightly anterior to the biceps tendon origin. Posterior or combined type II SLAP lesions can be secured by a mattress suture (or two simple sutures) passed on both sides of the biceps origin. When the labral separation extends more posteriorly, a second suture anchor inserted even more posterior to the one at the biceps origin may be required to firmly stabilize the posterior superior labrum.

The optimal placement for SLAP repair suture anchors is evolving as new data becomes available. There is no biomechanical advantage for placing two suture anchors anterior to the biceps attachment versus two anchors posterior to the biceps anchor (24). A comparison of three different posterior labral fixation methods demonstrated that a single anchor with one simple suture was as effective as a single anchor with a mattress suture or two anchors with simple sutures for posterior SLAP lesions (25). Therefore, placing a single stitch in a single anchor posterior to the biceps root should be sufficient for most posterior SLAPs and in fact may be sufficient for all SLAPs.

Variations exist in the anatomy of the biceps labral attachment. Approximately 50% of the long head attachments arise from the supraglenoid tubercle and 50% from the superior labrum with some variations. The labral contribution is primarily posterior. This further supports the posterior placement of a single vertical suture for the repair. This posterior placement may also decrease the development of postoperative stiffness often seen after SLAP repairs.

Arthroscopic evaluation and stabilization is the most accurate treatment for SLAP lesions, but the treatment depends on the type of SLAP encountered. The treatment for type I SLAP lesions is debridement of the labral fraying. Type II SLAP tears require reattachment of the superior labrum to achieve a stable biceps-superior labral anchor as described earlier. Debridement of the bucket handle is indicated for type III and type IV SLAP lesions, but a suture repair or a biceps tenodesis may also be required

for type IV lesions, depending on the severity the biceps pathology. Types V through VII are associated with glenohumeral dislocations or instability. The glenohumeral instability should be corrected along with repairing the superior labral detachment. Loose labral flaps associated with a type VI SLAP should be debrided. For types VIII through X, the labrum should be reattached with suture anchors and any labral flap debrided. The labral stabilization should seek to eliminate any associated peel-back and reduce the drive-through sign.

ARTHROSCOPIC EVALUATION

The arthroscopic identification of several types of SLAP lesions can be straightforward. Types III and IV are readily identifiable due to the associated bucket handle component and the extension into the biceps tendon. A type VI SLAP has an associated labral flap. The most difficult lesion to assess is the type II SLAP because of the many normal anatomic variations found in the superior labrum. Superior labral variations including sublabral holes are present in approximately 13% of patients. A cordlike middle glenohumeral ligament is the most common variation encompassing 8.6% and findings of a sublabral foramen are present in 3.3%. Another anatomical variation is the Buford complex, which consists of an absent anterior superior labrum and a cordlike middle glenohumeral ligament that inserts directly into the base of the biceps tendon. The Buford complex can be found in 1.5% to 6.5% of shoulders.

This underscores the importance of the patient's history and physical examination. The preoperative clinical presentation should be consistent with a symptomatic type II SLAP. Taken in the appropriate context, the arthroscopic evaluation is used to only confirm the diagnosis. In addition to some mobility of the superior labrum, the true type II SLAP lesion will demonstrate other components including sublabral chondromalacia at the superior glenoid, undersurface labral fraying, and a sulcus or gap present that separates the labrum and articular cartilage by more than 5 mm. Occasionally, sublabral hemorrhage may be observed.

A sublabral cyst is another condition that helps identify a type II SLAP (Fig. 14.16). This is created by a communication with the glenohumeral joint that can be identified after probing and elevation of the superior labrum. Repair of the labrum will treat both the SLAP lesion and the cyst.

The type II SLAP lesion has three variations: anterior, posterior, and combined anterior and posterior (17). The anterior is the most common variety seen in nonthrowers. The anterior microinstability created by the anterior type II SLAP lesion can exacerbate the laxity of the SGHL. This can lead to increasing contact by the humeral head with the anterior supraspinatus tendon with resultant fraying. This creates damage to the anterior cuff and has been termed a superior labrum anterior cuff lesion. The posterior type II SLAP is more common in overhead,

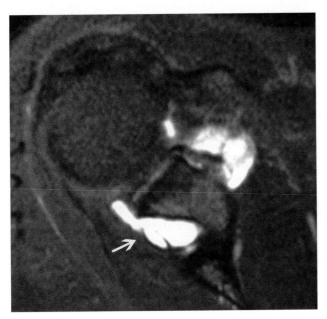

FIGURE 14.16. A sublabral cyst is another condition that helps identify a type II SLAP and can be identified with a gadolinium-enhanced MRI study. (Photograph © F. Alan Barber MD.)

throwing athletes, and represents greater than 50% of the type II SLAP lesions in that population. The last subtype, the combined anterior and posterior, is the least common.

COMPLICATIONS, CONTROVERSIES, AND SPECIAL CONSIDERATIONS

Stiffness is the most commonly encountered problem after performing a SLAP repair. Postoperative protocols that include prolonged immobilization should be avoided. Instead, using only a sling for comfort for the first 3 weeks is recommended. Operating on a patient for an incorrect diagnosis can also be considered a complication. One of the clear challenges with this condition is making an accurate diagnosis. With increasing age, the labrum undergoes degenerative changes, which can be mistaken for a pathologic biceps-labral attachment requiring treatment. Patients with rotator cuff tears, glenohumeral arthritic changes, and those older than 40 years should be considered carefully. Often the complaints are not due to superior labral lesions. Operative fixation of the labrum which does not address the principal pathology results in a poor outcome.

The fixation device used may be a source of poor outcomes. Poly Levo Lactic Acid (PLLA) tacks have been linked to continued pain and postoperative dysfunction. Complications seen at second look arthroscopy ranged from chondral injury, inadequate tissue healing, foreign body reaction, granuloma formation, stiffness, and device breakage. Metal anchors which become proud can be problematic resulting in chondral damage.

Finally, portal placement can be associated with night pain, lower functional scores, poorer patient satisfaction,

and decreased postoperative pain relief (22). However, recent reports do not support the disadvantages of a trans-cuff portal (23, 26). In contrast, piercing the rotator interval does not seem to be associated with portal complications. Failure to perform subacromial decompression for associated subacromial impingement may also result in poor result (22).

PEARLS AND PITFALLS

Probably the greatest potential pitfall associated with the treatment of a SLAP injury is in making an inaccurate diagnosis. The patient's history is the most important element in this process. Both the physical examination and understood mechanism of injury should be consistent with a SLAP lesion. Preoperative imaging studies usually correlate with the examination, but can provide false-positive results and should not be the only basis for the diagnosis. Patient age is another important element in the diagnosis. Patients older than 40 years often have naturally occurring degenerative changes, which can be confused with pathology. Another important pearl is that an unexpected superior labral abnormality found at the time of surgery is unlikely to be a clinically significant SLAP lesion causing the patient's complaints.

When probing the SLAP lesion, it is important to understand the morphology of anatomical variations. Be mindful not to consider a meniscoid type lesion pathological. The superior labrum and biceps anchor can attach up to 5 mm medial to the glenoid articular surface. Three specific clues for pathological lesions include sublabral fraying, superior glenoid chondromalacia, and SGHL injury. Sometimes, there is an associated biceps tendon injury.

Once the proper diagnosis has been made, anchor placement can be done from the anterior superior portal just off the acromion onto the glenoid rim directed into an area of adequate bone stock. This avoids penetrating the rotator cuff tendon. The angle of anchor insertion is important because too shallow an angle will result in chondral damage and too deep an angle may result in the anchor cutting out posteriorly. Recent biomechanical testing suggests that a single suture anchor posterior to the biceps anchor is sufficient for most SLAPs and may be sufficient for all posterior SLAPs.

Suture passage after anchor insertion can be a challenge. Many methods can be used, but using a large bore spinal needle placed into either the portal of Wilmington or the Neviaser portal areas can simplify this process and avoid an accessory portal. If the needle is passed high enough so that its entry into the joint is clearly visible before it passes under the labrum, a twisted wire suture passer (the Chia Percpasser, DePuy-Mitek, Rayham, MA) or some other suture-passing device can be inserted through this needle. The passing device is then retrieved anteriorly, the needle removed, one suture also pulled out the anterior cannula, and this suture attached to the suture-passing device. When the suture passer is pulled back out the Neviaser portal, it carries the labral repair suture through the labrum. Both sutures can then be retrieved from the anterior portal cannula and a simple stitch ties. This method removes the need for additional portals, while providing the surgeon with improved access to the lesion.

Finally, it is important to know the chosen cannula sizes and which instruments will fit through each of them. It is much easier and time efficient if the proper cannula is inserted first rather than having to replace it for a larger one.

One final point is that there are three nerves that innervate the shoulder: the axillary, SSN, and lateral pectoral (LPN) nerve. Intraoperative and postoperative pain can be decreased by a percutaneous block of the SSN and LPN before prepping the patient. At this point, we do not block the axillary nerve in this manner. Both blocks are performed with 0.25% bupivacaine without epinephrine. The SSN block is administered through an 18G spinal needle placed about 8 cm medial to the lateral border of the acromion near the Neviaser portal (Fig. 14.17). The needle is advanced toward the coracoid until it contacts the scapula and then walked anteriorly until it "falls off" the supraspinatus fossa. The needle is moved posteriorly until it touches bone again, an aspiration is performed, and 20 cc of bupivacaine solution are injected. The LPN block is performed by the infiltration of 10 cc inserted anterior to the clavicle at the level of the deltopectoral groove aiming for the medial border of the coracoid process.

REHABILITATION

Prevention of stiffness is the primary challenge during the postoperative period. Internal rotation, external rotation,

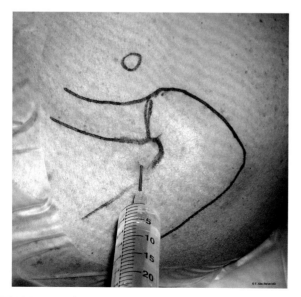

FIGURE 14.17. The suprascapular nerve block is administered through an 18G spinal needle placed near the Neviaser portal to flood the area of the supraspinatus fossa near the base of the coracoid process. (Photograph © F. Alan Barber MD.)

and humeral translation are significantly decreased after type II SLAP repair. A sling is used for comfort for approximately 3 weeks and immobilization avoided. Pendulum exercises and elbow motion are permitted at 3 weeks, but no flexion above the horizon is allowed. The patient is also restricted from elbow flexion with greater than 1 lb (greater than 0.45 kg) for 6 weeks to minimize tension on the repaired tissue. After a period of 6 weeks, strengthening of the rotator cuff, scapular stabilizers, biceps, and deltoid muscles is initiated. Posterior capsule stretching (sleeper stretches) should continue to be performed until complete recovery occurs.

Throwing athletes may begin an interval throwing program on a level surface at 4 months. Posterior capsule stretches continue to be emphasized as well as a continued strengthening program. Pitchers may begin throwing from the mound at 6 months and are released to full activity at 7 months. Contact athletes may return to their sports at 3 months without restrictions if they are not involved in throwing or overhead activities. Recent evidence has shown that overhead throwing athletes do not have as good an outcome after SLAP repair as nonthrowing athletes. Unfortunately, gymnasts are in a category of their own and do worse than throwing athletes.

CONCLUSIONS

SLAP lesions have been found in less than 10% of all shoulder arthroscopies and may be confused with normal anterior labral variations that occur in 13% of patients. They are unlikely to occur except in the young active population, overhead throwing athletes, or after significant trauma. A SLAP lesion should be suspected before surgery rather than discovered. Both clinical and imaging tests are inconsistently accurate for the diagnosis of a SLAP lesion. Arthroscopy should only be a final diagnostic confirmation of a clinical diagnosis.

Glenohumeral instability may be associated with SLAP lesions, but abnormal labral attachment associated with glenohumeral arthritic changes or a rotator cuff tear is unlikely to be clinically significant. The typical pathologic SLAP lesion is found in the dominant arm of a male, overhead or throwing athlete, who is younger than 40 years; or it can be found after a shoulder dislocation, a fall on an outstretched arm, or in a patient involved in a motor vehicle accident while wearing a shoulder-lap belt.

REFERENCES

1. Andrews JR, Carson WG Jr, McLeod WD. Glenoid labrum tears related to the long head of the biceps. *Am J Sports Med.* 1985;13:337–341.
2. Snyder SJ, Karzel RP, Del Pizzo W, et al. SLAP lesions of the shoulder. *Arthroscopy.* 1990;6:274–279.
3. Maffet MW, Gartsman GM, Moseley B. Superior labrum-biceps tendon complex lesions of the shoulder. *Am J Sports Med.* 1995;23:93–98.

4. Powell SE, Nord KD, Ryu RK. The diagnosis, classification and treatment of SLAP lesions. *Oper Tech Sports Med.* 2004;12:99–110.

5. Burkhart SS, Morgan CD, Kibler WB. The disabled throwing shoulder: spectrum of pathology. Part II: evaluation and treatment of SLAP lesions in throwers. *Arthroscopy.* 2003;19:531–539.

6. Burkhart SS, Morgan CD. The peel-back mechanism: its role in producing and extending posterior type II SLAP lesions and its effect on SLAP repair rehabilitation. *Arthroscopy.* 1998;14:637–640.

7. Pfahler M, Haraida S, Schulz C, et al. Age-related changes of the glenoid labrum in normal shoulders. *J Shoulder Elbow Surg.* 2003;12:40–52.

8. Ruotolo C, Nottage WM, Flatow EL, et al. Controversial topics in shoulder arthroscopy. *Arthroscopy.* 2002;18:65–75.

9. O'Brien SJ, Pagnani MJ, Fealy S, et al. The active compression test: a new and effective test for diagnosing labral tears and acromioclavicular joint abnormality. *Am J Sports Med.* 1998;26:610–613.

10. Stetson WB, Templin K. The crank test, the O'Brien test, and routine magnetic resonance imaging scans in the diagnosis of labral tears. *Am J Sports Med.* 2002;30:806–809.

11. McFarland EG, Kim TK, Savino RM. Clinical assessment of three common tests for superior labral anterior-posterior lesions. *Am J Sports Med.* 2002;30:810–815.

12. Holtby R, Razmjou H. Accuracy of the Speed's and Yergason's tests in detecting biceps pathology and SLAP lesions: comparison with arthroscopic findings. *Arthroscopy.* 2004;20:231–236.

13. Reuss BL, Schwartzberg R, Zlatkin MB, et al. Magnetic resonance imaging accuracy for the diagnosis of superior labrum anterior-posterior lesions in the community setting: eighty-three arthroscopically confirmed cases. *J Shoulder Elbow Surg.* 2006;15:580–585.

14. Westerheide KJ, Karzel RP. Ganglion cysts of the shoulder: technique of arthroscopic decompression and fixation of associated type II superior labral anterior to posterior lesions. *Orthop Clin North Am.* 2003;34:521–528.

15. Chen AL, Ong BC, Rose DJ. Arthroscopic management of spinoglenoid cysts associated with SLAP lesions and suprascapular neuropathy. *Arthroscopy.* 2003;19:E15–E21.

16. Gobezie R, Zurakowski D, Lavery K, et al. Analysis of interobserver and intraobserver variability in the diagnosis and treatment of SLAP tears using the Snyder classification. *Am J Sports Med.* 2008;36:1373–1379.

17. Morgan CD, Burkhart SS, Palmeri M, et al. Type II SLAP lesions: three subtypes and their relationships to superior instability and rotator cuff tears. *Arthroscopy.* 1998;14:553–565.

18. Burkhart SS, Morgan C. SLAP lesions in the overhead athlete. *Orthop Clin North Am.* 2001;32:431–441, viii.

19. Barber FA, Field LD, Ryu RK. Biceps tendon and superior labrum injuries: decision making. *Instr Course Lect.* 2008;57:527–538.

20. Snyder SJ, Banas MP, Karzel RP. An analysis of 140 injuries to the superior glenoid labrum. *J Shoulder Elbow Surg.* 1995;4:243–248.

21. Handelberg F, Willems S, Shahabpour M, et al. SLAP lesions: a retrospective multicenter study. *Arthroscopy.* 1998;14:856–862.

22. Cohen DB, Coleman S, Drakos MC, et al. Outcomes of isolated type II SLAP lesions treated with arthroscopic fixation using a bioabsorbable tack. *Arthroscopy.* 2006;22:136–142.

23. Oh JH, Kim SH, Lee HK, et al. Trans-rotator cuff portal is safe for arthroscopic superior labral anterior and posterior lesion repair: clinical and radiological analysis of 58 SLAP lesions. *Am J Sports Med.* 2008;36:1913–1921.

24. Morgan RJ, Kuremsky MA, Peindl RD, et al. A biomechanical comparison of two suture anchor configurations for the repair of type II SLAP lesions subjected to a peel-back mechanism of failure. *Arthroscopy.* 2008;24:383–388.

25. Yoo JC, Ahn JH, Lee SH, et al. A biomechanical comparison of repair techniques in posterior type II superior labral anterior and posterior (SLAP) lesions. *J Shoulder Elbow Surg.* 2008;17:144–149.

26. O'Brien SJ, Allen AA, Coleman SH, et al. The trans-rotator cuff approach to SLAP lesions: technical aspects for repair and a clinical follow-up of 31 patients at a minimum of 2 years. *Arthroscopy.* 2002;18:372–377.

Biceps Instability and Tendinitis

Keith D. Nord • Paul C. Brady • Bradford Wall

Biceps pathology has been recognized for centuries, but the function of the biceps has been controversial and its treatment varied. Neer described the long head of the biceps (LHB) tendon as a depressor of the humeral head. Even this early observation is still questioned. Pathology of the biceps tendon is frequently associated with other conditions such as impingement, Superior Labrum Anterior and Posterior (SLAP) tears, and supraspinatus or infraspinatus tears. The anatomy of the biceps has been studied extensively, yet only recently have we begun to understand the significance of the medial sling. Monteggia recognized instability of the biceps tendon, yet identification of this condition has been difficult and often unrecognized or incidentally noted. Treatment of this condition has been rapidly improving, as we begin to understand the progression of and the restraints to instability.

Arthroscopy has shed more light on the anatomy and biomechanics of the biceps and pulley system. In this overview of the LHB tendon, we will review the well-accepted anatomy and more controversial topics such as its function, pathophysiology, and treatment of instability, tendinitis, and tears.

BASIC SCIENCE

Anatomy

The anatomy of the LHB is well described, yet our understanding of its function is still progressing. The LHB originates at and around the supraglenoid tubercle. The LHB is intra-articular, yet extrasynovial, because it is lined by a synovial sheath. The proximal and middle portions receive blood supply from branches of the anterior humeral circumflex artery by the vincula, which move with the tendon in the groove. The distal third of the tendon receives nourishment from branches of the deep brachial artery. Despite the vincula, the blood supply in the portion of the tendon within the groove is still markedly reduced.

The LHB has been observed to originate primarily from the posterosuperior labrum 48% of the time by Habermayer et al. (1) and 70% by Pal et al. (2) Origin from the supraglenoid tubercle was reported to occur 20% and 25%, respectively, and Habermayer et al. noted that in

28% of the specimens the biceps originated from both the labrum and the tubercle.

The tendinous portion of the LHB measures approximately 9 cm in length, and the musculotendinous junction is at the level of the deltoid and pectoralis major insertions. Its shape is relatively flat at its origin, becoming more tubular as it proceeds distally and into the intertubercular groove. The LHB tendon is weakest at its midpoint and this is the site of most ruptures.

The LHB courses from the posterosuperior glenoid obliquely over the top of the humeral head. This oblique course is at a 30° angle, which decreases its effectiveness in comparative anatomy and increases the pressure on the medial side of the bicipital (intertubercular) groove. This groove is formed by the confluence of the lesser tuberosity (anteriorly) and the greater tuberosity (posterosuperiorly). The depth of the groove is typically 4 mm. Ueberham and Le Floch-Prigent (3) described a ridge on the upper portion of the lesser tuberosity (termed a supratubercular ridge) in 45% of anatomic specimens, which was postulated to "push" the biceps anteriorly and could be a cause of primary biceps lesions. Whereas some authors have suggested that a shallow inclination of the groove predisposes to dislocation (1) others have found no such association (3).

The most critical anatomic consideration regarding the LHB is its stabilizing structures. Specifically, a thorough understanding of the rotator interval (RI) and medial pulley system is essential. The RI is the triangular interval bordered superiorly by the anterior margin of the supraspinatus, inferiorly by the superior margin of the subscapularis, and medially by the anterior aspect of the glenoid. Within this triangular space exists the anterior glenohumeral capsule as well as the coracohumeral ligament (CHL) and the superior glenohumeral ligament (SGHL). The SGHL and the medial head of the CHL join to form a medial sling, or pulley system, for the LHB, and this is the major restraint to medial subluxation/dislocation of the LHB (4) (Fig. 15.1).

The CHL originates from the base of the coracoid process and divides into two bands—a superior band, which inserts into the anterior supraspinatus to form the

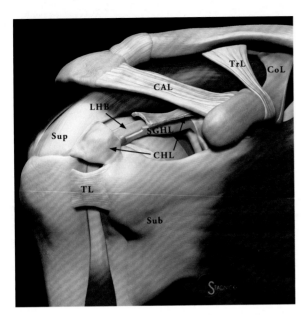

FIGURE 15.1. Tendons, ligaments labeled showing intimate relationship of CHL, SGHL forming a sling or pulley around the *LHB* tendon. Coracoacromial *(CAL)*, transverse humeral *(TL)*, trapezoid *(TrL)* and conoid *(CoL)* ligaments, supraspinatus *(Sup)*, and subscapularis *(Sub)* tendons are labeled.

lateral or superior pulley, and an inferior band whose medial head inserts into the superior subscapularis and then onto the superior aspect of the lesser tuberosity. The SGHL also contributes to this medial sling as it courses from the anterior labrum (just anterior to the biceps origin) and inserts onto the superior aspect of the lesser tuberosity (Fig. 15.2). The fibers of the medial head of the CHL are much more robust and structurally important to the medial sling than the fibers of the SGHL. This medial sling or reflection pulley, is critical in preventing the LHB from displacing medially onto the lesser tuberosity. In this way, the sling protects the proximal insertion of the subscapularis

from the stresses that would result from a medially displaced LHB.

The medial sling and its relationship to the biceps tendon have been described as "the comma sign" by Lo and Burkhart (5). This comma sign is an arthroscopic description of the medial sling based on its appearance. The comma sign consists of the medial head of the CHL and SGHL (medial sling of the biceps) intersecting with the superior border of the subscapularis. Although the comma sign is visible in the absence of pathology, it is much more prominent, recognizable, and useful in the presence of a torn and retracted subscapularis tendon. When the subscapularis is torn from its insertion on the lesser tuberosity, the medial sling of the biceps is also pulled off and its association maintained with the subscapularis. Identification of this comma structure is critical when searching for the subscapularis tendon because it is always located at the superolateral border of the subscapularis tendon (Fig. 15.3).

Historically, it was felt that the transverse humeral ligament was the vital structure in regard to retaining the biceps within the bicipital groove (BG). However, this view is no longer well accepted. Ruotolo et al. (6) described the arthroscopic release of the sheath of the biceps tendon and dividing the transverse humeral ligament. Yet postoperative dislocation or subluxation of the biceps tendon did not occur. Ruotolo et al. emphasized that the CHL must be preserved with this technique to prevent biceps instability.

Biomechanics

The critical role of the biceps brachii at the elbow joint and its function has been well documented. It is the LHB's role at the shoulder that causes arguments. Many authors have suggested that the LHB has a role in humeral head depression—particularly with shoulder external rotation. Andrews et al. (7) observed the biceps arthroscopically while electrically stimulating the biceps muscle and saw

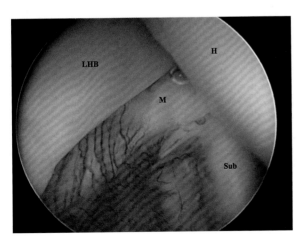

FIGURE 15.2. Posterior view of the right shoulder demonstrating the medial sling *(M)* of the *LHB* tendon and its confluence with the superolateral border of the subscapularis *(Sub)*. Patient is in the lateral decubitus position.

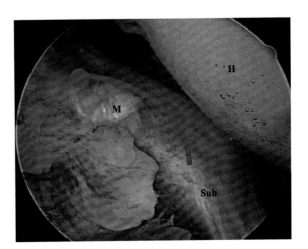

FIGURE 15.3. Posterior view of a right shoulder in the lateral decubitus position with a torn subscapularis *(Sub)* tendon. The comma sign is created by the intersection of the medial sling *(M)* and the subscapularis.

the labrum lift superiorly and compression of the gleno-humeral joint. However, other studies showed no humeral head motion with active biceps contraction.

Electromyography (EMG) studies have also demonstrated varying findings. Basmajian (8) demonstrated that the LHB did have EMG activity during active shoulder flexion. The LHB was estimated to contribute 7% of the power of shoulder flexion. Jobe et al. (9) showed peak biceps activity during follow through and deceleration in the throwing motion. However, in separate studies, Yamaguchi et al. (10) modified the EMG experiment to control (limit) elbow flexion and showed minimal to no EMG activity during isolated shoulder flexion. Another intriguing EMG finding has been an increase in EMG activity of the LHB in patients with rotator cuff deficiency. This increased activity may result in increased tendon diameter. Although still somewhat controversial, there is current literature that suggests the LHB has a depressing function in the shoulder and helps stabilize the humeral head in the glenoid. Even so, these effects are not dramatic.

Pathophysiology

Multiple classification schemes have been developed to describe disorders of the LHB tendon. These divisions have been only marginally useful with regard to diagnostic and treatment decisions. Understanding the various pathologic processes involving the biceps tendon and how to treat each process is more important. The three biceps tendon pathologies discussed here are biceps tendinitis, rupture, and instability.

BICEPS TENDINITIS

Biceps tendinitis can be referred to as primary or secondary. Primary tendinitis involves inflammation of the tendon within the BG. To be considered primary, no other pathologic findings (such as impingement, bony abnormalities within the groove, or biceps subluxation) should be present. It is considered an uncommon condition, and Habermayer and Walch (11) felt that this diagnosis could only be made during arthroscopy. Visualization of that part of the LHB in the groove is facilitated by pulling the tendon into the joint with a probe or advancing the scope into the BG (Fig. 15.4).

Secondary biceps tendinitis is more common and well recognized. The LHB coexists with the anterior supraspinatus and superior subscapularis under the anterolateral acromion and, therefore, is affected by the same forces. Although subacromial impingement produces undue forces on the anterior rotator cuff, it also compresses the underlying LHB and produces concomitant pathology (and thereby symptoms) in this structure. In fact, the impingement upon the LHB worsens as a rotator cuff tear progresses and increased contact between the LHB and the coracoacromial arch occurs. Up to one-third of patients with rotator cuff disease will have biceps involvement.

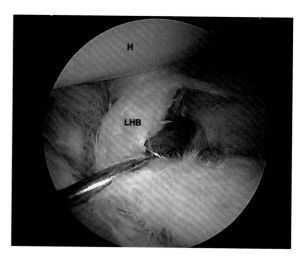

FIGURE 15.4. MRI axial view showing subscapularis tendon tear (white arrow) and biceps tendon dislocation medially (black arrow). The bicipital groove is empty (gray arrow) and tendon is medial to groove, posterior to subscapularis.

Another potential cause of secondary biceps tendinitis is the presence of bony anomalies of the proximal humerus. Most commonly these bony anomalies are secondary to malunion or nonunion of a proximal humerus fracture. If a fracture extends into the BG, significant irritation of the LHB can occur. Younger patients with biceps tendinitis may be more likely to have groove anomalies such as narrowing or osteophytes, but it is difficult to determine the sequence of events in such conditions.

BICEPS TENDON RUPTURE

While acute ruptures of the LHB do occur, they are more commonly the end result of chronic biceps tendinitis and impingement and frequently associated with rotator cuff disease. Acute ruptures can occur with a fall on an outstretched hand or with rapid deceleration of the arm during throwing activities. In this case, the deceleration force can result in trauma to the origin of the LHB resulting in a SLAP lesion. If the force is great enough from a single traumatic event or on a repetitive basis, it can result in LHB rupture with or without an associated SLAP tear.

Chronic biceps tendinitis is a more common cause for LHB rupture and tends to occur from repetitive overuse with the arm in adduction and internal rotation or from multidirectional or inferior instability. The LHB becomes attenuated and weakened by the continued impingement between the humeral head and the coracoacromial arch. In the case of impingement causing a rupture, the rupture typically occurs around the area of the rotator cuff interval (a weak point for the LHB) rather than at its origin.

BICEPS INSTABILITY

Biceps instability takes the form of either frank dislocation or more subtle subluxation. As previously noted, the primary restraining structures holding the LHB in the BG are the medial sling and subscapularis tendon. Habermayer and Walch (11) divided LHB tendon dislocations into extra-articular and intra-articular. The much less common extra-articular dislocations dislodge from the BG and travel over (anterior to) an intact subscapularis tendon. Extra-articular dislocations are extremely uncommon and occur with roof disruption due to CHL and supraspinatus tears.

The more common intra-articular LHB dislocation is associated with a partial or complete tear of the subscapularis tendon, which allows the LHB to dislocate posterior to the subscapularis. The medial sling remains attached to the superolateral border of the subscapularis tendon—even when that tendon retracts medially. This arthroscopic anatomic landmark has been termed the "comma sign" (5). It is a critical arthroscopic finding because the comma easily guides the surgeon to the superolateral border of the subscapularis tendon, thereby assisting in anatomic arthroscopic repair of the tendon back to the lesser tuberosity bone bed (8) (Fig. 15.3).

Biceps tendon subluxation can be a much more subtle diagnosis and is frequently missed even during arthroscopy. Walch has referred to this as the "hidden lesion." As with dislocation, the critical anatomic components that prevent biceps subluxation are the medial sling and subscapularis tendon. In the early phases of biceps subluxation, the medial sling structures may remain largely intact while creating mechanical wear to the anteromedial portion of the LHB, which resides in the BG. It is, therefore, quite important to thoroughly examine the anteromedial portion of the LHB by pulling the structure intra-articularly with a probe while visualizing "over the top." As the pathology progresses, the medial sling becomes detached from its insertion on the superior aspect of the lesser tuberosity and the LHB begins to act as a knife cutting its way through the subscapularis tendon insertion, detaching it from the lesser tuberosity. Early findings of this phenomenon can only be seen with the 70° scope visualizing "over the top" to look down at the bone bed of the lesser tuberosity. Lo and Burkhart (5) have described this view with the 70° scope as the "aerial view."

As the humerus is internally and externally rotated the biceps tendon can be seen "breaking" posterior to the plane of the anterior border of the subscapularis (Fig. 15.5). As a normal biceps tendon should remain anterior to the plane of the subscapularis, this "broken plane" phenomenon is a sure sign of early biceps instability and if not recognized will likely progress to LHB dislocation and complete tearing of the upper subscapularis insertion.

CLINICAL EVALUATION

Pertinent History

Anterior shoulder pain (particularly in the region of the BG) is the hallmark of biceps tendon problems. With biceps

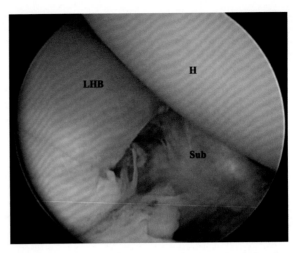

FIGURE 15.5. The *LHB* tendon is seen cutting posterior to the plane of the torn anterior subscapularis *(Sub)*.

tendinitis, the pain is usually described as a chronic aching pain, which is worsened by lifting and overhead activities. The pain frequently radiates distally to approximately the mid-arm level, but seldom radiates proximally. There is such a close association between subacromial impingement and biceps tendinitis that the two conditions have closely overlapping symptoms. They can be very difficult to distinguish and generally occur in tandem. Biceps instability may present with a painful click with arm elevation and/or rotation. Symptoms can be very similar to biceps tendinitis and are frequently seen at the same time.

Patients who present with rupture of the LHB are usually much easier to diagnose. These patients complain of a history of chronic anterior shoulder pain consistent with biceps tendinitis and/or impingement. Then, they usually report an episode of a painful "pop" in the shoulder, which was followed by partial or complete relief of their impingement symptoms. Subsequently, they may develop ecchymosis in the arm and an associated muscular deformity in the arm—frequently termed the "Popeye" muscle (Fig. 15.6). Sometimes, the "Popeye" deformity does not develop because the LHB becomes incarcerated in a stenotic BG.

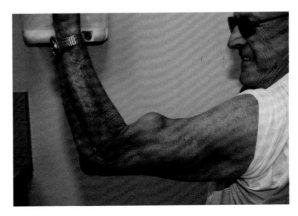

FIGURE 15.6. Popeye deformity with biceps retracted distally.

Physical Examination

Distinguishing anterior shoulder pain caused by biceps tendon disorders as opposed to subacromial impingement can be difficult, as these two entities usually coexist. Although there are some exam maneuvers that attempt to isolate the biceps tendon, there is still a fair amount of overlap and the definitive diagnosis of isolated biceps tendon pathology is extremely difficult based on history and physical exam alone. Often selective injections are helpful in differentiating the etiology of the pain.

The hallmark of biceps tendon pathology is point tenderness in the BG. Without this finding, it is extremely unlikely the LHB is involved in the patient's symptoms. The BG is best palpated approximately 3 below the acromion with the arm in 10° of internal rotation. As the arm is internally and externally rotated, the pain should move with the arm (Bennett rotation test). This is distinct from subacromial bursitis where the pain location remains relatively constant despite the position of the arm. This "tenderness in motion" sign can be quite specific for biceps tendon disorders. In the situation in which it is unclear whether the pain is secondary to the LHB or to possible impingement/bursitis, selective injections of these areas can help make the diagnosis.

There are several provocative tests, which can be helpful in the diagnosis of LHB pathology. However, the sensitivity and specificity of these tests intended for the diagnosis of LHB pathology are questionable.

Speed's test (12) (Fig. 15.7)—With the elbow in extension, the patient flexes the shoulder against resistance from the examiner. Pain in the BG is considered positive.

Yergason test (13)—The patient attempts to supinate the wrist against resistance (with the elbow flexed at the side). Pain in the BG is considered positive.

Bear hug test (14) (Fig. 15.8)—This test was developed by Barth et al. to better isolate upper subscapularis lesions. Since these lesions are almost always associated with LHB instability, it is a good test for LHB pathology.

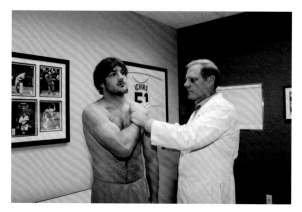

FIGURE 15.8. Bear Hug test: The patient places the palm of the affected extremity on the contralateral shoulder with the fingers held straight and the elbow kept in front of the patient. The examiner applies an upward force to the extremity while the patient resists this force and tries to keep the palm on the shoulder. If the examiner is able to lift the palm off the shoulder, this is a positive test.

The patient places the open palm of the affected extremity on the contralateral shoulder. In so doing, the ipsilateral elbow is held well anterior to the plane of the patient's body. As the examiner tries to lift the hand off the shoulder (resisted internal rotation), the patient tries to keep the palm on the shoulder. Weakness (in comparison with the contralateral side) is a positive test and indicative of a tear of the upper subscapularis (and thereby likely LHB instability). In general, the examiner should not be able to lift the hand off the contralateral shoulder unless there is tearing of the upper subscapularis, in which case there is usually concomitant subluxation of the biceps tendon.

Napoleon test (15, 16) (Fig. 15.9)—This test also attempts to assess the integrity of the subscapularis. The patient

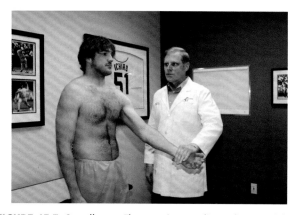

FIGURE 15.7. Speed's test: The examiner applies a downward force to the patients extended arm while the patient resists the downward force. Pain in the region of the biceps tendon is positive.

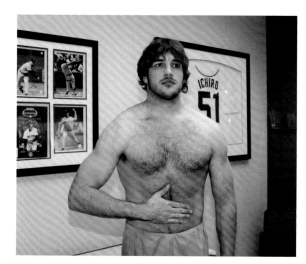

FIGURE 15.9. Napoleon test: The patient places the hand of the affected extremity on the abdomen and tries to keep the wrist straight. Inability to keep the wrist straight while performing this test is a positive finding.

pushes on the abdomen with the palm of the affected extremity and tries to keep the wrist completely straight. If the patient is unable to keep the wrist straight, but rather flexes the wrist to perform the test, this is considered a positive or intermediate test and suggestive of a subscapularis tear.

Belly-press test (16, 17) (Fig. 15.10)—This test is similar to the Napoleon test in that the patient places the palm on the abdomen with the wrist held straight. The physician then tries to pull the hand off the abdomen. If the physician is able to pull the hand off easily, this is considered a positive test and suggestive of a subscapularis tear.

Lift-off test (18) (Fig. 15.11)—This is the fourth test to assess subscapularis integrity. The patient places the back of the hand of the affected extremity on the ipsilateral buttock. The examiner then lifts the hand posteriorly and asks the patient to hold it in that position. Weakness or inability to lift the hand off the lower back is considered positive and suggestive of a subscapularis tear.

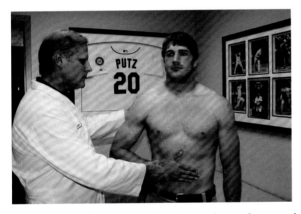

FIGURE 15.10. Belly-press test: Examiner resists patient pressing against his abdomen. If the examiner is able to lift hand from abdomen, this is a positive test.

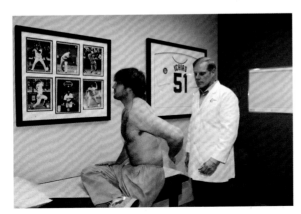

FIGURE 15.11. Lift-off test: The patient is asked to place the hand behind the back and then lift the dorsum of the hand off the back. Inability to do so is considered a positive test.

The biceps instability test (18)—This test is performed to demonstrate biceps subluxation. It is performed with the shoulder abducted 90° and with full external rotation while palpating over the BG. As the arm is internally rotated, an audible or palpable click occurs as the biceps subluxates over the lesser tuberosity.

The Ludington test—This test is utilized when a biceps rupture is not clearly visible. The patient places both hands behind his head and flexes the biceps. The contour of the muscle can be better appreciated in this position.

The described tests can be useful in assisting the clinician with the diagnosis of biceps tendon disorders. However, the sensitivity/specificity of most of these tests has not been examined. The exceptions include Speed's test, which Bennett (19) determined to be 90% sensitive for shoulder pain but only 13% specific for bicipital pathology. Its positive predictive value was 23%, whereas its negative predictive value was 83%. The bear hug test was determined to have a sensitivity of 60% and specificity of 92% for tears of the upper subscapularis (17).

Given the intimate relationship between biceps tendon pathology and concomitant subacromial impingement and/or rotator cuff tear, it is important to examine the remainder of the shoulder in this patient population. Specific tests for range of motion, impingement, rotator cuff integrity, and instability should be performed.

Imaging

The examination should begin with a complete series of radiographs. These should include an AP view, axillary view, and outlet view (or scapular-Y view). We also include a 30° caudal tilt view to better assess the AC joint. Others have described radiographic projections that are more specific for the BG region of the proximal humerus. These include the Fisk projection and the BG view. The Fisk method has the patient hold the cassette while leaning forward on their elbows and the beam is projected perpendicular to the floor (and cassette) (Fig. 15.12). This view looks down the bicipital tunnel.

The BG method has the patient lie supine with the shoulder slightly abducted and the arm in external rotation. The cassette is placed on the top of the shoulder and the beam is directed up the patient's axilla (parallel to the long axis of the humerus) and perpendicular to the plate (Fig. 15.13). This view can elucidate the depth of the BG, the inclination of the walls of the groove, as well as any associated spurs within the groove.

Prior to the advent of magnetic resonance imaging (MRI), arthrography was a commonly utilized method for evaluation of the rotator cuff. It was also useful in the evaluation of the biceps tendon. The loss of a sharp delineation of the tendon can indicate biceps tendon pathology. Arthrography remains an invasive technique with possible contrast complications, and this constitutes its main disadvantage.

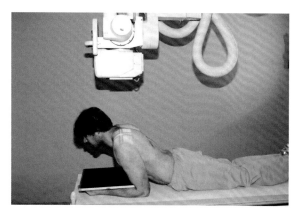

FIGURE 15.12. Fisk Projection: the patient holds the cassette while leaning forward on his elbows. The beam is projected perpendicular to the X-ray cassette.

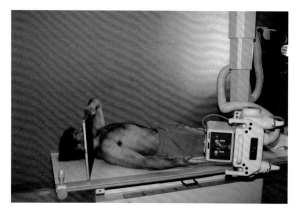

FIGURE 15.13. Bicipital Groove (BG) view: The patient lies supine with the arm in slight external rotation. The X-ray cassette is held on top of the patient's shoulder and the X-ray beam is aimed perpendicular to the cassette along the axis of the patient's humerus.

Ultrasound has emerged as a potentially effective, noninvasive technique in the evaluation of biceps tendon pathology. Ultrasound compared with arthrography are equally effective in the diagnosis of rotator cuff problems, but ultrasound may be superior in the evaluation of the biceps tendon. Ultrasound (20) demonstrated an 86% sensitivity for the diagnosis of LHB subluxation (as confirmed surgically). Ultrasound also has the added benefit of being a dynamic study and permits evaluation with shoulder motion. In comparison with other imaging modalities, ultrasound is more operator dependent. Therefore, a well-trained technician is essential to obtain meaningful and helpful studies.

MRI is another effective diagnostic tool. The anatomy (or pathoanatomy) of the biceps tendon and the BG, as well as associated findings such as rotator cuff pathology, is well delineated with MRI. Making the diagnosis of biceps tendon rupture or dislocation is relatively simple with MRI; however, biceps tendinitis and degenerative changes within the tendon are difficult to determine. Increased fluid around the biceps may suggest biceps tendinitis, but

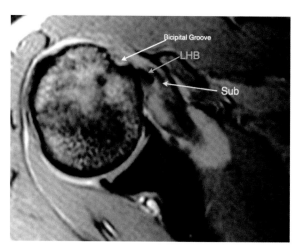

FIGURE 15.14. MRI axial view showing subscapularis tendon tear and biceps tendon dislocation medially. BG is empty and tendon is medial to groove, posterior to subscapularis.

this has been challenged. Edema can be readily seen on T2-weighted images in the presence of bicipital tendinitis. Biceps tendon subluxation and dislocation are well visualized on axial MRI views of the shoulder. MRI remains our favored test for evaluating biceps pathology. MR arthrography does not provide any additional benefit in assessing the biceps (Fig. 15.14).

TREATMENT

Nonoperative Treatment

The initial treatment of bicipital tendinitis is conservative using the traditional methods of rest, ice, and nonsteroidal anti-inflammatory medications. As symptoms improve, range of motion exercises and strengthening can be added. Mechanical flaws in sports should be addressed, and trunk, torso, and scapular stabilization should be stressed. Instruct the patient not to reproduce the click, if present, except in the office. The actual treatment is frequently directed more toward the treatment of underlying rotator cuff pathology. Subacromial, intra-articular, or bicipital sheath injections may also be utilized. Caution should be exercised in injecting the bicipital sheath. Intratendinous injection should be avoided due to the risk of tendon rupture or atrophic changes. Bicipital sheath injections can achieve up to 74% good to excellent results. It can be difficult to inject directly into the bicipital sheath; therefore, intra-articular injections are our preferred method since the proximal portion of the tendon is directly accessible and some of the fluid can track down the BG.

We prefer an intra-articular injection using a standard posterior portal approach. The joint line is palpated and entered approximately 4 cm inferior and 3 cm medial to the posterolateral corner of the acromion. A 22G, 1½-in (3.8 cm) needle is aimed toward the coracoid and a pop is felt as the needle perforates the posterior capsule. This is the same direction as inserting a posterior cannula for glenohumeral arthroscopy. Four milliliters of Betamethasone (6 mg per mL) and 6 mL of 0.5% bupivacaine are instilled into the glenohumeral joint. In addition to the rapid therapeutic effects of bupivacaine on the intra-articular portion of the biceps, its added volume aids in travel of the mix down the BG.

Injections of a corticosteroid should be limited to two or three injections due to the risk of tendon rupture, fluid retention, osteoporosis, avascular necrosis, and weight gain. The patient is started on a rotator cuff rehabilitation program consisting of internal and external rotation strengthening with elastic bands, scapular-stabilizing exercises, and shoulder shrugs. The patient is seen back at monthly intervals for re-evaluation and possibly a repeat injection. If symptoms progress or the condition worsens, a further workup with MRI, ultrasound, or CT arthrogram may be indicated. If symptoms improve with initial conservative therapy, gradual increase in activities is allowed, still limiting any inciting activity until the patient is relatively symptom free.

If no other pathology is present, greater than 80% of patients can be expected to achieve good results with nonoperative treatment. If patients continue to have significant pain and further work-up including MRI is negative, other sources of pain must be considered such as cervical radiculopathy, instability, glenohumeral or acromioclavicular (AC) arthritis, coracoid impingement, adhesive capsulitis, lung conditions with referred pain such as Pancoast tumor (malignancy in the upper lobe of the lung), or medical conditions including cardiac or gallbladder referred pain. The senior author has diagnosed a Pancoast tumor on routine shoulder X-rays, demonstrating the importance of a thorough radiographic evaluation.

Associated SLAP tears may be present, but little information regarding success rates with nonoperative treatment of SLAP lesions is available. The same conservative treatments may be employed, but many SLAP tears may ultimately require surgical intervention or may not be definitively diagnosed until arthroscopy is performed. The important subject of SLAP tears will be addressed elsewhere in this text.

Instability lesions of the biceps including subluxations or dislocations are frequently associated with rotator cuff tears. Treatment should be directed toward treatment of the rotator cuff tear and such treatment is frequently operative. Conservative treatment strategies should initially be employed, but surgical intervention is often necessary.

Ruptures of the LHB tendon typically do not require surgical intervention. Patients with proximal biceps ruptures regain function and have substantial pain relief. The functional deficit is typically slight. Many patients with pain before a biceps rupture will report pain relief once the rupture occurs. An associated cosmetic defect may be present in greater than 20% of proximal biceps ruptures, and patients should be provided information regarding the minimal strength loss if surgical intervention is avoided. Mariani et al. (21) reported on 26 patients (27 shoulders) undergoing

biceps tenodesis versus 30 patients undergoing nonsurgical treatment. Residual arm pain was minimal in both groups. Biomechanical analysis showed a 21% loss of forearm supination strength and 8% loss of elbow flexion strength in the nonsurgical group. The nonsurgical group had no weakness in pronation, elbow extension, or grip. The surgically treated patients had no loss of strength in elbow flexion, extension pronation, supination, or grip. Additionally, surgically treated patients returned to work later than nonsurgical patients, but 11 in the nonsurgical group were not able to return to full work capacity with weakness as their primary complaint. Only two patients in the surgically treated group could not return to full work capacity. Warren (22) tested 10 patients with chronic biceps ruptures and reported no loss of flexion strength and 10% loss of supination strength.

Operative Treatment

Indications

If conservative treatment measures fail and the patient continues to have biceps-associated symptoms for more than 3 months, surgical management should be considered. The imaging studies previously discussed should be utilized prior to considering surgical treatment because of the significant overlap of biceps disorders and other shoulder conditions.

Biceps tendinitis is commonly associated with impingement syndrome and rotator cuff tendinitis or tears (11). Biceps tendon ruptures can result from trauma, which is also often associated with rotator cuff tears or SLAP lesions. Overload flexion force or flexion with forced extension may cause a biceps tendon rupture. Other maladies associated with the biceps tendon involve medial dislocation, spontaneous dislocation, and pathologic lesions.

Treatment options for biceps tendon disorders include tendon debridement (with or without subacromial decompression), a de Quervain's type release, biceps tenotomy, or biceps tenodesis. Only limited reports are available on the effectiveness of a de Quervain's type release of the transverse humeral ligament. If this is performed, care must be taken not to damage the medial sling. The decision regarding tenotomy versus tenodesis is still a controversial one. A tenotomy of the proximal biceps has been reported to carry a 21% incidence of a "Popeye" deformity with distal retraction of the biceps, resulting in a larger muscle mass contracted distally and the loss of proximal muscle bulk. More recent studies by Kelly et al. have shown the "Popeye" deformity to occur in 70% of biceps tenotomies.

Simple debridement of the biceps tendon is of questionable value. If fraying or partial tearing of the biceps tendon is encountered during arthroscopy, its cause should be thoroughly explored. Even a small amount of fraying is suggestive of a mechanical abnormality within the shoulder joint and likely needs further arthroscopic evaluation and treatment (Fig. 15.15). Debridement of biceps tendon tears involving less than 50% of the tendon thickness is frequently recommended, but we feel tendon debridement

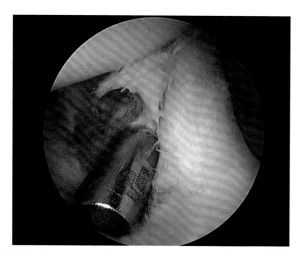

FIGURE 15.15. Minimal fraying and partial tearing of the LHB tendon.

is, in essence, treating the end result of the mechanical problem and not addressing the source of the problem. Arthroscopic subacromial decompression should be considered if the biceps pathology is felt to be secondary to impingement.

The debate over biceps tenotomy versus tenodesis is still quite controversial. Many factors should be weighed when making the decision to perform a tenotomy or tenodesis. These factors include the patient's age, body habitus, activity level, as well as the extent and location of biceps tendon degeneration. Typically, tenotomy is reserved for elderly patients, sedentary patients with a larger body habitus, or patients with significant tendon degeneration that extends into the BG. Tenodesis, in the latter situation, may result in persistent pain due to pathology extending distal to the tenodesis site.

Biceps tenodesis is indicated in active patients younger than 50 who require full elbow flexion and supination strength and in cases of biceps subluxation or dislocation. Chronic biceps tendinitis with stage II or III impingement may also be managed with tenodesis. Many open techniques have been described for the tenodesis of the LHB tendon. One commonly used open procedure is the keyhole technique. Alternative methods of open tenodesis involve soft tissue and periosteal tenodesis within the BG, subpectoral tenodesis with a screw and washer, or a Bio-Tenodesis screw. For chronic retracted ruptures of the LHB, open techniques are usually required although Richards and Burkhart (23) reported an arthroscopic-assisted tenodesis technique (the Cobra procedure) for dealing with selected retracted tears of the biceps tendon. The remainder of this chapter will describe several arthroscopic biceps tenodesis techniques.

TENODESIS TECHNIQUE

Operative intervention for biceps pathology begins with arthroscopic inspection of the glenohumeral joint and debridement. The proximal biceps tendon is easily visualized during standard glenohumeral arthroscopy from the posterior portal. The tendon should be inspected from its origin on the superior glenoid tubercle and superior labrum all the way into the bicipital sheath. It should be examined for fraying, degenerative changes, thickening, and synovitis. The tendon should be pulled from inside the bicipital sheath into the joint with a probe to assess its integrity. Flexing the elbow, supinating the forearm, externally rotating, and abducting the arm can decrease the tension on the biceps and increase the tendon length brought into the joint. This maneuver can expose lesions of the biceps that might otherwise be missed and is important to assess the integrity of the tendon. Any fraying of the biceps tendon adjacent to the medial sling can be an important clue to early tendon subluxation. Arthroscopic biceps tenodesis can obviate the need for a repeat surgery to deal with a much more difficult problem such as tendon dislocation with associated subscapularis tears.

The next portion of the diagnostic arthroscopy is the assessment of the medial sling. This is best done using a 70° arthroscope. The scope is directed to obtain an "aerial" view of the confluence of the subscapularis, the biceps tendon, and the medial sling of the biceps (composed of the medial head of the CHL and the SGHL). This view is maintained while an assistant rotates the humerus internally and externally. Special attention should be paid to the relationship between the biceps and the superior border of the subscapularis. In a normal shoulder, the biceps tendon should never cut posterior to the plane of the superior subscapularis tendon during arm rotation. If the biceps does slip posterior to this plane, it is a sure sign of early biceps instability (Fig. 15.5). If the biceps is not addressed by tenotomy or tenodesis, the patient will eventually develop frank biceps instability and an associated subscapularis tear.

At the completion of the diagnostic arthroscopy, if biceps pathology exists the surgeon must make the decision between biceps tenotomy and tenodesis as outlined previously. Tenotomy can easily be performed using arthroscopic scissors or a radiofrequency probe. The tendon should be cut at its base being sure not to damage the superior glenoid labrum during this procedure. The tendon will usually retract into the bicipital sheath, but if it does not the shaver should be used to excise the intra-articular portion of the biceps tendon so it does not impinge during shoulder motion.

The Bio-Tenodesis Screw System

We perform all-arthroscopic shoulder procedures in the lateral decubitus position under general anesthesia. Five to ten pounds of balanced suspension are used with the arm in 30° of abduction and 20° of forward flexion. Diagnostic glenohumeral arthroscopy is performed through a standard posterior portal with an arthroscopic pump maintaining pressure at 60 mm Hg. An anterosuperolateral (ASL) portal is created using a spinal needle to localize the portal site. A cannula is inserted above the biceps at the superior edge of the safe zone bordered by the biceps superiorly, subscapularis tendon inferiorly, and the glenoid medially. The biceps/labrum complex and the LHB are assessed. A complete assessment of the biceps tendon is performed by pulling the intertubercular portion of the biceps tendon intra-articularly and assessing the amount of degeneration, partial tearing, and instability. Any damage to the subscapularis tendon requires a thorough evaluation of biceps stability.

We prefer the technique described by Lo and Burkhart (24) that utilizes a bioabsorbable PLLA (poly-L-lactic acid) cannulated screw (the Bio-Tenodesis Screw System, Arthrex, Inc., Naples, FL). This uses a uniquely designed driver for inserting an interference screw. The cannulated driver (Fig. 15.16) is specially designed with a reverse-threaded sleeve and thumb piece on the driver shaft. The pitch of the threads on the sleeve is equal and opposite in direction to the pitch of the threads on the Bio-Tenodesis screw. This design allows the biceps tendon to be maintained at the bottom of the bone socket under tension as the Bio-Tenodesis screw is advanced in the bone socket by the hex-driver and by the reverse-threaded pitch of the thumb sleeve. These Bio-Tenodesis screws are available in three diameters (7 to 9 mm) and are 23 mm in length.

After completion of diagnostic arthroscopy, any tendon degeneration is debrided. If a concomitant rotator cuff tear is present, a lateral portal is established directly through the defect created by the torn rotator cuff. Two racking stitches are placed into the biceps tendon (Fig. 15.17). Sutures are placed approximately 1 to 1.5 cm distal to the biceps origin from the superior labrum and are then retrieved through the lateral or ASL portal. The racking sutures tightly grip the degenerative biceps tendon. The biceps tendon is then severed from the superior labrum using electrocautery or arthroscopic scissors (Fig. 15.18). The tagged end of the tendon is then brought out through the ASL portal. The excursion of the tendon is short. Flexion of the elbow allows a greater length of

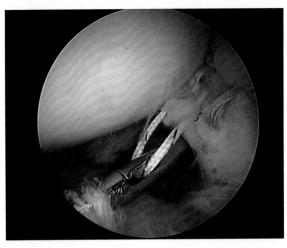

FIGURE 15.17. Arthroscopic view of the right shoulder biceps tendon demonstrating two racking sutures being placed. A Penetrator (Arthrex, Inc., Naples, FL) is used to penetrate the biceps tendon. The Penetrator then grabs the suture and the loop is pulled out of the cannula. The free ends of the suture are brought through the looped end and the free ends are pulled, which creates a tight racking suture around the biceps tendon. The knot pusher allows the racking suture to be tightened.

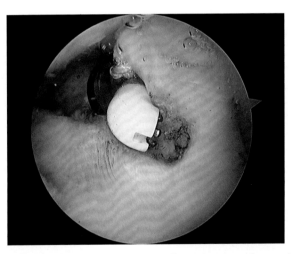

FIGURE 15.18. The biceps tendon is cut from its origin on the superior labrum/glenoid with the cautery device. If increased length is needed, the pencil tip cautery allows maximal retention of biceps tendon length.

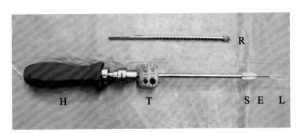

FIGURE 15.16. Bio-Tenodesis cannulated driver (Arthrex, Inc., Naples, FL) with driver handle (H), reverse-threaded sleeve and thumb piece (T), bioabsorbable Bio-Tenodesis screw (S), and a loop of suture (L) loaded through the cannulated tip. Turning the handle (H) and holding the thumb piece (T) advances the screw (S) by means of the reverse-threaded sleeve that advances on the driver shaft while the driver end (E) remains stationary at the base of the bone socket. The measuring guides on the thumb piece (T) are used to size the biceps tendon. The reamer for making the bone socket is also shown and is marked (R).

tendon to be pulled through the skin. The diameter of the tendon is then measured using the slotted measuring plate on the Bio-Tenodesis driver.

Typically, the tendon measures approximately 8 mm in men and 7 mm in women. If the tendon will not fit easily through the 8-mm hole, the end of the tendon is tapered such that it will fit through the 8-mm slotted measuring plate. It is important that the tendon fit rather easily through the plate, as this will make insertion into the bone socket much easier later in the case. A Krakow whipstitch is placed in the tendon such that the suture ends exit the superior surface of the tendon 5 mm from its free end and then the racking sutures are removed (Fig. 15.19).

Next, a bone socket is created in the greater tuberosity, approximately 5 mm posterolateral to the top of the BG. A 2.4-mm guide wire is initially placed and is then overreamed with a cannulated headed reamer. The bone socket is reamed to the size of biceps tendon previously measured (usually 7 or 8 mm in diameter) and to a depth of 25 mm to accommodate a screw length of 23 mm (Fig. 15.20). If there is not an associated rotator cuff tear involving the supraspinatus tendon, the bone socket should be drilled at the top of the BG. After the biceps tenodesis portion of the procedure, two or four suture tails (depending on the technique) will be exiting the Bio-Tenodesis screw construct.

The whipstitch sutures are then passed through a loop of suture at the end of the cannulated driver (Fig. 15.21). Alternatively, the suture ends may be passed directly through the cannulated driver. The driver tip is advanced to the end of the tendon (on its superior surface) and the suture loop is used to snare the whipstitched tendon 2 mm from the end of the graft. The sutures are tensioned and wrapped around the "O" ring on the driver. In this position, the biceps tendon can be manipulated and controlled by the cannulated driver tip.

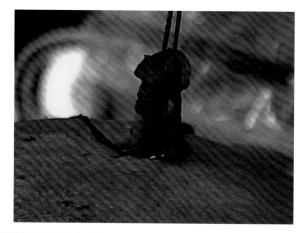

FIGURE 15.19. The biceps stump is seen here exteriorized. A Krakow whipstitch is placed in the tendon and the racking sutures will be removed. The thumb piece from the Bio-Tenodesis driver (Arthrex, Inc. Naples, FL) will be used to size the tendon.

The driver tip is used to push the biceps tendon down to the base of the previously drilled bone socket (Fig. 15.22B). A Bio-Tenodesis screw (the same size as

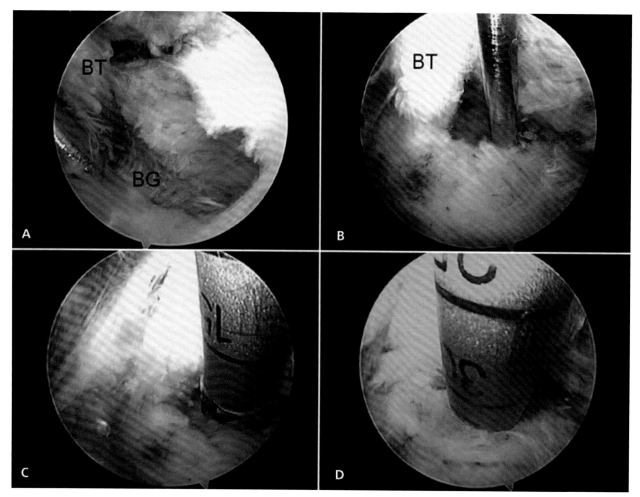

FIGURE 15.20. A: The LHB tendon is seen within the BG. **B:** The guide wire is placed at the top of the BG in this case (without an associated rotator cuff tear). **C:** The cannulated reamer is then advanced over the guide wire. **D:** The reamer is advanced to a depth of 25 mm.

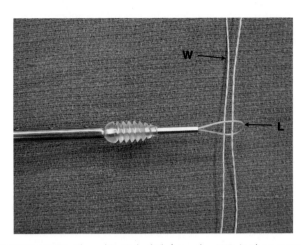

FIGURE 15.21. The whipstitch *(W)* from the LHB is then passed through the loop of suture *(L)* passing through the Bio-Tenodesis driver (Arthrex, Inc., Naples, FL). The whipstitch can be thread through the middle of the cannulated Bio-Tenodesis driver (Arthrex, Inc., Naples, FL). This makes manipulation with the end of the driver easier.

the drilled socket) is then advanced by turning the driver handle while holding the thumb plate that is attached to the reverse-threaded sleeve. This allows the screw to be advanced while the tendon is maintained in a stationary position at the base of the bone socket (Fig. 15.22C).

This assures an adequate bone–tendon–screw interface within the bone socket (Fig. 15.22D) and eliminates the need for transosseous drilling. We prefer to avoid transosseous drilling in order to eliminate any potential risk to the axillary nerve. The two (or four) sutures exiting the Bio-Tenodesis screw (Fig. 15.23) should be used in place of a suture anchor to augment the rotator cuff repair or can simply be cut if no cuff tear is present.

The Biceptor Tenodesis System

An alternative method for utilizing an interference screw without having to whipstitch the biceps tendon has been developed. It attempts to simplify the biceps tenodesis by not requiring the tendon to be brought outside the body

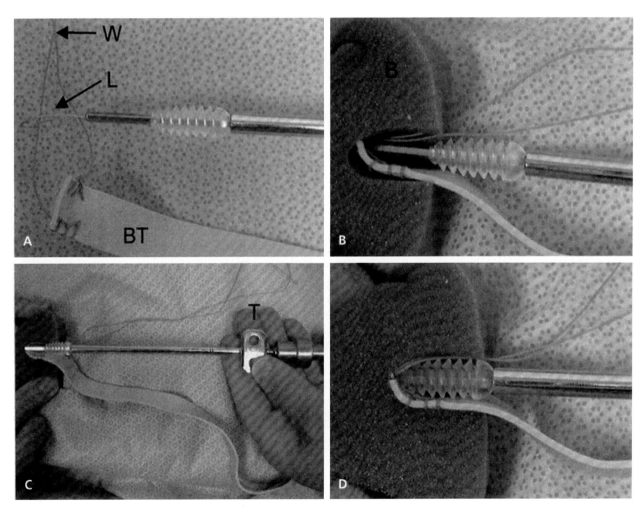

FIGURE 15.22. This is a dry lab demonstration of the Bio-Tenodesis system. **A:** The whipstitch *(W)* from the biceps tendon is then passed through the loop of suture *(L)* passing through the Bio-Tenodesis driver (Arthrex, Inc., Naples, FL). **B:** The biceps tendon is pushed to the base of the prepared bone socket with the tip of the Bio-Tenodesis driver. **C:** The screw is advanced by holding onto the thumb piece while turning the driver clockwise. **D:** The screw is advanced until it is flush with the bone surface.

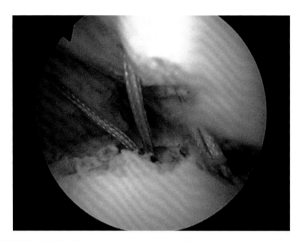

FIGURE 15.23. The Bio-Tenodesis screw is advanced to the point it is flush with the bone surface. The LHB tendon is now secure in the bone socket. Two sutures from the Bio-Tenodesis screw can be used for rotator cuff repair.

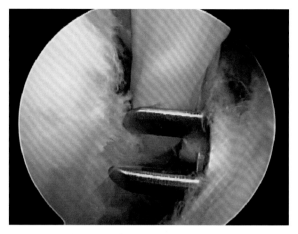

FIGURE 15.24. The tendon fork is used to size the LHB tendon.

for whipstitching, thereby creating an all-arthroscopic technique. We have had good success with this technique and it can be used above or below the BG.

When using the BICEPTOR Tenodesis System (Smith & Nephew, Andover, MA), standard arthroscopic portals may be utilized, which include the posterior, lateral, ASL, and an anterior portal. Intra-articular pathology within the glenohumeral joint should be assessed before biceps tenodesis can begin. We utilize a racking hitch performed through the ASL portal in the same fashion that we described in the Bio-Tenodesis technique. Although the BICEPTOR tenodesis has also been performed in situ without a suture on the LHB, this may tighten the tendon slightly. We prefer to cut the LHB with an electrocautery device or arthroscopic scissors proximal to the two racking hitches close to the labral attachment. Debridement of the biceps stump on the labrum can be completed at this time. The lateral portal is then utilized to remove any bursal tissue found in the subacromial space. We typically visualize with the arthroscope in the posterior portal if the tenodesis is performed above the BG and through the ASL or lateral portal if the tenodesis is performed below or in the groove. A needle is placed anteriorly to verify the intertubercular BG location; a cannula is inserted into this portal to be viewed in the subacromial space.

Once a bursectomy down the humeral face is completed and the suprapectoralis location is visualized, the transverse ligament should be cut between the lesser and the greater tuberosity to identify the LHB in the BG. To determine the size of the BIOSURE PK (PEEK is polyetheretherketone) interference screw (Smith & Nephew, Andover, MA), a tendon fork should be inserted (Fig. 15.24), and the tendon should be captured.

If the tendon is situated easily into the tendon fork, then a 7.0-mm Endoscopic XL drill bit (Smith & Nephew, Andover, MA) and a 7.0-mm BIOSURE PK interference screw should be utilized. However, if the tendon is too

large for the fork then a medium (8.0 mm) or large (9.0 mm) fork should be used. Line-to-line sizing is proper for drilling the socket, that is, 8.0-mm hole for an 8.0-mm screw. A guide pin is placed in the appropriate location and an Endoscopic XL drill bit is used to make the recipient site for the LHB. This socket may be made at the top of the BG, within the groove itself after the transverse humeral ligament is cut, or below the groove. An extra 5 mm of depth should be drilled (typically 30 mm for a 25-mm screw), and the drill bit and guide wire removed. A tap can be used if the bone is hard. The perimeter of the socket should be debrided with a shaver of any remaining soft tissue, which improves the insertion of the tendon and screw. The whipstitch sutures are used to tension the biceps tendon to achieve the desired tension in the LHB. The tendon fork is then utilized to position the LHB into the socket, a 2.4-mm guide wire is introduced through the fork and the fork is then removed. The tendon is now pinned into the recipient socket (Fig. 15.25) and no tension should be present on the suture or tendon when removing the tendon fork. The appropriate BIOSURE PK interference screw is then placed on the driver that is inserted over the guide pin (Fig. 15.26). The driver and pin are removed and excess tendon is cut away. The anchor firmly holds the tendon in the socket (Fig. 15.27).

Suture Anchor Technique

Tenodesis with suture anchors was previously described by Gartsman and Hammerman (25) and subsequently by Nord et al. (26) Each used suture anchors inserted in different locations to obtain fixation to the proximal humerus or the greater tuberosity. Two suture anchors are inserted through the subclavian portal (Nord) or from the anterior portal (Gartsman). The method described by Gartsman and Hammerman (25) requires debridement of the CHL and requires more extensive anterior debridement to allow insertion of the anchors into the intertubercular groove.

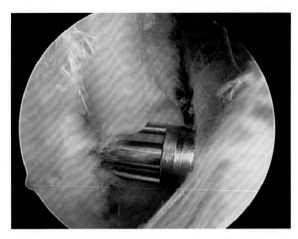

FIGURE 15.25. The tendon is pushed into the socket, the tendon is pinned, and the tendon fork is removed.

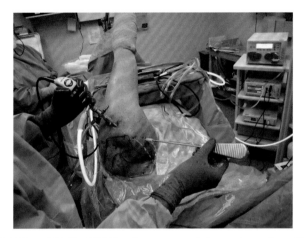

FIGURE 15.26. The PEEK interference screw is inserted over the guide wire, which is holding the LHB tendon in the drill hole. This eliminates the need for whipstitching the end of the tendon.

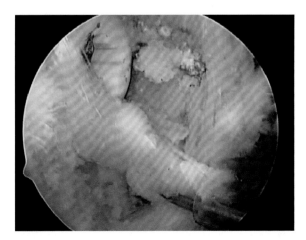

FIGURE 15.27. The PEEK interference screw firmly wedges the LHB tendon into the drill hole.

The Nord Technique

Glenohumeral arthroscopy is performed in the lateral decubitus position under 10 lb of traction as described in the preceding paragraphs. The arm is suspended at approximately a 30° angle of abduction and 10° forward flexion. This allows for external and internal rotation of the distracted shoulder; however, it can be performed in the beach chair position if the surgeon desires. Four to six portals are utilized during the procedure. The anterosuperior, posterior, and lateral portals are made to obtain visualization of anatomical structures and defects. These portals are also used as working portals and cannulas are utilized. When a rotator cuff repair is necessary, the subclavian, anterolateral, and modified Neviaser portals are utilized as necessary for passing sutures through the tendon. Anchors for rotator cuff repair are typically inserted through an anterolateral portal without a cannula. To facilitate biceps tenodesis, the subclavian portal is used for anchor insertion. The subclavian portal is located 1 to 2 cm medial to the AC joint, above and slightly medial to the coracoid, and directly inferior to the clavicle (Fig. 15.28). A cannula is not needed or recommended for this portal. Instruments or anchors are passed inferior and anterior to the AC joint before entering the subacromial bursa. Subacromial decompression optimizes the use of the subclavian portal.

The scope is introduced into the glenohumeral joint through a standard posterior portal. An ASL portal is made following the path of a spinal needle. The anatomical structures are visualized and any abnormalities are assessed. Treatment of other pathology is performed as indicated. A lateral portal is created and subacromial decompression is performed, which relieves shoulder impingement and facilitates the use of the subclavian portal. The scope is utilized through the posterior portal below the rotator cuff to gain visualization of the biceps tendon. Using a burr through the lateral portal, a small area of the articular and bony surface is abraded under the biceps tendon, just proximal

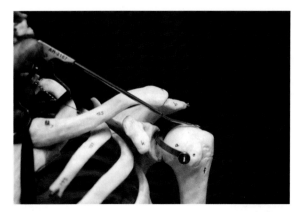

FIGURE 15.28. Skeleton demonstrating the proper orientation for the subclavian portal passing anterior and inferior the AC joint and into the subacromial bursa. The Penetrator (Arthrex, Inc., Naples, FL) is utilized in this fashion to retrieve sutures through the supraspinatus tendon. For insertion of an anchor during biceps tenodesis, the anchor in aimed slightly caudal. The exact location is identified with a spinal needle prior to insertion of the anchor.

to the BG. A spinal needle is inserted through the subclavian portal in order to identify the tract through the CHL to the biceps tendon. A 3-mm incision is made for the subclavian portal and no cannula is used. A metal suture anchor, 5 mm (preferred) or 3.5 mm, is passed through the subclavian portal entering the joint through the RI. Then, the suture anchor is placed through the biceps tendon slightly proximal to the BG. Lifting the biceps tendon with a probe will help facilitate visualization of the anchor through the biceps tendon and embedding into bone (Fig. 15.29).

The subclavian approach allows fixation of the tendon "in situ" just proximal to the point at which the tendon enters the BG. The anchor can be placed directly through the biceps or adjacent to it. Sutures are passed with a penetrating suture grasper or with suture passers. The sutures can be passed through the subclavian or ASL portal—whichever provides a better angle. The biceps is left attached while the suture anchor is inserted through the tendon. If a rotator cuff tear is present, the sutures in the biceps may be tied through the lateral portal. However, if a rotator cuff tear is not present, sutures are tied through the anterior portal. One limb of the suture is pulled underneath and over the biceps tendon and then out the appropriate portal with a crochet hook and the sutures tied. Knot security and loop security are assessed. A second suture anchor is introduced through the subclavian portal, passed through the biceps tendon slightly proximal to the other suture anchor, and sutures retrieved. The biceps tendon is found to be firmly attached by testing the tenodesis with a hook probe.

The residual intra-articular biceps tendon is released from a site just proximal to the sutures using a basket cutter, and the remaining stump is excised at the point of attachment at the superior glenoid labrum utilizing a basket cutter and shaver. Arthroscopic rotator cuff repair is performed as necessary after the completion of the biceps tenodesis. The tenodesis will not add any significant

bulk beneath the rotator cuff repair and allows for normal shoulder motion. During range of motion testing of the shoulder and elbow, stability of the biceps tenodesis is arthroscopically assessed.

The Cobra Procedure

Richards and Burkhart (23) described an arthroscopic-assisted repair of the LHB titled the "Cobra procedure" in honor of the tattoo of a king cobra (Figure 15.30). First, a standard arthroscopic shoulder procedure is performed, intra-articular pathology is addressed, and the cuff thoroughly examined. Subscapularis pathology (which is common since when the LHB ruptures it can disrupt the upper subscapularis) is addressed and repaired arthroscopically. Proper ASL portal placement is essential since this portal will be utilized extensively to perform the tenodesis. Next, the subacromial space is cleared and the anterior, lateral, and posterior gutters are cleared. The scope is then removed and attention is turned toward preparing the LHB.

The inferior border of the pectoralis major is palpated, and a small incision (2 to 3 cm) is made a few centimeters distal to this landmark in line with the lower boarder of the pectoralis major (Figure 15.31). Typically, blunt dissection with the finger easily palpates the cord-like tendon of the ruptured LHB. If the rupture is relatively acute, delivering the tendon from the wound is not difficult. However, if the rupture is more than a few weeks old it may be necessary to free adhesions between the torn LHB and the surrounding structures. The fingertip is used to release these adhesions proximally and distally until the tendon can be delivered from the incision. Once the LHB tendon is freed of adhesions, the length and excursion are assessed. For the Cobra procedure to be effective, the surgeon should be able to stretch the LHB tendon up to the ASL portal (off the anterolateral

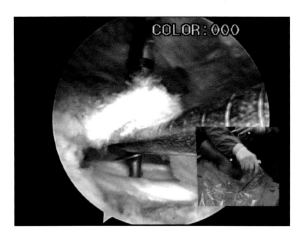

FIGURE 15.29. Arthroscopic view looking from posterior showing the metal suture anchor passing through the RI/CHL and directly through the biceps tendon just proximal to the BG. The area under the biceps has been abraded with a shaver to improve healing of the tendon to bone.

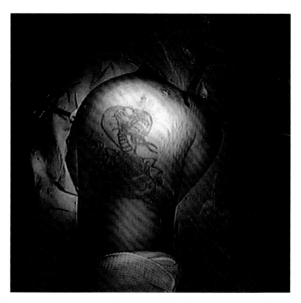

FIGURE 15.30. Tattoo on the arm of the first patient to undergo the Cobra procedure.

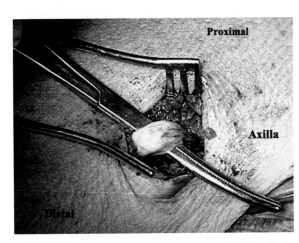

FIGURE 15.31. Incision is made a few centimeters distal to the lower border of the pectoralis major. Tendon of LHB is palpated and delivered from the wound.

tip of the acromion Figure 15.32). This will allow an arthroscopic biceps tenodesis with a bio-interference screw. Next, a Krakow whip-suture is placed in the proximal 3 cm of the LHB tendon. The tendon is sized with the Bio-Tenodesis driver apparatus. The tendon is typically a size of 7 or 8 mm.

A blunt switching stick is then inserted from the arm incision proximally up into the BG. The switching stick is placed underneath the pectoralis major tendon and along the BG and then pushed proximally until the switching stick exits the ASL portal (Figure 15.33). The switching stick is modified slightly such that on one end (the distal end) there is a small slit in the metal for the insertion of the Krackow whip-sutures in the biceps tendon. A beath pin with the pointed tip cutoff will also work in this situation.

Once the whip-sutures are loaded into this slit, the switching stick is advanced proximally and the whip-sutures will be pulled out the ASL portal (Figure 15.34). The elbow is then flexed to release the tension of the biceps

muscle. The whip-sutures pull the biceps tendon into the BG and out the ASL portal. The scope is then reinserted into the intra-articular space. A guide pin is placed through the ASL portal (adjacent to the LHB tendon) and into the BG between the greater and the lesser tuberosities. Once it is positioned, a reamer that corresponds to the size of the biceps tendon is advanced over the guide pin and drilled to a depth of 25 mm (Figure 15.35). The reamer and guide pin are both removed and a shaver is utilized to remove any loose tissue and allow for adequate visualization of the bone socket. Sometimes it is helpful to use a 70° arthroscope in this process.

The Krakow whip-suture is then advanced through the middle of the Bio-Tenodesis screwdriver (using a nitinol guide wire), and the tip of the screwdriver is positioned directly on the tip of the LHB tendon. Tension is held on the whip-suture to allow the surgeon good control of the tendon with the tip of the screwdriver. The tendon is then "pushed" into the bone socket with the tip of the screwdriver. Once it is well seated such that the tendon is pushed all the way to the base of the bone socket, the 23-mm Bio-Tenodesis screw is advanced with the driver such that the top of the screw is flush with the bone (Figure 15.35). Finally, the scope is inserted through the ASL portal, and the Bio-Tenodesis screw visualized. The blue Krakow sutures can be visualized all the way to the base of the bone socket. The ends of the whip-sutures are then cut flush with the top of the screw.

Although this procedure is absolutely not indicated for most LHB ruptures, it offers a minimally invasive approach to this problem for a select subset of patients. Functional and cosmetic outcomes are generally excellent.

Soft Tissue Tenodesis Technique

Suture tenodesis to soft tissue has been advocated due to its simplicity. Two methods have been described. One involves open suturing of the biceps tendon to the transverse

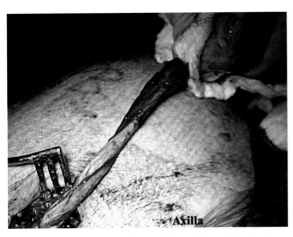

FIGURE 15.32. The biceps tendon is delivered out of the incision and stretched to ASL portal (off the anterolateral tip of the acromion).

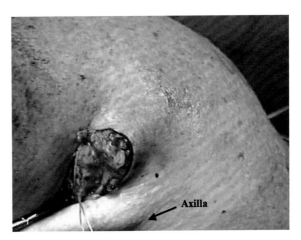

FIGURE 15.33. A switching stick is inserted through the incision, proximally into the bicipital groove, underneath the pectoralis major tendon, and out the ASL portal.

humeral ligament, and the other involves arthroscopic suturing of the tendon to the CHL or the anterior supraspinatus tendon.

The arthroscopic suture tenodesis technique begins with an anterosuperior portal being made for the introduction of a suture-passing device. Alternatively, a spinal needle can be used to pass PDS suture through the biceps after passing the needle through the rotator cuff using an anterolateral portal. If the tendon is of poor quality, racking sutures provide better purchase on the tendon. A second suture can then be placed in a similar manner. The biceps is released from its attachment to the labrum and supraglenoid tubercle using a radiofrequency device or arthroscopic scissors. The edge of the superior labrum is smoothed.

Once the tendon is released from the labrum, it retracts slightly and the sutures are passed through the CHL or anterior supraspinatus with a suture-passing device. If a spinal needle was used to pass the no. 1 PDS suture, the sutures have already passed through the supraspinatus. With the camera in the subacromial space, the sutures are retrieved through the lateral cannula and then securely tied. This anchors the biceps to the supraspinatus or the CHL. The authors seldom perform this soft tissue tenodesis technique and prefer to securely anchor the biceps to bone with a suture anchor or interference screw.

The senior author (K.D.N.) uses this technique only in the case of an extremely degenerative tendon. In such cases, Bio-Tenodesis interference fixation or suture anchor fixation is sometimes not secure, and two racking sutures more distal in the degenerative biceps provide relatively secure purchase on the tendon. More recently, methods of balling up the LHB or detaching the biceps tendon with a section of the labrum to allow the thickened end to catch at the entrance of the groove have been described. Reservations exist about sacrificing part of the superior labrum or having a more prominent tissue ball under the anterolateral acromion.

Pulley Repair

Direct pulley repair is not typically advocated unless associated with a comma sign and a retracted subscapularis tendon repaired at the same time. Direct pulley repair may be considered in young patients (teens), acute trauma, and a healthy tendon. Postoperative shoulder stiffness with loss of external rotation is the typical consequence. This occurs because of tightening the capsular structures including the CHL and SGHL, as well as tethering of the biceps tendon that normally has some excursion through the BG.

We routinely perform a biceps tenodesis in this situation to effectively resolve the biceps symptoms. This allows end range of motion with no consequences to shoulder function. Most of the time the medial sling or pulley is still attached to the subscapularis. In this situation, repair of the subscapularis and the medial pulley is

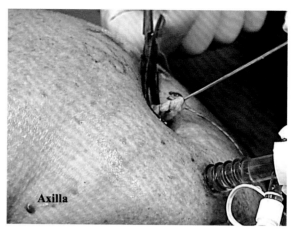

FIGURE 15.34. The whip-sutures pull the biceps tendon into the BG and out the ASL portal.

performed with two suture anchors placed from medial to lateral. The 30° scope is placed in the ASL portal and the lesser tuberosity is roughened with the burr or shaver to stimulate healing to a bleeding bone bed. Suture anchors are inserted through the anterior inferior portal into the lesser tuberosity. The sutures are passed through the subscapularis tendon and medial pulley utilizing a Penetrator or Scorpion through an anteroinferior portal. Simple sutures work fine in this situation, and the sutures are tied through the ASL portal. If the superior portion of the CHL and supraspinatus are torn, they are repaired in the standard fashion with suture anchors, and sutures are tied in the subacromial space.

REHABILITATION

Rehabilitation is similar for a patient undergoing a tenotomy or tenodesis. This is due to the risk of developing a "Popeye" deformity in a tenotomy patient with more aggressive flexion of the shoulder or elbow or with supination. If there is no additional pathology, the patient is placed in a sling for 4 to 5 weeks. Full elbow flexion and extension is encouraged with no resistance. Gentle shoulder motion is permitted, and elbow extension and passive flexion are allowed. At 4 weeks, the sling is discontinued, and a full shoulder and elbow range of motion program is permitted.

Grip strengthening, pendulums, and shoulder shrugs are permitted immediately. External shoulder rotation is permitted to 25° with a tenodesis, to neutral with a subscapularis or pulley repair. At 4 weeks, gradual supine external rotation to 30° and supine forward flexion are permitted. At 8 weeks, cross-chest stretches are started and early extension behind the back below waist level is encouraged. Isometric strengthening is started at 8 weeks. During weeks 10 to 12, rotator cuff and scapular strengthening are started. By 4 to 6 months sport-specific exercises are started and gradual return to activities is permitted.

COMPLICATIONS AND SPECIAL CONSIDERATIONS

Complications of the biceps tenotomy primarily involve the risk of a "Popeye" deformity as the biceps muscle retracts distally (up to a 70%). Men may not be concerned over this deformity, but it may not be cosmetically acceptable to women or bodybuilders. Patients should be counseled about this risk and if this is unacceptable to the patient, a tenodesis performed. Arthroscopic biceps tenotomy is otherwise a relatively safe procedure with very minor risks of infection, blood clots, or neurovascular injury.

The portals used for a tenotomy are the standard arthroscopy portals, and the risks are comparable to diagnostic shoulder arthroscopy risks. Pain relief is generally very good although occasionally a patient may have some residual pain or cramping with activities involving forceful elbow flexion. Risks of shoulder arthroscopy include infection, blood vessel or nerve injury, upper extremity deep venous thrombosis, neuropraxia of the ulnar nerve secondary to compression of the nerve at the cubital tunnel, and brachial plexus traction injuries, which are usually a result of head and neck positioning.

Complications associated with the Bio-Tenodesis screw technique include the same risks associated with tenotomy except a Popeye deformity would not be expected unless failure of fixation occurred. If not adequately seated in the bone bed, prominence of the Bio-Tenodesis screw could potentially cause impingement upon the acromion. Therefore, the surgeon must advance the screw head until it is flush with the bone surface. The tendon may not be pulled down into the drill hole enough, resulting in a lax tendon or fixation of the tendon with sutures alone. Close attention to the technique will prevent this problem. Fractures could potentially occur depending on the location of screw insertion, but we have not seen this complication. Osteoporotic bone may not allow rigid fixation, but the Bio-Tenodesis screw would be expected to have better

fixation than suture anchors in osteoporotic bone. If the Bio-Tenodesis screw appears somewhat loose after insertion into osteoporotic bone, its stability may be improved by inserting a 5-mm Bio-Corkscrew suture anchor directly adjacent to it, thereby achieving an interference-fit by the suture anchor against the Bio-Tenodesis screw.

The question of whether it is necessary to release the LHB from the glenoid labrum when a tenodesis has been performed has been raised by Franceschi et al. (27) They utilized a suture anchor tenodesis technique. This is a fascinating concept that does allow incorporation of the intra-articular biceps into a rotator cuff repair with no functional deficit, yet improving the rotator cuff repair. In techniques utilizing a biotenodesis or interference screw, we would recommend still performing a tenotomy since a segment of the tendon will be inserted into the drill hole, thereby functionally shortening the tendon.

Complications associated with suture anchors carry all the standard arthroscopy risks. Additionally, failure of fixation can occur in the form of anchor pullout or suture breakage. When postoperative anchor pullout occurs, an additional procedure may be required to retrieve the anchor. Failure of fixation of the biceps tendon results in a biceps tenotomy with the potential "Popeye" deformity, so the surgeon should discuss this possibility with the patient.

CONCLUSIONS AND FUTURE DIRECTIONS

Treatment for ruptures and instability of the LHB continues to progress aided by new instrumentation and techniques. The function of the SGHL and CHL as stabilizing structures is becoming better understood. This has improved our ability to recognize and treat biceps instability. Subscapularis repairs will fail if the biceps instability is not addressed with a tenotomy or tenodesis. Long-term patient outcome studies comparing alternative treatment modalities are needed. Arthroscopic treatment is rapidly becoming the standard of care for the treatment of disorders of the biceps tendon.

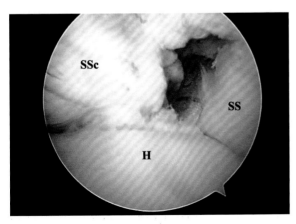

FIGURE 15.35. Intra-articular view of reamer at BG. The Bio-Tenodesis screw is advanced to the point it is flush with the bone surface. The LHB tendon is now secure in the bone socket.

REFERENCES

1. Habermayer P, Kaiser E, Knappe M, et al. Functional anatomy and biomechanics of the long biceps tendon. *Unfallchirurg.* 1987;90:319–329.
2. Pal GP, Bhatt RH, Patel VS. Relationship between the tendon of the long head of biceps brachii and the glenoid labrum in humans. *Anat Rec.* 1991;229:278–280.
3. Ueberham K, Le Floch-Prigent P. Intertubercular sulcus of the humerus: biometry and morphology of 100 dry bones. *Surg Radiol Anat.* 1998;20:351–354.
4. Bennett WF. Subscapularis, medial and lateral head coracohumeral ligament insertion anatomy: arthroscopic appearance and incidence of "hidden" rotator interval lesions. *Arthroscopy.* 2001;17:173–180.

5. Lo IK, Burkhart SS. The comma sign: an arthroscopic guide to the torn subscapularis tendon. *Arthroscopy.* 2003;19:334–337.

6. Ruotolo C, Nottage WM, Flatow EL, et al. Controversial topics in shoulder arthroscopy. *Arthroscopy.* 2002;18:65–75.

7. Andrews J, Carson W, McLeod W. Glenoid labrum tears related to the long head of the biceps. *Am J Sports Med.* 1985;13:337–341.

8. Basmajian JV. *Muscles Alive.* 5th ed. Baltimore, MD: Williams & Wilkins; 1985.

9. Jobe FW, Tibone JE, Tibone JE, et al. An EMG analysis of the shoulder in pitching. A second report. *Am J Sports Med.* 1984;12:218–220.

10. Yamaguchi K, Riew KD, Galatz LM, et al. Biceps during shoulder motion. *Clin Orthop Relat Res.* 1997;336:122–129.

11. Habermayer P, Walch G. The biceps tendon and rotator cuff disease. In: Burkhead WZ Jr, ed. *Rotator Cuff Disorders.* Media, PA: Williams & Wilkins; 1996:142.

12. Gilcreest EL, Albi P. Unusual lesions of muscles and tendons of the shoulder girdle and upper arm. *Surg Gynecol Obstet.* 1939;68:903–917.

13. Yergason RM. Rupture of biceps. *J Bone Joint Surg.* 1931;13:160.

14. Barth JR, Burkhart SS, De Beer JF. Barth JR, Burkhart SS, De Beer JF. The bear-hug test: a new and sensitive test for diagnosing a subscapularis tear. Arthroscopy. 2006;10:1076-1084. *Arthroscopy.* 2006;22:1076–1084.

15. Schwamborn T, Imhoff AB. Diagnostik und klassifikation der rotatorenmanchettenlasionen. In: Imhoff AB, Konig U, eds. *Schulterinstabilitat-Rotatorenmanschette.* Darmstadt, Germany: Steinkopff Verlag; 1999:193–195.

16. Burkhart SS, Tehrany AM. Arthroscopic subscapularis tendon repair: technique and preliminary results. *Arthroscopy.* 2002;18:454–463.

17. Gerber C, Krushell RJ. Isolated rupture of the tendon of the subscapularis muscle: clinical features in 16 cases. *J Bone Joint Surg Br.* 1991;73:389–394.

18. Abbott LC, Saunders LB de CM. Acute traumatic dislocation of the tendon of the long head of biceps brachii: report of 6 cases with operative findings. *Surgery.* 1939;6:817–840.

19. Bennett WF. Specificity of the Speed's test: arthroscopic technique for evaluating the biceps tendon at the level of the bicipital groove. *Arthroscopy.* 1998;14:789–796.

20. Farin PU, Jaroma H, Harju A, et al. Medial displacement of the biceps brachii tendon: evaluation with dynamic sonography during maximal external shoulder rotation. *Radiology.* 1995;195:845–848.

21. Mariani EM, Cofied RH, Askew LJ, et al. Rupture of the tendon of the long head of the biceps brachii. Surgicalversus nonsurgical treatment. *Clin Orthop Relat Res.* 1988; 228:233–239.

22. Warren RF. Lesions of the long head of the biceps tendon. *Instr Course Lect.* 1985;34:204–209.

23. Richards DP, Burkhart SS. Arthroscopic-assisted biceps tenodesis for ruptures of the long head of the biceps brachii: the Cobra procedure. *Arthroscopy.* 2004;20:201–207.

24. Lo IK, Burkhart SS. Arthroscopic biceps tenodesis using a bioabsorbable interference screw. *Arthroscopy.* 2004;20:85–95.

25. Gartsman GM, Hammerman SM. Arthroscopic biceps tenodesis: operative technique. *Arthroscopy.* 2000;16:650–652.

26. Nord KD, Smith GB, Mauck BM. Arthroscopic biceps tenodesis: using suture anchors through the subclavian portal. *Arthroscopy.* 2003;19:24.

27. Franceschi F, Longo UG, Ruzzini L, et al. To detach the long head of the biceps tendon after tenodesis or not: outcome analysis at the 4-year follow-up of two different techniques. *Int Orthop.* 2007;31:537-545.

Anterior Shoulder Instability: Suture Anchor

Benjamin Shaffer • Jonas R. Rudzki • Patrick Birmingham

Anterior shoulder instability is a common problem, particularly in the young athletic population, with a prevalence of anterior shoulder dislocation between 2% and 8% (1). Although most of these instability events are traumatic dislocations, some patients experience an initial subluxation. Recurrent instability (dislocations and subluxations) is often age-dependent, with the risk among patients younger than age 20 averaging between 50% and 65%, although in some series it can be as high as 90% with nonoperative treatment. (1) This recurrence rate drops below 50% in patients greater than 25 years old (2).

The high recurrence rate, combined with the significant athletic impairment in patients with anterior instability, has led us to consider operative intervention as the definitive treatment for most young athletes. For nearly a century, stabilization has been achieved through an open surgical technique, the Bankart repair, with reported success rates up to 97% (1, 3, 4). However, with the advent of less invasive technology, arthroscopic techniques for anterior instability have flourished and over time evolved to become the de facto standard for many physicians treating this condition. In comparison to traditional open approaches, arthroscopic repair offers the potential advantages of decreased postoperative pain, stiffness, recurrent instability, and a faster functional recovery. Although there is current dispute whether arthroscopic repair affords better stability results than open, the practical benefits of arthroscopic repair have been well established.

Arthroscopic stabilization has seen a dramatic evolution in technology over the last few decades, transitioning from a simple reapproximation of the detached labrum with a metal staple to a more stable fixation technique using suture anchors. Suture anchors offer numerous advantages over other current techniques including flexibility in number and type of suture used, and the ability to individually titrate capsular patholaxity in each case.

Today's operative success rates of 90% to 95% are attributable in part to advances in technology but can also be traced to refinements in our indications, recognition and treatment of contributory pathology (especially concomitant capsular patholaxity), and advances in surgical technique and experience. The purpose of this chapter is to provide an overview of our understanding and approach to treating the patient with anterior instability, emphasizing the clinical evaluation and indications, and to provide a detailed map for the successful arthroscopic repair technique using suture anchors.

NORMAL SHOULDER FUNCTIONAL ANATOMY

The shoulder is a highly unconstrained ball and socket joint, which relies upon both static and dynamic mechanisms for stability. Its intrinsic lack of constraint allows for its wide range of motion, translation, and function, although these render it vulnerable to instability. Architecturally, the glenoid is a shallow socket whose concavity and depth are increased 50% to 80% by the surrounding labrum. The fibrocartilaginous labrum helps to increase the diameter of the socket by up to 57% in the transverse direction and 75% vertically (5). In conjunction with adjacent capsular ligaments, the labrum significantly enhances glenohumeral stability.

Viewed arthroscopically, the shoulder capsule comprises three discrete glenohumeral ligaments, which serve as static stabilizers (Fig. 16.1). Selective cutting and biomechanical studies have shown that their individual contributions vary depending upon arm position, rotation, and magnitude of the applied force. The superior glenohumeral ligament (SGHL) serves to resist inferior translation with the arm in the adducted position and is thought to play a significant role in patients with inferior laxity and multidirectional instability (MDI). The middle glenohumeral ligament (MGHL) varies in size and shape but resists external rotation and translation with the arm abducted 45°. The most important of the glenohumeral ligaments is the inferior glenohumeral ligament (IGHL) complex, which is the primary stabilizer to anterior humeral translation at 90° of abduction (6). This complex consists of anterior and posterior bands with an intervening sling cradling the

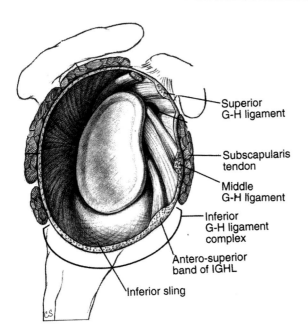

FIGURE 16.1. The shoulder capsule is composed of discrete glenohumeral ligaments, including superior, middle, and inferior. The inferior glenohumeral ligament complex (IGHL), including the anterosuperior band and inferior sling (posterior band not shown) serves as important static stabilizers to normal stability.

humeral head inferiorly. The bands have been described to function as a hammock, with the anterior band reciprocally tightening in abduction and external rotation whereas the posterior band comes under tension with forward elevation and internal rotation. Together with the glenoid labrum, these ligaments form a capsulolabral complex, which serves as the primary static stabilizer of the glenohumeral joint (6).

Dynamic stability is provided by the rotator cuff muscles, which through concavity-compression center the humeral head on the glenoid (6). The interaction between these static and dynamic stabilizers helps to maintain glenohumeral stability through a broad range of motion.

Anterior shoulder instability is typically thought to occur subsequent to injury to the static stabilizers, specifically to the anteroinferior labrum and capsule (6,7). Detachment of the labrum from the anterior glenoid in the setting of recurrent anterior shoulder instability was originally described in 1938 (Fig. 16.2) These lesions have been reported in 65% to 95% of shoulders, undergoing surgical treatment for anterior instability (3); however, there is likely no single "essential lesion" in anterior shoulder instability. Basic science data have shown that isolated labral detachments are in fact uncommon, and most instability has some element of associated capsular pathology. This underscores the importance of addressing concomitant capsular patholaxity along with labral repair.

In addition to soft tissue injury, bony pathology is not uncommon in patients with shoulder instability. Osteochondral injury to the posterior humeral head, known

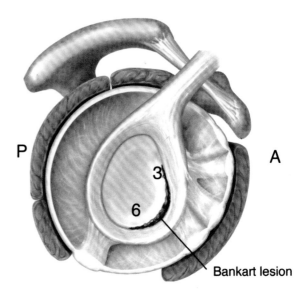

FIGURE 16.2. The Bankart lesion describes a detachment of the labrum and capsuloligamentous sleeve, usually from the approximately 3 o'clock to 6 o'clock position; A, anterior; P, posterior.

as a Hill–Sachs lesion, is common resulting from humeral head impaction against the anterior-inferior (AI) glenoid at the time of subluxation or dislocation (Fig. 16.3). Several studies have reported a considerable increase in recurrence rate following arthroscopic stabilization in patients with significant "engaging" Hill–Sachs lesions.

On the glenoid side, osseous Bankart lesions with fracture of the adjacent anterior-inferior glenoid rim may occur in up to 73% of cases (3) (Fig. 16.4). The avulsed fracture fragment typically remains attached to the capsulolabral tissue. This bony injury is significant because it may result in compromise of the normal articular arc and decrease the threshold of force necessary for humeral head translation, leading to recurrent subluxation and/or dislocation. Soft tissue procedures that repair the labrum

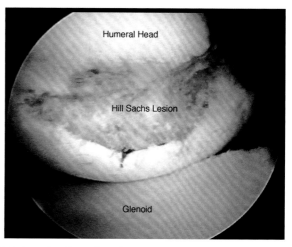

FIGURE 16.3. The Hill–Sachs lesion, a hatched-shaped defect in the posterolateral head, is seen in this arthroscopic photo of a right shoulder in the lateral decubitus position.

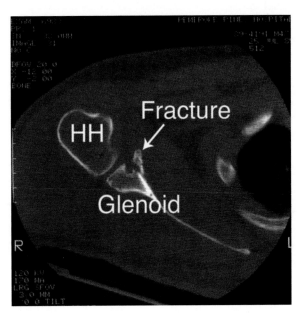

FIGURE 16.4. Fracture of the anterior-inferior glenoid rim is assessed via CT scan, in this axial section demonstrating greater than 25% compromise; HH, humeral head.

and/or address capsular patholaxity are not likely to be effective in the face of articular arc deficiency.

Less commonly, instability can occur subsequent to other structural injuries. Tears of the rotator cuff can occur with shoulder dislocation and can predispose to recurrence either in isolation or accompanying a labral detachment. Subscapularis tendon disruptions are uncommon but require consideration in traumatic instability among contact/collision athletes. Capsular failure on the humeral side, known as a HAGL (humeral avulsion of the glenohumeral ligament) lesion, can cause instability without labral injury.

CLINICAL EVALUATION

The clinical evaluation of the patient with anterior shoulder instability begins with a thorough history, paying particular attention to the patient's age at the time of initial injury, mechanism of injury, hand dominance, and desired occupational and/or recreational activity level. Age at the time of acute shoulder dislocations has been shown to influence the subsequent risk of recurrent instability with patients under 20 years of age at greatest risk. Eliciting the mechanism helps with understanding the likely injury pattern and possible presence of concomitant pathology.

One should determine the severity of the instability, episode and its precipitating cause. Did the shoulder completely dislocate or just sublux? How many instability episodes have occurred, have the instability episodes changed over time, and have they required manipulative reductions or recurred with less provocation? In what position has the arm been positioned at the time of these instability episodes? Was the dislocation documented with X-rays? All these considerations affect understanding

the significance of the problem and influence both the evaluation and the treatment decision-making.

Physical exam must include standard tests for active and passive range of motion, deltoid and cuff strength, and neurovascular status. In the acutely dislocated shoulder, physical examination may be of limited value because of pain and apprehension. Patients with recurrent instability offer an easier exam.

Tests specific for instability include glenohumeral translation and functional instability testing, which help determine the direction and extent of the instability pattern and may suggest concomitant pathology. It is important to distinguish laxity, an objective measurement of joint translation, from instability, which is symptomatic laxity.

In laxity, assessment loads are applied to the glenohumeral joint, noting the degree of humeral head translation. Because of variable laxity in the population, comparison with the opposite shoulder is important. Occasionally, translation testing will reveal mechanical catching or grinding consistent with labral pathology, or elicit symptoms that occur with the patients' instability episodes.

Several grading classifications for translation testing have been described. In one such scale, Grade 0 represents no translation. Grade 1 is mild translation, in which the humeral head moves slightly up the face of the glenoid 0 to 1 cm. Grade 2 refers to moderate translation, in which the humeral head rides up the glenoid face to but not over the rim (1 to 2 cm translation). In Grade 3, there is severe (greater than 2 cm) translation, in which the humeral head rides up and over the glenoid rim (though it usually reduces when stress is removed).

Subjective functional instability tests attempt to elicit symptoms by placing the arm in provocative positions and under various loads. The time-honored apprehension test may be of greatest value, placing the arm in the abducted, externally rotated (i.e., throwing) position. Some patients require some translation force in this position to elicit the sense of instability. This can be performed either in the supine position with gentle anterior load applied to the posterior shoulder or in an upright seated position. Prior to applying the translation force, the humeral head is loaded in the glenoid and then shifted, thus the name "load-and-shift" tests. Our preference is to perform the test supine, which provides for a more relaxed exam.

The "relocation" test may be of value in detecting subtle anterior instability, particularly in patients without a history of overt dislocations. In this test, the arm is placed in the abduction, external rotation position, and a gentle anterior load applied to the humeral head. This test is considered positive when the patient feels subjective apprehension or discomfort under anterior load, alleviated by posterior translation to the humeral head with presumed reduction of the joint.

Tests that facilitate detection of other pathology include an apprehension and load-and-shift test for posterior instability, and the active-compression test (among others) for detection of superior labral (SLAP) pathology. Inferior instability can occur in conjunction with anterior instability, and has traditionally been assessed using the sulcus sign in adduction, repeated again in external rotation. The sulcus sign is considered more significant if it persists with external rotation. Because the sulcus sign may be normal in some patients with generalized laxity, it is important to assess overall soft tissue laxity such as metacarpophalangeal (MCP) hyperextension, elbow recurvatum, and the "thumb-to-forearm" tests.

Evaluation of the rotator cuff is important particularly in contact, collision sport athletes with a traumatic dislocation in which compromise of the cuff may coexist with labral pathology. Conventional tests for supraspinatus strength (empty-can position against resistance) and infraspinatus strength (external rotation of the adducted arm at the side against resistance) are standard. Evaluation for occult subscapularis injury includes the abdominal compression and lift off tests. In the patient with recurrent instability, observation of scapulothoracic mechanics is an important component of a comprehensive exam as scapulothoracic dysfunction may contribute to instability in some patients. Finally, the neurovascular status of the upper extremity (e.g., axillary nerve) and a cervical spine examination complete a thorough assessment of the shoulder.

Diagnostic imaging of anterior shoulder instability includes standard anterior–posterior (AP) and axillary views.

Abnormalities may warrant more specialized radiographs, such as a Stryker view for evaluation of a Hill–Sachs lesion and a West-Point axillary view to better assess an osseous Bankart lesion (Fig. 16.5). In cases where there is a significant Hill–Sachs or bony Bankart lesion, a CT scan with three-dimensional reconstruction can better quantify the extent of articular-arc compromise and the potential need for alternative surgical strategies (Fig. 16.6).

Magnetic resonance imaging is not routinely necessary in the evaluation of shoulder instability, though it may be appropriate in specific circumstances. These include patients with first time instability over age 40 to evaluate the cuff integrity and following significant trauma to assess possible subscapularis tendon rupture. An MRI can be helpful in evaluating the location and extent of the capsulolabral injury. Enhanced-imaging techniques with chondral sequencing have enabled some magnets to provide vivid detail of the capsulolabral complex and osteochondral anatomy without contrast. MR arthrography is not usually necessary, though may be of value in some cases with unclear instability patterns.

TREATMENT DECISION-MAKING

Following reduction (spontaneously or with manipulation) of an anteriorly dislocated shoulder, most patients with acute shoulder instability are managed

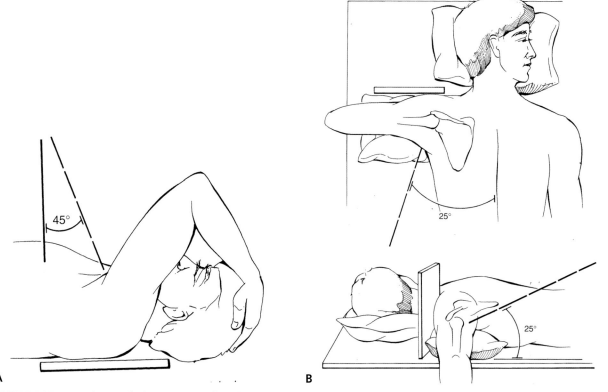

FIGURE 16.5. A: Stryker Notch view to assess Hill–Sachs lesion. **B:** West-Point view to assess the anterior glenoid for a bony Bankart lesion or glenoid insufficiency.

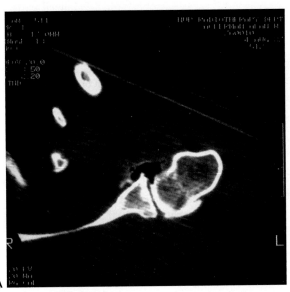
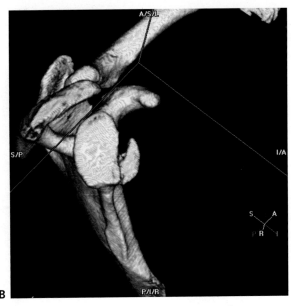

FIGURE 16.6. A: A CT scan shows an avulsion injury of the anterior-inferior glenoid rim. **B:** This cutaway 3D CT scan has digitally removed the humeral head, permitting assessment of the size and location of the glenoid defect. This type of computer-generated imaging is critical in preoperative planning.

nonoperatively. Nonoperative treatment should focus on a rehabilitation program that avoids the provocative position and incorporates a strengthening program designed to enhance the dynamic shoulder stabilizers. Patients with recurrent instability following nonoperative treatment may be surgical candidates. Studies have shown that in the young athlete, nonoperative treatment is largely ineffective with recurrence rates approaching 90% in those under 20 years of age (1). Because of the high risk of recurrence in some groups, surgical treatment of the first-time dislocator in the younger athlete has gained traction. Other factors that may influence primary repair of the first-time dislocator include arm dominance, type of sport or activity, level of participation and performance, goals, timing with respect to their athletic season, and factors related to the instability episode itself such as the presence of a repairable bony Bankart lesion.

The threshold for operative intervention in patients with recurrent instability and functional impairment is considerably lower. Painful instability episodes, repeated stints in physical therapy, athletic disability, and impairment in activities of daily living all contribute to the surgical decision-making.

INDICATIONS

The current ideal indication for arthroscopic stabilization is a patient with recurrent posttraumatic anterior instability who has a Bankart lesion, good quality labral tissue, and no evidence of significant bony pathology. From an athletic standpoint, arthroscopic stabilization has been particularly emphasized over open procedures

in the throwing population in which motion preservation is critical.

CONTRAINDICATIONS

Current contraindications to arthroscopic stabilization include patients with "significant" bony pathology and poor quality capsulolabral tissue. "Significant" bony defects include glenoid insufficiency in which greater than 25% of the anterior-inferior glenoid surface is deficient and/or an "engaging" Hill–Sachs on the humeral side, typically constituting greater than 30% of the articular surface (Fig. 16.7). Yet even these guidelines are not absolute and some authors have reported successful outcomes with arthroscopic management of anterior shoulder instability even in the face of a deficient glenoid (termed an "inverted pear" (8)). In addition, several procedures have been introduced that arthroscopically address articular arc deficiency. These include soft tissue advancement of the infraspinatus tendon into the humeral head (Hill–Sachs) defect ("Remplissage" technique (9)) and bone grafting of the humeral head defect (10). However, most authors would agree that significant bony pathology warrants open reconstruction by an anatomic open Bankart repair that addresses the bony defect directly, or a nonanatomic open repair such as the Bristow-Latarjet procedure.

Compromised soft tissue capsulolabral tissue is relatively uncommon but may be a limiting factor in patients who have undergone thermal capsulorrhaphy or revision surgery. In these cases, open repair using soft tissue augmentation may be necessary.

Until recently, other contraindications included patients with HAGL lesions (more easily fixed open),

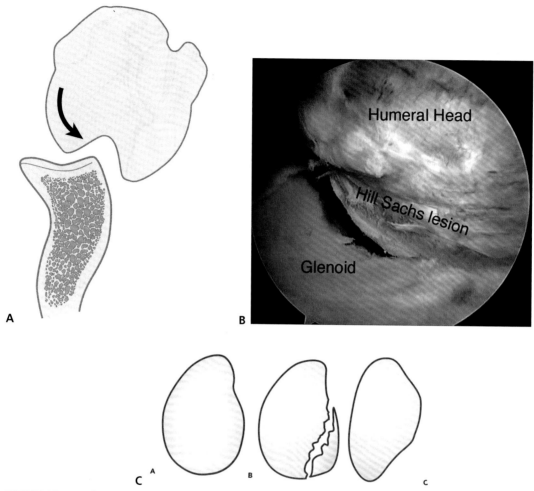

FIGURE 16.7. A: This aerial perspective shows the significant osteochondral Hill–Sachs defect, which when the arm is positioned in external rotation, "engages" (*arrow*) the anterior glenoid rim (here shown somewhat blunted as often seen in shoulders with recurrent instability). **B:** Arthroscopic photo of Hill–Sachs lesion engaging anterior glenoid rim as the arm is externally rotated. **C:** The "pear-shaped" glenoid is shown here in profile; A, normal glenoid; B, acute fracture to anterior-inferior glenoid; C, pear-shaped appearance due to erosion of the anterior-inferior glenoid glenoid from recurrent instability.

those undergoing revision surgeries, and those playing contact or collision sports. As arthroscopic techniques have evolved and experience is accrued, each of these have become only "relative" contraindications with operative decision making influenced by the presence of concomitant pathology, technical experience, and surgeon preference.

The optimal approach for treatment of contact and collision-sports athletes remains a controversial topic. Historically, open anterior stabilization has been advocated as the "gold standard" or treatment of choice for this patient population. Arthroscopic stabilization in a contact and collision sport athlete has been contraindicated because of reports suggesting a higher risk of failure. Some authors have advocated open stabilization in this group of athletes citing low recurrence rates. But outcome data have recently called this conclusion into question. Stratifying the data based on factors other than simply the sport have shown that recurrence is more likely due to bone

deficiency, which is more common in contact athletes, rather than the surgical technique (11). Mazzocca reported an 11% rate of recurrent dislocation in their series of collision and contact athletes treated with arthroscopic suture anchor shoulder stabilization.

Many studies have shown satisfactory outcomes with revision surgery following failed open or arthroscopic surgery. The key is the quality of the soft tissue and bone integrity, expectations of the patient, and skill of the surgeon. Patients with voluntary instability in which there may be secondary gain or psychological issues are not appropriate candidates for arthroscopic stabilization and are probably inappropriate candidates for open surgical repair as well. Likewise, patients who are unable to comply with the postoperative immobilization or rehabilitation risk a compromised outcome and may be better treated without surgery. Favorable surgical outcomes can follow conservative management, rehabilitation, and bracing (position dependent) until the completion of the season (11).

SURGICAL TECHNIQUE

Instrumentation, Implants, and Cannula Selection

In addition to the standard setup for shoulder arthroscopy, stabilization requires specific instrumentation (Fig. 16.8). This includes a 70° arthroscope and cannulas with internal diameters sufficient to accommodate anchor and suture passing instruments. An angled arthroscopic elevator (Liberator rasp, ConMed Linvatec, Largo, FL) is required to mobilize the capsulolabral complex. Shaver blades that both debride and abrade are necessary for glenoid preparation. Several different types of suture passing instruments are helpful to minimize struggling during this step. A soft tissue grasper, suture retriever, knot pusher, and knot cutter complete the instrumentation.

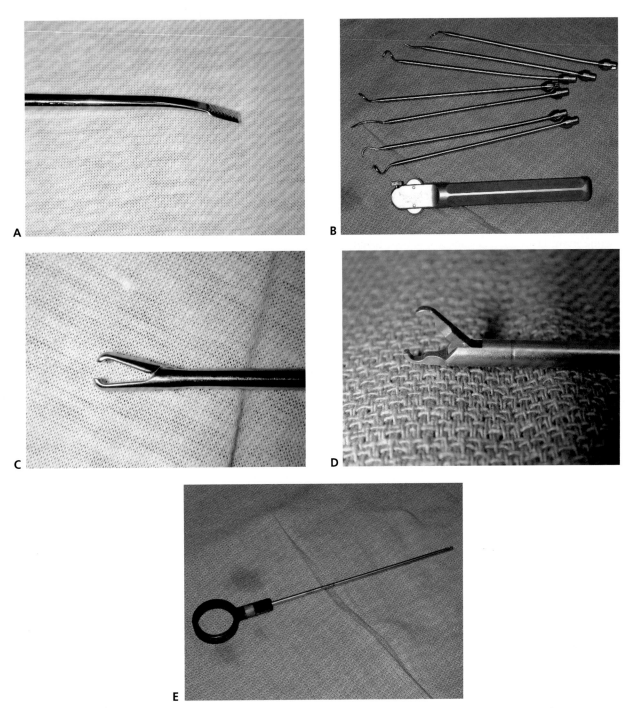

FIGURE 16.8. A: Liberator Rasp for mobilization of capsulolabral tissue off glenoid. **B:** Spectrum device with associated tips for suture passage. **C:** Soft tissue grasper for atraumatic soft tissue manipulation. **D:** Suture retriever device for retrieving and shuttling sutures. **E:** Knot tyer.

Several considerations influence the physician's preference and choice of a suture anchor, including the composition, size, number and type of sutures per anchor, and ease of use. Pullout strength is probably sufficient for most anchors currently on the market, so this biomechanical factor is of little significance when choosing an implant. Some surgeons still favor metallic implants due to their comfort level, low cost, ability to visualize on X-ray, and lack of osteolysis. However, limitations of metal implants include possible suture abrasion through the eyelet (depending upon eyelet design), difficulty with anchor extraction if improperly placed or proud, and the potential for devastating chondral wear in cases of suboptimal positioning or migration. Metal anchors are also visible on X-rays which depending upon one's perspective may or may not be advantageous; and, in cases of recurrent instability or postoperative complications may interfere with MR interpretation due to artifact.

The trend in stabilization surgery is away from metal and today most implants are made of either a bioabsorbable material most commonly poly-L-lactic acid (PLLA), or nonabsorbable biologically inert plastic, polyetheretherketone (PEEK) (12). Recently, there has been interest in the use of tricalcium-phosphate derivatives, which have osteoconductive properties and may incorporate into the host bone more favorably. The most practical benefit of bioabsorbable anchors is that they may be overdrilled for new implant placement in cases of suture compromise or suboptimal anchor position.

Most implants come with proprietary suture materials, which have evolved to provide greater strength than braided polyester suture, while retaining the handling properties of smooth monofilament suture. Anchors come preloaded with one to three sutures. We usually use an anchor that has two sutures so that the option for redundant fixation is available, particularly at the site of the most inferior glenoid anchor. Regardless of your preference in anchor selection, consider the value of having more than one type of implant available to accommodate intraoperative implant malplacement, eyelet failure, and for cases of revision surgery.

Positioning/Anesthesia/EUA

Arthroscopic anterior stabilization can be carried out either under a general anesthesia, interscalene block and sedation (requires anesthesia expertise and experience), or all three. A careful examination under anesthesia is carried out on both shoulders prior to positioning, assessing laxity, and motion. Positioning is based on surgeon preference, with both lateral decubitus and beach-chair positions well established. When using an interscalene block technique, the beach-chair position is better tolerated.

AUTHORS' PREFERRED TECHNIQUE

Our preferred approach is the lateral decubitus position under general anesthesia (Fig. 16.9). Once anesthetized, the patient is placed in the lateral decubitus position on a

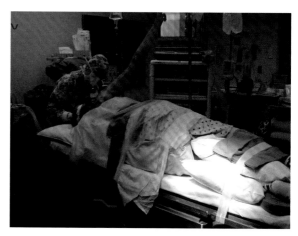

FIGURE 16.9. The lateral decubitus position, with careful padding of the downside extremity, an axillary roll, use of a vacuum beanbag to maintain position, and elevation/flexion of the affected shoulder.

vacuum beanbag, carefully padding the downside extremity and using an axillary roll. Care is taken to ensure the patient is rolled back about 10° to 15° from vertical, ensuring adequate access to the front of the shoulder. Five-pound sand bags wedged in front and behind the beanbag maintain patient position. The bed is then rotated so that when viewing from the posterior portal, the monitor is directly in-line with the surgeon's view. A dual monitor setup permits visualization when or if the scope is placed anteriorly. After prepping and draping, the operative arm is placed in a commercial traction device with 7 to 10 pounds of distraction, positioning the arm in approximately 35° of abduction, and 15° of forward flexion.

Portal Placement and Diagnostic Arthroscopy

Anatomic landmarks are outlined, and the arthroscope is introduced through a standard posterior scope portal. The anterior portal is established using an outside-in technique, first targeting the intended approach with an 18G spinal needle. Precision in anterior portal placement is critical to facilitate several steps during stabilization. If placed too high in the interval, the anterior portal may not permit easy targeting for suture anchor placement along the anterior-inferior glenoid. If positioned too inferiorly, labral mobilization and preparation, and at times suture passage, can be difficult (Fig. 16.10).

When first performing arthroscopic stabilization, these pitfalls can be avoided by using a "twin-portal" technique (AS and AI portals), which also facilitates suture management (Fig. 16.11). The AS portal is established just off the anterolateral corner of the acromion entering the joint under cover of the biceps long head tendon. This portal permits "in-line" instrumentation along the anterior glenoid, facilitating easy capsulolabral mobilization and glenoid preparation. When placing this portal it is also important to try to place it more medially than laterally within the rotator interval. Doing so enhances

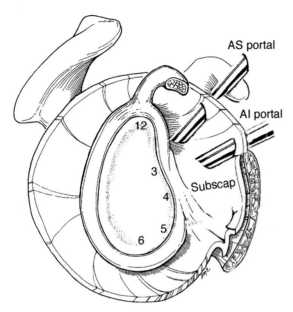

FIGURE 16.10. "Twin" anterior portals are seen in this cutaway illustration. The anterosuperior portal (AS) is seen coming in under cover of the biceps and in line with the anterior glenoid. The anterior-inferior (AI) portal enters immediately above the subscapularis tendon and facilitates targeting the anterior-inferior glenoid rim.

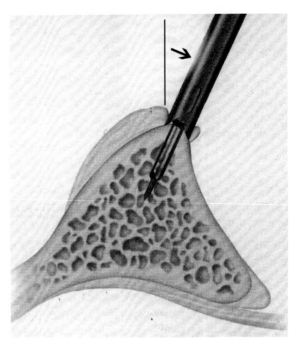

FIGURE 16.12. Cannula-targeting angle is important for secure implant fixation. Ensure the drill sleeve engages the glenoid rim and is angled such that it engages good glenoid bone.

navigating suture passing instruments underneath the humeral head (which can sometimes be an obstruction).

The AI portal should enter the joint just above the upper subscapularis tendon edge (Fig. 16.11). The more inferior placement of this portal permits better targeting of the inferior aspect of the anterior glenoid, accessing the otherwise difficult-to-reach 6 o'clock position (the apex of the Bankart lesion tear). The portal should be angled from

lateral to medial to ensure targeting of the glenoid margin and face during anchor placement (Fig. 16.12). When establishing twin anterior portals, care must be taken to ensure that externally they are sufficiently separated to avoid instrument crowding (Fig. 16.13). With experience, arthroscopic stabilization can be achieved using a single anterior portal, whose placement should be closer to the AI portal, and sufficiently angled to target the glenoid during anchor placement. In this surgical technique description, a twin-portal approach will be described.

An accessory posterior-inferior portal (13) can be of great value in arthroscopic stabilizations, particularly

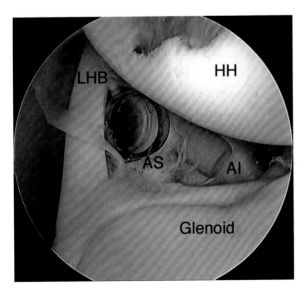

FIGURE 16.11. Arthroscopic view of "twin" anterior portals, with the anterior-superior (AS) portal established with an 8.25-mm "fishbowl" (Arthrex) cannula entering under the long head biceps (LHB). The lower anterior-inferior (AI) portal is positioned inferiorly, just above the subscapularis tendon; HH, humeral head.

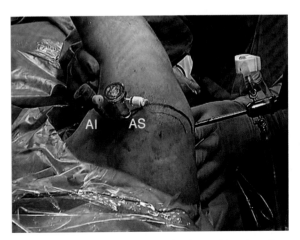

FIGURE 16.13. Avoid instrument crowding by ensuring the twin anterior cannulae are separated externally; AI, anterior-inferior portal; AS, anterior-superior portal.

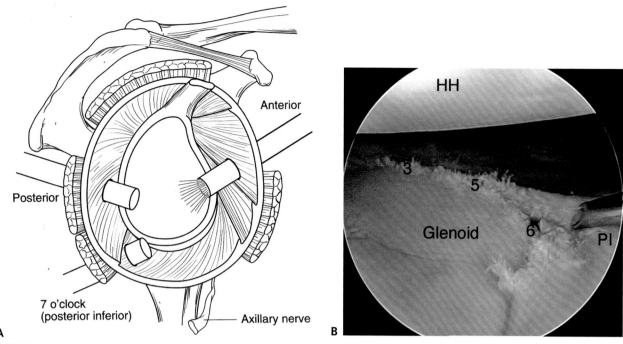

FIGURE 16.14. A: An accessory posterior-inferior portal (13) (shown here at 7 o'clock) can be of great value in arthroscopic stabilizations, particularly when the labral detachment extends beyond the 6 o'clock position. **B:** Establishing this posterior-inferior portal is achieved by spinal needle targeting, aiming toward the 6 o'clock position, the typical apex of the Bankart lesion (right shoulder, lateral decubitus position, scope posterior portal); PI, posterior-inferior; HH, humeral head.

when the labral detachment extends beyond the 6 o'clock position (Fig. 16.14). Access through this portal permits targeting of the inferior and posterior-inferior glenoid as well as facilitating suture passage through the inferior part of the IGHL. This is particularly helpful in cases where access anteriorly is tight, and when capsular patholaxity requires a superior shift of the inferior capsule. Because suture passing instruments, particularly the Spectrum hook (ConMed Linvatec), are used during this part of the procedure we use an 8.25-mm diameter cannula to accommodate the various tips.

There are many different cannulas that can be used during stabilization. When using a twin anterior portal approach, we prefer an 8.25-mm disposable clear (fish bowl) cannula (Arthrex, Naples, FL) for the AS portal to accommodate suture passing. The AI portal is established using a 5-mm diameter disposable cannula sufficient to accommodate shaver tips and anchor drill, sleeve, and implants. In cases where only a single anterior portal is used, we prefer the 8.25-mm cannula.

A thorough diagnostic arthroscopy is performed to confirm the expected diagnosis and evaluate for concomitant pathology. This includes the glenoid articular surface, cuff undersurface, circumferential labrum, biceps tendon, and subscapularis tendon. The labrum should be examined and probed for integrity, degree of displacement, and extent around the glenoid face. Probe palpation may reveal labral detachment that is not displaced, as well as GLAD (glenohumeral labral articular defect) lesions (Fig. 16.15).

Cases of instability in which a Bankart lesion is not seen must be examined for a possible HAGL lesion, which is best seen when viewing from either an anterior portal or by using a 70° arthroscope from the posterior portal.

Subtle lesions may require probe palpation to identify occult detachments sometimes masquerading as a

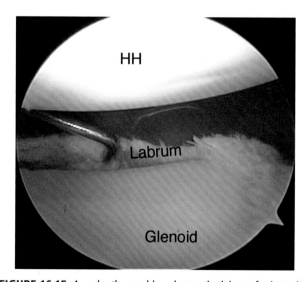

FIGURE 16.15. A probe thoroughly palpates the labrum for integrity, extent and degree of displacement around the glenoid face. Probe palpation may reveal labral tears that are not displaced, or glenohumeral labral articular defects (GLAD) lesions; HH, humeral head, right shoulder, lateral decubitus position, scope posterior portal.

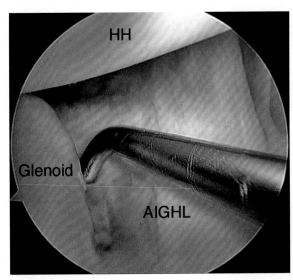

FIGURE 16.16. An anterior labral periosteal sleeve avulsion (ALPSA) is seen in this right shoulder, lateral decubitus position, viewing from posterior portal. Instead of arising from the glenoid rim, the capsulolabral sleeve has fallen down on the glenoid neck, and healed in this nonanatomic position; HH, humeral head; AIGHL, anterior-inferior glenohumeral ligament.

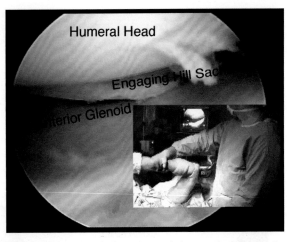

FIGURE 16.17. Removal of traction and placement of the arm in the "throwing position" shows "engagement" of the lesion, (8) which may contraindicate a simple capsulolabral repair (right shoulder, lateral decubitus position, scope posterior portal).

"fissure" at the chondro–labral junction. Cases of chronic instability may have an ALPSA lesion (anterior labral periosteal sleeve avulsion) lying displaced medially along the glenoid neck (Fig. 16.16). This lesion can be deceptive in appearance and only careful mobilization renders this Bankart-equivalent evident.

Assessment for capsular laxity is important. The drive-through sign, or ease with which the camera passes between the humeral head and glenoid, has been described as a tool to quantify the extent of anterior-inferior laxity. This finding varies and can be normal in patients with and without instability. Because a deficiency in the rotator interval has been implicated in some cases, particularly those with MDI and posterior instability, examination of this area has value, though there are no established criteria for grading interval pathology.

The humeral head must be evaluated for a Hill–Sachs lesion. Removal of traction and placement of the arm in the "throwing position" may show "engagement" of the Hill–Sachs lesion, (8) which may contraindicate a simple capsulolabral repair (Fig. 16.17). The glenoid is examined for any bony deficiency relying on a technique described by Burkhart, in which he describes the "inverted pear" shape of the deficient anterior-inferior glenoid. (8) In this technique, a calibrated probe is used to assess the percentage of bone loss (Fig. 16.18). While viewing from an anterior portal (achieved by using switching sticks or scope placement through an established cannula), the probe is placed across the glenoid from the posterior portal and the glenoid width measured. The probe then measures the distance from the posterior glenoid rim to the glenoid's central thin spot. Since the thin spot is considered the center of the inferior

glenoid equator, twice this measurement corresponds to what should be the normal glenoid width. By comparing the measured width to what has been calculated as the normal width, one can estimate the degree of compromise of the anterior-inferior glenoid bone stock. Loss of 20% to 25% or more of the inferior glenoid bone stock may contraindicate arthroscopic stabilization.

Capsulolabral Mobilization

The labrum and attached tissue (capsulolabral complex) must be thoroughly mobilized from the anterior-inferior glenoid. This step is critical both to assess soft tissue integrity and to facilitate anatomic reapproximation to the glenoid. The capsulolabral complex must be sufficiently mobile to permit easy approximation to the glenoid, and in cases of capsular patholaxity, capable of being shifted superiorly to restore normal tension.

With the arthroscope in the posterior portal, a spatula-like elevator (Liberator Rasp) is placed through the anterior-superior portal and used to develop the plane between the capsulolabral complex and the anterior-inferior glenoid (Fig. 16.19). Care should be used to avoid damage to the capsule itself. More extensive lesions may be better accessed by approaching from the AI portal, continuing mobilization along the inferior glenoid rim until reaching the tear's apex. Adequate mobilization is confirmed by grasping the soft tissue sleeve, seeing that it translates superiorly without tension, and visualizing the underlying subscapularis muscle fibers.

Glenoid Preparation

Soft tissue healing to the glenoid requires bone preparation to achieve a "healing response." A motorized shaver or burr passed through the anterior-superior portal removes soft tissue and abrades the glenoid rim and neck. For more inferior lesions, the AI portal may provide better

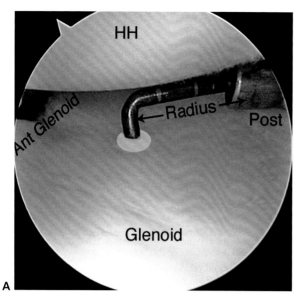
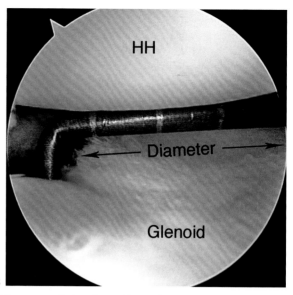

A   **B**

FIGURE 16.18. A: The glenoid is examined for any bony deficiency, relying on a technique by Burkhart, which he used to describe the "inverted pear" shape of the deficient anterior-inferior glenoid. (8) In this technique, a calibrated probe is used to assess the percentage of bone loss. While viewing from the anterior-superior portal, the calibrated probe is used to measure the glenoid radius, the distance from the posterior rim to the central thin spot on the glenoid face (*white circle*) (right shoulder, lateral decubitus position, scope anterosuperior portal; HH, humeral head). **B:** The calibrated probe is then advanced to the anterior-inferior glenoid rim and this distance measured and compared with that expected of the normal glenoid (twice the radius measured in **A**) (right shoulder, lateral decubitus position, scope anterosuperior portal; HH, humeral head).

access. Use of a 70° arthroscope in the posterior portal or viewing from either anterior portal confirms adequate preparation (Fig. 16.20).

Anchor Placement

Anchor placement begins at the inferior glenoid as close as possible to the 6 o'clock position or at the axilla of the detachment, which can sometimes extend beyond this point. Gentle lateral translation of the humeral head will facilitate drill guide placement. Anchor placement on the glenoid rim is important to reestablish normal anatomy but can be technically challenging in some cases. With the arthroscope in either the posterior or anterior-superior portal and the drill sleeve in the AI portal, the first anchor pilot hole is drilled (Fig. 16.21). Even when targeting from the AI portal, the 6 o'clock position on the rim may not be easily achieved. There are several strategies to adjust for this technical limitation. The first is to "cheat" the drill guide for the most inferior anchor up onto the glenoid face by a few millimeters. Placement a few millimeters onto the glenoid face ensures secure anchor implant fixation within good glenoid bone stock and facilitates restoration of the "buttress" effect achieved when the labrum is rolled up on the glenoid. (Fig. 16.22).

A second alternative is to use an additional AI accessory portal to directly target the 5 to 6 o'clock position (Fig. 16.23). Described as a "5 o'clock" portal (14), this accessory portal penetrates the subscapularis and allows

targeting directly on the inferior glenoid rim. Because of technical difficulties in placing a large diameter cannula through the subscapularis and to minimize any risk to the adjacent neurovascular structures, we prefer to use a percutaneous technique using a small-diameter drill sleeve (Fig. 16.24). A spinal needle from outside-in is used to target the intended anchor site. A small percutaneous stab incision is then made next to the spinal needle, and a long hubless spinal needle is positioned adjacent to the spinal needle. A drill sleeve with a cannulated obturator is then passed over the hubless needle and advanced into the joint. Upon removal of the needle and obturator, the drill and anchor can be placed very low at the glenoid margin. Because this technique requires use of anchor implants that are specific to this sleeve/obturator system, we use 3.0-mm Bio-SutureTaks (Arthrex) for this purpose.

A third alternative to achieve anchor placement inferiorly is through an accessory posterior-inferior portal (Fig. 16.25). This is especially relevant in cases where the Bankart lesion extends posteriorly along the inferior rim. A posterior-inferior portal is best established by viewing from the anterior-superior portal. The cannula is inserted approximately 1 to 2 cm inferior to the conventional posterior scope portal. Conversely, a percutaneous "7 o'clock" technique (for the right shoulder) using an accessory posterior-inferior portal can also be performed using the small diameter drill sleeve/obturator combination.

Once the most inferior anchor has been placed, the suture limbs are retrieved out the AI portal (if they were

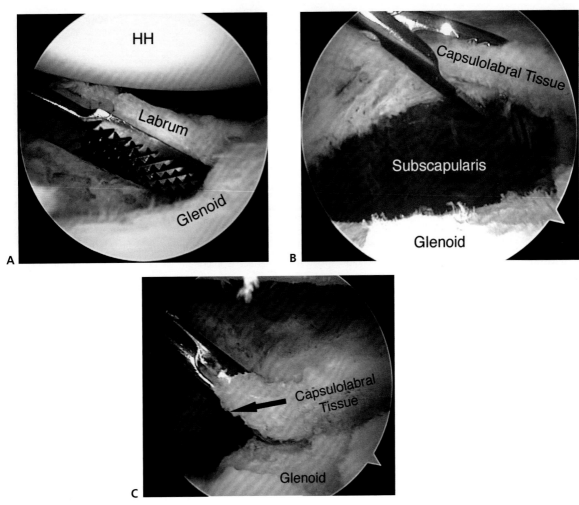

FIGURE 16.19. A: With the arthroscope in the posterior portal, a spatula-like elevator (Liberator Rasp, ConMed Linvatec, Largo, FL) through the anterior-superior portal is used to develop the plane between the capsulolabral complex and the anterior-inferior glenoid (right shoulder, lateral decubitus position, scope posterior portal; HH, humeral head). **B:** The capsulolabral tissue must be thoroughly mobilized to permit restoration of normal tension, including, when necessary, a capsular shift superiorly. A good mobilization is confirmed by visualizing the subscapularis muscle fibers below the tissue sleeve (right shoulder, lateral decubitus position, scope posterior portal). **C:** This arthroscopic view demonstrates a soft tissue grasper successfully translating (shifting) the capsulolabral complex superiorly (right shoulder, lateral decubitus position, scope posterior portal).

not placed through this portal during implantation), followed by suture passage and knot tying for this anchor (Fig. 16.26). We then place subsequent anchors in order up the glenoid, pass the sutures, and tie the knots. Placing all anchors at one time can lead to suture mismanagement, so we prefer repeating each of these steps (anchor implantation, suture passage, knot tying) for each anchor. Subsequent anchor placement is less technically demanding. We usually space anchor placement approximately 4 to 5 mm apart and use, on average, three implants. However, the number of anchors used depends on the length of the labral detachment, so this determination is made intraoperatively (Fig. 16.27).

Anchor placement must be on the glenoid rim or up on the glenoid face. If this is not done and the capsulolabral complex is attached medially along the glenoid neck, an

iatrogenic ALPSA lesion is created, which precludes the creation of a "bumper" effect, may not restore appropriate capsular tension, and risks repair failure. Suboptimal anchor implantation at the peripheral margin of the glenoid face may also result in suboptimal anchor purchase in bone and implant migration. The angle for targeting good glenoid bone stock has been shown to be smallest at the anteroinferior glenoid (45° ± 7°) (15).

Suture Passage and Knot Tying

Suture passage can be the most challenging part of arthroscopic shoulder stabilization. Proper restoration of normal capsulolabral tension requires the accurate assessment of patholaxity and precise suture placement for anatomic reapproximation. Technical passage can also be difficult, particularly in tight shoulders. Once passed,

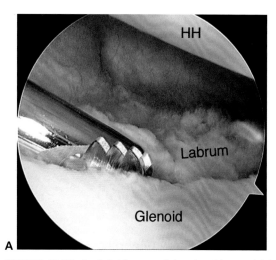
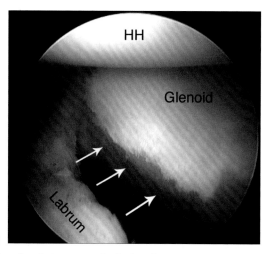

FIGURE 16.20. A: Debridement of the glenoid–capsulolabral interface is important for both soft tissue mobilization and for glenoid preparation (right shoulder, lateral decubitus position, scope posterior portal). **B:** Viewing from the anterior-superior portal, or with a 70° lens in the posterior portal, confirms adequate preparation, including petechial bleeding from abraded anterior glenoid (*white arrows*). Soft tissue healing to the glenoid requires preparation to achieve a "healing response" (HH, humeral head; right shoulder, lateral decubitus position).

suture mismanagement looms as yet another potential impediment to progress.

Ideal suture placement should restore normal anatomic positioning of the capsulolabral complex. After placing the most inferior anchor, the first suture limb must be passed so that when tied, it approximates the soft tissue against the glenoid rim anatomically and incorporates any soft tissue laxity to restore normal tension. This step requires some experience and may require several passes to ensure accurate placement and adequate tissue capture.

Our preferred technique is a "two-step" approach to suture passage, first passing a monofilament suture followed by "shuttling" the anchor's suture limb through the tissue (Fig. 16.28). The instrument we most commonly use is the Spectrum suture hook (ConMed Linvatec). It has a curved needle tip that facilitates suture passage. While viewing from the posterior scope portal, the suture passer is introduced through the anterior-superior portal and negotiated under the humeral head toward the axilla. Lateral humeral head translation by an assistant helps visualization of this inferior apex. Because it is detached, there

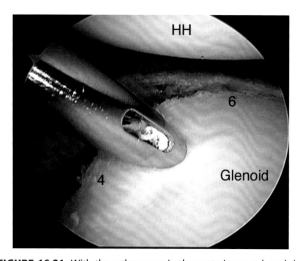

FIGURE 16.21. With the arthroscope in the posterior portal, and the drill sleeve in the anterior-inferior portal, the first anchor pilot hole is drilled as close to the 6 o'clock position (or at axilla of the detachment, which can extend beyond this point) as possible. In this arthroscopic view, the sleeve cannot be positioned lower than about 5 o'clock and has to come up onto the glenoid face to ensure bone purchase (HH, humeral head).

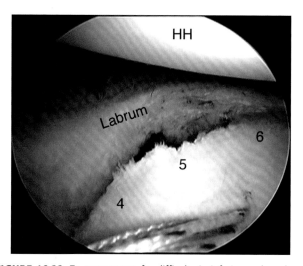

FIGURE 16.22. To compensate for difficulty in inferior anchor placement, the implant is moved up onto the glenoid face. This ensures secure anchor implant fixation within good glenoid bone stock and facilitates restoration of the "buttress" effect achieved when the labrum is rolled up on the glenoid (HH, humeral head; viewing from posterior scope portal, right shoulder, and lateral decubitus position).

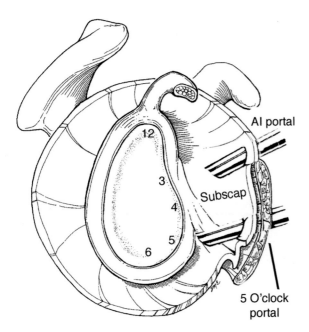

FIGURE 16.23. The 5 o'clock portal (14) penetrates the subscapularis and allows targeting directly on the inferior glenoid rim; (AI, anterior inferior).

may not be sufficient tension on the capsulolabral tissue to easily penetrate it with the Spectrum suture hook tip and shuttle the monofilament suture (No. 1 PDS) through the tissue. In this case, the tissue can be independently grasped through the accessory AI portal and the suture passage reattempted. The disadvantage here is instrument crowding with the grasper interfering with the spectrum-passing device. Alternatively, the instruments can be exchanged, grasping the sleeve from the anterosuperior portal and passing the sutures using the AI cannula.

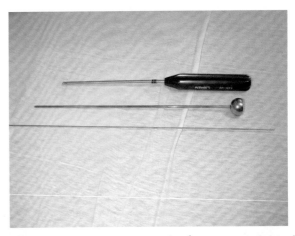

FIGURE 16.24. Instruments necessary for percutaneous technique for inferior glenoid rim targeting and anchor placement. The set includes a long hubless spinal needle (bottom), a cannulated obturator (middle) that slides through the drill sleeve (top) (Arthrex).

In situations where suture passage is still not easily achievable using the spectrum device, a Caspari tissue-grasping suture passer (ConMed Linvatec) may be more effective. The tissue is grasped at the appropriate site and the suture shuttled through. The disadvantage of this device is that its needle is not always long enough or sharp enough to penetrate the capsule and can require back-and-forth "toggling" to penetrate. Although it is fine for the most inferior suture placement, this technique cannot be repeated for subsequent suture anchors without risking the security of the lowest suture anchor repair.

An alternative useful tool is the Needle Punch (Arthrex), which can grasp the tissue and shuttle a suture through into its capturing jaw (Fig. 16.29). Although not routinely used

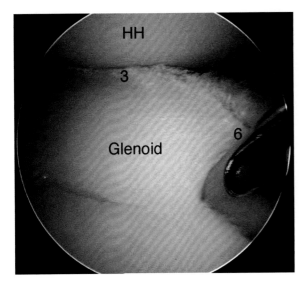

FIGURE 16.25. Anchor placement inferiorly can also be achieved using the accessory posterior-inferior portal. Here, the drill sleeve directly targets the rim just past 6 o'clock in this right shoulder (scope posterior, lateral decubitus position; HH, humeral head).

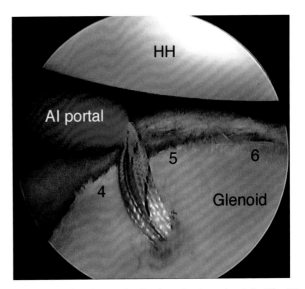

FIGURE 16.26. The first anchor has been implanted and the FiberWire sutures exit the anterior-inferior cannula in preparation for tying; HH, humeral head; right shoulder, lateral decubitus, viewing from antero-superior portal.

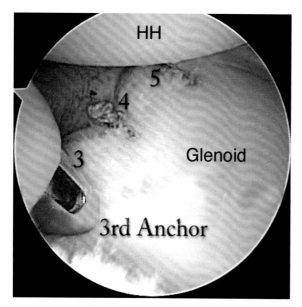

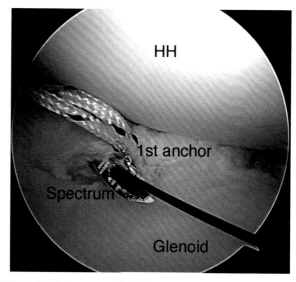

FIGURE 16.27. In this scope photo, the two most inferior anchors have been implanted, and their sutures passed and tied. The drill sleeve has been positioned to place the third and in this case, final repair anchor (right shoulder, lateral decubitus, viewing from anterosuperior portal; HH, humeral head).

FIGURE 16.28. A spectrum hook (Linvatec) has penetrated the inferior capsulolabral tissue and has begun to shuttle no. 1 PDS monofilament suture into the joint, adjacent to a limb of the first suture anchor (right shoulder, lateral decubitus, scope posterior; HH, humeral head).

because of its wide jaw and occasional difficulty navigating under the humeral head, it is an excellent backup tool when facing difficult inferior suture passage. Another strategy that can facilitate suture passage is to use the accessory posterior-inferior portal, which provides a direct shot to the anterior-inferior capsulolabral tissue (Fig 16.30).

Once the monofilament suture has been passed, it is grasped and withdrawn through the cannula containing the anchor suture limb(s). The first limb of the anchor's suture

is now ready for passage. Using a suture retriever, the limb of the anchor suture (closest to the tissue through which the monofilament suture has been shuttled) is grabbed along with a limb of the monofilament suture (Fig. 16.31). The monofilament and anchor suture are withdrawn together out the cannula, ensuring that they cannot be crossed or tangled with any other sutures occupying the cannula. The monofilament suture is tied to the anchor suture and then shuttles the anchor suture through the tissue.

The second suture limb is then retrieved through the same cannula and a simple knot is tied, using the suture limb passed through the soft tissue as the post (Fig. 16.32).

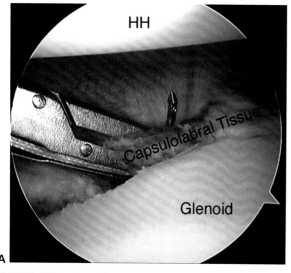

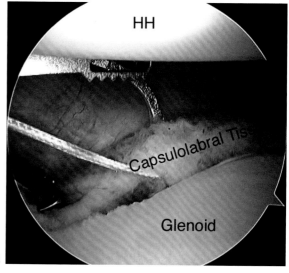

FIGURE 16.29. A: An alternative strategy for suture passage is via a device like this needle punch (Arthrex, Naples, FL), which can grasp the tissue and penetrate a needle through it (right shoulder, lateral decubitus, scope posterior; HH, humeral head). **B:** The needle has been captured into its jaw and the FiberWire will now be shuttled through the tissue (right shoulder, lateral decubitus, scope posterior, HH).

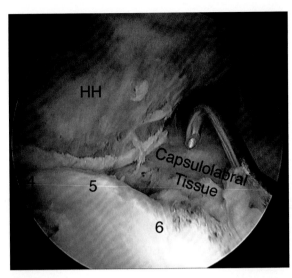

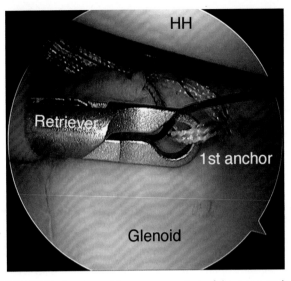

FIGURE 16.30. Another strategy that can facilitate suture passage is through the use of an accessory posterior-inferior portal, which provides a direct shot for the suture-passing device to the anterior-inferior capsulolabral tissue (right shoulder, lateral decubitus, scope posterior; HH, humeral head).

FIGURE 16.31. A suture retriever secures a limb of the suture anchor and a limb of the monofilament and withdraws them together out the anterior-inferior cannula. Securing the monofilament and anchor sutures together avoids crossing or entanglement (right shoulder, lateral decubitus, scope posterior; HH, humeral head).

We prefer a sliding "Fisherman's" knot followed by three alternating half-hitches. Attention is placed on ensuring the labrum is pushed up onto the glenoid face to restore the buttress, and the knot kept away from the glenoid rim.

Anchors may be single- or double-loaded with suture. The latter offers additional fixation for the capsulolabral repair, and backup in case of first suture compromise by inadequate knot or loop security, or suboptimal suture placement. When using a double-loaded anchor, the first passed

suture and its paired limb are positioned and clamped outside the cannula and kept untied. Another monofilament suture is passed approximately 3 to 5 mm from the first shuttled suture. The first limb (of the second suture) is now shuttled through the tissue, and this limb, along with its paired nonpassed suture limb, is retrieved together and clamped outside the cannula.

The suture pairs can then be tied using a simple suture configuration. Care is taken to use the knot pusher to

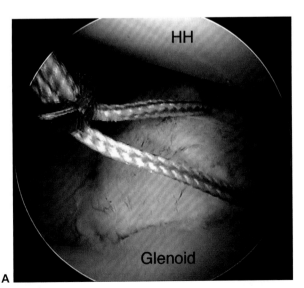

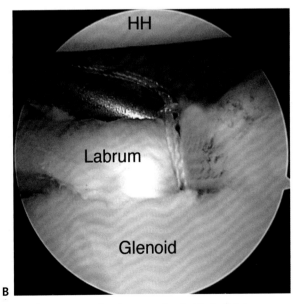

FIGURE 16.32. A: Both limbs of the same FiberWire suture are now retrieved, again, grasping them together inside the joint so that they do not get crossed or tangled with any other suture (right shoulder, lateral decubitus, scope posterior; HH, humeral head). **B:** A simple knot is now tied, using the suture limb passed through the soft tissue as the post. Attention is directed to ensure the labrum is pushed up onto the glenoid face to restore the buttress, keeping the knot away from the glenoid rim (right shoulder, lateral decubitus, scope posterior, and HH).

separate the two sutures so that they secure a breadth of tissue over 3 to 4 mm in length, rather than capture the tissue with two side-to-side sutures (Fig. 16.33). On occasion, a simple suture will be passed first, followed by passing both limbs of the second suture. When tied, a combination of simple and mattress suture has been achieved, which results in excellent tissue apposition and secure fixation.

Identifying and Addressing Capsular Patholaxity

When capsular patholaxity is thought to be present, a "shift" superiorly of the inferior capsular tissue (using the sutures already established with the suture anchor) is important. Axillary nerve proximity requires limiting the depth of the suture passing through tissue at the inferior area of the glenoid. One strategy is to pass the suture in two "bites." First, selectively grabbing a pinch of capsule and then advancing the tissue to penetrate the labrum. Care is taken to avoid an "East–West" shift of capsule, which can inadvertently tighten the shoulder, but rather shift redundant/lax inferior capsule superiorly. The amount of superior shift is titrated individually based on the perception of capsular patholaxity.

Suture Management

Successful stabilizations can be achieved by following the steps outlined above. But, accomplishing this in an efficient and reproducible manner depends upon mastering some of the more subtle details of suture management. Some specific recommendations to optimize the repair experience and result are listed below.

PEARLS AND PITFALLS

1. Avoid crossing sutures from the same anchor. When preparing to retrieve an anchor suture limb for shuttling

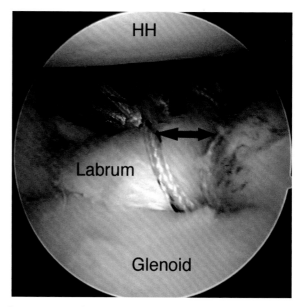

FIGURE 16.33. When using double-loaded anchors, suture passage of the two sutures should ideally be sufficiently separate to capture a bridge of tissue (*double arrow heads* show 3 to 4 mm bridge of captured tissue [right shoulder, lateral decubitus, scope posterior; HH, humeral head]).

through the capsule/labrum, select the limb closest to the site of capsular passage, and ensure it does not cross over or under its other limb. When the suture is tied, it will not cross on itself underneath the soft tissue, which can otherwise prevent good tissue apposition (Fig. 16.34).

2. When preparing to shuttle an anchor suture limb through soft tissue, grab the shuttling suture and the anchor limb suture together at their point of origin within the joint. By withdrawing them together out the cannula and keeping

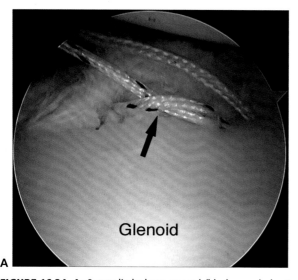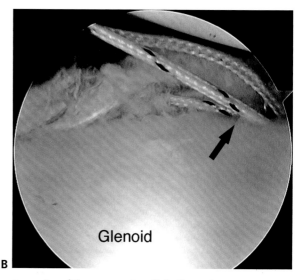

FIGURE 16.34. A: Suture limbs have crossed (*black arrow*), due to errant grasping of the wrong suture limb. Crossed sutures prevent secure tissue apposition against the glenoid during knot tying. Always check for suture crossing before knot tying (right shoulder, lateral decubitus, scope posterior). **B:** Uncrossed (*black arrow*), sutures can now be securely tied (right shoulder, lateral decubitus, scope posterior).

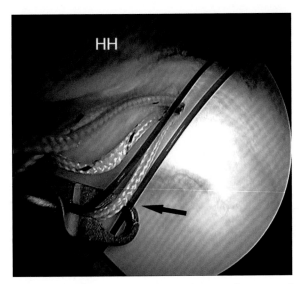

FIGURE 16.35. When preparing to shuttle an anchor suture limb through soft tissue, grab the shuttling suture, and the anchor limb suture together at their point of origin within the joint. By withdrawing them together out of the cannula, and keeping them together, they cannot cross or be crossed by any other sutures in the cannula, no matter how many are present. (right shoulder, lateral decubitus, 70° lens with scope posterior; HH, humeral head).

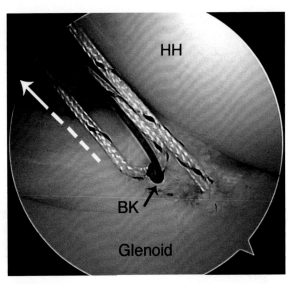

FIGURE 16.36. Unloading of the anchor suture limb during shuttling can be avoided by using either a Shuttle Relay (ConMed Linvatec, Largo, FL), or a "blocking knot" (BK), in which a knot is tied in a monofilament suture (no. 1 PDS), which dilates the tissue at the site of suture passage (dotted white arrow shows direction of shuttle suture pull, right shoulder, lateral decubitus, scope posterior; HH, humeral head).

them together, they cannot cross or be crossed by any other sutures in the cannula (Fig. 16.35).

3. Avoid inadvertent unloading of the anchor suture limb during shuttling. This can be minimized by either using a Shuttle Relay (ConMed Linvatec), or when using monofilament suture (no. 1 PDS) tying a "blocking knot," which dilates the tissue at the site of suture passage (Fig. 16.36).
4. Avoid suture tangling by placing sutures in accessory cannulae.
5. Keep the knots away from the articular surfaces of the joint. This is done by using a past-pointing technique with the knot pusher, advancing it toward the capsule and away from the articular margin. By pulling on the postlimb and with the knot pusher directed into the soft tissue, the knot will serve to "roll" the capsulolabral tissue up against the glenoid face restoring the buttress. This will also decrease the risk of a "squeaky" knot at the articular margin.
6. Ensure you have evaluated the repair by inspection and palpation of the reconstructed labral buttress (Fig. 16.37).

REHABILITATION

The rehabilitation protocol for arthroscopic shoulder stabilization should be tailored for surgeon preferences, concomitant pathology, and patient-specific concerns. It can be subdivided into four phases.

The initial recovery, or Phase I, typically lasts 4 to 6 weeks and focuses on sling immobilization for three weeks, active-assistive elbow/wrist/hand range-of-motion exercises, and gentle protected passive forward elevation in the plane of the scapula with care taken to protect the anterior capsulolabral repair from stress. Phase II (beginning at weeks 4 to 6 through weeks 10 to 12) incorporates the addition of gentle motion exercises as the patient weans from the sling and begins to gradually include passive external rotation and pendulum exercises. Deltoid and rotator cuff isometrics are incorporated further as are posterior glide joint mobilizations—all in an arc and manner that emphasize protection of the anterior capsule.

By 12 weeks, as the patient progresses to Phase III, full motion has usually been achieved and the emphasis is on resistance exercises for the cuff and the scapular rotators. A functional progression follows and at weeks 16 to 20, the patient transitions to Phase IV, where muscle strengthening and endurance activities progress, and functional and sport-specific exercises and activities are incorporated. Return to sports is predicated on the type of activity (e.g., contact/collision, overhead athlete, etc.) and patient-specific motion and strength. In our experience, most contact/collision athletes are able to return to their sport between 4 and 6 months after surgery.

RESULTS

The results of arthroscopic stabilization for anterior glenohumeral instability are comparable to those of open stabilization. Two recent randomized controlled trials have presented more relevant data based on using contemporary

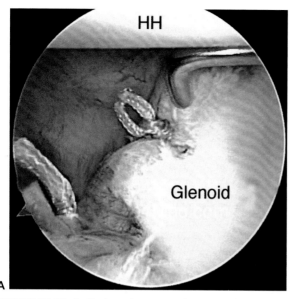
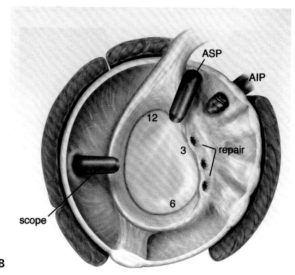

FIGURE 16.37. A: Final repair construct is examined, looking from anterosuperior portal, probing from the posterior portal (right shoulder, lateral decubitus position; HH, humeral head). **B:** Illustration of final repair with labrum restored at three points of fixation; ASP, anterosuperior portal; AIP, anteroinferior portal).

techniques. Bottoni et al. reported the results of 61 patients randomized to arthroscopic or open stabilization evaluated at a mean of 32 months, reporting two failures in the open and one failure in the arthroscopic group (16). A recent systematic review of anterior shoulder instability treatment by Brophy and Marx found comparable rates of recurrent instability after arthroscopic (6.4%) and open (8.2%) stabilization (17). The one parameter consistently found in the literature to be significantly different is greater motion loss in the open stabilization groups.

COMPLICATIONS

Complications after arthroscopic stabilization include recurrent instability, stiffness, infection, neurovascular injury, implant migration, chondrolysis, and glenoid fracture or compromise of the osseous rim. Recurrent instability using suture anchors has been reported to occur between 5% and 10%, although this rate is higher in some series, particularly those involving contact athletes. Though uncommon, stiffness can occur following Bankart repairs. Care must be taken to avoid overtightening and to ensure that any shift is in the North–South, rather than in the East–West direction.

Neurovascular injury, though fortunately a rare event, typically involves the axillary or musculocutaneous nerves. The axillary nerve travels in proximity to the inferior capsule and is at risk when placing sutures inferiorly (18). Careful attention to suture passage and a pinch-tuck technique to avoid an overexuberant bite of inferior capsule can help avoid this injury. Implant migration, glenoid fracture, or osseous rim compromise may be related

to anchor placement and has the potential for devastating consequences for the articular cartilage and function of the glenohumeral joint. Chondrolysis has been reported after thermal capsulorrhaphy as well as with the use of intraarticular pain pumps (19,20).

CONCLUSIONS AND FUTURE DIRECTIONS

Arthroscopic stabilization using the suture anchor technique has proven effective in the surgical treatment of anterior shoulder instability. Attention to careful preoperative planning, appropriate patient selection, and meticulous intraoperative technique will lead to good results in most patients. Advances in technology and experience have narrowed those ineligible for arthroscopic reconstruction. Current strong contraindications include those with articular arc compromise on the humeral side, glenoid side, or both. Although current recurrence rates with the suture anchor technique are comparable to those achieved with open methods, there is room for improvement. The next phase in the evolution of this procedure will likely be in the biologic realm, incorporating bioactive substances into the implants and suture materials to enhance the speed, degree, and strength of healing.

REFERENCES

1. Hovelius L. Anterior dislocation of the shoulder in teen-agers and young adults. Five-year prognosis. *J Bone Joint Surg Am.* 1987;69:393–399.
2. McLaughlin HL, MacLellan DI. Recurrent anterior dislocation of the shoulder. II. A comparative study. *J Trauma.* 1967;7:191–201.

3. Rowe CR, Patel D, Southmayd WW. The Bankart procedure: a long-term end-result study. *J Bone Joint Surg Am.* 1978;60:1–16.

4. Speer KP. Anatomy and pathomechanics of shoulder instability. *Clin Sports Med.* 1995;14:751–760.

5. Howell SM, Galinat BJ. The glenoid-labral socket. A constrained articular surface. *Clin Orthop Relat Res.* 1989;243:122–125.

6. O'Brien SJ, Neves MC, Arnoczky SP et al. The anatomy and histology of the inferior glenohumeral ligament complex of the shoulder. *Am J Sports Med.* 1990;18:449–456.

7. Speer KP, Deng X, Borrero S, et al. Biomechanical evaluation of a simulated Bankart lesion. *J Bone Joint Surg Am.* 1994;76:1819–1826.

8. Burkhart SS, De Beer JF. Traumatic glenohumeral bone defects and their relationship to failure of arthroscopic Bankart repairs: significance of the inverted-pear glenoid and the humeral engaging Hill–Sachs lesion. *Arthroscopy.* 2000;16:677–694.

9. Purchase RJ, Wolf EM, Hobgood ER, et al. Hill–Sachs "remplissage": an arthroscopic solution for the engaging Hill–Sachs lesion. *Arthroscopy.* 2008;24:723–726.

10. Gerber C, Lambert SM. Allograft reconstruction of segmental defects of the humeral head for the treatment of chronic locked posterior dislocation of the shoulder. *J Bone Joint Surg Am.* 1996;78:376–382.

11. Mazzocca AD, Brown FM Jr, Carreira DS, et al. Arthroscopic anterior shoulder stabilization of collision and contact athletes. *Am J Sports Med.* 2005;33:52–60.

12. Barber FA, Herbert MA, Beavis RC, et al. Suture anchor materials, eyelets, and designs: update 2008. *Arthroscopy.* 2008;24:859–867.

13. Difelice GS, Williams RJ III, Cohen MS, et al. The accessory posterior portal for shoulder arthroscopy: description of technique and cadaveric study. *Arthroscopy.* 2001;17:888–891.

14. Davidson PA, Tibone JE. Anterior-inferior (5 o'clock) portal for shoulder arthroscopy. *Arthroscopy.* 1995;11:519–525.

15. Lehtinen JT, Tingart MJ, Apreleva M, et al. Variations in glenoid rim anatomy: implications regarding anchor insertion. *Arthroscopy.* 2004;20:175–178.

16. Bottoni CR, Smith EL, Berkowitz MJ, et al. Arthroscopic versus open shoulder stabilization for recurrent anterior instability: a prospective randomized clinical trial. *Am J Sports Med.* 2006;34:1730–1737.

17. Brophy RH, Marx RG. The treatment of traumatic anterior instability of the shoulder: nonoperative and surgical treatment. *Arthroscopy.* 2009;25:298–304.

18. Ball CM, Steger T, GalSatz LM, et al. The posterior branch of the axillary nerve: an anatomic study. *J Bone Joint Surg Am.* 2003;85-A:1497–1501.

19. Busfield BT, Romero DM. Pain pump use after shoulder arthroscopy as a cause of glenohumeral chondrolysis. *Arthroscopy.* 2009;25:647–652.

20. Coobs BR, LaPrade RF. Severe chondrolysis of the glenohumeral joint after shoulder thermal capsulorrhaphy. *Am J Orthop.* 2009;38:E34–E37.

I. The Shoulder

Anterior Shoulder Instability: Suture Plication

Robert M. Lucas • Anthony A. Romeo • Scot A. Youngblood • Neil Ghodadra • Matthew T. Provencher

Anterior instability is the most common type of shoulder instability with an estimated incidence of 2% for traumatic anterior dislocation over the lifetime of the general population. It can lead to significant functional disability and decreased quality of life. Numerous anatomic lesions can be responsible, including disruption of the glenoid labrum from its attachment at the glenoid, stretching or disruption of the glenohumeral ligaments, poor dynamic control of the shoulder girdle, rotator cuff tears, and osseous lesions of the glenoid rim and humeral head. By arthroscopically repairing the pathology present in the capsuloligamentous complex and glenoid labrum, the biomechanics of the glenohumeral joint are reliably restored (1, 2).

Open repair of the unstable shoulder has previously been considered the gold standard given its high success rate. However, recent advances in arthroscopic procedures have shown that if performed correctly, arthroscopic repair of shoulder instability can equal the success of open repair. Arthroscopic stabilization by suture anchor fixation with capsular plication has shown failure rates ranging from 5% to 11%, comparable with open repair (3). Arthroscopic repair has several advantages over open repair, including reduced postoperative morbidity and pain, shorter hospitalization, improved range of motion, more complete inspection of the glenohumeral joint, and less damage to surrounding soft tissue, including the subscapularis tendon. However, certain cases of anterior instability repair, especially those patients with significant bony deficiencies, are better approached by an open technique (4). The keys to the successful arthroscopic treatment of anterior shoulder instability are to first properly identify pathology amenable to arthroscopic repair and then ensure that the capsulolabral structures are adequately repaired and tensioned to the glenoid.

PATHOLOGY

Biomechanically, the glenohumeral joint is a shallow ball and socket joint with stability maintained by both static and dynamic anatomic mechanisms. The dynamic stabilizers consist of the muscle–tendon units of the rotator cuff, tendon of the long head of the biceps, superficial muscle layer, and scapulothoracic muscles. Static stabilizers include the concavity of the glenoid fossa, adhesion-cohesive properties of synovial fluid, negative intra-articular pressure, and soft tissue structures consisting of the glenoid labrum and capsular ligaments. The glenohumeral capsuloligamentous complex consists of collagenous bands, which originate from the glenoid labrum and attach to the humerus. They serve to statically restrain the glenohumeral joint against excessive translation in varying positions of arm rotation and may also have a proprioceptive role in shoulder stability. The anterior band of the inferior glenohumeral ligament (IGHL) attaches to the glenoid at the anteroinferior labrum and is the primary static restraint to anterior translation in the abducted and externally rotated shoulder.

The glenoid labrum is a fibrocartilaginous ring, which lines the glenoid fossa and is a critical static stabilizer of the shoulder (Fig. 17.1). The labrum itself acts to support the glenohumeral joint by increasing the surface area and concavity of the joint and by acting as a bumper to prevent translation of the humerus on the glenoid. It also serves as a fibrocartilage transition zone where the glenohumeral ligaments and long head of the biceps tendon attach to the glenoid rim. The Bankart lesion, which is an avulsion of the anterior inferior glenoid labrum from the bony glenoid rim, is commonly encountered in anterior shoulder instability and often involves a fracture of a piece of the inferior glenoid (Fig. 17.2). As mentioned, the anterior band of the IGHL attaches to the glenoid at the anteroinferior labrum, and disruption of this attachment can lead to excessive anterior humeral translation. It is often disrupted during a traumatic dislocation event.

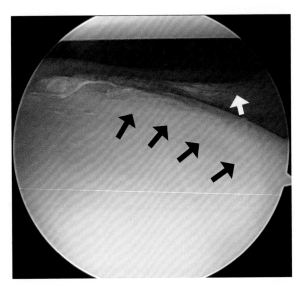

FIGURE 17.1. The glenoid labrum is shown including the chondro-labral junction on the glenoid (*black arrow*). The IGHL (*white arrow*) is also shown.

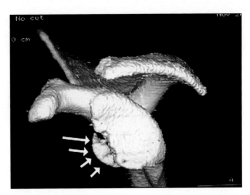

FIGURE 17.3. A bony Bankart injury is demonstrated on a sagittal oblique CT scan, demonstrating an avulsed anterior portion of the glenoid.

While the Bankart lesion has been referred to as the essential lesion of anterior instability, Speer et al. (5) demonstrated that an isolated Bankart lesion was insufficient to cause significant increased translation and instability and surmised that in addition to the Bankart lesion, plastic deformation of the IGHL must also occur for instability to exist. A previous study by Bigliani et al. (6) showed that the IGHL undergoes strain injury during an anterior shoulder instability event and may become permanently stretched even without detachment from the anterior glenoid labrum. Open revisions of failed arthroscopic instability repairs have shown marked capsular laxity even in the presence of healed Bankart lesions (7) due to permanent deformation of the glenohumeral ligaments and anterior capsule. This emphasizes the need for appropriate retensioning of capsular laxity in addition to repair of the glenoid labral lesion in order to achieve successful results.

Bony lesions associated with anterior instability are typically located in the anteroinferior quadrant and consist of a displaced fracture fragment or an attritional bone loss due to bone erosion from repetitive episodes of subluxation or dislocation (Fig. 17.3). This can lead to the glenoid taking on the shape of an inverted pear, which has been shown to correlate with a bone loss of 25% to 30% (Fig. 17.4) (8). Another common lesion encountered in instability is at the rotator interval, which is the triangular space bordered superiorly by the supraspinatus tendon and inferiorly by the subscapularis tendon. Widening of this interval can lead to a voluminous capsule and a resultant decrease in glenohumeral stability. It has been shown that in select patients adjunct treatment with closure of the rotator interval can improve anterior instability (9).

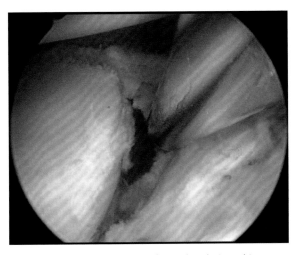

FIGURE 17.2. Typical appearance of a Bankart lesion. This represents a soft tissue type of Bankart tear—with an avulsed anterior labrum from the glenoid.

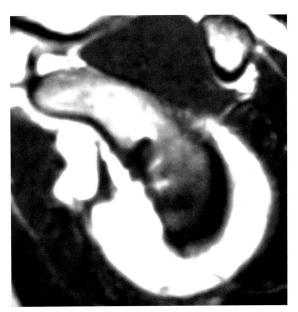

FIGURE 17.4. An inverted-pear type of glenoid, with attritional loss seen on the sagittal oblique MRI arthrogram image. This represents glenoid bone loss of approximately 25% to 30% and is attritional in nature (the bone fragment is no longer present).

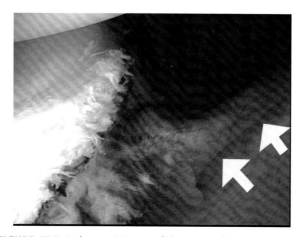

FIGURE 17.5. Arthroscopic image of the anteroinferior glenoid demonstrating an anterior labral periosteal sleeve avulsion (ALPSA). The anterior glenoid labrum is healed medially approximately 1 cm down the glenoid neck. The IGHL is shown attaching to the labrum and medially down the glenoid neck (*white arrows*).

Other articular lesions associated with anterior instability include a superior labral anterior posterior (SLAP) lesion, which is a detachment of the glenoid labrum at the insertion of the long head of the biceps tendon, the medial displacement of the labrum and glenoid sleeve of the anterior glenoid (anterior labral periosteal sleeve avulsion or ALPSA) and the humeral avulsion of the glenohumeral ligament (HAGL lesion). The presence of these lesions can lead to significant instability and future dislocations if not properly addressed. Therefore, care must be taken to identify their presence (Fig. 17.5).

CLINICAL EVALUATION

History

When evaluating the patient with recurrent anterior instability, the history should include a complete description of symptoms and any previous shoulder dislocations, injuries, or previous surgery. A full history of glenohumeral instability should also be obtained and includes the nature of previous dislocations (voluntary vs traumatic), the nature of the reduction (self-reductions vs reduction by a healthcare professional), the number and duration of dislocations or instability events, and any previous therapy or treatments to the affected shoulder.

The type of activity in which the patient is engaged and the specific activities that cause instability should be noted. Patients with anterior shoulder instability most often present with feelings of subluxation or impending dislocation with apprehension during certain shoulder positions (namely, abduction and external rotation and with overhead activities). In addition, they may also complain of pain and weakness in the affected shoulder. Subjective feelings of instability are often experienced during repetitive overhead activities, such as throwing and swimming. Patients may also complain of sudden, transient, sharp pain, numbness, or weakness that usually resolves spontaneously as the only symptom of instability.

Physical Examination

Physical examination should include a comprehensive evaluation of the shoulder to include visualization, palpation, ranges of motion, strength, neurologic exam, and specific stability testing. An evaluation of posture and gross examination of shoulder symmetry should be performed in comparison with the contralateral shoulder. Active and passive range of motion should be measured bilaterally in external rotation, internal rotation, flexion, and abduction, with attention also directed to scapular function during range of motion. Instability encountered during mid-range of motion may indicate significant bony defects. The affected shoulder should be palpated to assess for inflammation, deformity, muscle wasting, and tenderness with attention to AC joint and biceps tendon involvement. Strength testing should be performed for each motion and compared with the contralateral shoulder. Differences in active versus passive range of motion may be evidence of an associated rotator cuff tear or nerve injury. A complete neurologic examination of the extremity should be performed to rule out injury to the brachial plexus, axillary nerve, or any cervical or peripheral nerve involvement.

Apprehension testing recreates the position of anterior instability with an abduction external rotation force placed on the humerus. The apprehension test is positive when the patient senses an impending dislocation. With the relocation test, the feeling of dislocation is alleviated with a posteriorly directed force to the humeral head. The presence of pain is not indicative of a positive test.

Translational load and shift tests should be performed to assess the degree and direction of instability and to rule out multiple direction instability (MDI). These tests may be performed in the lateral decubitus position and compared with the contralateral side in the anterior and posterior planes, documenting the presence of pain or instability throughout the exam. A directional force is applied to the concentrically loaded humeral head and the amount of translation of the humerus on the glenoid is then graded zero (minimal translation), 1+ (translation of the humeral head up to the face of the glenoid labrum without subluxation), 2+ (translation with subluxation over the glenoid rim and spontaneous reduction), and 3+ (translation over the glenoid rim completely without spontaneous reduction) (10, 11).

An inferior translation (sulcus test) should also be performed to look for MDI by placing an inferiorly directed force on the adducted arm in both the neutral and the externally rotated positions measuring the amount of separation in centimeters between the humeral head and the acromion to evaluate for inferior laxity. This can be graded according to the measured distance of the sulcus ranging from 0 to 3+ (10, 11). If a large sulcus persists in external rotation, it is likely that a rotator interval lesion is contributing to a component of the patient's overall instability pattern (Fig. 17.6).

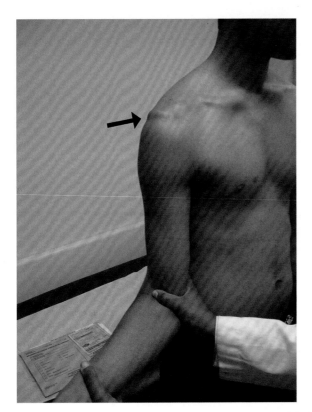

FIGURE 17.6. A sulcus finding that persists in external rotation (*black arrow*) is indicative of an incompetent rotator interval.

Other joints should be evaluated for laxity including the contralateral shoulder and tests to evaluate for global joint hyperlaxity such as the ability of the patient to bring the thumb to the wrist. Specific tests such as the cross-body adduction, Neer's and Hawkin's impingement tests, O'Brien's active compression test, and Speed's test may help in identifying other possible causes of shoulder pain.

Radiologic Evaluation

Anterior glenoid bony defects may be present in most anterior instability cases. Plain film radiographs of the shoulder in the anterior–posterior (AP), supraspinatus outlet, and axillary views can help assess the integrity of the glenoid rim and humeral head and can rule out other osseous lesions. The West Point, Garth, and Stryker notch views are also helpful in determining the extent of bone loss of the glenoid rim and the presence of Hill–Sachs lesions.

Imaging with a computed tomography (CT) scan can help to better visualize bony defects or abnormalities and can further aid in the diagnosis and operative planning. If a significant bony glenoid lesion is suspected, a CT scan with 3D reconstruction and digital subtraction of the humeral head can be used to evaluate the extent and location of bone loss. A 3D CT can be used to accurately measure anterior bone loss and aid in preoperative planning, ensuring that an arthroscopic repair is a viable option for the patient (12). The extent of bone loss on imaging studies is an important

consideration before choosing arthroscopic management of shoulder instability as those with significant bony defects of the glenoid and/or humeral head may have higher rates of recurrence without open augmentation (4).

Magnetic resonance imaging (MRI) can also be used to visualize bony lesions and soft tissue injuries and to evaluate labral and capsuloligamentous integrity. MRI should be considered in patients over age 40 with anterior shoulder instability due to the high incidence of associated rotator cuff tearing in this population. MR arthrogram provides additional sensitivity in the detection of capsulolabral pathology, and it has been shown that MR arthrogram can successfully measure capsular volume in relation to the degree of instability (Figs. 17.7 and 17.8) (13).

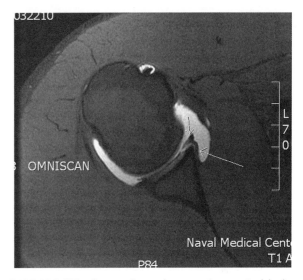

FIGURE 17.7. MR arthrogram image demonstrating anterior labral tear.

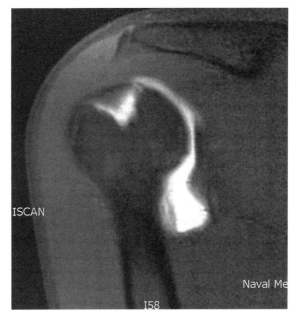

FIGURE 17.8. A sizable Hill–Sachs injury is demonstrated on the coronal MR arthrogram sequence. This patient also had a 20% glenoid bone loss lesion and was treated with a Latarjet procedure.

Classification

Anterior shoulder instability can be classified according to four criteria: frequency, cause, degree, and direction. The frequency of subluxation and instability events is an important indicator of the degree of structural tissue damage. The cause of instability can be divided to include traumatic, microtraumatic, and atraumatic. This can provide clues about the nature of the intra-articular pathology present with traumatic more likely to have glenoid rim damage and atraumatic instability more likely to have capsular laxity. The degree of instability refers to complete dislocation of the glenohumeral joint versus excessive translation of the humerus on the glenoid with associated symptomatic instability. The direction of instability refers to anterior, posterior, and multidirectional.

Decision Making

The natural history of acute anterior instability events has been evaluated through numerous prospective studies with age at the time of initial dislocation being the most significant prognostic factor for future instability events. Physically active patients under the age of 30 treated nonoperatively with a supervised physical therapy program have had recurrence rates ranging from 38% to 80%, whereas those treated with arthroscopic repair have had failure rates ranging from 3% to 20% (25). Additionally, quality of life assessments have shown superior outcomes with early arthroscopic repair. However, postoperative activity level is also a risk factor for recurrent dislocation, and several of these studies were of a military population engaging in physical activity levels that may not be seen in the general population. These data indicate early arthroscopic repair following first time dislocation is applicable for young, highly active patients or those engaged in activities involving overhead use of their arms.

Additional studies of the general population have shown that for patients with primary anterior shoulder dislocations, over half of the patients at followup periods ranging from 4 to 25 years after the initial event did not have a repeat instability event, and of those that did only half ultimately requested surgery (14, 26). Despite lower outcome scores, nonoperatively treated patients were able to cope with their symptoms and many did not request surgery. It is therefore likely that immediate surgical stabilization is indicated for only a small subset of highly active young individuals or those in whom a redislocation event would be catastrophic. Nonoperative treatment may be applicable for the general population. Nonoperative treatment through focused physical therapy should also be recommended to older, less active patients with comorbidities that would increase surgical risk.

TREATMENT

Nonoperative

Nonoperative treatment for anterior shoulder instability consists of physical therapy tailored toward the acuity and mechanism of instability.

Acutely dislocated shoulders should be initially treated with urgent reduction of the shoulder, which is best accomplished by experienced individuals to limit any further damage. If any question exists regarding the extent of damage, it should be postponed until radiographs can be obtained to rule out significant fractures. Postreduction treatment consists of a short period of immobilization followed by the gradual progression of physical therapy. Recent studies have shown immobilization is only necessary until pain control is achieved, typically 1 to 3 weeks. Of additional importance may be the position in which the shoulder is immobilized. Shoulder immobilization in 10° to 20° of external rotation has been shown to have superior results (15). However, this assertion has recently been challenged by others (16).

Physical therapy for chronic instability consists initially of relative rest, including avoidance of activities that increase pain or cause feelings of instability, anti-inflammatory medications, and progressive exercises emphasizing early return of motion and strengthening of the dynamic shoulder stabilizers for up to 6 months. Strength training should begin with isometric exercises and progress to isotonic exercises with light resistance exercises focusing on the rotator cuff, deltoids, and scapulothoracic muscles.

The criteria for a return to sports should include a physical examination with the patient showing full range of motion and strength compared with the contralateral shoulder, and an absence of pain and instability on provocative maneuvers.

Operative

Indications

Operative indications for the repair of anterior shoulder instability include the patient's age, activity level, symptoms, and failure of physical therapy. Age was determined to be the most important prognostic indicator of future dislocations with a recurrence rate of up to 95% in patients under the age of 20 (17, 27). Patients with increased physical demands and those who perform overhead activities are also at high risk for recurrent dislocation and are considered operative candidates. Other indications for operative repair are patients who desire an early return to physical activity, patients who have symptoms at rest or symptoms interfering with activities of daily living, and patients with recurrent subluxations and dislocations.

Arthroscopic repair is not indicated when the patient has a large bony defect of the glenoid greater than 20% to 25%, or a large Hill–Sachs lesion. Other contraindications to arthroscopic repair include significant soft tissue injury such as ligament and tendon ruptures and HAGL lesions, although these rarer instability injuries have been approached using arthroscopic techniques. The presence of bony defects of the anterior glenoid rim has been the subject of controversy. Several studies have shown that patients with an inverted pear glenoid defined as a loss of

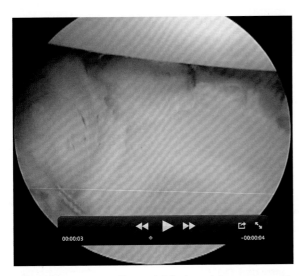

FIGURE 17.9. A "balanced" capsulolabral repair in a patient with recurrent anterior shoulder instability. Posterior plication sutures to an intact posterior labrum are utilized after repair of the primary injury to the anteroinferior capsulolabral structures.

at least 25% (8) have shown a failure rate of 67% to 89% when treated with arthroscopic repair. However, a recent study has shown failure rates of 13.3% in patients with bony defects of up to 30% (18). In this study, all the failures were in patients with a chronic attritional bone loss pattern versus bony fragments of the anterior glenoid, suggesting this pattern of bone loss may be more appropriate for open bone graft procedures.

Examination Under Anesthesia

With the patient under general anesthetic an examination to evaluate motion, laxity, and stability should be performed in comparison with the contralateral shoulder. Range of motion should address forward elevation, external rotation with the arm at the side and in abduction, internal rotation in abduction, and cross-body adduction. Load and shift tests should be performed to measure anterior, posterior, and inferior translation and graded according to previously mentioned criteria to evaluate for MDI.

SURGICAL TECHNIQUE

When deciding upon the best technique for anterior instability repair, the lesions responsible for the instability must be considered. Multiple techniques for arthroscopic repair have been developed with varying success rates, including staple capsulorrhaphy, transglenoid suturing, bioabsorbable tack fixation, suture anchor fixation, and capsulorrhaphy by thermal means or with suture plication. The technique with the best current success rate is suture anchor fixation with capsular plication. For treatment of lesions of the anteroinferior glenoid labrum, this technique has shown success rates comparable with open repair. We have demonstrated that plication sutures attached to an intact labrum may have strength comparable with anchor fixation, which may obviate the need for anchor placement

when there is a patulous capsule with an intact labrum (19). In a patient with anterior instability, this will generally be in the posteroinferior quadrant of the shoulder to provide what Snyder and Romeo have termed a "balanced repair" (Fig. 17.9).

AUTHORS' PREFERRED TREATMENT

The patient is positioned in the lateral decubitus position with the operative extremity suspended in an overhead traction sleeve (Fig. 17.10). The arthroscope is inserted through a standard posterior portal and an anterosuperior portal established from outside-in high in the rotator interval adjacent to the biceps tendon. A diagnostic arthroscopy is performed to evaluate the joint and identify all lesions present.

If a Bankart lesion is present, a midglenoid portal is made in the lower portion of the rotator interval just above the subscapularis tendon, and a posterolateral portal in the 7 o'clock position is made. Anterior glenoid bone loss (if present) may be estimated by viewing from the anterior superior portal (4, 8).

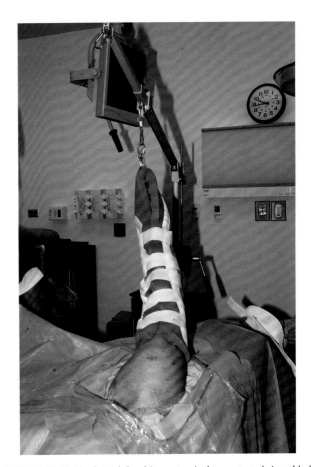

FIGURE 17.10. The lateral decubitus setup is demonstrated. A padded suspension sleeve is shown to carefully suspend the arm in approximately 45° of abduction, 15° of forward flexion, and a small amount of direct lateral translation at the axilla to easily open up and provide access to the glenohumeral joint.

With the arthroscope either in the anterosuperior portal or posterior portal, the capsulolabral tissue is mobilized. The glenoid neck and surface are then debrided with a combination of an elevator device, a high-speed burr (on reverse) or bone-cutting shaver, and a rasp to obtain adequate bony preparation and elevation of the labrum from its injured and healed position. The preparation of the glenoid and labrum is a critical step in order to obtain an adequate mobilization of the labrum to the native position on the glenoid and to facilitate healing by preparing the bone of the anterior glenoid neck. The labrum is then repaired to the glenoid by placement of absorbable suture anchors. If the labrum is healed in a medially displaced position, this is termed as ALPSA and

has been associated with lower outcome scores and a higher redislocation rate versus non-ALPSA tears treated arthroscopically. (Fig. 17.11).

The key to a successful repair is obtaining access for optimal anchor placement on the glenoid. It is difficult to obtain an anchor position much below 5:30 on the glenoid from the usual midglenoid portal, which enters the glenohumeral joint just superior to the subscapularis tendon. In order to place an anchor inferiorly on the glenoid near the 6 o'clock position, the anchor may be inserted either through the posterolateral 7 o'clock portal or from anteriorly, often through a trans-subscapularis stab incision with the inserter device. For the posterolateral portal, a percutaneous incision is utilized to insert the anchor

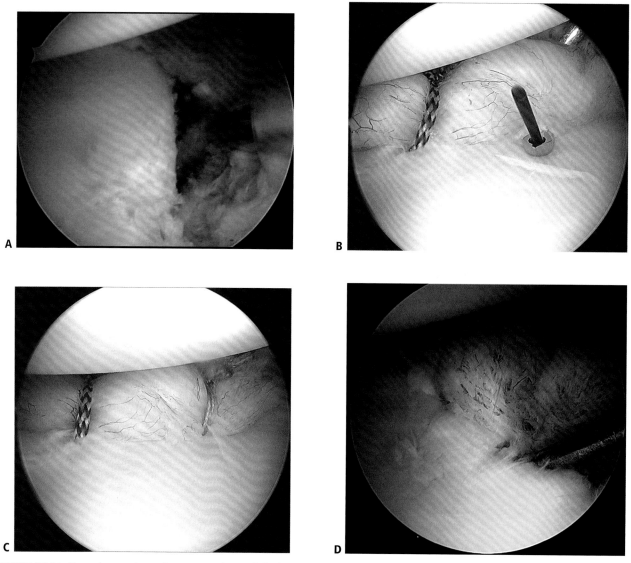

FIGURE 17.11. The arthroscopic repair steps are shown. **(A)**. The labrum is elevated sharply off the anterior glenoid neck with a combination of an elevator device, a rasp, and a shaver. Care is taken to preserve glenoid bone stock during the preparation **(B)**. The progressive repair is started from inferiorly using various available capsulolabral repair devices **(C and D)**. The repair progresses until three to four anchors are placed and sutures appropriately tensioned. Ideally, these anchors are below the 3 o'clock position and adequately tension the anteroinferior capsulolabral structures

device after the trajectory is identified with an 18 G spinal needle. The anchor inserter device is then placed at the inferior aspect of the glenoid and drilled. Prior to drilling, the anchor inserter device may be gently tapped in place with a mallet in order to avoid scuffing of the cartilage due to inserter slippage.

Once the first anchor is placed inferiorly, the capsulolabral repair is performed with various commercially available repair devices. The inferior tissue is easily repaired with a curved hook inserted in the original posterior portal through a cannula large enough to accommodate it. No matter which device is utilized, the goal is to obtain a caudal to cephalad shift of capsule and labral tissue, ensuring that an adequate amount of capsular tissue is imbricated into the repair. It remains unknown how much capsule to imbricate with the repair; however, it is usually in the realm of 5 to 10 mm of capsule. This decision is based upon the patient's instability, the magnitude of translation, and range of motion obtained on the examination under anesthesia (EUA). The repair may be accomplished with the arthroscope either in the anterosuperior portal or in the posterior portal. However, visualization of the anterior glenoid labrum and capsule is greatly enhanced in the anterosuperior portal.

A temporary outside traction suture (TOTS) can be a useful adjunct to help hold the labrum in a reduced position and then perform the capsulolabral repair. As each anchor is inserted and the capsule and labrum repaired, the sutures are tied with a secure arthroscopic knot and then additional anchors are placed at intervals of 5 to 7 mm. It should be noted that the glenoid bone length measures approximately 30 to 35 mm in a superior to inferior direction. A repair performed in the inferior portion of the glenoid has approximately 15 to 20 mm of bone available into which these anchors may be placed. Thus, anchor placement needs to be carefully planned out in this important area of the glenoid.

If an excessively patulous capsule is noted, a multiple-pleated plication can be performed, which has shown capsular volume reductions similar to an open repair. In this technique, a repair stitch is passed two or more times through the capsule to reduce capsular volume. This is especially useful if you do not feel enough capsule was plicated with the initial capsulolabral repair stitch.

Often, patients with anterior instability have a tear that extends inferiorly and posteriorly. Suture anchors placed posteriorly are also helpful to repair the torn labrum. In this case, a smaller amount of posterior capsule is repaired (compared to the anterior capsule) in order to prevent motion loss, especially if the primary direction of instability is anterior.

Some have advocated a "balanced" repair construct in order to balance the posterior aspect of the shoulder in an anterior instability repair. Plication sutures are utilized to repair the posterior capsule to an intact labrum by having the suturing device exit at the chondrolabral junction (Fig. 17.12). Provencher et al. (19) has shown that an intact

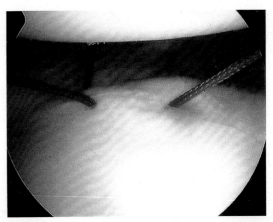

FIGURE 17.12. An inferior capsular plication is demonstrated here with repair stitches through the inferior capsule and through the capsulolabral junction. These are tied with standard arthroscopic knots. This patient had multidirectional instability and was repaired with a total of four inferior, anteroinferior, and posteroinferior capsulolabral repair sutures without anchors in order to decrease capsular volume.

labrum has strength similar to suture anchors and can act as an excellent point of fixation (9, 20). A similar technique of suture plication to an intact labrum without anchors is used for patients with multidirectional instability without labral tears. A balanced inferior 180° repair in a patient with true multidirectional instability is effective at reducing capsular volume and providing reliable results (13). If a Kim's lesion is present or there is damage to the posterior labrum, suture anchor labroplasty with a posterior capsule shift in the cephalad direction should be performed. In patients with multidirectional instability, an inferior capsule shift may also need to be performed with suture plication depending on the amount of laxity present.

After the repair is completed, the joint is then taken through a range of motion. A rotator interval closure can improve anterior stability if an increased amount of anterior translation remains after capsulolabral repair (9, 20). If no posterior labral tear or Kim's lesion is identified and laxity persists, a suture plication of the posterior inferior glenohumeral ligament may also be performed (Fig. 17.13).

REHABILITATION

The arm is immobilized postoperatively in a sling in neutral rotation for between 4 and 6 weeks. Patients are allowed forward flexion in the scapular plane from 90° to 120°, external rotation to 30°, and abduction to 90° during this time. After this 6-week period, patients are started on full active range of motion and begin a strengthening program of the rotator cuff and scapular-stabilizing muscles. At the 6-month point, patients are returned to full unrestricted activities. Prior to returning to sports, the patients should be evaluated clinically. The criteria for clearance include full range of motion, full strength, and negative provocative maneuvers.

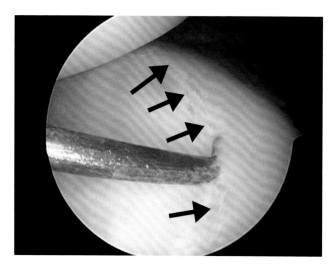

FIGURE 17.13. A posteroinferior "Kim" lesion or a marginal crack in the posteroinferior labrum. This patient had anterior instability with extension of the anterior labral tear posteriorly, ending in a "Kim" lesion. This was taken down and subsequently repaired with a total of three anchors anteriorly and one anchor posteriorly to address the "Kim" lesion.

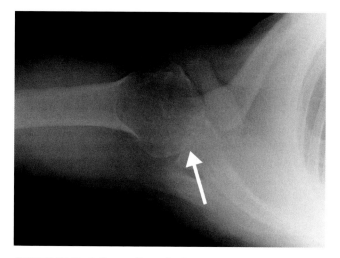

FIGURE 17.14. Axillary radiograph of a 22-year-old patient 8 months after an arthroscopic instability procedure demonstrating cystic degenerative changes in the glenoid and humeral head, with near bone-on-bone obliteration of the joint space.

COMPLICATIONS

Infections from arthroscopic surgery are a relatively uncommon occurrence; however, precautions must be taken to minimize this risk by the use of appropriate preoperative antibiotics and gentle handling of soft tissues. Iatrogenic injury can also occur, usually to the articular cartilage, cuff, or labral tissue, and can be prevented by careful surgical technique, appropriate portal placement and proper placement of implants. Placing the suture anchor cannula at less than 45° relative to the glenoid articular surface predisposes to anchor displacement into the joint with resultant cartilage injury. Proper tensioning at the time of placement can prevent proud or loose suture anchors.

Nerve injury is another complication associated with shoulder arthroscopy and most commonly involves the cutaneous nerves during portal placement. By making superficial incisions and bluntly spreading subcutaneous tissue, these injuries can be avoided.

Proper portal placement is also important to prevent nerve injuries. The posterior portal should be placed approximately 1 to 3 cm inferior and 1 cm medial to the posterolateral edge of the acromion in order to avoid damaging the axillary and suprascapular nerves. Axillary nerve damage can also be minimized with the arm kept in abduction-neutral rotation during the procedure. This provides the greatest distance between the inferior glenoid and the nerve. The closest position of the axillary nerve to the capsule is in the 6 o'clock position. Care should be taken to ensure that only the capsule is plicated during the repair and to avoid deep tissue penetration. The capsule is only 2- to 4-mm thick at this position and care should be taken not to penetrate below this depth in order to protect the axillary nerve.

Damage to the brachial plexus can occur from excess traction in the lateral decubitus position. This can be avoided by minimizing the amount of weight and providing a balanced suspension setup.

Chondrolysis has been reported as a rare but devastating complication of shoulder arthroscopy (21). Currently, the causes of chondrolysis remain to be elucidated; however, it has been speculated that young age, high temperatures during thermal treatment, and the postoperative use of continuous intra-articular bupivacaine pain pump catheters may be causal factors. It has been suggested that such devices be avoided for postoperative pain control and patients should be informed of the small but serious risk of chondrolysis preoperatively. Additional work is necessary in this area to elucidate the multifactorial issues that have been implicated in the development of postarthroscopic glenohumeral chondrolysis (Fig. 17.14).

CONTROVERSIES

Suture Anchor Versus Stitch Plication

Current techniques of arthroscopic repair have incorporated suture anchor fixation of the glenoid labrum in addition to capsular plication. This method has shown success and is reasonable in patients with defects in the glenoid labrum junction. However, if there is an intact labral attachment to the glenoid, it may either be taken down fully and repaired with a suture anchor construct or left intact and plicated with a labral repair stitch only. Suture plication through an intact labrum in the anteroinferior and posteroinferior quadrants has been shown to provide comparable fixation strength with suture anchors (19).

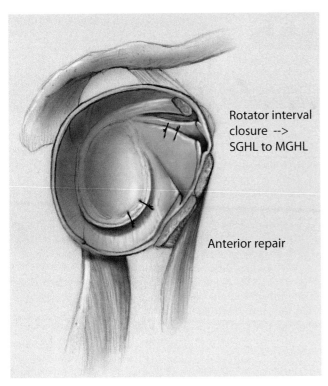

Rotator interval
closure -->
SGHL to MGHL

Anterior repair

FIGURE 17.15. A rotator interval closure has been shown to improve anterior stability after an anterior instability repair although improvement in posterior and inferior stability with rotator interval closure remains more controversial.

Amount of Capsule to Plicate

An advantage of arthroscopic capsular plication is the ability to precisely adjust the amount of tissue plicated based on intraoperative findings. It is therefore necessary to be able to predict the amount of capsular volume reduction, which will result from different amounts of plication. Two studies (22, 23) showed capsular volume reductions of 16.2% with four plications of 5 mm of tissue and 19% to 33.7% volume reductions with four 10-mm plications. These studies examined capsular volume reduction after placement of sutures in four locations and showed predictable capsular volume loss with specific amounts of tissue plication. Further studies will be necessary to analyze how the amount of tissue plicated in different capsular areas affects capsular volume and how this will affect clinical stability and postoperative range of motion. It is paramount to successful repair to provide sufficient capsular volume reduction without overtensioning the capsule.

Location of Plication and Subsequent Effect on Range of Motion

An important consideration in performing capsular plication is the effect of suture placement on postoperative range of motion. Gerber et al. (24) demonstrated that localized capsular plication leads to a predictable loss of

passive range of motion of the glenohumeral joint in cadaveric specimens. Knowing the pattern of motion loss associated with certain capsular plication locations aids the surgeon in addressing specific shoulder pathologies and directions of laxity. There is also the potential for loss of external rotation with rotator interval closure especially with external rotation at the side (9, 20). Further research must provide clinical correlation as the effects of dynamic shoulder stabilizers, course of healing, and symptomatic response to specific plication locations remain unknown.

Adjuncts to Anterior Plication

Anterior labral repair with suture anchor plication has proven successful in anterior shoulder instability; however, other defects may be present such as capsular laxity and rotator interval widening. Successful adjuncts to suture anchor fixation of the labrum in appropriate settings include posterior capsular plication to an intact posterior inferior labrum and rotator interval closure (Fig. 17.15) (9, 19, 20).This highlights the importance of recognizing and addressing all lesions present in the unstable shoulder and the evaluation of stability, following anterior labral repair.

REFERENCES

1. Shafer BL, Mihata T, McGarry MH, et al. Effects of capsular plication and rotator interval closure in simulated multidirectional shoulder instability. *J Bone Joint Surg Am.* 2008;90:136–144.
2. Black KP, Schneider DJ, Yu JR, et al. Biomechanics of the Bankart repair: the relationship between glenohumeral translation and labral fixation site. *Am J Sports Med.* 1999;27:339–344.
3. Freedman KB, Smith AP, Romeo AA, et al. Open Bankart repair versus arthroscopic repair with transglenoid sutures or bioabsorbable tacks for Recurrent Anterior instability of the shoulder: a meta-analysis. *Am J Sports Med.* 2004;32:1520–1527.
4. Burkhart SS, De Beer JF. Traumatic glenohumeral bone defects and their relationship to failure of arthroscopic Bankart repairs: significance of the inverted-pear glenoid and the humeral engaging Hill–Sachs lesion. *Arthroscopy.* 2000;16:677–694.
5. Speer KP, Deng X, Borrero S, et al. Biomechanical evaluation of a simulated Bankart lesion. *J Bone Joint Surg Am.* 1994;76:1819–1826.
6. Bigliani LU, Pollock RG, Soslowsky LJ, et al. Tensile properties of the inferior glenohumeral ligament. *J Orthop Res.* 1992;10:187–197.
7. Cole BJ, L'Insalata J, Irrgang J, et al. Comparison of arthroscopic and open anterior shoulder stabilization. A two to six-year follow-up study. *J Bone Joint Surg Am.* 2000;82-A:1108–1114.
8. Lo IK, Parten PM, Burkhart SS. The inverted pear glenoid: an indicator of significant glenoid bone loss. *Arthroscopy.* 2004;20:169–174.
9. Mologne TS, Zhao K, Hongo M, et al. The addition of rotator interval closure after arthroscopic repair of either anterior or posterior shoulder instability: effect on

glenohumeral translation and range of motion. *Am J Sports Med.* 2008;36:1123–1131.

10. Gerber C, Nyffeler RW. Classification of glenohumeral joint instability. *Clin Orthop Relat Res.* 2002;400:65–76.

11. Altchek DW, Warren RF, Skyhar MJ, et al. T-plasty modification of the Bankart procedure for multidirectional instability of the anterior and inferior types. *J Bone Joint Surg Am.* 1991;73:105–112.

12. Chuang TY, Adams CR, Burkhart SS. Use of preoperative three-dimensional computed tomography to quantify glenoid bone loss in shoulder instability. *Arthroscopy.* 2008;24:376–382.

13. Dewing CB, McCormick F, Bell SJ, et al. An analysis of capsular area in patients with anterior, posterior, and multidirectional shoulder instability. *Am J Sports Med.* 2008;36:515–522.

14. te Slaa RL, Wijffels MP, Brand R, et al. The prognosis following acute primary glenohumeral dislocation. *J Bone Joint Surg Br.* 2004;86:58–64.

15. Itoi E, Hatakeyama Y, Sato T, et al. Immobilization in external rotation after shoulder dislocation reduces the risk of recurrence. A randomized controlled trial. *J Bone Joint Surg Am.* 2007;89:2124–2131.

16. Miller BS, Sonnabend DH, Hatrick C, et al. Should acute anterior dislocations of the shoulder be immobilized in external rotation? A cadaveric study. *J Shoulder Elbow Surg.* 2004;13:589–592.

17. Kralinger FS, Golser K, Wischatta R, et al. Predicting recurrence after primary anterior shoulder dislocation. *Am J Sports Med.* 2002;30:116–120.

18. Mologne TS, Provencher MT, Menzel KA, et al. Arthroscopic stabilization in patients with an inverted pear glenoid: results

in patients with bone loss of the anterior glenoid. *Am J Sports Med.* 2007;35:1276–1283.

19. Provencher MT, Verma N, Obopilwe E, et al. A biomechanical analysis of capsular plication versus anchor repair of the shoulder: can the labrum be used as a suture anchor? *Arthroscopy.* 2008;24:210–216.

20. Provencher MT, Mologne TS, Hongo M, et al. Arthroscopic versus open rotator interval closure: biomechanical evaluation of stability and motion. *Arthroscopy.* 2007;23:583–592.

21. Greis PE, Legrand A, Burks RT. Bilateral shoulder chondrolysis following arthroscopy. A report of two cases. *J Bone Joint Surg Am.* 2008;90:1338–1344.

22. Flanigan DC, Forsythe T, Orwin J, et al. Volume analysis of arthroscopic capsular shift. *Arthroscopy.* 2006;22:528–533.

23. Karas SG, Creighton RA, DeMorat GJ. Glenohumeral volume reduction in arthroscopic shoulder reconstruction: a cadaveric analysis of suture plication and thermal capsulorrhaphy. *Arthroscopy.* 2004;20:179–184.

24. Gerber C, Werner CM, Macy JC, et al. Effect of selective capsulorrhaphy on the passive range of motion of the glenohumeral joint. *J Bone Joint Surg Am.* 2003;85:48–55.

25. Brophy RH, Marx RG. The Treatment of traumatic anterior instability of the shoulder: nonoperative and surgical treatment. Arthroscopy. 2009;25:298–304.

26. Hovelius L, Olofsson A, Sandstrom B, et al. Nonoperative treatment of primary anterior shoulder dislocation in patients forty years of age and younger. A Prospective twenty-five-year follow-up. J Bone Joint Surg Am. 2008;90:945–952.

27. Rowe CR, Sakellarides HT. Factors related to recurrences of anterior dislocations of the shoulder. Clin Orthop Relat Res. 1961;20:40–48.

Multidirectional and Posterior Shoulder Instability

Alan S. Curtis • Suzanne L. Miller • Aaron Gardiner

KEY POINTS

- Posterior and multidirectional instability represent a spectrum of disease encompassing posterior instability with dislocation, posterior unidirectional instability with recurrent posterior subluxation, bidirectional instability with posterior and inferior subluxation, and multidirectional instability with global laxity.

- Nonoperative approaches are the mainstay of treatment for most cases.

- History and physical examination, especially examination under anesthesia, are critical to selecting the proper diagnosis and treatment, as imaging studies are often nondiagnostic.

- Arthroscopic approaches allow a thorough evaluation of intra-articular pathology and a pathology-specific treatment approach.

- Arthroscopic treatment allows the surgeon to address labral tears, capsular laxity, capsular tears, and the rotator interval.

- Open procedures may be preferred in cases of bone loss and in certain revision cases.

Posterior and multidirectional shoulder instability represent a spectrum of disease from posterior instability with dislocation to posterior unidirectional instability with recurrent posterior subluxation, bidirectional instability with posterior and inferior laxity, and multidirectional instability with global laxity. Posterior instability is uncommon, representing approximately 5% of all glenohumeral instability. However, more subtle cases of posterior subluxation or multidirectional instability are likely often undiagnosed. Classically, these patterns of instability have been treated with an open surgical approach (1). However, arthroscopic techniques have progressed to the point where they are an excellent option for treating these conditions. This chapter will review the diagnosis and treatment of posterior and multidirectional instability with an emphasis on arthroscopic surgical techniques.

POSTERIOR INSTABILITY

Clinical Evaluation

Pertinent History

Acute posterior dislocation is a rare event, much less common than anterior dislocation. Many times the dislocation is self-reduced immediately or shortly after the event. A history of seizures or electrocution should alert the clinician to the possibility of posterior dislocation secondary to the severe muscular contractions which occur in these conditions. Acute posterior dislocations are often missed in the emergency department as anterior–posterior (AP) radiographs may look relatively normal to the unsuspecting eye and patients will be relatively comfortable in a sling with the arm internally rotated. There is a delay in diagnosis in many cases of posterior dislocation, leading to delayed diagnosis in a larger percentage of chronic dislocations in comparison with anterior dislocations (2). In these cases, any history of seizures or alcohol abuse should be elicited.

Physical Examination

The most dramatic finding with a posterior dislocation is the severe limitation of external rotation. Most patients will have a range of motion limited to approximately 90° of forward flexion and external rotation to neutral. Many patients find the sling position tolerable while dislocated. A careful neurologic and vascular examination should be performed both before and after any reduction attempts.

Imaging

Plain X-rays are generally sufficient to make the diagnosis. Three orthogonal views, consisting of AP, outlet, and axillary views, should be obtained in all cases. Poor quality or inadequate X-rays are the most common cause of a missed diagnosis. Axial imaging with a CT scan is very helpful to assess any bone impaction or defects as well as in cases where adequate axillary X-rays cannot be obtained (Fig. 18.1).

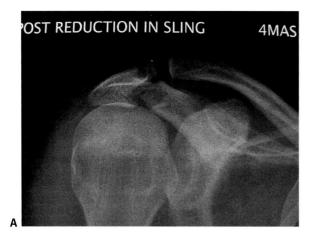

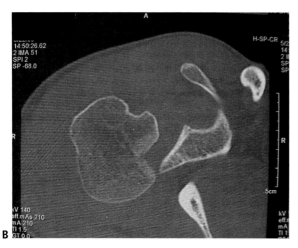

FIGURE 18.1. A: Postreduction radiograph of a right shoulder obtained in the emergency department. **B:** CT scan of the same patient showing a posterior dislocation.

Treatment

Acute Dislocation

Treatment of acute posterior dislocation is generally nonoperative. Closed reduction is generally successful in the emergency department with sedation. An external rotation or "gunslinger" brace is often useful immediately after reduction. A small impaction defect in the humeral head (greater than 20%) generally will not need operative treatment. In these cases, operative treatment is reserved for patients with dislocations not reducible with closed means or for cases with recurrent instability.

Missed or Chronic Dislocation

Treatment of missed or chronic posterior dislocations is difficult and often requires open surgical techniques (2). A thorough examination of this topic is beyond the scope of this chapter. In general, relatively acute dislocations (greater than 6 months) with smaller impaction defects (approximately 20% to 40% of the humeral head) may be treated with an open reduction and a repair of the pathology present. This may consist of an allograft to the humeral head or a partial arthroplasty to fill the defect.

A McLaughlin procedure, consisting of transfer of the lesser tuberosity to the humeral head defect, may also be performed. More chronic dislocations and larger bone defects are often best treated with arthroplasty. In rare cases, such as in patients with high surgical risk and minimal symptoms, the preferred course of action may be to treat chronic dislocations nonoperatively.

RECURRENT POSTERIOR SUBLUXATION AND MULTIDIRECTIONAL INSTABILITY

Clinical Evaluation

History

Recurrent posterior subluxation is more common than posterior dislocation. In many cases, this condition is the sequela of a traumatic event or of repetitive trauma. This is often the case in football players or weightlifters. Classically, patients will sustain contact with the arm outstretched in front of their body or will fall on an outstretched hand. Cases without a history of trauma are also common. This is often the case in athletes who perform overhead activities who have underlying capsular laxity such as swimmers, gymnasts, or volleyball players.

With multidirectional instability, patients usually present with a complaint of pain in the affected shoulder. Patient age typically ranges from teenage to middle age. In some cases, patients will report a history of a subluxation or dislocation, often with spontaneous reduction. Symptoms often present gradually, however, with no traumatic inciting event. Repetitive microtrauma may lead to symptomatic instability such as in competitive swimmers and volleyball players. The activities and arm positions that lead to symptoms should be elucidated. Also, the level of activity during which instability occurs should be determined. For example, symptoms may only occur during the overhead activity of spiking a volleyball or may occur while carrying light objects with the arms at the patient's side. Occasionally, patients may report neurologic symptoms in the affected arm, which may be due to the inferiorly subluxing humeral head stretching the brachial plexus. A history of connective tissue disorders should be sought. Patients with Ehlers–Danlos or Marfan's syndrome may have a predisposition for increased joint laxity and instability.

It is essential to differentiate between laxity and instability. Patients have varying degrees of laxity, which is often asymptomatic. Instability is laxity that is causing dysfunction. With multidirectional instability, the patient may often report varying levels of symptoms in both shoulders. This, especially in cases without a history of significant trauma, is consistent with the generalized capsular laxity that can be present with multidirectional instability.

Classification

Classification of instability is usually by the direction of the instability. Patients may have unidirectional instability (anterior or posterior), bidirectional instability (anterior or posterior and inferior), or multidirectional instability. Patients may also be classified by their mode of instability, which may be involuntary, positional, or voluntary. Patients with involuntary instability are unable to demonstrate their instability in the office. Their instability is usually elicited by trauma, often during their sport of choice. Patients with positional instability are able to demonstrate their instability in the office by positioning their shoulder appropriately. However, this causes discomfort to the patient and the patient generally goes to great lengths to avoid this position of instability during their daily activities and during sports. Patients with voluntary instability are able to demonstrate their instability at will in the office, often with little or no discomfort. These cases should be approached with caution. Often the instability is either habitual or associated with secondary gain. Surgery should be avoided in these cases.

Physical Examination

Physical examination should begin with a visual inspection of the affected shoulder to evaluate for any skin changes, swelling, or atrophy. Palpation can identify any localized areas of tenderness. A thorough examination should be performed to exclude other causes of shoulder pain such as cervical spine pathology, and complete peripheral neurologic and vascular exams should be performed. Active and passive range of motion should be determined and compared with the unaffected side. Muscle strength should also be documented as many patients with multidirectional instability can have some degree of weakness from neurologic injury.

The scapula is often overlooked during shoulder examination. The scapula has a large arc of motion on the thoracic wall, which allows the glenoid to maintain an efficient link to the humeral head during athletic activity. Scapular winging may be present in association with instability. In these cases, the winging is often secondary, and due to pain and inhibition of the scapular stabilizers. Primary scapular winging due to long thoracic or spinal accessory nerve palsy is rare but should be excluded.

Several specialized tests exist to evaluate instability and determine the direction of instability. The sulcus test is used to evaluate inferior instability. This test is performed by placing an inferiorly directed force on the affected arm with the shoulder adducted. In a positive test, the humeral head is translated inferiorly, leaving a hollow area or "sulcus" between the lateral edge of the acromion and the humeral head. The sulcus test may be performed in both neutral rotation and external rotation. If the sulcus sign decreases or disappears with external rotation, this suggests a competent rotator interval.

Anterior instability is evaluated by the apprehension test and the Jobe relocation test. These examinations are performed with the patient supine on the exam table. The affected shoulder is abducted to 90°, and the shoulder is externally rotated. A positive test produces a sense of impending instability. The Jobe relocation test involves placing a posteriorly directed force on the shoulder while the anterior apprehension test is performed. In cases of anterior instability, this posterior force should relieve the apprehension from abduction and external rotation.

Posterior instability may be evaluated with the jerk test. This may be performed in the sitting or standing position. The shoulder is forward flexed to 90° and internally rotated. The examiner then applies a posteriorly directed force while moving the arm across the body. In a positive test, as the arm is adducted, a "jerk" will be observed as the humeral head subluxes posteriorly out of the glenoid. The test may also be positive when there is a palpable "jerk" when the posteriorly subluxed humeral head reduces back into the glenoid with external rotation of the shoulder.

The load and shift test can be used to evaluate both anterior and posterior instability. This test is performed in the supine position. The shoulder is abducted slightly and an axial load as well as either an anterior or a posterior force is applied. This exam is graded from 1+ to 3+. 1+ is the ability to translate the humeral head to the edge of the glenoid, 2+ is the ability to subluxate the humeral head over the glenoid rim and have it spontaneously reduce, and 3+ is a dislocation that does not spontaneously reduce.

In addition to the previous tests, all patients with suspected multidirectional instability should be evaluated for generalized ligamentous laxity with an examination for elbow, thumb, and metacarpophalangeal joint hyperextension.

Imaging

In cases of recurrent posterior subluxation or multidirectional instability, X-rays and CT scans are usually normal. The CT scan is very useful if there is a small glenoid rim fracture present. If there is any question of bone loss or bone deficit such as in glenoid hypoplasia, then a CT scan is useful for evaluation. CT scans are also useful in revision cases where hardware may be present.

MRI is useful for evaluation of capsule, labral, and other soft tissue pathology. In cases of posterior instability, a posterior Bankart or labral tear may be seen (Fig. 18.2). Capsular injuries such as a reverse humeral avulsion of the glenohumeral ligaments (RHAGL lesion) may be seen in cases of posterior instability. MRI may be performed with or without intra-articular contrast. Some authors have reported an increased sensitivity for detecting labral pathology with MR arthrogram compared with conventional MRI. It is important to remember that ultimately the diagnosis of instability is clinical, and many patients, especially those with multidirectional instability, will have normal MRI exams. MRI may still be useful in these cases for excluding other causes of shoulder pain or dysfunction.

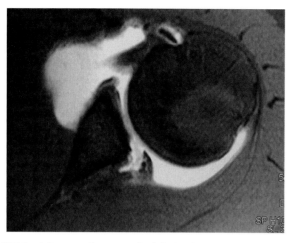

FIGURE 18.2. MR arthrogram of a left shoulder showing a posterior labral tear.

Treatment

Many cases of posterior instability and most cases of multidirectional instability are successfully treated nonoperatively (3,4). In almost all cases, nonoperative treatment is the appropriate initial treatment. Nonoperative treatment consists of initial activity modification and formal physical therapy focusing on strengthening and scapular stabilization. Especially in cases of multidirectional instability, a progressive exercise program that gradually strengthens the scapular stabilizers, deltoid, and rotator cuff muscles has been successful in returning patients to normal activity.

Operative treatment is usually reserved for the failure of a thorough course of nonoperative treatment. It is important to assess preoperatively, which patients need to have their pathology addressed with an open surgical technique. This is the case for patients with bone loss that will require bone grafting. Selected revision cases also may be better served by an open surgical approach. A failed arthroscopic stabilization may sometimes be salvaged by an open capsular shift. A failed thermal capsulorrhaphy may also be an indication for open treatment with capsular augmentation.

Arthroscopic treatment of posterior or multidirectional instability consists of a pathology-specific approach that is tailored to the individual patient. After completion of an examination under anesthesia and diagnostic arthroscopy, the entire capsule and labrum as well as rotator interval may be addressed as needed to recreate a balanced capsule and a stable glenohumeral joint. Arthroscopic techniques have been published with excellent success rates, comparable with open techniques for both posterior and multidirectional instability (5–12).

OPERATIVE TECHNIQUES

In all cases, an examination under anesthesia is performed both of the affected and of the unaffected shoulder. In many cases, an accurate load and shift exam can only be adequately performed while under anesthesia. Prior to beginning surgery, the instability pattern should be clearly defined and the magnitude of instability in the anterior, posterior, and inferior directions quantified.

A thorough diagnostic arthroscopy is then performed in order to clearly define any intra-articular pathology. A major advantage of arthroscopic treatment of posterior and multidirectional instability is the ability to tailor the treatment to the patient after a thorough diagnostic arthroscopic evaluation.

In general, two or three portals are required for these techniques. For posterior work, an anterior superior portal is used for viewing and a posterior portal for working. An accessory portal, either anterior or posterior, is also sometimes required for suture management. Similarly, for anterior work, three portals are used, with the viewing portal posterior and the working and accessory portal anterior.

Unidirectional Posterior Instability with Posterior Bankart

In the case of unidirectional posterior instability with a posterior Bankart lesion, the labrum is repaired to the glenoid using suture anchors in a technique analogous to the arthroscopic Bankart repair performed in cases of anterior instability (5, 6, 10, 11). Viewing from an anterior portal and working from a posterior portal, the torn labrum is elevated from the neck of the glenoid using an elevator. During initial portal placement, it is important that the posterior portal is placed as far lateral to the glenoid as possible to facilitate work on the torn labrum. A cannula of adequate size to allow passage of instruments should be used. We use a 7-mm cannula as our main working cannula. As with cases of anterior instability, it is essential to adequately mobilize the labrum. Care should be taken with the elevator not to damage or tear the labrum or capsular tissue.

After adequate mobilization, the glenoid is prepared using an arthroscopic shaver or burr to remove any scar tissue and prepare an area of bleeding bone to improve healing of the labral repair. A small area of articular cartilage from the posterior rim of the glenoid may also be removed to facilitate proper anchor placement. We use a small ring curette for this purpose as it gives more precise control than a mechanical shaver or burr. Suture anchors are placed in the posterior glenoid at the 7, 8, and 9 o'clock positions when looking at a right shoulder. After placement of the most inferior suture anchor, the sutures are removed through the accessory portal. Next, an arthroscopic suture passer is used to pass a polydioxanone (PDS) through the capsule and labral tissue starting on the capsule side and exiting next to the prepared bony surface of the glenoid. If this suture is passed inferior to the anchor position, when the suture is tied it will tighten the inferior glenohumeral ligament and increase stability. If a double-loaded anchor is used, the second suture is then passed. The sutures are tied with the post for the arthroscopic knot on the capsular side, keeping the knot away from the articular surfaces. Alternatively, knotless anchors can be used if the surgeon desires. The procedure is repeated with two additional anchors proceeding from inferior to superior at the 8 and 9 o'clock positions on a right shoulder. Generally, three anchors are used; however, in some patients with a small glenoid only two anchors need to be used. In these cases, double-loaded anchors may increase the strength of the repair.

In patients with isolated unidirectional posterior instability, the rotator interval is usually not addressed. However, in these patients, the posterior portals are closed at the conclusion of the case. The technique for portal closure involves backing out the cannula to just outside the capsule. A slightly curved arthroscopic suture passer is then used to pass a PDS suture through the capsule from outside to inside, adjacent to the portal. Next, a tissue-penetrating suture grasper is used to pierce the capsule on the opposite side of the portal. This grasper is used to retrieve the PDS suture from the inside of the joint. A knot is then tied blindly down the cannula outside the capsule to close the portal. During this technique, it is essential to keep the cannula just outside the capsule during the closure.

Capsular Plication for Instability and Capsular Laxity Without a Bankart Lesion

In patients with capsular laxity and instability without a Bankart lesion, the surgical technique focuses on balancing a pathologically lax capsule using plication sutures (7,12). Cadaver studies have shown arthroscopic suture plication to result in a significant volume reduction of the glenohumeral joint capsule (13,14). This technique may be used if a pathologically lax capsule is identified for unidirectional, bidirectional, as well as multidirectional instability.

Capsular plication can be performed using a single anterior and single posterior portal (Fig. 18.3). A posterior portal is established first. As with a posterior Bankart repair, this posterior portal is more lateral than the standard posterior portal used for rotator cuff work in the shoulder. Keeping the portal closer to the humeral head allows for better access with instrumentation to the capsule and labrum. An anterior portal is then established with an outside-in technique using a spinal needle to localize the precise location. This portal is typically in the rotator interval beneath the biceps tendon and above the superior border of the subscapularis. With the spinal needle in the joint, access to the anterior inferior and anterior superior portion of the capsule labral complex is checked before actually making the portal. Once the position is confirmed with the spinal needle, a 1-cm skin incision is made and a cannula is placed anteriorly. A complete arthroscopic examination of the shoulder is then performed.

Posterior Capsular Plication

In cases of multidirectional instability, the posterior inferior capsule is typically plicated first. To accomplish this,

the arthroscope and working cannula must be switched. A switching stick is placed through the anterior cannula across the joint and through the cannula of the arthroscope posteriorly. The cannulas may now be switched and the arthroscope is placed anteriorly and a 7-mm cannula is placed posteriorly. Prior to beginning suture plication, an arthroscopic rasp is used to roughen the capsule and create a bleeding surface in order to improve soft tissue healing.

The arthroscopic suture passer is then loaded on the back table with either no. 1 or no. 0 PDS suture. These suture passers are available in various shapes and sizes. For posterior capsular plication in a right shoulder, a suture passer with a 45° left curve works best, and for anterior capsular plication a 45° right curve works best. A curved suture passer without a left or right twist also will often be used, depending on the patient's anatomy.

The repair is started working on the posterior-inferior glenohumeral ligament. Approximately 1 cm from the labrum the capsule is penetrated using the arthroscopic suture passer. If the labrum is competent, the capsule is sewn to the labrum using a second pass of the suture passer. Several inches of PDS suture is shuttled into the joint and the suture passer is removed from the posterior portal.

The suture retriever is then used to retrieve the end of the PDS suture from the joint. The PDS suture can be left in place and tied to begin arthroscopic plication or can be exchanged for a nonabsorbable braided suture. We generally perform arthroscopic capsular plication with absorbable suture. If exchanged for a nonabsorbable braided suture, the PDS suture can simply be tied with a single knot to the end of a nonabsorbable suture and shuttled through capsule labral complex. Tying a leading knot in the PDS will often help facilitate the passage of the nonabsorbable suture. After suture passage, an arthroscopic knot is tied with the post placed on the capsular tissue side as opposed to the labral side of the plication. This allows the capsule to be advanced up to the labrum and reduces the likelihood that the knot will contact the articular surface.

After plication of the posterior inferior capsule, the plication is then continued superiorly with a second suture using the same technique (Fig. 18.4). This technique can be repeated as needed. Usually from two to four sutures are needed to adequately tighten the capsule.

Anterior Capsular Plication

Once the posterior capsule is plicated, a switching stick is used as before to move the arthroscope posteriorly and the working cannula anteriorly. The technique is the same for suture passage except if a right or left curved suture passer tip has been used, the tip should be switched for the opposite direction. As with the posterior capsule, the sutures are tied progressively from inferior to superior. Generally, two to four sutures are used. The determination of how many plication sutures to place involves visualizing the capsule and humeral head, and adding

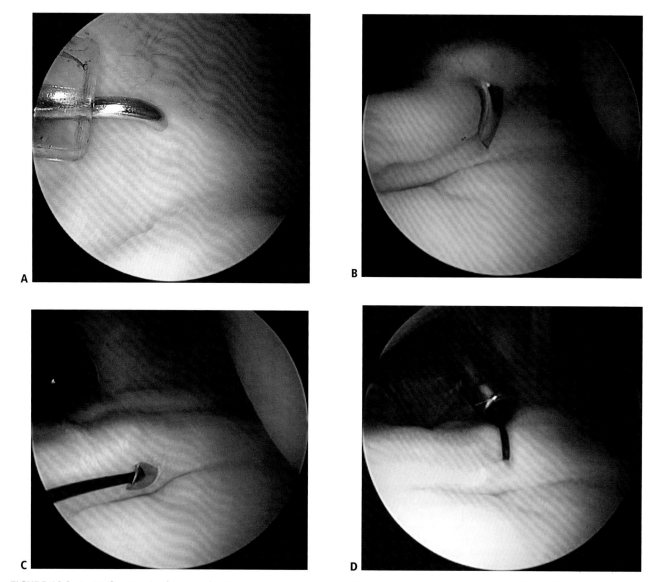

FIGURE 18.3. A–D: The steps in placing a plication suture are shown here. All views are of the posterior capsule of a left shoulder viewing from an anterior portal. First, a tissue-piercing suture passer is used to pass a suture through the capsule approximately 1 cm from the labrum **(A)**. Next the instrument is passed back through the capsule and into the joint **(B)**. The instrument is then passed through the labrum and the suture is fed into the joint **(C)**. In the final step, both ends of the suture are retrieved through the cannula and an arthroscopic knot is tied, with the post on the capsular tissue **(D)**.

plication sutures until the humeral head is centered in the glenoid and the capsule is balanced both anteriorly and posteriorly (Fig. 18.5).

Rotator Interval Closure

In order to close the rotator interval, the superior glenohumeral ligament is sutured to the middle glenohumeral ligament. The technique is similar to the technique for closing portals described earlier. A suture passer is used to pass a PDS suture through the superior glenohumeral ligament and coracohumeral ligament at the superior margin of the rotator interval. This can be retrieved using a tissue-penetrating suture grasper through the middle glenohumeral ligament. With both suture ends in the

anterior cannula, the cannula is backed out of the joint and the sutures tied outside the joint capsule (Fig. 18.6). One to two stitches can be placed, depending on the degree of laxity. Rotator interval closure will improve stability in multidirectional patterns of instability, but will not improve isolated unidirectional posterior instability (15). Rotator interval closure also has the risk of reducing external rotation.

Capsular Laxity with Bankart Lesion

Occasionally, in cases with capsular laxity, the labrum is detached either anteriorly or posteriorly. In these cases, the labrum must be repaired first with a standard Bankart or reverse Bankart repair using bioabsorbable suture

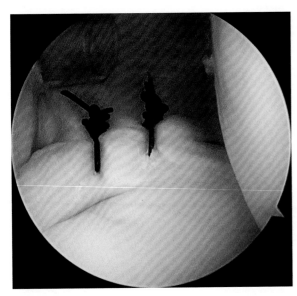

FIGURE 18.4. Completed posterior capsular plication with two plication sutures. Figure shows a left shoulder viewed from the anterior–superior portal.

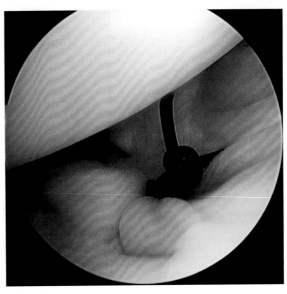

FIGURE 18.5. Completed anterior capsular plication with two plication sutures. Figure shows a left shoulder viewed from the posterior portal.

anchors for fixation. After fixation of the labrum, if there is still capsular redundancy, proceed with plication as described above.

Capsular Rent

Occasionally, instead of a pathologically lax capsule, the surgeon will instead find a torn capsule. These capsular rents can sometimes be identified preoperatively by MRI. In these cases, the rent can be repaired with a series of side-to-side sutures placed with an arthroscopic suture passer (Fig. 18.7).

AUTHOR'S PREFERRED TREATMENT

Surgery is reserved for the patient who has failed a good nonoperative program. The procedure begins with an examination under anesthesia of both shoulders with the patient in the supine position. This allows the surgeon to confirm the diagnosis and to assess the degree and direction of laxity present. A comparison exam of the unaffected shoulder is important to determine what normal laxity is for the individual patient.

We perform instability surgery in the lateral decubitus position. When positioning, care should be taken to ensure that the peroneal nerve is protected on the dependent leg. The area around the head should be clear for easy access to both the anterior and the posterior portals. The arm is placed in a padded arm holder and between 5 and 7 lb of weight is used for suspension. The idea is not to pull the shoulder out of the joint but to balance the humeral head over the glenoid. An arthroscopic pump is used with the pressure set initially at 30 mm Hg.

Prior to making an incision, a spinal needle is used to insufflate the glenohumeral joint with 30 cc of normal

saline from the posterior side. This helps to protect the articular surfaces when entering the joint. The posterior portal is established first. This portal should be made slightly more lateral than the standard portal used during rotator cuff surgery. Keeping the portal lateral and closer to the humeral head allows for easier access to the posterior capsule and labrum and allows for insertion of anchors into the glenoid if needed. A complete diagnostic arthroscopy is performed. Careful attention should be paid to the entire capsule–labral complex. The rotator interval is examined for signs of a stretch injury.

After the arthroscope is introduced posteriorly, an anterior portal is precisely located with an outside-in technique using a spinal needle. The spinal needle can confirm that the planned portal position allows access to all necessary areas of the joint. Precise localization is especially important if two anterior portals are to be used, in order to prevent the portals from being placed too close to one another.

After diagnostic arthroscopy, if the posterior capsule or labrum needs to be addressed, this is done prior to any anterior work. If needed, labral repairs are performed prior to capsular plication. The arthroscope is switched to the anterior superior portal and a 7-mm working cannula is placed posteriorly. If labral work is performed posteriorly, an accessory portal is needed for suture management. The senior author (A.S.C.) uses an anterior portal for this purpose in order to minimize trauma to the pathologic posterior capsule. If the posterior labrum is torn, this is repaired first since an intact labrum is necessary to anchor plication sutures. We prefer double-loaded 3.0-mm bioabsorbable suture anchors to reconstruct the inferior portion of the inferior glenohumeral ligament. Single-loaded 2.4-mm bioabsorbable anchors are used for the superior

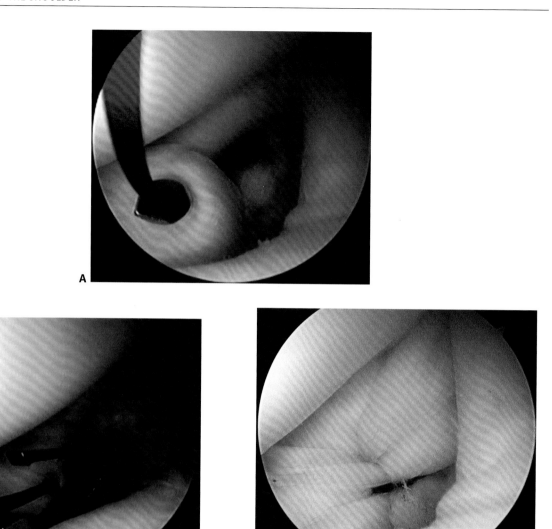

FIGURE 18.6. A–C: The steps in closing the rotator interval are shown. All views are of a left shoulder viewed from the posterior portal. A suture passer is used to place a suture through the inferior tissue of the rotator interval **(A)**. Next a tissue-penetrating suture grasper is passed through the superior tissue of the rotator interval and the suture is retrieved **(B)**. The suture is tied blindly inside the cannula on the outside of the capsule to complete the rotator interval closure **(C)**.

portion of the repair or to augment a dysplastic labrum prior to placing plication sutures.

Once any labral pathology has been addressed, the capsular plication is performed. The amount of plication needed is determined by the examination under anesthesia and the diagnostic arthroscopy. The goal is to finish the case with a reduced capsular volume and the humeral head balanced over the glenoid. PDS suture passed with a suture passing device is typically used for plication. If desired, the PDS may be used to shuttle a permanent suture. The first suture is placed at the level of the posterior inferior glenohumeral ligament. An approximately 1-cm capsular pass is made with the suture passer and this is brought to the labrum and sewn into the labrum. This is tied with the postsuture on the capsular side, keeping the knot away from the articular surface. This also allows the knot to push the capsule up to the labrum.

This first suture is not the most inferior of the plication sutures. The first suture creates a fold that extends inferiorly, which makes passage of a subsequent inferior plication suture much easier. It also serves to draw that capsule up and away from the axillary nerve, especially the more vulnerable posterior branch, which is a risk near the inferior aspect of the glenoid. A series of plication sutures are placed in the posterior capsule to reduce capsular laxity to the point where the capsule is balanced. Typically three to four sutures are placed in the posterior capsule during this procedure.

In cases of multidirectional instability, after completing the posterior plication, the arthroscope is then replaced in the posterior portal and the anterior capsule and labrum are addressed in a similar manner to achieve a balanced capsule. As with the posterior capsule, the first plication suture is placed at the level of the inferior glenohumeral

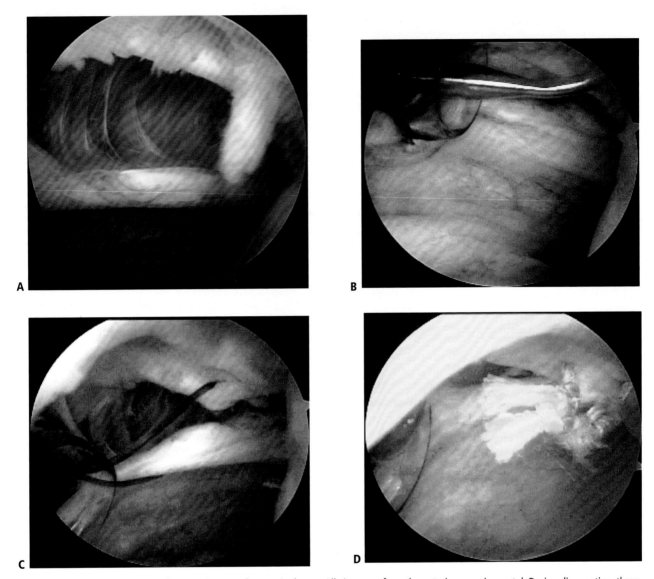

FIGURE 18.7. A–D: The repair of a posterior capsular rent is shown. All views are from the anterior-superior portal. During diagnostic arthroscopy, a posterior capsular rent is seen **(A)**. A curved suture passer is used to pass a PDS suture across the capsular rent **(B)**. The PDS suture is retrieved through the posterior cannula **(C)**. The PDS is used to shuttle a permanent suture, which is then tied with a standard arthroscopic knot. In this picture, two permanent sutures have been placed across the capsular rent **(D)**.

ligament and additional sutures are placed inferiorly and superiorly as required. After the sutures are placed, the arm is often taken out of suspension to ensure that a balanced capsule with a centered humeral head is achieved.

If necessary, based on the examination under anesthesia and diagnostic arthroscopy, the rotator interval is addressed next using the technique described earlier. One or two sutures are generally used for rotator interval closure.

As a final step, the posterior portal is closed. This is done in the fashion of the rotator interval closure. After the cannula is backed out to level of the capsule, an arthroscopic suture passer is used to pass one limb of a PDS suture through the capsule adjacent to the portal from outside to inside. A tissue-penetrating suture grasper is then passed from outside to inside on the other side of the portal and the suture is retrieved. Both suture limbs

are now exiting in the cannula and the cannula is backed up to just outside the capsule and the sutures are tied blindly. The pathology-specific repairs are summarized in Table 18.1.

REHABILITATION

Rehabilitation is progressed slowly in these patients. Stiffness is uncommon and an overzealous rehabilitation program puts the patient at increased risk of recurrent instability. Postoperatively, the patient is maintained in a pillow brace in neutral position for 5 weeks following surgery. At 5 weeks, they are allowed to begin active range of motion. The patients are assessed at the 5 and 8-week point to make sure they are regaining motion appropriately.

Table 18.1

Pathology-Specific Repairs

• Unidirectional posterior instability with posterior Bankart	• Repair posterior Bankart, ± posterior capsular plication
• Unidirectional posterior instability without Bankart	• Posterior capsular plication
• Bidirectional instability (posterior and inferior)	• Posterior capsular plication (especially inferior ligament) • Rotator interval closure
• Multidirectional instability	• Posterior and anterior capsular plication (especially inferior ligament) • Rotator interval closure
• Capsular rent	• Side-to-side suture repair
• RHAGL	• Suture anchor repair to humerus
• All cases	• EUA determines direction and degree of laxity • Close portals • Labral repair prior to capsular plication if labrum is torn

At 8 weeks, a formal physical therapy program working on active and active-assisted range of motion is started. Passive range of motion is not allowed. We like to have the patient in control of regaining their motion. In the third month, isometrics and scapular work are started, and the patients progress to full strengthening in the fourth month. It is typically 5 to 6 months before these patients return to full athletic activity.

COMPLICATIONS, CONTROVERSIES, AND SPECIAL CONSIDERATIONS

Fortunately, the complications after these arthroscopic procedures are rare. Recurrence of instability is perhaps the most common problem, especially in patients with multidirectional instability and generalized ligamentous laxity. We feel that a slow rehabilitation and adequate preoperative counseling are essential in these patients. Overtightening the capsule is a theoretical risk; however, in these patients with lax tissue it is rarely a problem.

Rotator interval closure is an area of controversy, and the exact indications for this procedure are unclear at this time. Rotator interval closure certainly can increase stability but may do so by limiting external rotation. Caution should be exercised prior to performing this procedure in athletes such a baseball pitchers and other overhead throwing athletes who require significant external rotation for their sport.

Neurologic injury is a possible complication. The axillary nerve is theoretically at risk during the placement of the most inferior capsular plication sutures. This risk can be minimized by keeping the suture passer just behind the capsular tissue in order to avoid injury to any deeper structures.

Thermal capsulorrhaphy was used extensively in the recent past to reduce capsular volume. Due to the significant complications associated with this technique, it is no longer recommended.

Perhaps the most important consideration prior to an arthroscopic stabilization procedure is recognizing the cases that are not amenable to arthroscopic treatment. Any case with significant bone loss should be treated open. Also, certain revisions, especially in the case of failed thermal capsulorrhaphy with the loss of capsular tissue, may benefit from an open reconstruction.

PEARLS AND PITFALLS

1. The examination under anesthesia of both shoulders is essential to define the magnitude and direction of instability.
2. The goal of the procedure is to balance the capsule in order to create a stable glenohumeral joint.
3. In each case, pathology-specific procedures can be employed to address the specific areas of pathology and the degree of laxity in each structure. Both the anterior and the posterior capsule and labrum can be addressed, as well as the rotator interval.
4. The posterior portal should be placed lateral away from the labrum to improve access to the posterior capsule and labrum.

5. Be alert to the possibility of a posterior dislocation in the emergency department or in follow-up as these are often missed, especially with inadequate radiographs.
6. Avoid surgical intervention in patients who have voluntary instability as it is difficult to achieve satisfactory results.

CONCLUSIONS

Arthroscopic techniques allow a greater understanding of the pathology and offer surgical treatments which have less morbidity for with posterior and multidirectional instability. Despite this fact, it is important to remember that most cases can be treated nonoperatively. If patients fail conservative treatment and require surgery, the key to a successful outcome is to tailor the procedure to the specific capsule, labral, or rotator interval pathology that is present in each case.

REFERENCES

1. Neer CS, Foster C. Inferior capsular shift for involuntary inferior and multidirectional instability of the shoulder. *J Bone Joint Surg Am.* 1980;62:897–908.
2. Hawkins RJ, Neer CS, Pianta RM, et al. Locked posterior dislocation of the shoulder. *J Bone Joint Surg Am.* 1987;69:9–18.
3. Burkhead WZ, Rockwood CA. Treatment of instability of the shoulder with an exercise program. *J Bone Joint Surg Am.* 1992;74:890–896.
4. Misamore GW, Sallay PI, Didelot W. A longitudinal study of patients with multidirectional instability of the shoulder with seven- to ten-year follow-up. *J Shoulder Elbow Surg.* 2005;14:466–470.
5. Bottoni CR, Franks BR, Moore JH, et al. Operative stabilization of posterior shoulder instability. *Am J Sports Med.* 2005;33:996–1002.
6. Bradley JP, Baker CL III, Kline AJ, et al. Arthroscopic capsulolabral reconstruction for posterior instability of the shoulder: a prospective study of 100 shoulders. *Am J Sports Med.* 2006;34:1061–1071.
7. Gartsman GM, Roddey TS, Hammerman SM. Arthroscopic treatment of multidirectional glenohumeral instability: 2- to 5-year follow-up. *Arthroscopy.* 2001;17:236–243.
8. Gartsman GM, Roddey TS, Hammerman SM. Arthroscopic treatment of bidirectional glenohumeral instability: two- to five-year follow-up. *J Shoulder Elbow Surg.* 2001;10:28–36.
9. Kim SH, Kim HK, Sun JI, et al. Arthroscopic capsulolabroplasty for posteroinferior multidirectional instability of the shoulder. *Am J Sports Med.* 2004; 32:594–607.
10. Kim SH, Ha KI, Park JH, et al. Arthroscopic posterior labral repair and capsular shift for traumatic unidirectional recurrent posterior subluxation of the shoulder. *J Bone Joint Surg Am.* 2003;85:1479–1487.
11. Savoie FH III, Holt MS, Field LD, Ramsey JR. Arthroscopic management of posterior instability: evolution of technique and results. *Arthroscopy.* 2008;24:389–396.
12. Treacy SH, Savoie FH III, Field LD. Arthroscopic treatment of multidirectional instability. *J Shoulder Elbow Surg.* 1999;8:345–350.
13. Flanigan DC, Forsythe T, Orwin J, et al. Volume analysis of arthroscopic capsular shift. *Arthroscopy.* 2006;22:528–533.
14. Shafer BL, Mihata T, McGarry MH, et al. Effects of capsular plication and rotator interval closure in simulated multidirectional shoulder instability. *J Bone Joint Surg Am.* 2008;90:136–144.
15. Mologne TS, Zhao K, Hongo M, et al. The addition of rotator interval closure after arthroscopic repair of either anterior or posterior shoulder instability: effect on glenohumeral translation and range of motion. *Am J Sports Med.* 2008; 36:1123–1131.

I. The Shoulder

HAGL Lesion: Diagnosis and Repair

Curtis R. Noel • Robert H. Bell

Anterior shoulder instability, whether acute or recurrent, can be associated with numerous pathologic entities. These entities can be seen in isolation or in multiple combinations, with the most commonly encountered deficit being the detachment of the anterior glenohumeral ligament–labral complex off the glenoid (the Perthes–Bankart lesion). Although disruption of the ligament–labral complex off the glenoid is the most common, avulsion of the glenohumeral ligament off its humeral insertion may also occur. Increasing knowledge about the mechanism of an anterior humeral avulsion of the glenohumeral ligament (HAGL), as well as advanced imaging and arthroscopic procedures, has led to better recognition and treatment of this pathologic entity. The diagnosis of a HAGL lesion requires a high index of suspicion along with the knowledge of the normal appearance of the glenohumeral ligament complex (Fig. 19.1) and the potential injury locations that may occur along its course.

The inferior glenohumeral ligament (IGHL) functions as the primary restraint to anterior, posterior, and inferior glenohumeral translation between 45° and 90° of humeral elevation or abduction. The IGHL has a defined anterior and posterior band with an interconnecting axillary pouch or hammock that rotates with respect to arm position. Therefore, in external rotation the complex tightens anteriorly and with internal rotation it tightens posteriorly. When viewing a right shoulder glenoid en face, the anterior band of the IGHL originates between the 2 and the 4 o'clock position and the posterior band originates from the 7 to 9 o'clock position (1). The IGHL complex attaches to the humerus just below the articular surface of the humeral head. Classically, this insertion has been described in two distinct variations: a collar-like attachment and a V-shaped attachment. (2, 20).

Bigliani et al. (3) tested the failure characteristics of the IGHL–labral complex. The labrum–ligament failed at the glenoid side 40% of the time, midsubstance of the IGHL 35% of the time, and from the humeral insertion 25% of the time. Gagey et al. (4) also studied shoulder dislocations in the laboratory and found a 63% incidence of humeral-sided ligament failure. Clinically, however, the incidence of HAGL lesions after anterior dislocations ranges from only 2% to 9.3% (5–7). To explain this disparity between the laboratory and the office, some authors have hypothesized that the dynamic shoulder stabilizers, specifically the subscapularis, protect the IGHL at its humeral insertion (8).

Nicola (1) was the first, in 1942, to identify (in four out of five surgically treated shoulder dislocations) the avulsion of the capsule from the neck of the humerus. Forty-six years later Bach et al. (9) described two more cases in which the inferior and lateral humeral insertions of the shoulder capsule were disrupted. In 1995, Wolf et al. coined the acronym HAGL for humeral avulsion of the glenohumeral ligaments. In their series of 82 patients, Wolf et al. (7) reported a 9.3% incidence of a HAGL lesion. In another large series, Bokor et al. (5) reported a HAGL incidence of 7.5% in 547 shoulders. When no Bankart lesion is identified in an anterior shoulder dislocation, the incidence of a HAGL lesion may be as high as 35% to 39% (5, 7), emphasizing the need to evaluate for HAGL lesions in shoulder injuries.

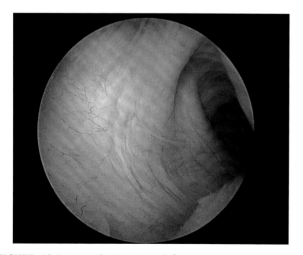

FIGURE 19.1. Normal IGHL viewed from posterior portal with a 30° scope.

CLINICAL EVALUATION

Pertinent History

The evaluation of the patient begins with obtaining the standard history and physical examination. Most patients will present with the complaint of shoulder instability after a violent traumatic event. However, there is one report of a HAGL lesion occurring after repetitive microtrauma associated with overhand throwing (10).

Physical Examination

The physical examination consists of the standard testing for shoulder instability including inspection, range of motion, strength testing, and special stability testing (apprehension test, load and shift, posterior jerk test, and inferior sulcus). Unfortunately, there is no single physical examination finding that will help differentiate a HAGL lesion from a more commonly encountered Bankart lesion and/or capsular laxity.

Imaging

Plain radiographs should be evaluated but are not often very useful in diagnosing a HAGL lesion. Occasionally, 20% of plain radiographs will reveal a bony sliver off the anterior humerus associated with a bony HAGL or BHAGL lesion (11). Otherwise, the standard shoulder radiographs should be obtained to evaluate adequate glenohumeral reduction, as well as bone loss and version on the humerus and glenoid.

A MRI study is recommended for the evaluation of the IGHL complex as well as the labrum and rotator cuff. A HAGL lesion will show up on the axial and coronal oblique images as irregularities in the humeral capsular attachment to the humerus. An MRI arthrogram will improve the specificity of the study and will demonstrate extravasation of contrast material through the region of the capsular avulsion from the humeral neck. On the sagittal oblique images, the normal axillary pouch is U-shaped, but when a HAGL is present, the axillary pouch may form a J-shape as the IGHL falls away from the humerus (11) (Fig. 19.2). In the acute setting, the increased intraarticular fluid may produce images similar to the arthrogram. Even though the MRI and MRI arthrogram are good at identifying capsular disruptions, they can miss up to 50% of the lesions (11). Once again, HAGL lesions can be associated with other pathologies (Hill–Sachs lesions, labral tear, and rotator cuff tears) and therefore, vigilance must be maintained whenever arthroscopically evaluating the glenohumeral joint.

Decision-Making Algorithms and Classification

Diagnostic arthroscopy allows for the inspection of entire glenohumeral complex and its insertions on the glenoid and humerus (18). A HAGL lesion can be identified

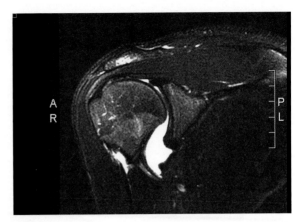

FIGURE 19.2. MRI showing a HAGL with the "J" sign of the inferior capsule.

through the posterior portal with the 30° arthroscope. The lesion can be further defined with a 70° scope and/or visualizing the capsule through the anterior portal. The HAGL lesion will appear as a defect in the anterior capsule, ranging from thin attenuation of the capsular fibers to complete ligament avulsion with visualization of the subscapularis muscle fibers (Figs. 19.3 and 19.4). Internal and external rotation of the humerus will also assist in the accurate diagnosis of a HAGL lesion, allowing the humeral capsular footprint to be visualized and demonstrating the lack of capsular movement during rotation due to the loss of humeral attachment.

Based on the patterns of injury, Bui-Mansfield et al. proposed a classification system for avulsions of the anterior humeral glenohumeral ligament complex. HAGL injuries can be described as capsular avulsions off the humerus (HAGL), bony avulsions off the humerus (BHAGL), and a combination of Bankart lesion and HAGL or floating HAGL (12, 18). Another subset of HAGL injury has been described in which the injury occurs in the mid-substance of the anterior glenohumeral ligament (13).

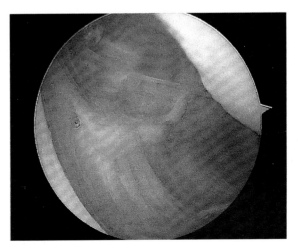

FIGURE 19.3. HAGL lesion seen through the posterior portal.

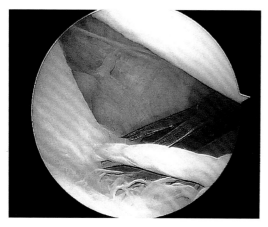
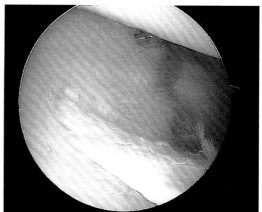

FIGURE 19.4. Reduction of a HAGL with a grasper.

Even though less frequently encountered, one must be ever vigilant for a HAGL lesion, and whenever identified the pathologic lesion must be anatomically repaired in order to restore stability to the shoulder. Over two-thirds of HAGL lesions occur with concomitant shoulder pathology (11), underscoring the importance of complete arthroscopic shoulder evaluations.

TREATMENT

Controversy exists on whether to treat first time dislocators, especially the young dislocator, operatively or with immobilization and physical therapy. We are unaware of any studies reporting the nonoperative treatment of HAGL lesions. Therefore, if identified by preoperative imaging, we recommend surgical repair of the avulsed ligament complex. As with most ligament or tendon injury, early intervention allows for easier repair before scarring and retraction sets in. Surgery may be performed in the beach chair or in the lateral decubitus position, and the lesion repaired with either open or arthroscopic techniques.

In 1988, Bach et al. (9) described the successful open repair of two patients with HAGL lesions. Bokor et al. (5) also repaired the HAGL lesions in their series through an open approach using either drill holes or suture anchors with good results. Similarly, Arciero and Mazzocca (14) described a mini-open technique for HAGL repair in eight patients in which the upper 50% of the subscapularis was spared and the ligament repaired with suture anchors. In their series, there were no recurrences and all patients returned to preoperative activity levels (14).

Wolf et al. first reported an arthroscopic repair of the HAGL lesion in four out of six patients. In this series, sutures were passed through the capsule and tied over the deltopectoral fascia. The other two patients underwent open repair with drill holes (7). Richards and Burkhart (15) described an all-arthroscopic repair using suture anchors in the lateral decubitus position in two patients, as did Spang and Karas (16). Kon et al. described using the beach chair position with their arthroscopic HAGL repairs.

AUTHORS' PREFERRED TREATMENT

We prefer using the lateral decubitus position and an all-arthroscopic technique when possible. Normally, the patient receives an interscalene block followed by a general anesthesia. Once anesthetized a formal examination under anesthesia is performed comparing the surgical shoulder with the nonoperative side. The patient is then placed in the lateral decubitus position and the arm sterilely prepped and draped. Dual traction is used to optimize joint distraction by using either a bump in the axilla or the STaR Sleeve (Arthrex, Naples, FL) (Fig. 19.5). Five to ten pounds of longitudinal traction is applied with the arm placed in 30° to 40° of abduction. The axillary bump or axillary strap of the STaR Sleeve is then placed in the armpit to apply lateral distraction of the glenohumeral joint.

A posterior portal is established by moving the standard portal slightly lateral and superior toward the posterior corner of the acromion. By moving this portal and aiming toward the superior aspect of the joint, we are better able to look around the humerus and visualize the capsular avulsion and its footprint without switching to a 70° arthroscope. Placing the portal "high" in the joint also makes it easier to treat posterior labral or capsular

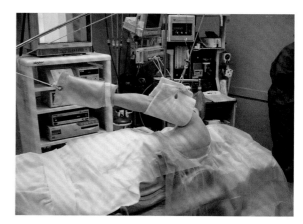

FIGURE 19.5. Dual traction system.

pathology when encountered. A diagnostic scope is then performed, carefully inspecting the rotator cuff, the biceps tendon, and the labrum (superior, anterior, inferior, and posterior). After assessing the bony anatomy of the glenoid and the potential Hill–Sachs lesion on the humerus, we routinely enter the axillary pouch. With rotation of the camera, the IGHL complex can be visualized from labrum to the humeral head insertion.

After performing a diagnostic scope, two anterior portals are established using an outside-in technique (Fig. 19.6). The anteroinferior portal is created just lateral to the coracoid, with the 18G spinal needle hugging

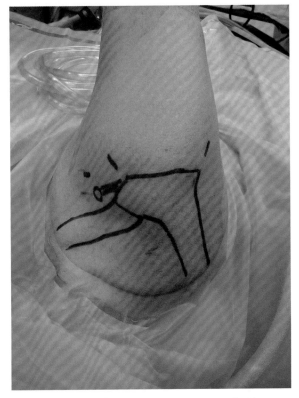

FIGURE 19.6. Portal placement: high posterior portal with an anteroinferior and anterosuperior portal.

the intra-articular portion of the subscapularis. The 18G needle can then be used to verify the appropriate approach to the humeral head for anchor placement. The anterosuperior portal is established off the anterior corner of the acromion with the 18G needle hugging the biceps tendon. An 8.25-mm cannula is placed in the anteroinferior portal, and a switching stick is placed in the anterosuperior portal. The camera is then switched to the anterosuperior portal and a 5.25-mm cannula is inserted in the posterior portal.

Occasionally, it is necessary to establish an anterior 5 o'clock portal or trans-subscapularis portal. This portal can be helpful for passing suture through the capsule and for allowing a better approach for anchor insertion on the humeral footprint. In addition, a separate posterior inferior portal may also be used as an additional working portal for suture management and to allow access to the more inferior aspect of the humeral head in large HAGL lesions (6).

Preparation of the capsular footprint begins by placing a motorized shaver or burr into the anteroinferior portal and a light decortication of the humeral surface is performed. Internal rotation of the shoulder brings the footprint into view, allowing for debridement of the footprint and creation of a trough (Fig. 19.7). Other authors have advocated external or neutral rotation when using a 5 o'clock portal, but we have found that internal rotation improves the visualization of the footprint and improves the angle of insertion of the anchors through the anteroinferior portal. The repair of the HAGL begins inferiorly and progresses superiorly toward the camera. The first anchor is placed either through the anteroinferior portal or through a trans-subscapularis portal, depending on which provides the optimum angle of insertion. Although we prefer suture anchors, knotless anchor systems can also be used.

A 3.0-mm anchor is inserted in the inferior aspect of the humeral footprint, and the suture limbs are retrieved out the posterior portal. The sutures can then be shuttled through the lateral edge of the avulsed ligaments using various instruments. We prefer using a Suturelasso (Arthrex, Naples, FL) or Spectrum suture passer (ConMed Linvatec, Largo, FL). If using a hooked suture-passing

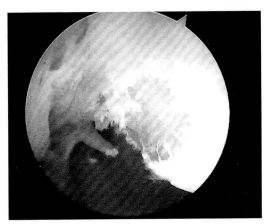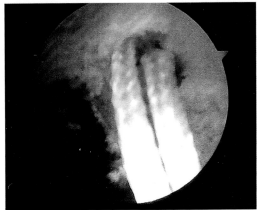

FIGURE 19.7. Debridement of humeral footprint and placement of anchor.

instrument, the suture (no. 1 monofilament) or nitinol wire is passed through the ligament and retrieved through the posterior portal. One limb of the anchor suture is then tied or placed in the nitinol loop and shuttled back through the tissue. The process can be repeated if a horizontal mattress suture knot is desired. Both limbs are then retrieved through the anteroinferior portal and tied using any combination of sliding knots or alternating half-hitches. These steps are repeated until adequate repair of the HAGL has occurred (Figs. 19.8 and 19.9A,B).

The camera is placed back in the posterior portal where the repair is further evaluated and the determination of whether or not to perform a rotator interval closure is made. If other shoulder pathology is present (rotator cuff tear, labral tear, or superior labral anterior posterior [SLAP] tear), then that pathology is addressed.

COMPLICATIONS AND SPECIAL CONSIDERATIONS

If at any time during the arthroscopic repair of a HAGL we feel that the pathology is not being adequately addressed, we do not hesitate to convert to a mini-open approach to

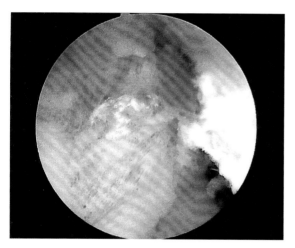

FIGURE 19.8. HAGL repair viewed through anterosuperior portal.

the shoulder as described by Arciero and Mazzoca (14). Through a mini-deltoid splitting or a deltopectoral approach, the upper one-third of the subscapularis is taken down and the ligament complex repaired with suture anchors or drill holes through bone.

As previously mentioned, the anterior glenohumeral ligament complex can be injured in association with other pathologic entities, such as a Bankart tear (19). If encountered in combination, the HAGL is repaired first, followed by the Bankart to avoid overtightening of the anterior capsule. Schippinger et al. (17) described a HAGL occurring after the successful repair of a Bankart tear. Mid-substance ligament tears may be encountered and treated arthroscopically as well (13). Similarly, the posterior glenohumeral ligament complex can be avulsed off the humeral head and can be repaired arthroscopically. The approach and steps are similar to an anterior HAGL repair, but is outside the scope of this chapter.

PEARLS AND PITFALLS

Identification is the key to the treatment of humeral avulsions of the glenohumeral ligament. One should become familiar with the normal appearance of the anterior capsule and its insertion on the humerus. Routine diagnostic arthroscopies should evaluate the labrum and the course of the anterior ligament to its insertion on the humerus. This can easily be done with a 30° arthroscope in the axillary pouch, directing the scope toward the humeral insertion. One may need to place the scope in the anterior portal or utilize a 70° scope to fully examine the anterior capsule. Because HAGL lesions occur along with other shoulder pathology up to two-thirds of the time, one must be vigilant for the possibility of humeral ligament avulsion. A thorough shoulder examination looking at all aspects of the shoulder should be routinely performed to decrease the possibility of missing other shoulder pathology.

Once identified, the next key component of the repair is obtaining the correct angle for anchor insertion. This is controlled by portal placement and rotation of the

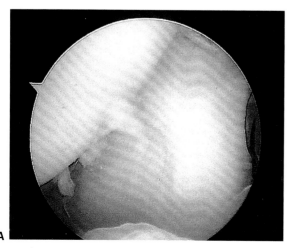
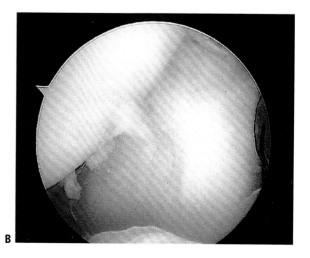

FIGURE 19.9. A, B: HAGL repairs viewed through posterior portal.

humerus. By using an outside-in technique with an 18G needle, one can verify the angle of the anchor placement. We have found that most of the work can be done through a properly positioned anteroinferior portal. With this portal, internal rotation helps bring the humeral footprint into view and ensures that anchor placement is more perpendicular to the humerus. When the anteroinferior portal approach is not adequate, then a trans-subscapularis or 5 o'clock portal may be used. When using this portal, Richards and Burkhart (15) emphasized that abduction and external rotation must be maintained.

REHABILITATION

After surgery the patient is placed in a sling and swathe and will continue the sling for approximately 6 to 8 weeks. For the first week, the shoulder is kept quiet in the sling, only removing the arm for gentle elbow range of motion and to shower and dress. Formal physical therapy begins after week 1, with active range of motion of the hand-wrist-elbow and Phase I (passive) exercises of the shoulder. Passive shoulder motion is limited to 0° of external rotation and 90° of forward elevation in the scapular plane for 4 weeks. Beginning at week 4 and continuing until week 8, motion is slowly increased to 40° of external rotation and 140° of forward elevation.

Phase II begins around week 6 with cane and pulley exercises. After 8 weeks, range of motion is increased to full and the sling is discontinued. Light resistance exercises begin around the eighth week and progress slowly. A more formal strengthening program is initiated around 12 weeks. Return to contact sporting activities occurs at 6 months after surgery.

CONCLUSIONS AND FUTURE DIRECTIONS

Shoulder arthroscopy has improved the recognition and treatment of various shoulder pathologies. Although infrequently encountered, surgeons need to be aware of injuries to the glenohumeral ligament on the humeral side. Although technically demanding, arthroscopic treatment of humeral avulsions of the glenohumeral ligament has produced excellent results. Future studies with larger patient populations and long-term follow-up will provide more information on the effectiveness of arthroscopic treatment of HAGL lesions.

REFERENCES

1. Nicola T. Anterior dislocation of the shoulder. *J Bone Joint Surg Am.* 1942;24:614–616.
2. Turkel SJ, Panio MW, Marshall JL, et al. Stabilizing mechanisms preventing anterior dislocation of the glenohumeral joint. *J Bone Joint Surg Am.* 1981;63:1208–1217.
3. Bigliani JU, Pollock RG, Soslowsky LJ, et al. Tensile properties of the inferior glenohumeral ligament. *J Orthop Res.* 1992;10:187–197.
4. Gagey O, Gagey N, Boisrenoult P, et al. Experimental study of dislocations of the scapulohumeral joint [in French]. *Rev Chir Orthop Reparatrice Appar Mot.* 1993;79:13–21.
5. Bokor DJ, Conboy VB, Olson C. Anterior instability of the glenohumeral joint with humeral avulsion of the glenohumeral ligament: a review of 41 cases. *J Bone Joint Surg Br.* 1999;81:93–96.
6. Rhee YG, Cho NS. Anterior shoulder instability with humeral avulsion of the glenohumeral ligament lesion. *J Shoulder Elbow Surg.* 2007;16:188–192.
7. Wolf EM, Cheng JC, Dickson K. Humeral avulsion of glenohumeral ligaments as a cause of anterior shoulder instability. *Arthroscopy.* 1995;11:600–607.
8. Parameswaran AD, Provencher MT, Bach BR, et al. Humeral avulsion of the glenohumeral ligament: injury pattern and arthroscopic repair techniques. *Orthopedics.* 2008;31:773–779.
9. Bach BR, Warren RF, Fronek J. Disruption of the lateral capsule of the shoulder: a cause of anterior shoulder instability. *J Bone Joint Surg Br.* 1988;70:274–276.
10. Gehrman RM, DeLuca PF, Bartolozzi AR. Humeral avulsion of the glenohumeral ligament caused by microtrauma to the anterior capsule in an overhand throwing athlete: a case report. *Am J Sports Med.* 2003;31:617–619.
11. Bui-Mansfield LT, Taylor DC, Uhorchak JM, et al. Humeral avulsions of the glenohumeral ligament: imaging features and a review of the literature. *AJR AM J Roentgenol.* 2002;179:649–655.
12. Bui-Mansfield LT, Banks KP, Taylor DC. Humeral avulsion of the glenohumeral ligaments. *Am J Sports Med.* 2007;35:1960–1966.
13. Mizuno N, Yoneda M, Hayashida K, et al. Recurrent anterior shoulder dislocation caused by a midsubstance complete capsular tear. *J Bone Joint Surg Am.* 2005;87:2717–2723.
14. Arciero RA, Mazzocca AD. Mini-open repair technique of the HAGL (humeral avulsion of the glenohumeral ligament) lesion. *Arthroscopy.* 2005;21:1152e1–1152e4.
15. Richards DP, Burkhart SS. Arthroscopic humeral avulsion of the glenohumeral ligaments (HAGL) repair. *Arthroscopy.* 2004;20:134–141.
16. Spang JT, Karas SG. The HAGL lesion: an arthroscopic technique for repair of humeral avulsion of the glenohumeral ligaments. *Arthroscopy.* 2005;21:498–502.
17. Schippinger G, Vasiu PS, Fankhauser F, et al. HAGL lesion occurring after successful arthroscopic Bankart repair. *Arthroscopy.* 2001;17:206–208.
18. Fiel LD, Bokor DJ, Savoie FH III. Humeral and glenoid detachment of the anterior inferior glenohumeral ligament: a cause of anterior shoulder instability. *J Shoulder Elbow Surg.* 1997;6:6–10.
19. O'Brien SJ, Neves MC, Arnoczky SP, et al. The anatomy and histology of the inferior glenohumeral ligament complex of the shoulder. *Am J Sports Med.* 1990;18:449–456.
20. Warner JJP, Beim GM. Combined Bankart and HAGL lesion associated with anterior shoulder instability. *Arthroscopy.* 1997;13:749–752.

Arthroscopic Approach to the Throwing Athlete

Milford H. Marchant Jr. • Ronald E. Glousman

The painful shoulder in the overhead-throwing athlete has been a remarkable challenge to orthopedic surgeons and researchers for over 25 years. Several injury mechanisms and multiple factors contributing to shoulder pathology have been recognized over time, yet numerous questions regarding the etiology and optimal treatment strategies are still unanswered.

Similar to other areas of orthopedics, research regarding the painful thrower's shoulder has undergone an evolution. Early investigations focusing on external impingent of the rotator cuff led to examination of the anterior capsule and the concept of microinstability. As clinical examination and arthroscopic techniques evolved, focus shifted toward the biceps anchor, labral injury secondary to internal impingement, and posterior capsular tightness in painful throwing shoulders. More recently, scapular kinematic alterations have received attention, and now there is more focus on trunk and pelvic stability. Although patient complaints and pathoanatomy present as joint-specific injury patterns, evaluation of the entire athlete is essential to appropriately guide the athlete back to preinjury participation, regardless of the need for surgical intervention. As arthroscopic surgeons, we cannot only aid in discovering and correcting the throwers' mechanical flaws that led to their injured shoulder, but we can also attempt to repair the pathoanatomic results of misguided biomechanics.

THROWING MECHANICS

While athletes in sports such as football, lacrosse, and tennis have injuries secondary to overhead stress, baseball, particularly pitching, serves as the prime example for throwing-related shoulder pathology. Shoulder injuries in baseball start early—the prevalence of shoulder pain has been reported to be as high as 35% in youth and adolescent pitchers.

Pitching is a complex series of motions that places tremendous repetitive stress on the athlete's shoulder and elbow joints. Energy generated in the lower extremities is amplified and transferred by the pelvis and trunk to the upper extremity where the shoulder acts as a force regulator to the arm, providing the delivery of force.

The pitching motion can be divided into six phases: windup, early cocking, late cocking, acceleration, deceleration, and follow through (Fig. 20.1).

Phase I, or windup, initiates the pitching cycle. The lead foot leaves the ground and the trunk and shoulders coil, storing energy for delivery. The center of gravity remains over the pivot foot. Both hands are in contact with the ball, and the pitching arm is relatively relaxed. The windup phase ends when the ball leaves the gloved hand.

Phase II is the early cocking phase. After the ball leaves the glove, the pitching arm begins to be positioned for delivery. The shoulder is abducted and begins external

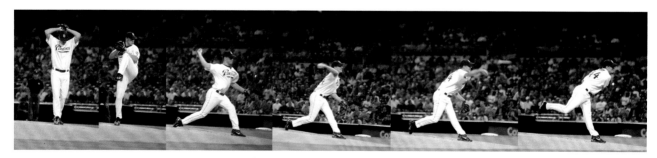

FIGURE 20.1. Six stages of throwing: (1) windup; (2) early cocking; (3) late cocking; (4) acceleration; (5) deceleration; and (6) follow through. (Reproduced with permission from Thomas WA, Hoenecke HR, Fronek J. Throwing injuries. In: Jonhson DH, Pedowitz RA, eds. *Practical Orthopaedic Sports Medicine and Arthroscopy*. 1st ed. Philadelphia, PA: Lippincott Williams & Wilkins; 2007:309–321.)

rotation, the elbow is high, slightly flexed, and the hand remains on top of the ball. The deltoid and rotator cuff muscles are active. Leading with the pelvis, the center of gravity shifts toward home plate, and the stride begins with the lead foot.

Phase III is the late cocking phase. The late cocking phase begins with lead foot contact toward home plate. The shoulders start closed, and the linear momentum gained during the stride shifts to rotational momentum during the trunk turn. The arm abducts to just above 90° so that the elbow is slightly above the shoulder, and the shoulder achieves maximum external rotation. The rotator cuff is highly active. It is not uncommon for a pitcher's shoulder to achieve 120° to 140° of external rotation. Although controversial, the humeral head position is thought to move in a posterior direction. During the same time, the anterior force on the shoulder approaches 400 N. The trapezius and the serratus anterior act as a force couple to stabilize the scapula. Late cocking ends at the point of maximum humeral external rotation.

Phase IV is the acceleration phase. Acceleration begins simply when the ball starts moving toward home plate. The potential energy built up in the lower extremities and trunk is finally transferred to the arm. This portion of the pitching cycle produces unparalleled forces in the shoulder. The force at the glenohumeral joint is estimated to be 860 N. Shoulder internal rotation exceeds 7,000° per second (1). The subscapularis exhibits high activity. Acceleration ends with ball release.

Phase V is the deceleration phase and compromises the first one-third of the time after ball release. Weight transfer from the pivot foot to the lead has finished. The shoulder is still hard at work as the rotator cuff initiates a strong eccentric contraction to slow down the internal rotation. The biceps and brachialis muscles have also been shown to initiate a strong eccentric contraction. Other muscles about the shoulder including the trapezius, serratus anterior, rhomboids, posterior deltoid, latissimus dorsi, and teres minor all activate to slow the shoulder and prevent subluxation.

Phase VI is the final follow-through stage. It compromises the latter two-thirds of the time after ball release. Shoulder adduction is followed by relaxation.

Every pitcher's delivery is different, and these differences can stress various parts of the shoulder. Regardless of pitching style, there are certain points in the pitching cycle that when executed poorly can cause pain or dysfunction. It is important to recognize that subtle differences in pitching form can translate into subtle differences in the shoulder pathology of injured players.

CLINICAL EVALUATION

History

The clinical evaluation of a thrower with shoulder pain starts with a detailed history. Patient age and the onset of

injury are important. It is also essential to know whether the patient had previous injuries or surgical interventions, as these factors can influence decision making.

In young players, particularly those with open physes, it is critical to know their level of competition. Do they pitch? How often do they pitch? Do they rest between outings? When they do not pitch what position are they playing? How many months out of the year do they not play baseball? What pitches are they throwing? Do they pitch in showcases? These questions are often difficult for children or parents to answer, but it is important to distinguish an acute injury from an overuse injury. Physeal injuries and capsular laxity are common in young overhead athletes, and typically, these patients can be treated without surgery.

In older adult players, the acuity of the problem is often difficult to ascertain. The patient may have trouble remembering the exact onset of symptoms, but it is important to know the last time the player participated fully without pain. In some instances, it may be months or years since the onset of symptoms, and this represents a completely different clinical picture than someone with pain for just a few weeks.

Other important questions to ask both young and older age groups include joint-specific and sport-specific questions. Where in the shoulder does pain occur? When in the throwing cycle does the pain occur? Posterior shoulder pain associated with late cocking or early acceleration can involve the labrum or rotator cuff. Is the pain present all the time or after throwing? During which inning does the arm start to hurt? Is the pain associated with the feeling of instability? Has there been any loss in velocity or control? Is the loss in velocity or control because of pain or fatigue? Are there mechanical symptoms such as clicking or grinding? Does the pain radiate down the arm? Does the patient experience the sensation of the arm "going dead"?

Finally, it is important to know why the patient came to see the doctor. Are you the first, second, or third opinion? After an acute injury, the problem is usually focused. However, in the patient with a long-standing problem, the reason for the visit may be more complex. For example, the goals of a patient coming in after a season of pain often differs from the patient coming in right at the onset of symptoms. It is important to understand not only the potential pathology in the patient but also the goals of the player with regard to future playing plans.

Physical Examination

Evaluation of a thrower with shoulder pain requires a global assessment, as pathology in the glenohumeral joint could be the result of breakdown anywhere in the kinetic chain. Although actual observation of the patient in action is not always possible in the clinic, a ground up approach should be taken. Asking the patient to simulate the throwing motion evaluates footwork and timing. The one-legged stance and squat can assess pelvic and core stability. For example, in the dynamic Trendelenburg test, a pitcher should be able to perform a single-leg half squat without ipsilateral femoral adduction, internal rotation, or contralateral pelvic drop and trunk lean (2). Proper pitching mechanics require a stable foundation.

Evaluating the upper extremity in a thrower expands the standard adult shoulder exam of inspection, palpation, range of motion, strength, and stability testing. Visual inspection of the thrower's posture, scapular position, and resting arm position is important. It is likely that the pitching or throwing arm will be overdeveloped in relation to the contralateral side, and slight asymmetry in scapular position may be present. While standing behind the patient, scapulothoracic motion should be assessed by having the patient perform active forward flexion of both upper extremities followed by a wall push-up. Gross asymmetry at rest and with motion or ipsilateral winging suggests scapular dyskinesis (Fig. 20.2). Prominence of the inferomedial border of the scapula at rest is often caused by weakness of the rhomboids, levator scapulae, and serratus anterior muscles that allow inferior displacement, lateral displacement, abduction, and protraction of the scapula in relation to the contralateral side (3). At the level of the glenoid, this produces an unbalanced platform for the humeral head, which can lead to injury of the glenohumeral joint.

Throwers often cannot point to the exact spot that elicits symptoms, particularly if labral pathology is involved. Instead, patients may complain of vague anterior or posterior pain, and very frequently complain of pain "deep" in the shoulder. Therefore, palpation may not pinpoint the diagnosis. However, thorough palpation of the shoulder region may identify periscapular crepitus or other associated symptoms such as tenderness over the biceps tendon or the acromioclavicular (AC) joint.

Standard range of motion testing should be followed by careful examination of glenohumeral rotation. Several longitudinal studies have shown that developmental changes in the shoulder capsule and an acquired proximal humeral retroversion lead to an arc shift that favors external rotation of the throwing arm. While supine with the arm abducted to 90°, throwing athletes, particularly pitchers, may have an additional 10° to 20° of external rotation and an equivalent loss of internal rotation in the throwing arm. However, the total arc should be within 10° to 15° of the contralateral limb. Loss of total arc with an associated glenohumeral internal rotation deficit (GIRD) >40° is pathologic and suggests a tight posterior capsule (Fig. 20.3).

Examination of shoulder strength involves testing the large motors (deltoid, pectoralis major, biceps, and triceps) as well as scapular and glenohumeral stabilizers. The rotator cuff is the primary dynamic stabilizer of the glenohumeral joint. Supraspinatus weakness or alterations in the force couple between the infraspinatus, teres minor, and the subscapularis can lead to altered kinematics throughout late cocking, acceleration, or deceleration phases. Although not entirely specific, supraspinatus strength is generally tested against resistance by comparison with the contralateral side, holding the arm in 90° of abduction and in the plane of the scapula. The infraspinatus is tested with resisted external rotation while the arm is held at the patient's side, and the teres minor is tested by resisting external rotation with the arm forward flexed approximately 45°. The subscapularis is tested

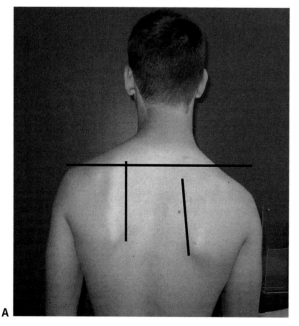
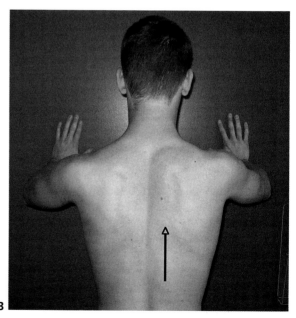

FIGURE 20.2. Scapular asymmetry. **A:** Sag of the dominant right shoulder with scapular abduction, inferior displacement, lateral displacement, and prominence of the inferior medial border. **B:** Prominence of the medial border of the scapula with wall press suggestive of dyskinesia.

I. The Shoulder

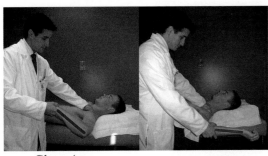

<u>Glove Arm</u>   Total Arc ≈ 150°

A

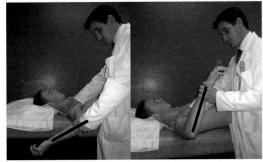

<u>Pitching Arm</u>   Total Arc ≈ 135°

B

FIGURE 20.3. Shoulder internal and external rotation. **A:** Glove-arm shoulder demonstrates relatively normal internal and external rotation with a total arc of approximately 150°. **B:** Pitching shoulder with increased external rotation, a loss of internal rotation, and a loss in total arc (135°) consistent with a tight posterior capsule.

with a posterior liftoff test and belly press maneuver (4). In addition to an abnormal wall push-up, scapular retraction with the belly press correlates with periscapular weakness.

Anterior and posterior stability testing should be performed routinely. In addition to load-shift maneuvers and sulcus testing, the Jobe relocation test is a provocative maneuver that can detect subtle anterior instability and internal impingement (5). While lying supine, the patient's arm is abducted to 90°, and maximum external rotation stress is applied. If anterior pain or apprehension is noted, it may be consistent with anterior instability symptoms. If a posteriorly directed force to the proximal humerus relieves the patient's symptoms, or if an anterior force to the humerus worsens the patient's symptoms (reverse relocation), the diagnosis of anterior instability is reinforced (Fig. 20.4). If posterior pain is elicited with abduction-external rotation testing, then internal impingement should be suspected.

Other provocative tests include the Neer forward flexion maneuver and the Hawkins abduction internal rotation exam for external impingement. The O'Brien active compression test examines the glenoid labrum and biceps anchor. Pain with resisted forward flexion, adduction, and internal rotation of the shoulder joint, relieved

with external rotation of the shoulder joint, is suspicious for superior labral pathology (Fig. 20.5). Speed's test, Yergason's maneuver, Andrew's clunk test, and the anterior slide test also stress the glenohumeral joint in an attempt to identify labral or biceps pathology (6). Currently, there is no single exam or test that can reliably delineate the solitary cause of internal derangement in the glenohumeral joint, but in combination, they can assist in formulating a differential diagnosis and orchestrating a treatment plan (7).

Imaging

Plain radiographs should be obtained to evaluate osseous abnormalities. Anterior–posterior (AP), scapular-Y, and axillary views should be routinely obtained. Glenohumeral rotation views can be ordered as necessary—the external rotation view is helpful in evaluating a young pitcher with proximal humeral epiphysiolysis. If patients have a current or past history of dislocation, the Stryker notch view is helpful in demonstrating the presence of a Hill–Sachs lesion. Standard radiographs can be helpful in identifying rotator cuff calcific tendinopathy, AC arthropathy, and exostosis of the posterior-inferior glenoid, or Bennett lesion. Although the Bennett lesion may be symptomatic, it is usually an incidental finding, and other sources of pathology should be ruled out prior to treatment of a Bennett lesion (8).

CT scanning, especially with three-dimensional reconstruction, provides enhanced evaluation of bony architecture but lacks the ability to assess the soft tissue envelope. CT scanning is not used routinely in the evaluation of throwers with shoulder pain. CT arthrography can be helpful in diagnosing full thickness rotator cuff tears and anterior labral injury but is not so reliable when evaluating partial thickness rotator cuff tears or injuries to the posterior or superior labrum.

MRI usually follows plain radiography and represents the diagnostic tool of choice for shoulder injuries in a thrower. MRI is helpful in the diagnosis of rotator cuff disease and labral pathology, including superior labrum anterior and posterior (SLAP) tears, anterior capsulolabral pathology, and perilabral cysts. Gadolinium-enhanced magnetic resonance arthrography (MRA) is thought to improve the reliability of diagnosing superior labral injuries and partial thickness rotator cuff tears. Extravasation of contrast under the superior labrum on the oblique, coronal, and axial views (Fig. 20.6) is indicative of a SLAP injury. The rotator cuff can be evaluated on several views; however, the oblique coronal provides an excellent view of the rotator cuff insertion. Anterior capsulolabral labral injury, perilabral cysts, and humeral avulsion injuries are best seen on the axial projections.

After the appropriate imaging studies, if there is any doubt as to the presence or the significance of the labral tear, other sources of pain should be considered.

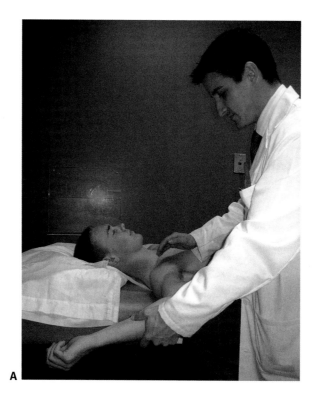

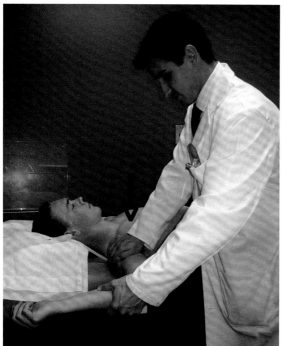

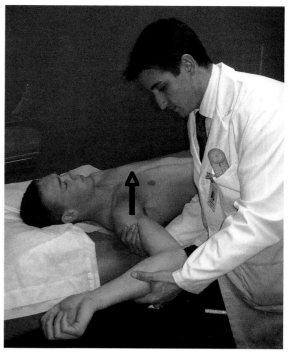

FIGURE 20.4. Jobe's relocation test. **A:** Lying supine, the arm is stressed in abduction and external rotation. Pain or apprehension is suggestive of instability. **B:** Next, a posteriorly directed force is applied to the proximal humerus. Pain relief is predictive of instability and/or internal impingement. **C:** The reverse relocation maneuver applies an anteriorly directed force that exacerbates the initial symptoms.

Subacromial bursitis, rotator cuff tear, AC-joint pathology, Bennett lesion, coracoid impingement, synovial cyst with suprascapular nerve dysfunction, adhesive capsulitis, acute cartilage injury, and degenerative arthropathy all may contribute to pain in the throwing shoulder. Noninvasive tests such as anesthetic injections or electromyographic (EMG) analysis can further help to distinguish the primary cause of discomfort.

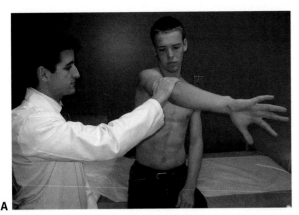 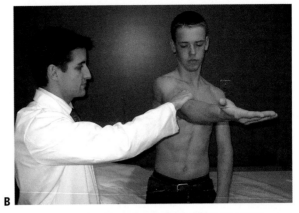

FIGURE 20.5. O'Brien's active compression test. **A:** The arm is maximally internally rotated, adducted, and forward flexed to 90° against resistance. **B:** The arm is then externally rotated and retested against resistance. Pain with internal rotation that is relieved with external rotation is suggestive of labral or biceps injury.

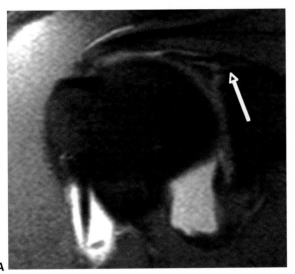 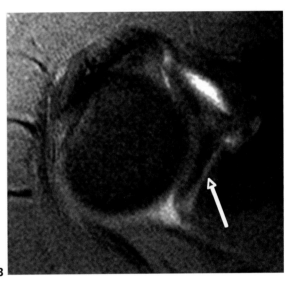

FIGURE 20.6. MRA demonstrating a SLAP lesion: SLAP tear visualized on the oblique coronal (**A**) and axial (**B**) views of a magnetic resonance imaging study with arthrography. The arrows in both planes demonstrate the Gadolinium traveling under the avulsed labrum along the glenoid neck.

BIOMECHANICS OF INJURY

The first step, or tipping point, in the disease process that causes pain and loss of performance in an elite thrower is still unknown. Static or passive motion biomechanical data that is currently available does not equal true active shoulder kinematics, and much is still unknown regarding the transition points between the late cocking, acceleration, and deceleration phases. Surgeons only see the resultant pathology, and since the findings are often similar, inferences have been made in attempts to complete the puzzle. Although often grouped separately, it is likely that the "dead arm" syndrome, internal impingement, SLAP lesions, posterior partial articular-sided rotator cuff avulsion (PASTA) lesions, posterior capsular contracture with GIRD, and anterior microinstability are all part of a spectrum of injury. The repetitive microtrauma associated with abduction-external rotation and traction stress induced during the throwing motion typically leads to injury (Fig. 20.7). While an injury to one solitary component can lead to injury in others, there are certain inherent characteristics that predispose a thrower to injury. Fatigue, game-time pressure, and a potential loss of focus can set the stage for altered kinematics leading to injury.

Throwers often complain of pain during the late cocking, acceleration, ball release, or deceleration phases. Acquired external rotation and posterior capsular tightness cause abutment of the greater tuberosity and undersurface of the rotator cuff with the posterior glenoid and posterior-superior labrum (9). The biceps tendon is also brought into a more vertical position with torsional force transmitted to the anchor at the superior glenoid tubercle and labrum (the peel-back phenomenon) (10). Although these may be normal occurrences, it predisposes

Internal Impingement Continuum

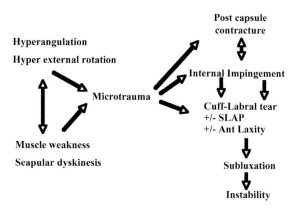

FIGURE 20.7. The interrelated factors of instability and internal impingement that lead to breakdown at various points of a thrower's shoulder.

the athlete to injury. Shoulder weakness or fatigue of the scapular stabilizers, seen in pitchers with chronic shoulder symptoms (11), causes internal rotation, abduction, and protraction. When combined with abduction-external rotation, this weakness causes hyperangulation between the glenoid neck and the proximal humerus (Fig. 20.8). Hyperangulation increases stress on the anterior capsule, and as the arm initiates forward acceleration, the likelihood or severity of abutment between the greater tuberosity and posterior-superior glenoid increases. This in turn places the posterior-superior labrum and undersurface of the rotator cuff at risk for impingement (Fig. 20.9). If perpetuated, the thrower may develop a tear of the posterior labrum or avulsion of the articular side of the rotator cuff. SLAP tears have been shown to increase glenohumeral external rotation and translation, which in turn increase anterior capsular stress and the potential for laxity and microinstability. Injury to the rotator cuff jeopardizes its ability to provide dynamic stability and places greater emphasis on the static stabilizers. Injury to the rotator cuff also has downstream consequences during ball release and deceleration phases, particularly on the biceps anchor and anterior-superior labrum. Therefore, injury to either the rotator cuff or the posterior-superior labrum potentiates the cycle and places the other structures at risk.

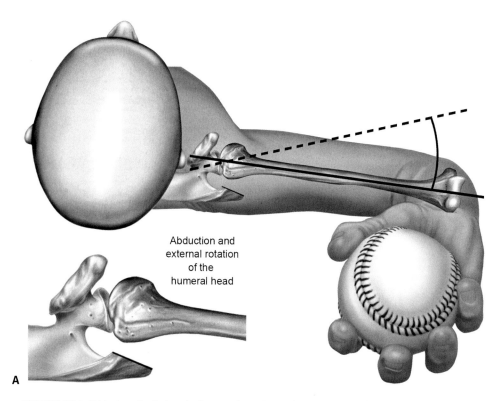

FIGURE 20.8. Critical angle. **A:** Acquired external rotation and posterior capsular tightness causes contact of the greater tuberosity and undersurface of the rotator cuff with the posterior glenoid and posterior-superior labrum. **B:** Weakness or fatigue of the scapular stabilizers causes internal rotation, abduction, and protraction of the scapula, which combined with the abduction-external rotation causes hyperangulation between the glenoid neck and proximal humerus. Hyperangulation increases stress on the anterior capsule, and as the arm initiates forward acceleration, the likelihood or severity of abutment between the greater tuberosity and posterior-superior glenoid increases. **C:** Composite vector diagram demonstrating the change in the critical angle between (**A**) and (**B**).

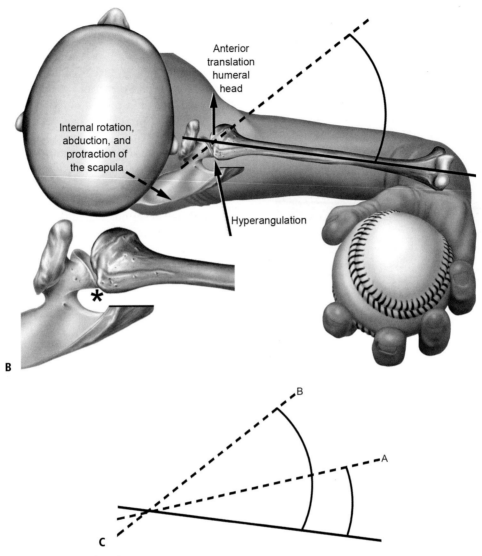

FIGURE 20.8. Continued

The biceps tendon is involved in both the windup and the delivery phases, and likely performs a secondary role to stabilize and control arm position during pitching. Loss of internal rotation beyond the standard arc secondary to a tight posterior capsule shifts the humeral head to a more posterior position on the glenoid during the late cocking phase (12). The origin of this capsular contracture is unknown, although it may be related to the inflammation secondary to posterior impingement, lack of stretching, or chronically poor mechanics. The additional stress on the biceps tendon secondary to the altered glenohumeral positioning exacerbates the peel-back phenomenon. Figure 20.10 demonstrates the pull on the biceps tendon during abduction-external rotation simulating the peel-back phenomenon. EMG analysis has shown the biceps to be active during the deceleration phase of the pitching cycle. In addition to posterior capsular contracture, weakness, fatigue, and injury of the rotator cuff muscles can also place increased demands on the biceps tendon, leading to tensile overload in the deceleration phase.

In summary, it is likely that labral pathology in a thrower originates from a combination of posterior internal impingement with associated microinstability followed by repetitive torsion and tension applied to the biceps tendon during the late cocking, acceleration, and deceleration phases. Based on whether the labral injury is primarily anterior or posterior, the development of an associated articular-sided rotator cuff lesion will likely follow. Furthermore, once the SLAP lesion has occurred, further glenohumeral translational instability, or pseudolaxity, is produced, thereby potentiating the cycle (13).

CLASSIFICATION OF SLAP TEARS

Superior labral lesions are suspected in a player with a positive history, physical exam, and imaging studies, but they are confirmed and classified with arthroscopy. Although first described by Andrews et al., (14) Snyder et al. (15) first classified SLAP tears based on their arthroscopic appearance. Type I SLAP lesions include fraying and an

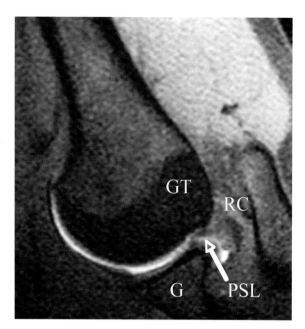

FIGURE 20.9. Specialized MRI image with the arm in abduction-external rotation demonstrating that the humeral greater tuberosity *(GT)* and posterior rotator cuff *(RC)* impinges on the glenoid *(G)* posterosuperior labrum *(PSL)*.

overall degenerative appearance of the labral tissue. Type II SLAP lesions are characterized by instability of the superior labrum and biceps anchor. Type III SLAP lesions are bucket handle tears. Type IV SLAP lesions involve a combination of a bucket handle or flap tear of the labrum with extension into the biceps tendon. Maffet et al. (16) extended Snyder's classification to include extension of the labral tear from the anterior-inferior capsulolabral junction up to the biceps anchor (type V), an unstable superior labrum with an associated flap tear (type VI), and a biceps anchor and labral detachment that extends into the middle glenohumeral ligament (MGHL) (type VII). Morgan et al. (17) further classified type II SLAP tears based on the location of the glenolabral disruption—anterior, posterior, or combined (Fig. 20.11). In their classification, they reported that most type II SLAP tears had a posterior component, and posterior type II SLAP tears were more than three times more prevalent in throwers versus nonthrowers.

NONOPERATIVE TREATMENT

Nonoperative treatment is the mainstay and should almost always be the first strategy in a high-level thrower, particularly a baseball pitcher. Even in the face of a documented SLAP tear, a trial of physical therapy is appropriate, particularly in a baseball pitcher. In contact sports such as football or lacrosse where glenohumeral stability is an issue and a traumatic component may also be present, operative treatment may be considered sooner for mechanical symptoms, but nonoperative care is still the first-line of care.

Ideally, the player is seen prior to anatomic breakdown. Rest from throwing is usually initiated for 4 to 6 weeks. Oral nonsteroidal anti-inflammatory medications can be helpful. Physical therapy is initiated to restore the glenohumeral motion (arc of motion) to normal. This includes an extensive posterior capsular stretching program and avoidance of excessive anterior or inferior capsular stress. Physical therapy should also assist with stretching and strength and endurance training of the rotator cuff and scapular rotators. A thorough recovery program should also emphasize lower extremity strength and core stability. The shoulder should not be making up for deficiencies in the lower extremities.

After the rest and rehabilitation period, a graduated throwing program is instituted, and the player advanced as long as he remains pain free. Finally, an evaluation of throwing mechanics should be performed, as subtle changes in arm position can have a dramatic impact on shoulder and elbow stress during delivery.

OPERATIVE TREATMENT

The decision to operate is the most challenging determination in the care of a throwing athlete. Even when pathology is confirmed diagnostically, restoring stability to a shoulder that requires 120° to 140° of external rotation for optimal performance is difficult.

SLAP Lesions

Superior labral pathology is often the suspected diagnosis when surgical intervention is considered. Indications for surgery start with a suspected diagnosis coupled with an inability to return to pitching because of persistent clinical symptoms not improved with rest, therapy, and addressing throwing mechanics. The decision to proceed with operative treatment is aided with a correlative MRI or MRA scan. Although many throwers have not returned to play after shoulder surgery in the past, the ability to correct pathology with less morbidity is possible with the advancement of arthroscopic techniques. When symptoms are career threatening, surgery does provide the possibility for a return to play. Ultimately, the goal is to restore balance within the shoulder and provide stability while allowing the shoulder to reach its maximum external rotation.

Arthroscopy provides the treating physician a diagnostic and operative tool to manage throwing injuries. Evaluation of the athlete's shoulder is traditionally performed using a standard posterior viewing portal and anterior rotator interval-working portal. Evaluation of the essential structures including the glenoid and humeral articular surfaces, rotator cuff, biceps anchor, labrum, and capsular ligamentous structures should all be visualized and palpated. Specific arthroscopic signs should be observed and noted, including the drive through sign suggesting instability (18), the peel-back test to evaluate biceps anchor instability (Fig. 20.12), and whether the anterior-superior

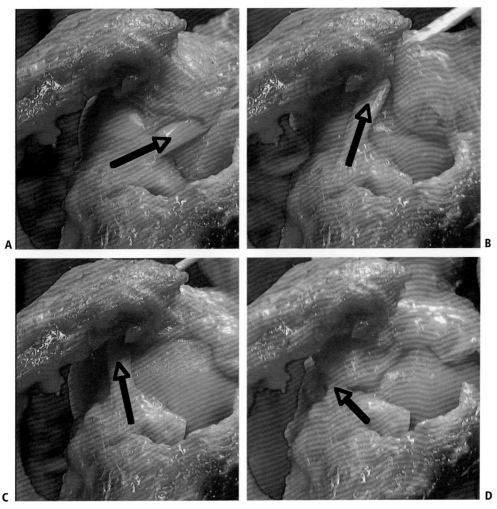

FIGURE 20.10. This cadaveric dissection demonstrates the pull on the biceps tendon during abduction-external rotation, simulating the peel-back phenomenon. The arrow follows the biceps from anterior **(A)** to posterior **(D)** as the humeral head rotates.

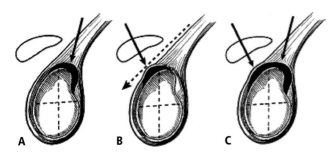

FIGURE 20.11. A: Anterior type II SLAP lesion has labral avulsion in the anterior-superior quadrant of the glenoid. **B:** Posterior type II SLAP lesion has labral avulsion in the posterior-superior quadrant of the glenoid. **C:** Combined anterior and posterior type II SLAP lesion has labral avulsion in both superior quadrants of the glenoid. (Reproduced with permission from Burkhart SS, Morgan CD. The peel-back mechanism: its role in producing and extending posterior type II SLAP lesions and its effect on SLAP repair rehabilitation. *Arthroscopy.* 1998;14:637–640.)

capsule is in direct contact with the biceps tendon after joint insufflation suggesting a full thickness rotator cuff lesion (19) (Fig. 20.13).

Degenerative lesions of the labrum and partial thickness tears of the rotator cuff should be carefully debrided. Rotator cuff fraying is debrided to assess the amount of damage to the cuff insertion (Figs. 20.14 and 20.15). In general, type I degenerative fraying of the labrum and unstable bucket-handles seen in type III tears should be debrided back to a stable border. Instability of the labral attachment seen with all other tear types should be repaired.

The general principles for fixation of SLAP lesions arthroscopically include the identification of labral instability, preparation of the labral reattachment site, and fixation of the capsulolabral tissue back to the glenoid neck. Figure 20.16 outlines identification and treatment of an anterior type II SLAP lesion using a two cannula technique with penetrating grasper and simple sutures. Identification

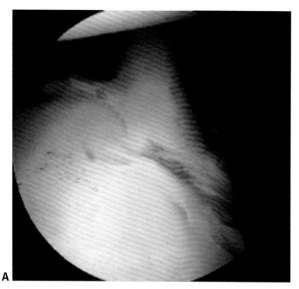
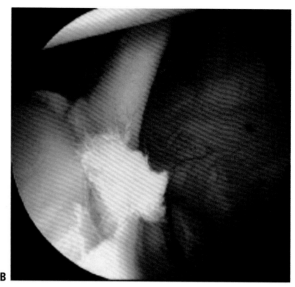

FIGURE 20.12. Peel-back mechanism. **A:** In this left shoulder in the resting (neutral) position, the posterior-superior labrum covers the corner of the glenoid. **B:** The arthroscopic view of the same shoulder in abduction and external rotation, which has caused the posterosuperior glenoid labrum to be peeled back and medially shifted over the corner of the glenoid. (Reproduced with permission from Burkhart SS, Morgan CD, Kibler WB. The disabled throwing shoulder: spectrum of pathology part I: pathoanatomy and biomechanics. *Arthroscopy.* 2003;19:404–420.)

of instability involves probing and displacing the biceps anchor and superior labrum medial to the articular margin. Depending on physician preference, available arthroscopic instruments, and the location of SLAP lesion, a third arthroscopic portal may be added. Posterior or large combined lesions usually require a portal that allows access to the posterior-superior glenoid. That portal is established under direct visualization using an outside-in technique. A skin incision off the lateral edge of the acromion allows

passage of a small cannula or instrument through the supraspinatus musculature medial to the rotator cuff cable into the joint (Fig. 20.17). The superior position allows for accurate anchor placement and suture passage on the posterior-superior glenoid neck. For anterior SLAP lesions, a second anterior portal may be established to allow for more accurate anchor placement or suture passage.

Preparation of the labral attachment site begins with the elevation of the scarred labrum from its recessed

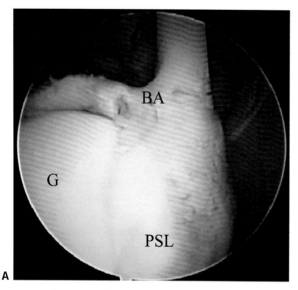
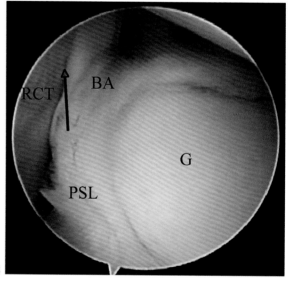

FIGURE 20.13. A: Arthroscopic image of the glenohumeral joint with an intact rotator cuff demonstrated by separation of the anterior-superior capsule and rotator cuff tendon *(RCT)* from the biceps anchor *(BA)*. **B:** Arthroscopic image of the glenohumeral joint with a full thickness rotator cuff tear demonstrated by the anterior-superior capsule in direct contact with the biceps tendon after joint insufflation. Posterior-superior labrum *(PSL)* and glenoid *(G)* are labeled for orientation.

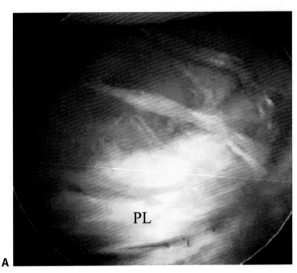
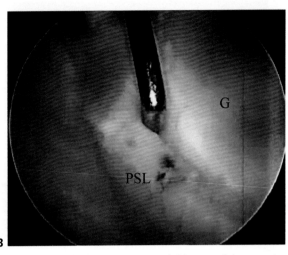

FIGURE 20.14. A: Degenerative fraying of the posterior labrum *(PL)* secondary to internal impingement. **B:** Debridement of degenerative labral tissue revealing a stable posterior-superior labrum *(PSL)*. Glenoid *(G)* and humeral head *(HH)* are labeled for orientation.

position. Further debridement of nonfunctional granulation tissue is performed as needed. An arthroscopic shaver or burr is used to roughen the articular junction and glenoid neck to promote healing. Figure 20.18 summarizes the identification, bone preparation with an arthroscopic shaver, and treatment of a combination anterior and posterior type II SLAP lesion, using a three cannula technique with two anchors and simple sutures.

Suture fixation has become the standard of care for securing the labrum to the glenoid. Suture anchors are used most commonly and require arthroscopic knot tying. Sliding knots such as the Westin and Tennessee slider are acceptable; however, the surgeon should use caution to avoid sawing through the labral tissue. Knots should also not be left on the glenoid surface but directed toward the capsulolabral

junction. Knotless systems are also available and effective, although tensioning the repair using knotless techniques can be difficult. The number of anchors used should be minimized in the throwing athlete. Overconstraint can be just as problematic as instability. Balance is the key.

Similar to arthroscopic rotator cuff fixation, variations in suture constructs exist for labral repairs. Simple and mattress suture designs are both effective. Sutures may be passed through the labral tissue with several different devices including sharp pointed suture graspers and suture shuttling devices. Figure 20.19 demonstrates a three cannula technique used to treat a posterior-based type II SLAP lesion, using a suture shuttling device and an alternative mattress suture technique. Physician preference, ability, and tear patterns should dictate the anchor choice, suture

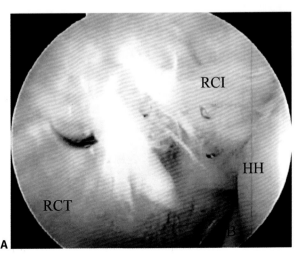
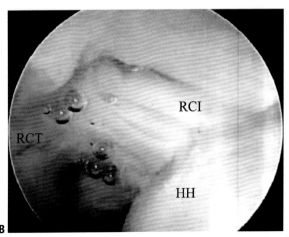

FIGURE 20.15. A: Posterior partial thickness articular-sided rotator cuff tear at the insertion onto the greater tuberosity *(RCI)* associated with internal impingement. **B:** Debridement of degenerative rotator cuff tissue reveals minimal damage to the tendon insertion, not requiring repair. Rotator cuff tendon *(RCT)*, biceps *(B)*, and humeral head *(HH)* are labeled for orientation.

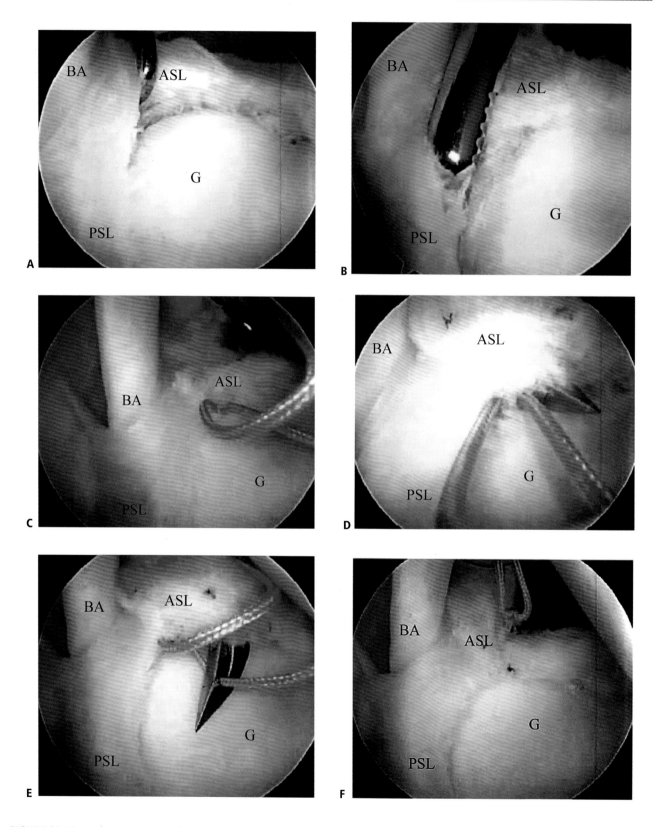

FIGURE 20.16. Single-anchor repair of an anterior-based type II SLAP lesion using a two-cannula technique. **A:** Arthroscopic probe identifies instability at the anterior-superior labrum *(ASL)* at the base of the biceps anchor *(BA)*. **B:** Arthroscopic shaver is used to debride granulation tissue and prepare the bone bed on the glenoid *(G)* neck for labral reattachment. **C:** A suture anchor is placed at the point of maximum instability right on the articular margin. **D:** The penetrating suture grasper pierces the capsulolabral junction at the anchor point and exits at the glenoid face. **E:** The suture is carefully retrieved. **F:** An arthroscopic knot secures the simple suture. The knot is directed away from the labral surface. **G:** A probe checks the stability of the construct and the repaired ASL. **H:** The probe also inspects the biceps anchor and posterior-superior labrum for stability after repair.

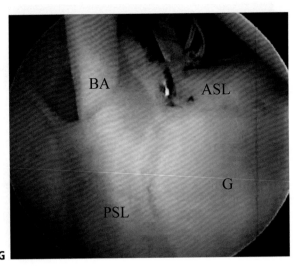

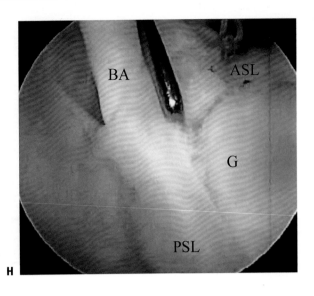

FIGURE 20.16. (continued)

passer, and overall design of the final construct. With the correct diagnosis and treatment, SLAP repair should improve glenohumeral stability.

Thermal capsular procedures have been used in the past to address capsular laxity. Thermal techniques should be avoided, as the capsular reduction typically stretches over time, and complications secondary to thermal chondrolysis and loss of capsular integrity have led to devastating outcomes in some patients.

Posterior Capsular Release

Posterior capsular release as part of the arthroscopic treatment is rarely required, but may be indicated. Conservative measures should be exhausted prior to proceeding with this procedure either in isolation or in combination

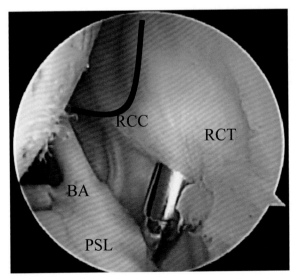

FIGURE 20.17. Transtendon rotator cuff portal. A small metal cannula is used to create a portal through the rotator cuff tendon (RCT) medial to the rotator cuff cable (RCC) to allow access to the posterior-superior labrum (PSL). The biceps anchor (BA) is labeled for orientation.

with a SLAP repair. Current indications call for a posterior capsular release in a patient with persistent symptoms, failure of prolonged therapy, and internal rotation of less than 20° when the arm is abducted. With the arthroscope placed in the anterior portal, the release may be performed with arthroscopic tissue punches and either a hooked intra-articular radiofrequency device through the posterior portal. Depending upon tissue compliance, the capsulotomy is made 1 cm away from the posterior labrum extending from the 6 o'clock to between the 9 and 11 o'clock position on the glenoid of a right shoulder. Figure 20.20 demonstrates the location and extent of the release necessary. To avoid possible injury to the infraspinatus muscle and axillary nerve, surgeons should be cautious not to penetrate too deeply or too inferiorly.

Anterior Capsulorrhaphy

Distinguishing between true anterior instability and pseudolaxity or micro-instability secondary to a SLAP lesion is often difficult. If a thrower has symptomatic instability without the presence of a SLAP lesion or anterior capsulolabral injury, then a suture capsular plication may be required. If a SLAP lesion is present in the thrower also symptomatic with anterior laxity, the anterior band of the inferior glenohumeral ligament (IGHL) should be probed before and after the SLAP repair. If tension in the anterior band of the IGHL has been restored after the SLAP repair (as is true in most instances), then a capsulorrhaphy should be avoided. However, if the lax anterior band of the IGHL is unchanged after SLAP repair, then a capsular plication procedure may be warranted.

Rotator Cuff Tears

Most tears in overhead throwers are partial thickness tears. For tears involving less than 50% of the footprint in a medial-lateral direction, limited debridement of the degenerative fraying is acceptable. Repairs, which typically involve tendon advancement onto the humeral greater tuberosity,

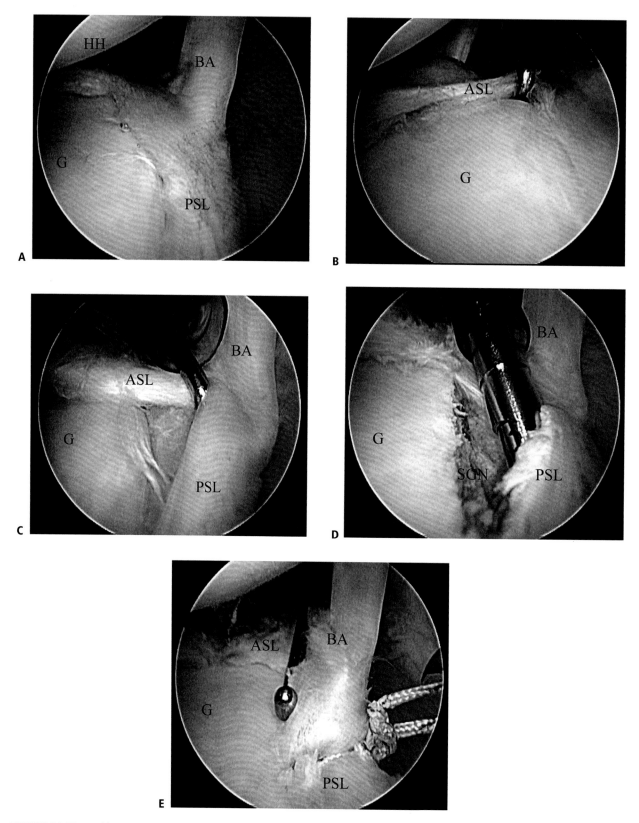

FIGURE 20.18. Double-anchor repair of a combination anterior- and posterior-based type II SLAP lesion using a three-cannula technique. **A:** Visualization of a loose appearing labrum during diagnostic arthroscopy. **B:** Probing the anterior-superior labrum *(ASL)* reveals anterior instability at the biceps anchor *(BA)*. **C:** Probing the posterior-superior labrum *(PSL)* reveals posterior instability at the biceps anchor. **D:** Preparation of the bone bed on the superior neck of the glenoid *(G)* using an arthroscopic shaver. **E:** Completed two-anchor repair with simple sutures anterior and posterior to the biceps anchor.

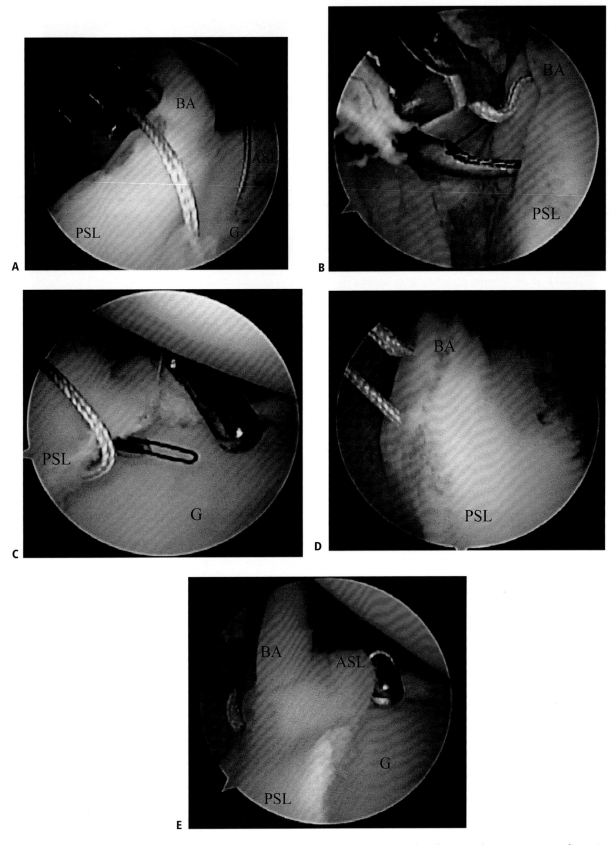

FIGURE 20.19. Single-anchor repair of a posterior-based type II SLAP lesion using a three-cannula technique and mattress suture configuration. **A:** Anchor is placed just posterior to the biceps anchor *(BA)*. **B:** A suture shuttling device is used through the transtendon portal to pierce the posterior-superior labrum *(PSL)* at the capsulolabral junction. **C:** The shuttling device exits the tissue underneath the labrum along the glenoid face *(G)* and the wire is used to shuttle the suture through the labral tissue. **D:** Both suture limbs are passed through the PSL. **E:** An arthroscopic knot is tied and the PSL, BA, and anterior-superior labrum *(ASL)* are rechecked for stability.

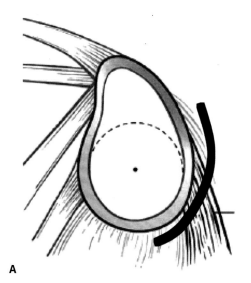
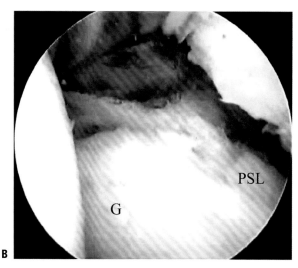

FIGURE 20.20. Selective posterior-inferior capsular release. **A:** The capsular contraction is located in the posterior-inferior quadrant of the capsule in the zone of the posterior band of the IGHL complex. Depending on tissue compliance, the capsulotomy is made 1 cm away from the posterior labrum *(PL)* from the 6 o'clock to between the 9 and 11 o'clock position on the glenoid *(G)*. **B:** An arthroscopic inspection of the posterior capsule after release with a hooked tip electrocautery device. The most inferior portion of the release was performed with an arthroscopic basket to avoid injury to the axillary nerve. (Adapted with permission from Burkhart SS, Morgan CD, Kibler WB. The disabled throwing shoulder: spectrum of pathology part I: pathoanatomy and biomechanics. *Arthroscopy.* 2003;19:404–420.)

are generally not well tolerated in the elite overhead-throwing athlete. For tears involving greater than 50% of the footprint (some argue greater than 75%), transtendon repair or debridement with full thickness repair are options. Surgeons in general should be very cautious when considering rotator cuff procedures as there is a high risk of the athlete not returning to competitive throwing following a repair.

AUTHORS' PREFERRED TECHNIQUE

For operative treatment of internal impingement and associated labral pathology in an overhead athlete, the patient is placed in the lateral decubitus position with the arm abducted 40° and forward flexed 15° to 20°. The arm is simply held in position using a 10-lb (4.53 kg) counterweight. Traction is not as important as the position of the arm. A three-portal technique is preferred utilizing suture anchors, small suture shuttling instruments, and arthroscopic knot tying. Far anterior tears focused primarily at the biceps anchor may be repaired with a single working portal placed through the rotator interval. Although a two-portal technique is also possible with anterior SLAP tears using penetrating suture grasping devices, it is felt that those instruments are larger and may cause greater trauma to the labral tissue during passage.

The posterior portal is placed 2 cm inferior to the posterolateral corner of the acromion, and the arthroscope is introduced into the shoulder. An anterior portal is immediately created through the subscapularis bursa with the use of a Wissinger rod. A complete intra-articular diagnostic arthroscopy is performed using a probe. The biceps anchor and superior labrum are examined for stability and degeneration. The rotator cuff is examined, particularly along the posterior insertion. After a SLAP tear is identified by elevating the labrum off of the articular margin, focus is placed on the biceps anchor and the direction of the labral injury. An intraoperative peel-back maneuver may be performed (Fig. 20.12).

An arthroscopic shaver is introduced to debride any fibrillated edges of the rotator cuff and the superior labrum. The superior glenoid rim is prepared with a shaver and a burr. The third lateral portal is created for the purpose of anchor placement. This portal is located anterolateral or posterolateral depending on extension of the tear. Passage through the cuff is delicate with care taken to identify the anterior–posterior suspension cable and pass medial to it. A suture anchor is placed into the superior glenoid either anterior or posterior to the biceps anchor. A sharp, low profile suture shuttling device is used to deliver one of the nonabsorbable sutures through the anterosuperior labrum. The simple suture construct is secured with caution using a sliding, locking knot (Westin) with three half hitches tied under direct visualization. Care is taken to seat the knot off the articular surface to avoid articular cartilage irritation. Occasionally, a second anchor is required to achieve balanced stability. The repair is probed to assess stability and repair integrity.

PEARLS AND PITFALLS

It is important to recognize that variations exist in normal glenoid labral anatomy. In patients with suspected SLAP injuries, a tear or instability must be differentiated from a recessed or meniscoid labral variant. A normal labrum should attach at the articular margin, regardless of the amount of overhang on the glenoid face.

Other anatomic variations are often found at the glenoid attachment of the MGHL. A cord-like MGHL or a sublabral hole with or without labral tissue may be present and should not be confused with a labral injury. Inadvertent arthroscopic imbrications of the MGHL tissue can cause a substantial limitation in shoulder abduction and external rotation.

Surgeons should be cautious in proceeding with a capsulorrhaphy after a SLAP repair, particularly in a pitcher without true episodes of subluxation or dislocation. Pitchers require a fine balance between laxity and constraint. They need stability yet also need to externally rotate their arm as much as 140°. Superior and anterior stabilization procedures may limit postoperative abduction-external rotation and prevent their return to competitive throwing.

On the other side of the glenoid, arthroscopic surgeons should avoid placing suture anchors too far posterior on the glenoid face. In a throwing athlete, posterior overtightening can exacerbate the posterior capsular contracture and worsen the internal rotation deficit and impingement process. This can be avoided by placing the suture anchor in a superior or anterior-superior position on the glenoid face. Also, by avoiding posterior anchor placement, the thrower's ability to stretch the posterior capsule during the rehabilitation phase will not be restricted.

Finally, in regard to rotator cuff pathology, surgeons should recall that the internal impingement mechanism for partial thickness rotator cuff lesions in throwers is markedly different than outlet impingement seen in degenerative rotator cuff tears. Tibone et al. (20) demonstrated poor results when treating pitchers with acromioplasty and related subacromial decompression procedures.

POSTOPERATIVE REHABILITATION

The goals of postoperative rehabilitation include protection of the repair during the healing phase followed by gradual restoration of capsular compliance and range of motion. This also involves reestablishing proprioception, strength, endurance, and finally scapulo-humeral synchrony and optimal throwing mechanics.

Patients are initially immobilized in a sling. Active elbow motion and elevation to the salute position are combined with Codman circumduction, scapular retraction, and scapular isometric exercises during the first 3 weeks. A progressive active-assisted range of motion program allowing overhead movements and external rotation up to 90° is performed from 3 to 6 weeks post-surgery. From 6 to 16 weeks, progression to full active range of motion is the goal, while incorporating scapular stabilization, rotator cuff strengthening, and posterior capsular stretching exercises. A progressive throwing

program is performed between 4 to 7 months, and a return to full competitive throwing can be expected in 8 to 12 months.

COMPLICATIONS

Surgical complications related to infections and neurovascular injuries are rare with arthroscopic shoulder surgery. However, labral repairs are challenging and errors are possible. Technical failures related to prominent implants, suture abrasion, and knot irritation can generate articular cartilage injury. Regardless of the suture-anchoring device chosen, a strong working knowledge of the implant is necessary, and practice in the laboratory environment is recommended prior to patient use. While returning to play after shoulder surgery is difficult in the elite overhead athlete, the challenge of returning after revision surgery is even more daunting.

Recurrent injury is also possible after labral reconstructions. Poor compliance with rehabilitation and mechanics training or accelerated recovery may lead to retear and continued symptoms.

SUMMARY

Internal impingement and related shoulder instability in throwers is a continuum, and symptomatic injury may be caused by a subtle breakdown in the kinetic chain. Injury to one or all elements of the restraint system likely occurs during the strenuous transitions between the late cocking, acceleration, and deceleration phases. It is important to understand the pieces involved in the injury process in order to identify the "shoulder at risk." Nonoperative care remains the treatment of choice in elite overhead athletes; however, with continued research and refinement of arthroscopic techniques, surgical intervention can be successful in treating those who have failed conservative measures.

REFERENCES

1. Fleisig GS, Barrentine SW, Zheng N, et al. Kinematic and kinetic comparison of baseball pitching among various levels of development. *J Biomech.* 1999;32:1371–1375.
2. Limpisvasti O, ElAttrache NS, Jobe FW. Understanding shoulder and elbow injuries in baseball. *J Am Acad Orthop Surg.* 2007;15:139–147.
3. Burkhart SS, Morgan CD, Kibler WB. The disabled throwing shoulder: spectrum of pathology part III: the SICK scapula, scapular dyskinesis, the kinetic chain, and rehabilitation. *Arthroscopy.* 2003;19:641–661.
4. Tokish JM, Decker MJ, Ellis HB, et al. The belly-press test for the physical examination of the subscapularis muscle: electromyographic validation and comparison to the lift-off test. *J Shoulder Elbow Surg.* 2003;12:427–430.
5. Kvitne RS, Jobe FW. The diagnosis and treatment of anterior instability in the throwing athlete. *Clin Orthop Relat Res.* 1993;291:107–123.

6. Jazrawi LM, McCluskey GM III, Andrews JR. Superior labral anterior and posterior lesions and internal impingement in the overhead athlete. *Instr Course Lect.* 2003;52:43–63.

7. Parentis MA, Glousman RE, Mohr KS, et al. An evaluation of the provocative tests for superior labral anterior posterior lesions. *Am J Sports Med.* 2006;34:265–268.

8. Wright RW, Paletta GA Jr. Prevalence of the Bennett lesion of the shoulder in major league pitchers. *Am J Sports Med.* 2004;32:121–124.

9. Jobe CM. Posterior superior glenoid impingement: expanded spectrum. *Arthroscopy.* 1995;11:530–536.

10. Burkhart SS, Morgan CD. The peel-back mechanism: its role in producing and extending posterior type II SLAP lesions and its effect on SLAP repair rehabilitation. *Arthroscopy.* 1998;14:637–640.

11. Glousman RE, Jobe FW, Tibone JE, et al. Dynamic electromyographic analysis of the throwing shoulder with glenohumeral instability. *J Bone Joint Surg Am.* 1988;70:220–226.

12. Grossman MG, Tibone JE, McGarry MH, et al. A cadaveric model of the throwing shoulder: a possible etiology of superior labrum anterior-to-posterior lesions. *J Bone Joint Surg Am.* 2005;87:824–831.

13. Panossian VR, Mihata T, Tibone JE, et al. Biomechanical analysis of isolated Type II SLAP lesions and repair. *J Shoulder Elbow.* 2005;14:529–534.

14. Andrews JR, Carson WG Jr, McLeod WD. Glenoid labrum tears related to the long head of the biceps. *Am J Sports Med.* 1985;13:337–341.

15. Snyder SJ, Karzel RP, Del Pizzo W, et al. SLAP lesions of the shoulder. *Arthroscopy.* 1990;6:274–279.

16. Maffet MW, Gartsman GM, Moseley B. Superior labrum-biceps tendon complex lesions of the shoulder. *Am J Sports Med.* 1995;23:93–98.

17. Morgan CD, Burkhart SS, Palmeri M, et al. Type II SLAP lesions: three subtypes and their relationships to superior instability and rotator cuff tears. *Arthroscopy.* 1998;14:553–565.

18. Pagnani MJ, Warren RF, Altchek DW, et al. Arthroscopic shoulder stabilization using transglenoid sutures. A four-year minimum followup. *Am J Sports Med.* 1996;24:459–467.

19. Temple JD, Sethi PM, Kharrazi FD, et al. Direct biceps tendon and supraspinatus contact as an indicator of rotator cuff tear during shoulder arthroscopy in the lateral decubitus position. *J Shoulder Elbow Surg.* 2007;16:327–329.

20. Tibone JE, Jobe FW, Kerlan RK, et al. Shoulder impingement syndrome in athletes treated by an anterior acromioplasty. *Clin Orthop Relat Res.* 1985;198:134–140.

Arthroscopic Treatment of Shoulder Fractures

Jesus Rey II • Sumant G. Krishnan

The appropriate management of shoulder fractures remains challenging. Therapeutic options for shoulder fractures include both conservative and surgical treatments. Indications for either treatment remain controversial and are often made based on surgeon experience rather than evidence-based algorithms. In recent years, the treatment of shoulder girdle fractures has evolved from extensive open reduction to minimally invasive surgery. Arthroscopy is increasingly being recognized as an important adjunct in treating periarticular fractures, especially to confirm accurate reduction of articular surfaces. Avoidance of large muscular dissections is attractive for potentially decreasing complications, reducing postoperative pain, enhancing healing potential, and shortening postoperative recovery time. These arthroscopic techniques also allow for complete joint inspection and more accurate assessment of concomitant injuries than conventional methods. Given the high incidence of associated injuries with proximal humerus fractures, arthroscopy may indeed be a useful diagnostic and treatment tool for associated labral lesions, rotator cuff injuries, and traumatic cartilage defects (1). However, the arthroscopic treatment of shoulder fractures requires a learning curve that depends on surgeon experience in shoulder arthroscopy. Long-term outcomes after all-arthroscopic management of shoulder fractures still remain elusive.

PROXIMAL HUMERUS FRACTURES

Overview

Proximal humerus fractures represent 4% to 5% of all fractures and are the most common fractures of the shoulder girdle. Nordqvist and Petersson, (2) in a review of all fractures treated in a single hospital during the course of a year, found that proximal humerus fractures accounted for 53% of all significant shoulder girdle injuries.

Greater and lesser tuberosity fractures can occur as isolated injuries or as a component of comminuted proximal humerus fractures. Despite the disagreement in the literature regarding the magnitude of displacement, when isolated, most authors advocate that 5 mm of

posterosuperior displacement of the greater tuberosity can lead to clinically significant impingement. With nondisplaced or minimally displaced (less than 5 mm) fractures, conservative management is an option (3). Management and outcomes for lesser tuberosity fractures are even more controversial since the incidence of this injury is far less common.

Clinical Evaluation

Pertinent History

The clinical history for proximal humerus fractures varies based upon which pattern of fracture is present. Although most of these fractures result from low-energy trauma usually following a fall in an elderly individual, isolated greater or lesser tuberosity fractures occur in younger patients. Tuberosity fractures usually occur in male patients between the second and the fifth decades of life (4) as well as adolescents with open humeral physis (5).

The mechanism of injury plays an important role in the pattern of fracture. It has been shown that over 50% of greater tuberosity fractures occur in the setting of an anterior shoulder dislocation (6). Eccentric loads on the tuberosities sustained by falling onto an outstretched arm can produce an avulsion-type fracture or propagate it with subsequent displacement. Lesser tuberosity fractures represent a rare injury that occurs in younger individuals. The arm is usually placed in an abducted and externally rotated position. Forceful contraction of the subscapularis muscle avulses the tuberosity. Another mechanism for lesser tuberosity fractures is a posterior dislocation of the shoulder.

Physical Examination

Acutely, the shoulder is often extremely swollen after a proximal humeral fracture. Ecchymosis tracks down the arm and into the chest and axilla. As most patients with proximal humeral fractures are elderly, assessment for concomitant injuries is paramount.

Electromyographic evaluation has demonstrated that approximately two-thirds (67%) of all patients with proximal humeral fractures suffer acute neurologic injury from the violence of the injury. Most commonly, this involves either the axillary nerve (58%) or the suprascapular nerve (48%) (7).

For isolated lesser tuberosity fractures, symptoms include pain with passive external rotation, pain with resisted internal rotation, and tenderness over the lesser tuberosity. Since the subscapularis tendon is attached to the fractured bony structure, insufficiency of the musculotendinous unit of the subscapularis muscle is present and lift-off and belly-press tests can be used to evaluate this pathology.

Imaging

Imaging is paramount in evaluating the proximal humerus fracture. Initial radiographic evaluation consists of a Neer trauma series with anteroposterior (AP), scapular "Y" and axillary roentgenographic views (Fig. 21.1). Because of the anatomy of the proximal humerus, it may be difficult to appreciate fracture lines and fragment displacement. If plain radiographs do not offer adequate visualization, the use of computed tomographic scans with three-dimensional (3D) reconstructions can be extremely helpful in assessing fracture pattern (Fig. 21.2). For fractures involving the greater tuberosity, it has been demonstrated that the most accurate displacement measurements are determined from the AP view in external rotation and the AP view with 15° caudal tilt (8). Displaced large lesser tuberosity fragments can usually be visualized on the AP images, whereas smaller fragments are better visualized on the axillary view.

MRI can detect occult nondisplaced fractures of the tuberosities. Zanetti et al (9). reported a 38% prevalence of occult fractures of the greater tuberosity in patients suspected of having traumatic rotator cuff tears.

Classification

Neer's four-part classification system of proximal humerus fractures has endured by virtue of its simplicity. Despite its poor interobserver reliability and intraobserver reproducibility, this classification allows a conceptual understanding of the fracture pattern by defining the fracture into separate parts.

Treatment

Nonoperative

Associated injuries, appropriate rehabilitation, and premorbid function may affect the final outcome once nonsurgical management has been established.

Good to excellent results have been reported with nondisplaced and minimally displaced greater tuberosity fractures (10). Every orthopedic surgeon should be mindful that patients who have persistent late pain after a greater tuberosity fracture treated conservatively may have rotator cuff injuries which should be evaluated and treated accordingly (11). Patients with lesser tuberosity fractures without significant displacement of the bony fragment can successfully be treated conservatively.

Operative Indications

Evidence-based indications for the operative management of proximal humeral fractures are based on various factors: fracture pattern, patient age, bone quality, medical comorbidities, level of activity, hand dominance, motivation for recovery, and timing from injury to evaluation. Despite objective evaluation parameters, surgeon experience in operatively managing these technically demanding and challenging injuries often supersedes all and plays the key role in decision making. The rationale for surgical

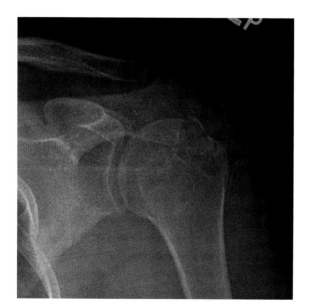

FIGURE 21.1. AP X-ray of a 35-year-old patient with a greater tuberosity fracture.

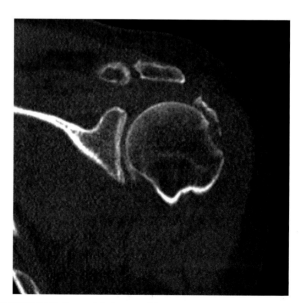

FIGURE 21.2. Coronal CT image of the same patient showing the comminuted pattern of the greater tuberosity fracture.

fixation of greater tuberosity fractures is prevention of nonunion, impingement, or mechanical blockage to abduction by a malpositioned tuberosity. The healing of the tuberosity in a malpositioned location alters the insertion of the rotator cuff tendons with subsequent weakness due to altered biomechanics.

Displacement of greater than 5 mm should be reduced surgically. For athletes and patients involved in overhead labor, fixation of even smaller displacements (3 mm) has been advocated.

Operative management of isolated lesser tuberosity fractures presents unique issues. Fixation techniques include heavy sutures, cannulated screws, cerclage wires, and all-arthroscopic suture anchor fixation. When these injuries are chronic, there is usually fibrous tissue interposed, which requires debridement to allow for bony healing to occur. Attention should be paid to the long head of the biceps tendon as well as the subscapularis tendon insertion as there is an intimate relationship between these structures. The superior glenohumeral ligament/coracohumeral ligament complex (pulley system) can be involved and destabilize the biceps tendon.

The arthroscopic treatment of proximal humeral fractures has been reported by different authors. Despite reports ranging from satisfactory to excellent outcomes, long-term results from randomized studies remain sparse.

Techniques

Tuberosity fractures can be approached either with open or with arthroscopic methods. All-arthroscopic procedures can be technically demanding and challenging and require the surgeon performing these procedures to be skilled in arthroscopic repair techniques. As with any other shoulder surgery, the positioning of the patient is key for proper visualization and access to the desired area of work. For the most part, instrumentation is the same used in arthroscopic rotator cuff and labral fixations, with the addition of cannulated screws or other implants based on the pathology to be treated. The use of fluoroscopy or C-arm X-ray is an adjunct to fracture management but not a requirement since (in most cases) direct visualization is obtained through the camera.

Authors' Preferred Treatment

Greater Tuberosity Fixation

The preferred way of treating these fractures is with the patient under general anesthesia. Patients are placed in a modified beach chair position with the involved extremity draped free and held by an arm holder. Fluoroscopic imaging is then performed to verify the position of the tuberosity and quality of the reduction. Provisional fixation can be achieved by placing a Kirschner wire percutaneously to temporarily fix the fragment until final fixation is accomplished.

Portal position is essential. The posterior portal should be placed more lateral and superior than in the classic soft spot as this will allow for better visualization of the greater tuberosity and rotator cuff insertion. It should be placed 10 mm inferior and 10 mm medial to the posterolateral corner of the acromion. The standard anterior portal is made at this time, and a cannula is introduced in the rotator cuff interval. Standard diagnostic examination of the shoulder should be performed, looking for associated injuries that could have been "missed" in the preoperative radiographic examination.

Special attention should be paid to soft tissue injuries, any such injuries should be addressed at the time of surgery. After all required work has been done in the glenohumeral joint, attention is turned to the subacromial space. A standard lateral or modified anterolateral portal is used to perform a bursectomy and minimal subacromial decompression. Once this has been achieved, a working cannula can be sutured into place.

The fracture should be identified and the fracture site cleaned of any interposed soft tissue with a burr and arthroscopic rasp (Fig. 21.3). The tuberosity fracture is reduced at this time using graspers usually placed through the anterior portal (Fig. 21.4). Once it is reduced into place it can be held in position by placing percutaneous guide wires (Fig. 21.5). Our preferred treatment uses arthroscopic transosseous tunnel fixation with sutures around the tuberosity fragment (Fig. 21.6). Fixation depends on the fracture pattern as well as surgeon preference. Taverna et al (12). reported on cannulated screw fixation. Heavy nonabsorbable rotator cuff incorporating sutures and anchors can also be used. Bhatia et al. (13) have reported on open reduction and internal fixation by use of double-row suture anchor fixation technique in 21 cases of comminuted greater tuberosity fractures, and the long-term results suggest a satisfactory outcome in most patients. Long-term follow-up results regarding

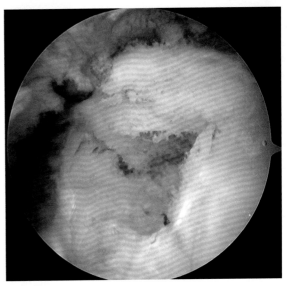

FIGURE 21.3. Arthroscopic view of an elevated greater tuberosity fracture fragment.

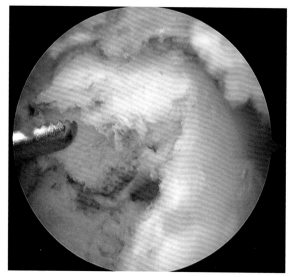

FIGURE 21.4. Arthroscopic reduction of a greater tuberosity with graspers.

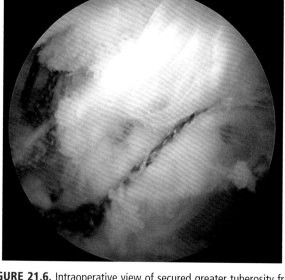

FIGURE 21.6. Intraoperative view of secured greater tuberosity fracture with final transosseous suture fixation.

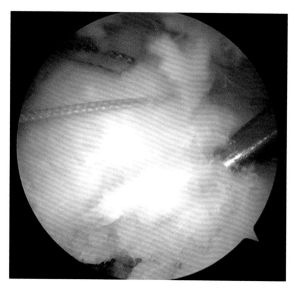

FIGURE 21.5. Provisional reduction and fixation of the greater tuberosity with K-wires. Transosseous sutures are placed around tuberosity fragment for later fixation.

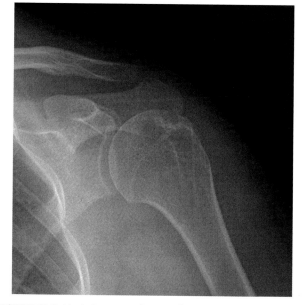

FIGURE 21.7. Healed greater tuberosity fracture at 6 months post-op.

all-arthroscopic management of greater tuberosity fractures are still needed (Fig. 21.7).

Lesser Tuberosity Fixation

The patient is placed under general anesthesia and in the beach chair position. Positioning of the patient should allow for arthroscopic as well as open surgery in case conversion to open surgery should be needed. Diagnostic arthroscopy is performed through a standard posterior portal. The subscapularis insertion zone is inspected from superior to inferior starting with the long head of the biceps and pulley system. The anterior glenohumeral ligaments should be inspected. The anterior and anterosuperior portals are then established to allow for mobilization of the tuberosity as well as for bone preparation. The subscapularis and lesser tuberosity fragment can be reconstructed with anchors at the fracture site. Penetrators are used to pierce the subscapularis tendon together with the lesser tuberosity which are then secured through vertical mattress stitches.

Rehabilitation

Postoperative management and rehabilitation are individualized and adapted to accommodate associated injuries, bone and soft tissue quality, strength of fixation, and anticipated patient compliance. Patients should be initially immobilized and begin passive range of motion (ROM) exercises during the first 6 weeks. Active ROM is started at this point for another 4 weeks. Strengthening is not begun until week 10.

Complications

Complications of tuberosity fractures include infection, malunion, nonunion, adhesive capsulitis, malreduction, and iatrogenic injury. All these can be minimized with meticulous preparation and anticipation, careful surgical technique, correct and early diagnosis, and prompt treatment of any such complications. Infection is a rare entity in the setting of arthroscopy, yet a possibility. Prevention of postoperative stiffness requires a properly conducted and followed course of physical therapy. Direct and constant communication should exist between the surgeon, the therapist, and the patient to ensure proper rehabilitation. Impingement and loss of cuff function from tuberosity malunion or malposition during surgery may result requiring corrective osteotomy or decompression.

GLENOID RIM AND FOSSA FRACTURES

Introduction

Fractures of the glenoid rim frequently occur in association with primary traumatic anterior dislocation of the shoulder, with a reported incidence of between 5% and 50% (14). Displaced articular fractures involving the glenoid rim and fossa are rare (15) and open reduction with stable internal fixation is the treatment of choice. Intra-articular fractures of the glenoid fossa are thought to result from impaction of the humeral head against the glenoid as the result of a medially directed force.

Clinical Evaluation

History and Physical Examination

Most patients with scapula fractures present to the emergency room following high-energy trauma. In this setting, concomitant life-threatening pulmonary, cardiac, or vascular injuries can be present and the patient should be carefully evaluated for them. A full physical examination for associated injury (especially head, chest, abdominal, and pelvic injuries) is mandatory. Due to the high incidence of associated ipsilateral rib fracture, physical examination of the involved shoulder may be extremely difficult in the setting of acute scapular fractures. Nevertheless, a complete neurovascular examination should be performed.

Imaging

Although plain radiographic evaluation using the standard trauma series is mandatory, the best imaging modality to evaluate glenoid fractures is a computed CT scan. These scans better demonstrate fracture displacement, comminution, and angulation.

For cases undergoing operative management, preoperative planning using CT scans is crucial to identify fracture fragments, plan the repair technique, and determine the optimal surgical approach. The use of 3D CT scan reconstructions has been found to augment standard radiographic views and allow for excellent preoperative evaluation of complex fractures.

Classification

Glenoid fossa fractures are classified by a functional modification of the existing Ideberg classification (13), depending on their location in the fossa and associated scapular body involvement requiring surgical fixation (14). Type I fractures involve the glenoid rim and type II fractures involve the superior 30% to 50% of the glenoid surface along with the coracoid base. Both type I and type II fractures invariably require surgical fixation.

Treatment

Nonoperative

The size of fragment that might predispose to recurrent instability is unknown. Most reports focus on small, so-called chip fractures. The most accepted current treatment for chip fractures is nonoperative. For larger, displaced fractures the most accepted current treatment is open reduction and fixation (15).

Maquieira et al. (16) have reported excellent results in a series of 14 patients treated conservatively. At a mean follow-up of 5.6 years (2.8 to 8.4), all patients reported a stable shoulder and rated their outcome as excellent. There were no complications, no redislocations, and no further intervention was necessary or planned. The mean subjective shoulder value was 97% (90% to 100%). There was minimal to no progression or development of osteoarthritis (OA). They concluded that nonoperative treatment of large anteroinferior glenoid rim fractures sustained during an episode of traumatic anterior shoulder instability leads to a stable, functional shoulder and high patient satisfaction. Moreover, at least within the first 5 years after injury, the development of OA is not a clinical problem. Traumatic anterior shoulder dislocation with a large, displaced glenoid rim fracture can be successfully treated nonoperatively, provided the glenohumeral joint is concentrically reduced.

Operative Indications

Guidelines for fixation of glenoid fractures have been well established. Fixation is recommended for fractures displaced more than 10 mm, involvement of at least 25% of the glenoid surface, and those that are associated with instability.

As in other joints, articular incongruity raises concerns about posttraumatic degenerative arthrosis and associated pain and disability. Glenohumeral subluxation and articular step-off are cited as the indications for surgical fixation, and we recommend fixation for any glenoid articular step-off or gapping greater than 2 mm. Any static humeral subluxation on radiographic evaluation also suggests a component of instability, which should be stabilized. We follow the Itoi evaluation of glenoid rim fractures to determine what potential degree of instability may be present and, therefore, will necessitate surgical correction (17).

Authors' Preferred Treatment

There are multiple techniques for arthroscopic management of glenoid fractures. These range from arthroscopic-assisted reduction and percutaneous fixation, cannulated screw fixation, suture anchors, and/or plain sutures. Regardless of which technique is used, the surgeon performing these procedures should be experienced in arthroscopy. The possibility to converting to open surgery should be taken into account and the entire team prepared for this possibility.

As in any arthroscopic shoulder surgery, positioning of the patient is key in being able to properly visualize and access the desired area of work. We prefer the beach chair position for anterior and superior glenoid fractures as this will allow for a deltopectoral exposure should we need to convert to open surgery. Posterior rim fractures can be operated on in a lateral decubitus position, which allows for a Judet or reverse Judet type of approach. For the most part, instrumentation is the same as used in arthroscopic rotator cuff repairs, decompression, and labrum fixation, with the addition of K-wires, cannulated screws, or other implants based on the pathology to be treated. The use of fluoroscopy or C-arm X-ray is an adjunct to fracture management but not a requirement since in most cases direct visualization is obtained through the camera. Nonetheless, obtaining final X-rays is highly encouraged by the authors.

Depending on location, intra-articular glenoid fractures can be surgically managed with percutaneous fluoroscopically assisted and/or arthroscopically assisted methods. Percutaneous methods, while attractive, remain technically challenging in the treatment of these complex injuries. Adequate reduction can be achieved. While holding the fragment into place, K-wires are introduced from posterior to anterior. The position of the K-wire is confirmed with C-arm imaging. The K-wires are cut and buried under the skin for future removal after 4 to 6 weeks once there is evidence of bony healing. Cannulated screws can also be used, advancing them over threaded wires.

Rehabilitation

Postoperative management and rehabilitation are individualized and adapted to accommodate associated injuries, bone and soft tissue quality, strength of fixation, and anticipated patient compliance. It also depends on surgeon preference. The patient should be initially immobilized in a sling allowing for passive ROM exercises for the first 6 weeks. Active ROM is started at this point and continued for another 4 weeks. Strengthening is not begun until week 10.

Complications

Infection, malunion, nonunion, loss of fixation, and iatrogenic injury are all possible complications. All these can be minimized with meticulous preparation and anticipation, careful surgical technique, correct and early diagnosis, and prompt treatment of any complications. K-wire migration is a well-documented complication of any percutaneous approach, which can be minimized with the use of threaded pins. Frequent X-ray examination should be obtained to monitor K-wire position. Infection is a rare entity in the setting of arthroscopy, yet a possibility. Prevention of postoperative stiffness requires a properly conducted course of physical therapy. Direct and constant communication should exist between the surgeon, the therapist, and the patient to ensure proper rehabilitation.

CONCLUSIONS

Fractures of the proximal end of the humerus involving the lesser and greater tuberosities are amenable to both nonsurgical and surgical treatments.

Fractures of the glenoid cavity are rare and, despite occasional good results with nonoperative management, these intra-articular fractures can result in considerable morbidity because of chronic instability or degenerative joint disease. Anatomic restoration of the joint surface is the goal in the management of displaced intra-articular fractures. In the shoulder, visual inspection, lavage and fracture preparation, reduction of fracture fragments, and fixation conducted under arthroscopic control can restore the articular surfaces with the advantages of more accurate fracture reduction, reduced surgical trauma, minimal soft-tissue dissection, and shortened postoperative recovery. Arthroscopic techniques also allow for diagnostic and treatment alternatives for associated injuries because the injured shoulder can be totally visualized and conversion to an arthrotomy can be performed if necessary.

REFERENCES

1. Schai PA, Hintermann B, Koris MJ. Preoperative arthroscopic assessment of fractures about the shoulder. *Arthroscopy.* 1999;15:827–835.
2. Nordqvist A, Petersson CJ. Incidence and causes of shoulder girdle injuries in an urban population. *J Shoulder Elbow Surg.* 1995;4:107–112.
3. Park TS, Choi IY, Kim YH, et al. A new suggestion for the treatment of minimally displaced fractures of the greater tuberosity of the proximal humerus. *Bull Hosp Jt Dis.* 1997;56:171–176.
4. Kim E, Shin HK, Kim CH. Characteristics of an isolated greater tuberosity fracture of the humerus. *J Orthop Sci.* 2005;10:441–444.
5. Levine B, Pereira D, Rosen J. Avulsion fractures of the lesser tuberosity of the humerus in adolescents. *J Orthop Trauma.* 2005;19:349–352.

6. Bahrs C, Lingenfelter E, Fischer F, et al. Mechanism of injury and morphology of the greater tuberosity fracture. *J Shoulder Elbow Surg.* 2006;15:140–147.

7. Visser CP, Coene LN, Brand R, et al. Nerve lesions in proximal humerus fractures. *J Shoulder Elbow Surg.* 2001;10:421–427.

8. Parsons BO, Klepps SJ, Miller S, et al. Reliability and reproducibility of radiographs of greater tuberosity displacement. A cadaveric study. *J Bone Joint Surg Am.* 2005;87:58–65.

9. Koval KJ, Gallagher MA, Marsicano JG, et al. Functional outcome after minimally displaced fractures of the proximal part of the humerus. *J Bone Joint Surg Am.* 1997;79:203–207.

10. Kim SH, Ha KI. Arthroscopic treatment of symptomatic shoulders with minimally displaced greater tuberosity fractures. *Arthroscopy.* 2000;7:695–700.

11. Sugaya H, Moriishi J, Dohi M, et al. Glenoid rim morphology in recurrent anterior glenohumeral instability. *J Bone Joint Surg Am.* 2003;85:878–884.

12. Ideberg R, Grevsten S, Larsson S. Epidemiology of scapular fractures. Incidence and classification of 338 fractures. *Acta Orthop Scand.* 1995;66:395–397.

13. Idleberg R. Fractures of the scapula involving the glenoid fossa. In: Bateman JE, Welsh RP, eds. *Surgery of the Shoulder.* Philadelphia, PA: BC Decker; 1984:63–66.

14. Goss TP. Fractures of the glenoid cavity. *J Bone Joint Surg Am.* 1992;74:299–305.

15. Schandelmaier P, Blauth M, Schneider C, et al. Fractures of the glenoid treated by operation: a 5- to 23-year follow-up of 22 cases. *J Bone Joint Surg Br.* 2002;84:173–177.

16. Itoi E, Lee SB, Berglund LJ, et al. The effect of a glenoid defect on anteroinferior stability of the shoulder after Bankart repair: a cadaveric study. *J Bone Joint Surg Am.* 2000;82:35–46.

17. Zanetti M, Weishaupt D, Jost B, Gerber C, Hodler J. MR imaging for traumatic tears of the rotator cuff: high prevalence of greater tuberosity fractures and subscapularis tendon tears. AJR Am J Roentgenol. 1999; 172:463-467.

18. Taverna E, Sansone V, Battistella F. Arthroscopic treatment for greater tuberosity fractures: rationale and surgical technique. Arthroscopy. 2004; 20:e53–7.

19. Bhatia DN, van Rooyen KS, du Toit DF, de Beer JF. Surgical treatment of comminuted, displaced fractures of the greater tuberosity of the proximal humerus: a new technique of double-row suture-anchor fixation and long-term results. Injury. 2006; 37:946–952.

20. Maquieira GJ, Espinosa N, Gerber C, Eid K. Non-operative treatment of large anterior glenoid rim fractures after traumatic anterior dislocation of the shoulder. J Bone Joint Surg Br. 2007; 89:1347–1351.

I. The Shoulder

Arthroscopic Treatment of Anterior Glenoid Bone Loss: Latarjet Techniques

Ettore Taverna

The etiology of anterior-inferior glenohumeral instability is multifactorial. Successful treatment of this condition requires any surgical approach to be sufficiently flexible to allow the surgeon to identify and repair all clinically significant lesions, which may be causing shoulder instability.

At present, anterior-inferior shoulder instability associated with soft tissue lesions can be successfully treated arthroscopically and clinical outcomes are generally equivalent to those after open procedures.

A relationship has been shown between the extent of the glenoid bone loss and the results of the treatment of recurrent anterior shoulder instability. The osseous lesions may influence the results of arthroscopic soft tissue techniques for treating glenohumeral instability.

Glenoid erosion is quite common with chronic anterior shoulder instability and often coexists with a Hill–Sachs lesion. The reported prevalence of anteroinferior glenoid rim fracture or bone erosion ranges from 8% to 90% in shoulders with recurrent anterior dislocation. The lesions are caused by impaction of the posterior-superior humeral head on the anterior-inferior glenoid rim during a dislocation. Severe bony lesions (i.e., large Hill–Sachs lesions and/or glenoid bone loss) are associated with the failure of arthroscopic treatment and constitute the real limit for the arthroscopic approach.

Imaging has shown that 90% of recurrently unstable shoulders have a glenoid defect. Chronic glenoid fractures lead to glenoid bone loss, and the bony fragment tends to disappear with time.

Biomechanical studies have found an inverse relationship between the size of the glenoid defect and the stability of the shoulder: the larger the defect, the less stable the shoulder. The stability of the shoulder decreases as the osseous defect increases.

A large glenoid defect must be treated with glenoid bone grafting when a Bankart procedure is performed. Many authors recommend coracoid transfer if the glenoid rim deficiency involves 25% of the anteroposterior diameter of the glenoid. Others suggest that measures to restore the arc of the glenoid concavity may be beneficial in terms of both stability and motion for patients who have a glenoid defect whose width is at least 21% of the glenoid length. The exact size of the glenoid bone loss that contraindicates an open or an arthroscopic soft tissue repair is still unknown.

Dislocation of the shoulder can produce a wide variety of pathologic lesions. Patients with chronic anterior shoulder instability can be classified as having recurrent dislocations, recurrent subluxations, or a chronically painful shoulder. The reported incidence of bony lesions is variable throughout the existing literature and has been reported to occur in 11% to 90% of cases of recurrent anterior shoulder instability. In addition to an avulsion fracture of the inferior glenohumeral ligament, bony abnormalities of the glenoid associated with anterior instability include a loss of anterior-inferior glenoid bone (Fig. 22.1), probably related to resorption of an avulsion fracture fragment (Fig. 22.2) or a rounding off of the anterior-inferior glenoid bone caused by microimpaction fractures related to multiple dislocations or subluxations.

Arthroscopic techniques have advanced sufficiently so that the shoulder surgeon can successfully repair anterior-inferior glenohumeral instability. Optimally, however, the arthroscopic surgeon should be able to address all clinically relevant lesions, including bony defects, in all cases by incorporating techniques that allow restoration of both the anatomy and the biomechanical function of damaged structures.

The advantages of arthroscopic surgical stabilization include smaller incisions, less soft tissue dissection, the ability to completely inspect the glenohumeral joint, access to all areas of the joint for repair, and potentially, maximum preservation of external rotation. The greatest disadvantage of the arthroscopic procedures until very recently was the inability to successfully treat significant structural bony defects. These techniques continue to evolve, but despite progressive improvement, the results of the arthroscopic treatment of instability have not equaled those obtained with open techniques. The failure

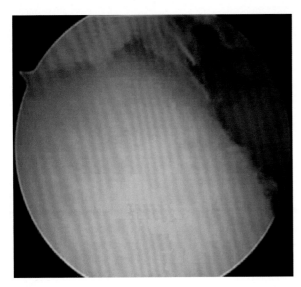

FIGURE 22.1. Arthroscopic view of an anterior glenoid bone loss.

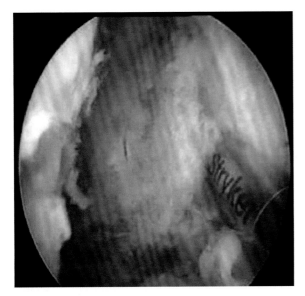

FIGURE 22.2. Arthroscopic view of a bony Bankart lesion.

rate of an arthroscopic soft tissue repair has been reported to be between 5% and 30%, especially when performed in a nonselected patient population.

Most authors agree that severe bony lesions in unstable glenohumeral joints are associated with the failure of an arthroscopic Bankart repair. If not properly addressed, plastic deformation of the capsule and ligaments and hyperlaxity could constitute another cause of failure of arthroscopic treatment.

HISTORICAL PERSPECTIVE

In 1923, Bankart proposed retensioning the anterior capsule and reinserting the labrum on the glenoid rim in order to restore the concavity of the glenoid surface. In 1932, Eden and Hybinette proposed the use of a bone block harvested from the iliac crest to increase the glenoid width. Later, the Bristow procedure was first done by Sir Rawley Bristow, who transferred a part of the coracoid process beneath the subscapularis muscle without any rigid attachment. The Bristow procedure transferred only the tip of the coracoid along with the attached conjoined tendon, but these were only sutured to the capsuloperiosteal elements through a short vertical incision made in the subscapularis.

In 1954, Michel Latarjet and Albert Trillat described two different procedures to stabilize the shoulder with the coracoid process and conjoint tendon. Trillat recommended a partial osteotomy of the coracoid process, which was then lowered and medialized before being secured on the anterior glenoid neck with a screw passing through the subscapularis. The main effect of this procedure was the sling created by routing the subscapularis by the conjoint tendon to act as a dynamic checkrein. Notably, the coracoid was not used as a bone block. The Latarjet procedure transfers most of the coracoid as a bone graft that usually measures 2 to 3 cm in length. The efficacy of the procedure is due to a double mechanism: a bone block effect provided by the coracoid, which increases the size of the concavity, and a sling effect provided by the lowering and crossing the subscapularis and conjoint tendon (Fig. 22.3). The success of the combined Trillat–Bristow–Latarjet procedure is from this double effect: a bone block (Latarjet) and a sling effect (Latarjet–Bristow–Trillat). The sling effect allows these procedures to be dynamic operations. The more the patient puts the arm in the throwing position, the more the conjoint tendon acts as a dynamic checkrein, pushing the humeral head backward and lowering the subscapularis. The Eden–Hybinette procedure provided only a bone block effect.

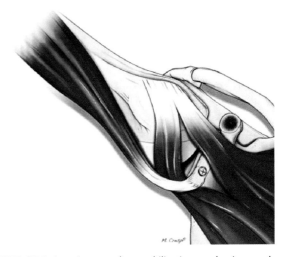

FIGURE 22.3. Latarjet procedure stabilization mechanisms: a bone block effect provided by the coracoid which increases the size of the glenoid and a sling effect provided by lowering and crossing the subscapularis with the conjoint tendon.

CLINICAL EVALUATION

Pertinent History

Patients presenting with glenohumeral anterior instability with bony lesions report various mechanisms of injury. These mechanisms often include individuals whose arm is taken into forcible external rotation when abducted 90°. A similar pattern can result from a fall on an outstretched, abducted arm. Direct distraction forces on the capsule and ligaments can be the mechanism of the injury. The amount of force required to create the instability is important. Atraumatic or minimally traumatic events lead generally to subluxation. In patients who sustain a dislocation, the force provoking the injury is generally greater and more likely results in capsule and ligament tearing and associated bony lesions.

Individuals who require reduction by a physician at the first dislocation episode are more likely to have a ligament insertion injury while with recurrent episodes bony defects are increasingly common. Patients who spontaneously reduce their shoulder at the first episode are more likely to have capsular elongation, interval enlargement, hyperlaxity, and no bony lesions.

Physical Examination

The diagnosis of shoulder instability is rarely made without a history given by the patient. Symptomatic instability is most often diagnosed by this history and then confirmed by the physical examination. Shoulder apprehension tests in all directions should be performed to confirm the clinical diagnosis. Hyperlaxity of the shoulder should be assessed. Anterior hyperlaxity is defined as external rotation greater than 85° with the arm at the side. Inferior hyperlaxity is defined when the result of the Gagey test test is positive. A positive test occurs when abduction of the affected arm with the scapula blocked by the physician is 20° greater than the other side.

Laxity must be differentiated from instability. Instability is defined as the symptomatic expression of excessive translation. The operative approach is aimed at the direction of the instability rather than all the directions of laxity. The presence of generalized ligamentous laxity is most likely in an individual with multidirectional instability. These patients rarely have any bony lesion associated with the instability. Hyperlaxity is one of the few contraindications for an open or arthroscopic Latarjet procedure.

Numerous instability tests have been described. In addition to the above-mentioned laxity tests, the drawer test should always be performed. The examiner stabilizes the scapula with one hand and grasps the humeral head with the other hand. Anterior and posterior stresses are applied. The amount of translation and pain must be recorded. In the presence of significant glenoid bone loss, anterior translation can cause a dislocation of the shoulder. The apprehension and relocation tests are also often positive in patients with glenoid bone deficits. With the patient supine, the arm is taken into abduction and external rotation, and an anterior stress is applied until the patient's apprehension is reproduced. Posterior stress is then applied by pressing against the humeral head with reduction of the anterior subluxation and an immediate decrease in the patient's apprehension.

Imaging

A standard radiographic series for instability should include anteroposterior views done in three rotations (internal, neutral, and external). The presence of a Hill–Sachs lesion should be noted for each rotation (present or absent). If present on the external rotation view, the lesion's location is more superior on the humeral head. Glenoid lesions are noted and a distinction should be made between an avulsion fracture and the loss of the anteroinferior sclerotic contour using an AP view (Fig. 22.4) or a glenoid profile view with a contralateral comparison view as described by Bernageau (Fig. 22.5).

Fractures are defined as an abnormality of the anterior glenoid rim characterized by a visible osseous fragment. The "cliff" sign is defined as a loss of the normal anterior triangle without a visible osseous fracture fragment. The "blunted angle" sign is defined as a rounding off of the normally sharp anterior angle of the triangle.

If a bone defect in the glenoid is shown with X-ray projections, it is important to determine the area and the percentage of the bone loss. In the past, the shape of the inferior glenoid has been described as a circle. Using this circle method with a 3D CT, spiral CT (Fig. 22.6), or MRI, it is possible to measure the bone defect of the glenoid. For detecting the lesions and the quality of the articular soft tissue, arthro-MRI and arthro-CT are needed.

Classification

Patients with anterior shoulder instability can be classified as having recurrent dislocations, recurrent

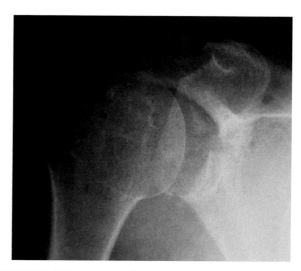

FIGURE 22.4. X-ray AP view: fracture with the loss of the anteroinferior sclerotic contour of the glenoid.

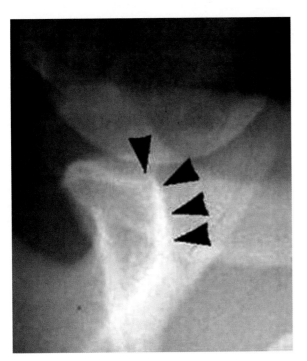

FIGURE 22.5. X-ray Bernageau view: loss of the anteroinferior sclerotic contour of the glenoid. Cliff sign positive (loss of the normal anterior triangle without a visible osseous fracture fragment).

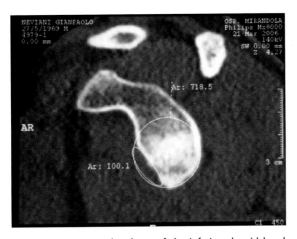

FIGURE 22.6. CT scan: the shape of the inferior glenoid has been described as a circle. The Pico method developed by Dr. Baudi from Mirandola (Italy) using a circle method in a CT scan can measure the bone defect of the glenoid.

subluxations, or an unstable painful shoulder. The incidence of bony lesions of the glenoid is higher in shoulders with a prior dislocation than in shoulders with a prior subluxation, and more common in shoulders with a prior subluxation than painful unstable shoulders. Using the classification of Rockwood and Matsen, the TUBS instability types are more likely to have glenoid bone defects than AIOS or AMBRI instability types. No clear classification system or guidelines exist to preoperatively select patients for arthroscopic or open shoulder stabilization.

Decision-Making Algorithms

Treatment algorithms depend on many factors, but the size and type (fragment or erosion) of the glenoid bone defect are paramount. If a mobile bone fragment is associated with the labral lesion, then despite the fragment size, the possibility for an arthroscopic reattachment exists (Fig. 22.7). If bone loss is present, no precise guidelines exist. If the percentage of bone loss is greater than 20% of the area of the intact contralateral glenoid, a bone grafting procedure (either open or arthroscopic) to fill the defect and restore the glenoid arc is recommended by most authors. If the missing glenoid area is less than 10% and there is no patulous soft tissue, an arthroscopic soft tissue reconstruction to restore joint stability is certainly an option. If the bone loss is between 10% and 20%, other factors should be considered. Certainly, a coexisting Hill–Sachs lesion could constitute an indication for a bony procedure. Table 22.1 outlines the treatment options based upon these factors.

In addition to an accurate preoperative assessment of a possible bone defect, other risk factors that could preclude arthroscopic soft tissue stabilization must be evaluated. If the instability severity index score (ISIS) (Table 22.2) is more than six points, an isolated soft tissue reconstruction could be insufficient to stabilize the shoulder.

In summary, the careful preoperative assessment of bony lesions, the ISIS scoring system, physical examination, and history may help the surgeon select patients who will benefit from arthroscopic anterior soft tissue stabilization and those who will not.

TREATMENT

Nonoperative

A great deal has been written on the management of anteroinferior shoulder dislocation. The shoulder should be protected against distraction for 6 weeks. One recent approach

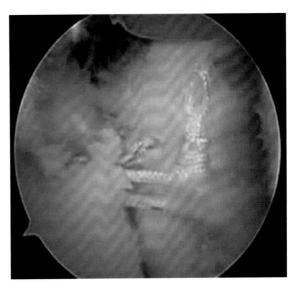

FIGURE 22.7. Arthroscopic bony Bankart repair.

Table 22.1

Decision-Making Algorithms for Operative Indications in Shoulder Instability

Glenoid Bone Loss	Decision-Making Algorithms in Shoulder Instability	
>20%	Bone grafting procedure	
<10%	Soft tissue procedure	
>10% <20%	Coexisting Hill–Sachs lesion	Bone grafting procedure
	ISIS score >6	Bone grafting procedure
	No Hill–Sachs—ISIS score <6	Soft tissue procedure

calls for constant immobilization of the shoulder in a sling in external rotation for a period of 6 weeks. As soon as the pain has subsided, the patient is started on a shoulder girdle rehabilitation program that includes strengthening of the deltoid, the scapular muscles, and the rotator cuff.

Nonoperative treatment for an athlete often is chosen based upon the specific sport's season. Operating on an athlete in the middle of the season can be a difficult choice, and surgery could be delayed until the end of the season. This may be less than ideal particularly if significant bony lesions are present. However, the decision should be made only after a comprehensive discussion of the injury, its prognosis, and the potential consequences of the various treatment options by the physician with the athlete, the coach, and the family.

Operative Indications

Individuals who sustain a dislocation as the result of significant trauma and who do not have generalized ligamentous laxity are more likely to benefit from surgical treatment. Recurrence of instability represents the leading complication of anterior shoulder stabilization. Currently, most surgeons use suture anchor techniques for arthroscopic soft tissue stabilization because of the more reproducible results. However, even with recent technical advances, a recurrence rate between 5% and 20% still persists. The best way would be to preoperatively identify patients whose risk factors preclude arthroscopic stabilization. Numerous prognostic factors have been reported in the literature. Younger patients are at risk, but no clear age limit is identified. Athletes who participate in contact or collision sports have higher recurrence rates after standard arthroscopic stabilization. Finally, patients with significant glenoid bone loss, which result in unacceptably high rates of recurrent dislocation and subluxation after arthroscopic soft tissue repair, are candidates for arthroscopic "bony procedures."

Table 22.2

Instability Severity Index Score (ISIS)

	Prognostic Factors		Points
Questionnaire	Age at surgery	≤20 y	2
		>20 y	0
	Degree of sport practice (preop)	Competition	2
		Recreational or no sports	0
	Type of sports (preop)	Contact or forced ABD-ER	1
		Other	0
Exam	Shoulder hyperlaxity	Shoulder hyperlaxity	1
		Normal laxity	0
AP X-ray	Hill–Sachs on AP X-ray	In external rotation	2
		Not visible in ER	0
	Glenoid loss of contour on AP X-ray	Loss of contour	2
		No lesion	0
Total			10 pts

TECHNIQUES

Arthroscopic Latarjet Procedure

In the arthroscopic Latarjet procedure first described by Lafosse, the whole horizontal part of the coracoid is transferred to the anterior glenoid rim in a horizontal manner reaching from the 2 to 3 o'clock position to the 5 to 6 o'clock position (Fig. 22.8). The coracoid is placed through a split in the subscapularis and fixed at antero-inferior part of the glenoid, preferably with two screws. The stabilization mechanism of this procedure includes bone restoration and augmentation and a dynamic musculotendinous sling effect created by the conjoint tendon passing over the inferior part of the subscapularis (Fig. 22.9). The latter creates dynamic tension in abduction and external rotation. In addition, the suture of the inferior glenohumeral ligament to the CA ligament, which is still attached to the coracoid, reinforces the stability. Owing to the enhanced arthroscopic visualization, the positioning of the coracoid fragment can have a perfect

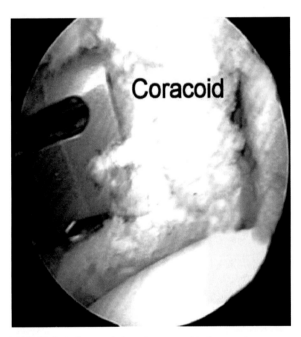

FIGURE 22.8. Arthroscopic Latarjet: coracoid placement.

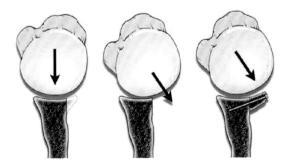

FIGURE 22.9. Principal stabilization mechanism of bone grafting procedures: increased diameter of the glenoid bone arc.

alignment with the glenoid rim and prevent medial placement of the graft in the joint.

Indications

1. Anterior-inferior glenoid bone loss
2. Poor quality ligaments
3. Revision surgery
4. Extreme sports participation

First step: Exposure of the coracoid

With visualization from the posterior portal, the anterior capsule together with the labrum is released between 2 and 5 o'clock through the anterior portal. The entire inferior glenohumeral ligament is detached. The rotator interval is opened with sectioning of the superior glenohumeral and coracohumeral ligaments. The coracoacromial ligament is cut, the lateral border of the conjoint tendon is released, and the coracoid is separated from the aponeurosis of the deltoid muscle.

Second step: Coracoid preparation

With the scope in a lateral portal, the rotator interval is opened until a good intra-articular view is achieved. The coracoid area is cleaned, and the subscapular nerve and axillary nerve are identified medially. A supracoracoid portal is created in the midpoint between the tip and the base of the coracoid. The pectoralis minor tendon is released (Fig. 22.10), and the medial border of the conjoint tendon is released. The plexus lies just behind the pectoralis minor, so the detachment should be as close as possible to the coracoid. Great caution should be exercised not to jeopardize the musculocutaneous nerve when the conjoint tendon is released.

Third step: Preparation of the coracoid holes and coracoid osteotomy

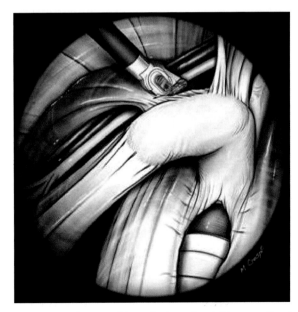

FIGURE 22.10. The coracoid area is cleaned and the pectoralis minor tendon is released. The plexus lies just behind the pectoralis minor.

Two 3.5-mm drill holes are placed vertically in the coracoid 8 mm apart (Fig. 22.11). A shuttle wire is passed through the holes in a U-shape and is retrieved through the coracoid portal (Fig. 22.12). A coracoid osteotomy is performed 2 to 2.5 cm above the tip of the coracoid, using a curved osteotome superiorly (Fig. 22.13) and straight osteotome laterally. The coracoid fragment is mobilized inferiorly, exposing the anterior subscapularis muscle fibers.

Fourth step: Coracoid transfer

With visualization through the anterior portal, the instrumentation passes through an anteroinferior portal.

An anterior axillary portal located in the anterior axillary fold is created. With the use of the ablation diathermy through the axillary portal, a horizontal split is created in the subscapularis between upper third and inferior two-thirds (Fig. 22.14). The split is created starting lateral to the axillary nerve and proceeding to the insertion stopping anterior to the biceps groove (Fig. 22.15). The split is opened using a switching stick from posterior in order to create room for the passage of the coracoid graft. Two cannulated guide screws are inserted with the aid of the

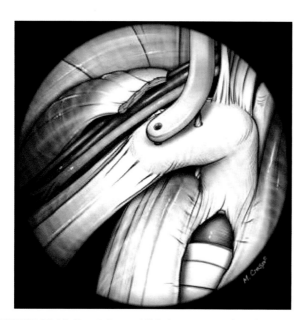

FIGURE 22.11. Two 3.5-mm drill holes are created in the coracoid vertically 8 mm apart.

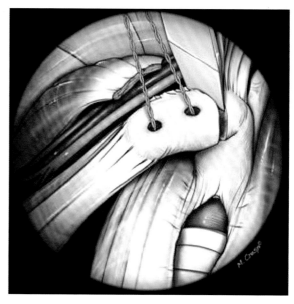

FIGURE 22.13. The shuttle wire is retrieved through the coracoid portal. A coracoid osteotomy is performed 2 to 2.5 cm above the tip of the coracoid using a curved osteotome.

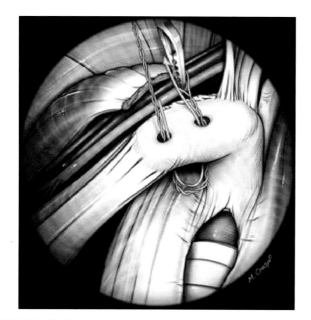

FIGURE 22.12. A shuttle wire is passed through the holes in a U-shape.

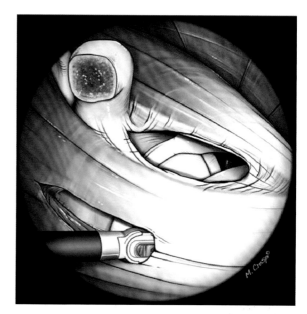

FIGURE 22.14. Ablation diathermy through the axillary portal creates a horizontal split in the subscapularis between upper one-third and inferior two-thirds.

sutures into the drill holes in the coracoid. The coracoid is fixed to a specific cannulated guide and transferred through the split and positioned on the anterior rim of the glenoid (Fig. 22.16).

Fifth step: coracoid fixation

With the scope in the anterior portal, instrumentation is introduced through the anterior-inferior portal. A guide wire is drilled through one of the guide screws, either superiorly or inferiorly, into the glenoid for temporary fixation. The guide screw is removed, and a 3.5-mm cannulated drill bit is advanced over the wire. The first screw is advanced until the head appears close to the anterior cortex of the coracoid but is not tightened completely. The second screw is inserted in the same

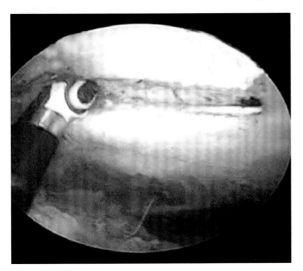

FIGURE 22.15. The split is created starting lateral to the axillary nerve and stopping anterior to the biceps groove.

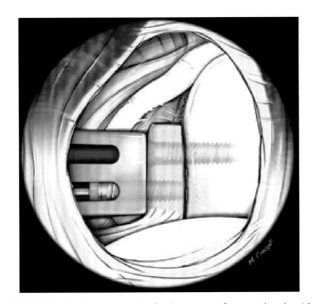

FIGURE 22.16. The coracoid is fixed to a specific cannulated guide and transferred through the split and positioned on the anterior rim of the glenoid.

way, and final compression of both screws is performed under arthroscopic visualization. The graft is fixed on the anterior glenoid from 2 to 6 o'clock at the level of the glenoid rim.

The arthroscopic Latarjet is a difficult surgical procedure. This procedure provides an anatomic solution for glenoid bone defects and a nonanatomic solution for soft tissue lesions utilizing the sling effect created by crossing the subscapularis with the conjoint tendon. Owing to the enhanced arthroscopic visualization, the positioning of the graft in the glenoid neck can be carefully assessed to prevent overhang. The Latarjet procedure with the transfer of the coracoid and the conjoint tendon through the subscapularis is a nonanatomic procedure. The damage of the subscapularis fibers is the greatest weakness of this procedure.

Arthroscopic Bristow—Latarjet Procedure

The arthroscopic Bristow–Latarjet procedure described by Boileau combines an arthroscopic Bankart repair with the transfer of the tip of the coracoid that is passed through the subscapularis and fixed on the glenoid rim below the equator. The efficacy of this procedure is related to a "triple locking" of the shoulder: the coracoid bone block increases the size of the glenoid surface, the sling effect provided by the conjoint tendon crossing the subscapularis, and the glenoid concavity re-creation provided by the labral repair. In this procedure, only the tip (10 to 15 mm) of the coracoid is harvested; the bone block is then positioned in the standing position.

Indications

1. Anterior-inferior glenoid bone loss
2. Poor quality ligaments
3. Revision surgery
4. Extreme sports participation

First step: Glenoid preparation

With the scope in the posterior portal, an anterior working portal is created. Once the thin capsule of the rotator interval is resected, the coracoid process can be clearly identified. The anterior labrum is detached and elevated from the glenoid neck from 2 to 6 o'clock. The capsule–labrum–ligament complex must be fully mobile. The scope is then inserted through the anterior-superior portal. The bony erosion is assessed and smoothed with a bur (Fig. 22.17). A specific guide is then introduced through the posterior portal. A guide pin is inserted through the guide from posterior to anterior and through the glenoid neck (Fig. 22.18A, B). Anteriorly, the pin is stopped by the anterior blade of the guide (Fig. 22.19). The guide pin is made of two parts: a female part 2.8 mm in diameter and a male part 1.5 mm in diameter (Fig. 22.20). The glenoid pin is positioned below the equator. The guide allows measurement of the drilling depth. Next, a blunt rod is introduced through the posterior portal and

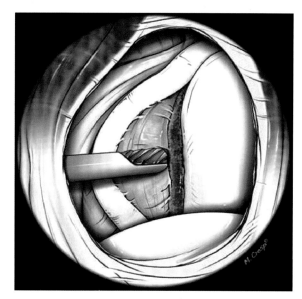

FIGURE 22.17. The thin capsule of the rotator interval is resected. The anterior labrum is detached and elevated from the glenoid neck from 2 to 6 o'clock until the complex capsule-labrum-ligaments are fully mobile. The bony erosion is assessed and smoothed with a bur.

is placed at the level of the equator and pushed under the labrum and through the subscapularis muscle fibers.

Second step: Coracoid harvesting

The scope is placed in the anterolateral portal. Using an outside-in technique, a spinal needle is aligned with the long axis of the coracoid, and an inferior portal is created. Then a medial portal perpendicular to the tip of the coracoid process is created (Fig. 22.21). At this point, the locations of the axillary nerve and the transglenoid rod are identified. The arm is placed in flexion, adduction, and full internal rotation in order to relax the axillary nerve. Using a blunt trocar, the axillary nerve is located and identified as it passes under the inferior rim of the subscapularis muscle. Once the axillary nerve has been identified and protected, the split of the subscapularis is started using a radiofrequency device from medial to lateral at the level of the transglenoid rod (Fig. 22.22). The muscle belly is usually divided in-line with its fibers. The more subscapularis that is taken inferiorly, the more external rotation may be limited. The coracoid process and the conjoint tendon are then separated from the deep surface of the deltoid muscle. The coracoacromial ligament is released from the lateral part of the coracoid, whereas the pectoralis minor insertion is released from its medial part. In order to not damage the brachial plexus, the releasing instrument must be kept in contact with the lateral side of the coracoid.

Once the coracoid is fully exposed, an additional portal is created at the level of the acromioclavicular joint. A spinal needle is used to verify that the direction of this portal is perpendicular to the coracoid process. The osteotomy harvests only the tip of the coracoid (approximately 15 mm). The osteotomy is carried out using an oscillating saw and is stopped before reaching the inferior

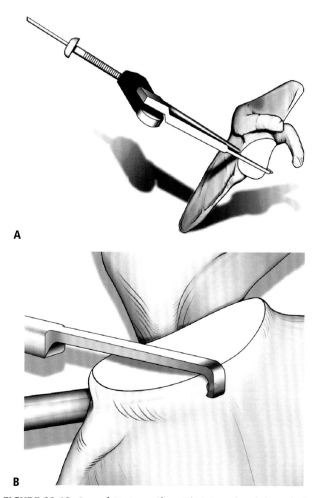

FIGURE 22.18. A and B: A specific guide is introduced through the posterior portal. A guide pin is inserted through the guide from posterior to anterior and into the glenoid neck. The glenoid pin is positioned below the equator.

cortex of the coracoid. Then a specific guide is introduced through the inferior portal and used to insert a guide pin along the longitudinal axis of the coracoid. The pin first hooks the center of the cancellous bone of the partially osteotomized coracoid.

The second part of the guide, the awl, is placed on the center of the tip of the coracoid. The guide pin, inserted along the axis of the coracoid, is used to insert a cannulated drill 3.5 mm in diameter. The coracoid guide allows measurement of the drilling depth of the coracoid graft. This is added to the glenoid drilling depth previously measured to give the length of the screw (Fig. 22.23). Once the cannulated drill has been engaged inside the coracoid, the guide pin is removed and replaced by a metallic suture passer. The loop end of the metallic suture passer is firmly held by a grasper introduced through the medial portal. The cannulated drill is disengaged from the coracoid process. The other end of the suture passer is also retrieved with the grasper and pulled through the same medial portal. The osteotomy of the coracoid process is

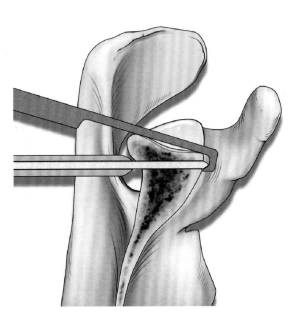

FIGURE 22.19. Anteriorly the pin is stopped by the anterior blade of the guide.

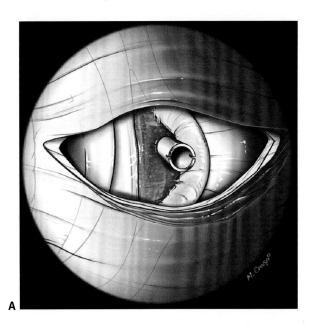

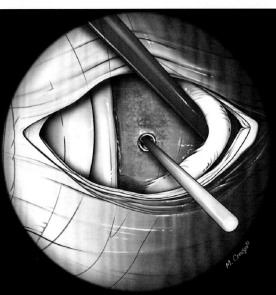

FIGURE 22.20. A and B: The guide pin is made of two parts: a female part 2.8 mm in diameter, and a male part of 1.5 mm in diameter.

then completed from inferior to superior. When the bone fragment is detached, both strands of the suture passer are pulled from the medial portal giving free access to the subscapularis muscle belly. The remaining coracoid process is smoothed with a bur.

Third step: coracoid transfer

The scope is placed in the anterior-inferior portal. Using a radiofrequency device introduced through the anteromedial portal, the muscle fibers of the subscapularis are split medially to the glenoid neck and laterally to the lesser tuberosity. A U-shaped retractor, introduced through the coracoid portal, is used to retract superiorly the upper two-third of the subscapularis. A second retractor, introduced through the anteroinferior portal inferiorly retracts the lower part of the muscle. At this moment, the anteroinferior margin of the glenoid is exposed, and the glenoid guide pin is visible. The female part of the guide pin is left in place, whereas the male pin is replaced with a longer pin sticking out of the anterior neck of the scapula. A reamer is then introduced over the male guide pin to create a socket of 2 to 3 mm deep that will receive the tip of the coracoid. The male glenoid guide pin is then removed and replaced with a suture retriever introduced from posterior to anterior. The distal loop of the coracoid suture passer is taken with the grasper from the lateral portal and connected to the suture retriever; it is then pulled through the glenoid. The suture passer is replaced with a wire driven through the coracoid, the glenoid, and retrieved posteriorly. At this point, a specific cannulated screw 36 to 40 mm in length is driven into the coracoid process over the wire. When the screw is engaged inside the coracoid, the wire is pulled posteriorly allowing the coracoid to be brought inside the glenoid socket. The bone block is inserted through the split fibers of the subscapularis and positioned on the anteroinferior

margin of the glenoid (Fig. 22.24). The scope is then placed through the anterior-superior portal to provide an intra-articular view of the bone block and verify that it is well positioned below the equator and flush to the glenoid surface.

Fourth step: Bankart repair

The scope is reintroduced through the posterior portal. A classic Bankart repair is performed using a suture anchors technique. This allows capsulo-ligamentous tensioning and recreation of the glenoid concavity. The advantages of the associated glenoid labrum repair are that the bone block is placed in an extra-articular position, preventing synovial fluid from coming in contact with the bone block; it avoids contact between the humeral head and the coracoid bone block with the screw, which can cause pain and glenohumeral osteoarthritis; and it avoids some of the pain

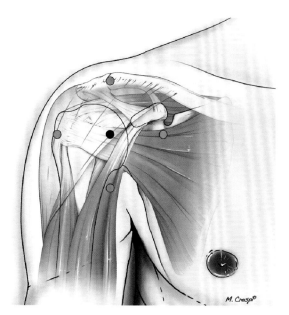

FIGURE 22.21. Portals for the arthroscopic Bristow–Latarjet procedure.

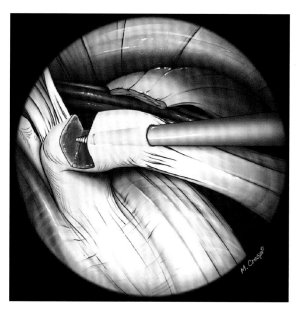

FIGURE 22.23. The guide pin, inserted along the axis of the coracoid, is used to insert a 3.5 mm in diameter cannulated drill.

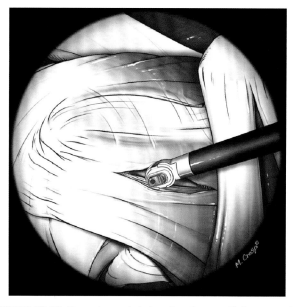

FIGURE 22.22. The subscapularis is split using a radiofrequency device from medial to lateral.

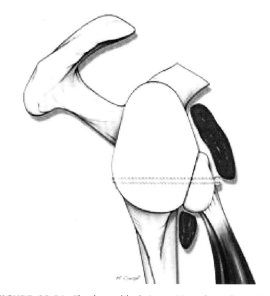

FIGURE 22.24. The bone block is positioned on the anteroinferior margin of the glenoid.

and persistent apprehension sometimes seen after a classical Bristow–Latarjet procedure. As for the arthroscopic Latarjet procedure, the transfer of the coracoid and the conjoint tendon through the subscapularis fibers define this operation as a nonanatomic procedure. The damage of the subscapularis fibers is also the weakest point of this procedure.

Arthroscopic Anterior Bone Block Procedure

The arthroscopic anterior bone block procedure first described by Taverna combines an arthroscopic Bankart repair with the transfer of the tip of the iliac crest graft that is passed

through a cannula placed in the rotator interval and fixed on the glenoid rim under the equator. The advantages of this procedure include the bone block effect provided by the tricortical bone graft that increases the glenoid surface size, the concavity re-creation provided by the labral repair, and the capsular and ligaments shift and repair. The goal of the procedure is to restore the normal anatomy of the unstable shoulder with bone defects on the glenoid.

Indications

1. Anterior-inferior glenoid bone loss
2. Revision surgery
3. Extreme sports participation

First step: bone graft harvest

With the patient in supine position, a tricortical bone graft measuring 1 cm by 2 cm is harvested from the iliac crest. Two holes are created by a 1-mm Kirschner wire 0.5 cm from the graft ends (Fig. 22.25A–C).

Second step: Glenoid preparation

With the patient in a beach chair position, the arthroscope is placed posteriorly, using an outside-in technique, a 10-mm cannula anterior-inferiorly, and a 5.5-mm cannula placed anterior-superiorly. The anterior capsuloligamentous complex is detached from the glenoid from 2 to 6 o'clock until it is possible to observe the muscular fibers of the subscapularis from the posterior portal, and the entire glenoid neck with the arthroscope in the anterior-superior portal (Fig. 22.26). The anterior bony glenoid defect is then smoothed with a motorized bur.

Third step: Bone graft transfer

Still viewing though the anterior-superior portal, two bioabsorbable suture anchors are placed 1 cm apart, 0.5 cm medial to the glenoid rim, and centered at the bone deficit of the anterior-inferior glenoid (Fig. 27). The sutures are retrieved out a 10-mm anterior-inferior cannula. The

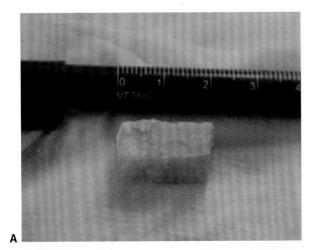

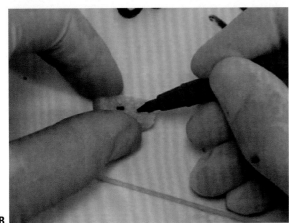

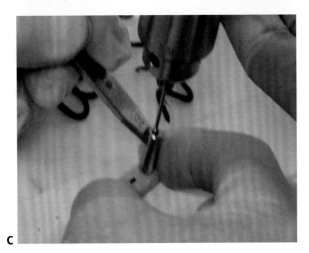

FIGURE 22.25. A–C: The tricortical bone graft measuring 1 cm by 2 cm is harvested from the iliac crest. Two holes at 0.5 cm from the ends are created with a 1-mm Kirschner wire.

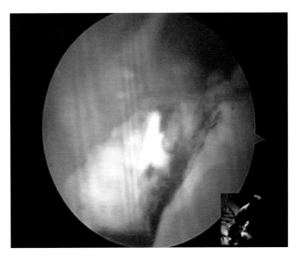

FIGURE 22.26. The anterior capsuloligamentous complex is detached from the glenoid from 2 to 6 o'clock.

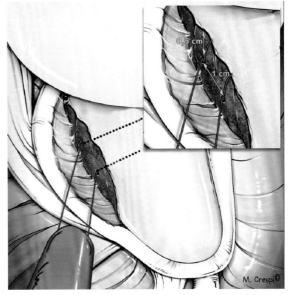

FIGURE 22.27. Two bioabsorbable suture anchors are placed 1 cm from each other, 0.5 cm medial to the glenoid rim, and centered on the bone deficit of the anterior glenoid.

four suture limbs are passed through the holes in the bone block graft. The bone block is rotated 90° with respect to the sutures coming out the cannula, and the sutures passed through the cannulated trocar of the cannula. The bone graft is introduced into the joint through the cannula by the cannulated trocar (Fig. 22.28) and under direct arthroscopic vision. The sutures that kept under gentle tension direct the bone graft precisely into the appropriate anterior-inferior position on the glenoid (Fig. 22.29). At this point, all four limbs of the suture anchors are retrieved out the posterior portal and are kept under tension in order to maintain the bone block parallel to the anterior glenoid neck and aligned with the glenoid rim.

Two 2-mm Kirschner wire are introduced percutaneously through the subscapularis fibers as in a 5 o'clock portal and are passed through the previously drilled point of the bone block and into the glenoid neck (Fig. 22.30). The tension in the sutures and a probe introduced through the anterior-inferior cannula prevent the bone block from rotating during the wire introduction. At this point, two 1-mm diameter Kirschner wires are introduced in the same fashion through the bone block immediately inferior to the superior sutures and immediately superior to the inferior sutures. After correct placement of the bone block is confirmed with a probe, the bone block and the glenoid are drilled using a 2.5-cannulated drill over the 1-mm Kirschner wires. Two 3.5-mm diameter half-threaded cannulated screws measuring 35 mm in length are introduced in the same fashion (Fig. 22.31). After the solidity of the graft is confirmed with an arthroscopic probe, the three Kirschner wires and the sutures from the glenoid neck anchors are removed.

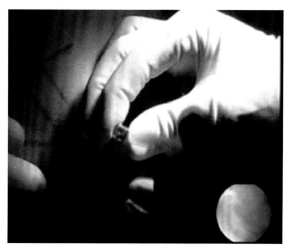

FIGURE 22.28. The bone graft is pushed through the cannula with the cannulated trocar.

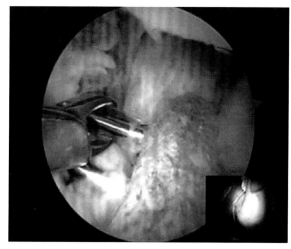

FIGURE 22.30. Two 2-mm Kirschner wires are introduced percutaneously through the subscapularis fibers as in a 5 o'clock portal and are passed through the previously drilled holes of the bone block into the glenoid neck.

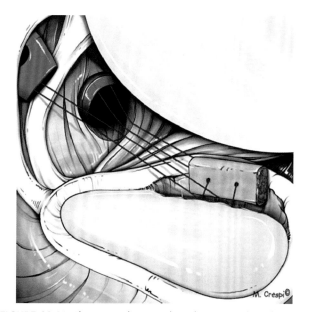

FIGURE 22.29. The sutures kept gently under tension drive the bone graft exactly into the anterior-inferior part of the glenoid.

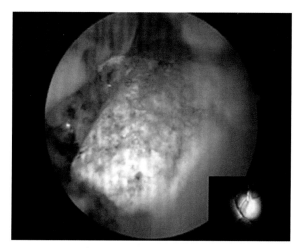

FIGURE 22.31. Arthroscopic fixation and compression of the bone block using two 3.5-mm diameter half-threaded cannulated screws measuring 35 mm in length.

Fourth step: soft tissue repair

Three suture anchors are then placed along the glenoid rim at the 3, 4, and 5 o'clock positions, and an anterior-inferior capsuloligamentous shift with an anterior labrum reattachment is performed. In this way, the graft becomes an extra-articular platform (Fig. 32A,B). The advantages of this procedure include the associated repair of the glenoid labrum and tensioning and shift of the capsule and ligaments. As with the Bristow–Latarjet procedure, the bone block is placed in an extra-articular position, preventing synovial fluid from coming in contact with the bone graft and avoids the potential contact between the humeral head and the coracoid bone block with the screw, which can cause pain and glenohumeral osteoarthritis. This is an anatomic procedure with the restoration of normal glenohumeral anatomy, increasing the damaged glenoid bony support and restoring the normal insertion of the labrum, ligaments, and capsule (Fig. 22.33A–E). Compared with the Bristow and Latarjet procedure, the damage of the subscapularis fibers is minimal. The weakest aspect of this procedure is the impossibility to address the rare combination of an unstable shoulder with glenoid bone defects and capsular–labrum–ligaments inconsistency. In such a case, the dynamic musculotendinous sling effect created by the conjoint tendon and the subscapularis of the Latarjet and Bristow procedures is mandatory.

REHABILITATION

Postoperatively the authors who have described "bony procedures" for shoulder instability recommend keeping patients in a sling for a period of 2 to 4 weeks. After the immobilization, there is no limitation in passive motion, and the patients are allowed to progressively recover full elevation and external rotation. After complete wound healing, active swimming pool exercises are recommended and working activities are resumed. Progressive strengthening exercises are started after 6 to 8 weeks. A return to overhead and contact sports is generally allowed at 4 to 6 months postsurgery.

CONCLUSION

The prevalence of fracture or erosion of the anteroinferior part of the glenoid rim in shoulders with recurrent anterior dislocations has been reported to range from 8% to 73%. Biomechanical studies have found an inverse relationship between the size of the glenoid defect and the stability of the shoulder: the larger the defect the less stable the shoulder.

The effect of a glenoid defect on shoulder stability after Bankart lesion repair continues to be investigated. Some have suggested that a defect involving at least one-third of the glenoid surface may necessitate a bone graft, whereas others have stated simply that bone grafting is necessary for the treatment of a "large glenoid defect." Many clinicians believe that a large defect of the glenoid must be treated with bone grafting to the glenoid when a Bankart procedure is performed. To date there is no consensus when and how bony procedures are needed to stabilize a glenohumeral joint. Further investigations are needed to determine the amount of bone loss that significantly affects the recurrence rate of an isolated soft tissue repair in an unstable shoulder.

Finally, the goal of any arthroscopic glenohumeral stabilizing procedure should be to restore the glenoid concavity arc along with a labrum repair and the proper restoration of the capsular and ligamentous tension.

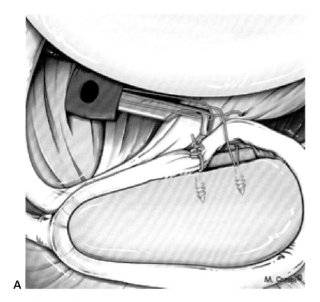

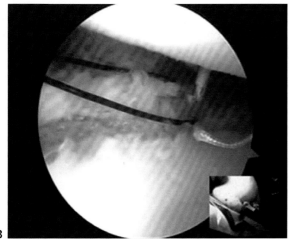

FIGURE 22.32. A and **B**: Three suture anchors are placed along the glenoid rim at the 3, 4, and 5 o'clock positions. Then an anterior-inferior capsuloligamentous shift and anterior labrum reattachment are performed. The graft becomes an extra-articular platform.

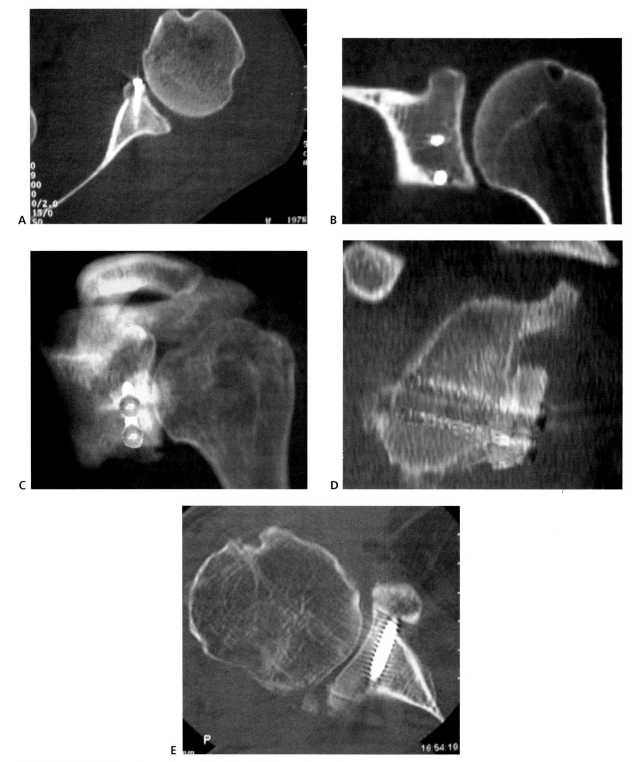

FIGURE 22.33. A–E: Imaging at 1-year after a bone block procedure.

SUGGESTED READINGS

Gartsman GM, Roddey TS, Hammerman SM. Arthroscopic treatment of anterior-inferior glenohumeral instability. Two to five-year follow-up. *J Bone Joint Surg Am.* 2000;82: 991–1003.

Bigliani LU, Pollock RG, Soslowsky LJ, et al. Tensile properties of the inferior glenohumeral ligament. *J Orthop Res.* 1992;10:187–197.

Taverna E, Sansone V, Battistella F. Arthroscopic rotator interval repair: the three-step all-inside technique. *Arthroscopy.* 2004;20:105–109.

Bigliani LU, Newton PM, Steinmann SP, et al. Glenoid rim lesions associated with recurrent anterior dislocation of the shoulder. *Am J Sports Med.* 1998;26:41–45.

Edwards TB, Boulahia A, Walch G. Radiographic analysis of bone defects in chronic anterior shoulder instability. *Arthroscopy.* 2003;19:732–739.

Sugaya H, Moriishi J, Dohi M, et al. Glenoid rim morphology in recurrent anterior glenohumeral instability. *J Bone Joint Surg Am.* 2003;85:878–884.

Itoi E, Lee SB, Berglund LJ, et al. The effect of a glenoid defect on anteroinferior stability of the shoulder after Bankart repair: a cadaveric study. *J Bone Joint Surg Am.* 2000;82:35–46.

Cassagnaud X, Maynou C, Mestdagh H. Clinical and computed tomography results of 106 Latarjet-Patte procedures at mean 7.5 year follow-up [French]. *Rev Chir Orthop Reparatrice Appar Mot.* 2003;89:683–692.

Hovelius L, Körner L, Lundberg B, et al. The coracoid transfer for recurrent dislocation of the shoulder: technical aspects of the Bristow-Latarjet procedure. *J Bone Joint Surg Am.* 1983;65:926–934.

Allain J, Goutallier D, Glorion C. Long-term results of the Latarjet procedure for the treatment of anterior instability of the shoulder. *J Bone Joint Surg Am.* 1998;80:841–852.

Vander Maren C, Geulette B, Lewalle J, et al. Coracoid process abutment according to Latarjet versus the Bankart operation: a comparative study of the results in 50 cases [Article in French]. *Acta Orthop Belg.* 1993;59:147–155.

Young DC, Rockwood CA Jr. Complications of a failed Bristow procedure and their management. *J Bone Joint Surg Am.* 1991;73:969–981.

Hybbinette S. De la transposition d'un fragment osseux pour remedier aux luxations recidivantes de l'epaule constatations et resultats opératoires. *Acta Chir Seand.* 1932;71:411–445.

Latarjet M. A propos du traitement des luxations récidivantes de l'Iepaule. *Lyon Chir.* 1954;49:994–1003.

Mochizuki Y, Hachisuka H, Kashiwagi K, et al. Arthroscopic autologous bone graft with arthroscopic Bankart repair for a large bony defect lesion caused by recurrent shoulder dislocation. *Arthroscopy.* 2007;23:677.e1–677.e4.

Nourissat G, Nedellec G, O'Sullivan NA, et al. Mini-open arthroscopically assisted Bristow-Latarjet procedure for the treatment of patients with anterior shoulder instability: a cadaver study. *Arthroscopy.* 2006;22:1113–1118.

Boileau P, Bicknell RT, El Fegoun AB, et al. Arthroscopic Bristow procedure for anterior instability in shoulders with a stretched or deficient capsule: the "belt-and-suspenders" operative technique and preliminary results. *Arthroscopy.* 2007;23:593–601.

Lafosse L, Lejeune E, Bouchard A, et al. The arthroscopic Latarjet procedure for the treatment of anterior shoulder instability. *Arthroscopy.* 2007;23:1242.e1–1242.e5.

Taverna E, Golanò P, Pascale V, et al. An arthroscopic bone graft procedure for treating anterior-inferior glenohumeral instability. *Knee Surg Sports Arthrosc.* 2008;16:872–875.

I. The Shoulder

The Stiff Shoulder: Planning and Treatment Options

John P. Goldblatt • Richard Woodworth • Bryan Mitchell

Shoulder stiffness is a common problem seen in orthopedic clinical practice. Limited active and passive motion of the glenohumeral joint can be seen with various causes, including adhesive capsulitis, trauma, or postsurgical changes. This chapter will outline and discuss the etiology, diagnosis, and treatment options for the stiff shoulder.

Primary adhesive capsulitis, or "frozen shoulder," is often not associated with an inciting event. Rather, the development of adhesive capsulitis may have various associated conditions. The prevalence in the general population is 2% to 5% (1) and can be as high as 20% in some patient subgroups such as diabetics (2). The incidence is approximately 2.4/1,000 people/year (3). Risk factors include female gender, thyroid disease, diabetes, stroke, myocardial infarction, and the presence of autoimmune disease (4). Age is another important risk factor. Most patients are between 40 and 60 years old. Not uncommonly, idiopathic primary adhesive capsulitis can occur without identifiable risk factors (5).

Post-traumatic or postsurgical shoulder stiffness is defined as acquired or secondary shoulder stiffness. The important distinction from primary adhesive capsulitis is that for the acquired form there is a known event that precipitated the onset. These triggers may cause changes around the shoulder joint affecting intra- and extra-articular structures.

HISTORICAL NOTE

Adhesive capsulitis has been variously described and named. Codman in 1934 wrote that the "frozen" shoulder is difficult to define, treat, and explain from a pathologic perspective. Additional early investigators include McLaughlin, Asherman, Moseley, Neviaser, and DePalma.

Quigley outlined the characteristic findings of adhesive capsulitis in his classic article on the "checkrein shoulder" (6). This condition occurs most commonly in middle life, more often in women than in men. There is no obvious predisposition, including a lack of an association between arthritis, rotator cuff tears, and other metabolic diseases. The inciting event can be "a minor contusion or wrench, or an episode of inflammation ... there apparently is no initiating episode except pain. Invariably, the onset is followed by a period of disuse, imposed by pain." Quigley described a limited arc of both active and passive motion, with the passive motion pain free up to a limit, at which point motion is sharply checked.

Treatment recommendations at that time consisted of a gradual stretching program followed by active exercise, heat therapy, X-ray therapy, or repeated procaine infiltration. This was recognized as safe and effective; however, it often required months and "makes great demands on the patient's fortitude." Resolution of symptoms requires months or years and can result in permanent restrictions.

Various surgical options have been described. McLaughlin recommended surgical division of the subscapularis and anteroinferior joint capsule in refractory cases. Manipulation under anesthesia (MUA) was condemned as dangerous and futile, primarily because the pain after manipulation was so severe that active participation in rehabilitation was difficult or impossible.

Neviaser observed 15 shoulders manipulated after surgical exposure of the joint capsule. The adherent, contracted joint capsule was seen to tear and strip from its attachments to the humerus, and he described the condition as "adhesive capsulitis." Quigley found the reproducible block to motion present only in the anterior and inferior aspects of the joint and therefore coined the term "checkrein shoulder."

Quigley should be credited with his careful technique of manipulation, which allowed for a much more controlled release, as well as his attention to pain management postoperatively. His technique included the manipulation of the scapula after placing the well-supported humerus in varying positions of maximum flexion, abduction, and rotation. He emphasized avoiding the use of the humerus as a lever. This was preoperatively and postoperatively accompanied by adrenocorticotropic hormone (ACTH) administration for pain management. Quigley's technique was able to effectively obtain and maintain a nearly normal range of motion.

CLINICAL EVALUATION

Stiff shoulders can be classified into three main types: primary adhesive capsulitis, secondary adhesive capsulitis, and acquired stiffness. Defining the cause of stiffness will help guide the treatment.

Pertinent History and Physical Exam by Stages of Disease

Primary Adhesive Capsulitis

Primary adhesive capsulitis is the progressive loss of motion in the shoulder associated with inflammation and subsequent fibrosis. The pathogenesis of adhesive capsulitis has long been debated and is still not fully understood. In addition to the clinical symptoms, histopathologic changes in the synovium and subsynovium are observed (7). The histology suggests both an inflammatory and fibrosing etiology, evident to varying degrees during the separate stages of the disease. There is significant evidence to support the hypothesis that adhesive capsulitis is caused by a synovial inflammation, with subsequent reactive capsular fibrosis, leading to loss of motion.

Adhesive capsulitis is described as a condition of shoulder stiffness that progresses through four stages originally described by Neviaser and Neviaser (7). Table 23.1 summarizes each stage. It is critical to recognize that accurate identification of the stage will guide treatment and that the presentation of the disease represents a continuum rather than a discrete stage. Each stage can be identified by duration of symptoms, arthroscopic features, range of motion limitations both clinically and under anesthesia, and histopathology. Neviaser described the arthroscopic changes of adhesive capsulitis (1).

Stage I is described as the painful phase, with limited active motion secondary to painful inflammation. Passive motion is preserved when the patient is examined under anesthesia, either with a local anesthetic block or with a general anesthesia. This finding confirms the early stage of disease, as the motion loss is secondary to pain caused by inflammation rather than fibrosis. Loss of active motion occurs in forward flexion, abduction, and internal rotation, with minimal external rotation deficit. Symptoms last up to 3 months. Arthroscopic examination of the glenohumeral joint reveals diffuse synovitis, most pronounced in the anterosuperior capsule and rotator

Table 23.1

Stages of adhesive capsulitis

Stage I
Duration of symptoms: 0–3 months
Pain with active and passive ROM
Limitation of forward flexion, abduction, internal rotation, external rotation
EUA: normal or minimal loss of ROM
Arthroscopy: diffuse synovitis, most pronounced in the anterosuperior capsule
Pathology: hypertrophic, hypervascular synovitis, inflammatory cell infiltrates, normal capsule

Stage II ("Freezing Stage")
Duration of symptoms: 3–9 months
Chronic pain with active and passive ROM
Significant limitation of forward flexion, abduction, internal rotation, external rotation
EUA: ROM essentially identical to awake ROM
Arthroscopy: diffuse, pedunculated synovitis
Pathology: hypertrophic, hypervascular synovitis, perivascular, subsynovial, and capsular scar

Stage III ("Frozen Stage")
Duration of symptoms: 9–15 months
Minimal pain except at end ROM
Significant limitation of ROM with rigid "end feel"
EUA: ROM identical to awake ROM
Arthroscopy: remnants of fibrotic synovium, diminished capsular volume
Pathology: minimal synovium, underlying capsule with dense scar formation

Stage IV ("Thawing Phase"):
Duration of symptoms: 15–24 months
Minimal pain
Progressive improvement in ROM
Examination under anesthesia: data not available

interval (Fig. 23.1). The histology of biopsy specimens in the painful phase reveals hypertrophic, hypervascular synovitis, with inflammatory infiltrates, but normal-appearing capsular tissue.

Stage II, the freezing phase, is associated with more chronic shoulder pain and significant loss of motion in all planes. The duration of symptoms is typically from months 3 to 9. An exact definition of this stage is debated based on actual degree of motion loss; however, examination under anesthesia will demonstrate only a partial loss of motion. This reflects a loss of capsular volume secondary to the onset of fibrosis. Arthroscopy reveals diffuse, dense, proliferative and hypervascular synovium (Fig. 23.2). Cellular changes identified in biopsy specimens include new collagen deposition with disorganized collagen fibrils and no inflammatory infiltrates.

Stage III, the frozen phase, occurs between months 9 and 15. Patients in this phase report a history of improvement in their shoulder pain over time, yet continue to demonstrate stiffness. When the shoulder is examined under anesthesia, there is no improvement in passive range of motion when compared with the active motion while awake. Arthroscopic inspection reveals resolution of the hypervascular synovitis, persistent loss of capsular volume, and a residual synovial layer with patches of thickened, injected, waxy tissue (Fig. 23.3). Biopsy of stage III capsule shows dense hypercellular, organized collagenous tissue.

Stage IV, the resolution phase, is characterized by a gradual return of motion, with no associated pain. The histologic characteristics of this phase have not been characterized, as the need for arthroscopy and biopsy is obviated.

Post-traumatic or Postsurgical Shoulder Stiffness

The layers of tissue surrounding the shoulder joint each permit a fixed amount of motion as they glide over each other. The ligaments, tendons, and muscles all have variable lengths depending on tissue elasticity and the

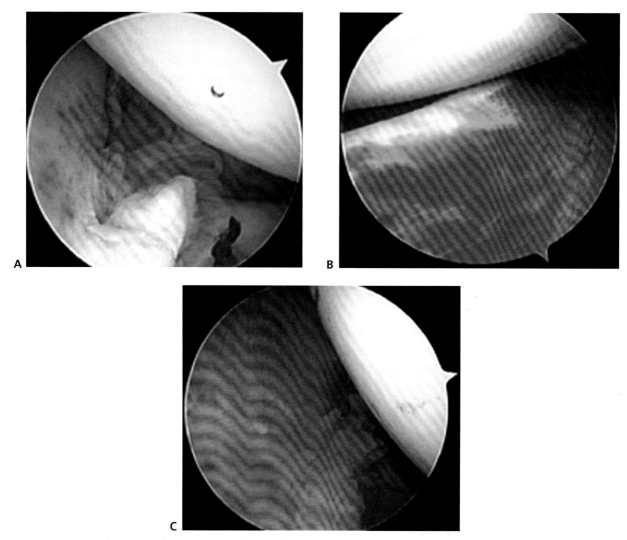

FIGURE 23.1. Stage I adhesive capsulitis. **A:** Hypertrophic synovitis in rotator interval. **B:** Posterior-inferior capsule and synovium. **C:** Posterior-superior capsule and hypertrophic synovium.

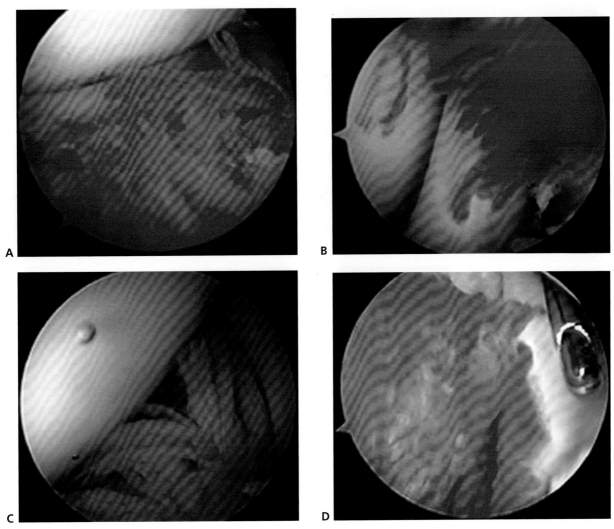

FIGURE 23.2. Stage II adhesive capsulitis. **A:** Hyperemic, hypertrophic, frond-like synovium. **B:** Hypertrophic synovium posterior to biceps tendon. **C:** Frond-like synovitis in rotator interval. **D:** Thick, hyperemic synovium posterior-superior capsule.

distances between skeletal structures. Acromion morphology has not been associated with adhesive capsulitis (8). When any of these layers or parts is injured, inflamed, or deformed, it can result in loss of motion.

The glenoid and humeral head articulation can have altered anatomy from trauma, surgery, or arthritis (9). This can have various effects on joint capsule volume. The effect on the capsule can be global, affecting all planes of motion. Alternatively, joint capsule tightness can involve specific locations of the capsule, with resultant effects on the individual ligaments, producing recognizable patterns of deficiency.

Contracture of the rotator interval, which is comprised in part by the coracohumeral ligament and superior glenohumeral ligament, typically limits forward flexion, extension, and external rotation when the shoulder is in the adducted position. The anteroinferior ligament complex is a restraint to external rotation in abduction. The postero-inferior complex limits internal rotation and forward flexion. Isolated contracture of these ligaments will produce

limits in motion in a predictable fashion. The restraint to motion results in an increase in the translation of the humeral head opposite the side the lesion.

Capsulorrhaphy arthropathy is an example of a condition in which the humeral head is translated posteriorly by a tight anterior capsule. This results in increased joint reactive forces on the posterior glenoid and subsequent arthropathy. When both limbs of the inferior glenohumeral ligament complex are affected, the result is a superior migration producing what some have termed "non outlet impingement."

Rotator cuff injuries and repairs have the potential to cause stiffness. In the setting of rotator cuff tear or tendinopathy, patients lose the action of dynamic stabilization. A voluntarily decreased glenohumeral motion in an effort to reduce the pain of impingement may lead to a compensatory increase in scapulothoracic motion. After surgical repair, or in the setting of a chronic, contracted tear, the rotator cuff muscle–tendon units may actually be shorter. This can result in restricted motion. It is critical to fully mobilize the

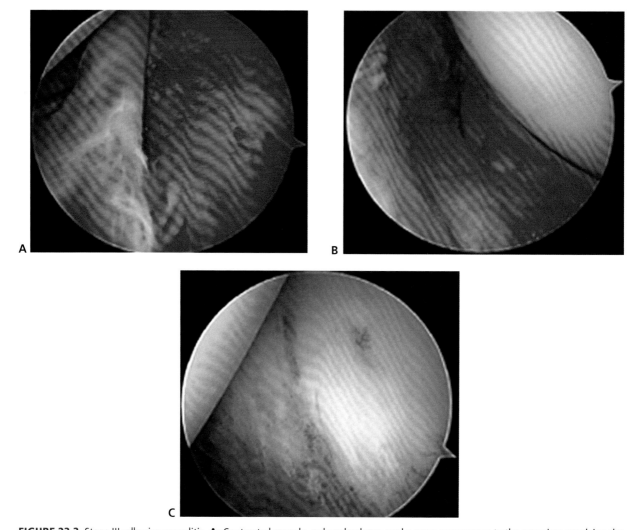

FIGURE 23.3. Stage III adhesive capsulitis. **A:** Contracted capsule, reduced volume, and a waxy appearance to the synovium overlying the biceps tendon. **B:** Posterior capsular contracture and waxy appearance. **C:** Contracted capsule and less hyperemic synovium.

tendons from adhesions during the procedure, as well as perform appropriate releases. During the postsurgical rehabilitation, it is also important to perform early passive mobilization of the joint to prevent adhesion formation.

Intra-articular deformity is less well tolerated than extrinsic contracture in shoulder stiffness. This deformity can be caused by erosion of bone secondary to osteoarthritis or from fractures. Fractures alter the anatomy directly and potentially indirectly in the setting of post-traumatic arthritis.

In arthritis, the joint incongruity leads to global capsular thickening and scarring, secondary to an inflammatory component of the disease. Fractures of the proximal humerus can also lead to stiffness either by intra-articular incongruity or by malpositioning of the tuberosities and subsequent poor function of dynamic stabilization. Even after arthroplasty, nonanatomic reconstruction such as oversizing and poor orientation of components can lead to stiffness. Procedures to treat instability such as arthroscopic capsular plication, Bristow, Latarjet, or Trillat can successfully treat instability; however, this can be at the expense of limited motion.

TREATMENT

The treatment of adhesive capsulitis and acquired shoulder stiffness remains controversial. Support can be found in the literature for addressing these conditions using benign neglect, physical therapy, nonsteroidal anti-inflammatory drugs (NSAIDs), injections, brisement, (MUA), or with surgical interventions. Surgical options include direct manipulation or can include open or arthroscopic releases. All these modalities have relevance for treatment under the appropriate conditions. It is paramount to make an accurate diagnosis, including the etiology, and know the current stage of disease. Notably, staging will help to direct the appropriate course of treatment.

Nonoperative Management of Adhesive Capsulitis

The mainstay of the treatment for adhesive capsulitis is with conservative measures. Most patients with this condition will experience a complete resolution of symptoms without surgical intervention. Adhesive capsulitis is felt to be a self-limited disease with predictably good to excellent results (18). Surgical intervention should typically not be considered unless a patient shows no response or worsening symptoms after 3 to 6 months of nonoperative management.

Approach to Stages I and II Adhesive Capsulitis

A significant pain component exists in the inflammatory phases of stages I and II adhesive capsulitis. Neviaser and Neviaser (7) underscore the importance of refraining from MUA or other surgical intervention during this painful phase. Such intervention carries the potential to exacerbate the condition and contribute to a further decrease in range of motion. Various modalities should be utilized to address the patient's pain and to potentially shorten the inflammatory state.

Physical therapy is the mainstay for patients with stage I and II disease. Most patients with early-stage primary adhesive capsulitis can be managed successfully with physical therapy. Therapy needs to be closely monitored to ensure appropriate technique and patient compliance. Strengthening exercises should be avoided until the pain component has resolved, and the majority of the range of motion restored. Therapy may include a home-based program, formal outpatient visits, or a combination of the two, depending upon the preference of the treating physician. Regardless of the setting, it is important to avoid aggressive therapy in a patient with significant pain, as this may potentiate symptoms and discourage patient participation. Diercks and Stevens (10) compared intensive physical therapy with supervised neglect. They found that 89% of patients treated with supervised neglect reach a constant score of 80 at a final follow-up of 2 years versus only 63% in the intensive physical therapy group. They concluded intensive therapy likely has an adverse effect on the natural course of the disease. When used appropriately, however, physical therapy has shown significant benefits in patient outcomes.

Oral NSAIDs may be used regardless of the stage of disease. The NSAIDs can effectively alleviate pain and inflammation in the inflammatory stages and can shorten the course to recovery. Patients must be counseled on appropriate dosing in order to achieve and maintain therapeutic levels.

Injection therapy has been used extensively to treat adhesive capsulitis and varies in both content and location of delivery. Injections can be beneficial in both diagnosing the stage of disease and providing therapeutic effects. Evaluation of the shoulder range of motion following a local anesthetic injection will help determine the exact stage of disease and help guide decisions in the approach to treatment. In the early, painful phases of capsulitis, the shoulder range should improve after the elimination of pain. If passive and active ranges of motion remain unchanged, the stage of disease by definition is later in the fibrosing stage.

Most commonly injections involve the delivery of corticosteroid into the subacromial space and/or directly into the

glenohumeral joint. As with the use of oral NSAIDs, injection of a steroid is thought to decrease synovial inflammation as well as to inhibit the development of fibrosis. Ultimately, this will decrease pain and improve range of motion.

The natural course of the disease can be shortened with appropriate use of anti-inflammatory medications. Marx et al. (11) concluded that the administration of intra-articular corticosteroid allowed for a more rapid reduction of pain and recovery of range of motion. A significantly more rapid response was demonstrated in patients with stage I versus stage II disease. This emphasizes the importance of early intervention in order to prevent the onset of fibrosis.

Hazleman (12) found a similar trend in his review of several studies. Most patients treated with an intra-articular injection of corticosteroid within 1 month of the onset of symptoms recovered fully within 1.5 months. Injection 2 to 5 months after the onset of symptoms allowed recovery in 8.1 months. Finally, patients treated 6 to 12 months from the time of symptom onset had full recovery at an average of 14 months. This demonstrates the utility of early intervention to significantly shorten the time to recovery.

Capsular distention, also known as brisement, is another modality that has been used to treat the stiff shoulder. Intra-articular injection of fluid under pressure is performed to cause disruption of the joint capsule. Capsule disruption is intended to decrease pain and improve range of motion. The fluid injected can be a combination of saline, local anesthetic, and corticosteroid. Buchbinder et al. (13) randomized 46 patients into either an arthrographic distention or a sham distention group. They concluded that arthrographic distention with normal saline and corticosteroid resulted in a reduction of pain and disability and improved overall range of motion. However, as with other forms of treatment, the results from brisement have been variable.

Approach to Stages III and IV Adhesive Capsulitis

In later-stage disease, the patient's pain component has largely resolved. Significantly limited range of motion as well as altered scapulohumeral mechanics remains. The inflammatory component has resolved, and the fibrosis of the capsule is established. Activities of daily living are often difficult.

Steroid injection is no longer warranted. The focus of treatment is on physical therapy and modalities to help restore motion. At this stage, the patient is often frustrated with his or her lack of progress despite compliance with physical therapy. It may be beneficial to review again the natural history of the disease with the patient in order to facilitate continued active participation in therapy. Stretching exercises should be continued until most shoulder motion has returned. Once this occurs, strengthening exercises can be implemented to target specific areas of weakness. Restoration of the normal scapulohumeral rhythm should be emphasized. If the patient shows no improvement or worsening symptoms despite genuine efforts in therapy, surgical intervention can be discussed.

Surgery is typically not offered prior to 3 to 6 months of failed conservative measures.

Nonoperative Management of the Acquired Stiff Shoulder

Acquired shoulder stiffness develops most commonly in the post-traumatic or postsurgical setting. The limited range of motion experienced can be due in part to prolonged immobilization. Regardless of the cause, treatment of the stiff shoulder is usually more aggressive than that used for adhesive capsulitis, as it tends to be less responsive to conservative measures. This is especially true for stiffness that occurs after a surgical procedure for instability. In this case, loss of motion and humeral head subluxation may be the result of overaggressive capsular tightening. Care must be taken to avoid this complication, as persistent subluxation has been shown to predispose the joint to accelerated cartilage wear.

Despite resistance to conservative measures, the treatment of acquired shoulder stiffness should first begin with supervised physical therapy. The goals are to alleviate pain and improve range of motion. As with adhesive capsulitis, surgery is then considered if no improvement is noted after 3 to 6 months. Surgery includes the release of adhesions, as well as the limited release of an overtightened capsule if identified.

Operative Management of Adhesive Capsulitis

Operative intervention for adhesive capsulitis includes MUA as well as various open and arthroscopic releases. Such procedures are not typically performed prior to stage III of the disease. As with aggressive physical therapy, surgical intervention during the acute pain phases may lead to poor outcomes and even worsen the condition (7).

Manipulation Under Anesthesia

MUA can be attempted with or without a formal arthroscopic or open release (14, 19). Closed manipulation is performed after an interscalene block and/or induction of general anesthesia. A regional block may be beneficial to allow the patient to note the improvement in range of motion directly after the manipulation. In either case, best results are obtained with complete muscular paralysis.

Manipulation is performed while stabilizing the scapula with one hand or with help from an assistant to maintain the scapula in a fixed position. The arm is initially taken into external rotation in an adducted position. The shoulder is next abducted while pressure is maintained on the scapula. With the shoulder now abducted, it is then brought into internal rotation. Next, the shoulder is flexed. Finally, the shoulder is brought back into adduction and then internally rotated (7). A palpable and even audible release of soft tissue may be noticed. Several manipulation techniques have been described over the years. The author's preferred technique is presented later in the chapter.

MUA is not a benign process and can result in injury. Loew et al. (15) reported on intra-articular lesions noted during arthroscopy after closed manipulation. Iatrogenic injuries noted in this study were superior labrum anterior and posterior (SLAP) tears, subscapularis tears, and anterior labral avulsions. Additional injuries reported by others include fractures of the humerus, as well as intratendinous or intramuscular ruptures of the biceps and rotator cuff. In order to decrease the risk to these structures, the hand used to manipulate the extremity should never be placed distal to the patient's elbow. Doing so creates a large lever arm and increases risk of iatrogenic injury. MUA should be avoided altogether in patients with documented osteopenia or a recent upper extremity surgery. In these cases, arthroscopic or open releases are preferred.

ARTHROSCOPIC SURGICAL RELEASE

Arthroscopic release is often performed prior to MUA (16). Advantages of this procedure include the identification of concomitant intra-articular lesions and the precise control of surgical releases. In addition, the use of arthroscopy avoids the morbidity associated with an open procedure. Arthroscopic release prior to MUA reduces the force needed to perform the manipulation.

Introduction of the arthroscope into the glenohumeral joint can be difficult as a result of capsular scarring and decreased joint volume. Care must be taken to avoid injury to the articular surfaces. A smaller 3.8-mm arthroscope may be utilized if entry into the joint is difficult. Once inside the joint, it may be difficult to navigate the arthroscope as a result of reduced joint volume. Intra-articular distension with forced injection of normal saline can be useful to maximally distend the capsule prior to attempting to introduce the arthroscope.

Attention is first directed to the rotator interval. Through an anterior portal, and with the use of an electrocautery device, the capsule is released just inferior to the biceps tendon and the release is extended inferiorly to the superior edge of the subscapularis. Release of the rotator interval improves visualization by allowing the humeral head to move inferiorly and laterally.

The anterior capsular release is continued inferiorly from the superior edge of the subscapularis to the 5 o'clock position (right shoulder). Full-thickness capsule release is performed approximately 1 cm from the capsulolabral junction. Visualization of the muscle fibers of the subscapularis confirms a full-thickness release has been performed. The capsule thickness is quite variable and may be dramatic. Effective release, however, requires care and patience to ensure that it is complete.

Many surgeons avoid release from the 5 to 7 o'clock position in order to avoid iatrogenic injury to the axillary nerve. However, with the avoidance of electrocautery and attention to detail, cutting instruments such as a curved basket forceps can facilitate a careful release between these locations.

The posterior capsule is similarly released from the 7 to the 11 o'clock position (right shoulder). To facilitate the posterior release, the arthroscope is switched to the anterior portal location and the working portal is switched to the posterior portal. Improvement in internal rotation can be expected from a complete posterior release. At this point, the arthroscopic instruments are removed and a MUA is performed.

OPEN SURGICAL RELEASE

If arthroscopy is contraindicated or fails to restore range of motion, an open surgical release may be performed. Failure of an arthroscopic release is noted most commonly in the setting of acquired shoulder stiffness as a result of extra-articular soft tissue contractures and adhesions. The procedure is typically done through a deltopectoral approach. Abducting the shoulder results in deltoid relaxation and allows easier entry into the subdeltoid space. Release of adhesions is performed with care to avoid injury to the axillary nerve. Once this has been accomplished, adhesions in the subacromial space are then released. Next, adhesions between the conjoined tendon and the subscapularis are released. It is important to stay lateral to the conjoined tendon in order to avoid injury to the musculocutaneous nerve and other neurovascular structures located nearby. The rotator interval is then released.

If the subscapularis tendon is contracted, a Z-plasty lengthening of the tendon can be performed. The anterior capsule is also released. External rotation should now be restored. If internal rotation and flexion are still limited, a release of the posterior capsule may then be performed. This release can be accomplished through the deltopectoral approach with the use of a humeral head retractor to obtain appropriate exposure.

OPERATIVE MANAGEMENT OF THE ACQUIRED STIFF SHOULDER

As with adhesive capsulitis, options for operative intervention of acquired shoulder stiffness include MUA and arthroscopic as well as open releases. These options should be avoided in the context of acquired capsulitis that can occur with overuse injuries, trauma, or surgical intervention (7, 9). Instead, a combination of pain management and gentle physical therapy should be used.

Fractures and prior surgical procedures about the shoulder may cause acquired shoulder stiffness as a result of scarring between soft tissue planes. Prolonged immobilization after these events likely contributes to the development of this stiffness. The techniques used are the same as those described earlier. An open release is often necessary as the pathology in this form of acquired shoulder stiffness is extra-articular and difficult to address arthroscopically.

Acquired shoulder stiffness may also be the result of subscapularis shortening seen with bone block procedures used to treat shoulder instability. Examples include the Putti-Platt or Magnuson-Stack procedures. In these instances, external rotation may be severely limited. Other procedures used to address shoulder instability, such as the Latarjet procedure, may disrupt articular congruity leading to decreased range of motion. Shoulder stiffness as a result of these interventions is best treated with open surgical lengthening of the subscapularis and correction of articular incongruity (9, 17).

AUTHORS' PREFERRED TECHNIQUE

Certainly, the initial management of a shoulder with adhesive capsulitis should be nonoperative. It is important to determine the stage of disease to assist in the decision as to how aggressive to be in terms of a conversion to operative intervention. The history provided by the patient is critical. History includes the duration of symptoms, progression of symptoms (improving, static, or worsening), inciting event if present, and underlying medical history.

Nonoperative interventions should begin with physical therapy. The focus of therapy is on the restoration of motion with a guided stretching program. Toning with light progressive resistance exercises can be included; however, this needs to be tailored to avoid aggravation of pain. At the early stages of adhesive capsulitis, persistent pain will undoubtedly result in the persistence of stiffness. Additionally, an oral NSAID medication, such as nabumetone, is added.

Early in the treatment, the patient is seen frequently. This serves to establish a definitive diagnosis for staging, assess the devotion of the patient to recovery, and determine whether progress is underway. Frequent visits also provide the opportunity to educate the patient about the expected course and, finally, to see if progress has plateaued. As long as the patient is making progress, I am careful not to proceed to surgical intervention too quickly. Any progress prior to surgical intervention will typically not be lost at surgery and will potentially serve to hasten a full recovery if surgery becomes necessary.

Injection therapy with corticosteroid is the next level of intervention. In cases that present with an established case of adhesive capsulitis, thought to be stage I or II disease, an injection can be considered at the first visit. The injection is performed as a combined intra-articular and subacromial treatment. I use 80-mg Depo-Medrol with 6 cc 1% lidocaine equally divided between the two sites. The injection is performed from a posterior approach. The intra-articular component can be delivered as if initiating a standard posterior portal for arthroscopy, approximately 2 cm distal and 2 cm medial to the posterolateral corner of the acromion. The needle can then be redirected to the subacromial space through the same skin location or a second needle insertion closer to the acromion depending on patient size.

Diagnostic studies should include a radiographic evaluation (true AP, outlet, and axillary views). The information gained by radiographs includes a determination of potential confounding factors, as well as a potential etiology for the adhesive capsulitis. Calcific tendonitis can be seen with plain films. A massive rotator cuff can be inferred by noting a high-riding humeral head and potentially acetabularization of the acromion. Furthermore, advanced arthritic changes may be seen on radiographs.

In the typical case of adhesive capsulitis, other than a hook-shaped acromion and arthritic changes at the acromioclavicular joint, the images would be expected to be normal. If radiographs reveal arthritis or a massive rotator cuff tear, the approach should be modified to treat these conditions and abort the typical approach to adhesive capsulitis.

I do not routinely obtain MRI examinations of the shoulder. My indications for MRI include patients not progressing with the nonoperative approach, patients that present with an established adhesive capsulitis for greater than 6 months, and patients for whom a more aggressive course of intervention may be indicated (those whose employment may be jeopardized by a protracted recovery). The MRI findings are utilized to discuss with the patient what can be expected at surgery if operative intervention is required.

Concurrent rotator cuff tears require a careful discussion with the patient. The incidence of this finding is not unusual and can be seen in up to 20% of cases. My preference is to address the rotator cuff at a second surgery. Although published studies recommend a combined release with a rotator cuff repair at the same setting, I am not inclined to do the combined procedure. It has been my experience that the best results from a capsular release require an aggressive postoperative stretching program. This program is much more aggressive than that prescribed after rotator cuff repair. If the repair fails during the postoperative period, the requirement for a revision repair becomes more challenging with a potentially poor outcome.

If surgery is required for a failed nonoperative course, usually between 4 and 6 months of formal therapy, or for extenuating circumstances such as a patient who presented at a later stage or for return to work considerations, I then approach this with an arthroscopic lysis of adhesions and manipulation. I prefer the lateral decubitus position to allow easy access for a circumferential release. The beach chair position can be utilized; however, it has been my experience that the lateral decubitus position allows unobstructed access to the anterior and posterior shoulder, as well as the ability to perform the manipulation in all planes.

Surgery is performed under general anesthesia. I supplement this preoperatively with an interscalene block. The block serves to control postoperative pain, reduce postoperative nausea by minimizing intraoperative narcotic requirements and allow immediate motion postoperatively. The demonstration of a full range of motion when the patient is awake, yet still under the block, is often motivating to the patient.

The prerelease range of motion is documented prior to the initiation of arthroscopy. This serves to determine where particular attention is required during the release. As noted earlier, the particular pattern of lost motion is specific to the portion of the capsule most involved with fibrosis.

The patient is placed in the lateral decubitus position, and intra-articular viewing is initiated from a posterior portal. Almost routinely, a circumferential release is performed. Limited release can be performed in the setting of isolated anterior or posterior stiffness, such as after previous anterior capsulorrhaphy or posterior contracture in throwing athletes. Postoperative instability has been documented in the literature after circumferential release; however, if patient selection is based on appropriate indications, I have not found that a complete release of the capsule has been detrimental. Further, the circumferential release can be done safely without risk to the axillary nerve if care is taken in the region of the axillary recess.

The greatest initial gain in capsular volume, and thus visualization, is achieved from a thorough release of the rotator interval (Fig. 23.4). All inflammatory synovium

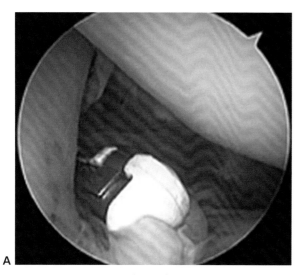
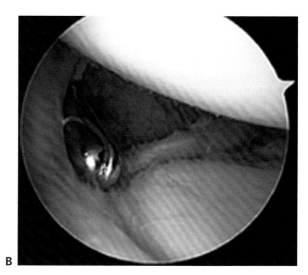

FIGURE 23.4. Arthroscopic release of rotator interval. **A:** Ablation of hypertrophic synovium. **B:** Complete release of rotator interval.

should be removed, either with a shaver or with an electro-cautery device. The capsular tissues, including the superior glenohumeral ligament, can be resected. Additionally, a thorough synovectomy should be performed prior to release, to remove the inciting inflammatory tissue and to assist in visualization during capsular release (Fig. 23.5).

The capsular release can proceed either anteriorly or posteriorly. This is determined based on ease of visualization. The easiest to visualize should be approached first. This will allow a progressive release and an incremental increase in capsular volume, then to assist in the approach to the opposite side.

The release is initiated at approximately 1 cm from the labrum. A full-thickness capsular release is required. This is confirmed by the visualization of the fibers of either the subscapularis muscle anteriorly or the infraspinatus posteriorly. I use an electrocautery device to carry the release from the rotator interval anteriorly and posteriorly (Fig. 23.6).

The posterior release can begin from the anterior working portal, above the biceps insertion, to approximately the 10:00 position (right shoulders). At that point, the remaining posterior approach requires switching the viewing portal anteriorly and utilizing a posterior working portal (Fig. 23.7).

The anterior and posterior release can safely be continued with electrocautery to below the equator, to approximately the 5:00 and 7:00 position. At these locations, the release should be completed with a curved basket forceps or other mechanical biting device. Gentle traction is applied by an assistant, and again full-thickness release is accomplished with the basket forceps to complete the release from 5:00 to 7:00. This typically requires both an anterior and a posterior approach, to reach, and connect at the 6:00 position (Fig. 23.8).

After the circumferential release, the arm is taken down from traction, and a manipulation is performed. Careful manipulation using scapular rotation with the arm positioned in varying degrees of maximal forward elevation, abduction, external, and internal rotation is sufficient to restore motion to full. The manipulation procedure is described in detail in the Pearls section.

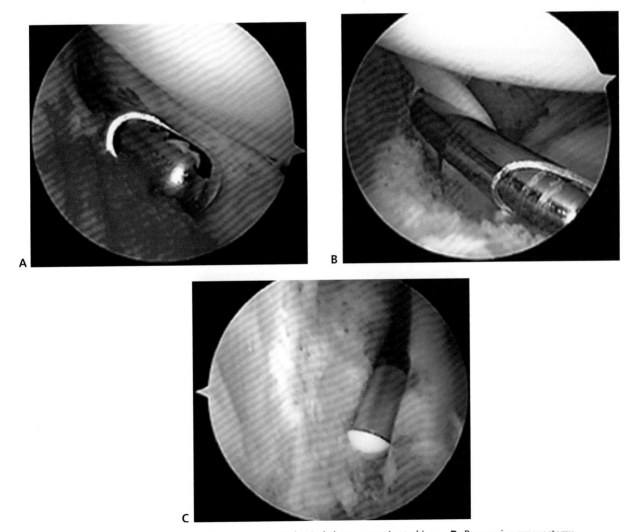

FIGURE 23.5. Synovectomy prior to capsule release. **A:** Mechanical shaver posterior to biceps. **B:** Progressive synovectomy from anterior working portal. **C:** Thermal ablation of synovium.

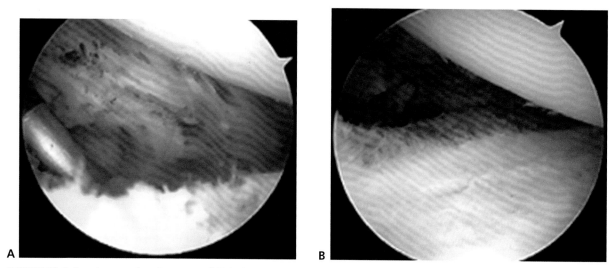

FIGURE 23.6. Anterior capsular release. **A:** A full-thickness release over the subscapularis with a thermal device. **B:** Completed anterior release with visible subscapularis muscle fibers.

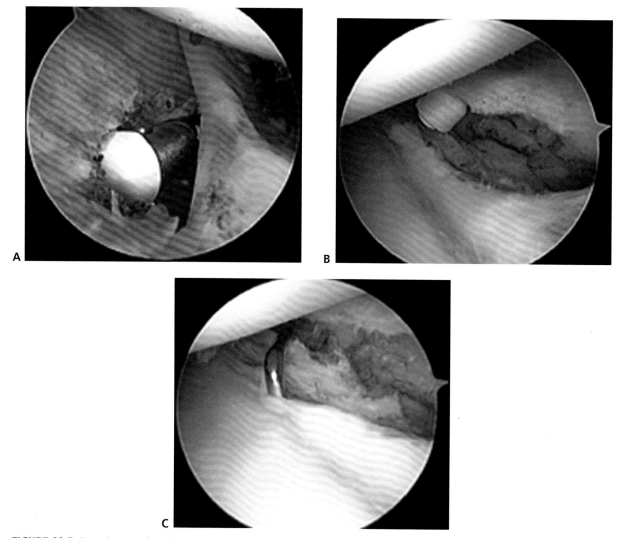

FIGURE 23.7. Posterior capsular release. **A:** Thermal release of the posterior-superior capsule. **B:** The posterior release from the posterior working portal. **C:** Completed posterior release with visible infraspinatus muscle fibers.

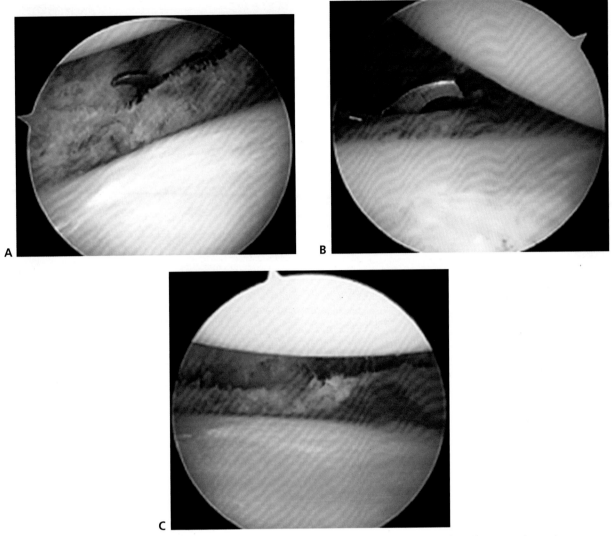

FIGURE 23.8. Inferior capsular release in the axillary recess. **A:** Posterior-inferior release with Shutt biter from posterior working portal. **B:** Anterior-inferior release from anterior working portal. **C:** Completed inferior release.

PEARLS

Shoulders with extreme capsular contracture may need additional measures to allow initiation of visualization. If the joint cannot be entered safely, or once the arthroscope is in place does not allow visualization of the rotator interval, two options are available: distension arthrography and manipulation.

First, a trial of distension arthrography can be useful. A forced introduction of up to 60 cc of saline through an 18G spinal needle may be sufficient to obtain distension of the capsule to allow sufficient visualization of the rotator interval. If after distension the rotator interval can now be safely viewed from posteriorly, no prerelease manipulation is required.

For a very tight capsule, a gentle manipulation can be performed prior to arthroscopy in order to initiate the capsular release. This will create an initial release of the capsule and will allow better distension of the capsule and

visualization. The manipulation is performed only to the degree necessary to allow visualization within the joint. The final manipulation is performed after completion of the arthroscopic release in order to avoid risk of fracture.

The technique for manipulation utilizes scapular rotation, after placing the capsule on maximal stretch through arm positioning. Initially, the arm is placed at maximal forward elevation and is held firmly by an assistant. The scapula is then manipulated by rotating the winged edge of the scapula along the thoracic cage. A palpable release will be noted (Fig. 23.9). This is repeated with the arm in abduction in the scapular plane (Fig. 23.10). The arm is then positioned at 90° of abduction and maximal external rotation, and again the scapula is manipulated. Finally, at 90° of abduction and maximal internal rotation, the last manipulation of the scapula is performed (Fig. 23.11). This is sufficient to gain a full range of motion and minimizes any risk of fracture. The final range of motion is demonstrated and should be full.

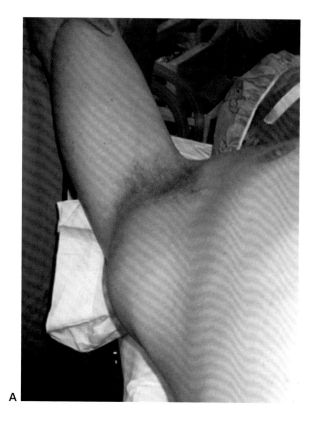

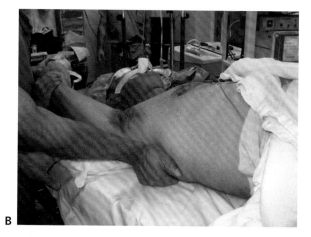

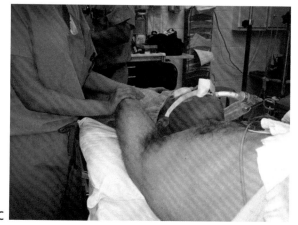

FIGURE 23.9. MUA in supine position. **A:** Arm in maximal abduction with notable winging of scapula. **B:** Scapula manipulation along the thoracic cage. **C:** After manipulation, winging absent and arm maximally abducted.

In order to maintain motion postoperatively, the capsular release should include complete debridement of any inflamed synovium. All erythematous or frond-like synovium is removed with a shaver or electrocautery. This serves to remove the inflammatory mediators that potentiate the disease.

Subacromial decompression is performed to remove all subdeltoid bursa, as well as release any extra-articular adhesions. The coracoacromial ligament is also released, as this can be a source of rotator cuff irritation (Fig. 23.12). Acromioplasty is not routinely performed as part of the decompression. The bleeding accompanying the bone resection can result in a reactive inflammation and can be a source for poor response to the release.

In cases where rotator cuff pathology is noted, including undersurface fraying or full-thickness tearing, a debridement is performed. The torn fibers of the cuff should be resected and the tear margin refreshed. The subdeltoid bursa should then be fully resected and the undersurface of the acromion is stripped of all soft tissue if the space remains quite narrow. Again, I do not perform any bone resection at this time.

It is my preference to not repair rotator cuff tears identified at the time of release and manipulation. I recommend a careful discussion with any patient suspected of having a rotator cuff tear or with a tear identified by preoperative MRI, about a two-stage approach. After motion is restored, the rotator cuff tear can be addressed arthroscopically. I have found little resistance to this two-stage approach as long as the discussion has taken place prior to the initial surgery. This allows for a reliable restoration of motion through an aggressive postoperative stretching program, without fear of disruption of a repair.

Patients that do not progress postoperatively on a steady basis will potentially require further intervention. NSAIDs can be added for patients with failure to progress after 2 weeks. If motion plateaus despite adherence to physical therapy stretching guidance, I perform a combined intra-articular and subacromial injection of corticosteroid at postoperative week 4. Finally, if motion is not satisfactory at 8 weeks postoperatively, I offer a repeat arthroscopic release and manipulation. I do not routinely utilize postoperative continuous passive motion devices; however, I do use them for shoulders requiring repeat procedures.

Patients with a limited adhesive capsulitis, typically throwing athletes, can be considered for a limited release and manipulation. Throwers can present with a

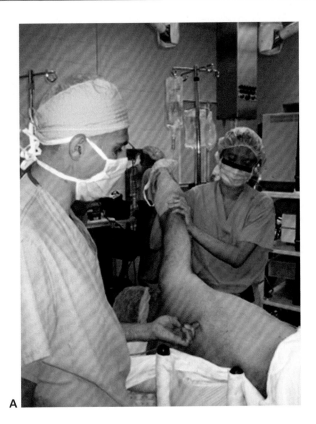

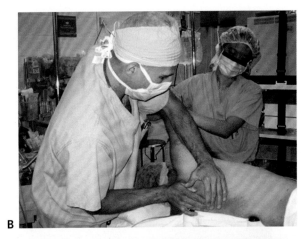

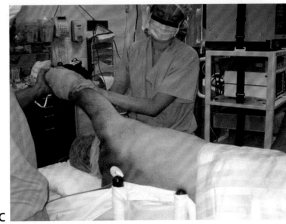

FIGURE 23.10. MUA in lateral decubitus position. **A:** Pre manipulation positioning with maximal abduction and notable winging of the scapula. **B:** Scapula manipulation along thoracic cage. **C:** After manipulation, winging absent and arm maximally abducted.

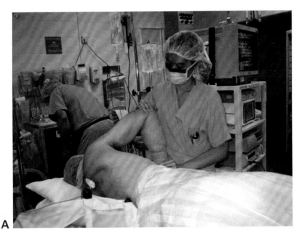

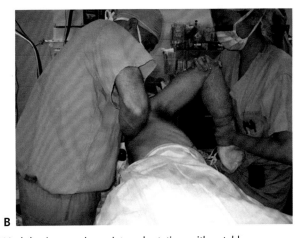

FIGURE 23.11. Manipulation to regain internal rotation. **A:** Arm at 90° abduction, maximum internal rotation, with notable winging of scapula. **B:** Scapula manipulation to restore internal rotation.

painful shoulder and limited internal rotation. This is commonly associated with internal impingement. These individuals can benefit from a limited posterosuperior release, along with appropriate intra-articular debridement. The primary etiology for the internal rotation deficit is a tight posterior capsule. I would only consider a limited release after failure of a structured posterior capsular stretching program over a course of several months.

PITFALLS

Patience is a virtue, but many patients do not have the time. A careful approach is the cornerstone of a successful

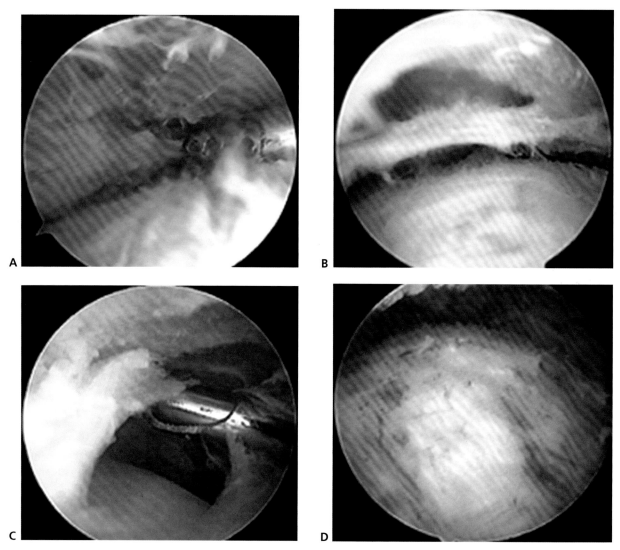

FIGURE 23.12. Subacromial appearance in setting of adhesive capsulitis. **A:** Hypertrophic, thickened bursa. **B:** Subacromial adhesions. **C:** Release of adhesions. **D:** Final appearance after decompression without acromioplasty. Injected rotator cuff tendons.

recovery from shoulder stiffness, whether acquired or primary adhesive capsulitis. Overzealous stretching, strengthening, or even surgical intervention can potentiate the disease and delay recovery. Care must be taken to establish an accurate diagnosis and stage of the disease. Interventions need to be based on disease stage. Surgical interventions or manipulations performed during the inflammatory phase are very likely to fail or prolong the recovery.

MUA without premanipulation release must be done cautiously. Manipulation of the shoulder by use of the arm as a lever risks fracture of the humerus, particularly manipulation with rotation. Manipulation in this fashion should be limited or not done at all. An alternate method of manipulation has been outlined earlier.

Frequent interaction with the patient is imperative. Any suggestion postoperatively of failure to progress needs to be recognized early to allow appropriate intervention prior to

reestablishment of firm scar tissue. I recommend a minimum of three visits during the first 8 postoperative weeks.

Patient education is paramount to patient satisfaction. An explanation of the expected course of the disease is the best method to achieve good results. Lack of understanding on the patient's part will undoubtedly result in frustration and potentially a failure to achieve the desired result.

REFERENCES

1. Binder AI, Bulgen DY, Hazleman BL, et al. Frozen shoulder: a long-term prospective study. *Ann Rheum Dis.* 1984;43:361–364.
2. Thomas S, McDougall C, Brown ID, et al. Prevalence of symptoms and signs of shoulder problems in people with diabetes mellitus. *J Shoulder Elbow Surg.* 2007;16:748–751.
3. van der Windt DA, Koes BW, de Jong BA, et al. Shoulder disorders in general practice: incidence, patient characteristics, and management. *Ann Rheum Dis.* 1995;54:959–964.

4. Hand C, Clipsham K, Rees JL, et al. Long-term outcome of frozen shoulder. *J Shoulder Elbow Surg.* 2008;17:231–236.

5. Warner JJ. Frozen shoulder: diagnosis and management. *J Am Acad Orthop Surg.* 1997;5:130–140.

6. Quigley TB. Checkrein shoulder; a type of frozen shoulder; diagnosis and treatment by manipulation and ACTH or cortisone. *N Engl J Med.* 1954;250:188–192.

7. Neviaser RJ, Neviaser TJ. The frozen shoulder. Diagnosis and management. *Clin Orthop Relat Res.* 1987;223:59–64.

8. Richards DP, Glogau AI, Schwartz M, et al. Relation between adhesive capsulitis and acromial morphology. *Arthroscopy.* 2004;20:614–619.

9. Warner JJ, Greis PE. The treatment of stiffness of the shoulder after repair of the rotator cuff. *J Bone Joint Surg Am.* 1997;79:1260–1269.

10. Diercks RL, Stevens M. Gentle thawing of the frozen shoulder: a prospective study of supervised neglect versus intensive physical therapy in seventy-seven patients with frozen shoulder syndrome followed up for two years. *J Shoulder Elbow Surg.* 2004;13:499–502.

11. Marx RG, Malizia RW, Kenter K, et al. Intra-articular corticosteroid injection for the treatment of idiopathic adhesive capsulitis of the shoulder. *HSS J.* 2007;3:202–207.

12. Hazleman BL. The painful stiff shoulder. *Rheumatol Phys Med.* 1972;11:413–421.

13. Buchbinder R, Green S, Forbes A, et al. Arthrographic joint distension with saline and steroid improves function and reduces pain in patients with painful stiff shoulder: results of a randomised, double blind, placebo controlled trial. *Ann Rheum Dis.* 2004;63:302–309.

14. Farrell CM, Sperling JW, Cofield RH. Manipulation for frozen shoulder: long-term results. *J Shoulder Elbow Surg.* 2005;14:480–484.

15. Loew M, Heichel TO, Lehner B. Intraarticular lesions in primary frozen shoulder after manipulation under general anesthesia. *J Shoulder Elbow Surg.* 2005;14:16–21.

16. Berghs BM, Sole-Molins X, Bunker TD. Arthroscopic release of adhesive capsulitis. *J Shoulder Elbow Surg.* 2004;13:180–185.

17. MacDonald PB, Hawkins RJ, Fowler PJ, et al. Release of the subscapularis for internal rotation contracture and pain after anterior repair for recurrent anterior dislocation of the shoulder. *J Bone Joint Surg Am.* 1992;74:734–737.

18. Levine WN, Kashyap CP, Bak SF, et al. Nonoperative management of idiopathic adhesive capsulitis. *J Shoulder Elbow Surg.* 2007;16:569–573.

19. Andersen NH, Søjbjerg JO, Johannsen HV, et al. Frozen shoulder: arthroscopy and manipulation under general anesthesia and early passive motion. *J Shoulder Elbow Surg.* 1998;7:218–222.

I. The Shoulder

Arthroscopic Approach to Glenohumeral Arthritis

Felix H. Savoie III • Michael J. O'Brien

Arthritis of the shoulder is not as commonly seen as arthritis of the knee and hip. However, the shoulder is the third most common joint where prosthetic replacement is performed, and the incidence of osteoarthritis of the shoulder appears to be on the rise (1). Additionally, more patients of a younger age are presenting with degenerative changes of the glenohumeral joint. These patients are less willing to tolerate or accept the decrease in activity level required for longevity of total shoulder arthroplasty. Young patients with degenerative joint disease of the shoulder are increasingly requesting alternative treatments to shoulder arthroplasty in order to maintain a physically active lifestyle.

Younger patients have shown dissatisfaction at adopting a restrictive lifestyle following shoulder replacement. Sperling et al. (2) have shown a very high subjective dissatisfaction rate with total shoulder arthroplasty in these young patients and have projected a loosening rate of over 50% by 10 years. These finding have led to an investigation into alternative measures for the active individual with degenerative joint disease of the shoulder. Early pioneer work by Ellman et al. (3) indicated little usefulness for arthroscopy in the degenerative shoulder. However, Guyette et al. (4) found value to arthroscopic subacromial decompression in patients with both low-grade glenohumeral arthritis and impingement syndrome. Weinstein et al. (5) also found benefit to arthroscopic debridement in the degenerative shoulder with a 1-to 5-year follow-up. Richards and Burkhart (6) found some benefit to capsular release in the arthritic shoulder, postulating the decrease in compressive forces from the release provided some benefit. Dews et al. have reported the results of capsular release and decompression in a subset of patients with arthritis and impingement with promising early results (Dews R, Field LD, Savoie FH, et al. Early arthroscopic contracture release for severe postoperative shoulder stiffness. unpublished data).

Arthroscopic resurfacing of the glenoid in the degenerative shoulder was initially proposed by Brislin et al., (7) with additional reports by Bhatia et al., (8) and by Pennington and Bartz (9). Savoie et al. later reported midterm follow-up of the procedure first reported by Brislin (10).

These procedures were based on open work performed at the Carrell clinic by Krishnan et al. (11). Although each has utilized various resurfacing tissues, the early results have been quite encouraging. However, other reports by Elhassan et al. (12) and others have delineated less than satisfactory results with a similar procedure, calling into question whether this is a reasonable treatment protocol. More encouraging is the recent report by Wirth (13) on biologic resurfacing of the glenoid with good early results (13).

The purpose of this chapter is to describe the role of arthroscopy and arthroscopic-assisted surgery in the management of glenohumeral arthritis. It should be understood that shoulder replacement remains the gold standard and is the treatment of choice for most patients requiring surgery for arthritis of the shoulder.

CLINICAL EVALUATION

History

The patient with degenerative joint disease of the shoulder usually presents with pain and loss of motion. The usual complaints are those of stiffness in the early morning along with pain during activities requiring a full arc of motion. Occasionally difficulty with sleeping may be reported although this is more commonly noticed during changes of position. In those patients with coexisting pathology in the subacromial area, the symptoms may be more of impingement and rotator cuff tendonitis rather than arthritis. There may be additional symptoms related to the degenerative acromioclavicular joint in addition to the problems in the glenohumeral joint.

Physical Examination

The initial aspects of the physical examination center on inspection and palpation. The shoulder is evaluated for atrophy and bone contours. The neurovascular status of the extremity is similarly evaluated. Passive and active range of motion is checked, and the amount of loss is compared with the opposite side. In these patients, there is always a loss of internal rotation in abduction. In the more severe cases, a global loss of motion that mimics adhesive capsulitis can be detected even with the arm in adduction. The differentiating factors between the two of these, besides the normal radiographic appearance of adhesive capsulitis, include the lack of tightness in palpating the rotator interval and the lack of pain on inferior glide testing. Even in the early arthritic shoulder, there may be crepitation associated with movement of the humeral head on the glenoid.

It is important to check for additional pathology. Concomitant impingement, biceps tendonitis, or acromioclavicular arthritis may be present in addition to the glenohumeral arthritis. All these can be detected by the usual examination findings.

Imaging

Standard PA (posterior to anterior), scapular Y, and axillary lateral radiographs are essential on the initial visit. Common findings may include small inferior spurs on the humerus noticed in the PA (posterior to anterior) view, slight posterior subluxation on the Y view, and narrowing of the joint on the axillary lateral view (Fig. 24.1). Determination of asymmetrical glenoid wear may also be assessed on the axillary lateral radiograph.

MRI testing is often performed. Current MRI units provide less than optimal assessment of the status of the articular cartilage but may be helpful in detecting additional

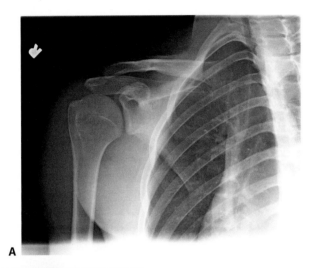

A

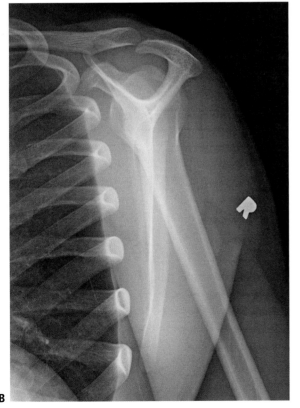

B

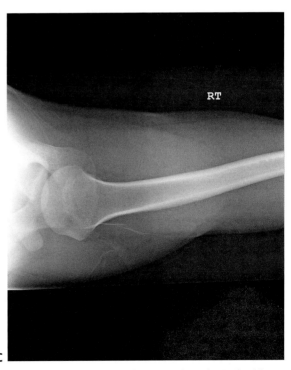

C

FIGURE 24.1. A–C: The standard three-view shoulder radiographs demonstrate various commonly seen findings in the arthritic shoulder.

I. The Shoulder

pathology in the labrum, biceps, and rotator cuff. There are technologic advances in the current systems that may allow better determination of the amount of damage to the articular cartilage. The addition of saline or gadolinium may be helpful in outlining suspected defects in the articular surface.

Classification

The most useful initial classification is the radiographic one of Weinstein et al. (5) In this system, the grading is based on radiographs. Stage I has normal radiographs. Stage II demonstrates joint narrowing with a concentric humeral head and glenoid. Stage III has moderate joint space narrowing with early inferior osteophyte formation. Stage IV includes severe joint space narrowing with osteophyte formation and loss of concentricity between the humeral head and the glenoid (Fig. 24.2).

The morphology of the glenoid can be determined by radiographic appearance utilizing the system described by Walch et al. (14) In this classification, a Type A glenoid shows concentric wear, which is either minor (Type A1) or major with substantial central wear causing a glenoid cup (Type A2). Type B has asymmetrical posterior glenoid wear with loss of joint space and sclerosis that is predominantly posterior (Type B1); or a posterior cup that gives the appearance of a double concavity or biconcavity (Type B2). Type C is defined as glenoid retroversion of greater than 25° and represents posterior glenoid hypoplasia.

The most common classification system grading articular cartilage injuries is that of Outerbridge (15). This system is based on direct inspection of the surface. Grade 1 change shows softening or blistering. Grade 2 shows fibrillation or superficial fissures of less than 1 cm, whereas Grade 3 shows deep fissuring extending to the subchondral bone and measuring more than 1 cm. Grade 4 shows exposed bone.

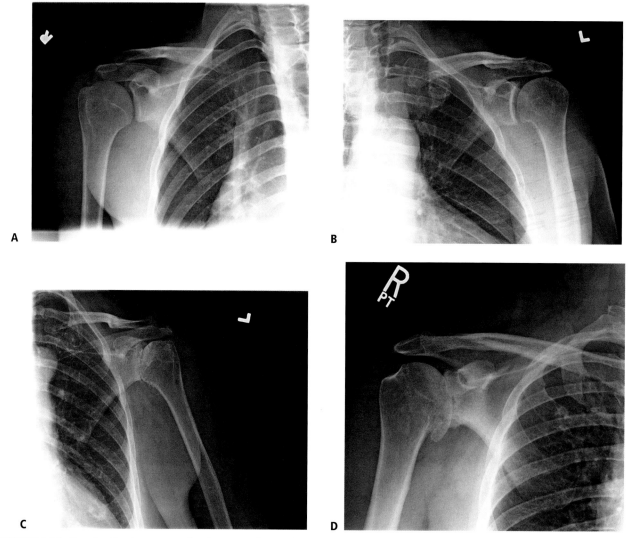

FIGURE 24.2. The classification system of Weinstein et al. is useful in the preoperative assessment of arthritis. **A:** Stage I showing no arthritic changes. **B:** Stage II with mild changes of arthritis. **C:** Stage III is significant arthritic change. **D:** Stage IV with bone-on-bone articulation.

The systems of Weinstein et al. and Walch et al. are useful in preoperative planning, whereas that of Outerbridge is helpful in determining treatment options while visualizing the articular surface during arthroscopy.

TREATMENT OPTIONS

Nonoperative Management

The hallmark of the treatment for shoulder osteoarthritis is a slow and stepwise progression through conservative to aggressive management. The initial treatment involves the use of anti-inflammatory medication and physical therapy. Therapy should involve distraction of the joint while mobilizing, rather than the standard stretching and joint mobilization, in order to avoid increased irritation of the shoulder. This distraction-stretching program should be combined with scapular retraction and rotator cuff exercises to rebalance the shoulder. The next step involves the use of selective intra-articular injections to decrease the inflammation. If effective, these may sometimes be followed by the off-label use of intra-articular lubricants.

Operative Management

Operative treatment of arthritis of the shoulder is defined by the success of total shoulder arthroplasty. Shoulder replacement is considered the treatment of choice in older glenohumeral arthritic patients willing to accommodate a change in lifestyle to preserve the longevity of the replacement. In many cases, however, patients are interested in a much more active lifestyle that may jeopardize the long-term results. This discrepancy has been noted by Sperling et al. (2) In their excellent study of total shoulder arthroplasty in the young active patient, the objective results were excellent in almost all of their cases; however, subjectively 50% were dissatisfied with the outcome of the operation.

This subjective dissatisfaction and the multiple advantages of arthroscopy have led to an interest in the arthroscopic management of the degenerative shoulder. In this section, we have divided the potential surgeries into five main groups based upon lesion and surgical procedure.

Group 1 patients are those whose lesions involve a small area on one side of the joint. These lesions are almost always discovered during arthroscopy for other reasons. The area of damage is relatively small and is managed by abrasion and/or microfracture of the defect when first encountered (Fig. 24.3). These patients will usually have a contracture of the inferior capsule, which can be released, and additional biceps pathology, subacromial impingement, and acromioclavicular arthritis, which can be managed in the usual fashion. Restoration of motion and rebalancing of the shoulder through postoperative therapy often leads to a successful result for many years.

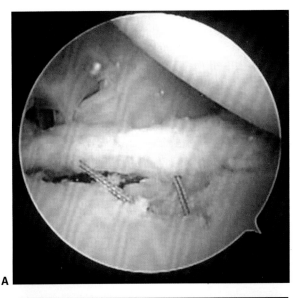

A

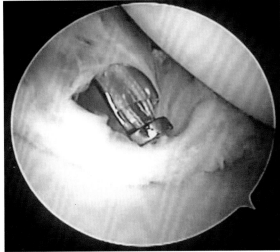

B

FIGURE 24.4. A, B: Full-surface articular cartilage defects can be managed by various measures.

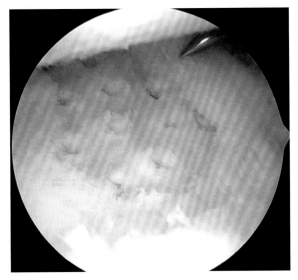

FIGURE 24.3. A small full-surface defect managed by microfracture.

I. The Shoulder

Group 2 patients are those with panarticular but congruent arthritis with associated symptoms of a tight capsule, biceps tendonitis, impingement, and sometimes AC (acromioclavicular) joint problems. In these patients, a chondroplasty of the loose cartilage along with a capsular release, biceps tenotomy or tenodesis, decompression and, when necessary, excision of the distal clavicle will achieve a satisfactory result for a number of years. The restoration of motion and decrease in joint contact forces from the capsular release seems to slow the progression of the disease while the creation of space in the subacromial area along with postoperative rehabilitation will restore scapular kinematics with associated improved function.

Group 3 patients are those group 1 patients in whom the above-described treatment fails. In these individuals, there are several options. Peripheral lesions of the glenoid can be resurfaced by mobilization of the labrum over the defect (Fig. 24.4A). Central defects are managed by biologic resurfacing with a small patch of tissue (Fig. 24.4B). On the humeral side, defects are usually managed by limited resurfacing operations through an enlarged anterior-superior portal and a splitting of the rotator interval. In older patients, a limited metal resurfacing option is available, whereas in young patients fresh articular osteochondral allograft may be a better option (Fig. 24.5A).

Group 4 patients are those with primary disease on one or the other side of the joint without deformity or significant involvement of the other surface. Unlike group 2 patients these patients have "bone-on-bone" contact between the two surfaces without a concentric tracking pattern. In these patients with a concentric humeral head and a glenoid devoid of articular cartilage, an arthroscopic biologic glenoid resurfacing procedure may be performed (Fig. 24.6). It is essential that the humeral head is not deformed in

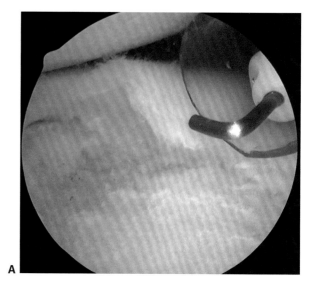

A

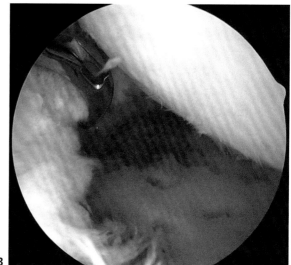

B

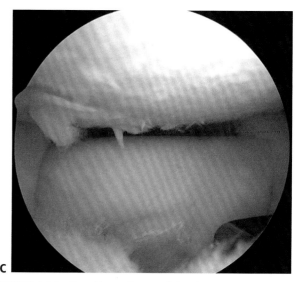

C

FIGURE 24.6. Glenoid resurfacing of the shoulder: **A:** The arthritic glenoid is debrided and correct version created. **B:** The surface of the glenoid is microfractured. **C:** The graft covering the glenoid is placed and sutured down.

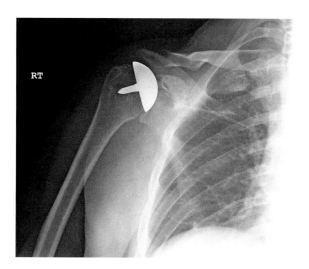

FIGURE 24.5. A limited Grade 4 articular surface defect managed by limited resurfacing of the defect with an implant.

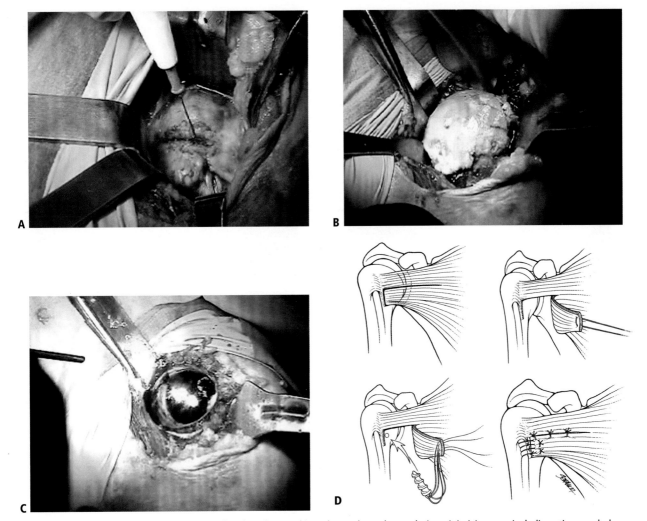

FIGURE 24.7. The humeral head can be resurfaced without taking down the subscapularis, minimizing surgical dissection, and decreasing the risk of complications. **A:** The initial split in the subscapularis. **B:** The exposure of the humeral head. **C:** The humeral head resurfaced. **D:** Illustration of the subscapularis-sparing approach.

any way for this to be effective. In a relatively concentric shoulder joint with squaring of the humeral head, an arthroscopically assisted surface replacement is the treatment of choice. This is performed through a small window formed by taking down only the inferior one-third of the subscapularis (Fig. 24.7).

Group 5 patients are those with significant deformity in both the humeral head and the glenoid. These patients require resurfacing of both sides of the joint. Arthroscopically, the release, biceps tenotomy, glenoid smoothing, and suture placement can be performed intra-articularly, followed by deltoid elevation, subacromial decompression, and distal clavicle excision in the subacromial area as indicated. An axillary or deltopectoral approach can be used, and the biologic glenoid resurfacing and humeral head resurfacing performed through a partial inferior subscapularis takedown.

Obviously, many patients in groups 4 and 5 with low demand activity will be candidates for standard total shoulder arthroplasty achieving a satisfactory result.

AUTHORS' PREFERRED TECHNIQUES

Glenoid Resurfacing

Indications: Grade 4 degenerative changes with a spherical humeral head on the axillary radiographs. This situation is commonly seen in failed instability surgery patients with DJD (degenerative joint disease) and also in chondrolysis patients (Fig. 24.8).

The patient is placed in the surgeon's favored position. The glenohumeral joint is approached through a standard posterior portal. An anterior-inferior and an anterior-superior portal are each established, far apart on the skin but both entering the shoulder through the rotator interval. Once the presence of severe arthritis is confirmed, a complete 360° capsular release is performed. In most cases, the biceps tendon is also released at this time. The glenoid is then measured from anterior to posterior using a graduated probe or a multi-knotted suture in order to prepare the graft. The AP (anterior to posterior) length is usually two-third the distance of the superior inferior

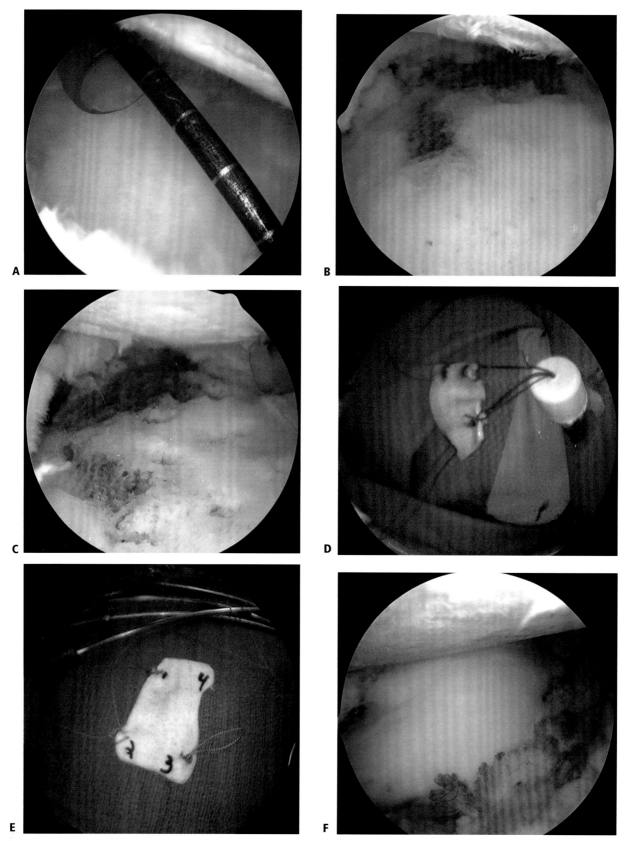

FIGURE 24.8. The steps in the technique of glenoid resurfacing of the glenoid: **A:** The arthritic glenoid is visualized and measured. **B:** The glenoid is coplaned to a smooth surface in correct version as determined by the preoperative CT scan. **C:** Vascular channels are created in the glenoid through a microfracture technique. **D:** The anterior-superior and anterior-inferior sutures are placed in preparation for graft placement. **E:** The graft is prepared outside the shoulder. **F:** The graft is placed down the cannula and into the joint, then sutured in place.

height. The glenoid is then prepared by coplaning it to a smooth surface. Any retroversion or biconcavity of the glenoid is corrected at this time. A 90° microfracture awl is then used to deeply penetrate the subchondral bone, releasing any increased pressure and allowing access of pleuripotential cells into the graft area.

If the posterior labrum is hypertrophic, it is preserved and used to sew the graft into position. If absent or damaged, then anchors are placed into the posterior glenoid neck at the 7 and 11 o'clock positions. A suture or additional anchor is placed anterior inferiorly into the capsule or glenoid neck at the 5 o'clock position and an additional anchor into the anterior-superior glenoid neck at the 1 o'clock position.

The graft is then prepared by placing sutures into the posterior edge at the 7 and 11 o'clock positions. If anchors have been placed posteriorly, STIK (short tailed interference knot) knots are used to deliver the graft and retrieve sutures. If anchors have not been utilized, these are barrel stitched to give added hold on the graft. The anterior sutures are then placed through the graft in the correct position (1 and 5 o'clock) and held with some tension. The posterior sutures are then individually passed down the anterior cannula, retrieved under the posterior labrum, and out the posterior cannula in the position corresponding to their location on the graft. These sutures are used to pull the graft down the anterior cannula and into the joint.

Once in the joint, the anterior-inferior suture is tied (after ascertaining there are no tangles or inadvertent suture twists) and then the anterior-superior suture is tied. If the posterior labrum has been preserved, the two posterior sutures are tied together. If anchors have been used, the STIK knots are used to pass the anchor sutures through the graft and these sutures are then individually tied, securing the posterior fixation. The subacromial portion of the procedure is then completed as per the surgeon's preference.

Humeral Resurfacing

Indications: Any Grade 4 DJD with humeral head deformity in a patient who wishes to maintain a high-activity level (heavy weight lifting, throwing sports, combative sports, etc.) (Fig. 24.9).

The patient is placed in the preferred position for arthroscopy. A standard posterior portal is created and a diagnostic arthroscopy is performed. A 360° capsular release and biceps tenotomy are performed. The glenoid is evaluated and any deformity or irregularity is removed or abraded down to a smooth surface. A subacromial and subdeltoid bursectomy, decompression, and distal clavicle excision are performed as determined on the preoperative radiographs. The arthroscopic procedure is then terminated and the arm positioned for the open procedure. A small incision is made in the anterior axillary fold and the deltopectoral interval developed. The subscapularis muscle and tendon are split horizontally from lateral to medial and then the inferior one-third is taken down from the humerus as a periosteal flap beginning just medial to the biceps tendon. This flap is continued medially around the medial aspect of the humerus to the posterior aspect while externally rotating the humerus. The head is then delivered into the wound by abducting and externally rotating the arm. If necessary, a Cobb elevator may be placed into the joint to help lever the head out below the still-attached superior part of the subscapularis. All the spurs are then removed from the humeral head and the head is sized, reamed, and resurfaced. The resurfaced head is reduced into the joint and the subscapularis repaired with a double-row technique. The biceps is tenodesed as a part of the subscapularis repair.

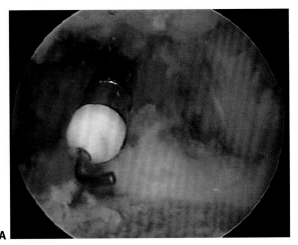
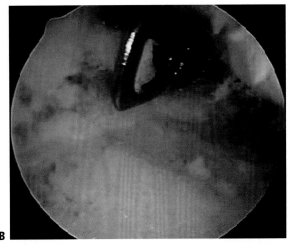

FIGURE 24.9. The steps in the technique of arthroscopically assisted humeral head resurfacing. **A:** A 360° capsular release is performed. **B:** A biceps tenotomy is performed. **C:** The subdeltoid bursa is released, freeing the deltoid from the underlying humerus. **D:** A subacromial decompression is performed. **E:** If necessary excision of the distal clavicle are performed. **F:** Through a mini-open subscapularis-sparing approach, the humeral head is replaced. **G:** The lower one-third of the subscapularis is closed in a double-row technique.

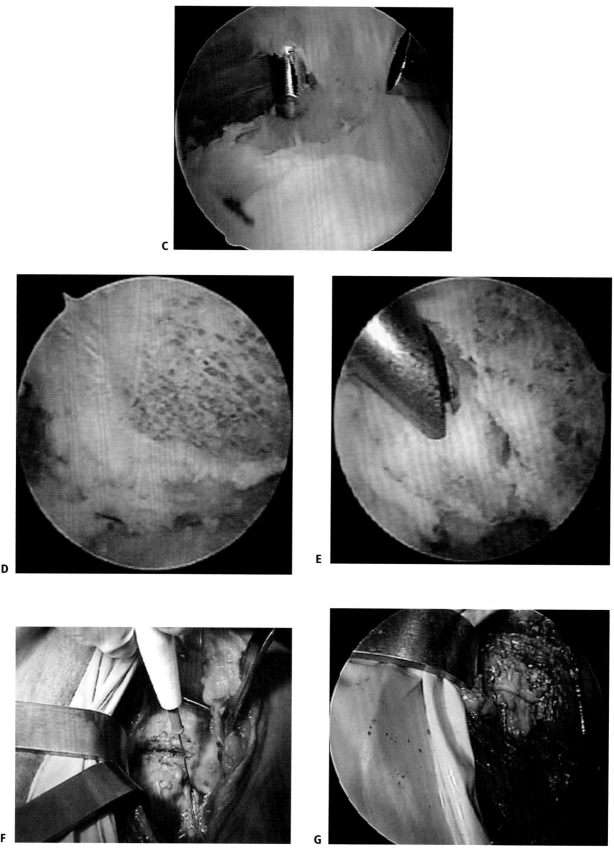

FIGURE 24.9. (continued)

COMPLICATIONS, CONTROVERSIES, AND SPECIAL CONSIDERATIONS

The primary complication of any treatment for arthritis is progression of the disease. The second is loosening or failure of the prosthesis. These two problems often go together, in that as the disease progresses, it produces changes in the underlying bone that lead to prosthetic failure. In arthroscopic glenoid resurfacing, the most common complication was an error in patient selection, leading to an unsatisfactory result due to lack of motion. In these patients, the humeral head was too deformed for an isolated glenoid procedure to provide a satisfactory result. Once the patient selection criteria were refined, the primary complication was progression of the humeral deformity leading to the need for a humeral resurfacing. This occurred in 5% of patients during the 6-year follow-up period.

In humeral resurfacing, very few complications have been reported. When an arthroscopic acromioplasty was not performed at the time of the index operation, the most common complication in these patients was impingement with tendonitis of the supraspinatus muscle. Most of these resolved with nonoperative treatment, but in 2 of the 100 cases reviewed, surgery was required to eliminate the problem.

There is considerable disagreement in the literature about the role of both open and arthroscopic resurfacing with biologic materials on the glenoid. In the open literature, positive reports by Wirth and Krishnan et al. are balanced by negative ones by Elhassan et al. Similarly, there have been variable results reported with arthroscopic debridement, with the best summary of effectiveness being the report of Weinstein. The glenoid resurfacing procedure is a relatively new one, with a recent midterm report by Savoie providing a promising start. Much work remains to be done to make its use widespread.

The controversies on humeral head replacement versus total shoulder are well described in the literature and beyond the scope of this chapter. However, it should be noted that the activities pursued by the patients in the subscapularis splitting surface replacement arthroplasty (SRA) group would not be allowed by most total shoulder surgeons if a prosthetic glenoid had been implanted.

PEARLS AND PITFALLS

1. Suture management is essential in glenoid resurfacing. The use of a different-colored or marked suture for each of the four quadrant sutures is helpful to prevent tangling.
2. Pass a lobster claw-type retractor around the set of sutures to be tied before actual tying to make sure there are no additional sutures wrapped around the ones to be tied.
3. Perform all the procedures under gravity or a very low flow setting to prevent excessive distension and edema of the shoulder.

4. When performing the subscapularis split, remain on the bone of the humerus to prevent inadvertent damage to the axillary nerve, or dissect out the nerve and protect it.

REHABILITATION

In patients without resurfacing, the initial rehabilitation consists of aggressive manual glides to stretch out the IGHL (inferior glenohumeral ligament) complex. Stretching and scapular rehab are emphasized immediately and strengthening initiated as flexibility improves.

In the glenoid resurfacing group, the patient is placed in an abduction sling for the first 4 weeks. During this time, scapular exercises are initiated, and gentle, pain-free home exercises are allowed. Four weeks post surgery, manual therapy emphasizing distraction of the joint, with mobilization while the distraction force is maintained, is started and progressed as tolerated. Resistive rehabilitation is started at 6 weeks and also progressed. In most patients, 85% of normal motion and function is achieved by 4 months.

In the humeral resurfacing through the subscapularis split, the patient is placed in an abduction sling for the first week. Passive motion is initiated in the first week. Active external rotation and use of just a sling starts in the second week. The sling is discontinued in week 3 and therapy starts without restriction in weeks 3 or 4. Most patients are utilizing the arm for activities of daily living by 4 weeks and are back in their sporting activities within 6 to 12 weeks. We have noted continued improvement for up to 5 years in these patients without any deterioration of the glenoid. There are no activity restrictions placed on these patients.

CONCLUSIONS AND FUTURE DIRECTIONS

The arthroscopic management of the arthritic shoulder has had varied success. The new management algorithms seem to allow a more accurate prediction of expected results, with overall improvements in patient care and satisfactory results. The midterm results of biologic resurfacing and the preservation of the subscapularis during humeral resurfacing allow for a significant decrease in potential complications along with an improvement in function.

The future is promising. Advances in the materials used for biologic resurfacing and the future use of articular cartilage growth factors to coat the material will hopefully make the need for plastic or metal glenoid replacement a historical footnote. The continued advances in humeral resurfacing should allow improved longevity without sacrificing function. Advances in technology may someday allow a prosthetic implant to be placed down a cannula and unfurled to cover the humeral head without any incision on the shoulder. Hopefully, the greatest advance yet to come will be a way to prevent or reverse the osteoarthritic process and restore a normal joint without surgical intervention.

REFERENCES

1. Bohsali K, Wirth M, Rockwood C. Complications of total shoulder arthroplasty. *J Bone Joint Surg Am.* 2006;88:2279–2292.

2. Sperling JW, Cofield RH, Rowland CM. Minimum fifteen-year follow-up of Neer hemiarthroplasty and total shoulder arthroplasty in patients aged fifty years or younger. *J Shoulder Elbow Surg.* 2004;13:604–613.

3. Ellman H, Harris E, Kay SP. Early degenerative joint disease simulating impingement syndrome: arthroscopic findings. *Arthroscopy.* 1992;8:482–487.

4. Guyette TM, Bae H, Warren RF, et al. Results of arthroscopic subacromial decompression in patients with subacromial impingement and glenohumeral degenerative joint disease. *J Shoulder Elbow Surg.* 2002;11:299–304.

5. Weinstein DM, Bucchieri JS, Pollock RG, et al. Arthroscopic debridement of the shoulder for osteoarthritis. *Arthroscopy.* 2000;16:471–476.

6. Richards DP, Burkhart SS. Arthroscopic debridement and capsular release for glenohumeral osteoarthritis. *Arthroscopy.* 2007;23:1019–1022.

7. Brislin KJ, Savoie FH III, Field LD, et al. Surgical treatment for glenohumeral arthritis in the young patient. *Tech Shoulder Elbow Surg.* 2004;5:165–169.

8. Bhatia DN, van Rooyen KS, du Toit DF, et al. Arthroscopic technique of interposition arthroplasty of the glenohumeral joint. *Arthroscopy.* 2006;22:570.e1–570.e5.

9. Pennington WT, Bartz BA. Arthroscopic glenoid resurfacing with meniscal allograft: a minimally invasive alternative for treating glenohumeral arthritis. *Arthroscopy.* 2005;21:1517–1520.

10. Savoie FH III, Brislin KJ, Argo D. Arthroscopic glenoid resurfacing as a surgical treatment for glenohumeral arthritis in the young patient: mid-term results. *Arthroscopy.* 2009;25:864–871.

11. Krishnan SG, Nowinski RJ, Harrison D, et al. Humeral hemi-arthroplasty with biologic resurfacing of the glenoid for glenohumeral arthritis. Two to fifteen-year outcomes. *J Bone Joint Surg Am.* 2007;89:727–734.

12. Elhassan B, Ozbaydar M, Diller D, et al. Soft-tissue resurfacing of the glenoid in the treatment of glenohumeral arthritis in active patients less than fifty years old. *J Bone Joint Surg Am.* 2009;91:419–424.

13. Wirth MA. Humeral head arthroplasty and meniscal allograft resurfacing of the glenoid. *J Bone Joint Surg Am.* 2009;91:1109–1119.

14. Walch G, Badet R, Boulahia A, et al. Morphologic study of the glenoid in primary glenohumeral osteoarthritis. *J Arthroplasty.* 1999;14:756–760.

15. Outerbridge RE. The etiology of chondromalacia patellae. *J Bone Joint Surg Br.* 1961;43:752–757.

Calcific Tendinitis

Brian R. Wolf • Jonathan A. Donigan

Calcific tendinitis (also referred to as calcifying tendinitis and calcific tendinopathy) of the shoulder is a common disorder of unknown etiology. It is characterized by the multifocal accumulation of basic calcium phosphate crystals within the rotator cuff tendons. The deposition of calcium itself may cause mild-to-moderate chronic discomfort in some patients, but during the resorption of these calcifications many patients have significant acute pain. This acute and chronic pain can lead to restriction of range of motion and function. Various treatment modalities have been found beneficial in the management of this disorder, and many patients do well with conservative measures alone.

INCIDENCE AND EPIDEMIOLOGY

The reported incidence of tendon calcification varies, with 2.7% to 20% of asymptomatic shoulders found to have radiographic calcifications. It has been estimated that 35% to 45% of patients with deposits eventually become symptomatic. Fifty-one to ninety percent of calcifications have been reported to be located in the supraspinatus tendon.

It is important to note, however, that not all calcifications in the rotator cuff, even in a symptomatic shoulder, are due to calcific tendinitis. Dystrophic calcifications can be seen around the torn edges of a complete tear and portend a different prognosis than calcific tendinitis. Significant calcifications can also be seen in patients with rotator cuff arthropathy.

Women are more commonly affected than men, with studies finding that 57% to 76% of the calcific tendinitis occurs in female patients. The age distribution with the highest incidence has been reported in various studies to be in 31-to 50-year-olds, and there have been some reports of ethnic variation with an increased average age in Asians. Calcifications are uncommon in patients over 70 years old, and calcifications have been reported in a 3-year-old child. The right side is more commonly affected than the left, and bilateral involvement was present in 24% in one report.

There is good agreement that calcific tendinitis is not part of a generalized disease process. It is not believed that there is a relationship between trauma and calcific tendinitis, nor is there evidence of a correlation between tendon tears and calcific tendinitis. An association with diabetes and gout has been suspected, but no significant evidence of such has been documented. One study showed an association between calcific tendinitis and endocrine disorders; however, 65% of the patients with calcific tendinitis carried a diagnosis of a specific endocrine disorder (16). In that study, those with endocrine disorders had a higher rate of failure of conservative management leading to surgical intervention (47% underwent surgical intervention vs. 23% in patients without endocrine disorders).

PATHOLOGY AND PATHOGENESIS

In most cases, the multifocal calcifications are located 1 to 2 cm from the insertion of the supraspinatus tendon on the greater tuberosity (in the "critical zone"). Gartner and Heyer (1) analyzed calcific deposits and found that they consist of hydroxyapatite crystals $(Ca_{10}[PO_4]_6(OH)_2)$ with a varying amount of H_2O, CO_3, and PO_4 (1). The macroscopic appearance changed from a granular conglomerate during the chronic or formative phase to a milky emulsion in the acute or resorptive phase. The etiology of calcific tendinitis is still a matter of controversy. Degenerative calcification and reactive calcification are the two fundamentally different processes proposed as the cause of formation of calcium deposits in rotator cuff tendons.

Codman (2) believed that degeneration of the tendon fibers precedes calcification, with necrosis of fibers followed by dystrophic calcification. Degeneration occurs through "wear and tear" with aging. This wear and tear is accentuated by a diminution in the vascularity of the tendons with age. Fascicles become thin and fibrillated. Tendon fibers split and fray and are hypocellular. These changes begin at the end of the fourth or fifth decade. Since Codman's description of degenerative calcification, there has been some evidence supporting this sequence of degeneration, necrosis, and calcification.

However, as Uhthoff et al. (3) argue this degenerative process does not accurately describe the clinical and morphologic aspects of calcific tendinitis. A purely degenerative etiology does not explain the peak of calcific tendinitis in the fifth decade when degeneration is known to increase in incidence as aging continues. In addition, a degenerative process would not include the self-healing that is seen in calcific tendinitis. Thus, they concluded that there is a separate entity appropriately called *degenerative calcification*, and another process of *reactive calcification*, which cause calcific tendinitis.

Reactive calcification occurs in a viable environment and is a cell-mediated process that is felt to occur in three distinct stages: precalcific, calcific, and postcalcific.

Precalcific stage: During this first stage, a portion of the tendon undergoes fibrocartilaginous transformation with metaplasia of tenocytes into chondrocytes. There is a concomitant elaboration of proteoglycan. Histologic evaluation reveals areas of fibrocartilaginous metaplasia that are generally avascular.

Calcific stage: The calcific stage is broken down further into formative, resting, and resorptive phases. During the formative phase, calcium crystals are deposited in matrix vesicles that coalesce to form large deposits. The enlarging deposits erode the fibrocartilaginous septa. Histologic examination shows this deposition of calcium crystals in the fibrocartilaginous matrix. The resting phase describes the period of fibrocollagenous tissue bordering the foci of calcification, indicating that deposition has ceased. The length of this period is variable. During the resorptive phase, spontaneous resorption of the calcium deposits occurs. Thin walled vascular channels appear at the periphery of the deposit. Macrophages and giant cells phagocytose and remove the calcium. Histologic examination shows this cell-mediated resorption of the calcific deposit (Fig. 25.1).

Postcalcific stage: As the calcifications are resorbed, granulation tissue with fibroblasts and vascular channels remodels the space that was occupied by the deposits. These scars remodel with fibroblasts and collagen aligned along the longitudinal axis of the tendon and type I collagen replaces type III collagen. Of note, not all foci of calcification are in the same phase in a given patient at a single point in time, but in general, one phase predominates (3).

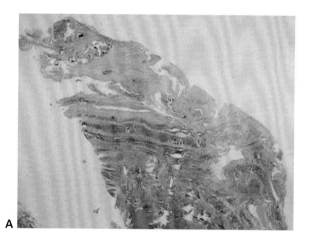
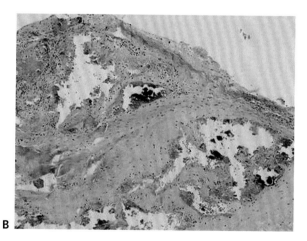
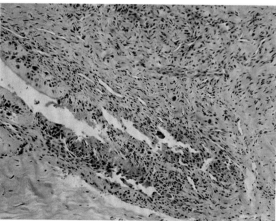

FIGURE 25.1. A: Low-power view demonstrating multiple calcific deposits throughout the supraspinatus. **B:** Higher power view of calcific deposits. **C:** Calcifications, giant cells, and chronic inflammation.

In spite of the pathogenesis being thus described, the triggering event of the precalcific stage is unknown. It is thought by many to be related to tissue hypoxia. There is some evidence that there is a genetic component, with an increased incidence of HLA-A1 identified in patients with calcific tendinitis although other studies dispute this.

CLINICAL EVALUATION

Pertinent History

Patients with calcific tendinitis will complain of pain and a loss of range of motion. The most significant pain generally occurs during the resorptive phase, with some milder symptoms present in some patients during the formative and the postcalcific phases. The pain is believed to be caused during the resorptive phase by raised intratendinous pressure from exudation of cells and vascular proliferation. Patients are usually able to localize the pain and the point of maximal tenderness although there is often a radiation of pain with referral to the deltoid. Patients often have difficulty sleeping on the shoulder, and many complain of an increase in the pain at night. Patients often indicate that they sense catching in the shoulder as they go through an arc of motion.

Physical Exam

In cases of long-standing symptoms, patients may show atrophy of the supraspinatus or infraspinatus. Some authors have reported swelling and redness, but this has not been found by all reporters. Patients will exhibit significant tenderness in the area of the affected tendon. As mentioned above, patients usually show a loss of range of motion and may have a sensation of catching. In severe cases in the acute phase, patients may refuse to move their arms at all, and they may insist on maintaining their arms in internal rotation against their bodies. Impingement signs are frequently present although bursitis is a minor and infrequent feature based on surgical findings.

Imaging

Plain radiographs will demonstrate calcifications beginning in the formative phase (Fig. 25.2). In addition to standard AP and optional axillary views, internal and external rotation views have also been recommended for identification and evaluation of deposits (4). Deposits become less dense and homogenous during the acute or resorptive phase and may become difficult to visualize with plain films. In addition, during the resorptive phase, a crescent of calcification may be seen in the overlying bursa due to rupture into the bursa. Serial radiographs are helpful in following the progression of the resolution of pathology (Fig. 25.3). Calcifications from arthropathies are associated with degenerative articular changes and are adjacent to the bony insertion and thus can be differentiated from calcific tendinitis.

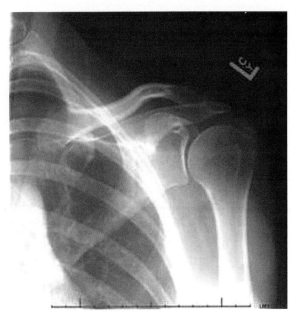

FIGURE 25.2. AP view of a 56-year-old woman with left shoulder pain. There is calcification along the superior-lateral aspect of the humeral head consistent with calcific tendinitis of the supraspinatus.

Some associations between particular radiographic features and the phase of disease have been advanced. It has been suggested that during the formative or chronic phase, the deposit is homogenous, well defined, and dense (Fig. 25.2) and then becomes fluffy and heterogenous during the resorptive or acute phase (Fig. 25.3).

MRI and ultrasound have been used to visualize calcifications in those cases (10). MRI is rarely indicated, but when obtained, deposits appear as areas of decreased signal intensity on T1-weighted images, whereas on T2-weighted images they often show a perifocal band of increased signal intensity (Fig. 25.4). Ultrasound has been found to be more sensitive than plain radiographs by some authors, with 100% ultrasound compared with 90% radiographic identification of histologically proven calcific tendinitis. It should be noted, as with any ultrasound technique, that these results are very operator dependent.

Classification

Bosworth (4) divided deposits into three sizes, which he felt correlated with the increasing likelihood of clinical significance: small, measuring up to 0.5 mm; medium, measuring 0.5 to 1.5 mm; and large, measuring greater than 1.5 mm. Calcific tendinitis has also been described based on the duration of symptoms as acute (up to 2 weeks), subacute (3 to 8 weeks), and chronic (3 months or more) (5). The chronic presentations are likely to occur during the formative phase, whereas the acute phase occurs during resorption. Calcific tendinitis has also been described as localized or diffuse, with the diffuse form generally causing symptoms that are more severe and of longer duration. Rowe (6) described a chronic asymptomatic stage correlating with the gross finding of dry, powder-like calcific

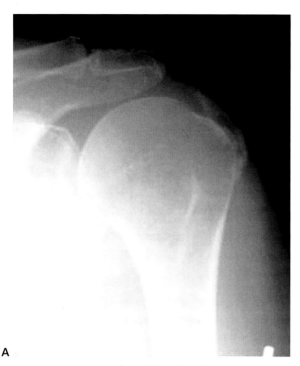
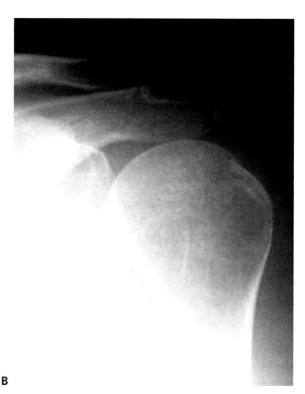

A
B

FIGURE 25.3. A, B: Serial AP radiographs taken 3 months apart demonstrating resorption of calcifications. **A:** the initial image. **B:** the same view taken 3 months later.

deposits, a mild chronic pain correlating with the gross finding of soft toothpaste-like deposits, and a milky or creamy consistency in the extremely painful period. Harvie et al. (7) recommended classifying calcific tendinitis as idiopathic (type I) or secondary (type II) based on whether patients had an endocrine disorder. In their study, those with endocrine disorders (type II) had a higher rate of failure of conservative management leading to surgical intervention compared with those without an endocrine diagnosis (type I), with 47% surgical intervention required in type II versus 23% in type I patients.

Gartner and Heyer (1) created a radiographic classification, which is often referenced, with type I referring to a homogenous deposit on X-ray with a sharp outline, type II an inhomogenous structure with a sharp outline or a homogenous structure without a defined outline, and type III an inhomogenous structure without a defined outline. He reported that response to needling is related to the appearance of the deposit, with 85% of fluffy accumulations (type III) resorbed at 3 years versus only 33% of sharply defined calcifications (type I). Patte and Goutallier (8) also classified deposits radiographically.

A French classification system (9) that is commonly used is based on the radiographic appearance as well: type A is dense, rounded, and sharply delineated; type B is multilobular in appearance, radiodense, and with sharp outlines; type C is more radiolucent and heterogenous with irregular outlines; and type D has dystrophic calcific

lesions at the tendon insertion, which many would say is separate from true calcific tendinitis.

TREATMENT

Conservative Management

The natural history of calcific tendinitis is variable. Bosworth (4) reported a yearly resolution rate of 3%, with vanishing of the deposits seen in 9% of his patients at 3 years (4). The first line of treatment is conservative. The patient is instructed to do range of motion exercises to avoid the loss of mobility of the glenohumeral joint. Pendulum exercises can be advanced to muscle strengthening as the patient's symptoms allow. In patients with chronic symptoms, this may be initiated immediately, while those with acute symptoms may benefit from waiting a week to allow symptoms to decrease. It has been recommended that patients keep their arms abducted for symptomatic relief. Heat provides symptomatic relief to some patients. NSAIDs are often utilized although there is no evidence that they affect the natural history of calcific tendinitis. In general, corticosteroids are not recommended unless there is a concomitant impingement syndrome although some reports confirm their routine use for symptomatic relief. Some authors advise a single intrabursal cortisone injection during the acute phase (3). Patients are assessed clinically and radiographically approximately every 4 weeks. There have been widely variable rates of success, with reports ranging from 6% to 99% success with conservative management.

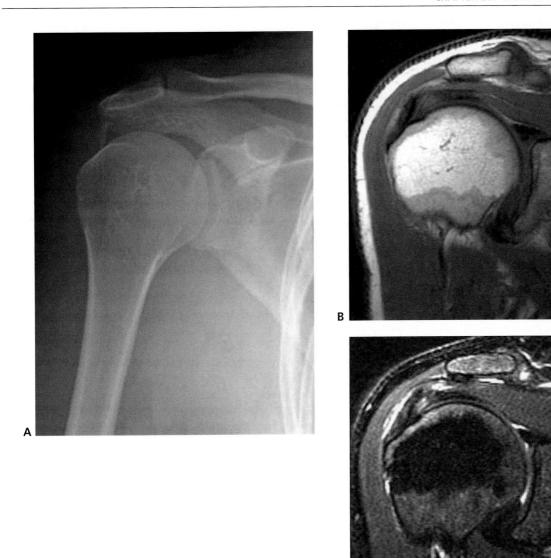

FIGURE 25.4. A: AP, **B:** T1-, and **C:** T2-weighted coronal MRI slices. The deposit visualized on the radiograph is seen to demonstrate low signal intensity on T1-weighted images and also very low T2 signal intensity with intermediate T2 signal in the surrounding tendon compatible with calcific tendinitis.

Needling and Lavage

During the resorptive phase, when symptoms are acute, some authors advocate lavage of deposits using two large bore needles and lidocaine. Radiographs have been used to guide needling the deposits, and recent literature supports the use of ultrasound guided needling when available with rates of elimination reported between 28% and 76%. Gartner and Heyer (1) reported that response to needling is related to the appearance of the deposit, with 85% of fluffy accumulations resorbed at 3 years versus only 33% of sharply defined calcifications.

Some authors have advocated combining ultrasound-guided needling and extracorporeal shock wave

therapy (ESWT). When compared with ESWT alone, the combined treatment group has shown significantly better clinical improvement (constant shoulder scoring system), radiographic improvement (disappearance of deposits on plain radiographs), and a lower rate of required surgical intervention without any increase in complications.

Ultrasound

The use of ultrasound to treat calcific tendinitis is controversial and has not been widely accepted. However, Ebenbichler et al. (10). conducted a randomized, double-blind comparison of ultrasonography and sham insonation in

54 consecutive patients with symptomatic calcific tendinitis. At 9 months, they found resolution or significant decrease in the size of deposits in 65% of patients treated with ultrasound compared with 20% of the sham group. The ultrasound patients had greater decreases in pain and greater improvements in quality of life at 6 weeks, but at 9 months there was no clinical difference between the two groups. Thus, perhaps the best evidence supports the use of ultrasound for a short-term benefit, but evidence of a long-term clinical benefit is lacking.

Extracorporeal Shock Wave Therapy

The use of high-energy ESWT has been reported as a non-invasive alternative prior to surgical intervention in patients with symptomatic calcific tendinitis that has failed conservative management. Shock waves are acoustic waves associated with a sudden rise in pressure. They are produced by electrohydraulic, piezoelectric, and electromagnetic devices, and the amount of energy is measured as millijoules per millimeter. ESWT has been used successfully in the lithotripsy of various types of kidney stones. Its effects are felt to be primarily related to the transfer of energy, causing disintegration of the deposit or at least affecting a change in the consistency of the deposit with subsequent cellular resorption.

A trial of conservative management of 3 to 6 months is usually recommended before referring a patient for ESWT. Contraindications are infection, pacemaker use, pregnancy, local tumor, avascular necrosis of the humeral head, heterotopic ossification, osteomyelitis, and open growth plates. Various protocols have been published for the use of ESWT in treating calcific tendinitis, with some evidence that high-energy ESWT has significantly better clinical efficacy than low-energy ESWT (8). High-energy shock waves are more painful, but usually tolerated by most patients. Many protocols include the use of local anesthesia at the site of ESWT. Local hematomas also occur but there have not been any reports of significant sequelae. Most studies report no complications from ESWT although there have been two reports of humeral head osteonecrosis, which may be related to nonstandard indication and application. Maier et al. (11) looked at the MRIs of shoulders after ESWT and found no bony or tendinous changes.

Most of the recent published studies show a degree of efficacy, with the rate of elimination of deposits quoted as between 15% and 75%. Included in this group are several randomized, controlled trials showing a significant treatment response to ESWT compared with placebo. Gerdesmeyer et al. (12) performed a double-blind, randomized, placebo-controlled trial of ESWT involving 144 patients. They found higher constant scores, better pain relief, and diminished calcification size at 6 months (complete disappearance in 60% of the high-energy group) in the ESWT groups compared with placebo group. Rompe et al. (13). performed a prospective, quasi-randomized study comparing ESWT with open surgery for 79 patients with chronic calcific tendinitis. Overall, the surgery group had a higher percentage of good or excellent results at 1 year (75% vs. 60%) and 24 months (90% vs. 64%). However, when they subdivided the groups based on radiographic appearance, patients with homogenous deposits had superior results with surgery, whereas patients with inhomogenous deposits had equivalent results with ESWT.

Operative Treatment

There is no agreed upon time frame at which point conservative management is abandoned for surgical intervention, with some authors recommending early open treatment, whereas most authors advise operating only when conservative measures have failed. Surgical intervention can be considered when symptoms are progressive, the patient has constant pain interfering with the activities of daily living, and there has been no improvement after conservative therapy. Surgical intervention should be considered with continued symptoms after 6 to 12 months of nonoperative treatment. Ark et al. (14). reported their series with arthroscopic treatment for those patients who failed to respond to at least 1 year of conservative management. Uhthoff et al. recommend surgical intervention when patients have chronic symptoms consistent with the formative phase and fail to respond to conservative management. They recommend against surgical intervention during the resorptive or acute phase, as those patients generally improve over the course of weeks (3). The best method of operative treatment is not clearly defined.

Arthroscopy has become a commonly used method to treat refractory calcific tendinitis. The advantages are those of arthroscopy in general, including a shorter rehabilitation period, better cosmesis, the ability to identify and potentially treat other pathology, and better preservation of adjacent tissue. Failure to identify the deposit arthroscopically has been reported as 12%, which is similar to the 15% failure reported in open management. Several authors have published their outcomes with arthroscopic management. Ark et al. (14) reported on 23 patients at 26 months with good results in 50%, with full motion and complete pain relief, satisfactory results in 41% with full motion and occasional episodes of pain, and unsatisfactory results in 9% with those patients reporting persistent pain. Acromioplasty does not appear to affect outcome, but patients with the postoperative elimination or reduction of deposits had better outcomes than those patients who had no radiographic change. Mole (15) and colleagues reported on 112 patients treated arthroscopically and reported 89% clinical and 88% radiographic success at 21 months. Patients returned to work at an average of 3 months, and full functional recovery occurred by 6 months, which was similar to their results from open surgery. More recently, Seil et al.(16) reported on 54 patients treated arthroscopically, with constant score improvement from 33 to 91 and 92% patient satisfaction at 2 years. Sixty-five percent of patients took at least 6 months to reach their minimum pain level although 78% of patients returned to work within 6 weeks.

Bosworth (4) opined that the quickest and most dependable way of relieving patients with large and troublesome deposits was by open surgery (4). Vebostad (17) obtained excellent and good results in 34 of 43 patients treated with open excision of deposits. Gschwend (18) reported excellent and good results in 25 of 28 patients. DePalma and Kruper (5) reported 96% good results. Many authors have noted, as did Seil in their arthroscopic series, that postoperative symptoms persist for longer than anticipated, and some have noted that the recovery from surgery is longer than the convalescence in many conservatively managed patients. This lends further support to initial nonoperative management.

ARTHROSCOPIC TECHNIQUE

The patient is positioned in a beach chair or lateral decubitus position per the surgeon's preference with general anesthesia and optional regional anesthesia for postoperative pain relief. A standard diagnostic arthroscopic examination of the glenohumeral joint is performed with posterior and anterior portals. If the location of a deposit is identified during glenohumeral examination, it can be marked with a nonabsorbable dark suture, 0 PDS (polydiaxonone sulfate), for example, percutaneously introduced using a spinal needle to allow localization on the bursal side. (Fig. 25.5) However, it is unusual to identify the deposit on the articular side of the rotator cuff in the authors' experience. The scope is removed from the glenohumeral joint and introduced into the subacromial space using the same posterior skin incision. A lateral portal is created, and a subacromial bursectomy is performed to allow for adequate visualization and for the examination of the subacromial space. The rotator cuff is examined methodically by palpation to identify any hardening indicative of a calcific deposit. Preoperative and intraoperative imaging can also be helpful to localize deposits. A spinal needle can be used to help locate calcific deposits as well by using the needle to stab into the cuff tissue. Once a deposit is needled, calcific material will usually emerge into the subacromial space (Fig. 25.6). Once the deposit is identified, if the deposit is not readily accessible, some authors recommend making a longitudinal incision in line with the tendon fibers. A probe, hook, or shaver can then be used to release the deposit (Fig. 25.5). Alternatively, other authors recommend using arthroscopic resectors and curettes to remove deposits. The subacromial space is then irrigated to remove as much of the deposit as possible as calcific material can float out into the subacromial space during removal (Fig. 25.7). After removal of the deposit, a careful inspection is performed of the cuff from the bursal and articular sides to ensure that no significant tear has resulted or been created during the removal process. Significant tears can be repaired either arthroscopically or using open techniques.

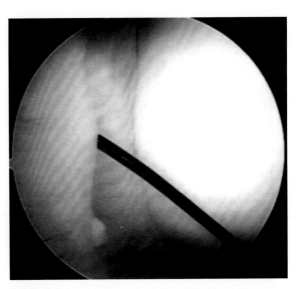

FIGURE 25.5. Arthroscopic image within the glenohumeral joint with a marking suture placed adjacent to visualized calcific deposit for better localization in the subacromial space. (Courtesy Suzanne Miller, MD.)

OPEN TECHNIQUE

The patient is placed in either the lateral decubitus or the beach chair position, and general anesthesia is induced. Adjunctive regional anesthesia is optional for postoperative pain management. A sandbag can be placed under the affected shoulder. An incision is made from the lateral or anterolateral aspect of the acromion. The deltoid fibers are split for a distance no more than 5 cm from the acromion to avoid injury to the axillary nerve, the bursa is opened, and the undersurface of the acromion is palpated to identify potential spurring. Anterior acromioplasty can be performed, but is not routinely done. The tendon is inspected and incised as necessary in the direction of the fibers, and the calcific mass is treated with curettage. Copious lavage is performed. The tendon edges are approximated if necessary, and the wound is closed in layers.

AUTHORS' PREFERRED TREATMENT

After the diagnosis of symptomatic calcific tendinitis is made, treatment is started with conservative measures. Patients with acute bursal inflammation are offered an injection of corticosteroid into the subacromial space. Patients are sent to physical therapy for rotator cuff-focused rehabilitation. Ultrasound is used at the discretion of the physical therapist, and some patients have attributed symptomatic improvement to this modality. NSAIDs are usually prescribed unless contraindicated.

Patients return at 6 weeks for repeat clinical evaluation. In many cases, patients respond well to these conservative measures, and a conservative course is continued with a repeat visit in 6 weeks. In cases in which the outcome of conservative measures is not satisfactory, we discuss arthroscopic management with the patient. In our experience,

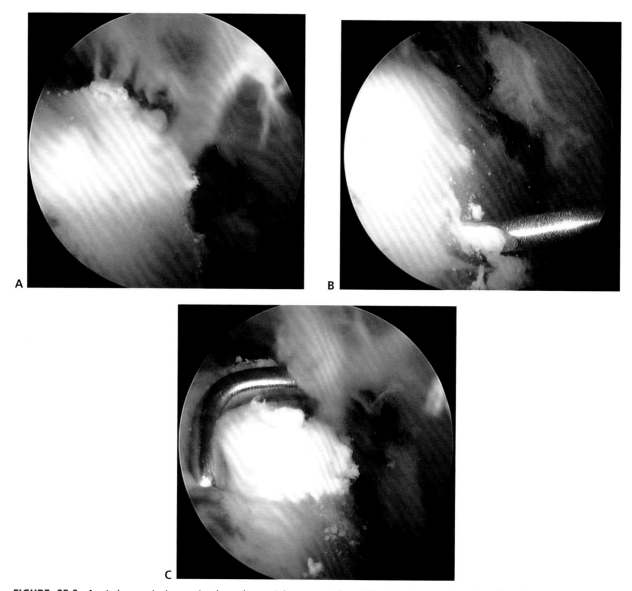

FIGURE 25.6. A: Arthroscopic image in the subacromial space with calcific deposit noted on bursal surface of rotator cuff. **B:** A percutaneous spinal needle is used to identify the calcific deposit in the rotator cuff. **C:** A probe being used to remove calcific material from the rotator cuff. (Courtesy Michael Codsi, MD.)

many of these patients are extremely symptomatic and are anxious to have an intervention performed.

If surgery is indicated, calcium deposits are removed arthroscopically under general anesthesia usually accompanied with regional anesthesia for improved postoperative pain control. The authors find preoperative plain X-ray and MRI imaging useful to help localize the deposits and therefore these studies should be accessible and visible for review within the operating room. The patient is positioned in the beach chair position, and a standard diagnostic examination of the glenohumeral joint and its structures is performed using an arthroscopy pump for distention. Any intra-articular pathology is treated. It is unusual in the authors' experience to identify deposits from within the glenohumeral joint. However, if identified, then the location of a deposit identified during glenohumeral

examination can be marked with a nonabsorbable dark suture (0-PDS) introduced percutaneously through an 18 G spinal needle to allow localization on the bursal side.

The scope is removed and introduced into the subacromial space using the same posterior skin incision. A lateral portal is created, and a bursectomy is performed to allow for an adequate visualization for examination of the subacromial space. The rotator cuff is examined methodically by palpation to identify any hardening indicative of a calcific deposit. After the bursectomy is completed, the scope is placed in the lateral portal or through an accessory posterolateral portal for better direct visualization of the rotator cuff. Working instruments are placed through the anterior or posterior portal. The bursal side of the rotator cuff is gently debrided with an arthroscopic shaver to try to identify deposits. A probe or a percutaneously placed

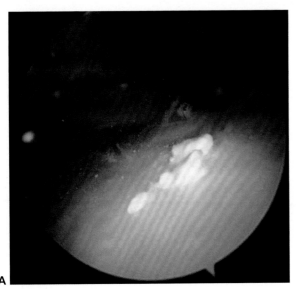
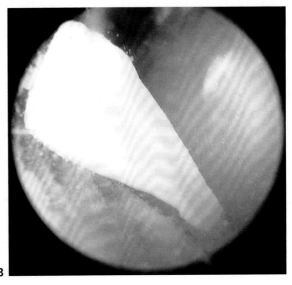

A   B

FIGURE 25.7. A and B: Calcific debris within the subacromial space following debridement of deposits within the rotator cuff. (Courtesy Michael Codsi, MD.)

18 G spinal needle is used to identify deposits within the rotator cuff. If not readily apparent, fluoroscopy or mini fluoroscopy can be used to locate hidden deposits. Location is confirmed using a spinal needle.

Occasionally deposits are very superficial within the bursal cuff tissue and are removed during bursectomy. Buried deposits are opened using a superficial incision of the rotator cuff with an arthroscopic knife or percutaneously with a 15 blade through an established portal under arthroscopic visualization. A probe or 4.5-mm shaver is then used to release and debride the deposit (Fig. 25.5). The subacromial space is then irrigated to remove any free-floating deposit material. Fluoroscopy is used to confirm the complete removal of all calcific material when necessary. After removal of the deposit(s), a careful inspection is performed of the cuff from the bursal and articular sides to ensure that no tear exists.

Partial and full-thickness tears are treated in a standard fashion. Tears 5 mm or greater in depth are repaired using a tendon-to-tendon or tendon-to-bone technique. Tears of minimal depth are smoothed and debrided with a 4.5-mm shaver. An acromioplasty is not performed unless there are obvious signs of wear and impingement on the coracoacromial ligament, or a very large acromial spur is present. The patient is placed in a sling and is generally discharged home the same day as the surgery.

COMPLICATIONS AND CONTROVERSIES

Complications

Overall, reported complications from the management of calcific tendinitis are rare. In the series by Rompe et al. they had one deep infection in 29 patients treated with open removal of deposits and no adverse events other than a transient subcutaneous hematoma in the 50 patients treated with high-energy ESWT. They used MRI or ultrasound to rule out rotator cuff pathology after shock wave therapy (8). In the larger trial of ESWT by Gerdesmeyer, local skin complications including petechiae, bleeding, and erythema were reported in 68 of 90 patients, with slightly higher rates in the higher energy group. No other clinically significant adverse effects were found, including neurologic disorders, tendon injury, infection, aseptic necrosis, or muscle hematoma. There have been two reports of humeral head osteonecrosis in patients treated with ESWT, which may be related to nonstandard indication and application. Maier et al. looked at MRIs of shoulders after ESWT and found no bony or tendinous changes.

No significant complications have been consistently reported from the arthroscopic management of calcific tendinitis although the risks of shoulder arthroscopy in general, including infection, nerve, and soft tissue damage are certainly applicable. In the study by Jacobs and Debeer, they reported an 18% rate of frozen shoulder in their arthroscopically treated patients, but this has not been reported in other series. Rotini had one case of frozen shoulder in 126 shoulders treated arthroscopically. In their series of 54 patients treated arthroscopically, Seil et al. reported a subcutaneous hematoma in one patient and secondary stiffness in two patients that resolved over 3 months with corticosteroid injections.

Controversies

Pathogenesis

The cause of calcifications of the rotator cuff is unclear. Relative ischemia as a result of hypovascularization in the "critical zone," metabolic disturbances, and degeneration of the rotator cuff tendons has been suggested as etiologies. Although the cycle and stages have been well described by Uhthoff and others, the factor that triggers metaplasia has not yet been identified. Hypoxia is thought by many to be the primary factor, but this remains an area that requires further study (3).

Importance of Deposit Removal and Subacromial Decompression

Most studies have confirmed the importance of complete removal of the calcific deposits. Rompe et al. (8) found a strong association between complete disintegration of deposits and good outcome in both surgically treated and ESWT-treated patients (8). Porcellini et al. (19) found in their series of arthroscopically treated patients that those with residual deposits consistently had lower postoperative constant scores, with higher scores in the presence of small calcifications and the highest scores in the absence of deposits. They also found, as have others, that the addition of a subacromial decompression did not affect the outcome. Similarly, Jerosch et al. (20) found that acromioplasty did not affect the outcome, but patients with postoperative elimination or reduction of deposits had better outcomes than those patients who had no radiographic change.

However, there have been a minority of studies that found that excellent results did not depend on deposit removal. Tillander et al. (21) suggested that calcific deposits could be left untouched based on their retrospective review of arthroscopic subacromial decompressions performed on patients with radiographic calcific deposits. They found similar outcomes for pain, constant score, range of motion, and patient satisfaction in those with deposits and those without deposits who underwent arthroscopic subacromial decompression. At 2 years, 79% of deposits had either disappeared (54%) or decreased in size (25%) on radiographic evaluation. The persistence of calcifications at 2 years did not correlate with constant scores. Jacobs and de Beer (22) also concluded from their study of arthroscopic treatment that the presence of residual calcifications did not influence the functional outcome. They recommended accepting residual calcifications in order to preserve tendon integrity.

PEARLS AND PITFALLS

1. Patient presentation is often similar in nature to patients with acute subacromial bursitis, rotator cuff tendinitis, or impingement syndrome. It is imperative to closely scrutinize plain radiographs for any sign of calcific deposits in these patients.
2. Fluoroscopy can be a valuable tool during surgical intervention for calcific deposits. It is useful to locate the deposit using a spinal needle in the rotator cuff as a reference. This can help avoid cutting into the rotator cuff to explore for deposits. It is also useful to confirm complete removal of calcific material.
3. Most series have not shown acromioplasty to add benefit to calcific deposit removal.

REHABILITATION

The initial conservative management includes a daily program of exercise to maintain full shoulder mobility.

With both the arthroscopic and the open techniques, early mobilization is recommended. The patient meets with a physical therapist preoperatively to ensure that appropriate postoperative rehabilitation occurs. Range of motion exercises begin 24 to 48 hours after surgery. These exercises begin with pendulums, and then active assisted exercises are initiated after approximately 3 days. This is advanced to active exercises as tolerated. A sling is used only during the first 1 to 3 days for comfort and is then discontinued. If a rotator cuff repair was necessary after deposit removal, then rehabilitation is modified accordingly with longer sling use and a slower return to activities consistent with rotator cuff repair.

CONCLUSIONS AND FUTURE DIRECTIONS

The diagnosis and management of calcific tendinitis can be satisfying for both the patient and the physician. Successful management depends on understanding what is known about the pathogenesis and the disease process. In many patients, spontaneous resorption takes place. There are various management options, and many interventions have been shown to be effective. No one protocol for management has been shown to be best. Most patients have excellent outcomes with a course of management that starts with a trial of conservative measures followed by one or more of various noninvasive tools like ultrasound and ESWT if needed, with surgical intervention preserved for those patients who have persistent symptoms affecting their activities of daily living.

Further research on the pathogenesis of calcific tendinitis could lead to the potential prevention and improvements in management. The process that initiates the fibrocartilaginous metaplasia and the factors that lead to the initiation of the resorptive process are two particular areas that should be at the forefront of research efforts on this topic. Continued reports of clinical outcomes will also help the practitioner in selecting the best possible treatment option for the patient.

REFERENCES

1. Gartner J, Heyer A. Calcific tendonitis of the shoulder. *Orthopade.* 1995;24:284–302.
2. Codman EA. *The Shoulder: Rupture of the Supraspinatus Tendon and Other Lesions in or About the Subacromial Bursa.* Boston, MA: Thomas Todd; 1934:178–215.
3. Uhthoff HK, Sarkar K, Maynard JA. Calcifying tendinitis: a new concept of its pathogenesis. *Clin Orthop Relat Res.* 1976;118:164–168.
4. Bosworth BM. Examination of the shoulder for calcium deposits. *J Bone Joint Surg Am.* 1941:23:567–577.
5. DePalma AF, Kruper JS. Long term study of shoulder joints afflicted with and treated for calcific tendinitis. *Clin Orthop Relat Res.* 1961;20:61–71.

6. Rowe CR. Calcific tendinitis. *Instr Course Lect.* 1985;34:196–198.

7. Harvie P, Pollard TC, Carr AJ. Calcific tendinitis: natural history and association with endocrine disorders. *J Shoulder Elbow Surg.* 2007;16:169–73.

8. Patte D, Goutallier D. Periarthritis of the shoulder. Calcifications. Rev Chir Orthop Reparatrice Appar Mot. 1988; 74:277–278.

9. Mole D, Kempf JF, Gleyze P, Rio B, Bonnomet B, Walch G. Resultat du traitement arthroscopique des tendinopathies non rompues, II: les calcifications. Rev Chir Orthop 1993; 79:532–41.

10. Ebenbichler GR, Erdogmus CB, Resch KL, et al. Ultrasound therapy for calcific tendinitis of the shoulder. *N Engl J Med.* 1999;340:1533–1538.

11. Maier M, Stäbler A, Lienemann A, et al. Shockwave application in calcifying tendinitis of the shoulder--prediction of outcome by imaging. Arch Orthop Trauma Surg. 2000;120:493–498.

12. Gerdesmeyer L, Wagenpfeil S, Haake M, et al. Extracorporeal shock wave therapy for the treatment of chronic calcifying tendonitis of the rotator cuff: a randomized controlled trial. JAMA. 2003; 290:2573–2580.

13. Rompe JD, Zoellner J, Nafe B. Shock wave therapy versus conventional surgery in the treatment of calcifying tendinitis of the shoulder. *Clin Orthop Relat Res.* 2001;387:72–82.

14. Ark JW, Flock TJ, Flatow EL, et al. Arthroscopic treatment of calcific tendinitis of the shoulder. *Arthroscopy.* 1992;8:183–188.

15. Molé D, Kempf JF, Gleyze P, et al. Results of endoscopic treatment of non-broken tendinopathies of the rotator cuff. 2. Calcifications of the rotator cuff. Rev Chir Orthop Reparatrice Appar Mot. 1993; 79:532–541.

16. Seil R, Litzenburger H, Kohn D, et al. Arthroscopic treatment of chronically painful calcifying tendinitis of the supraspinatus tendon. Arthroscopy. 2006; 22:521–527.

17. Vebostad A., Calcific Tendinitis in the shoulder region. Acta Orthop Scand. 1975;46:205–210.

18. Gschwend N, Patte D, Zippel J. Therapy of calcific tendinitis of the shoulder. Arch Orthop Unfallchir. 1972; 73:120–135.

19. Porcellini G, Paladini P, Campi F, et al. Arthroscopic treatment of calcific tendinitis of the shoulder: clinical and ultrasonographic follow-up findings at 2 to 5 years. *J Shoulder Elbow Surg.* 2004;13:503–508.

20. Jerosch J, Strauss JM, Schmiel S. Arthroscopic treatment of calcific tendinitis of the shoulder. *J Shoulder Elbow Surg.* 1998;7:30–37.

21. Tillander BM, Norlin RO. Change of calcifications after arthroscopic subacromial decompression. *J Shoulder Elbow Surg.* 1998; 7:213–217.

22. Jacobs R, Debeer P. Calcifying tendinitis of the rotator cuff: functional outcome after arthroscopic treatment. Acta Orthop Belg. 2006; 72:276–281.

I. The Shoulder

Scapulothoracic Endoscopy and the Snapping Scapula

Laurence D. Higgins • Michael J. DeFranco • Benjamin Sanofsky

Since its first description in the mid-19th century (1), the diagnosis and management of the snapping scapula has been a challenge for orthopedic surgeons. The snapping scapula is commonly referred to by the symptoms it produces, namely, retroscapular pain and retroscapular cracking. Each of these descriptions implies a clinical syndrome consisting of a painful tactile acoustic phenomenon localized to the scapulothoracic space. Although this condition is frequently localized to the superomedial corner of the scapula, it can occur in other areas as well and is particularly associated with overhead activity (2). Snapping may arise from soft tissue and/or osseous lesions in the scapulothoracic space, but in some cases, there is no definitive lesion. The purpose of this chapter is to review the pathoanatomy and clinical assessment of a snapping scapula and to describe the current treatment options for this condition.

SCAPULOTHORACIC ANATOMY

The scapulothoracic articulation consists of the ventral (anterior), concave surface of the scapula and the convex posterior thoracic wall. The stability of the scapula on the posterior thoracic cage is provided by 10 periscapular muscles. The acromioclavicular joint is the only other attachment of the scapula to the rest of the skeleton. At rest, the normal position of the scapula is approximately 2 cm lateral from the spine and between the second and the seventh ribs (3). The plane of the scapula is a static position defined as 30° to 40° in the frontal plane with 10° to 20° of anterior inclination (4). The soft tissue and osseous structures of the scapulothoracic space determine the congruity of movement.

The soft tissue structures surrounding the scapula consist primarily of muscle and bursae. More importantly, the scapulothoracic articulation consists of three muscular layers: superficial, intermediate, and deep. Table 26.1 defines these layers with respect to muscles and bursae (5). Understanding this anatomy is critical to determining the etiology of a symptomatic scapulothoracic articulation, to establishing an adequate treatment plan, and to planning

operative procedures. Several bursae exist not only between the muscles but also between the muscles and the chest wall (Fig. 26.1). Table 26.2 provides a summary of the scapulothoracic bursae, which are critical to the normal function of the scapula and a common source of pain and crepitus.

The osseous anatomy of the scapula and the ribs is also important in understanding the etiology of a snapping scapula. The surfaces of these structures must be smooth in order for there to be normal motion between the scapula and the thorax. Bony abnormalities of the scapula or the ribs may create incongruity and lead to a symptomatic scapulothoracic motion.

Etiology of the Snapping Scapula

Snapping of the scapula occurs during rotation of the anterior scapula on the posterior surface of the chest wall. In general, the etiology of the snapping scapula can be classified according to the pathologic lesion, which is usually a soft tissue or bony prominence that disrupts the congruity of the scapulothoracic space (Table 26.3). In some cases, there may be no identifiable lesion. Clinically, the snapping may be described as physiologic (nonpathologic/asymptomatic) or pathologic (symptomatic). Patients with physiologic snapping have scapulothoracic crepitus but are asymptomatic. In these patients, treatment is rarely necessary. However, the onset of symptoms, such as pain, reflects a transition to a pathologic articulation that requires further assessment and treatment. In most cases, this transition represents either a change in the intervening soft tissue between the scapula and the chest wall or the development of an osseous lesion that causes a loss of congruity between the scapula and the thorax. In some patients, pain may occur without audible or palpable crepitation or snapping (6).

The most common soft tissue abnormalities involve bursae and muscles. Similar to bursae near other joints, the scapulothoracic bursae can become inflamed and symptomatic. In chronic cases, the development of adhesions and scar tissue in the scapulothoracic space significantly affects scapular function (7).

Table 26.1

Three layers of the scapulothoracic articulation

Structure	Superficial	Intermediate	Deep
Muscles	Latissimus dorsi	Levator scapulae	Subscapularis
	Trapezius	Rhomboid minor	Serratus anterior
		Rhomboid major	
Bursae	Inferior angle (number 1) four of eight specimens	Superomedial angle (number 2) eight of eight specimens	Serratus space (number 3) eight of eight specimens
			Subscapularis space (number 4) five of eight specimens
Nerves	—	Spinal accessory	—

Trauma, disuse, or nerve injury may lead to damage, weakness, and atrophy of the periscapular muscles (8, 9). As a result, there is often an associated decrease in the soft tissue cushion interposed between the scapula and the rib cage. The loss of soft tissue decreases the congruency of the scapulothoracic space and contributes to the development of a painful, snapping scapula. For example, the serratus anterior atrophy occurs secondary to paralysis of the long thoracic nerve. Likewise, the subscapularis atrophy occurs secondary to surgical fusion of the glenohumeral joint or from damage of motor branches to the subscapularis during open surgery. The serratus anterior and subscapularis are two of the most important muscles that prevent scapular winging and provide a mechanical cushion between the scapula and the ribs. Atrophy and loss of function of these muscles are relevant factors in the development of a snapping scapula. Furthermore, the superior angle, inferior angle, and medial border are relatively poorly cushioned compared with the rest of the scapula. As a result, these locations are common areas of increased friction that lead to symptomatic snapping. In addition, muscle

fibrosis can develop secondary to traumatic injuries and disrupt the normal motion of the scapulothoracic space. Muscle tightness (pectoralis minor and levator scapulae) may cause abnormal scapulothoracic rhythm and produce a snapping scapula.

Less common causes of a snapping scapula include infection, congenital deformity, and tumors. Infectious lesions of the ribs or scapula may develop, in rare cases, secondary to tuberculosis or syphilis (10). Sprengel's deformity is present at birth and may lead to symptomatic

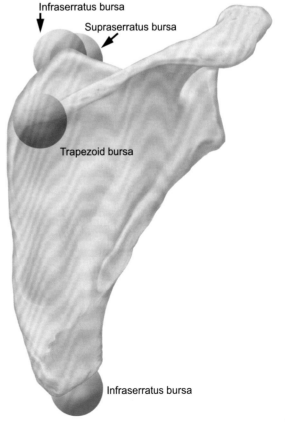

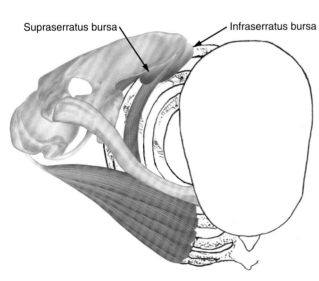

A

B

FIGURE 26.1. A, B: Anatomical bursae.

Table 26.2

Bursae around the scapula

Major/anatomical bursae
Infraserratus bursae: between the serratus anterior muscle and the chest wall
Supraserratus bursae: between the subscapularis and the serratus anterior muscles
Scapulotrapexial bursae: between the superomedial scapula and the trapezius
Minor/adventitial bursae
Superomedial angle of the scapula
Infraserratus bursae: between the serratus anterior muscle and the chest wall
Supraserratus bursae: between the subscapularis and the serratus anterior muscles
Inferior angle of the scapula
Infraserratus bursae: between the serratus anterior muscle and the chest wall
Spine of the scapula
Trapesoid bursae: between the medial spine of scapula and the trapezius

From Kuhn JE, Hawkins RJ. Evaluation and treatment of scapular disorders. In: Warner JP, Iannotti JP, Gerber C, eds. *Complex and Revision Problems in Shoulder Surgery*. Philadelphia, PA: Lippincott-Raven Publishers; 1997:357–375.

scapular motion later in life. Tumors, such as elastofibromas, may also develop in the scapulothoracic space (11, 12). In some patients, the scapulothoracic symptoms may be out of proportion to the expected level of discomfort for a snapping scapula. In these cases, secondary gain, workers' compensation issues, and psychiatric conditions should be considered as relevant factors in the development of a diagnosis and treatment plan.

Osseous Anatomy

The gliding motion of a bony prominence over the ribs provokes the sounds associated with a snapping scapula. The morphology of the superomedial border of the scapula is a common factor contributing to the development of this condition (13, 14). Several reports have described variations in this morphology ranging from a thickened bulbous corner to a hook-shaped bony prominence (7, 10, 14).

More specifically, Luschka's tubercle is a fibrocartilagenous nodule on the anterior aspect of the superomedial angle of the scapula. The prominent nature of the tubercle within the scapulothoracic space can become a significant source of pain contributing to the development of a snapping scapula. Being aware of its role in the development of a snapping scapula is essential to creating a treatment plan that addresses all sources of pain within the scapulothoracic space.

Bony prominences also develop secondary to fractures, dislocations, and tumors. Fractures of the ribs and/or scapula may heal with exuberant callus or as a malunion or nonunion that causes a painful, snapping scapula (15). An osseous tumor, such as an osteochondroma, may form on the anterior surface of the scapula and, depending on its size, become a significant irritant during scapular motion. Another source of osseous irritation in the scapulothoracic space is a bone spur that develops from the traction

Table 26.3

Etiology of the snapping Scapula

Changes in Bony Structure	Changes in Intervening Muscle	Scapulothoracic Bursae
Luschka's tubercle	Tendinitis of scapular stabilizers	Inflammation
Increased curvature superior medial angle	Anatomic muscle variations	—
Exostosis	Muscle insertion avulsions/ traction spurs	—
Rare bony tumors of ribs/scapula	—	—
Tuberculosis/syphilis	—	—
Sprengel's deformity	—	—

of muscles on the scapula during movement. This process most commonly occurs at the inferolateral portion of the scapula at the attachment site for the teres minor (13). Overall, soft tissue or bony lesions in the scapulothoracic space most commonly contribute to the development of a symptomatic snapping scapula. Scapulothoracic pain may also occur secondary to cervical spondylosis, cervical radiculopathy, glenohumeral pathology, and periscapular muscle strain. These conditions should be considered in the differential diagnosis of all patients with a snapping scapula.

CLINICAL ASSESSMENT

History

The clinical assessment of a snapping scapula consists of a thorough history, physical examination, and imaging studies. Patients with a snapping scapula frequently report a crepitant sound associated with the movement of their scapula. The crepitus may be associated with pain, but this is not always the case. Types of crepitus (froissement, frottement, and craquement) have been described and correlated with clinical patterns (Table 26.4) (16). Although the validity of this classification has not been proven, it provides a guide by which to assess crepitant sounds originating in the scapulothoracic space. Patients may have a family history of this disorder, and it may occur bilaterally (17). Asymptomatic crepitus rarely requires treatment, but the onset of symptoms requires further evaluation and management.

Physical Examination

Physical examination should begin with evaluating the patient's posture and spinal alignment. In some cases, structural spinal deformities (scoliosis and thoracic kyphosis) can contribute to the development of a snapping scapula. The periscapular muscles should be assessed for tone, atrophy, and strength (trapezius, rhomboids, serratus anterior, latissimus dorsi, levator scapulae, rotator cuff muscles, and deltoid). Patients will often experience tenderness over inflamed areas, such as the superomedial border or inferior angle of the scapula. As the arm is brought through a range of motion, crepitus and pain should be noted at specific locations. The position of the scapula on the posterior thoracic wall should be evaluated for winging. The normal ratio of glenohumeral to scapulothoracic motion is 2:1 (scapulothoracic rhythm). However, this rhythm can be disrupted by pathologic lesions and pain. Pseudo- or compensatory winging of the scapula, which develops secondary to patients avoiding painful scapulothoracic motion, should be differentiated from true scapular winging caused by muscle weakness or nerve injury. A thorough neurovascular examination will help distinguish these two conditions, but electromyogram and nerve conduction studies can be used as adjuncts to provide objective evidence of neurologic injury.

Scapulothoracic injections of local anesthetic with or without corticosteroid assist in making diagnostic conclusions and providing therapeutic pain relief (Fig. 26.2). Accurate injections into specific sites of the scapulothoracic space may confirm the diagnosis if there is significant pain relief. The addition of corticosteroid offers a longer-acting anti-inflammatory effect, which can help patients tolerate physical therapy. During these injections, care must be taken to avoid penetration into the thoracic cavity to prevent a pneumothorax.

Imaging Studies

Imaging studies of the scapulothoracic articulation include plain radiographs (tangential scapular views), computed tomography (three-dimensional reconstructions), and MRI. These studies are useful to further define specific pathology when there is a high suspicion for osseous or soft tissue lesions (18). Anteroposterior radiographs, however, do not always reveal scapulothoracic bony lesions. Therefore, oblique views of the scapula are

Table 26.4		
Chart IV scapulothoracic crepitus		
Type of Crepitus	**Sound Description**	**Clinical Presentation**
Froissement	A gentle friction sound, which may arise from normal muscular action and which may be considered physiologic	Patients usually present with no clinical symptoms or if they do they are minimal. The snapping sounds are discovered accidentally during the course of routine examinations
Frottement	A somewhat louder sound, which may be grating or snapping and indicates some underlying pathologic condition	Patients may present complaining of pain, annoying scapula sounds, or prominence of the scapula on the involved side
Craquement	A loud typically snapping sound, which is invariably of pathologic significance	Patients may present complaining of pain, annoying scapula sounds, or prominence of the scapula on the involved side

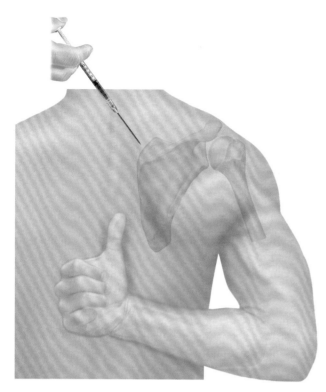

FIGURE 26.2. Patient positioning and needle placement for scapulo-thoracic injection.

recommended. In some patients, radiographs of the glenohumeral joint and cervical spine may be necessary to rule out unrelated disorders (such as glenohumeral pathology and cervical radiculopathy) that can influence the scapulothoracic motion.

TREATMENT OPTIONS

Conservative Treatment

The most successful response to nonoperative management is in patients with an identifiable soft tissue abnormality, altered posture, scapular winging, and scapulothoracic dyskinesis (19). Conservative treatment options include skillful neglect, activity modification, physiotherapy, systemic nonsteroidal anti-inflammatory medication, and corticosteroid injection into scapulothoracic bursae (8, 20, 21). Pain relief is critical to the success of nonoperative management. Nonsteroidal anti-inflammatory medications, local injections, thermal modalities, diathermy, ultrasound, and iontophoresis may be used to accomplish this goal (22). The other essential element of nonoperative care is therapy. The overall goal of therapy is a full functional recovery for the patient. The specific aims are to correct abnormal posture, to improve range of motion (scapulothoracic rhythm), to stretch tight muscles, to strengthen periscapular muscles, and to improve endurance. Strengthening the serratus anterior and subscapularis is critical in cases where atrophy and

loss of function of these muscles contributed to the development of a snapping scapula. The therapy program for a snapping scapula is reviewed in detail by other authors (19). Overall, therapy should progress from correcting posture to restoring motion and scapular strength using open and closed chain exercises. There should then be a gradual progression into functional patterns of movement (activities of daily living, occupational activities, and athletic activities). Failure to adequately train the patient in functional activities is a common reason for poor results (19).

Operative Treatment

Patients who have a nerve deficit, bony incongruity in the scapulothoracic space, or voluntarily snapping scapula are more likely to fail nonoperative management. If the nonoperative treatment program fails to relieve pain and return the patient to satisfactory function after 3 to 6 months, then surgery may be indicated and will be most successful when there is a definitive diagnosis. However, some patients, who do not respond to conservative management and have no identifiable lesion on imaging studies, can also respond favorably to arthroscopic surgery (2, 22–24). The range of surgical options includes open (7, 10, 23, 25–28) and arthroscopic (2, 23, 24, 29, 30) procedures for the resection of soft tissue (21, 22, 24, 25, 31) and/or bony lesions (2, 9, 23, 27, 28, 31, 32). A combined open and arthroscopic approach may be the most effective technique (6).

Essential to performing a successful open or arthroscopic procedure is understanding the periscapular anatomy. Previous authors have reviewed this anatomy in detail (5). For open procedures, it is useful to understand the periscapular area in terms of three layers (Fig. 26.3A–F) (5). In open procedures, the incision is made along the medial border of the scapula. Determining where to make the incision is based on the location of the pathologic lesion. For example, at the superomedial aspect of the scapula after subperiosteal dissection of the serratus anterior (anterior surface) and the levator scapular (posterior surface) muscles off of the superomedial angle of the scapula, the prominent tubercle can be removed. Once the pathologic tissue is resected, the periscapular muscles are repaired back to the medial border of the scapula through drill holes. The skin may be closed over a drain, but this is usually determined based on surgeon preference. Open procedures that involve repair of the periscapular muscles require immobilization during the postoperative period. Rehabilitation focuses first on restoring range of motion; strengthening begins in the subsequent 8 to 12 weeks (31).

Recently, arthroscopic procedures have been advocated as an alternative to open techniques. Proponents of scapulothoracic arthroscopy suggest that it minimizes the morbidity associated with open dissection and that it allows for earlier rehabilitation and return to improved function (2, 22, 23, 33, 34). The disadvantages are the technical difficulty, limited visualization of the superior

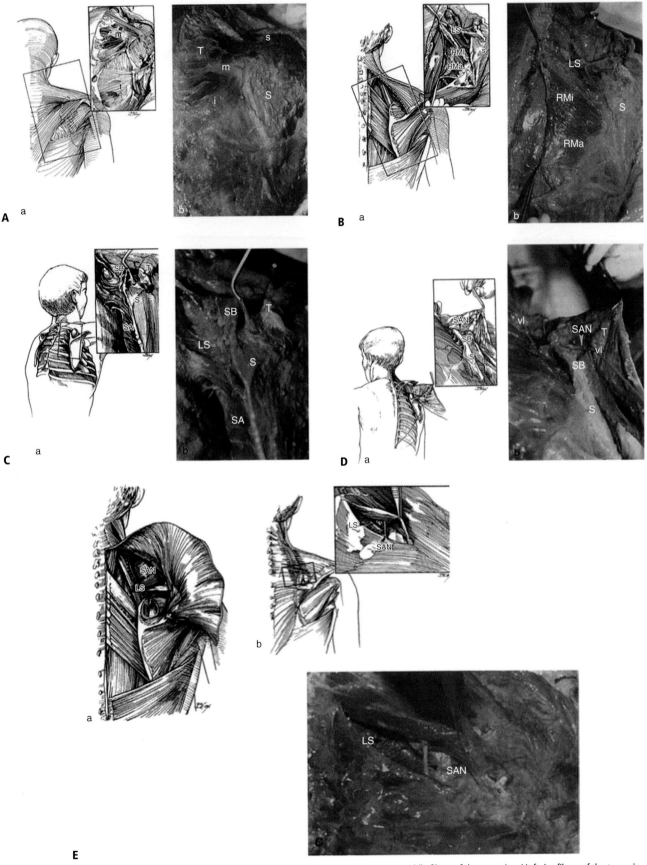

FIGURES 26.3. A-F: Three layers of periscapular anatomy. **A:** T trapezius, L latissimus dorsi, m middle fibers of the trapezius, i inferior fibers of the trapezius, S scapula **B:** LS, levator scapulae; RMi, rhomboid minor; RMa, rhomboid major; T, trapezius; S, scapula. **C:** SB, scapulotrapezial bursa; T, trapezius; S, scapula; LS, levator scapula; SA, serratus anterior. **D:** SAN, spinal accessory nerve; T, trapezius; SB, scapulotrapezial bursa; S, scapular spine; vl vessel loops. **E:** SAN, spinal accessory nerve; LS, levator scapulae. **F:** SA, serratus anterior; S, medial scapular border; STB, scapulothoracic bursa; SSB, subscapularis bursa. (From Williams GR Jr, Shakil M, Klimkiewicz J, et al. Anatomy of the scapulothoracic articulation. *Clin Orthop Relat Res.* 1999;(359):237–246, with permission.)

313

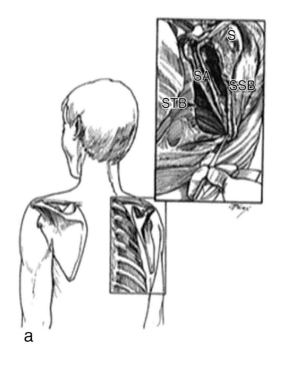

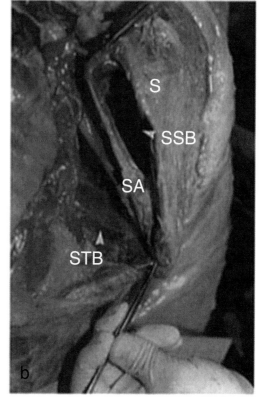

F
FIGURES 26.3. (continued)

angle and superomedial border of the scapula (35), and the risk of missing pathologic tissue (25). Furthermore, arthroscopic procedures do not allow for the reattachment of the complex insertion of the levator scapulae and serratus anterior after resection of the superomedial angle of the scapula (5).

Surgical Anatomy

The important anatomic factors relevant to a scapulothoracic arthroscopy have been reviewed by other authors (29). The principles of the procedure will be reviewed here. The arthroscopic tower (monitor and pump) is placed on the patient's operative side. The surgeon stands on the side of the table opposite to the patient's operative side. Arthroscopic surgery on the scapulothoracic space is best done with the patient in the prone position. Attention should be directed to proper positioning of the head and extremity in order to protect neurovascular structures from excessive compression during the procedure. The operative arm is placed in a "chicken-wing" position with the arm placed behind the back in extension and internal rotation (Fig. 26.4). This position lifts the medial border of the scapula off of the posterior thorax and facilitates access into the scapulothoracic space.

Two consistent spaces exist between the scapula and the posterior thoracic wall that can be used for portals. One of the spaces is between the ribs and the serratus anterior, and the other one is between the serratus anterior and the subscapularis (5, 29). In general, portal placement

is recommended at or below the scapular spine to avoid injury to the spinal accessory and dorsal scapular neurovascular bundle.

Standard arthroscopic portals are used to begin the procedure. The initial "safe" portal is placed 2 cm medial to

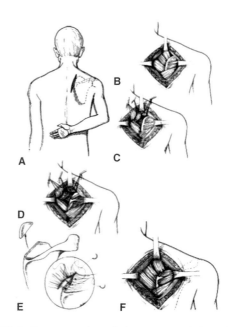

FIGURE 26.4. Open resection of the superomedial angle of the scapula.

the medial scapular edge at the level of the scapular spine. This location is between the serratus anterior and the posterior thoracic wall. The dorsal scapular nerve and artery run along the medial border of the scapula. The more medial position of the "safe" portal helps avoid injury to these structures. The subserratus space is localized with a spinal needle and distended with 30 cc of saline. The arthroscope is inserted and arthroscopic fluid distends the space. Fluid extravasation should be minimized by keeping the arthroscopy pump pressure low (30 mm Hg). A second "working" portal is then established using a spinal needle. The working portal is established 4 cm inferior to and in-line with the first portal. A 6-mm cannula may be used in the "working portal." A motorized shaver and bipolar radiofrequency device are used to remove bursal tissue. Because there are few landmarks to help orient the arthroscopist, a methodical approach is essential to performing an adequate decompression of the scapulothoracic space. A 70° arthroscope should be available in case improved visualization is needed during the procedure. Spinal needles and a probe should be used throughout the procedure to orient the surgeon to the thoracic cage and to the borders of the scapula. Care should be taken not to penetrate the posterior thoracic wall as instruments are passed into the scapulothoracic space. Puncturing the posterior thoracic wall can result in pneumothorax and injury to the lung.

A superior portal above the spine of the scapula may be required in order to remove pathologic bone and/or bursae. Portals in this area place the dorsal scapular neurovascular structures, accessory spinal nerve, suprascapular nerve, and transverse scapular artery at risk. With correct placement of the portals, the mean distance to the accessory spinal nerve beneath the trapezius is approximately 35 mm (35). The position for the superior portal is marked out at the junction between the medial and the middle thirds of the line between the superomedial angle of the scapula and the lateral border of the acromion (Fig. 26.5) (23).

A safe zone exists for arthroscopic resection of the superomedial scapular border (Fig. 26.6A,B) (36). This portal is a minimum distance of 12 mm from the suprascapular nerve (35). Even though 12 mm may be a safe distance for establishing the portal, it may be inadequate when operating the shaver or burr with suction. The zone of resection is situated equidistant between the inferior scapular angle and the scapular spine or more lateral to the inferior angle of the scapula (36). During scapulothoracic arthroscopy,

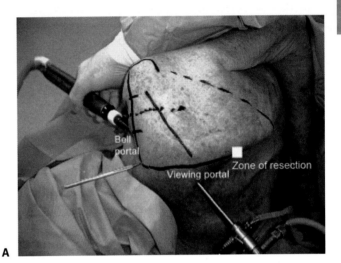

A

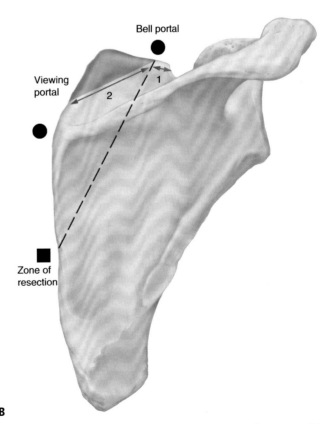

B

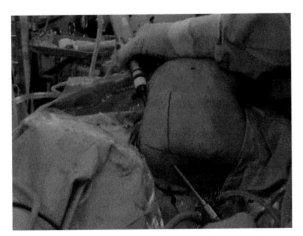

FIGURE 26.5. Superomedial portal viewing portal is used to place the arthroscope into the space of this right scapula. The superior "Bell portal" shows an inserted shaver

FIGURE 26.6. A, B: The safe zone for resection of superomedial scapular is outlined on this right scapula.

the burr or shaver should be directed toward the zone of resection landmark to maintain a minimum distance of 25 mm between the resected bony edge and the suprascapular nerve (36). Overall, soft tissue resection should not be performed beyond the medial border of the scapula in order to avoid neurovascular injury. Swelling from arthroscopic fluid may make it difficult to completely define the superior border of the scapula. In these cases, a small incision can be made to resect the superomedial border of the scapula (6, 30). After the arthroscopic procedure, patients are placed in a simple sling for comfort only. Gentle passive range of motion is started immediately to avoid stiffness. At 4 weeks, active-assisted range of motion begins with isometric exercises. At 8 weeks after the surgery, strengthening of the periscapular muscles begins. Complications of scapulothoracic arthroscopy include failure to resect all pathologic tissue, pneumothorax, and neurovascular injury.

AUTHORS' PREFERRED TREATMENT

A thorough clinical assessment helps to determine the definitive diagnosis. For patients with soft tissue lesions or without a definable lesion in the scapulothoracic space, nonoperative management should be used for a period of 3 to 6 months. Both asymptomatic and symptomatic snapping scapulas should be treated in this manner. Patients who do not respond to conservative management become candidates for surgery. At the initial evaluation, some patients may have a definitive lesion (soft tissue or bony) that would prevent nonoperative management from being successful. For example, a large osteochondroma on the anterior surface of the scapula would most likely not respond well to nonoperative treatment modalities. In these cases, surgical intervention may be the first line of treatment. Several factors determine whether the surgery should be performed as an open or arthroscopic procedure. The size, location, and composition of the lesion as well as the skill of the surgeon are primary factors that determine how pathologic lesions should be removed from the scapulothoracic space. Larger (greater than 1 cm) osseous lesions and unfamiliarity with scapulothoracic arthroscopic surgery would favor an open procedure. However, for soft tissue lesions, such as chronically inflamed bursae, arthroscopic surgery is a reasonable choice provided that the surgeon is comfortable with the anatomy and skills required to perform the procedure. In some cases, a combination of open and arthroscopic procedures may be the best option. Overall, treatment plans should be individualized to the patient depending on the pathologic lesion, response to nonoperative treatment, and level of surgical skill.

CONCLUSION

The snapping scapula is a diagnostic and therapeutic challenge. In most cases, patients are responsive to nonoperative care. However, some patients require operative treatment to alleviate symptoms and to restore congruity to the scapulothoracic space. Historically, open procedures have been the gold standard for treating patients who do not respond favorably to nonoperative management. The evolution of arthroscopy has allowed surgeons to address pathologic lesions in the scapulothoracic space with less invasive procedures. With either approach, an understanding of the periscapular anatomy is essential to avoid neurovascular injury, to completely remove the pathologic lesion, and to achieve a successful outcome for the patient.

REFERENCES

1. Boinet W. Snapping scapulae. *Bulletin de la Societe Imperiale de Chirurgie de Paris*, 2nd Series. Vol 8. 1867: 458.
2. Harper GD, McIlroy S, Bayley JI, et al. Arthroscopic partial resection of the scapula for snapping scapula: a new technique. *J Shoulder Elbow Surg*. 1999;8:53–57.
3. Kapandji I. *The Physiology of Joints*. Vol 1. 5th ed. London, England: Churchill Livingstone; 1982.
4. Johnston T. The movements of the shoulder joint: a plea for the use of the plane of the scapula as the plane of reference in movements occurring at the humero-scapular joint. Br J Surg. 1937;(25):252.
5. Williams GR Jr, Shakil M, Klimkiewicz J, et al. Anatomy of the scapulothoracic articulation. *Clin Orthop Relat Res*. 1999; 359:237–246.
6. Lehtinen JT, Macy JC, Cassinelli E, et al. The painful scapulothoracic articulation. *Clin Orthop Relat Res*. 2004;(423):99–105.
7. Milch H. Partial scapulectomy for snapping of the scapula. *J Bone Joint Surg Am*. 1950;32:561–566.
8. Percy EC, Birbrager D, Pitt MJ. Snapping scapula: a review of the literature and presentation of 14 patients. *Can J Surg*. 1988;31:248–250.
9. Strizak AM, Cowen MH. The snapping scapula syndrome. A case report. *J Bone Joint Surg Am*. 1982;64(6):941–942.
10. Milch H. Snapping scapula. *Clin Orthop*. 1961;20:139–150.
11. Kuhn JE, Plancher KD, Hawkins RJ. Symptomatic scapulothoracic crepitus and bursitis. *J Am Acad Orthop Surg*. 1998;6:267–273.
12. Haney TC. Subscapular elastofibroma in a young pitcher. A case report. *Am J Sports Med*. 1990;18(6):642–644.
13. Edelson JG. Variations in the anatomy of the scapula with reference to the snapping scapula. *Clin Orthop Relat Res*. 1996;(322):111–115.
14. Avlik I. Snapping scapula and Sprengel's deformity. *Acta Orthop Scand*. 1959;(29):10–15.
15. Takahara K, Uchiyama S, Nakagawa H, et al. Snapping scapula syndrome due to malunion of rib fractures: a case report. *J Shoulder Elbow Surg*. 2004;13:95–98.
16. Mauclaire M. Craquements sous-scapulares pathologiques traits par l'interposition musculaire interscapulo-thoracique. *Bull et Mem Soc Chir*. 1904;(30):164–169.
17. Cobey MC. The rolling scapula. *Clin Orthop Relat Res*. 1968;60:193–194.
18. Mozes G, Bickels J, Ovadia D, et al. The use of three-dimensional computed tomography in evaluating snapping scapula syndrome. *Orthopedics*. 1999;22:1029–1033.

19. Manske RC, Reiman MP, Stovak ML. Nonoperative and operative management of snapping scapula. *Am J Sports Med.* 2004;32:1554–1565.

20. Cameron HU. Snapping scapulae: a report of three cases. *Eur J Rheumatol Inflamm.* 1984;7:66–67.

21. Sisto DJ, Jobe FW. The operative treatment of scapulothoracic bursitis in professional pitchers. *Am J Sports Med.* 1986;14:192–194.

22. Ciullo JV, Jones E. Subscapular bursitis: conservative and endoscopic treatment of snapping scapula or washboard syndrome. *Orthop Trans.* 1993;(60):193.

23. Pavlik A, Ang K, Coghlan J, et al. Arthroscopic treatment of painful snapping of the scapula by using a new superior portal. *Arthroscopy.* 2003;19:608–612.

24. Pearse EO, Bruguera J, Massoud SN, et al. Arthroscopic management of the painful snapping scapula. *Arthroscopy.* 2006;22:755–761.

25. Nicholson GP, Duckworth MA. Scapulothoracic bursectomy for snapping scapula syndrome. *J Shoulder Elbow Surg.* 2002;11:80–85.

26. Parsons TA. The snapping scapula and subscapular exostoses. *J Bone Joint Surg Br.* 1973;55:345–349.

27. Wood VE, Verska JM. The snapping scapula in association with the thoracic outlet syndrome. *Arch Surg.* 1989;124:1335–1337.

28. Chan BK, Chakrabarti AJ, Bell SN. An alternative portal for scapulothoracic arthroscopy. *J Shoulder Elbow Surg.* 2002;11:235–238.

29. Ruland LJ III, Ruland CM, Matthews LS. Scapulothoracic anatomy for the arthroscopist. *Arthroscopy.* 1995;11:52–56.

30. Lien SB, Shen PH, Lee CH, et al. The effect of endoscopic bursectomy with mini-open partial scapulectomy on snapping scapula syndrome. *J Surg Res.* 2008;150:236–242.

31. McClusky GM, Bigliani L. Partial scapulectomy for disabling scapulothoracic snapping. *Orthop Trans.* 1990;(14):252–253.

32. Richards RR, McKee MD. Treatment of painful scapulothoracic crepitus by resection of the superomedial angle of the scapula. A report of three cases. *Clin Orthop Relat Res.* 1989;(247):111–116.

33. Matthews L, Poehling G, Hunter D. *Operative Arthroscopy.* 2nd ed. Philadelphia, PA: Lippencott-Raven; 1996.

34. Bizousky DT, Gillogly S. Evaluation of the scapulothoracic articulation with arthroscopy. *Orthop Trans.* 1992;16:822.

35. Chan BK, Chakrabarti AJ, Bell SN. An alternative portal for scapulothoracic arthroscopy. *J Shoulder Elbow Surg.* 2002;11:235–238.

36. Bell S, van Riet RP. Safe zone for arthroscopic resection of the superomedial scapular border in the treatment of snapping scapula syndrome. *J Shoulder Elbow Surg.* 2008;17:647–649.

Arthroscopic Suprascapular Nerve Release

F. Alan Barber • James A. Bynum

Suprascapular nerve disorders are an often overlooked source of shoulder pain and dysfunction and are estimated to comprise 1% to 2% of all shoulder complaints (1). Since Thompson and Kopell (2) first described this condition in 1959, many authors have sought to characterize the diagnosis and treatment of suprascapular nerve entrapment. Based upon a greater appreciation of this pathology, effective treatments have been described, providing symptomatic relief and the return of function.

ANATOMY

The suprascapular nerve is a peripheral sensory motor nerve arising from the upper brachial plexus that receives contributions from the fifth, sixth, and, occasionally, fourth cervical nerve roots (3). It provides motor innervation to the supraspinatus and infraspinatus muscles as well as sensory innervation around the shoulder (4). From its origin in the superior trunk of the brachial plexus, the nerve passes through the posterior cervical triangle and arises deep to the trapezius and omohyoid muscles where it then follows the suprascapular artery to enter the suprascapular notch. While the artery passes over the transverse scapular ligament (TSL), the nerve passes beneath it before entering the supraspinatus fossa (Fig. 27.1). A superior articular branch arises from the main trunk of the nerve at or near the ligament and travels with the main nerve through the notch. This branch supplies sensory innervation to the coracoclavicular and coracohumeral ligaments, the acromioclavicular joint, and the subacromial bursa. Within 1 cm of passing through the notch, two motor branches arise, which terminate in the supraspinatus muscle. The main nerve then courses inferiorly through the spinoglenoid notch, giving rise to yet another small sensory branch that innervates the posterior glenohumeral joint capsule. The remaining nerve enters the infraspinatus fossa, terminating as multiple motor branches to the infraspinatus muscle (4).

There are two locations of suprascapular nerve entrapment (the suprascapular notch and the spinoglenoid notch). Six types of supra scapula notches have been described (5). The most common types are a wide, a shallow

"v"- (type II, 31%), and a "u"-shaped notch (type III, 48%) (Fig. 27.2). Although it has been suggested that entrapment may be associated with a calcified, bifid, trifid, or hypertrophied TSL, no studies have linked nerve entrapment to scapular notch morphology.

In contrast, the spinoglenoid notch is a fibro-osseous tunnel composed of the spinoglenoid ligament and the spine of the scapula. Cadaveric studies have placed the actual occurrence of a spinoglenoid ligament to range from 3% to 80%, but Plancher et al. (6) attributed this variation to be due to errors in specimen preparation and reported the spinoglenoid ligament to be a distinct anatomic structure present in 100% of specimens. This ligament originates from the lateral aspect of the scapular spine and the deep fibers insert distally into the posterior aspect of the glenoid neck, whereas the superficial fibers insert into the posterior glenohumeral joint capsule (Fig. 27.1).

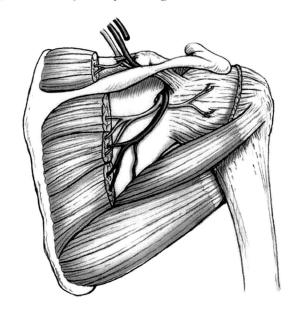

FIGURE 27.1. After passing under the TSL, the suprascapular nerve gives off motor branches to the supraspinatus muscle before passing around the spinoglenoid notch. (From Iannotti JP, Williams GR. *Disorders of the Shoulder: Diagnosis and Management.* Philadelphia, PA: Lippincott Williams & Wilkins; 2007, with permission.)

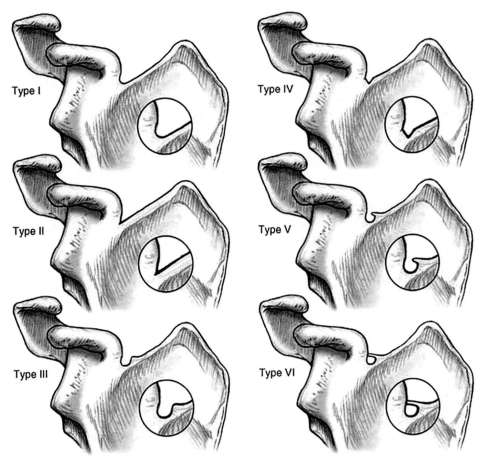

FIGURE 27.2. Six morphologic types of suprascapular notches described by Rengachary. (From Iannotti JP, Williams GR. *Disorders of the Shoulder: Diagnosis and Management.* 2nd ed. Philadelphia, PA: Lippincott Williams & Wilkins; 2007, with permission.)

PATHOPHYSIOLOGY

The suprascapular nerve, like all peripheral nerves, is susceptible to injury from compression or stretching, resulting in nerve ischemia, edema, and decreased conduction. Previous animal studies have shown that as little as 6% increase in length causes conduction abnormalities, and 15% or more may cause irreversible damage.

Normal shoulder girdle motion does not result in a translational motion of the suprascapular nerve through the suprascapular notch and thus frictional injury does not appear to contribute to nerve damage (5). However, the nerve pass through a sharp turn around the TSL while passing through the notch, making it susceptible to compression against the sharp, inferior margin of the ligament. The term "sling effect" describes this potential source of nerve injury (5), which can be exacerbated by shoulder depression, retraction, or hyperabduction. This mechanism is often associated with overuse or athletic injuries and is thought to be the most common cause of suprascapular nerve impingement at the suprascapular notch.

Direct traumatic injury to the nerve is not common due to its relatively protected position underneath the trapezius muscle. Injury from scapular or clavicle fracture,

shoulder dislocation, or penetrating trauma has been reported. Iatrogenic injury from procedures such as distal clavicle excision greater than 1.5 cm has also been reported. A cadaveric study by Warner et al. (7) suggested that a nerve traction injury may occur in massive rotator cuff repairs when the supraspinatus or infraspinatus tendons are mobilized more than 3 cm, but no clinical studies have demonstrated nerve damage from this mechanism.

Distal suprascapular nerve injury at the spinoglenoid notch is often the result of direct compression from a mass, most commonly a ganglion cyst (Fig. 27.5A, B), or from repetitive overhead or throwing activity. Injury at this level spares the supraspinatus muscle, but affects conduction to the infraspinatus. Ganglion cysts near the spinoglenoid notch result from synovial fluid extravasating into the tissues through a posterior capsulolabral tear, creating a one-way valve effect. At this location, the sensory fibers have already branched and the nerve is mainly a motor nerve. Consequently, posterior shoulder pain often associated with these lesions may be a result of the posterior labral tear itself. Other reported but rare causes of compression include synovial sarcoma, Ewing's sarcoma, chondrosarcoma, renal cell carcinoma, and schwannoma.

In addition to compression, nerve injury at this level can occur secondary to repetitive overuse such as that seen with overhead-throwing athletes. Plancher et al. (8) conducted a cadaveric study involving pressure measurements in the spinoglenoid notch, as the shoulder was taken through the six phases of the throwing motion. The spinoglenoid ligament insertion on the posterior capsule made the ligament susceptible to the same dynamic forces that act on the posterior capsule itself during the throwing motion. The pressure measurements within the spinoglenoid notch increased during every phase of the throwing cycle, peaking at the follow-through phase with shoulder adduction and internal rotation (8). This explains why atrophy and electromyographic changes in the infraspinatus muscle are often observed in pitchers and in the dominant arm of competitive volleyball players. A subsequent release of the spinoglenoid ligament resulted in relief of the high pressure readings throughout the entire throwing cycle (8). Another theory of distal nerve injury in overhead athletes involves repetitive microtrauma to the intimal lining of the suprascapular artery, ultimately leading to microemboli to the *vaso vasorum* of the suprascapular nerve and nerve injury (9). However, the clinical data to support this is currently insufficient.

CLINICAL EVALUATION

History

Patients with suprascapular nerve entrapment are typically between 20 and 50 years of age and commonly have deep, aching posterior and lateral shoulder pain in their dominant arm. While occasionally associated with trauma, the usual onset is insidious and often exacerbated by overhead activity. Weakness in external rotation or abduction may be reported. Isolated infraspinatus weakness without significant pain is not uncommon with distal spinoglenoid notch lesions since most sensory fibers branch more proximally. Alternate diagnoses to consider include cervical radiculopathy, brachioplexopathies, rotator cuff pathology, and other glenohumeral joint pathology.

Physical Exam

Proximal lesions at the suprascapular notch result in atrophy of both the supraspinatus and the infraspinatus muscles. Tenderness at the notch, located posterior to the clavicle in the trapezius muscle belly overlying the scapular spine can often be elicited. Weakness in external rotation and abduction compared with the uninvolved side is not uncommon. Distal suprascapular nerve compression at the spinoglenoid notch results in isolated atrophy of the infraspinatus muscle (Fig. 27.4). Posterior shoulder tenderness overlying the spinoglenoid notch and isolated weakness in external rotation may be present.

Diagnostic Studies

Plain cervical or glenohumeral radiographs are usually normal but should be obtained to rule out other causes of shoulder pain. Magnetic resonance imaging is useful in diagnosing these lesions and may show fatty infiltration and atrophy of the supraspinatus and infraspinatus muscles resulting from muscle denervation. Posterior ganglion cysts arising from the glenohumeral joint are also readily apparent on MRI, appearing as a high-intensity signal on T2 images and low on T1 images (Fig. 27.5). The MRI alone is less sensitive in detecting associated posterior capsulolabral tears, but with the use of MR arthrography sensitivities of 91% and specificities of 93% have been achieved for these labral tears. Electromyographic studies can help determine the location of the nerve entrapment by distinguishing between combined supraspinatus and infraspinatus and isolated infraspinatus changes. Fibrillations and positive sharp waves may be observed as early as 3 weeks after injury.

TREATMENT

Nonoperative

The initial treatment for all suprascapular nerve injuries is nonoperative. This should include 4 to 6 weeks of anti-inflammatory medication, avoidance of repetitive overhead activity, and a physical therapy program involving scapular stabilizer and rotator cuff strengthening exercises. Even ganglion cysts of the spinoglenoid notch may resolve spontaneously; however, these patients should be closely monitored in the event that their symptoms worsen. Operative treatment is indicated for those who fail nonoperative treatment or those with electrodiagnostically proven nerve compression. Nerve decompression is associated with high rates of pain relief, but recovery of muscle atrophy is less predictable.

Operative Treatment: Open Ligament Release

Open approaches for TSL and spinoglenoid ligament releases have been described in the literature and can be performed through a single skin incision using a posterior or superior approach. To do this, the operative extremity is draped free with the patient in the semi-prone position. The superior trapezius-splitting approach involves a skin incision 2 cm medial to the medial border of the acromion parallel to Langer's lines (Fig. 27.6). The overlying trapezius muscle is then split in line with its fibers. The supraspinatus muscle is bluntly retracted inferiorly, exposing the suprascapular notch and the TSL. Careful isolation of the overlying artery and underlying nerve is required to provide clear visualization before the ligament is sharply released.

Originally described by Post and Mayer (10), the posterior approach involves a skin incision over the scapular spine, detaching the trapezius muscle from the spine of the scapula, and opening the space overlying the suprascapular ligament (Fig. 27.3). The trapezius muscle is retracted superiorly. The supraspinatus muscle is carefully retracted inferiorly, exposing the suprascapular notch and allowing release of the suprascapular ligament under direct visualization.

A similar posterior incision may be utilized for release of the spinoglenoid ligament and decompression of any spinoglenoid ganglion cyst present. Starting 3 cm medial to the posterolateral corner of the acromion, a skin incision is made along the scapular spine. The deltoid muscle is then split in line with its fibers to expose the infraspinatus muscle. Retracting the infraspinatus muscle inferiorly exposes the spinoglenoid notch, allowing removal of any underlying ganglion cyst and release of the spinoglenoid ligament. A burr may be used to deepen the notch if necessary, but the resection should be limited to less than 1 cm to avoid scapular spine fracture.

ARTHROSCOPIC TRANSVERSE SUPRASCAPULAR LIGAMENT RELEASE

Multiple arthroscopic techniques have been described to address nerve compression at the suprascapular (11, 12) and

spinoglenoid notches (8). Proponents of these techniques report superior visualization of the neurovascular structures, more precise dissection due to arthroscopic magnification, and decreased postoperative pain since there is less dissection and the trapezius muscle attachment is left intact.

Arthroscopic TSL release may be performed in the lateral decubitus or beach chair positions, utilizing the standard posterior "soft spot," lateral subacromial, and anterolateral portals with an additional "SSN" portal placed directly over the suprascapular notch (Fig. 27.7). A complete subacromial decompression is initially performed with special attention to removing the anteromedial bursa. Continuing the dissection of the fibrofatty tissue medial and posterior to the distal clavicle allows visualization of the posterior aspect of the coracoclavicular ligaments, which are seen coursing inferiorly, 90° to the clavicle.

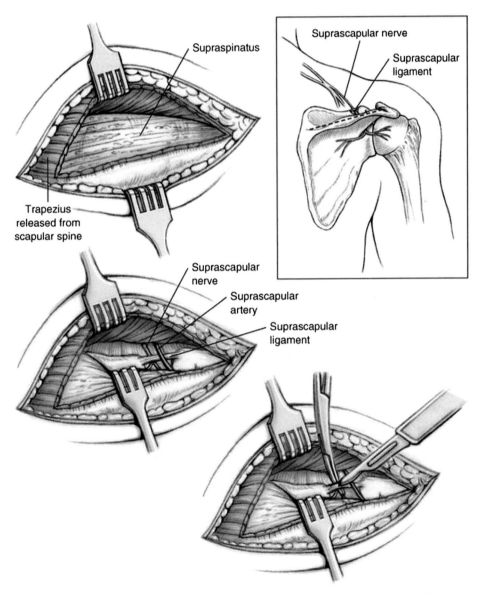

FIGURE 27.3. The posterior surgical approach to the suprascapular notch. (From Iannotti JP, Williams GR. *Disorders of the Shoulder: Diagnosis and Management.* 2nd ed. Philadelphia, PA: Lippincott Williams & Wilkins; 2007, with permission.)

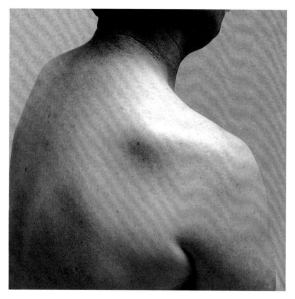

FIGURE 27.4. Distal suprascapular nerve compression at the spinoglenoid notch results in isolated atrophy of the infraspinatus muscle. (Photo copyright by F. Alan Barber, MD.)

They may also be localized by following the coracoacromial ligament to its insertion on the coracoid. The supraspinatus muscle belly is "retracted" by use of the shaver in the lateral portal to depress it away from the coracoclavicular ligaments, allowing the medial border of the conoid ligament to be defined (Fig. 27.8). The medial aspect of the conoid ligament insertion into the coracoid base is visualized, and these fibers are confluent with the lateral insertion of the TSL. The TSL can then be seen coursing horizontally across the field of view in a medial direction over the scapular notch (Fig. 27.9).

The superior and inferior edges of the ligament are then defined by gently dissecting the fibrofatty tissue above and below the ligament with a probe or blunt obturator to avoid damaging the suprascapular artery and nerve. Extensive dissection and visualization of the nerve itself is not necessary and may actually result in injury. Once the entire ligament is well visualized, the SSN portal is localized by placing an 18G spinal needle through the skin between the clavicle and the spine of the scapular directly over notch, approximately 7 cm medial to the lateral border of the acromion or 2 cm medial to the Neviaser portal. The needle tip should enter the field of view immediately above the TSL, just anterior to the supraspinatus muscle belly. A small skin incision is made and soft tissue dissection down to the ligament is performed with a blunt obturator (Fig. 27.7).

Basket forceps or up-cutting scissors may then be inserted through this incision or through an accessory portal placed 1.5 cm medial or lateral to it (Fig. 27.10). The ligament should be incised with caution to avoid damage to the neurovascular structures (Fig. 27.11). Adequate release is confirmed by manipulation with a probe of the two cut ends of the TSL. In the presence of a partially ossified ligament, a small burr may be required to perform a notchplasty (Fig. 27.12).

AUTHORS' PREFERRED TECHNIQUE: PERCUTANEOUS TRANSVERSE SUPRASCAPULAR LIGAMENT RELEASE

The previously described procedure for visualizing the TSL is performed. Instead of using an 18G spinal needle for localization of the SSN portal, a 14G beveled

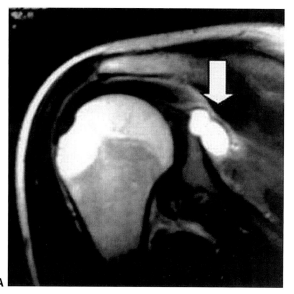

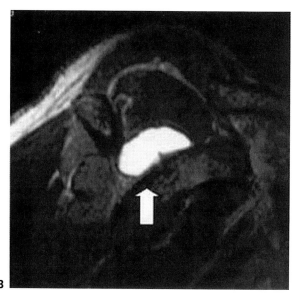

A   B

FIGURE 27.5. Magnetic resonance imaging of a ganglion cyst. Coronal **(A)** and sagittal **(B)** views of the cyst, which can cause compression of the suprascapular nerve at the spinoglenoid notch. (From Iannotti JP, Williams GR. *Disorders of the Shoulder: Diagnosis and Management.* 2nd ed. Philadelphia, PA: Lippincott Williams & Wilkins; 2007, with permission.)

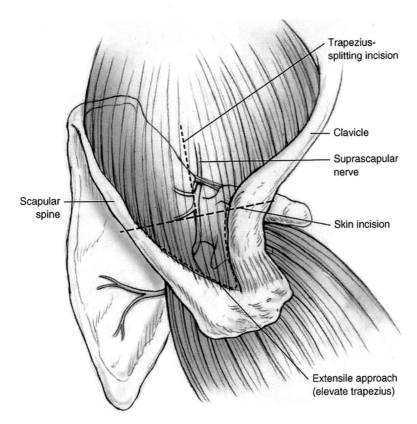

FIGURE 27.6. The superior trapezius-splitting approach to the suprascapular notch. (From Iannotti JP, Williams GR. *Disorders of the Shoulder: Diagnosis and Management.* 2nd ed. Philadelphia, PA: Lippincott Williams & Wilkins; 2007, with permission.)

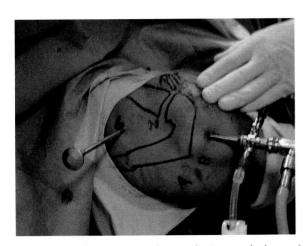

FIGURE 27.7. Arthroscopic TSL release utilizes a standard posterior, lateral subacromial, and anterolateral portals with an additional suprascapular nerve portal placed directly over the suprascapular notch. (From Lafosse L, Tomasi A. Technique for endoscopic release of suprascapular nerve entrapment at the suprascapular notch. *Tech Shoulder Elbow Surg.* 2006;7:1–6, with permission.)

needle (taken from an intracath) measuring at least 10-cm long is inserted through the skin (Fig. 27.8). The tip of the needle is visualized as it enters the field of view immediately above the TSL, just anterior to the supraspinatus muscle belly. The tip of this needle is positioned immediately above the TSL attachment to the conoid ligament and used to incise the ligament with a gentle anterior to posterior sweeping motion (Fig. 27.13). The ligament is usually less than 5-mm thick, so overpenetration and of the needle tip and potential nerve injury should be avoided by grasping the needle immediately adjacent to the skin to facilitate a smooth sweeping motion. Once the TSL is divided, complete separation of the two ends can be confirmed using the shaver blade previously used to retract the supraspinatus muscle belly (Fig. 27.14). This technique avoids an additional portal, is technically simple, and results in shorter operative times. This technique is of limited value in the treatment of an ossified ligament and an actual portal may be required to allow the use of a burr.

TREATMENT OF DISTAL SUPRASCAPULAR NERVE COMPRESSION SECONDARY TO A GANGLION CYST

Suprascapular nerve compression secondary to an MRI confirmed ganglion cyst requires decompression of the cyst and careful attention to any intra-articular pathology to prevent recurrence. A thorough diagnostic arthroscopy of the glenohumeral joint is initially performed to identify the posterior capsulolabral tearing, which is almost

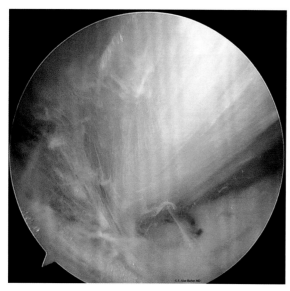

FIGURE 27.8. The supraspinatus muscle belly is depressed by a shaver from the lateral portal to demonstrate the coracoclavicular ligaments. The conoid ligament is demonstrated here. (Photo copyright by F. Alan Barber, MD.)

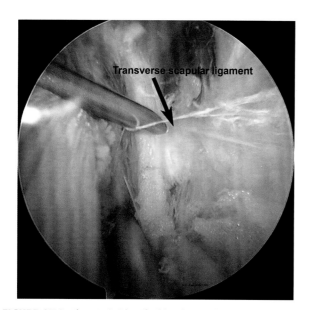

FIGURE 27.9. The TSL is identified by the needle pointing to it as it courses horizontally across the field of view from the conoid ligament (on the *right*). A shaver blade (in the *foreground*) is depressing the supraspinatus muscle for better visualization. The suprascapular artery passes over the TSL. (Photo copyright by F. Alan Barber, MD.)

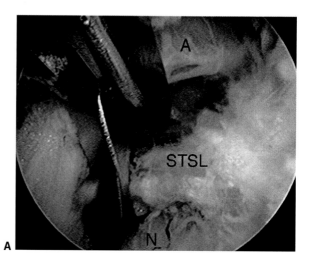

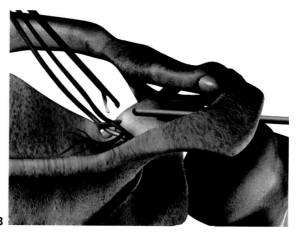

FIGURE 27.10. A, B: A basket forceps or arthroscopic scissors is then inserted through the suprascapular nerve portal or an accessory portal placed 1.5 cm medial or lateral to it. (From Lafosse L, Tomasi A. Technique for endoscopic release of suprascapular nerve entrapment at the suprascapular notch. *Tech Shoulder Elbow Surg.* 2006;7:1–6, with permission.)

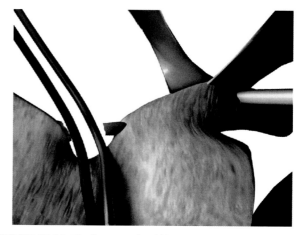

FIGURE 27.11. The ligament should be incised with caution to avoid damage to the neurovascular structures. (From Lafosse L, Tomasi A. Technique for endoscopic release of suprascapular nerve entrapment at the suprascapular notch. *Tech Shoulder Elbow Surg.* 2006;7:1–6, with permission.)

always present. The tearing may be obscured by a thin synovial membrane, but gentle manipulation with a probe will often expose the lesion. A motorized shaver is then inserted into the tear, which communicates with the cyst. It is not unusual to see amber-colored, gelatinous fluid from the cyst extravasate into the joint. The shaver is then used to decompress the cyst and debride the lining. Care is taken not to insert the shaver more than 1 cm medial to the posterior glenoid labrum to avoid injury to the distal

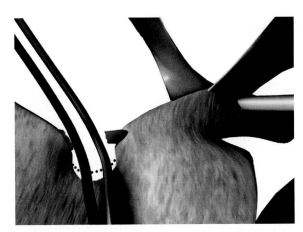

FIGURE 27.12. In the presence of a partially ossified ligament, a small burr may be required to perform a notchplasty. (From Lafosse L, Tomasi A. Technique for endoscopic release of suprascapular nerve entrapment at the suprascapular notch. *Tech Shoulder Elbow Surg.* 2006;7:1–6, with permission.)

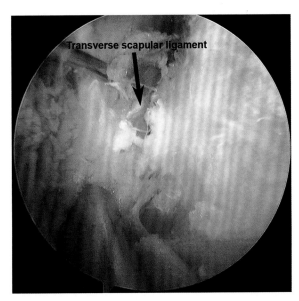

FIGURE 27.13. A 14G needle is utilized to divide the TSL. (Photo copyright by F. Alan Barber, MD.)

suprascapular nerve, which has been found in anatomical studies to lie approximately 2 cm medial to the labrum. The capsulolabral tear is then repaired using suture anchors in the standard technique. A report of 42 patients with symptomatic spinoglenoid ganglion cysts treated with labral repair alone described complete cyst resolution in 88% of the patients (13). Good or excellent results were reported in 40 of 42 patients.

ENDOSCOPIC SPINOGLENOID LIGAMENT RELEASE

Plancher et al. (8) described an endoscopic technique for release of the spinoglenoid ligament. Two portals are made 1 to 2 cm inferior to the scapular spine. A lateral portal is placed 4 cm medial to the posterolateral tip of the

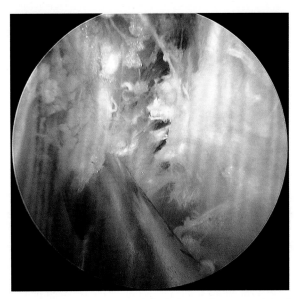

FIGURE 27.14. Once the TSL is divided, complete separation of the two ends can be confirmed by probing with the shaver blade previously used to retract the supraspinatus muscle belly. (Photo copyright by F. Alan Barber, MD.)

acromion and a second, more medial portal placed 4 cm medial to the first portal (Fig. 27.15). Two blunt trochars are then inserted along the inferior aspect of the scapular spine being careful to stay against the bone of the scapula.

A working space is blindly created by triangulating the two trochars. Next, a standard 30° scope is inserted in the medial portal and the lateral portal is used for instrumentation. The initial dissection may be carried out dry with occasional irrigation to clear the field of vision. A vessel from the infraspinatus to the scapula is often encountered and may require cauterization. The dissection is carried out toward the spinoglenoid notch, which is typically located 1 to 2 cm inferior to the lateral portal. Ultimately, the nerve, artery, and vein can all be visualized as they course through the notch and under the ligament. A probe is inserted through the lateral portal into the notch to confirm its identity by palpation of a firm, bony surface. The probe is then rotated superiorly and laterally to engage the spinoglenoid ligament. To aid in this visualization, a third accessory portal may be created between the two existing portals, which allows for enhanced retraction of soft tissue. After the neurovascular structures and the ligament are thoroughly visualized, an arthroscopic cutting device is inserted and the ligament is incised under direct visualization. The probe is reinserted to confirm that an adequate release has been performed.

POSTOPERATIVE CARE AND REHABILITATION

These procedures can be performed in the outpatient setting and are often associated with other arthroscopic procedures including rotator cuff and labral repairs. Except

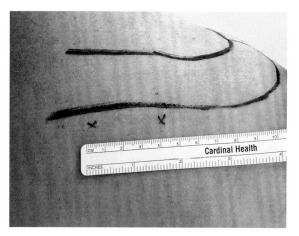

FIGURE 27.15. Two portals are placed for an endoscopic spinoglenoid ligament release. A lateral instrumentation portal is placed 4 cm medial to the posterolateral tip of the acromion and a second, viewing portal is placed 4 cm medial to the first portal. (Photo copyright by F. Alan Barber, MD.)

where associated procedures dictate otherwise, a sling is worn for comfort for the first 2 to 3 days after surgery. Pendulum and range-of-motion exercises are started immediately, and patients are allowed to progress to full activity as soon as pain permits.

COMPLICATIONS

The most common complications are continued symptoms due to incomplete ligament releases, damage to underlying neurovascular structures, or irreversible changes in the nerve from preoperative pressure. Adequate visualization and a firm understanding of the anatomy involved are keys to safely performing these procedures. Meticulous hemostasis in achieved by the use of an arthroscopic pump providing and adequate pressure and flow levels as well as the use of hypotensive anesthesia. Careful, blunt dissection of the soft tissues around the neurovascular structures also minimizes the risk to these structures.

PEARLS

1. Maintain hemostasis through hypotensive anesthesia and adequate water pressure.
2. Release the TSL before repairing a massive retracted rotator cuff tear. Otherwise, mobilization of the massive tear may place undue tension on nerve and prolong its recovery.
3. If a distal clavicle excision is necessary, it should be performed after the TSL release to avoid problems with visualization due to soft tissue extravasation.

CONCLUSION

Suprascapular nerve entrapment, whether isolated or associated with other shoulder pathology such as rotator cuff tears, is now recognized as an important contributor to shoulder pain and dysfunction. This entrapment can occur at either the suprascapular notch or the spinoglenoid notch. Compression at the suprascapular notch results in atrophy of both the supraspinatus and the infraspinatus muscles, whereas compression at the spinoglenoid notch limits the damage to the infraspinatus. It is important to perform a thorough diagnostic workup and include these disorders in the differential diagnosis to ensure patients reach an optimal clinical outcome.

REFERENCES

1. Zehetgruber H, Noske H, Lang T, et al. Suprascapular nerve entrapment. A meta-analysis. *Int Orthop.* 2002;26:339–343.
2. Thompson WA, Kopell HP. Peripheral entrapment neuropathies of the upper extremity. *N Engl J Med.* 1959;260:1261–1265.
3. Lee HY, Chung IH, Sir WS, et al. Variations of the ventral rami of the brachial plexus. *J Korean Med Sci.* 1992;7:19–24.
4. Cummins CA, Messer TM, Nuber GW. Suprascapular nerve entrapment. *J Bone Joint Surg Am.* 2000;82:415–424.
5. Rengachary SS, Burr D, Lucas S, et al. Suprascapular entrapment neuropathy: a clinical, anatomical, and comparative study. Part 2: anatomical study. *Neurosurgery.* 1979;5:447–451.
6. Plancher KD, Peterson RK, Johnston JC, et al. The spinoglenoid ligament. Anatomy, morphology, and histological findings. *J Bone Joint Surg Am.* 2005;87:361–365.
7. Warner JP, Krushell RJ, Masquelet A, et al. Anatomy and relationships of the suprascapular nerve: anatomical constraints to mobilization of the supraspinatus and infraspinatus muscles in the management of massive rotator-cuff tears. *J Bone Joint Surg Am.* 1992;74:36–45.
8. Plancher KD, Luke TA, Peterson RK, et al. Posterior shoulder pain: a dynamic study of the spinoglenoid ligament and treatment with arthroscopic release of the scapular tunnel. *Arthroscopy.* 2007;23:991–998.
9. Ringel SP, Treihaft M, Carry M, et al. Suprascapular neuropathy in pitchers. *Am J Sports Med.* 1990;18:80–86.
10. Post M, Mayer J. Suprascapular nerve entrapment. Diagnosis and treatment. *Clin Orthop Relat Res.* 1987;223:126–136.
11. Lafosse L, Tomasi A, Corbett S, et al. Arthroscopic release of suprascapular nerve entrapment at the suprascapular notch: technique and preliminary results. *Arthroscopy.* 2007;23:34–42.
12. Barber FA. Percutaneous arthroscopic release of the suprascapular nerve. *Arthroscopy.* 2008;24:236.e1–236.e4.
13. Schroder CP, Skare O, Stiris M, et al. Treatment of labral tears with associated spinoglenoid cysts without cyst decompression. *J Bone Joint Surg Am.* 2008;90:523–530.

Periarticular Ganglion Cysts of the Shoulder

Ronald P. Karzel • David W. Wang

As MRI has become commonly utilized to diagnose shoulder pathology, scans may reveal the presence of periarticular ganglion cysts in some patients with shoulder pain. Many of these cysts are small and of uncertain significance. However, larger ganglion cysts can cause significant shoulder pain and weakness, particularly if the cyst compresses the suprascapular nerve.

Compression neuropathy of the suprascapular nerve is rarely included in the differential diagnosis by health care providers. Compression of the nerve at the suprascapular notch was first described in 1959. By the 1980s, entrapment at the spinoglenoid notch had been recognized as a more common cause of suprascapular neuropathy. Later authors noted that compression at the spinoglenoid notch could be caused by a ganglion cyst. However, prior to the advent of newer radiographic and surgical techniques, the diagnosis was generally made incidentally while performing an open procedure to decompress the nerve. Shoulder MRI studies now allow surgeons to confirm the diagnosis preoperatively and noninvasively and to plan the best approach to decompress the cyst. Likewise, many surgeons have described advances in arthroscopic techniques that now allow less invasive treatment of the cysts and associated labral pathology. In this chapter, we will review the relevant pathology and anatomy, diagnostic findings, and current trends in the treatment of ganglion cysts.

PATHOGENESIS

The pathogenesis of ganglion cysts has not been clearly defined. Ganglion cysts are characteristically found in close proximity to joints, leading some to postulate that injury to the capsule may lead to the formation of the ganglion. A ganglion may develop when a capsulolabral tear allows synovial fluid to enter the adjacent soft tissues but not return, creating a one-way valve mechanism. This mechanism is well accepted in the formation of cysts around the knee and wrist and is gaining support in the shoulder since capsulolabral pathology is commonly noted adjacent to cysts (1). Several authors have described the association of ganglion cysts with glenoid labral tears (1–4). Piatt

(3) identified posterosuperior labral tears using MRI in 65 of 73 patients with spinoglenoid cysts. Moore et al. (2) found a labral tear in 10 of 11 patients undergoing arthroscopy for the treatment of a ganglion cyst causing suprascapular nerve compression. In our study of 14 patients at the Southern California Orthopedic Institute (SCOI) who had superior glenoid cysts associated with suprascapular nerve palsy, all had labral pathology, and seven required superior labral reattachment (4).

The presence of small ganglion cysts on shoulder MRI studies is not uncommon. Our study at SCOI of ganglion cysts about the shoulder found that cysts less than 1 cm in size rarely caused symptoms, except that such cysts may be a sign of associated labral tearing. If the labral tears are large enough to cause mechanical symptoms or instability, then treatment might be required for the labral tear itself. Generally, cysts greater than 1 cm can be symptomatic when they cause nerve compression.

The suprascapular nerve is particularly susceptible to compression by a ganglion cyst at the spinoglenoid notch because the nerve is relatively immobile as it traverses the lateral edge of the scapular spine and is in close proximity to the posterior glenoid. Also, the scapular spine forms a rigid medial border to this space, providing a block to further expansion of the cyst. This leads to a progressive increase in cyst pressure, which compresses the nerve between the cyst and the bone ultimately causing nerve dysfunction. Bigliani et al. (5) showed in their cadaveric study that the average distance from the posterior glenoid rim to the suprascapular nerve was 1.8 cm. Similarly, Warner et al. (6) demonstrated in a cadaver model that the motor branches to the infraspinatus were 2.1 ± 0.5 cm from the posterior glenoid rim. Not surprisingly considering these findings, Tung et al. (7) found that cysts associated with denervation had an average diameter of 3.1 cm and were significantly larger than cysts not associated with muscle denervation (7).

Authors have theorized that ganglion cysts follow the paths of least resistance causing the cysts to dissect along the fibrofatty tissue overlying the suprascapular nerve and between the infraspinatus and the supraspinatus muscle bellies. This dissection directs the cysts toward the spinoglenoid notch and the adjacent suprascapular nerve (Fig. 28.1). Given the relatively high frequency of superior labral tears compared with other labral tears, cysts may also be more likely to arise in this location. Presumably, an inferior labral injury could similarly result in fluid dissecting into the quadrilateral space. In fact, a case report showed a patient who developed axillary nerve compression from a paralabral cyst associated with an inferior labral tear (8). Successive MRIs over 5 years showed an increase in the size of the cyst associated with progressive muscle atrophy and fatty infiltration of the teres minor muscle.

ANATOMY

A knowledge of the anatomy of the suprascapular nerve is critical to interpretation of this clinical presentation. The suprascapular nerve is a mixed motor and sensory peripheral nerve derived from the upper trunk of the brachial plexus formed by the C5 and C6 roots at Erb's point. The nerve travels through the posterior triangle of the neck, deep to the brachial plexus and trapezius muscle, and enters the supraspinatus fossa through the supraspinatus notch. The nerve passes below the superior transverse scapular ligament, whereas the suprascapular artery and vein travel above the ligament. The space available for the suprascapular nerve at this location depends on the shape of the suprascapular notch and the size and structure of the transverse scapular ligament. This is a common location for suprascapular nerve compression to occur, and several authors have recently advocated arthroscopic techniques to decompress the notch.

The suprascapular nerve then supplies motor innervation to the supraspinatus muscle and receives sensory afferent signals from the coracoclavicular and coracohumeral ligaments, the acromioclavicular joint, and the subacromial bursa. Next, the suprascapular nerve travels toward the lateral border of the scapular spine, where it receives sensory input from the glenohumeral joint capsule.

The suprascapular nerve continues around the scapular spine, through the spinoglenoid notch, where it is relatively fixed in location by the inferior transverse scapular ligament. This ligament, also referred to as the spinoglenoid ligament, has been reported to have variable morphology and prevalence. When present, the ligament causes the suprascapular nerve to be relatively immobile as it passes through fibro-osseous tunnels at the spinoglenoid notch.

After the nerve passes through the spinoglenoid notch, it then terminates by giving two to four motor branches to the infraspinatus muscle belly (Fig. 28.2). A thorough knowledge of the anatomy of the suprascapular nerve allows the surgeon to correctly interpret the clinical findings and to determine the appropriate site for surgical intervention.

CLINICAL EVALUATION

History and Physical Examination

The diagnosis of suprascapular nerve compression by a ganglion cyst can be difficult to make on clinical exam alone because findings on the history and physical exam overlap significantly with other more common disorders, such as rotator cuff or labral pathology. However, some clinical findings are suggestive of suprascapular nerve compression due to a ganglion cyst. Cysts compressing the nerve at the spinoglenoid notch cause denervation of the infraspinatus muscle only. This may be seen clinically as isolated atrophy of the infraspinatus muscle. In contrast, compression of the nerve at the suprascapular notch causes denervation of both the supraspinatus and

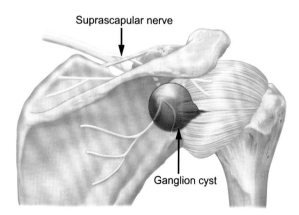

FIGURE 28.1. Cysts arising from the posterior superior labrum can enlarge and compress the suprascapular nerve against the spinoglenoid notch.

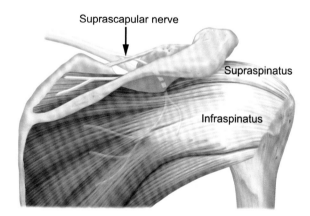

FIGURE 28.2. The suprascapular nerve innervates the supraspinatus muscle before passing around the spinoglenoid notch and sending branches to the infraspinatus muscle.

the infraspinatus. For this reason, patients should always be examined in attire that will allow the inspection of both shoulder girdles to search for asymmetry in muscle bulk that may be present with nerve entrapment (Fig. 28.3).

There is often a history of trauma or some type of overuse, particularly overhead activity. Sports activities that have been implicated include volleyball, baseball, tennis, swimming, weightlifting, and other types of throwing. Regardless of the mechanism, most patients develop a capsulolabral injury that allows a cyst to develop. The presenting complaint is often nonspecific pain that is exacerbated by overhead activity. The pain may radiate medially and upward into the neck and laterally down the arm due to pressure on the sensory nerve branches. Suprascapular neuropathy often presents as vague, aching shoulder pain with varying degrees of abduction, and external rotation weakness. Although these complaints are more commonly due to rotator cuff disease or impingement syndrome, the orthopedist must consider neuropathy of the suprascapular nerve in the differential diagnosis. However, given its rarity, the lack of reproducible signs on physical exam, and the overlapping symptoms with other shoulder problems, this disorder is easily overlooked.

As the nerve compression progressively increases, the patient will often describe chronic pain and weakness that become constant, severe, and interrupt sleep. Patients may have pain to palpation in the spinoglenoid notch posteriorly or the suprascapular notch superiorly. Cross-body adduction has been described to localize pain to the posterior shoulder as the nerve is placed on stretch (9). If there is an associated labral tear, signs such as painful catching or locking may be present. Patients may present with painless infraspinatus wasting because the sensory portion of the suprascapular nerve may be unaffected in the distal spinoglenoid notch. A very common finding in these patients is marked weakness to resisted external rotation, tested with the arm at the side, without significant pain. In contrast to the patient with a rotator cuff tear, these same patients generally exhibit good strength to resisted supraspinatus testing with the arm in a forward elevated position. Such

problems are relatively infrequent in women compared with men. This may be due to the generally lower incidence of superior labrum anterior and posterior (SLAP) lesions in women compared with men or with differences in the anatomy at the spinoglenoid notch.

Diagnostic Imaging

Plain radiographs, including AP, axillary, and supraspinatus outlet views, should be obtained to rule out any fracture, osseous compression, or erosion that might be present. The increasing use of MRI to evaluate shoulder conditions has demonstrated the presence of cystic lesions in patients with and without symptoms of suprascapular neuropathy. A cyst appears as a well-defined, smoothly marginated mass with low signal intensity on T1 images, which are better seen as high signal intensity masses on T2 images (Figs. 28.4 to 28.6). MRI is also helpful for detecting associated intra-articular lesions such as labral pathology. Tirman et al. (1) found that all 20 patients reviewed retrospectively after arthroscopy had abnormal signal intensity of the labrum near the cyst. Another study found 89% of MRI scans of patients with cysts had associated pathology of the superior labrum, usually posterosuperior.

The sensitivity of MRI for associated labral pathology can be improved with MR arthrography (MRA). MRA has been shown to be the most sensitive technique for detecting labral tears. In a study by Chandnani et al., (10) MR arthrography with gadolinium injected intra-articularly was shown to have a sensitivity of 96% for detecting both labral tears and detachments in comparison with 93% and 46%, respectively, with standard MR imaging. Tung identified 60% of labral tears with paralabral cysts by standard MRI. However, with MR arthrography, contrast dissected into discrete labral tears in 100% of these patients (7). These findings support the theory that the paralabral cyst is probably a secondary sign of a labral tear in most patients, requiring treatment of the labral pathology to minimize recurrence.

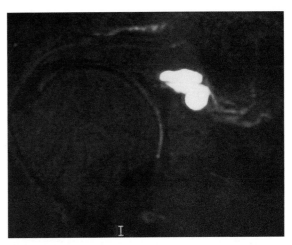

FIGURE 28.4. MRI T2-weighted coronal view of a large, multiloculated cyst that extends to the spinoglenoid notch, where it compresses the suprascapular nerve.

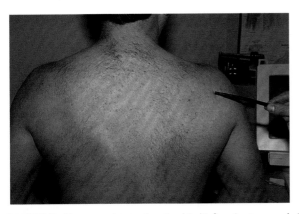

FIGURE 28.3. The pen points to the atrophied infraspinatus muscle in this patient with suprascapular nerve entrapment by a ganglion cyst.

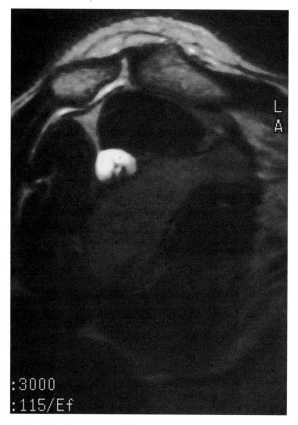

FIGURE 28.5. This sagittal MRI view shows the characteristic location of the superior labral ganglion cyst as it passes between the supraspinatus and the infraspinatus muscle bellies.

Although MRI is an accurate tool for demonstrating the location and size of ganglion cysts and labral pathology, the presence of a ganglion cyst on MRI does not necessarily indicate suprascapular neuropathy. Sometimes, abnormal signal intensity within the infraspinatus muscle can suggest compression of the suprascapular nerve. Subacute denervation will cause increased signal intensity

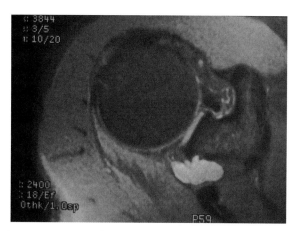

FIGURE 28.6. An axial MRI view showing the classic cyst location posterior to the glenoid.

with normal muscle mass. This is best seen on T2, fast spin echo with fat saturation, and is thought to be caused by neurogenic edema. Chronic denervation will often manifest on MRI as muscle atrophy with fatty change. This is best seen on T1 spin-echo images as increased signal intensity within the muscle (11).

Electromyography/Nerve Conduction Studies

The diagnosis of nerve compression, however, can only be confirmed by electromyography (EMG) and nerve conduction studies (NCS) with a directed exam to evaluate for the presence of suprascapular neuropathy. When the suprascapular nerve is compressed by a cyst at the spinoglenoid notch, nerve tests will generally show decreased innervation of the infraspinatus muscle with preserved innervation of the supraspinatus muscle. In contrast, decreased muscle function in both the supraspinatus and the infraspinatus muscles generally indicates compression at or proximal to the suprascapular notch. Electrophysiologic evaluation of the suprascapular nerve is based on stimulation at Erb's point and measuring motor distal latency and motor response amplitude at the supraspinatus and infraspinatus muscles. A side-to-side difference is usually compared, but the acceptable variance is debated in the literature. Positive findings such as delayed conduction velocity and fibrillation potentials are decisive. However, the only early finding may be increased nerve conduction time (11). This finding is still important, because it localizes the lesion beyond the cervical spine and brachial plexus and can identify the level of compression and the chronicity of damage to the nerve.

Unfortunately, in some cases NCS can be normal despite suprascapular nerve compression. Moore et al. (2) described four patients who had obvious infraspinatus atrophy with normal studies. Upon repeat testing and a discussion with the neurologist, a diagnosis was confirmed. There are several possible explanations for EMG/NCS inaccuracies. Stimulation of other periscapular muscles leads to volume interference; therefore, needle recording is preferable to surface recording (12). There are three to four motor branches that supply the infraspinatus muscle; therefore, multiple locations should be tested with the needle. Lastly, the suprascapular nerve is a mixed sensory and motor nerve, which makes it more difficult to detect a partial compression. The limitations of EMG/NCS reinforce the importance of good communication with the neurologist to focus on the suprascapular nerve. The neurologist should be informed about physical exam findings, MRI findings, and the location of the cystic mass to improve the accuracy of the study.

TREATMENT

The initial treatment for paralabral cysts of the shoulder depends upon whether the suprascapular nerve is compressed. As discussed previously, if a cyst is small and not causing nerve dysfunction and if no treatment is indicated for symptoms of any associated labral pathology, initial treatment should be nonoperative. As with ganglion cysts around other joints, it is possible for these to spontaneously shrink and resolve. However, if the patient presents with severe suprascapular neuropathy or disabling pain, then operative decompression should be undertaken as soon as possible to avoid permanent nerve loss.

Nonoperative treatment includes advising patients to avoid repetitive overhead activities and other actions that might aggravate the condition. In addition, a physical therapy program may be prescribed that improves flexibility and strengthens the scapular stabilizers and the rotator cuff muscles. These patients should be monitored closely for signs of nerve compression, because it is possible for the cysts to become larger. For the patient that continues to have pain despite conservative therapy or has confirmed nerve compression, there are several nonsurgical treatment options that have been described in the literature. Image-guided aspiration assisted by ultrasound, CT, or MRI has been reported with mixed results. Piatt et al. (3) reported an 18% failure rate for aspiration of spinoglenoid cysts and 48% recurrence rate for those cysts that were aspirated successfully. The disadvantage of aspiration techniques is the inability to assess and treat the associated capsulolabral lesion, which is presumably the cause of the cyst in the first place. Leaving these lesions untreated increases the risk of recurrence. Aspiration may be a viable treatment option for those patients who would like a chance at pain relief without undergoing a significant surgery, as long as they understand the lower success rate and the higher chance of recurrence compared with surgical intervention.

Surgical options for a more definitive treatment of ganglion cysts of the shoulder include open and arthroscopic techniques. The traditional open posterior approach for decompression of spinoglenoid cysts has been used with success (13). The advantage of an open decompression is direct visualization of the cyst and suprascapular nerve, which allows direct confirmation that the cyst has been completely excised and the nerve protected and decompressed. However, disadvantages include the morbidity of the incision, muscle detachment, and, again, the lack of capsulolabral assessment and treatment, which may lead to recurrence.

Arthroscopic techniques have gained considerable traction, as multiple authors have reported case series yielding comparable results without the morbidity of an open approach. Numerous ways to treat these cysts have been described, including (1) cyst decompression alone or (2) cyst decompression in combination with labral debridement or (3) cyst decompression in combination with labral repair and, more recently, (4) labral repair without cyst decompression. Some have advocated arthroscopically repairing the labral lesion and then immediately performing an open cyst excision if the cyst could not be decompressed arthroscopically (3). It is important to note that all these treatments have been reported only in retrospective studies. No prospective, randomized trials have been performed to compare these different treatment options.

Studies have shown that debridement or repair of the glenoid labrum was required in most patients with spinoglenoid ganglion cysts for the best outcome and lowest recurrence (2–4,13–15). Moore et al. described a patient treated with a combined arthroscopic evaluation and open decompression who subsequently had a recurrence documented by MRI. At the time of repeat arthroscopy, a labral tear was identified and treated, the cyst was decompressed, and the patient was pain free (2). Iannotti described three patients treated entirely arthroscopically with a posterior-superior capsulotomy. At 1 year, there were no recurrences by MRI, and all the patients had complete relief of pain and return of external rotation strength (14). Romeo et al. (9) reported six patients successfully treated arthroscopically using an accessory posterolateral portal to access the spinoglenoid cyst. Similarly, Westerheide et al. (4) reported 14 patients successfully treated with arthroscopic cyst excision. All had rapid return of suprascapular nerve function. No patient had recurrence of the cyst on postoperative MRI scans (Fig. 28.7).

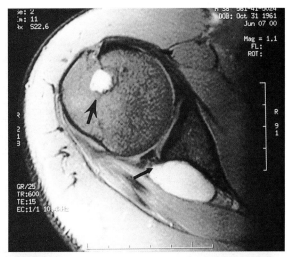

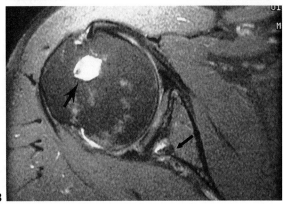

FIGURE 28.7. A: T2-weighted magnetic resonance image of a ganglion cyst. *Small arrow*, ganglion cyst; *large arrow*, incidental intraosseous bone cyst. **B:** T2-weighted image of the same patient 1 year after arthroscopic resection of a ganglion cyst and repair of the posterior labrum. Notice that the cyst is completely resolved and only the suture anchor used to repair the labrum remains *(small arrow)*.

AUTHORS' PREFERRED TREATMENT

A complete 15-point diagnostic arthroscopic shoulder exam is performed, paying particular attention to the posterior and superior labrum. We feel that decompression of the cyst is important at the time of surgery, particularly if the patient has significant neuropathy with infraspinatus atrophy. While fixing the labral lesion should prevent the cyst from growing in size, it will still take the body some months to resorb the cyst contents and decompress the nerve. Therefore, we prefer to immediately decompress the nerve at the time of surgery.

If a SLAP lesion or posterior labral detachment is found, the cyst occasionally can be decompressed through this lesion. If the labrum is well attached, however, a shaver is used to create a 1-cm capsulotomy posterior and superior to the glenoid rim. The capsulotomy is based on the anatomic location surmised from careful study of the preoperative MRI scan. Under direct visualization from the posterior portal, a shaver is inserted through the anterior portal and used to carefully develop the capsulotomy until the cyst is located (Fig. 28.8). Following identification of

the cyst, the shaver is placed within the cyst, the characteristic amber-colored fluid evacuated with suction, and the cyst wall removed off the undersurface of the supraspinatus muscle (Fig. 28.9). Careful control of the suction is maintained at all times to modulate the excision of the cyst and its contents. The shaver is kept pointing at the glenoid neck at all times, and no attempt is made to remove the cyst capsule from the area about the spine of the scapula in order to avoid damage to the suprascapular nerve. Dissection should not extend beyond 1 cm medial to the superior capsule attachment to the glenoid to avoid the nerve as it courses through the spinoglenoid notch. Frequently, fat surrounding the suprascapular nerve is noted deep in the cyst cavity. We avoid dissection in this area and make no attempt to dissect out the nerve or perform a neurolysis.

The arthroscope is next moved to the anterior portal, and the shaver is introduced through the posterior portal. With the shaver again directed at the glenoid neck, the capsulotomy is further developed to remove the posterior portion of the cyst. Following removal of the cyst, the remaining intra-articular pathology is addressed. This usually includes either debridement of type I SLAP lesions or stabilization of type II SLAP lesions. SLAP lesions are classified by the status of the biceps anchor to the superior labrum and the condition of the superior labrum as described by Snyder et al. (16) A type I SLAP has significant fraying of the superior labrum, but the biceps anchor is well attached. These are treated with debridement. Type II SLAP lesions have a detached superior labrum and biceps anchor, such that when traction is applied to the biceps, the labrum arches away from the glenoid and the superior and middle glenohumeral ligaments are unstable. Often, patients with cysts have a small posterior-superior cleft in the capsulolabral attachment that is the entrance to the cyst cavity, but this does not pull away significantly from the glenoid when probed. In our experience, such a lesion is satisfactorily

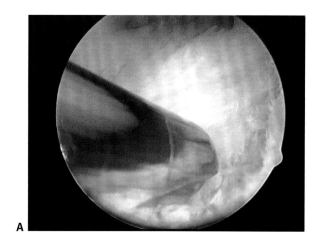

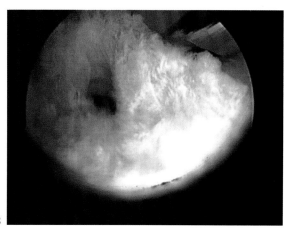

FIGURE 28.8. A: A shaver is used to open the superficial capsule beneath the posterior and superior labral attachment to enter the ganglion cyst. **B:** Once the cyst is entered, the capsule over the cyst and the synovial lining are opened further.

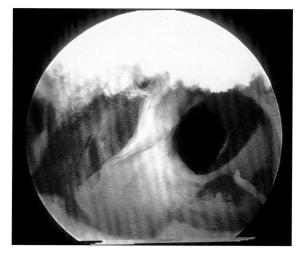

FIGURE 28.9. The capsulotomy is expanded and the cyst is widely opened, revealing several chambers.

treated with debridement alone and does not require reattachment.

Unstable type II SLAP lesions are repaired using a single anchor with a double-loaded suture. Two anterior portals are created from outside in: one just anterior and superior to the biceps tendon and the second just above the subscapularis tendon. The soft cartilage and fibrous tissue are debrided from the superior glenoid neck below the detached superior labrum with a shaver. A pilot hole is made just below the biceps/superior labrum anchor. It is very important to visualize this hole to ensure that it is in bone and does not skive posteriorly. This pilot hole is not placed on the articular surface rim as it is for anterior instability, but just below the articular margin. A suture anchor loaded with two strands of no. 2 high-strength polyethylene suture is inserted into the superior glenoid just below the biceps tendon. Systematic steps are followed to avoid suture tangling, moving sutures outside the cannulas. Using the crescent suture hook and suture Shuttle Relay, the sutures are passed through the labrum, one posterior and one anterior to the biceps. The sutures are tied using an sliding–locking knot with the knot situated on the glenoid neck, so that it is located away from the humeral head articular cartilage (Fig. 28.10). Occasionally, a posterior superior labrum "peel back" lesion is present and may need to be stabilized with a single posterior anchor.

COMPLICATIONS

Although this complication has not been reported in the literature, suprascapular nerve injury could occur during decompression or excision of the spinoglenoid cyst. The knowledge of the anatomy is essential to avoid nerve injury. As discussed above, the average distance from the posterior glenoid rim to the suprascapular nerve is 1.8 cm and the motor branches to the infraspinatus are 2.1 ± 0.5 cm from the posterior glenoid rim. Avoiding cyst resection greater than 1 cm medial to the glenoid rim is the safest way to prevent injury to these nerves. If nerve injury does occur, the patient will develop progressive atrophy of the infraspinatus muscle. An EMG/NCS should be performed to confirm the diagnosis and determine the extent of the injury. If the injury is a neuropraxia, then renervation of the infraspinatus should occur over several months. If the injury is more severe, complete recovery may be impossible, and depending on the patient's work, hobbies, and desire for active external rotation, a latissimus dorsi transfer could be considered.

Recurrence of the cyst has also been reported. Recurrence may be due to failure of the SLAP repair to heal or due to inadequate initial resection of the cyst. Failure of healing of a SLAP repair correlates with the quality of the labral repair and the innate healing potential of the patient. It is essential to debride all the tissue off the glenoid neck and prepare a bleeding bony surface to give the labrum the best chance for the bone marrow mesenchymal stem cells, growth factors, and vascular channels to heal the labrum back to the glenoid rim. If the patient's symptoms are not improving postoperatively, a repeat MRI, preferably with gadolinium contrast, should be performed to evaluate both the labral repair and the presence of a cyst. If a repeat procedure is necessary, care should be taken to evaluate the entire capsulolabral attachment to confirm that the communication between the cyst and the joint is found. The surgeon should then repair the labrum solidly with adequate fixation and ensure that the cyst has been adequately decompressed.

CONTROVERSIES

Although studies of arthroscopic treatment of ganglion cysts associated with suprascapular nerve entrapment have generally shown good results with low complication rates, some aspects of arthroscopic treatment remain controversial.

One controversy concerns the method used to decompress the cyst. We generally perform a capsulotomy to decompress the cyst. Others debride the cyst through the interval resulting from the detachment of the superior labrum from the glenoid with a type II SLAP lesion. Some even recommend creating a type II SLAP lesion to drain the cyst when the superior labrum is still well attached. Although these authors believe that decompressing the cyst through a SLAP lesion potentially decreases the risk of suprascapular nerve injury compared with a capsulotomy, this assumption remains unproved. It may, in fact, be more difficult to determine the appropriate depth of resection when resecting a cyst at an oblique angle through the tight space between the glenoid and the superior labrum compared with creating a capsulotomy at a known position

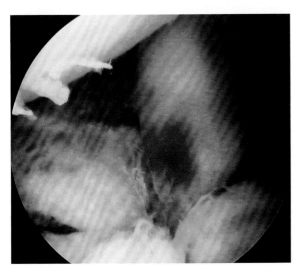

FIGURE 28.10. A completed type II SLAP repair using a single, double-loaded anchor.

under direct vision. Creating a type II SLAP lesion to drain a cyst strikes us as undesirable, as a capsulotomy also has been shown to be a safe and effective method and one-half of our patients with cysts had a well-attached superior labrum not requiring repair. In these patients, creating a type II SLAP lesion risks the possibility of incomplete healing of the repair. Also, SLAP repair requires postoperative immobilization that lengthens the recovery period and increases the chance of stiffness. We believe, therefore, that capsulotomy remains the best option in these patients.

Some authors have recently questioned whether the cyst actually needs to be decompressed. These authors advocate treating the capsulolabral injury alone and not decompressing the cyst. They cite the complication of suprascapular nerve injury during arthroscopic excision of the spinoglenoid cyst as a deterrent for that procedure. Youm et al. (17) described decompressing the cyst if the contents extruded during the preparation of the glenoid bone bed for the labral repair. But no attempt was made to excise any portion of the cyst medial to the fibers of the superior labrum. Schroder et al. (18) reported 42 patients treated with labral repair alone. No attempt was made to decompress or excise the cyst and only in a "few patients" were any cyst contents encountered. All patients in these studies had successful outcomes. All patients in the Schroder study had a follow-up MRI performed at least 1 year postoperatively. Five of the 42 patients in Schroder's study continued to have a cyst present, but all were reduced in size compared with preoperatively. None of these patients complained of pain, and all reported good or excellent satisfaction. The authors conclude that spinoglenoid cyst excision is unnecessary and avoids undue risk of injury to the suprascapular nerve during surgery. Although good results have been reported with this approach, we are concerned that some of their patients were noted to still have residual cysts on postoperative MRI scans over 1 year after surgery, despite recovery of nerve function. Studies with longer follow-up will be necessary to determine if these residual cysts subsequently resolve or whether they may increase again in size and lead to recurrence of the nerve injury. Also, some of our patients exhibited only a small labral tear with an adjacent small hole at the capsulolabral junction leading into the cyst. Although such a hole could be significantly enlarged to allow drainage of the cyst, the enlarged hole may then be unstable and require repair. This again results in the need for a more prolonged postoperative course.

Simply debriding the labral tear and decompressing the cyst through a capsulotomy appear to us to offer a better and more predictable treatment option. Finally, the goal of surgery is to decompress a nerve that has already sustained injury. If the cyst is not decompressed directly but instead allowed to resorb over time after addressing the labral pathology, the nerve remains under pressure for a more prolonged time as the cyst slowly disappears. Thus, the nerve function may recover more slowly, and in some cases, the more prolonged pressure on the nerve might ultimately lead to incomplete nerve recovery. For these reasons, our preferred method remains an arthroscopic capsulotomy with decompression of the cyst and appropriate treatment of any concomitant labral pathology.

PEARLS AND PITFALLS

Often, the most difficult part of the procedure is finding the cyst. The cyst is frequently not visible below the capsule or may present as only a slight capsular bulge. However, knowing the characteristic location of these cysts makes them easy to locate. The best area to find the cyst is under the capsule, adjacent to the posterior and superior quadrant of the glenoid (approximately at the 10:30 position in a right shoulder) (Fig. 28.11). The capsule is opened in this area, beginning just below the medial glenoid attachment of the posterior-superior labrum. Once the cyst is entered, dissection of the thin superficial cyst wall progressively outward can be performed under direct vision.

POSTOPERATIVE REHABILITATION

Postoperative rehabilitation depends on whether stabilization of the labrum was performed. If a concomitant SLAP repair was performed, the patient is supported in a padded immobilizing sling for approximately 3 to 4 weeks. Elbow, wrist, and hand exercises and gentle pendulum exercises are begun in the first week. Active range of motion exercises are started at 3 weeks. Biceps strengthening is delayed until 6 weeks postoperatively. Full activities are resumed when motion and strength are normal, usually about 4 months postoperatively. If no SLAP repair was performed, patients briefly use a sling for comfort only. They resume progressive strengthening exercises as tolerated. Full return to activities is often possible within 6 weeks.

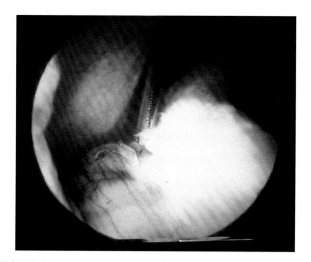

FIGURE 28.11. An intraoperative view shows the characteristic posterior-superior location of the cyst beneath the capsule in this right shoulder. The cyst has been injected with methylene blue to illustrate its location below the glenoid labral attachment.

SUMMARY

Ganglion cysts of the shoulder causing suprascapular nerve compression should be considered in the differential diagnosis of shoulder pain. These cysts are commonly associated with labral tears, especially SLAP lesions. Although the history and physical examination may suggest the diagnosis, diagnostic tests are necessary for confirmation. MRI scans can diagnose the presence of a cyst abutting the spinoglenoid notch, whereas the EMG/NCS tests confirm the suprascapular nerve entrapment.

A trial of nonoperative management is warranted if the cyst is not causing nerve entrapment. However, when the cyst causes documented nerve entrapment and infraspinatus weakness, surgical intervention is indicated. Recent studies document a high success rate with arthroscopic decompression of these cysts combined with appropriate treatment of any labral pathology. It is critical during these procedures to be aware of the location of the suprascapular nerve and to avoid resection in this area that might cause injury to the nerve.

Arthroscopic excision avoids much of the morbidity of an open approach and allows intra-articular pathology to be addressed concomitantly, thereby reducing the risk of cyst recurrence due to unrecognized intraarticular pathology. Furthermore, because of the limited surgical dissection, postoperative pain is lessened, cosmesis is improved, and rehabilitation is able to begin earlier with less patient discomfort and a quicker return to normal activities. Further studies should reveal the long-term success rate of these procedures, and whether decompression of the cyst is necessary in addition to treating the underlying labral pathology.

REFERENCES

1. Tirman PFJ, Feller JF, Janzen DL, et al. Association of glenoid labral cysts with labral tears and glenohumeral instability: radiologic findings and clinical significance. *Radiology*. 1994;190:653–658.
2. Moore TP, Fritts HM, Quick DC, et al. Suprascapular nerve entrapment caused by supraglenoid cyst compression. *J Shoulder Elbow Surg*. 1997;6:455–462.
3. Piatt BE, Hawkins RJ, Fritz RC, et al. Clinical evaluation and treatment of spinoglenoid notch ganglion cysts. *J Shoulder Elbow Surg*. 2002;11:600–604.
4. Westerheide KJ, Dopirak RM, Karzel RP, et al. Suprascapular nerve palsy secondary to spinoglenoid cysts: results of arthroscopic treatment. *Arthroscopy*. 2006;22:721–727.
5. Bigliani LU, Dalsey RM, McCann PD, et al. An anatomical study of the suprascapular nerve. *Arthroscopy*. 1990;6:301–305.
6. Warner JP, Krushell RJ, Masquelet A, et al. Anatomy and relationships of the suprascapular nerve: anatomical constraints to mobilization of the supraspinatus and infraspinatus muscles in the management of massive rotator-cuff tears. *J Bone Joint Surg Am*. 1992;74:36–45.
7. Sanders TG, Tirman, PFJ. Paralabral cyst: an unusual cause of quadrilateral space syndrome. *Arthroscopy*. 1999;15:632–637.
8. Tung GA, Entxian D, Stern JB, et al. MR imaging and MR Arthrography of paraglenoid labral cysts. *AJR Am J Roentgenol*. 2000;174:1707–1715.
9. Romeo AA, Rotenberg D, Bach BR Jr. Suprascapular neuropathy. *J Am Acad Orthop Surg*. 1999;7:358–367.
10. Chandnani VP, Yeager TD, DeBerardino T, et al. Glenoid labral tears: prospective evaluation with MR imaging, MR arthrography, and CT arthrography. *AJR Am J Roentgenol*. 1993;161:1229–1235.
11. Bredella MA, Tirman PFC, Fritz RC, et al. Denervation syndromes of the shoulder girdle: MR imaging with electrophysiologic correlation. *Skeletal Radiol*. 1999;28:567–572.
12. McCluskey L, Feinberg D, Lolinskas C. Suprascapular neuropathy related to a glenohumeral joint cyst. *Muscle Nerve*. 1999;22:772–777.
13. Fehrman DA, Orwin JF, Jennings RM. Suprascapular nerve entrapment by ganglion cysts: a report of six cases with arthroscopic findings and review of the literature. *Arthroscopy*. 1995;11:727–734.
14. Iannotti JP, Ramsey ML. Arthroscopic decompression of a ganglion cyst causing suprascapular nerve compression. *Arthroscopy*. 1996;12:739–745.
15. Chochole MH, Senker W, Meznik C, et al. Glenoid-labral cyst entrapping the suprascapular nerve: dissolution after arthroscopic debridement of an extended SLAP lesion. *Arthroscopy*. 1997;13:753–755.
16. Snyder SJ, Karzel RP, Del Pizzo W, et al. SLAP lesion of the shoulder. *Arthroscopy*. 1990;6:274–279.
17. Youm T, Matthews PV, El Attrache NS. Treatment of patients with spinoglenoid cysts associated with superior labral tears without cyst aspiration, debridement, or excision. *Arthroscopy*. 2006;22:548–552.
18. Schroder CP, Skare O, Stiris M, et al. Treatment of labral tears with associated spinoglenoid cysts without cyst decompression. *J Bone Joint Surg Am*. 2008;90:523–530.

I. The Shoulder

Clavicle Fractures

R. Cole Beavis • F. Alan Barber

The clavicle acts as a strut suspending the shoulder girdle from the thorax facilitating upper extremity function and placement of the hand in space. It is vulnerable to injury due to this unique role, its subcutaneous location, and unusual bony geometry. This is particularly true in the athletic population with sports injuries being the most common mechanism of injury, leading to clavicle fracture in younger patients. These common fractures have historically been treated nonoperatively with reports of uniformly favorable outcomes. More recently, this has been questioned. However, considerable debate exists about the indications for operative management as well as the clinical benefit and cost-effectiveness of surgical treatment of clavicle fractures.

Early descriptions of clavicle fracture management date back to Hippocrates; however, only recently has scientific enquiry led to reproducible descriptions, classification, and treatment recommendations. As the era of evidence-based medicine using patient-oriented outcomes has emerged, investigation into the role of surgical treatment of clavicle fractures has regained a newfound vigor.

Clavicle fractures have been reported to be the most common adult fracture accounting for up to 5% of all fractures. The most comprehensive study of clavicle fracture epidemiology followed more than 1,000 patients with this injury and information about age, gender, mechanism of injury, fracture type, and outcome was collected (1). Review of these cases led the development of a comprehensive classification system. The reported incidence is 29.14/100,000 population/year with a mean age of 33.6 and a male to female ratio of 2.6:1. There are two incidence peaks with males aged 13 to 20 and those in their seventh decade most at risk. The most common mechanism of injury in younger male patients is sports while simple falls account for the most injuries overall. Fracture of the middle third of the clavicle is the most common type accounting for 69% to 81% of all clavicle fractures, whereas distal third injuries account for 16% to 28% (1,2).

CLINICAL EVALUATION

Pertinent History

Assessment of all injured patients must be individualized based on the mechanism of injury and potential for associated injury. Appropriate trauma assessment according to the Advanced Trauma Life Support (ATLS) protocol is mandatory in all patients with a high-energy mechanism. A high index of suspicion for associated injuries is particularly important for patients with open fractures, medial third fractures, and clavicle fractures with associated scapular fractures or scapulothoracic dissociation. In these cases, additional imaging to rule out associated chest injury is mandatory. For all clavicle fracture patients, the history typically yields the primary complaint of shoulder pain; however, a comprehensive evaluation requires specific questions about cervical spine, chest, and neurologic symptoms due the potential for additional injuries. Finally, a thorough assessment of an injured upper limb requires assessment of the entire arm distal to the injury. Additional history should include inquiry about previous shoulder injury, level of activity, and expectations regarding return to sport or laboring occupations.

Physical Examination

Examination should begin with the exposure and inspection of both shoulders. In cases of displaced fractures, there is a typical deformity with prominence of the medial fragment due to the weight of the arm, displacing the lateral fragment and the pull of the sternocleidomastoid on the medial fragment. Shortening of the fracture fragments may result in a visible loss of shoulder width associated with protraction of the scapula. Noting the condition of the skin is essential as surgical treatment is indicated in cases of open wounds or blanched skin from excessive tenting. Abrasions are commonly seen in patients who have fallen directly on their shoulder, particularly in cyclists. Typically, these are more lateral over the deltoid and acromion; however, they may have implications in patients where surgical treatment is being considered if the abrasions extend into the area of planned incisions.

Palpation should be performed systematically examining the sternoclavicular joint, subcutaneous surface of the clavicle, acromioclavicular (AC) joint, acromion and spine of the scapula. Identification of the specific areas of tenderness will allow for decision making regarding the necessary imaging as suspected medial clavicle fractures, sternoclavicular joint injuries, and scapular fractures generally require computed tomography to adequately define the injury. Range of motion is often limited due to pain; however, patients with isolated clavicle fractures will typically allow passive internal and external rotation. The presence of full passive rotation is a reassuring sign that an associated glenohumeral dislocation is unlikely. The proximity of the clavicle to the brachial plexus and subclavian vessels mandates a careful neurovascular examination of the arm. This should include pulse assessment and sensory and motor examination of the distal upper extremity.

Imaging

Radiographic evaluation should include a minimum of a frontal view of the entire clavicle including the AC joint. Additional oblique views including a 20° cephalic tilt may provide additional information about displacement or shortening. While not typically required for clinical decision making, computed tomography with reformats provides the most information about fracture configuration, displacement, and shortening. Any possibility of glenohumeral joint injury mandates AP and axially lateral views of the glenohumeral joint, whereas potential associated injuries to the chest or cervical spine require additional imaging as indicated by clinical suspicion.

Decision-Making Algorithms and Classification

In the 1960s, two clavicle fracture classification systems were published that have prevailed in the literature for over 30 years. The Allman (3) system described Group II (lateral third) and Group III (medial third) based simply on the location of the fracture. Neer (4) identified the unique nature of distal third fractures and subclassified these based upon the integrity of the coracoclavicular (CC) ligaments. Neer type I fractures have intact ligaments, which keep the fracture fragments relatively well aligned, whereas Neer type II fractures have preserved soft tissue attachments only to the distal fragment with detachment of the CC ligaments from the proximal fragment. This allows the deforming forces of the weight of the arm and pull of the pectoralis musculature to displace the distal fragment inferior and medial due to its intact ligamentous attachments, whereas the proximal fragment displaces posteriorly into the trapezius muscle.

The AO/OTA comprehensive fracture classification system is a very detailed system, which divides the clavicle (identified as bone number 15) into medial end (A), diaphyseal (B), and lateral end (C) segments. Medial and lateral end fractures are then divided into extra-articular (1) or intra-articular (2), whereas diaphyseal fractures are classified as simple (1), wedge (2), or complex (3). Additional subclassification is also possible with this system based upon specific fracture configuration and characteristics. This complex classification system has not been studied for intraobserver agreement and does not have any specific prognostic value and as such is primarily used for research purposes.

A more practical and evidence-based classification system was described by Robinson (1). This *Edinburgh classification* includes displacement and comminution as key features with therapeutic and prognostic significance and has shown substantial interrater reliability. Table 29.1 outlines the details of this system, which describes type I fractures involving the medial one-fifth (medial to the first rib), type II involving the central three-fifths, and type III involving the lateral one-fifth (lateral to the coracoid). All types are then subclassified based upon displacement with *subtype A* being less than 100% displaced and *subtype B* being greater than 100% displaced. Additional

Table 29.1

Edinburgh classification of clavicle fractures

Type 1—Medial 1/5
- 1A: Undisplaced
  - 1A1: Extra-articular
  - 1A2: Intra-articular
- 1B: Displaced
  - 1B1: Extra-articular
  - 1B2: Intra-articular

Type 2—Middle 3/5
- 2A: Cortical alignment
  - 2A1: Undisplaced
  - 2A2: Angulated
- 2B: Displaced
  - 2B1: Simple
  - 2B2: Comminuted/segmental

Type 3—Lateral 1/3
- 3A: Cortical alignment
  - 3A1: Extra-articular
  - 3A2: Intra-articular
- 3B: Displaced
  - 3B1: Extra-articular
  - 3B2: Intra-articular

groupings are based upon the amount of comminution or intra-articular involvement.

TREATMENT

The once commonly heard adage *the only clavicle fractures which don't heal are the ones that get operated on* is no longer valid. Expert opinion and historical information from textbooks have been supplanted by high-level evidence including prospective randomized controlled trials examining the management of midshaft clavicle fractures. In addition, improved understanding of the natural history of lateral third fractures and malunited middle third fractures allows for greater appreciation of these fractures, which were once considered benign with infrequent long-term sequelae (5).

Nonoperative Treatment

Although the management of clavicle fractures now clearly requires the consideration of surgical indications, most clavicle fractures can be managed successfully with nonoperative treatment. Options for nonoperative management include a simple sling or figure-of-8 bandage. Neither has been shown to be effective in reducing displaced fractures and a comparative study revealed greater patient satisfaction and fewer complications with sling immobilization (6). Figure-of-8 bandages have been associated with pressure sores and neurovascular compression, particularly when overtightened in hopes of obtaining a closed reduction. Most authors recommend use of the sling full-time for a minimum of 10 to 14 days to allow resolution of acute pain before introducing range of motion exercises. Typically, patients gradually progress their range of motion such that the sling is discontinued by 4 to 6 weeks, and overhead activities are permitted. A return to full noncontact activities is allowed once progression toward radiographic union begins and when full motion has returned which is typically 6 to 8 weeks. A return to contact sports and repetitive overhead activities typically is delayed until 12 weeks. It should be noted that radiographic

union often lags behind clinical improvement and that a combination of these factors must be considered in deciding upon the return to activity.

Operative Indications, Timing, and Technique

In rare situations, clavicle fractures require urgent or emergent surgical treatment. These include open fractures and impending open fracture from displaced fragments threatening the skin or neurovascular compromise. In these circumstances, rapid evaluation and operative treatment are required to prevent serious complications such as chronic infection, skin necrosis, or permanent impairment of the distal upper extremity. Additional indications for early operative management include multiply injured patients where fixation of the clavicle facilitates mobilization and the rare case of concomitant ipsilateral fractures of the clavicle and scapula. This double disruption of the superior shoulder suspensory complex can be addressed by stabilizing either or both of the clavicular and scapular fractures.

More commonly, treatment decisions are guided by optimizing functional outcome. Inherent in the assessment are the principle goals of minimizing the risk of nonunion and symptomatic malunion, which are the primary adverse events associated with isolated clavicle fractures. The available literature and classification systems provide a guide for predicting, which fractures are at greatest risk of developing these late complications (7,8). Indications for surgery are summarized in Table 29.2.

MIDSHAFT CLAVICLE FRACTURES

Fractures of the midshaft clavicle (Edinburgh type II) are the most common fracture pattern and account for 69% to 81% of all clavicle fractures in adults (Fig. 29.1). Undisplaced and minimally displaced fractures (Edinburgh type IIA) can be treated nonoperatively with predictably good functional results and low risk on nonunion. Controversy exists regarding the management of displaced diaphyseal fractures (Edinburgh type IIB.) This is

Table 29.2

Indications for surgery

• Absolute	• Relative
– Open fractures	– High risk of non-union • Displaced lateral third • Midshaft with greater than 2 cm displacement
– Impending open fractures threatening skin	– High risk of symptomatic malunion • Midshaft with 2 cm shortening
– Neurovascular compromise	– Concomitant scapular fracture – Polytrauma patient

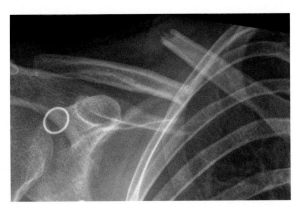

FIGURE 29.1. Displaced middle third clavicle fracture (Edinburgh 2B1).

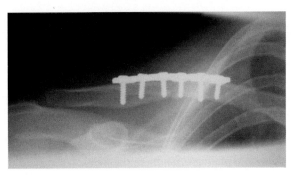

FIGURE 29.2. Open reduction and internal fixation with superior 3.5 mm dynamic compression plate.

particularly true in cases with significant displacement (greater than 2 cm), shortening (greater than 2 cm), or comminution, as there has been an increased advocacy for surgical management in these cases. While most of these fractures do go on to unite, there is increased awareness of the potential for functional deficits related to malunion with three-dimensional deformities including shortening, displacement, and rotation. Nonoperative treatment and the resultant malunion have been associated with pain, neurologic symptoms, diminished strength, patient dissatisfaction, and impairment documented by patient-oriented outcome measures (5).

A systematic review of 2,144 midshaft clavicle fractures revealed a nonunion rate of 15.1% with nonoperative treatment of displaced fractures compared with 5.9% for all clavicle fractures treated without surgery (9). Factors associated with nonunion included displacement, female gender, comminution, and advanced age. Based upon these data, a relative risk reduction of 86% for nonunion can be achieved by using plate fixation compared with nonoperative treatment for displaced fractures. This is further supported by a recent prospective, randomized, multicenter trial comparing plate fixation with nonoperative treatment for adults with completely displaced midshaft clavicle fracture, which demonstrated improved patient-oriented outcomes scores and lower rates of malunion and nonunion with surgical treatment (10).

The most common technique for the management of displaced middle third clavicle fractures is open reduction and internal fixation with plates and screws (Fig. 29.2). This can be done through either superior or anteroinferior approaches and can take the form of compression or bridge plating. The most common alternative surgical technique is intramedullary fixation, and various devices have been used for this, including titanium flexible nails and stainless steel pins.

Plate fixation of middle third clavicle fractures is supported by biomechanical studies, which have demonstrated that superior placement of either a 3.5-mm low contact, dynamic compression plate, or locked plate

has the greatest stability (11). Previously reconstruction plates were commonly used to facilitate plate contouring; however, these have been associated with a high rate of fixation failure. Anatomic precontoured plates are available to aid plate positioning on the curved clavicle, yet a biomechanical advantage has not been demonstrated. While superior plate position does have a biomechanical advantage, some advocate the anteroinferior plate position to minimize hardware prominence and minimize risk to neurovascular structures during fixation.

Some evidence exists to support intramedullary fixation of displaced midshaft clavicle fractures over nonoperative treatment; however, no comparison between plate fixation and intramedullary fixation exists (12). Proponents of intramedullary fixation advocate the benefits of the minimally invasive procedure and high rate of union. However, complication rates of up to 70% have been reported. Furthermore, the inability to statically lock intramedullary constructs does not allow control of length or rotation. As a result, open reduction and plate fixation remains the most commonly advocated treatment for the surgical management of displaced clavicle shaft fractures (8).

Operative Technique

Optimal access for superior plating of the clavicle is facilitated by the beach-chair or semisitting position without the need for additional positioning devices. The patient's head should be tilted slightly toward the opposite shoulder, and the endotracheal tube placed away from the operative side to facilitate access to the medial fragment. A sandbag can be placed under the ipsilateral shoulder to protract the scapula and deliver the shoulder forward. This contrasts with some recommendations to place a sandbag between the shoulder blades, which retracts the scapula. This may facilitate reduction but has been shown to reduce the distance between the subclavian vein and the undersurface of the medial third of the clavicle. Anatomic studies have shown a distance of less than 5 mm between the vessels and the medial third, increasing to 19 mm in the midclavicular line. This must be foremost in the surgeon's mind during dissection and fixation to minimize the risk of inadvertent vascular injury.

Preliminary infiltration with 0.25% bupivacaine with epinephrine provides preemptive local anesthesia and aides in hemostasis. A horizontal incision centered at the level of the fracture affords the most extensile exposure. Attempts should be made to identify and protect the supraclavicular nerves in the subcutaneous layer to minimize risk of neuroma formation. In cases of simple fracture patterns where compression plating is planned, the fracture site should be exposed directly to allow for anatomic reduction and interfragmentary lag screw fixation if possible. Conversely, in more comminuted fracture patterns, subperiosteal dissection at the fractures site should be avoided and a bridge-plating technique employed. Reduction is facilitated by positioning and direct manipulation of the fractures with reduction clamps. Once length and alignment are restored, an appropriate length plate is applied to the superior surface of the clavicle such that a minimum of six cortices of purchase on either side the fracture is achieved. If the fracture pattern allows, the plate should be applied in compression mode. In highly comminuted fracture patterns, consideration should be given to use of a longer plate if a bridge-plating technique is required. While newer plate designs allow for a combination of compression and locking screw placement, principles of internal fixation dictate that in simple fracture patterns, compression must first be applied. Locking screws are an option in poor quality bone, when bridge-plating techniques are used or to augment construct stiffness after compression has been applied.

Following fracture fixation, closure is performed with care to meticulously repair the myofascial layer. Restoring the soft tissue envelope helps minimize hardware prominence and wound complications. Subcuticular closure is followed by application of a compressive dressing and shoulder sling. Postoperative activity includes sling used for comfort with immediate pendulum and gentle active-assisted range of motion exercises. Range of motion as tolerated with progression to strengthening is begun at 6 weeks postoperatively. Return to sports and unrestricted activity typically occurs at 12 weeks.

LATERAL THIRD CLAVICLE FRACTURES

Fractures of the outer third (Edinburgh type III) account for 20% to 28% of all clavicle fractures but result in a disproportionately high complication rate. Neer (4) reported this phenomenon and related it to the greater incidence of nonunion secondary to the deforming forces unique to the lateral third of the clavicle. Others have implicated the higher incidence of this fracture type in middle-aged or elderly patients, in contrast to middle third fractures, which are more common in children and young adults. Advancing age has been linked to an increased incidence of nonunion but has also been associated with frequent asymptomatic nonunion (7,13).

Undisplaced lateral clavicle fractures (Edinburgh type IIIA, Neer type I) have favorable outcomes with nonoperative treatment and can be treated in a similar fashion to undisplaced midshaft fractures. Fractures that extend into the AC joint (Edinburgh type IIIA2) may be associated with future AC joint pain and osteolysis of the distal clavicle. However, it is unclear that acute surgical treatment alters this outcome and those patients who develop late AC joint pain or arthrosis can be effectively managed with an arthroscopic distal clavicle excision once the fracture has united.

Significant controversy exists in the management of displaced lateral clavicle fractures (Edinburgh type IIIB, Neer type II) due to the relatively higher incidence of nonunion (Fig. 29.3). A level-I study examining nonunion risk demonstrated an 11.5% nonunion rate for lateral fractures; however, many of these patients were pain free and did not require treatment (7). Asymptomatic nonunion is particularly common in elderly and lower demand patients. As a result, some authors have recommended a protocol of primary nonoperative treatment recognizing that union rates exceed 85%, and many of those which do not unite will be asymptomatic. However, the presence of a completely displaced lateral third clavicle fracture in a younger, active patient represents a relative indication for early surgical management. In these cases, an informed discussion should be undertaken with the patient and appropriate treatment can proceed recognizing the relative risks of operative compared with nonoperative management (14).

Various fixation options have been described for lateral third clavicle fractures, and little evidence exists to support any particular method. Commonly described constructs include clavicular hook plates, tension band wires, CC screws, and CC suture slings. More recently available implants have led to increased popularity of suture anchors repairs, CC button fixation, and anatomic plates designed for the distal clavicle (8) (Figs. 29.4 to 29.7). Conventional plate designs do not allow adequate fixation into the distal fragment due to their typically small size and associated comminution. In response to this, clavicular hook plates were developed, which allow rigid plate

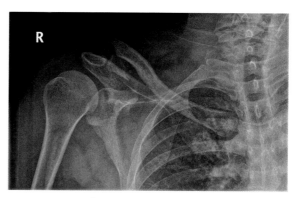

FIGURE 29.3. Displaced lateral third clavicle fracture (Neer II, Edinburgh 3B1).

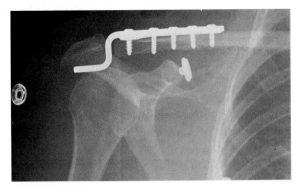

FIGURE 29.4. Clavicular hook plate. Note position of hook in subacromial space.

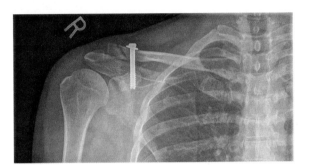

FIGURE 29.5. Coracoclavicular screw fixation of Edinburgh 3B1 fracture.

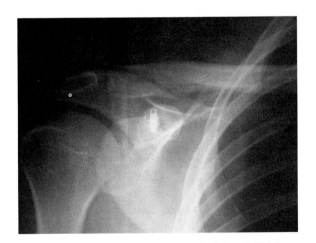

FIGURE 29.6. Suture anchor stabilization of Edinburgh 3B1 fracture.

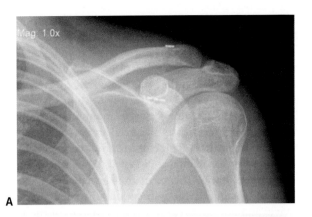

A

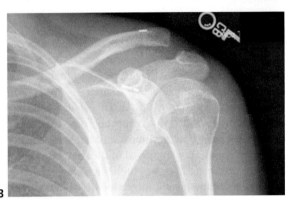

B

FIGURE 29.7. A: Coracoclavicular stabilization with Tightrope. **B:** Note delayed loss of fixation.

and screw fixation into the clavicle but require a metallic hook to be placed under the acromion into the subacromial space (Fig. 29.4). This is effective in preventing superior displacement of the medial fragment but is associated with a very high incidence of subacromial impingement necessitating plate removal. Recently, specialized distal clavicle plates have been designed to allow for placement of multiple screws into the small distal fragments. Often these designs utilize locking screw technology to optimize fixation in small, comminuted distal fragments.

The alternative to plate fixation is to stabilize the distal clavicle through CC fixation. This most commonly requires implants such as screws, sutures, suture anchors, or buttons but can also include biologic stabilization options such as coracoacromial (CA) ligament transfer or CC ligament reconstruction. Based upon the typical pathology associated with distal third fractures, the primary goal is to reapproximate the fractured bone ends and provide provisional stability while bony union occurs. Ligament repair or reconstruction is not required for a successful result provided fracture healing occurs.

As movement does normally occur between the scapula and the clavicle, it is understood that CC fixation must either allow some motion or it will ultimately fail. As a result, rigid fixation devices such as screws are typically removed after 12 to 16 weeks once union has occurred. Newer high strength suture constructs allow some motion and have demonstrated adequate stability to allow bony union to occur. Once fracture healing has taken place, normal CC motion may lead to attritional construct failure either by suture breakage or cutout without the need for reoperation to remove the hardware. By this time, construct failure is inconsequential as fracture union has occurred. However, this mode of failure is more problematic when these devices are used for AC joint injuries due to delayed soft tissue healing in contrast to the more rapid bony union that occurs with fractures (Fig. 29.7A,B). As a result, newer devices that have been marketed for AC joint reconstruction may

I. The Shoulder

actually be more ideally suited to CC stabilization in the setting of distal clavicle fracture.

CA ligament transfer has been a commonly employed procedure for the management of chronic distal clavicle instability, and some authors have advocated its use in the setting of acute distal clavicle fracture (14). Advantages include the ability to simply resect comminuted distal bone fragments, which obviates the need to obtain fixation in the lateral fragment and preemptively addresses any future AC joint arthrosis, which could occur. However, evidence has emerged that CA ligament transfer alone is likely inadequate to support the tremendous forces at the distal clavicle and does not reproduce the strength of the intact CC ligaments. Loss of reduction following CA ligament transfer has been commonly reported and newer techniques of anatomic CC reconstruction have been recently popularized for AC joint reconstruction. As a result, CA ligament transfer can no longer be recommended for the management of distal clavicle fractures.

Additional techniques for distal clavicle stabilization that should be included in a comprehensive list are transacromial Kirschner wire and tension band wire constructs. These were commonly employed in the past; however, both have been associated with a high incidence of hardware problems including distant migration of broken wires (Fig. 29.8). This potentially catastrophic complication combined with the relative lack of construct stability has led to the mention of this technique for historical interest only (8).

The role of arthroscopy is evolving in the management of distal clavicle fractures, particularly as surgeons have become more familiar with arthroscopic visualization of the coracoid. Techniques have been described to arthroscopically pass subcoracoid sutures, which can then be tied through an open superior incision. Instrumentation has been recently developed to permit arthroscopically assisted placement of CC fixation devices (15, 16). As surgeons gain experience with these novel techniques, arthroscopy is likely to play an increased role in the management of distal clavicle fractures.

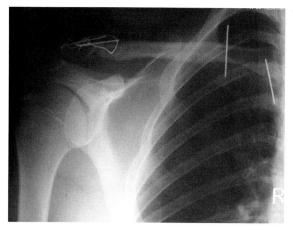

FIGURE 29.8. Dangerous hardwire migration from Kirschner wire fixation of distal clavicle. Wires required mediastinoscopy for removal.

Operative Technique

The patient should be positioned nearly upright in the beach chair to allow surgical access and aid with image intensifier positioning. Draping the limb free facilitates indirect reduction with superiorly directed force on the ipsilateral elbow. Preliminarily infiltration of long-acting anesthesia with epinephrine is beneficial before making a shoulder strap incision centered over the distal clavicle. A longitudinal incision may be favored if a hook plate or anatomic distal clavicle plate fixation is being used. The delto-trapezius fascia overlying the fracture site should be incised carefully as meticulous closure of this layer is critical at the end of the procedure. Similar to diaphyseal clavicle fractures, the degree of dissection at the fracture site depends upon the type of fixation to be employed. Most distal clavicle fractures cannot be reduced anatomically enough to allow interfragmentary fixation and absolute stability. As a result, minimizing any dissection at the fracture site is preferable to preserve the periosteal blood supply and promote union in the setting of relative fracture stability. Fracture reduction is achieved through upward displacement of the arm and the distal fragment and facilitated by use of reduction clamps. Provisional Kirschner wire fixation can be helpful to maintain reduction while the definitive fixation is placed.

The extent of additional dissection depends upon the chosen fixation device. Plate and screw constructs require additional medial exposure, and the technique proceeds in a similar fashion for the management of midshaft clavicle fractures. Access to the coracoid for CC fixation can be achieved through direct exposure, arthroscopic visualization or radiographic control. Extending the incision distally to allow access to the upper portion of the delto-pectoral interval allows access for direct exposure to the coracoid if necessary.

In the case of CC fixation, image guidance can be combined with tactile feedback as instruments are passed through a drill hole in the clavicle to the *base of the coracoid*. It is essential to ensure that screws, anchors, or cortical buttons are passed through this portion of the coracoid rather than the more easily palpable but far less robust coracoid tip. Secure CC fixation can be achieved with various screws, cortical button devices such as the Tightrope (Arthrex, Naples, FL), or suture anchors using high-strength sutures or tape passed through clavicular drill holes.

No specific attempts are made to repair the torn CC ligaments unless the surgical approach has left them obviously visible in the wound. In these rare cases, CC repair can be performed using high-strength nonabsorbable suture through drill holes in the clavicle or around the heads of CC screws, which can act as a suture post. Closure is performed in layers with particular attention paid to the myofascial layer directly over the site of fixation. A compressive dressing and shoulder sling are applied before the patient is awakened from anesthesia. Postoperatively, full-time sling use for 6 weeks is recommended to protect against downward displacement from the weight of the arm. Early passive and active-assisted range of motion exercises are encouraged with the arm supported while pendulum exercises are avoided. Unrestricted range of motion is permitted after 6 weeks and anticipated return to full activities and sports is between 12 and 16 weeks. In cases where CC screw fixation is used, providing radiographic healing progression is noted, implant removal under local anesthesia is performed after 12 weeks to prevent screw breakage or cutout. Clavicular hook plates should also be removed to prevent late impingement, but there is less urgency as these devices do not rigidly transfix the scapula to the clavicle. Hook plate removal requires a formal anesthetic and is typically performed after complete radiographic union has occurred.

AUTHORS' PREFERRED TREATMENT

Based upon the available evidence, nonoperative treatment is prescribed for all undisplaced and minimally displaced clavicle fractures. In addition, displaced lateral third fractures in elderly or lower demand patients are treated without surgery considering that even if the fracture fails to unite the nonunion is often asymptomatic. Nonoperative treatment consists of simple sling immobilization for comfort followed by the initiation of a gentle range of motion program after 2 weeks. Activity then progresses based upon patient comfort and a return to unrestricted activities is permitted after 8 weeks if the patient is pain free with full range of motion and radiographic healing is visible.

Surgical treatment is reserved for healthy, adult patients with displaced midshaft fractures, demonstrating any of the following features: complete lack of cortical contact, shortening of 2 cm, or a high degree of comminution such that it is anticipated that further shortening or displacement will occur. In these cases, open reduction with plate and screw fixation is recommended. In most cases, patients have reasonable bone quality and standard compression-plating techniques are utilized with attempts made to achieve interfragmentary lag screw fixation when possible. Only infrequently is a bridge-plating technique necessary, and in these cases, the use of locked plating systems is advantageous. The superior plate position is preferred for its biomechanical benefits recognizing the greater potential need for hardware removal in the future. Following stable plate fixation, early range of motion and light activity is permitted immediately; however, a return to aggressive activity and sports is delayed for a minimum of 12 weeks.

Active patients with displaced lateral third fractures are treated with open reduction and either anatomic distal clavicle plate fixation or CC fixation. The fixation choice is based upon the ability to gain purchase in the distal fragment. A hybrid technique can be employed if distal clavicle plate fixation is questionable as stability can be augmented by securing the plate to the coracoid by placing a long CC screw through the plate hole lying directly over the coracoid. If the fracture is far lateral, then CC fixation alone is preferred. Until recently, CC screw fixation with a 7.0-mm short thread cancellous cannulated screw was utilized with good results. However, improved implant design and possible arthroscopic options have led to a switch to a cortical button-based CC high-strength suture fixation. Activity is progressed more slowly following operative treatment of distal clavicle fractures due to less rigid attainable fixation. A full-time sling is prescribed and only gentle passive and active assisted range of motion is permitted for the first 6 weeks. Based upon radiographic progression toward union and maintenance of fixation integrity, activity is advanced on an individualized basis.

COMPLICATIONS AND SPECIAL CONSIDERATIONS

Undisplaced fractures are rarely associated with long-term sequelae. Common adverse events associated with the nonoperative treatment of displaced fractures have been discussed and include nonunion or symptomatic malunion. Some authors have reported brachial plexus compression or thoracic outlet syndrome in association with malunited clavicle fractures; however, this diagnostic entity remains elusive and difficult to confirm. While the proponents of aggressive surgical indications argue that the complications of nonoperative treatment are preventable, the potential complications of surgery must also be considered. The most feared intraoperative complication is iatrogenic vascular injury. There are no reports detailing the incidence of this complication; however, significant vascular injury is very rare and particularly infrequent in the setting of acute fracture fixation. Delayed surgical management and treatment of nonunions does increase the risk due to the distorted anatomy and scar formation. Careful attention to surgical technique and an awareness of the regional vascular anatomy is essential. Bleeding related to a minor injury caused by a sharp instrument will typically stop with direct pressure and no additional treatment required. These injuries can be likened to those which occur following subclavian vascular line insertion. More significant injuries warrant emergent intraoperative vascular surgical consultation.

The most dreaded early postoperative complications include infection and wound dehiscence. Postsurgical infection rates of up to 18% have been reported and are most commonly caused by *Propionibacterium* or *Staphylococcs aureus*. These are particularly problematic when associated with wound dehiscence and inadequate soft tissue coverage. In addition to antibiotic therapy, the principles of wound management involve adequate debridement of all devitalized and contaminated tissue and establishment of adequate soft tissue coverage (17). This can occasionally require plastic surgical consultation for local or free tissue transfers. Controversy exists regarding the removal or retention of implants. While hardware can act as a nidus of ongoing infection, a strong argument can be made that maintaining bony stability is essential for optimizing the soft tissue environment and facilitating wound healing. Symptom control can be achieved with antibiotics, debridement, and wound care such that implants can be retained until union occurs and then removed at a later time to definitely eradicate any residual infection.

Delayed complications following clavicle fracture surgery include failure of fixation, nonunion, and symptomatic hardware prominence. Patients who demonstrate loss of reduction and fixation failure must be carefully assessed to determine the cause of the complication. Infection must be ruled out before implicating other causes such as an inadequate construct stability or patient noncompliance. Management should proceed based upon the patient's symptoms and preferences and can include nonoperative treatment, implant removal, or revision internal fixation with or without bone grafting.

Medial Third Clavicle Fractures

Limited data exists to guide management of these very rare injuries with account for less than 5% of all clavicle fractures. A recent review demonstrated that these injuries are highly associated with multisystem injury and over half occurred from motor vehicle accidents (18). In patients under age 25, medial clavicle fractures represent a physeal injury and have tremendous healing and remodeling potential with conservative treatment. In all ages of patients, most cases can be treated nonoperatively with satisfactory results. Similar to posteriorly displaced sternoclavicular dislocations, mediastinal compromise has been described. This warrants urgent reduction with the assistance of a cardiothoracic surgeon. Closed reduction may be successful; however, if open reduction is required, stabilization should be performed with interosseous sutures due to the risk of hardware migration with other forms of fixation.

Open Clavicle Fractures

Open clavicle fractures are often secondary to high-energy mechanisms of injury and frequently are associated with many other injuries. Up to 75% have associated pulmonary injury and 35% spinal column injury in addition to a high frequency of other fractures. Some authors have raised concerns about the increased risk of nonunion and infection due to the soft tissue disruption and high-energy mechanism. However, the largest reported series demonstrated 100% union with both open reduction and plate fixation or irrigation and debridement followed by nonoperative fracture treatment. Despite the intuitive concern about infection and soft tissue complications with these injuries, this has been rarely reported (19).

Pediatric Clavicle Fractures

Nonoperative treatment of all clavicle fractures is associated with rapid progression to union with no documented sequelae in newborns and infants. Young children with thick periosteum have tremendous remodeling potential and management should be focused exclusively on symptom control with a brief period of protected activities. Nearly all children and young adolescents can be treated without surgery with successful results, and published data regarding adult fracture management cannot be extrapolated to this group (20). However, as adolescents reach skeletal maturity, their remodeling potential lessens, and consideration of more aggressive surgical indications is warranted.

PEARLS AND PITFALLS

1. Most clavicle fractures can be effectively treated without surgery; however, level I evidence now supports open reduction and internal fixation for some displaced fractures.
2. While most clavicle fractures heal without surgery, symptomatic malunion is an increasingly recognized complication, which is preventable by recognizing the need for fixation of significantly shortened or displaced clavicle shaft fractures.
3. When nonoperative treatment is prescribed, it should include simple sling immobilization for comfort and once pain allows early range of motion.
4. When surgery is indicated, open reduction and internal fixation with a strong compression or locking plate provides the most reliable results.
5. Reconstruction plates are biomechanically inadequate and are associated with a high rate of fixation failure.
6. Subclavian vascular structures are intimately opposed to the undersurface of the medial one-third of the clavicle and must be protected during clavicle fracture surgery.
7. Displaced distal third clavicle fractures in adults are at greater risk of nonunion; however, in elderly and sedentary patients many of these are asymptomatic.

CONCLUSIONS AND FUTURE DIRECTIONS

Modern day fracture management requires careful consideration of patient factors and expectations in addition to the specific fracture characteristics. The findings of this clinical evaluation must then be appraised with the best available evidence in order to optimize outcomes and minimize complications. Thanks to ongoing study, the science of clavicle fractures is advancing and high-level evidence exists to guide the treatment of many fractures. In particular, it has become clear that midshaft clavicle fractures with significant displacement or shortening are at risk for complications with nonoperative treatment. Furthermore, it has been shown that displaced distal third fractures are at greater risk of nonunion, which is likely to be symptomatic in younger or active adults.

Technically, clavicle fracture fixation has benefitted from the emergence of anatomically designed plates with locking options to optimize fixation in small fragments or osteoporotic bone. Nevertheless, standard principles of interfragmentary fixation and compression plating remain the ideal mode of fixation when the fracture pattern allows. Minimally invasive methods such as intramedullary fixation have become popular in some centers; however, the future of these techniques will depend upon the scientific rigor with which they are tested. Finally, arthroscopy has emerged as a useful means to aid in the management of distal third clavicle fractures. Undoubtedly, as arthroscopists become increasingly comfortable with visualization of the coracoid process and CA ligaments, the use of arthroscopic clavicle fracture fixation techniques will increase.

REFERENCES

1. Robinson CM. Fractures of the clavicle in the adult. Epidemiology and classification. *J Bone Joint Surg Br.* 1998;80:476–484.
2. Postacchini F, Gumina S, De Santis P, et al. Epidemiology of clavicle fractures. *J Shoulder Elbow Surg.* 2002;11:452–456.
3. Allman FL Jr. Fractures and ligamentous injuries of the clavicle and its articulation. *J Bone Joint Surg Am.* 1967;49:774–784.
4. Neer CS II. Fractures of the distal third of the clavicle. *Clin Orthop Relat Res.* 1968;58:43–50.
5. McKee MD, Pedersen EM, Jones C, et al. Deficits following nonoperative treatment of displaced midshaft clavicular fractures. *J Bone Joint Surg Am.* 2006;88:35–40.
6. Andersen K, Jensen PO, Lauritzen J. Treatment of clavicular fractures. Figure-of-eight bandage versus a simple sling. *Acta Orthop Scand.* 1987;58:71–74.
7. Robinson CM, Court-Brown CM, McQueen MM, et al. Estimating the risk of nonunion following nonoperative treatment of a clavicular fracture. *J Bone Joint Surg Am.* 2004;86:1359–1365.
8. Khan LA, Bradnock TJ, Scott C, et al. Fractures of the clavicle. *J Bone Joint Surg Am.* 2009;91:447–460.
9. Zlowodzki J, Zelle BA, Cole PA, et al. Treatment of acute midshaft clavicle fractures: systematic review of 2144 fractures: on behalf of the Evidence-Based Orthopaedic Trauma Working Group. *J Orthop Trauma.* 2005;19:504–507.
10. Canadian Orthopaedic Trauma Society. Nonoperative treatment compared with plate fixation of displaced midshaft clavicular fractures. A multicenter, randomized clinical trial. *J Bone Joint Surg Am.* 2007;89:1–10.
11. Celestre P, Roberston C, Mahar A, et al. Biomechanical evaluation of clavicle fracture plating techniques: does a locking plate provide improved stability? *J Orthop Trauma.* 2008;22:241–247.
12. Smekal V, Irenberger A, Struve P, et al. Elastic stable intramedullary nailing versus nonoperative treatment of displaced midshaft clavicle fractures—a randomized, controlled, clinical trial. *J Orthop Trauma.* 2009;23:106–112.
13. Robinson CM, Cairns DA. Primary nonoperative treatment of displaced lateral fractures of the clavicle. *J Bone Joint Surg Am.* 2004;86:778–782.
14. Anderson K. Evaluation and treatment of distal clavicle fractures. *Clin Sports Med.* 2003;22:319–326.
15. Checchia SL, Doneaux PS, Miyazaki AN, et al. Treatment of distal clavicle fractures using an arthroscopic technique. *J Shoulder Elbow Surg.* 2008;17:395–398.
16. Pujol N, Philippeau JM, Richou J, et al. Arthroscopic treatment of distal clavicle fractures: a technical note. *Knee Surg Sports Traumatol Arthrosc.* 2008;16:884–886.
17. Duncan SF, Sperling JW, Steinmann S. Infection after clavicle fracture. *Clin Ortho Relat Res.* 2005;439:74–78.
18. Throckmorton T, Kuhn JE. Fractures of the medial end of the clavicle. *J Shoulder Elbow Surg.* 2007;16:49–54.
19. Taitsman LA, Nork SE, Coles CP, et al. Open clavicle fractures and associated injuries. *J Orthop Trauma.* 2006;20:396–399.
20. Bishop JY, Flatow EL. Pediatric shoulder trauma. *Clin Orthop Relat Res.* 2005;432:41–48.

Arthroscopic Knot Tying

Michell Ruiz-Suárez

Knot tying is an essential skill that every surgeon should master before actually participating in a surgery, whatever this may be. Arthroscopic surgery, especially shoulder arthroscopy, represents a challenge for a good knot tying technique. The challenges are because of the limited surgical space and the distance that a knot has to travel in order to be delivered before fulfilling its purpose. Therefore, an adequate arthroscopic knot tying technique is a sine qua non requirement for a successful arthroscopic shoulder reconstruction procedure.

Most surgical knots have their roots in fishing and sailing activities. More than 1,400 different knots are known, but only a few are suitable for arthroscopic surgery. A knot must meet the following criteria in order to be considered surgically adequate: (1) its technique has to be feasible and compatible with an arthroscopic OR setting, (2) it has to be as simple as possible, (3) it must adequately approximate two tissues, and (4) it must lock with no or minimal slippage. The ideal surgeon's knot is a square knot. As stated before, shoulder arthroscopy provides a limited surgical space. Owing to this characteristic, tying square knots is not possible. Therefore, all the arthroscopic techniques try to approximate the clinical and biomechanical characteristics of the square knot.

The arthroscopic setting presents several challenges to good knot tying technique. First, it is a fluid environment that modifies the "dry" characteristics of the suture and makes suture handling considerably more difficult in comparison with conventional open surgery. Second, most of the knots must pass through a cannula. This increases the fluid flow in the space in which the knot has to be developed. There is the significant potential for soft tissue entanglement if suture management is not adequate, suture twisting (that may be overlooked), and the loss of suture tension that may jeopardize the efficacy of the knot. Third, not all surgeons are familiar with the use of a knot pusher. This instrument, although extremely helpful, requires specialized training in order to be proficiently used.

It is important to mention some alternatives to arthroscopic knot tying. Suture welding of monofilament suture has been described. Although there are some studies that claim clinical results similar to that of knots, welding is very seldom performed. Another option is the use of knotless suture anchors to approximate the tissues. Although, knotless anchors may offer the benefit of technique simplicity, they are not exempt from complications. At the end of the day, we have to remember that we are surgeons. A surgeon must master all surgical techniques in order to consider himself a professional.

TERMINOLOGY

When a suture passes through a tissue or an implant (most frequently a suture anchor), there are two free ends. These ends are termed suture limbs. As previously stated, it is not possible to create square knots arthroscopically. Therefore, most of the knots consist of half-hitch knots. In half-hitch knots, one of the limbs is called the post. This is the limb around which the knot is going to be tied. The other limb is called the loop. This is the limb that is tied around the post limb. Tension is maintained on the post limb during the construction of the knot.

A complex knot can be created by alternating the post limb or the loop limb during the knot construction. The surgeon arbitrarily chooses the post and loop limbs. As a general rule, the post limb is the farthest from the center of the joint. It is possible to alternate post limbs during the construction of the knot. The loop limb may be tied over or under the post limb. The direction of the loop limb determines the knot configuration. Releasing the tension on the suture limb that is functioning as a post and pulling up the loop limb can do this. Once this is done, traction can be placed on the former loop limb and the former post limb is then advanced as a half hitch. Once the post is switched, the direction of the half hitch is also reversed.

In a knot diagram, a half hitch is represented with the symbol "S." This half hitch can be created by moving the loop limb under and then over the post limb (Fig. 30.1), or as an alternate in an over and then under direction (Fig. 30.2). No matter which is the case, the symbol is the same. In the case of identical half hitches around the same post, the symbol is S=S (Fig. 30.3). This symbol represents passing two half hitches in the same direction around the post limb.

When two sequential half hitches go in opposite directions around the post limb, this is represented with the symbol SxS (Fig. 30.4) and defined as reversed half

hitches on the same post. Finally, when two sequential half hitches are passed in opposite directions around opposite posts, this is represented with the symbol S//S (Fig. 30.5). This is referred to as reversed half hitches on alternating posts and is commonly abbreviated as RHAP. This knot configuration has been considered the gold standard for backing up an arthroscopic knot.

There are other knot tying terms that should also be clarified. The term "turn" refers to the several twists in a given throw. The term "throw" refers to the specific step

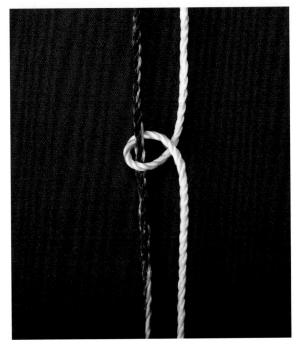

FIGURE 30.1. A half hitch can be created by moving the loop limb *(white)* under and then over the post limb *(black)*.

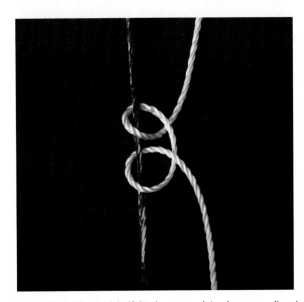

FIGURE 30.3. Identical half hitches passed in the same direction around the post limb.

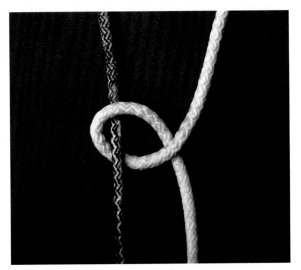

FIGURE 30.2. An alternate half hitch can be created by moving the loop limb *(white)* over and then under the post *(black)*.

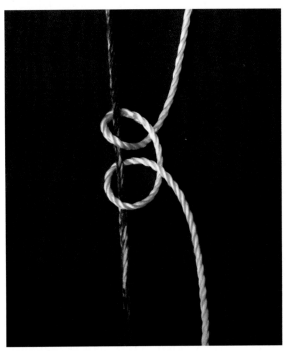

FIGURE 30.4. When two sequential half hitches go in opposite directions around the post limb, they are defined as reversed half hitches on the same post.

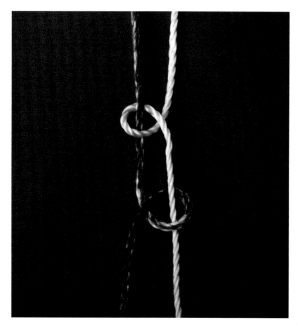

FIGURE 30.5. Two half hitches passed in opposite directions around opposite posts are referred to as reversed half hitches on alternating posts and commonly abbreviated RHAP.

in tying a particular knot. The term "slack" refers to the loose configuration of the loop limb around the post.

KNOT TYING PRINCIPLES

There are principles that should be followed in order to have a successful result. Instrumentation plays a vital role in knot tying. The suture itself is vital, but the cannula through which it is tied and delivered, the knot pusher that carries the suture to the surgical site, and the surgeon are also vital. The principles can be summarized as follows:

1. There should only be one pair of limbs through an arthroscopic cannula. These limbs are the post and the loop limb of the same suture. If for some reason, there are two pairs of sutures exiting through the same portal, each pair must be handled independently. In other words, one of the pairs should run inside the cannula, and the other pair should be taken through the portal, outside the cannula. Another possibility is retrieving the nonworking pair of sutures through another portal. By doing this, the possibility of suture entanglement, especially in the cases of suture anchors loaded with multiple sutures, is reduced.

2. The tip of the cannula should be as close to the fixation point as possible. The purpose is two-fold. First, it reduces the possibility of soft tissue interposition. Second, this reduces the possibility of suture entanglement.

3. Always maintain tension in the first loop. This is particularly crucial in stacked half-hitch knots, or while constructing nonlocking sliding knots. Some sliding knots are self-locking; therefore, the chance of knot slippage is diminished. If slack is observed after the first half hitch,

one method to eliminate it is to deliver a second throw with a reverse half hitch without switching posts.

4. Pass the knot pusher down the post limb to the fixation point, in-line with the cannula, to "clear" the limb before starting to construct the knot. This double-checks for soft tissue interposition and suture entanglement.

5. To prevent suture twisting outside the cannula, the post limb should be tagged with a hemostat while constructing the knot. The suture limbs are not to be crossed with subsequent throws. Always keep the suture limbs apart as they exit the cannula. Unplanned, additional suture twisting may lead to knot failure or premature knot locking.

6. It is not adequate to tie a knot by placing all its throws around the same post. Several studies have demonstrated that the best method of preventing suture slippage and of having good knot and loop security is to back up all knots with at least three reversed half hitches using alternating posts. This is applicable to all knots and all suture materials.

7. Use a sliding knot (locking or nonlocking) whenever possible. Before constructing and delivering the knot, the surgeon should check the suture anchor eyelet orientation and the depth of the eyelet with respect to the bone surface. Although the newest suture eyelets decrease suture friction, suture rubbing against a bone ridge because of over sinking the suture anchor into the bone should be avoided.

INSTRUMENTATION

The instrumentation for arthroscopic knots consists of three basic elements: suture material, arthroscopic cannulas, and knot pushers.

Suture Material

The purpose of the suture is to hold soft tissue to bone or to keep in close contact two soft tissue edges during its healing period. Once the healing process has concluded, the goal of the suture has been achieved. We are experiencing an evolution of suture materials. This evolution is reflected in increased biomechanical strength, resistance to breakage, as well as diminished elongation during the healing process. The optimal suture material must have excellent handling properties (optimal knot sliding, minimal surgeon finger discomfort, and good griping ability), optimal suture strength, and optimal knot strength without slippage.

The most commonly used suture materials can be divided into monofilament sutures and braided sutures. The most representative monofilament suture is polydioxanone. This is an absorbable suture material that provides a slippery surface for sliding knots. This suture material is stiffer than braided ones, thus it makes it more difficult to adequately tighten as a knot. This suture material is weaker when compared with braided sutures, and it tends to elongate over time and with repeated cyclic loads.

Consequently, its use is limited to only a few arthroscopic procedures. It is important to mention that with polydioxanone sutures S×S×S×S and S//S//S//S knot configurations have equal knot security.

Previously, the most commonly used braided suture material in arthroscopic applications was made from nonabsorbable polyester. Braided polyester suture has increased pliability and ductility in comparison with the monofilament absorbable sutures. However, it is more difficult to handle with sliding knots, and it may become frayed with handling. Coating polyester suture with polybutylate improves the suture handling and sliding properties, but this does not increase the biomechanical strength. The loops of braided polyester suture with S//S//S//S have greater knot strength than S×S×S×S knot configurations.

Recently, new stronger suture have emerged. These all contain ultrahigh-molecular weight polyethylene (UHMWPE) in either strand or woven forms. These new sutures have been termed "super sutures" or "high-strength sutures." Although they are definitely stronger than braided polyester sutures, there is a concern regarding slippage of knots tied using this suture at submaximal loads. The knots constructed with these sutures are stronger (2 to 2.5 times compared with polydioxanone and braided polyester) and do not break when cinching knots by hand.

Arthroscopic Cannulas

Arthroscopic shoulder surgery requires cannulas for tying and effectively delivering knots to the fixation site. Cannulas come in a wide variety of diameters and designs. They can be divided into clear and nonclear cannulas. Nonclear cannulas are routinely used for fluid management and for passing shaving, burring, or radiofrequency instruments. These are generally nonthreaded cannulas. The cannulas most widely used for arthroscopic knot tying are clear, screw-in cannulas that provide self-retention at the fixation site and a clear visual field for delivering the knot. When the cannulas are intended for suture management, an 8-mm minimum diameter cannula is used. The arthroscopic cannula always should be directed in-line with the suture to avoid significant chafing of the suture by the cannula's edge, which may lead to suture breakage.

Knot Pusher

The knot pusher serves two purposes: prevent suture twisting prior to knot tying and to tie nonsliding and sliding knots. It is a common practice to construct the knot outside the cannula and advance it to the surgical site with a knot pusher. The single-hole knot pusher is the most widely used. This type of knot pusher is the ideal design for novice surgeons. It is easy to use, easy to past-point, and helps untangling suture limbs better than any other design. A double-hole knot pusher was originally intended for creating arthroscopic square knots. Since most arthroscopic square knots change to a half-hitch knot, this knot pusher design has been almost completely discarded. On the other hand, this knot pusher design is the best for avoiding suture twisting prior to knot tying.

Another design is the double-diameter knot pusher (Sixth-Finger Knot Pusher, Arthrex, Naples, FL). This design is intended to increase loop and knot security. Although this may be theoretically true, it is not easy to use in the OR setting. It requires previous arthroscopic experience to handle it adequately. A less popular, but apparently effective design is an end-splitting knot pusher (Arthrotek, Warsaw, IN). It is designed to create tight knots as strong as those in open surgery. While promising, it too has a significant learning curve before it can be used proficiently.

KNOT AND LOOP SECURITY

Knot and loop security are two basic principles in arthroscopic knot tying. Loop security refers to the ability of the suture loop to hold tissue and maintain the initial tension as the knot is tied and tightened. Loop security is influenced by the mechanical properties of the suture and by the tension applied while tightening the knot. Knot security refers to the ability of the knot to withstand slippage and maintain the initial tension.

These two principles are vital when considering the type of knot to tie and the particular suture material. Not all knots can be adequately tightened with all suture materials.

The principles of knot and loop security can be summarized as follows:

1. Surgeon's square knot (five open throws) has the best knot and loop security regardless the suture material that is used. It remains the gold standard.
2. A sliding knot should be backed up with at least three RHAP in order to increase its knot and loop security.
3. Knot and loop security is greater with sliding knots using high-strength sutures in comparison with knots tied with conventional braided suture material. Nevertheless, some studies have reported increased slippage with sliding knots using high-strength sutures.
4. Applying heat to increase knot and loop security, especially in knots tied with high-strength suture, appears to increase the biomechanical properties. Nevertheless, there is not enough scientific information to fully support this conduct, and it should be done cautiously.
5. The use of multiply loaded suture anchors increases the strength at each fixation point, but it does not affect the knot or loop security of each suture.

Basic Knots and Tying Technique

There are basically two types of knot configurations: nonsliding and sliding knots. All surgeons should master at least one nonsliding and one sliding knot. Although many studies advocate advantages and benefits of some knots, the surgeon should use the one that he masters and with which he feels most comfortable.

Nonsliding knots are used when the suture does not slide freely through the suture anchor or soft tissue. Conversely, sliding knots can be used when the suture slides freely through the suture anchor and soft tissue. Sliding knots can be subdivided into nonlocking and locking. Sliding-locking knots can be further subdivided into proximal, middle, and distal locking. We will describe these characteristics in detail.

Nonsliding Knots

Arthroscopic Square Knot

Square knots are difficult to tie arthroscopically, because it is difficult to apply tension to both suture limbs simultaneously. Most attempts to tie a square knot convert the knot into two reversed half hitches. This may be the only case in which the knot pusher is placed on the loop limb.

Revo Knot

The Revo knot consists of multiple half hitches around alternating posts. The first two throws in the Revo knot have the same direction (under or overhand throws) on the same post. The third throw uses the same post but goes in a direction opposite to the first two throws. At this point, past-pointing is used to further tension the knot configuration. Subsequently, the post limb is alternated and an underhand throw is done. Finally, the post is again switched and an overhand throw is done. Once the knot is finished, the ends are cut 3 to 4 mm from the last throw. The final configuration can be seen in Figure 30.6.

Sliding Knots

The use of sliding knots has been advocated to oppose tissue under tension. Sliding knots are extremely helpful, but we must emphasize the need to verify that the suture limbs slide freely through the suture anchor and soft tissue before attempting to tie a sliding knot. Any sliding knot is assembled entirely outside the cannula.

To tie a sliding knot, the post strand should be shortened to half the length of the loop strand. As the post strand is pulled, the knot is delivered to the fixation site and the loop limb shortens. Once the knot has been delivered, the free suture ends must have adequate length to allow tying additional half hitches without crowding the cannula. The success of a sliding knot relies in its ability to maintain tension without slack until it is locked with the subsequent half hitches. As we mentioned before, sliding knots can be subdivided in nonlocking and locking knots, depending upon whether there is an internal locking mechanism.

A nonlocking sliding knot can be initially tensioned but not retain the tension until it is secured by subsequent half hitches. An example of a nonlocking sliding knot is the Duncan loop.

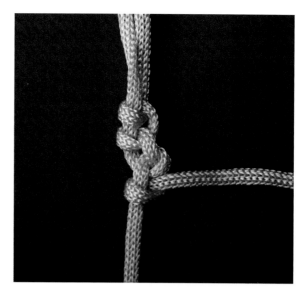

FIGURE 30.6. The Revo knot consists of multiple half hitches around alternating posts.

A self-locking knot can be tensioned in situ without the need to secure it. These self-locking knots can be further subdivided according to their internal locking mechanism into distal, middle, and proximal locking knots. Distal locking knots can prevent slippage better than proximal locking knots, but they are difficult to lock when high tension is applied to the knot. Proximal locking knots are easier to tension, but they can lose some tension while throwing subsequent half hitches. Middle-locking knots combine the advantages of ease of tensioning and prevention of slipping. The Roeder and Weston knots are examples of distal locking knots. The Samsung Medical Center (SMC) and Tennessee Slider knots are representatives of the middle locking knots, and the Nicky's knot is an example of a proximal locking knot.

Duncan Loop

The sutures are grasped between the thumb and index finger creating a loop by passing the loop strand over the post. This is followed by four subsequent overhand throws around the post of the loop limb. The free end of the loop limb is then passed through the original loop, and the knot tightened until the final knot formed. Once the knot is compacted, the post strand is pulled and the knot is advanced to the fixation point. It must be secured by at least three RHAP. The final configuration can be seen in Figure 30.7.

Roeder Knot

This is a variation of the Duncan loop. The first throw of the loop limb goes around the post strand, the second throw goes around both limbs, and the third throw goes around the post limb. The tail of the loop limb passes through the second and the third loop. The knot then is tensioned and passed into the joint. The knot is secured

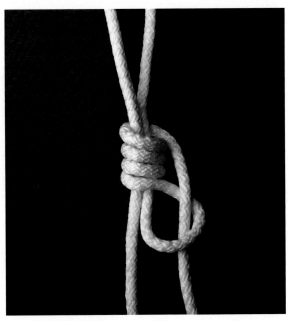

FIGURE 30.7. The Duncan loop knot has four overhand throws around the post. The loop limb is then passed through the original loop.

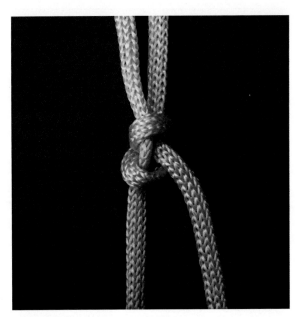

FIGURE 30.9. The Tennessee Slider starts with a buntline hitch on the post limb.

by at least three RHAP. The final configuration can be seen in Figure 30.8.

Tennessee Slider

This knot is a combination of a buntline hitch on the post limb followed by reversed half hitches on opposite post strands. The loop limb is thrown around the post and loop limb. A second throw goes around the post limb, and the free end is thrown between the parallel limbs through the first and second loop. It is secured with three RHAP. The final configuration can be seen in Figure 30.9.

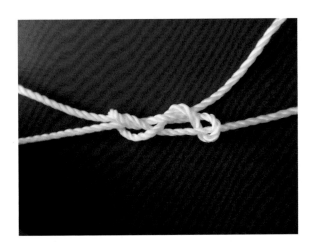

FIGURE 30.8. Roeder knot is a variation of the Duncan loop in which the first throw goes around the post, the second throw goes around both limbs, and the third throw goes around the post limb. The tail of the loop limb then passes through the second and the third loop.

SMC Knot

Pinch both free ends of the suture between the thumb and the index finger and cross the loop limb over the post. The loop limb goes under and then over both strands. Next, the loop limb goes under the post and then between both sutures and then over the top of the post strand away from the pinching fingers. A triangular interval will be formed between both throws over the post strand. The free end of the loop limb goes from the bottom of this interval under the post strand, and a locking knot is created. The thumb and index finger are released, and the locking loop kept open. As the post strand is pulled, the knot is formed. It is secured by three RHAP. The final configuration can be seen in Figure 30.10.

Weston Knot

Although not widely known in the arthroscopic field, the Weston knot is being used with increasing frequency. An underhand throw goes around the post strand, crossing over the same post and passing under the loop limb. Then a throw goes under the post strand and back over the two free limbs. The free suture end goes through the loop of the first throw, and the knot is formed. It is secured by three RHAP. The final configuration can be seen in Figure 30.11.

Nicky's Knot

An overhand half hitch is thrown around the post but not tightened preserving the hitch loop. The loop limb is then again thrown overhand around the post and through the hitch loop of the first throw. A third overhand half hitch is thrown between its own hitch loop and behind the

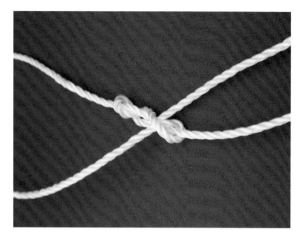

FIGURE 30.10. The SMC knot.

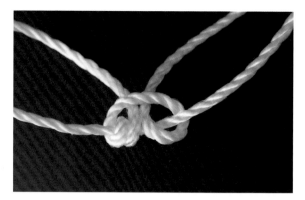

FIGURE 30.12. Nicky's knot.

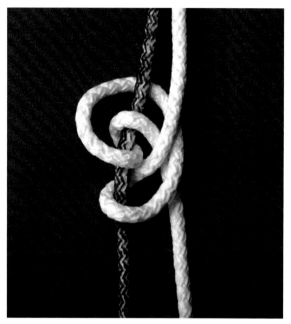

FIGURE 30.11. The Weston knot.

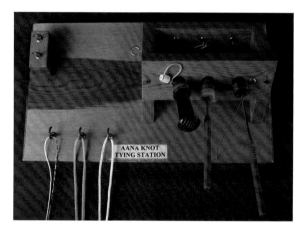

FIGURE 30.13. An arthroscopic knot tying board.

previous two throws around the post. The knot is formed and delivered. It is secured with three RHAP. The final configuration can be seen in Figure 30.12.

AVOIDING COMPLICATIONS

Complications are sometimes attributed to the surgeon and sometimes the suture material. It is obvious that the surgeon's lack of experience can alter the outcome. Success in arthroscopic tying comes with practicing in a dry-lab setting, starting with large suture or cords, and then progressing to tying standard sized sutures. The use of a knot training board (Fig. 30.13) is very helpful. The next step is acquiring the ability to pass sutures through cannulas in a dry-lab setting. Once the surgeon is comfortable in this setting, training in a wet-lab with cadaveric specimens should follow. This realistic training environment helps develop skill with cannula placement, suture handling in a fluid environment, managing suture entanglement, and learning the steps to avoid suture twisting, soft tissue entrapment, and/or loss of tension while tying a knot.

Each suture material has its own set of challenges, which affect knot tying. Knot failure occurs when there is a slippage or displacement of greater than 3 mm. This is recognized by the resultant loss of tissue apposition and a consequent clinical failure. Another frequent complication is breakage of a suture limb. The use of high-strength sutures is intended to avoid this problem.

TECHNIQUE OPTIMIZATION

Mastering arthroscopic knot tying is the cornerstone for a successful arthroscopic shoulder reconstruction. The surgeon can achieve consistently good results with the selection of an adequate suture, optimal knot configuration, and development of proficient surgical skills. The steps for an optimal tying technique include the proficient use of instrumentation. The surgeon must first avoid suture entanglement. Placing a clear, threaded cannula, seated just above the fixation point, helps do this. The cannula must not exit and then reenter the surgical site while tying the knot. The suture anchor eyelet must be oriented to face the direction the suture travels through the tissue. Do not tighten a knot that is not fully seated at the fixation point until you have verified that there is no suture entanglement. If at the end of these steps, the knot seems to have loosened or displaced, do not just trust your lucky stars, start all over again. Good teaching and a well-equipped training environment are essential for the development of adequate arthroscopic tying techniques. We have to remember that all our efforts are for the benefit of the patient.

SUGGESTED READINGS

Swan KG Jr, Baldini T, McCarty EC. Arthroscopic suture material and knot type: an updated biomechanical analysis. *Am J Sports Med.* 2009;37:1578–1585.

Barber FA, Herbert MA, Beavis RC. Cyclic load and failure behavior of arthroscopic knots and high strength sutures. *Arthroscopy.* 2009;25:192–199.

Ilahi OA, Younas SA, Ho DM, et al. Security of knots tied with ethibond, fiberwire, orthocord, or ultrabraid. *Am J Sports Med.* 2008;36:2407–2414.

Baumgarten KM, Brodt MD, Silva MJ, et al. An in vitro analysis of the mechanical properties of 16 arthroscopic knots. *Knee Surg Sports Traumatol Arthrosc.* 2008;16:957–966.

Williams DP, Hughes PJ, Fisher AC, et al. Heat treatment of arthroscopic knots and its effect on knot security. *Arthroscopy.* 2008;24:7–13.

Shah MR, Strauss EJ, Kaplan K, et al. Initial loop and knot security of arthroscopic knots using high-strength sutures. *Arthroscopy.* 2007;23:884–888.

Wüst DM, Meyer DC, Favre P, et al. Mechanical and handling properties of braided polyblend polyethylene sutures in comparison to braided polyester and monofilament polydioxanone sutures. *Arthroscopy.* 2006;22:1146–1153.

Kim SH, Yoo JC, Wang JH, et al. Arthroscopic sliding knot: how many additional half-hitches are really needed? *Arthroscopy.* 2005;21:405–411.

Milia MJ, Peindl RD, Connor PM. Arthroscopic knot tying: the role of instrumentation in achieving knot security. *Arthroscopy.* 2005;21:69–76.

Li X, King M, MacDonald P. Comparative study of knot performance and ease of manipulation of monofilament and braided sutures for arthroscopic applications. *Knee Surg Sports Traumatol Arthrosc.* 2004;12:448–452.

Lo IK, Burkhart SS, Chan KC, et al. Arthroscopic knots: determining the optimal balance of loop security and knot security. *Arthroscopy.* 2004;20:489–502.

Kim SH, Ha KI, Kim SH, et al. Significance of the internal locking mechanism for loop security enhancement in the arthroscopic knot. *Arthroscopy.* 2001;17:850–855.

Richmond JC. A comparison of ultrasonic suture welding and traditional knot tying. *Am J Sports Med.* 2001;29:297–299.

Loutzenheiser TD, Harryman DT II, Ziegler DW, et al. Optimizing arthroscopic knots using braided or monofilament suture. *Arthroscopy.* 1998;14:57–65.

Basics of Elbow Arthroscopy: Positioning, Setup, Anatomy, and Portals

William B. Stetson

Elbow arthroscopy is a technically demanding procedure. When performed with appropriate judgment and technique, elbow arthroscopy is an excellent tool for the correction of many lesions of the elbow joint and provides an opportunity for both diagnostic and therapeutic intervention with minimal risk (1). However, arthroscopy of the elbow joint is perhaps the most hazardous in terms of its potential for causing injury to important nearby nerves and vessels. The reason for this relates to the complex relationship of these structures to the joint (2) (Fig. 31.1). Because of the surrounding neurovascular structures, familiarity with the normal elbow anatomy and portals will decrease the risk of damage to important structures.

In 1985, Andrews and Carson (3) described the patient-supine technique and the use of various portals for elbow arthroscopy. In 1989, Poehling et al. (4) described the patient-prone position for elbow arthroscopy. Since then, the techniques and indications for elbow arthroscopy have expanded and there have been many more reports describing variations in operative technique. The purpose of this chapter is to give an overview of positioning, setup, anatomy, and the portals used for elbow arthroscopy.

ANATOMY

A clear understanding of the anatomy of the elbow is important before proceeding with arthroscopy. Important bony anatomic landmarks should be palpated, which include the lateral and medial epicondyle, the olecranon process, and the radial head (Fig. 31.2). On the lateral side, the lateral epicondyle, the olecranon process, and the radial head form a triangle. Located in the center of this triangle is a "soft spot" called the anconeus triangle. This is often used to inflate the joint with fluid before introducing any instruments or cannulas and can also be the landmarks for a direct lateral portal (Fig. 31.3). Posteriorly, important structures include the triceps muscle, tendon, and the tip of the olecranon.

Anteriorly, the antecubital fossa is formed by three muscular borders: laterally, by the "mobile wad of three"—the brachioradialis, the extensor carpi radialis brevis, and the extensor carpi radialis longus muscles; medially, by the pronator teres muscle; and, superiorly, by the biceps muscle. The anconeus muscle, which is located on the posterolateral aspect of the joint, originates on the lateral epicondyle and posterior elbow capsule and inserts on the proximal ulna.

Sensory nerves around the elbow include the medial brachial cutaneous, the medial antebrachial cutaneous, the lateral antebrachial cutaneous, and the posterior antebrachial cutaneous nerves. The medial brachial cutaneous nerve penetrates the deep fascia midway down the arm on the medial side and supplies skin sensation to the posteromedial aspect of the arm to the level of the olecranon. The medial antebrachial cutaneous nerve supplies sensation to the medial side of the elbow and forearm. The lateral antebrachial cutaneous nerve is a branch of the musculocutaneous nerve, which exits between the biceps and the brachialis muscles laterally to supply sensation to the elbow and lateral aspect of the forearm. Finally, the posterior antebrachial cutaneous nerve branches from the radial nerve and courses down the lateral aspect of the arm to supply sensation to the posterolateral elbow and posterior forearm (5).

The main neurovascular structures about the elbow are the median nerve, radial nerve, ulnar nerve, and brachial artery. The radial nerve spirals around the posterior humeral shaft, penetrates the lateral intermuscular septum, and descends anteriorly to the lateral epicondyle between the brachioradialis and the brachialis muscles. The radial nerve then branches to form the superficial radial nerve, which supplies sensation to the dorsoradial wrist and posterior surface of the radial three and one-half digits, and the posterior interosseous nerve, which provides motor branches to the wrists, thumb, and finger extensors. The ulnar nerve penetrates the medial intermuscular septum in the distal one-third of the arm, courses posteriorly to the median epicondyle, and then descends distally between the flexor carpi ulnaris and the flexor digitorum superficialis muscles. Finally, the brachial artery courses just medial to the biceps tendon in the antecubital fossa

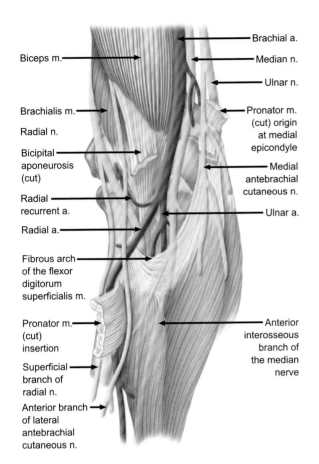

FIGURE 31.1. The antecubital fossa with important neurovascular structures.

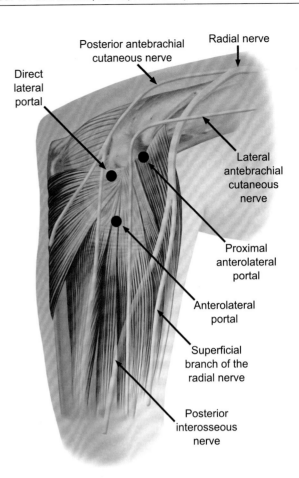

FIGURE 31.3. Lateral view in the prone position.

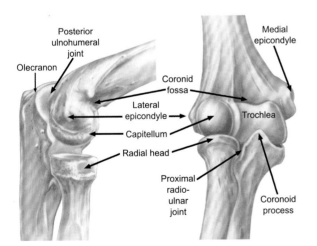

FIGURE 31.2. Bony landmarks of the elbow joint.

and then descends to the level of the radial head, where it bifurcates into the radial and ulnar arteries (5) (Fig. 31.1).

CLINICAL EVALUATION

History

A comprehensive history should be taken including the occupation of the patient, whether they are right or left handed, and the duration of their symptoms. It is also important to determine the details of whether their symptoms started with a single traumatic event or from repetitive activities. One should inquire about the presence and character of the pain, swelling, locking, and catching episodes, which can indicate intra-articular loose bodies. The location of the pain is also important as medial pain is most often medial epicondylitis, but can also be a medial epicondyle avulsion fracture, a medial collateral ligament sprain, ulnar neuritis, or ulnar nerve subluxation.

Symptoms in the lateral region of the elbow may be indicative of radiocapitellar chondromalacia, osteochondral loose bodies, radial head fracture, osteochondritis dissecans (OCD) lesions, and most commonly lateral epicondylitis.

The differential diagnosis for symptoms of the anterior elbow includes distal biceps tendon rupture, which can be partial or complete, an anterior capsular strain, and a brachioradialis muscle strain (6).

Symptoms in the posterior compartment can reflect valgus extension overload syndrome, posterior impingement, osteochondral loose bodies, triceps tendonitis, triceps tendon avulsion, or olecranon bursitis (7). Deep, aching pain in the posterior region of the elbow may also be indicative of an olecranon stress fracture (8).

II. The Elbow

A careful neurovascular history is also important as ulnar nerve paresthesias can be the result of cubital tunnel syndrome, a subluxing ulnar nerve, or a traction injury from valgus instability (5).

Throwing athletes are a unique patient population and it is important to gather information about prior injury and any changes in the throwing mechanism or rehabilitation regimen (6). A patient whose symptoms are related to throwing and are located medially may have an injury to the medial collateral ligament. Throwing athletes who report lost velocity and control or inability "to let the ball go" may have pain posterior on forced extension, which could be a sign of posterior olecranon impingement secondary to a medial collateral ligament injury. The typical patient is a baseball pitcher in his mid-20s who has posterior elbow pain during the acceleration and follow-through phases of pitching and complains of the inability to fully extend the elbow (5). Young throwing athletes (<18 years) with OCD lesions often report progressive lateral elbow pain during late acceleration and follow-through phases, with loss of extension and episodes of locking (7).

Physical Examination

A careful physical examination of all three compartments of the elbow is critical to determine the correct diagnosis. Each compartment should be examined individually in order to fully evaluate the elbow. The physical examination starts with careful inspection of the skin and soft tissues to make sure there are no scars, swelling, ecchymosis, soft-tissue masses, or bony abnormalities. The alignment of the elbow should also be inspected noting any significant varus or valgus deformities. Range of motion of the elbow in flexion, extension, supination, and pronation should be noted and compared with the contralateral side. Those with posteromedial impingement or valgus extension overload may reveal a flexion contracture and pain over the posteromedial olecranon tip (5).

Medially, pain along the medial aspect to palpation at the medial epicondyle usually indicates medial epicondylitis with provocative testing with the elbow extended and resisted wrist flexion reproducing the pain. In adolescents, pain medially can suggest a medial epicondyle avulsion fracture. It is important to differentiate medial epicondylitis from an injury to the ulnar or medial collateral ligament. Pain just distal to the medial epicondyle along the medial collateral ligament is usually indicative of an injury to the ligament. Palpation of the proximal flexor–pronator mass can indicate tendinopathy. The ulnar nerve should also be palpated, and a Tinel's sign demonstrates ulnar neuropathy. The elbow is also flexed and extended as the nerve is palpated to determine whether the nerve subluxates.

One should test for valgus instability with the elbow flexed to 30° to relax the anterior capsule and free the olecranon from its bony articulation in the olecranon fossa. A valgus stress is then applied with the elbow in full supination. Discomfort along the medial aspect of the elbow can indicate ulnar collateral ligament injury. Valgus laxity, however, is often difficult to discern, particularly if there is tearing of the undersurface of the ulnar collateral ligament (9). Comparing the contralateral elbow can help differentiate physiologic laxity from pathologic instability.

Posteriorly, the triceps muscle insertion and the posterolateral and posteromedial joint areas are palpated to assess for tenderness, bone spurs, and posterior impingement lesions. The so-called clunk test is performed to demonstrate posterior olecranon impingement. The upper arm is grasped and stabilized as the elbow is brought into full extension. Reproduction of pain at the posteromedial aspect of the joint suggests compression of the olecranon into the fossa and indicates valgus extension overload.

Laterally, the lateral epicondyle and extensor origin are palpated to assess for lateral epicondylitis. The radiocapitellar joint is palpated while the forearm is pronated and supinated to elicit crepitus or catching, which can be caused by chondromalacial lesions or impingement from a lateral synovial fringe. The "soft spot" is also inspected to determine whether there is synovitis or an effusion in the elbow joint (5).

Stability can be assessed with O'Driscoll's posterolateral rotatory instability test (10). The test is best done under general anesthesia because of the patient's apprehension while awake, which may give a false-negative result. However, it can be done with the patient awake with the extremity over the patient's head and the shoulder in full external rotation. During the test, a valgus, supination, and axial compression load is applied to the elbow, which is flexed approximately 20° to 30°. With the elbow in extension, subluxation or dislocation of the radius and of the proximal ulna creates a posterior prominence and sulcus sign. When the elbow is flexed, radiohumeral and ulnohumeral joints are visibly or palpably reduced (5).

A careful neurovascular examination should be done on every patient paying close attention to the ulnar nerve medially to differentiate cubital tunnel syndrome from concomitant medial epicondylitis or a medial collateral ligament injury.

Diagnostic Imaging

Routine diagnostic radiographs include an anterior–posterior (AP) view with the elbow in full extension and a lateral view with the joint in 90° of flexion. An axial view can also be obtained to outline the olecranon and its medial and lateral articulations. This is the best view for identifying and assessing a posteromedial osteophyte. When there is a history of trauma, an oblique view should also be done and careful attention should be paid to the radial head and the coronoid process for subtle fracture lines. Also, X-rays should be reviewed for more obvious anterior or posterior elbow dislocations along with more subtle degenerative changes, osteophytes, and loose bodies. However, plain radiographs are not always able to demonstrate all loose bodies.

A gravity stress test radiograph can be used to detect valgus laxity of the elbow. The patient is placed in a supine position and the shoulder is abducted and brought to maximum external rotation so that the elbow is parallel to the floor. If there is an injury to the ligament or bony attachment, increased joint space can be seen on radiographs (5).

Both MRI and CT arthrogram have been found to be accurate in diagnosing a complete tear of the ulnar collateral ligament (9). Early studies found CT arthrogram is more sensitive in detecting a partial undersurface tear of the ulnar collateral ligament (11). This was described as a "T sign" lesion by Timmerman and Andrews that represents dye leaking around the detachment of the deep portion of the ulnar collateral ligament (UCL) from its bony insertion, but remaining within the intact superficial layer, UCL, and capsule (9). MRI may not demonstrate subtle undersurface tears of the ulnar collateral ligament. Magnetic resonance arthrography with saline contrast or gadolinium, however, can increase the sensitivity for detecting undersurface tears of the ulnar collateral ligament and has now become the test of choice to detect these tears (9).

MRI is also useful for evaluating osteochondral lesions in the radiocapitellar joint and for demonstrating early vascular changes that are not yet apparent on plain radiographs and it can be used to assess the extent of the lesion and displacement of fragments (5). MRI is also helpful for evaluating the soft-tissue structures of the elbow including the tendinous insertions of the flexor and extensor musculature to help in diagnosing medial and lateral epicondylitis, the triceps insertion and associated musculature to evaluate for triceps tendonitis.

Decision-Making Algorithms

Appropriate conservative measures should always be tried before making the decision to proceed with elbow arthroscopy depending on the diagnosis. The indications include treatment for the diagnosis of intra-articular lesions of the elbow, the removal of loose and foreign bodies, irrigation of the joint, debridement of an infected joint, excision of osteophytes, treatment for lateral epicondylitis, and the treatment of intra-articular fractures. Each of these diagnoses has its own types of conservative treatments, which should be rendered before proceeding with elbow arthroscopy and are discussed in detail in later chapters.

TREATMENT

Nonoperative Treatment

Appropriate conservative measures should always be tried before making the decision to proceed with elbow arthroscopy. However, many times the diagnosis is not often clear until the time of diagnostic arthroscopy as loose bodies, articular cartilage damage, or other pathology cannot always be detected by physical examination, X-ray, or MRI.

Operative Indications

In 1992, O'Driscoll and Morrey (12) described the early indications for elbow arthroscopy, which was pain or symptoms that were substantial enough to interfere with work, daily activities, sports, or sleep and did not resolve after conservative treatment. In this early study, they analyzed their results of 71 elbow arthroscopies as the indications for such a procedure were evolving. Not surprising, the best early results were seen for arthroscopic removal of loose bodies, assessment of undiagnosed snapping, idiopathic flexion contractures, local debridement of damaged articular surfaces, and synovectomy. They found that the patients least likely to benefit were the ones in whom there was a disparity between objective and subjective findings.

Since then, the indications for elbow arthroscopy have evolved. In 1994, Poehling and Ekman (1) further refined the indications that included its use for the diagnosis of intra-articular lesions of the elbow, the removal of loose and foreign bodies, irrigation of the joint, debridement of an infected joint, excision of osteophytes, synovectomy, capsular release, excision of the radial head, and treatment of acute fractures of the elbow.

A number of authors have since reported on the usefulness of elbow arthroscopy for the removal of loose bodies (3, 5, 12–14), and this continues to be the primary indication for elbow arthroscopy. Several pathologic processes may initiate the formation of a loose body including trauma and synovial chondromatosis. Regardless of the etiology, the patients usually present with swelling, locking, pain, and loss of motion, all of which can be improved with the removal of loose bodies. These loose bodies can be found both in the anterior and posterior compartment and also in the posterior medial gutter and removing them can be a technically demanding procedure.

Elbow arthroscopy can also be an effective tool if the diagnosis of an infection is made or suspected. It is a less invasive way to enter into the joint with minimal trauma to confirm the diagnosis of an infection, irrigate the joint, debride infected tissue, and assess the condition of the underlying bone, cartilage, and synovial tissue (1).

The presence of osteophytes, or osseous spurs, is another condition that lends itself to arthroscopic management and removal (12–15). A true lateral radiograph of the elbow is useful for the identification of osteophytes that may limit full extension of the elbow with impingement of the posterior olecranon spur in the olecranon fossa (1, 12). An axial view may also show a posteromedial osteophyte (5). This can be easily removed arthroscopically.

The term "valgus extension overload" was coined to describe these findings, which can be found in baseball pitchers and other overhead athletes. The tremendous repetitive valgus forces generated during the acceleration and follow-through phases of pitching, as the elbow goes into extension, can result in osteochondral changes in the olecranon and distal humerus. A significant osteophyte forms on the posteromedial aspect of the olecranon fossa with continued pitching or overhead activities, creating an area of chondromalacia (5). The inability to reliably visualize the anterior bundle of the medial collateral ligament with the arthroscope limits the value of the arthroscope when assessing medial collateral ligament injuries (16, 17).

Chronic synovitis caused by inflammatory arthritis, which does not respond to nonoperative management and where there is minimal joint destruction, can also be an indication for elbow arthroscopy. Synovectomy can provide considerable relief of pain. Diagnostic elbow arthroscopy can also be used for synovial biopsy to establish the diagnosis of rheumatoid arthritis or other inflammatory arthritides, or a monoarticular or polyarticular arthritis of unknown etiology (12). The elbow joint is affected in approximately 20% to 50% of patients with rheumatoid arthritis, and 50% of these patients develop pain and associated loss of motion (12). Lee and Morrey achieved 93% good or excellent results in a short-term follow-up of 14 arthroscopic synovectomies in 11 patients. However, only 57% of their patients maintained good or excellent results at an average of 42 months after surgery. When performing elbow arthroscopy and synovectomy for rheumatoid arthritis and other inflammatory arthritides, it is important to set realistic expectations for the patient knowing that symptoms can recur.

OCD of the capitellum is characterized by pain, swelling, and limitation of motion and usually occurs during adolescence or young adulthood in a throwing athlete or gymnast. The underlying cause of this lesion is most likely repetitive microtrauma to a vulnerable epiphysis with a precarious blood supply. The lesion may progress to joint incongruity, loose body formation, and a locked elbow with chronic pain, all of which together are indications for elbow arthroscopy when conservative measures fail. The procedure involves the arthroscopic removal of osteophytes, excision of loose or detached cartilage, and curettement and drilling of the base of the lesion.

Panner's disease is an osteochondrosis of the entire capitellum in children and adolescents and may represent an early stage of OCD (5). Reconstitution of the capitellum usually occurs with rest without late sequelae or limitations.

The indications for arthroscopic debridement of the elbow for degenerative osteoarthritis are similar to those described for loose body removal, valgus extension overload, and OCD. Pain associated with swelling and mechanical symptoms of catching and locking respond well to arthroscopic debridement (13–15). Removal of loose bodies and osteophytes from the olecranon, olecranon fossa, and coronoid process can reduce pain, increase range of motion, and eliminate mechanical-like symptoms (13–15). Elbow arthroscopy has limited value in primary degenerative arthrosis where there are no significant osteophytes, loose bodies, or mechanical-like symptoms present.

Arthrofibrosis of the elbow treated arthroscopically can be a technically demanding procedure with an increased risk of complications because of the limited ability to distend the arthrofibrotic capsule and the close proximity of many neurovascular structures (1, 5, 13). Loss of elbow joint motion can be a result of bone or soft-tissue problems caused by trauma and degenerative or inflammatory arthritides. Patients can have a loss of flexion or extension or both. It is important to attempt to determine the cause of the contracture because this can influence treatment (5). If a nonoperative treatment of NSAID refers to non-steroidal anti-inflammatory (NSAID), stretching exercises, splinting, and other modalities fail, arthroscopic release and thorough joint debridement may be indicated in properly selected patients (13).

The indications for elbow arthroscopy have been extended to include the treatment of lateral epicondylitis. When conservative measures fail, arthroscopic release offers several potential advantages over open techniques (5). It preserves the common extensor origin by addressing the lesion directly and it also allows for intra-articular examination for possible chondral lesions, loose bodies, and other disorders such as an inflamed lateral synovial fringe. It also permits a shorter postoperative rehabilitation period and an earlier return to work or sports (5).

Radial head excision can be performed arthroscopically for post traumatic arthritis of the radiocapitellar joint secondary to a radial head fracture (1, 5, 13). Advantages of arthroscopic treatment include a more complete visualization of the articular surface of the elbow and associated chondral lesions or ligamentous disruptions (5). In addition to the entire radial head, as much as 2 to 3 mm of the radial neck can be removed. To maintain stability at the proximal radioulnar joint, the annular ligament must be left intact (1).

The arthroscopic management of selected fractures around the elbow with percutaneous pins and screws is evolving and includes the treatment of radial head fractures, capitellum fractures, and coronoid fractures. The arthroscopic-assisted treatment of coronoid fractures has shown promise in a small study group of seven patients. In addition, there are new frontiers of elbow arthroscopy including the treatment of olecranon bursitis, endoscopic repair of a torn distal biceps tendon, arthroscopic triceps repair, and arthroscopic ulnar nerve release.

Contraindications

The primary contraindication to elbow arthroscopy is any significant distortion of normal bony or soft-tissue anatomy that precludes safe entry of the arthroscope into the joint (12). For example, a previous ulnar nerve transposition either submuscular or subcutaneous would interfere with safe proximal, anterior medial portal placement and is a relative contraindication for safe introduction of the arthroscope through the medial side of the elbow (5, 18). In these cases, identification of the ulnar nerve is necessary before establishing a medial portal (18).

Another relative contraindication is a severely anky-losed joint may distort normal anatomy and place impor-tant neurovascular structures at risk. This may not allow for adequate joint distension and may not allow proper displacement of neurovascular structures away from por-tal sites and within the joint from instrumentation (5). As with any other procedure, a localized infection in the area of portal placement is also a contraindication to the elbow arthroscopy.

AUTHOR'S PREFERRED TREATMENT

When conservative measures have failed, elbow arthroscopy is a useful tool in the treatment of both simple and complex disorders of the elbow. However, it does not replace a care-ful history, physical examination, diagnostic testing, or an adequate course of nonoperative treatment. When the deci-sion is made to proceed with elbow arthroscopy, it is im-portant to discuss with the patient the risks and benefits of the procedure including the remote risk of blood vessel and nerve damage, and what realistic results can be expected after the surgery. The documentation of this discussion in the medical record and proper informed consent is critical before proceeding with this or any other surgical procedure.

Anesthesia

Most surgeons prefer to use general endotracheal anesthe-sia for patients undergoing elbow arthroscopy because it provides total muscle relaxation and is more comfortable for the patient (5, 18). The use of regional anesthesia is advocated by some including the use of an axillary nerve block or an interscalene nerve block. These can be admin-istered safely and successfully by a trained anesthesiolo-gist, but there is still inherent risk in these blocks not seen with general anesthesia.

There is apprehension among some surgeons about using local and intravenous blocks because the patient's postoperative neurologic status cannot be assessed and may be compromised by an extended axillary or intersca-lene nerve block (5). If there is a neurologic deficit found after the procedure, it may be difficult to determine how it occurred and there may be finger pointing between the anesthesiologist and the surgeon.

The use of local anesthetics for postoperative pain control is also not commonly used because of the diffi-culty in assessing the patient's postoperative neurologic status. However, there is no hard-and-fast rule against the use of local anesthetics for postoperative pain control and it should be left to the discretion of the operating surgeon.

Positioning

Traditionally, elbow arthroscopy was performed with the patient resting supine on the operating table, until use of the prone position was introduced in 1989 by Poehling et al. (4). The prone position improves the mobility of

the arthroscope within the joint, facilitates manipulation of the joint, provides for a more complete intra-articular inspection (especially in the posterior aspect of the joint), and eliminates the need for an overhead suspension device to support the elbow. The main disadvantage to this posi-tion is a more difficult access to the patient's airway (1).

After an appropriate level of anesthesia (general endo-tracheal or axillary block) has been achieved, the patient is placed prone, with large chest-rolls under the torso. It is important that these chest rolls are large enough to raise the patient's torso up from the operating room table. If these rolls are not large enough, it makes it difficult to position the arm and elbow in position to access the proxi-mal anterior medial portal. An arm board is placed on the operative side of the table and parallel to it. To increase the mobility of the upper extremity intraoperatively, a sand-bag, block, or firm bump of towels is placed under the shoulder to further elevate the arm away from the table. The forearm is then allowed to hang in a dependent posi-tion over the arm board at 90° (Fig. 31.4). A sterile tour-niquet may be placed around the proximal aspect of the arm to help to control bleeding during the procedure, but it is not always necessary to inflate when using a mechani-cal irrigation system (1). After the extremity is prepped and draped, a large sterile "bump" is placed under the arm proximal to the elbow to keep the shoulder abducted to 90° and also to keep the elbow at approximately 90° of flexion (Fig. 31.5).

Other authors prefer the lateral decubitus position because they feel it provides improved stability of the ex-tremity, is more convenient for the anesthesiologist and allows easier access to the airway, and allows posterior elbow joint access without compromising airway access (12, 18). The patient is placed in the lateral decubitus position with the involved extremity facing upward. The arm is then supported on a well-padded bolster with the

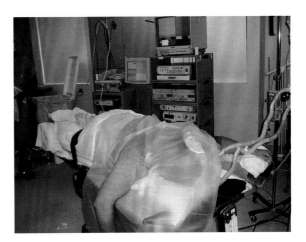

FIGURE 31.4. The prone position with the right elbow resting over an arm board, which is parallel to the operating room table. A nonsterile U-drape is placed proximally. A sterile bump is placed under the arm for support after the extremity is prepped.

II. The Elbow

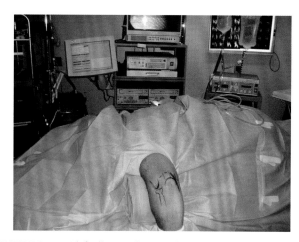

FIGURE 31.5. A left elbow is shown in the prone position. Anesthesia is at the head (*left*) of the patient and all equipments are on the opposite side of the table. Note the sterile bump under the arm, which helps stabilize the elbow during the procedure. This rests on the arm board that has been placed parallel to the table.

forearm hanging free and the elbow flexed to 90°. In this position, the elbow is supported in front of the surgeon who then has access to the various portal sites.

Whether using the prone or lateral decubitus position, the forearm is prepped from the proximal arm to the tip of the fingers and then the extremity is wrapped with an elastic bandage from the fingers to just below the elbow to minimize fluid extravasation into the forearm (18).

Operating Room Setup

When using the prone position, anesthesia is positioned at the head of the table and the surgeon stands directly lateral to the flexed elbow and the assistant stands toward the head of the patient. The ancillary scrub personnel stand toward the foot of the patient or behind the surgeon and the assistant. One Mayo stand is placed behind the surgeon and the other Mayo stand is on the opposite side of the table. All tubing and electrical cords run from this Mayo stand to run to the video monitor, recorder, light source, camera, fluid bags, and mechanical irrigation system, which are placed on the opposite side of the patient (Fig. 31.5).

Instrumentation

A standard 4.0-mm, 30° arthroscope permits excellent visualization of the elbow joint. A smaller 2.7-mm arthroscope is usually not necessary but can be useful for viewing small spaces, such as the lateral compartment from the direct lateral portal, and for arthroscopy in adolescent patients (5, 18). The use of cannulas allows one to switch viewing and working portals without repeated joint capsule injuries. This also minimizes the risk of injury to neurovascular structures and decreases the chance of fluid extravasation into the soft tissues, swelling, and possible compartment syndrome (5). A metal cannula is usually used for the arthroscope, and the working portal is usually a disposable plastic cannula with a diaphragm,

which allows instruments to be introduced without loss of joint distension.

Side-vented inflow cannulas should be avoided in elbow arthroscopy because the distance between the skin and the joint capsule is often very slight. With side-vented cannulas, the cannula can be intra-articular while the side vents remain extra-articular, resulting in fluid extravasation into the surrounding soft tissues. Inflow cannulas should be devoid of side vents, with fluid flow occurring directly at the end of the cannula (19).

All trocars should be conical and blunt tipped to decrease the possibility of neurovascular and articular cartilage injury. Various handheld instruments such as probes, grasping forceps, and punches along with motorized instruments such as synovial resectors and burrs are also used during elbow arthroscopy (5, 18).

If a mechanical pump is used, an inflow pressure of 35 mm Hg is usually used to maintain joint distension (5). Some authors prefer the use of gravity inflow and feel that it gives adequate joint distension without the risk of fluid extravasation. If a tourniquet is used, it can be set at 250 mm Hg and inflated if needed.

GENERAL SURGICAL TECHNIQUE

Elbow arthroscopy has a significant potential for complications, particularly neurovascular injury (5). The key to avoiding complications is to have a clear understanding of the relationship of the neurovascular structures to the soft-tissue and bony anatomy. With the patient positioned either in the lateral decubitus or in the prone position, it is important to identify and mark landmarks. This includes the tip of the olecranon, the medial and lateral epicondyle, the radial head, the soft spot of the elbow, the medial intermuscular septum, and the ulnar nerve (Fig. 31.6). Some authors recommend distending the joint with 20 to

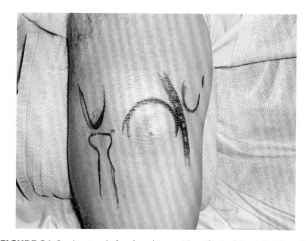

FIGURE 31.6. Anatomic landmarks are identified of the left elbow in the prone position including the medial epicondyle *(right)*, the lateral epicondyle *(left)*, the radial head, the olecranon, and the ulnar nerve *(dark blue line on right)*. The intermuscular septum is also identified on the medial aspect of the elbow, just anterior to the medial epicondyle.

40 cc of fluid through the lateral "soft spot" before establishing the initial portal (20). Other authors feel it is not necessary. Miller et al. demonstrated that there is a small distance (as narrow as 6 mm) between the joint capsule and the neurovascular structures, and that joint insufflation does not increase the capsule-to-nerve distance. We have found joint insufflation not necessary before making the proximal anterior medial portal, the first portal that we typically establish. If one pays close attention to anatomic landmarks, the elbow joint can be safely entered into without having to inflate the joint with fluid.

When creating portals, the surgeon should avoid penetrating the subcutaneous tissue, thereby helping to prevent injury to the superficial cutaneous nerves. A hemostat or mosquito clamp should be used to spread tissues down to the capsule (5). When the arthroscope is introduced, the elbow should be flexed to 90° to relax and protect the anterior neurovascular structures and only blunt trocars should be used.

Whether the anteromedial or anterolateral portal should be created first has been an issue of some debate. Many surgeons create a lateral portal initially and then establish a medial portal with a spinal needle by direct visualization from within the joint. Alternatively, an inside-out technique may be employed in which a switching stick is used to establish the medial portal from inside the joint. Other surgeons, using the same techniques, establish the medial portal first and cadaveric studies have found that it is safer to establish the proximal anterior medial portal first than the lateral portal.

I believe and many other authors agree that the proximal anterior medial portal should be created first as it is the safest as long as the surgeon has identified and outlined the important soft-tissue and bony landmarks including the intermuscular septum (5, 18). There is less fluid extravasation when starting medially because a superomedial portal traverses predominately tendinous tissue and a tough portion of the forearm flexor muscles. The thicker tissues minimize fluid extravasation more effectively than the softer, thinner, radial capsule. Finally, most elbow disorders are located in the lateral compartment, which is best visualized from the proximal anterior medial portal (5).

PORTAL PLACEMENT

Anterior Compartment

The proximal anterior medial portal is established first and was first described by Poehling et al. (4). It is located approximately 2 cm proximal to the medial epicondyle and just anterior to the intermuscular septum (Fig. 31.7). Prior to establishing this portal, the location and the stability of the ulnar nerve should be assessed. The prevalence rate of ulnar nerve subluxation anterior to the cubital tunnel is approximately 17%. Blunt dissection is carried out until the anterior aspect of the humerus is palpated, again, staying anterior to the intermuscular septum. The

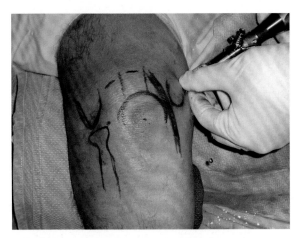

FIGURE 31.7. The proximal anteromedial portal is the first to be established, it is located just anterior to the intermuscular septum and 2 cm proximal to the medial epicondyle.

arthroscopic sheath is then inserted anterior to the intermuscular septum while maintaining contact with the anterior aspect of the humerus and directing the trocar toward the radial head. Use of the anterior surface of the humerus as a constant guide helps to prevent injury to the median nerve and the brachial artery, which are anterior to the capsule. The ulnar nerve is located approximately 3 to 4 mm from this portal, posterior to the intermuscular septum (Fig. 31.8). Palpating the septum and making sure that the portal is established anterior to the septum minimizes the risk of injury to the nerve while providing excellent visualization. This portal provides excellent visualization of the anterior compartment of the elbow, particularly the radiocapitellar joint, the humeroulnar joints, the coronoid fossa, and the superior joint capsule (1, 5).

The anteromedial portal as described by Lynch et al. is located 2 cm distal and 2 cm anterior to the medial epicondyle and is at or near the distal extent of the elbow capsule. Because of the location of this portal, the cannula can enter the joint only by being advanced straight laterally, toward the median nerve. Because of this, the proximal anterior medial portal is recommended as it is safer because the more proximal position allows the arthroscope to be directed distally, resulting in the arthroscope being almost parallel to the median nerve in the anteroposterior plane (5).

The anterolateral portal was originally described by Andrews and Carson (3). as being located 3 cm distal and 2 cm anterior to the lateral epicondyle. However, this portal location places the radial nerve at significant risk for iatrogenic injury. Lindenfeld demonstrated the radial nerve could be as close as 3 mm to this portal. To decrease the risk of injury to the radial nerve, several investigators have stressed the importance of avoiding the distal placement of this portal in favor of a more proximal placement of the anterolateral portal (2, 20). Field et al. (20) compared three lateral portals: a proximal anterolateral portal (located 2 cm proximal and 1 cm anterior to the lateral

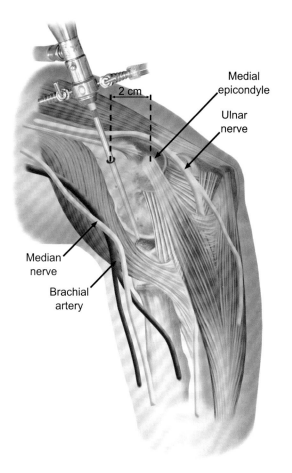

FIGURE 31.8. The arthroscope is inserted 2 cm proximal to the medial epicondyle and just anterior to the intermuscular septum on the medial aspect of the arm. In the prone position, the brachial artery and median nerve fall away from the joint capsule allowing for safe portal placement.

epicondyle), a distal anterolateral portal (as described by Andrews and Carson), and a middle anterolateral portal (located 1 cm directly anterior to the lateral epicondyle). The authors found that the proximal anterolateral portal was the safest and that the radiohumeral joint visualization was most complete and technically easiest using this most proximal portal.

After creating the proximal anteromedial portal and using it as viewing portal, we believe creating this proximal anterolateral portal is done best using an outside-in technique localizing the position with a spinal needle. This portal is created 2 cm proximal and 1 cm anterior to the lateral epicondyle as described by Field and coworkers (20). The exact entry can vary depending on the pathology to be addressed. Visualizing from the proximal anterior medial portal, the lateral capsule is visualized and palpation of the skin will help localize the exact location of the spinal needle to aid in portal placement (Fig. 31.9). It is important to direct the cannula toward the humerus while penetrating the capsule so that the portal placement is not too far anterior and medial. Viewing from the proximal anteromedial portal, the radiocapitellar joint is easily

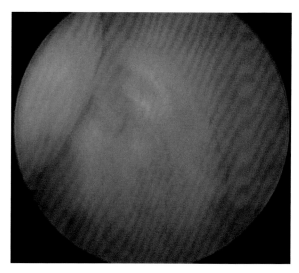

FIGURE 31.9. The lateral capsule is seen from the proximal antero-medial portal. This is the location where a spinal needle is introduced for the proximal anterolateral portal.

visualized (Fig. 31.10). The trochlea and the coronoid process can also be seen from the proximal anteromedial portal (Fig. 31.11).

The proximal anterolateral portal is often a working portal and is ideal for arthroscopic lateral epicondyle release and for debridement of the radiocapitellar joint. Viewing from this portal permits visualization of the anterior compartment (Fig. 31.12) and is particularly good in evaluating medial structures, such as the trochlea, the coronoid tip, and the medial capsule (Fig. 31.13).

Posterior Compartment

The straight posterior portal is located 3 cm proximal to the tip of the olecranon and can be used as a viewing portal or as a working portal. When it is the first portal created, a cannula

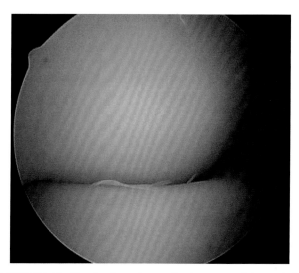

FIGURE 31.10. Viewing from the proximal anteromedial portal, the radial head, and the capitellum is easily visualized.

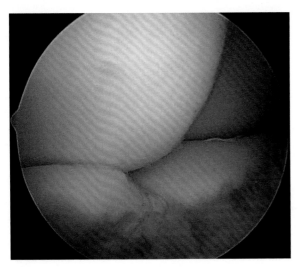

FIGURE 31.11. The trochlea *(top left)* and the coronoid process *(lower left)* can also be seen from the proximal anteromedial portal.

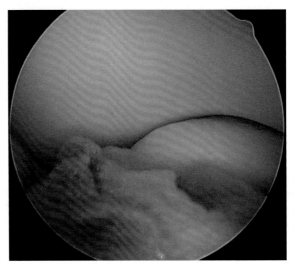

FIGURE 31.13. Viewing from the proximal anterolateral portal, the trochlea, and the coronoid process can also be seen.

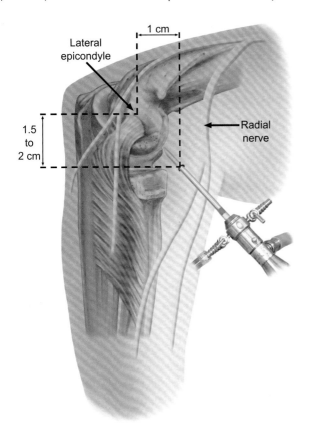

FIGURE 31.12. The proximal anterolateral portal is created 1 to 2 cm proximal to the lateral epicondyle and 1 to 2 cm anterior to the lateral epicondyle. Placing the arthroscope in the proximal anterolateral portal allows visualization of anterior compartment looking medially.

of impinging olecranon osteophytes and loose bodies from the posterior elbow joint. It is also needed when a complete synovectomy of the elbow is done (5). The straight posterior portal passes within 25 mm of the ulnar nerve and within 23 mm of the posterior antebrachial cutaneous nerve.

The posterolateral portal is located 2 to 3 cm proximal to the tip of olecranon at the lateral border of the triceps tendon. This is created while visualizing from the straight posterior portal using a spinal needle directed toward the olecranon fossa (Fig. 31.14). Initial visualization of the posterior compartment can be difficult because of synovitis, scar tissue, and fat pad hypertrophy. A trocar directed toward the olecranon fossa, passing through the triceps muscle to reach the capsule. A shaver is then introduced to improve visualization of the posterior compartment. It is important to patiently triangulate with your arthroscope and your shaver within the olecranon fossa to debride tissues in order

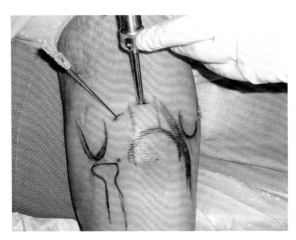

FIGURE 31.14. The arthroscope is introduced into the posterior compartment using a straight posterior portal, 3 cm proximal from the tip of the olecranon. A spinal needle is introduced lateral to the triceps tendon toward the olecranon fossa for the posterolateral portal.

with a blunt trocar is inserted. The cannula pierces the triceps muscle just above the musculotendinous junction and is bluntly maneuvered in a circular motion manipulating the soft tissues from the olecranon fossa for better visualization. When used as a working portal, it is helpful for the removal to gain adequate visualization. The tip of the olecranon is one of the first landmarks to be identified. Blindly debriding in the posterior compartment and straying outside of the olecranon fossa can cause severe iatrogenic nerve injury.

This portal permits visualization of the olecranon tip, the olecranon fossa, and the posterior trochlea and can be used a working portal to remove osteophytes and loose bodies from the posterior compartment (Fig. 31.15). However, the posterior capitellum is not well seen from this portal (5). The medial and posterior antebrachial cutaneous nerves are the two neurovascular structures at most risk; they are an average of 25 mm from this portal. The ulnar nerve is also approximately 25 mm from this portal also but as long as the cannula is kept lateral to the posterior midline, the nerve is not at risk.

The posterolateral anatomy of the elbow allows for portal placement anywhere from the proximal posterolateral portal to the lateral soft spot. Altering the portal position along the line between the posterolateral portal and the lateral soft spot changes the orientation of the portal relative to the joint (18). These portals are particularly useful for gaining access to the posterolateral recess.

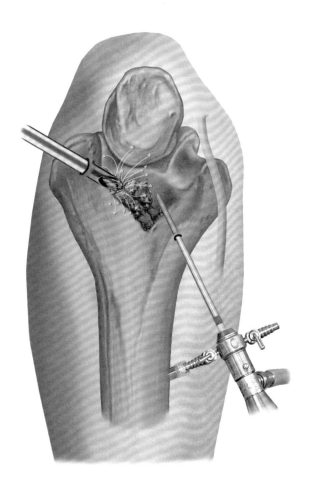

FIGURE 31.15. The posterior lateral portal is used as a working portal to remove osteophytes and loose bodies from the posterior compartment.

The direct lateral portal is located at the "soft spot," which is the triangle formed by the radial head, lateral epicondyle, and olecranon. It is developed under direct visualization using a spinal needle. It is useful as a viewing portal for working in the posterior compartment and viewing the radiocapitellar joint and for a working portal for radial head resection (13). This is the only portal that provides easy access to the posterior capitellum and radioulnar joint and can be useful for lesions of the radiocapitellar joint (5).

Diagnostic arthroscopy is useful when the clinical diagnosis is unclear and other studies have failed to lead to a diagnosis. Unexpected synovitis, osteoarthritis, loose bodies, and chondral defects may be discovered. It can also be used for the management of arthrofibrosis, osteoarthritis, and removal of olecranon spurs and for the management of OCD, fractures, and the treatment of lateral epicondylitis. Diagnostic arthroscopy along with the details of specific arthroscopic elbow procedures and rehabilitation is discussed by the many fine authors who have contributed to this section on elbow arthroscopy in the following chapters.

COMPLICATIONS

Complications due to elbow arthroscopy can be minimized if the surgeon has a sound knowledge of the anatomy of the elbow and uses proper equipment and meticulous operative technique. One of the most common complications is neurologic injury (1). including transient nerve palsies involving the radial nerve, posterior interosseous nerve, and ulnar nerve. Injury can be caused by direct laceration of a nerve by a knife penetrating deep to the skin or from the cannula trocar (6). Compression from a cannula, from fluid extravasation, or from the use of local anesthetics has also been reported to cause neurologic injuries (12) but is usually transient. Transection of the posterior interosseous nerve, the median nerve, the ulnar nerve, and the radial nerve has also been reported. In a 1986 review of 569 elbow arthroscopy procedures performed by members of the Arthroscopy Association of North America (AANA), only one neurovascular complication (radial nerve injury) was reported. In 2001, in a report of 473 elbow arthroscopies performed by experienced arthroscopists, four types of minor complications, including infection, nerve injury, prolonged drainage, and contracture, were identified in 50 cases. The most common complication was persistent portal drainage. This can be avoided by placing a box-like stay suture for closing the lateral portal.

Many of the complications associated with elbow arthroscopy are the result of inexperience, poor technique, and lack of knowledge in regard to the anatomy about the elbow. It is crucial that the surgeon who wishes to perform elbow arthroscopy safely and effectively adheres to strict surgical technique and portal placement to avoid preventable complications (6).

CONCLUSIONS AND FUTURE DIRECTIONS

Arthroscopic surgery of the elbow is a technically demanding procedure. Attention to detail including careful portal placement is necessary in order to avoid iatrogenic injury to neurovascular structures around the elbow joint. In every clinical case, the bony anatomy should be drawn on the patient's elbow and an 18G spinal needle should be used to confirm the correct portal location before introducing larger arthroscopic instruments (6). With new innovations in techniques and technology, it is possible to treat various lesions of the elbow. As with any operative procedure, careful preoperative planning including a detailed history and physical examination along with proper imaging studies is necessary along with sound clinical judgment to ensure a successful procedure. In addition, there are new frontiers of elbow arthroscopy including the treatment of olecranon bursitis, endoscopic repair of a torn distal biceps tendon, arthroscopic triceps repair, and arthroscopic ulnar nerve release.

REFERENCES

1. Poehling GG, Ekman EF. Arthroscopy of the elbow. *J Bone Joint Surg Am.* 1994;76-A(8):1265–1271.
2. Strothers D, Day B, Regan WR. Arthroscopy of the elbow: anatomy, portal sites, and description of the proximal lateral portal. *Arthroscopy.* 1995;11:449–457.
3. Andrews JR, Carson WG. Arthroscopy of the elbow. *Arthroscopy.* 1985;1:97–107.
4. Poehling GG, Whipple TL, Sisco L, et al. Elbow arthroscopy: a new technique. *Arthroscopy.* 1989;5:220–224.
5. Baker CL, Grant LJ. Arthroscopy of the elbow. *Am J Sports Med.* 1999;27(2):251–264.
6. Dodson CC, Nho SJ, Williams RJ, et al. Elbow arthroscopy. *J Am Acad Orthop Surg.* 2008;16(10):574–585.
7. Yadao MA, Field LD, Savoie FH III. Osteochondritis dissecans of the elbow. *Instr Course Lect.* 2004;53:599–606.
8. Cain EL, Dugas JR, Wolf RS, et al. Elbow injuries in throwing athletes: a current concepts review. *Am J Sports Med.* 2003;31:621–635.
9. Timmerman LA, Schwartz ML, Andrews JR. Preoperative evaluation of the ulnar ligament by magnetic resonance imaging and computed tomography arthrography. Evaluation in 25 baseball players with surgical confirmation. *Am J Sports Med.* 1994;22:26–32.
10. O'Driscoll SW, Bell DF, Morrey BF. Posterolateral rotatory instability of the elbow. *J Bone Joint Surg Am.* 1991;73A:440–446.
11. Timmerman LA, Andrews JR. Undersurface tear of the ulnar collateral ligament in baseball players. A newly recognized lesion. *Am J Sports Med.* 1994;22:33–36.
12. O'Driscoll SW, Morrey BF. Arthroscopy of the elbow. Diagnostic and therapeutic benefits and hazards. *J Bone Joint Surg Am.* 1992;74A:84–94.
13. Savoie FH, Nunley PD, Field LD. Arthroscopic management of the arthritic elbow: indications, technique, and results. *J Shoulder Elbow Surg.* 1999;8:214–219.
14. Thal R. Osteoarthritis. In: Savoie FH, Field LD, eds. *Elbow Arthroscopy.* New York, NY: Churchill Livingstone; 1996.
15. Steinmann SP, King GJ, Savoie FH. Arthroscopic treatment of the arthritic elbow. *J Bone Joint Surg Am.* 2005;87-A(9):2114–2121.
16. Field LD, Callaway GH, O'Brien SJ, et al. Arthroscopic assessment of the medial collateral ligament complex of the elbow. *Am J Sports Med.* 1995;23:396–400.
17. Field LD, Altchek DW. Evaluation of the arthroscopic valgus instability test of the elbow. *Am J Sports Med.* 1996;24:177–181.
18. Abboud JA, Ricchette ET, Tjoumakaris F, et al. Elbow arthroscopy: basic set-up and portal placement. *J Am Acad Orthop Surg.* 2006;14:312–318.
19. Ramsey ML, Naranja RJ. Diagnostic arthroscopy of the elbow. In: Baker CL Jr, Plancher DL, eds. *Operative Treatment of Elbow Injuries.* New York, NY: Springer-Verlag; 2002:162–169.
20. Field LD, Altchek DW, Warren RF, et al. Arthroscopy anatomy of the lateral elbow: a comparison of 3 portals. *Arthroscopy.* 1994;10:602–607.

SUGGESTED READINGS

Abboud JA, Ricchette ET, Tjoumakaris F, et al. Elbow arthroscopy: basic set-up and portal placement. *J Am Acad Orthop Surg.* 2006;14:312–318.

This is an up-to-date review of the basic setup and portal placement for elbow arthroscopy.

Baker CL, Grant LJ. Arthroscopy of the elbow. *Am J Sports Med.* 1999;27(2):251–264.

This "Current Concepts" is one of best reviews for elbow arthroscopy including a complete review of indications, surgical anatomy, preoperative evaluation including history, physical examination, and imaging. It also gives a detailed description of operating room setup and portal placement.

Field LD, Altchek DW, Warren RF, et al. Arthroscopy anatomy of the lateral elbow: a comparison of 3 portals. *Arthroscopy.* 1994;10:602–607.

This landmark article describes the research behind the proximal anterolateral portal and the risks of using other more distally placed anterolateral portals.

Poehling GG, Ekman EF. Arthroscopy of the elbow. *J Bone Joint Surg Am.* 1994;76-A(8):1265–1271.

This is an excellent review for the technique of elbow arthroscopy from positioning to portal placement.

Savoie FH, Nunley PD, Field LD. Arthroscopic management of the arthritic elbow: indications, technique, and results. *J Shoulder Elbow Surg.* 1999;8:214–219.

This is an excellent article for the technique of managing the arthritic elbow.

II. The Elbow

Diagnostic Elbow Arthroscopy and Loose Body Removal

Raymond R. Drabicki • Larry D. Field • Felix H. Savoie III

Despite what was thought a risky procedure, recent advances in elbow arthroscopy have enabled surgeons to treat a broad spectrum of disorders. An improved understanding of neurovascular anatomy, technologic improvements in arthroscopic equipment, and refined surgical procedures have made elbow arthroscopy safer and more effective.

Removal of loose bodies is perhaps the most common and rewarding arthroscopic procedure involving the elbow. Arthroscopic identification and removal of such impediments to joint motion have significant advantages. With careful portal placement, the arthroscope can be used to evaluate all compartments of the elbow. In addition, small portal incisions limit scar formation yet provide an outlet for easy loose body extraction.

CLINICAL EVALUATION

Pertinent History and Physical Examination

A careful history, physical examination, and appropriate imaging are imperative prior to arthroscopic excision of loose bodies and osteophytes within the elbow joint. Frequently, patients with loose bodies present with pain, stiffness, clicking, catching, and locking of the elbow joint. In some cases, these exam findings may present as subtle losses of flexion or extension accompanied with a small effusion, which is palpable in the posterolateral gutter (1).

Preoperative planning for elbow arthroscopy should always include a detailed history for prior elbow surgery, namely, ulnar nerve neurolysis or transposition. Physical examination for ulnar nerve subluxation cannot be overemphasized. A subluxated or dislocated ulnar nerve can be found in 16% of the normal population (1). Awareness of aberrant anatomy is imperative to prevent iatrogenic neural injury.

Imaging

Anteroposterior (AP) and lateral radiographs of the elbow should be routinely obtained. Figure 32.1 demonstrates the presence of a loose body in the anterior aspect of the elbow.

CT or MRI may be warranted as standard radiographs fail to demonstrate loose bodies in up to 30% of patients (1). Common locations for loose bodies include the coronoid fossa, olecranon fossa, and posterior aspect of the lateral gutter. It is important to note that loose bodies often migrate and may be difficult to see on imaging. In the absence of radiographic evidence of a loose body, high clinical suspicion should dictate arthroscopic inspection for a loose body.

Decision-Making Algorithms and Classification

Loose bodies within the elbow that cause pain, stiffness, or intermittently restrict motion are indications for surgical intervention. However, prior to surgical intervention, it is critical that the treating surgeon ascertain the etiology of these impediments to normal joint motion. Loose bodies may be the result of osteochondritis dissecans,

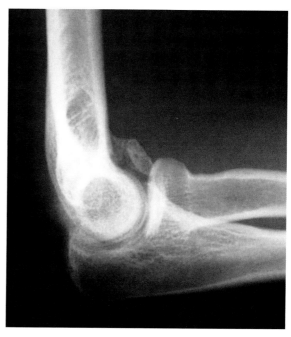

FIGURE 32.1. A large loose body can be seen in the anterior compartment of the elbow on this lateral radiograph.

degenerative arthritis, synovial chondromatosis, and trauma. A careful plan to address the primary, underlying pathology at the time of surgery serves to prevent the future formation of loose bodies (1).

At times, elbow arthroscopy may be contraindicated due to anatomic variations or prior surgery. Absolute contraindications to elbow arthroscopy include aberrant bony or soft tissue anatomy that precludes the safe portal creation. Other contraindications include ankylosis of the elbow, which precludes joint distension, and local soft tissue infection in the area of portal sites. Prior ulnar nerve transposition is a relative contraindication if it interferes with portal positioning. However, elbow arthroscopy can be utilized if the ulnar nerve is identified with open dissection and protected prior to portal creation.

TREATMENT OPTIONS

Nonoperative

Loose bodies in the elbow often present with mechanical symptoms that obstruct normal joint motion and predispose the joint to premature osteoarthritic wear. As a result, the role of conservative treatment is limited to asymptomatic loose bodies.

Operative Indications

Loose bodies in the elbow may restrict the patient's range of motion and render the joint cartilage prone to injury and arthritic degeneration. Loss of elbow motion, crepitus, pain, intermittent locking, and catching may be present on physical examination. Physical examination consistent with these findings in correlation with radiographic evidence suggestive of loose bodies in the elbow warrants arthroscopic intervention and loose body removal.

TECHNIQUE

Anesthesia

Anesthesia options include general anesthesia and regional blocks. General anesthesia is more commonly used, as it provides greater flexibility with respect to patient positioning and postoperative examination. The prone and lateral decubitus positions are poorly tolerated in an awake patient, and as a result, these positioning methods are most amenable to general anesthesia. General anesthesia also allows the surgeon to perform postoperative neurologic exams.

In patients who are unable to tolerate general anesthesia, interscalene, axillary, and regional intravenous (Bier) blocks can be used. Although these blocks can be used in combination with general anesthesia for postoperative pain management, their usage as the primary means of anesthesia has several disadvantages including limited tourniquet time, incomplete blockade of the surgical site, and pain from tourniquet constriction.

Patient Positioning

Supine

Once the patient is positioned supine on the operating table, the operative extremity is lateralized on the operating table, so that the shoulder is placed at the edge of the bed. The operative extremity is placed in 90° of shoulder abduction, 90° of elbow flexion, and neutral forearm rotation and a nonsterile arm tourniquet is applied (Fig. 32.2). Traction is applied with the use of a traction device.

The supine position offers several advantages to the elbow arthroscopist. The surgeon is easily able to convert to an open procedure if necessary. Lastly, this position enables quick access to the patient's airway and the choice of multiple effective anesthetic regimens. Disadvantages of the supine position include the necessity of a traction setup and the inability to easily visualize and work in the posterior compartment.

Prone

The prone position was described as an alternative method for positioning. Improved access to the posterior compartment of the elbow was realized, and the need for a traction apparatus was eliminated. Once the patient is intubated on a gurney, he/she are rolled to the prone position on the operating table. The face and chest are padded and supported by a foam airway/head positioner and padded chest rolls. The nonoperative extremity is positioned in 90° of shoulder abduction and neutral rotation with the elbow in 90° of flexion. The elbow and wrist are supported by a padded arm board. On the operative side, an arm board is placed parallel to the operating table centered at the shoulder level. A nonsterile arm tourniquet is applied, and the arm is placed in 90° of shoulder abduction and neutral rotation. The arm is supported at the midhumeral level by a padded bolster attached to the operating table or by a rolled towel bump, which is positioned on top of the arm board, which suspends the elbow in 90° of flexion (Fig. 32.2).

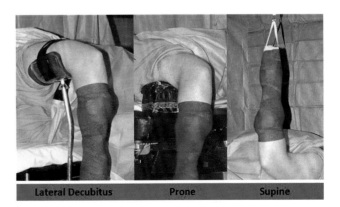

FIGURE 32.2. Three patient positions for elbow arthroscopy. Each position has inherent advantages and disadvantages with respect to anesthesia options, the need for positioning/traction devices, and the ease at which conversion to open procedures can be accomplished.

II. The Elbow

In the prone position, several advantages are realized. The elbow is easily manipulated from flexion to full extension. A traction setup and arm-positioning device are not necessary. The posterior compartment of the elbow is easily accessible. In addition, flexion of the elbow allows the neurovascular structures to sag anteriorly, providing a greater margin of error when establishing anterior portal sites. Lastly, as with the supine position, open procedures are easily performed if necessary. Drawbacks of the prone position primarily relate to patient positioning, ventilation, and anesthetic options. It is imperative to support the head and face with foam padding to secure the airway, and chest rolls are needed to facilitate ventilation. Regional anesthesia is poorly tolerated in most patients, and blocks may not provide adequate anesthesia, thus necessitating conversion to general anesthesia. In such cases, repositioning is necessary to establish an airway.

Lateral Decubitus

The aim of this position was to take advantage of the benefits of both the supine and the prone position while avoiding the major pitfalls inherent to each setup. A bean bag, sand bags, or kidney rests are used to place the patient in the lateral decubitus position. An axillary roll is appropriately placed. The operative extremity is positioned over an arm holder or over a padded bolster with the shoulder internally rotated and flexed to 90°. The elbow is maintained in 90° of flexion (Fig. 32.2).

The elbow is maintained in the prone position, thus affording the advantages of the prone position. Patient positioning is simplified with respect to prone positioning, and airway maintenance is easily monitored with adequate exposure for conversion from regional to general anesthesia. Disadvantages include the need for a padded bolster and the inconvenience of repositioning should the need for an open procedure arise.

Arthroscopic Portals

Establishing arthroscopic portals about the elbow requires a thorough understanding of the underlying neurovascular, bony, and intra-articular anatomy. Surface landmarks and their relation to underlying neurovascular anatomy should be utilized. Ten common portal sites, dictated by bony, neurovascular, and musculotendinous anatomy have been described in the literature. These portal sites can be used in various combinations to address pertinent pathology and surgical goals.

At the outset of any elbow arthroscopy procedure, it is imperative that various landmarks be localized and marked. The ulnar nerve, olecranon, radial head, medial epicondyle, and lateral epicondyle should all be traced with a marking pen. Palpating and outlining the course of the ulnar nerve cannot be overemphasized. An 18G spinal needle is then used to insufflate the elbow joint with approximately 30 cc of sterile saline. This can be accomplished either through a posterior injection into the

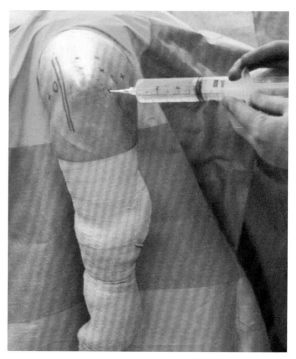

FIGURE 32.3. In the prone position, the elbow is seen with outlines of pertinent landmarks including the medial and lateral epicondyles (*circles*), ulnar nerve (*parallel lines*), and portal sites (x *marks*). Preinsufflation of the joint is demonstrated through the lateral soft spot portal.

olecranon fossa or through the lateral soft spot portal site, which is bounded by the radial head, lateral epicondyle, and olecranon (Fig. 32.3). Resistance to further inflow and often slight extension of the elbow seen as fluid is introduced confirms intra-articular injection. Distension of the joint capsule serves to protect the anterior neurovascular structures by displacing them anteriorly, and hence, further away from planned portal sites.

Proximal Anteromedial Portal

The proximal anteromedial has been recommended as the initial portal for elbow arthroscopy in the prone and lateral decubitus positions (2). Creation of this portal is suggested as it provides the best view of intra-articular structures and is less likely than the anterolateral portal to be affected by extravasation (2). The anterior elbow joint structures including the anterior capsule, coronoid process, trochlea, radial head, capitellum, and both the medial and the lateral gutters can be easily visualized.

The proximal anteromedial portal is established approximately 2 cm proximal to the medial epicondyle and just anterior to the intermuscular septum (Fig. 32.4). Placement anterior to the medial intermuscular septum reduces the risk of injuring the ulnar nerve, which courses posterior. The blunt trocar is introduced through a nick in the skin (alternatively a nick and spread technique can be employed with a small hemostat prior to trocar insertion) and advanced distally while maintaining contact with the anterior humerus. The trocar should be advanced toward

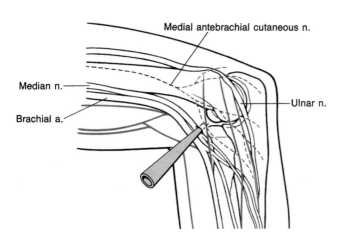

FIGURE 32.4. The position of the proximal anteromedial portal is approximately 2 cm proximal and 2 cm anterior to the medial epicondyle. The medial antebrachial cutaneous nerve is at risk when this portal is created.

the radiocapitellar joint. Maintaining contact with the humeral cortex during trocar advancement allows the brachialis muscle to serve as a partition between the trocar and the anterior neurovascular structures. The trocar enters the elbow through the tendinous origin of the flexor-pronator group and medial capsule.

Relative contraindications to creation of this portal include ulnar nerve subluxation or previous ulnar nerve transposition. It can, however, be used if open ulnar nerve localization and protection is conducted prior to portal creation. In the absence of ulnar nerve subluxation or history of transposition, the ulnar nerve is located between 12 and 23 mm from the portal site and is hence not at risk so long as the trocar entry site is placed anterior to the intermuscular septum (2).

The main neural structure at risk during creation of this portal site is the medial antebrachial cutaneous nerve as it courses approximately 2 mm from the entry site (Fig. 32.4). The median nerve is at risk as the trocar is advanced distally between the humerus and the brachialis muscle. The average distance from the trocar tip is 12 to 22 mm (2, 3).

Anteromedial Portal

The anteromedial portal is positioned 2 cm distal and 2 cm anterior to the medial epicondyle. This portal can be established with either an inside-out or an outside-in technique. The outside-in technique is accomplished by passing the blunt trocar toward the center of the joint while keeping the trocar in contact with the anterior humerus. The trocar tip is advanced through the flexor-pronator origin and into the joint at a position anterior to the medial collateral ligament.

The main neural structure at risk during creation of this portal site is the medial antebrachial cutaneous nerve as it lies within 1 to 2 mm from the portal site (3). The median nerve travels approximately 7 to 14 mm away from the portal site (3, 4). It is important to note that the safe

distance between the trocar and the nerve can be increased to 22 mm if the portal site is moved to 1 cm anterior to the medial epicondyle (2).

Proximal Anterolateral Portal

The proximal anterolateral portal is positioned approximately 2 cm proximal and 2 cm anterior to the lateral epicondyle (Fig. 32.5). As an alternative to the proximal anteromedial portal, it can be established as the initial portal in elbow arthroscopy. As the trocar is advanced distally, the brachioradialis and brachialis muscles are pierced prior to entering the lateral joint capsule toward the elbow joint. With the arthroscope placed into the cannula, the anterior capsule, lateral gutter, capitellum, radial head, coronoid, and anterolateral aspect of the ulnohumeral joint can be visualized.

Two neural structures are at risk with use of the proximal anterolateral portal. The development of the proximal anterolateral portal site was in response to the relative proximity of the radial nerve to the standard anterolateral portal (Fig. 32.5). Anatomic studies with the elbow in 90° of flexion and distended with fluid at the time of proximal anterolateral portal creation reveal a safe distance between 10 and 14 mm between the trocar and the radial nerve (3). This distance is markedly decreased to 5 to 9 mm when the standard anterolateral portal is created (3). Cutaneous sensation in the forearm can be disrupted if the posterior branch of the lateral antebrachial cutaneous nerve is injured. The pathway of this portal site lies an average of 6 mm distal from this sensory nerve (3).

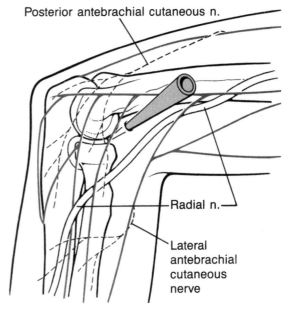

FIGURE 32.5. The position of the proximal anterolateral portal is approximately 2 cm proximal and 2 cm anterior to the lateral epicondyle. The radial nerve is at risk when this portal is created.

II. The Elbow

Anterolateral Portal

The anterolateral portal is created 3 cm distal and 1 cm anterior to the lateral epicondyle. As the blunt trocar is introduced, it passes through the extensor carpi radialis brevis muscle before transversing the lateral joint capsule. It permits visualization of the anteromedial aspect of the joint including the coronoid fossa, trochlea, coronoid process, and medial aspect of the radial head (5). In conjunction with the proximal anterolateral portal, the anterolateral portal can be utilized for procedures involving the radial head.

As with the anteromedial portal, the anterolateral portal site can be established with an inside-out technique. This can be accomplished with the aid of a proximal anteromedial or anteromedial viewing portal. In either case, the arthroscope tip is advanced to the capsule lateral to the radial head and held in this position as the arthroscope is removed from the cannula. A blunt switching stuck is then placed in the cannula and advanced through the joint capsule. The overlying tented skin is incised, the rod is advanced, and a cannula is introduced in a retrograde manner to create the anterolateral portal. Care must be taken to place the portal site lateral to the radial head as moving anterior to this position places the radial nerve at risk.

The primary structures at risk with creation of the anterolateral portal include the posterior antebrachial cutaneous and radial nerves. The distance of the portal site to these vital structures is approximately 2 mm and between 5 and 9 mm, respectively (3, 4).

Midlateral Portal

The midlateral portal can also be referred to as the direct lateral or the soft spot portal. The surface landmarks used to locate this portal are the lateral epicondyle, olecranon process, and the radial head. An 18G spinal needle can be inserted into the center of this triangular area for joint insufflation with sterile saline. When establishing this portal, the trocar is advanced through the anconeus muscle and entry to the lateral elbow joint is attained through the posterior elbow capsule. Visualization of the radioulnar joint, capitellum, and inferior aspect of the radial head can be achieved through this portal. In addition, this portal provides a safe entry site for instrumentation of the radiocapitellar joint and lateral gutter.

The midlateral portal is relatively safe. Injuries to the posterior antebrachial cutaneous nerve, which courses approximately 7 mm away, can occur (6). Drawbacks to creation of this include soft tissue fluid extravasation and the risk of iatrogenic articular cartilage damage, which stems from the limited space available for portal entry.

Straight Posterior Portal

The straight posterior portal is located 3 cm proximal to the tip of the olecranon in the midline (Fig. 32.6). In this position, the entire posterior compartment can be

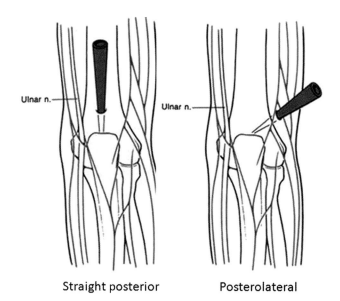

FIGURE 32.6. The straight posterior portal is established approximately 3 cm proximal to the olecranon tip, and the posterolateral portal is made 3 cm proximal to the olecranon tip and immediately lateral to the triceps tendon. These portals can be used interchangeably for working in the posterior compartment.

visualized in addition to the medial and lateral gutters. As the blunt trocar is advanced through the triceps tendon and joint capsule, it is placed directly upon the bone of the olecranon fossa. With the trocar held in place, the cannula is advanced to the bone. The extravasation of fluid with trocar removal confirms successful entry, and the arthroscope can subsequently be introduced. This portal also provides an alternative site for insufflation of the joint with an 18G spinal needle and sterile saline.

Posterolateral Portal

The location of the posterolateral portal is 3 cm proximal to the olecranon tip and immediately lateral to the triceps tendon (Fig. 32.6). Insertion of the trocar is directed toward the olecranon fossa passing just lateral to the triceps tendon and through the posterolateral joint capsule. Visualization of the olecranon fossa and both the medial and the lateral gutters is realized through this portal site.

The posterolateral portal can be used interchangeably with the straight posterior portal for viewing and instrumentation of the olecranon fossa and the lateral and medial gutters. It is imperative to be cognizant of the ulnar nerve location when instrumenting the medial gutter. The ulnar nerve is susceptible to injury posterior to the medial epicondyle where it transverses obliquely just superficial to the medial capsule of the elbow (4).

Accessory Posterolateral Portal

The posterolateral aspect of the elbow consists of the olecranon process and radiocapitellar joint. This portal is useful for the excision of a lateral olecranon spur or posterolateral plica. The placement of this portal can be accomplished in the area between the midlateral portal and the posterolateral portal, which is 3 cm proximal to the olecranon tip. Spinal needle localization under direct visualization is suggested for accurate portal placement to address pertinent pathology. Transillumination through the skin can be used to aid correct needle placement. Although there is limited risk to neurovascular structures, the triceps tendon and ulnohumeral articulation are at risk for iatrogenic damage with errant trocar or instrument placement (7).

AUTHORS' PREFERRED TREATMENT

The patient is positioned in the prone position with attention to pad all pertinent prominences and secure the airway. The shoulder is placed in 90° of abduction and neutral rotation with the elbow suspended in 90° of flexion (Fig. 32.2: prone). A nonsterile upper arm tourniquet is applied. An arm board, parallel to the operating table, centered under the shoulder supports a rolled towel bump and the operative extremity. A Duraprep solution is used to prep the arm and forearm. An impervious, sterile stockinette is applied to the hand and covered with self-adherent Coban to seal the hand and forearm contents from the operative field. Standard sterile draping is conducted followed by exsanguination of the limb with an esmarch bandage. The tourniquet is inflated.

All pertinent landmarks are outlined with emphasis upon locating the ulnar nerve, olecranon process, and medial and lateral epicondyles (Fig. 32.3). The course of the ulnar nerve is palpated, and it is evaluated for subluxation. An 18G spinal needle is introduced into the straight posterior portal site, and the joint is insufflated with 30 cc of sterile saline until resistance is felt (Fig. 32.3).

The proximal anteromedial portal site is established first 2 cm proximal to the epicondyle and immediately anterior to the intermuscular septum (Fig. 32.4). A blunt trocar and cannula for a 4.5-mm arthroscope are introduced through a nick made in the skin with a no. 11 blade knife and advanced distally toward the radiocapitellar joint. The trocar is advanced while in contact with the anterior aspect of the humerus, which ensures protection of the anterior neurovascular structures by the brachialis muscle. An egress of fluid with trocar removal confirms intra-articular placement. The 30° 4.5-mm arthroscope is introduced, and a diagnostic arthroscopy of the anterior compartment ensues.

The proximal anteromedial portal, if appropriately placed, permits a systematic evaluation of the lateral gutter, radial head, capitellum, anterior capsule, trochlea, coronoid process, and the medial gutter. The radiocapitellar joint is assessed for instability and articular cartilage damage with pronation and supination aiding the evaluation. Next, the 30° arthroscope lens is rotated to facilitate evaluation of the anterior capsule and extensor carpi radialis brevis tendon insertion. The coronoid and

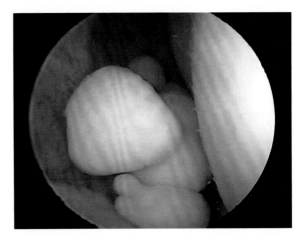

FIGURE 32.7. Multiple large loose osteochondral loose bodies are visualized in the anterior compartment of the elbow.

trochlea are then evaluated by withdrawing the scope and repositioning the lens of the arthroscope.

Loose bodies in the anterior compartment of the elbow are often found within the coronoid fossa (Fig. 32.7). Extraction of these osteochondral fragments is conducted after establishing a proximal anterolateral portal under direct spinal needle localization. The skin entry site for this portal is 2 cm proximal to the lateral epicondyle and 2 cm anteriorly. The spinal needle is removed and a no. 11 blade knife is used to incise skin only. A blunt trocar and cannula are inserted into the elbow while maintaining constant contact with the anterior humeral cortex, as the trocar is advanced. A meniscal grasper is introduced through the proximal anterolateral portal and used to remove any loose bodies (Fig. 32.8). If the size of the osteochondral fragment exceeds that of the cannula, it may be necessary to remove the fragment piecemeal with the use of a motorized shaver. In certain cases where the fragment is larger than the cannula, the grasper can be used to pull the cannula and fragment through the soft tissue and out of the body together. This can be accomplished by rotating

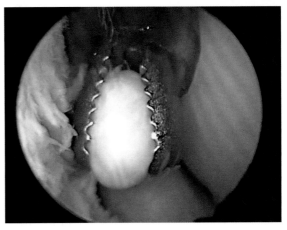

FIGURE 32.8. A meniscal grasper is utilized for the removal of a large loose body from the anterior compartment of the elbow.

II. The Elbow

the grasper as it is removed from the soft tissues while maintaining a firm grasp on the fragment. Alternatively, a spinal needle may be needed to skewer and stabilize the loose body for retrieval with a grasper (Fig. 32.9).

After a thorough evaluation and treatment of pathology in the anterior compartment, attention is focused on the posterior compartment. The water inflow is generally switched to the proximal anteromedial cannula (6). The straight posterior portal is established using a no. 11 blade knife 3 cm proximal to the tip of the olecranon (Fig. 32.6). After introducing the 30° 4.5-mm arthroscope into the straight posterior portal, the posterolateral portal is created 3 cm proximal to the olecranon tip just lateral to the triceps tendon under direct spinal needle localization (Fig. 32.6). Commonly, a motorized shaver in the posterolateral portal is used to remove soft tissue, obscuring the view to the olecranon fossa. The straight posterior portal and the posterolateral portal can be used interchangeably for removal of loose bodies. The olecranon fossa should be evaluated in its entirety, as it is a common source of loose bodies especially when osteoarthritis is present.

The arthroscope is then introduced into the medial gutter from the straight posterior portal. A milking maneuver can be performed from a distal to proximal direction on the medial side of the elbow, which often will propel loose bodies posteriorly and into view (8). In the lateral aspect of the elbow, entry through an accessory posterolateral portal or midlateral portal is needed for debridement. These portals are localized under direct visualization with a spinal needle. Transillumination of the skin can aid in correct spinal needle placement. A cannula, trocar, and then motorized shaver are introduced through the established portal. Often a soft tissue plica or synovial band may need to be excised with the shaver for adequate visualization. In this posterolateral location, loose bodies

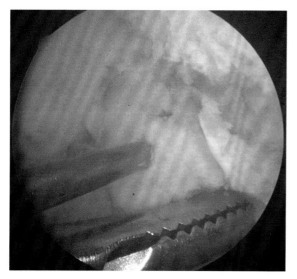

FIGURE 32.9. A spinal needle can be used to skewer a large loose body in the posterior compartment of the elbow to facilitate retrieval with a grasper.

are often "hidden," and it is imperative that a thorough evaluation be performed.

Following arthroscopic examination and removal of all loose bodies in the anterior and posterior compartments, the arthroscopic equipment is removed, steri-strips are applied to the portal sites, and the lateral portal sites are sutured with nylon suture to help prevent fistula formation. A sterile dressing is applied, allowing the elbow to move freely in an arc of flexion-extension and pronation-supination.

COMPLICATIONS, CONTROVERSIES, AND SPECIAL CONSIDERATIONS

Iatrogenic neurovascular injury is the most devastating complication of arthroscopic elbow surgery. Although most nerve palsies are transient, the reported complication rate for nerve injury in the literature ranges from 0% to 17%. Attributable causes include direct injury from trocars and motorized shavers, fluid extravasation, overaggressive joint distension, and inadvertent injury to cutaneous nerves when incising the skin for portal placement. These neural injuries are also more likely to occur with the usage of anteromedial and anterolateral portal sites, which inherently lie closer to neural structures. The anteromedial portal has been correlated with injuries to the median and anterior interosseous nerve, whereas the anterolateral portal has been associated with injuries to the radial, posterior interosseous, and superficial branch of the radial nerve. Other complications in elbow arthroscopy include iatrogenic injury to articular cartilage, draining portal sites, and arthrofibrosis.

PEARLS AND PITFALLS

Elbow arthroscopy and loose body removal can be safely and effectively performed if several key steps and clinical pearls are followed. Define and mark the course of the ulnar nerve and also assess whether or not it is dislocated or subluxable. If the location of the nerve is in question, dissect out the nerve prior to establishing portals. Preinsufflate the elbow prior to portal creation. Keep the elbow flexed at 90° when establishing portals to maximize the safe distance from neurovascular structures. Avoid the anteromedial and anterolateral portals when possible. Do not use pressurized insufflation pumps to avoid extravasation. Use sharp dissection through skin only, and use only blunt trocars. Lastly, avoid using suction, which can cause capsular collapse and inadvertent neurovascular injury.

REHABILITATION

In the postoperative period, the main goal is to restore a full range of motion. Usage of the patient's extremity should be encouraged immediately postoperatively. Splints should not be used. Surgical bandaging should not interfere with early flexion, extension, supination, and pronation. A home exercise program should be instituted. At 1-week time, patients should return to the office for a wound check and monitoring ranges of motion. Aggressive physical therapy should commence if improvements in motion are not attained.

CONCLUSIONS AND FUTURE DIRECTIONS

The success rates of arthroscopic loose body removal from the elbow approaches 90% when performed safely and methodically. It is critical to address the primary pathology that is responsible for loose body production, as failure to do so will likely result in limited patient improvement over time. This is especially true in the case of osteoarthritis.

REFERENCES

1. Field LD, Savoie FH. Management of loose bodies and other limited procedures. In: Morrey BF, Sanchez-Sotelo J, eds. *The Elbow and Its Disorders*. Philadelphia, PA: Saunders Elsevier; 2009:578–586.
2. Lindenfield TN. Medial approach in elbow arthroscopy. *Am J Sports Med*. 1990;18:413–417.
3. Stothers K, Day B, Reagan WR. Arthroscopy of the elbow: anatomy, portal sites, and a description of the proximal lateral portal. *Arthroscopy*. 1995;11:449–457.
4. Lynch GJ, Meyers JF, Whipple TL. Neurovascular anatomy and elbow arthroscopy: inherent risks. *Arthroscopy*. 1986;2:191–197.
5. Field LD, Altchek DW, Warren RF. Arthroscopic anatomy of the lateral elbow: a comparison of three portals. *Arthroscopy*. 1994;10:602–607.
6. Aboud JA, Ricchetti ET, Tjoumakaris F, et al. Elbow arthroscopy: basic setup and portal placement. *J Am Acad Orthop Surg*. 2006;14:312–318.
7. Savoie FH, Field LD. Anatomy. In: Savoie FH, Field LD, eds. *Arthroscopy of the Elbow*. New York, NY: Churchill Livingstone; 1996:3–24.
8. Plancher KD, Peterson RK, Breezenoff L. Diagnostic arthroscopy of the elbow: set-up, portals, and technique. *Oper Tech Sports Med*. 1998;6:2–10.

II. The Elbow

Arthroscopic Management of Osteochondritis Dissecans of the Elbow

Chris Pokabla • Felix H. Savoie III

KEY POINTS

- Osteochondritis dissecans (OCD) of the elbow is a disorder common in young repetitive-motion athletes.
- Although often characterized by inflammation, pain, and loss of motion, the pathologic changes within the bone itself have no inflammatory cells.
- Nonoperative management includes elimination of the secondary inflammatory changes by the use of anti-inflammatory modalities combined with elimination of the stress to the capitellum by rest and the use of an off-loading hinged elbow brace.
- Nonoperative management is most effective when the cartilage cap overlying the lesion is intact.
- Surgical intervention may take several forms when the disorder either does not respond to nonoperative management or is discovered in a later stage.
- Percutaneous fixation of nondisplaced lesions is an attractive option when there is enough bone in the loose fragment to allow purchase of the fixation device.
- Arthroscopic removal of loose bodies, excision of an inflamed posterolateral plica, and microfracture of the residual defect may be of benefit in the intermediate stages.
- In cases in which these options fail or in which there is extensive destruction of the bone and involvement of the extreme lateral cortex or "shoulder" of the capitellum, osteochondral grafting may be indicated.
- Results of each treatment modality are quite good, with success rates reported between 66% and 95%.
- The primary complications include loss of motion, early arthritis, and a failure to return to the same level of competition.

OCD is a localized condition involving the articular surface that results in the separation of a segment of articular cartilage and subchondral bone. Konig was the first to report on this condition in 1888 as an entity that produces loose bodies in the hip and knee in the absence of direct trauma. The term osteochondritis means an inflammation of bone and cartilage, whereas the word dissecans is derived from the Latin word "dissec," meaning to separate. The use of this term has persisted despite the absence of inflammatory cells in histologic sections of excised osteochondral fragments.

Panner first described OCD in the elbow as a lesion that appeared similar to Legg–Calves–Perthes disease. The most common site of OCD of the elbow is the capitellum, with the lesion typically involving the central or anterolateral portion. However, lesions have also been reported in the trochlea, radial head, olecranon, and olecranon fossa.

The exact etiology of OCD remains unproven; however, most research suggests that repetitive microtrauma plays an integral role in the pathophysiology. There is also evidence to support an ischemic theory for the development of OCD. Haraldsson demonstrated that the immature capitellar epiphysis is supplied by one or two isolated vessels that enter the epiphysis posteriorly and traverse the cartilaginous epiphysis to supply the capitellum. No contribution was detected from the metaphyseal vasculature. The structure of this blood supply may predispose the capitellum toward osteonecrosis.

Elbow OCD typically occurs in athletes aged 11 to 21 years who report a history of overuse. Adolescent athletes engaged in repetitive stress activities such as baseball, gymnastics, cheerleading, and swimming are at highest risk for the development of OCD. Males are affected more frequently than females and symptoms are typically seen in the dominant arm.

Several authors have commented on the relationship between this condition, baseball pitching, and competitive gymnastics. The creation of compressive and/or shearing forces in the radiocapitellar joint is believed to be the common denominator. The radiocapitellar joint acts as a secondary stabilizer of the elbow, in addition to accepting up to 60% of the force of compressive axial loads. The valgus stress on the elbow during the cocking phase of throwing creates a substantial compressive load at the radiocapitellar joint. This force may be responsible for the creation of subchondral fractures or the disruption of a tenuous blood supply to the capitellum.

CLINICAL EVALUATION

History

OCD is primarily a disorder of the young athlete. The usual age of presentation is 12 to 14 years of age, compared with 9 to 10 for Panner's disease. Males are affected more often than females, but there is a high prevalence in young female gymnasts and competitive cheerleaders. The dominant arm is most often involved with bilateral involvement in 5% to 20% of patients. There is usually a history of overuse, most commonly throwing, repetitive impact, or overhead sports. Early on, the symptoms may be obscure, with pain location difficult to determine. It most often begins with some mild aching after activity. Most patients will try self-medicating with anti-inflammatory medicine and ice, which may provide some temporary relief. Symptoms will often worsen very slowly. On presentation, the history is most often that of pain that increases with increased activity, loss of motion, and swelling on the lateral side of the elbow. Additional complaints of popping, clicking, or sudden "giving way," especially with load bearing, may also be present.

Physical Examination

The classic physical findings include loss of terminal extension and swelling along the posterolateral joint line along with inflammation of the normal posterolateral plica. Valgus extension overload testing will produce pain over the lateral aspect of the elbow and result in a measurable increase in the loss of terminal extension. This is one of the key differentiating factors in the physical examination of OCD. Most throwing or hyperextension overuse injuries when tested in valgus will have the primary component of pain along the medial aspect of the elbow: the medial apophysis, the medial ulnar collateral ligament, or the flexor-pronator muscle. These may coexist with the OCD, but in OCD patients these instability stress maneuvers, especially the moving valgus overload test, will result in pain more on the lateral than on the medial side.

Imaging

The initial testing involves standard PA and lateral radiographs. These will usually show the classic findings of radiolucency in the central aspect of the capitellum. There may be a small area of increased opacity in the center of the radiolucency (Fig. 33.1). In the later stages, loose bodies may be present.

Additional testing may be warranted early in the course of treatment. Computed tomography (CT), CT arthrograms, and ultrasound have all been utilized in the evaluation of these lesions. However, MRI has become the standard modality for evaluation of these lesions.

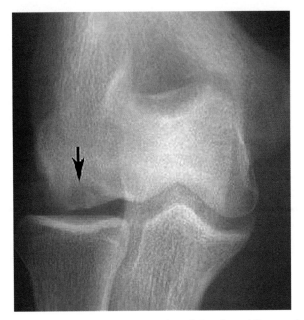

FIGURE 33.1. This posteroanterior view of the elbow delineates the area of radiolucency in the mid-capitellum, indicative of an early OCD lesion.

The key points to evaluate that will assist in determining appropriate management include the extent of the bone involvement, the integrity of the overlying cartilage cap, and the presence of loose bodies. Early lesions will show change on T1-weighted MRI images, but no change on T2 sequences. The cartilage covering will be intact, indicating an improved prognosis. Advanced lesions will show changes on both T1 and T2 images and may demonstrate a loose in situ bone fragment (Fig. 33.2). Assessment of the

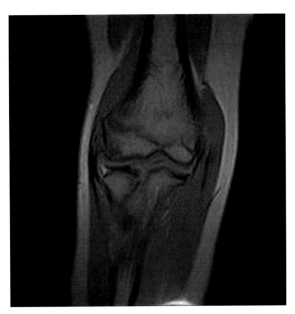

FIGURE 33.2. Magnetic resonance imaging may indicate either an intact or a disrupted cartilage cap as well as the presence of loose bodies within the defect.

integrity of the cartilage cap remains paramount. As the condition advances, the cartilage cap is violated, allowing synovial fluid between the fragment and the remaining capitellum. This jeopardizes any chance at union with fixation and may result in one or more loose fragments being shed into the joint. However, the simple presence of loose bodies does not definitively define a rupture of the cartilage, so MRI assessment remains necessary. The lesion that advances to the lateral edge or "shoulder" of the capitellum is a much more severe injury that requires more extensive reconstructive surgery (Fig. 33.3). In the most advanced cases, three-dimensional (3D) imaging may be helpful to define the loss of this critical lateral cortex (Fig. 33.4A–C).

Classification

The initial attempt at classification was a radiologic one by Minami et al. based on lateral radiographs: Grade I lesions demonstrate a shadow in the middle of the capitellum. Grade II lesions have a clear zone between the lesion and the adjacent subchondral bone. Grade III lesions are those with one or more loose bodies. Bradley and Petrie subdivided this classification to include MRI as a part of the classification. Baumgarten et al. classified the lesions according to the appearance on arthroscopy based on Ferkel's classification of similar lesions of the talus. However, none of these schemes have consistently been able to predict the course of the disease process and thus are of limited value.

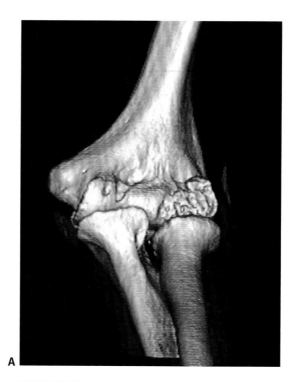

A

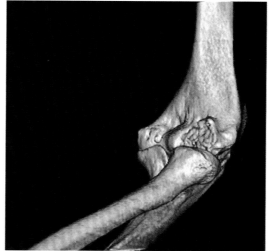

B

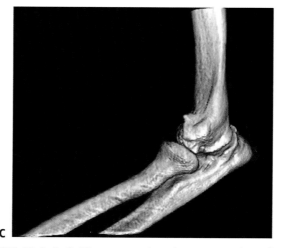

C

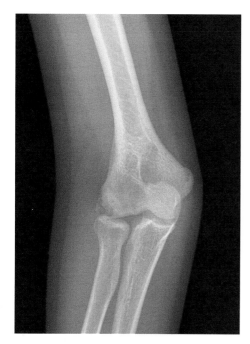

FIGURE 33.3. A late-stage OCD lesion as seen on a PA radiograph. Note the extension into the lateral aspect of the capitellum, usually indicative of a poor result with standard microfracture techniques. In these cases, osteochondral grafting may be utilized to reconstruct the "shoulder" or lateral cortical aspect of the capitellum.

FIGURE 33.4. A–C: 3D reconstructions demonstrating loss of the critical lateral cortex.

TREATMENT

Nonoperative

Treatment options for OCD remain controversial. Options vary from a total cessation of any irritating activities to immediate surgery. The current classification systems do not help in predicting the course of treatment or the prognosis. The critical determinant in the senior author's opinion is the presence or absence of an intact cartilage cap. Patients with intact articular cartilage should be managed nonoperatively. Patients with disruption of the articular cartilage cap may still be managed nonoperatively, but with less chance for a full recovery.

The hallmark of nonoperative treatment is rest and cessation of aggravating activities. This restriction is continued until symptoms resolve (usually 6 to 12 weeks) and radiographs or MRI shows complete healing of the lesion (6 to 12 months). This lengthy recovery may be too long for most patients and families to tolerate, resulting in a too early return to sports and recurrence and worsening of the problem.

One alternative method of management has been the protection of these lesions with an off-loading hinged elbow brace. The straight hinge changes the normal valgus tilt of the elbow and off-loads the lateral side, protecting the capitellum from injury. Initially the brace is set at the limits of pain-free range of motion, often as limited as 60° to 90°. As the inflammation in the plica decreases and pain-free motion increases, the brace is loosened to allow full range of motion. Sports and normal activities are allowed with the brace in place as long as symptoms do not occur during these activities. Utilization of this form of treatment allows the patient to continue normal activities without aggravating the lesion. In most cases, the patient is able to return to normal activities with the brace in place within 2 weeks of initiating treatment. The time of the normal healing process remains unchanged, and close monitoring with monthly radiographs and quarterly MRI is necessary to adequately follow the healing process if this treatment method is chosen.

Operative Indications

Progression of the disease process, the presence of symptomatic loose bodies, or disruption of the cartilage cap that continues despite rest, bracing, and cessation of activity may be considered indications for surgery. Arthroscopic evaluation of the lesion along with removal of the loose fragments and debridement of the base is currently the mainstay of operative management. Although much of the older literature focused on open management, most current studies delineate the efficacy of arthroscopic treatment.

OPERATIVE TECHNIQUE

The operative technique begins with a diagnostic arthroscopy of the anterior compartment of the elbow. In these cases, it is most useful to begin with a proximal anterior-medial portal for the arthroscope and visualize the radiocapitellar joint. In most cases, the anterior aspect of the capitellum is normal. In the case of a more anterior lesion, the 70° arthroscope may be utilized here to visualize and the anterolateral portal to manage the lesion, but the damage is usually more posterior and best treated by visualizing from posterior. The anterior compartment is then evaluated for loose bodies, which are removed through the anterolateral portal if necessary. The inflow is then left on the cannula in the proximal anterior medial portal and the posterior compartment of the elbow entered. The olecrenon fossa is also evaluated for loose bodies, which are removed through a posterior central or posterior lateral portal. The medial gutter is similarly evaluated for loose bodies and inflammation. Attention is then directed to the lateral gutter. The posterolateral plica is evaluated and removed through a soft spot posterolateral portal if there is any inflammation or thickening. The capitellum is then visualized from both the posterolateral and the soft spot portal and the degree of involvement of the capitellum assessed and documented. If operative management is indicated, the OCD lesion is best visualized through a superior posterolateral portal with a 70° arthroscope. This leaves the soft spot, straight lateral, and inferior straight lateral portals free for instrumentation (Fig. 33.5A, B). The cartilage cap may be probed through these portals for softness and fissures. Increasing the flexion of the elbow may be necessary to visualize the entire lesion.

Microfracture

In cases in which the preoperative workup has shown a large, repairable fragment, fixation in situ is accomplished through the inferior straight lateral portal under arthroscopic and fluoroscopic control using standard fixation techniques. In most cases, this is not an option, and a full-radius shaver is introduced and the necrotic bone debrided to a stable bed. All loose bodies are removed as well. A stable rim of cartilage is left in place. It is important to preserve the lateral aspect of the capitellum (the shoulder) as it provides both bone stability and the attachment of the lateral capsule and ligaments. Once the debridement has been completed, the base of the lesion is microfractured to stimulate increased blood flow.

Fragment Fixation

Occasionally one may encounter a large and viable fragment. In these cases, the fragment is "hinged" open and the base debrided. The fragment is then replaced into the defect and stabilized using a Kirschner wire. Many techniques for permanent stabilization have been described, including Herbert–Whipple screw fixation, retrograde suturing, cancellous screws, and bioabsorbable implants.

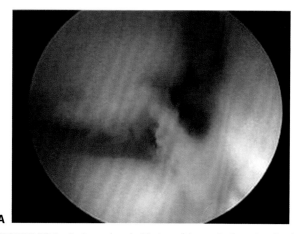
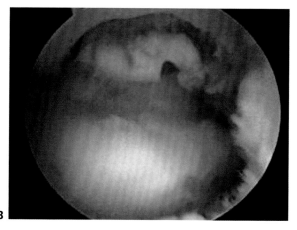

FIGURE 33.5. **A:** Osteochondral lesion of the capitellum visualized with a 30° arthroscope from the posterolateral portal with the patient in the prone position. The radial head is below and the lateral capsule to the right. The capitellum is at the top left of the figure. **B:** The OCD lesion of the capitellum as visualized from the same portal with a 70° arthroscope. Note the radial head below and the capitellum above with a loose lesion in the center.

Osteochondral Autograft Transfer and Synthetics

In the most severe cases osteochondral grafting from the knee, ribs, synthetics, or allograft has been reported. None of the synthetic implants have been approved for use in this area and their use should be considered experimental at this time. In these cases the procedure is as listed above for debridement and then the distal soft spot or distal lateral posterior portal is used to place the plugs. The elbow must be hyperflexed to allow correct orientation of the implants, which are then contoured to match the capitellar surface (Fig. 33.6A–D).

AUTHORS' PREFERRED METHOD

The senior author (F.H.S.) prefers nonoperative management in most cases of early lesions. If the radiographs and MRI reveal an intact cartilage cap or a relatively small (8 mm or less) lesion, then the patient is managed with full-time hinged elbow bracing and physical therapy. Once the elbow is pain free, the patient is allowed to return to sports with the brace in place and with improvement of core strength, posture, and correction of any improper sporting techniques that may produce increased stress on the elbow. The patient is allowed to return to sports with the brace in place once the elbow has regained a full and painless arc of motion. All activities are allowed with the brace in place until radiographic evidence of healing occurs. In the case of female gymnasts, we usually recommend quarterly MRI if possible and also will suggest radiographs and at least one MRI of the opposite, asymptomatic elbow.

If the patient has loose bodies, extensive involvement of the capitellum, or progression of the disease, then surgery is recommended. The procedure is performed arthroscopically with removal of loose bodies and debridement and drilling of the base of the lesion. Large lesions

are repaired with a cannulated Herbert–Whipple-type screw, but this type of lesion is rare in our practice. In the more extensive lesions with loss of the lateral cortex, we use osteochondral grafting with the proximal olecranon as the source of the graft.

COMPLICATIONS

Complications include recurrence or advancement of the lesion, arthrofibrosis, and heterotopic ossification. Advancement may occur despite adequate nonoperative treatment. Arthrofibrosis, or stiffness, is often present preoperatively and also may occur postoperatively. Most cases respond to nonoperative protocols, but capsular release or resection may be indicated in refractory cases. Heterotopic ossification occurs more frequently after open surgery. In the early stage, it may be addressed by arthroscopic excision and radiation. Later stages require open excision with exploration and protection of the nearby neurologic structures along with radiation therapy. In most studies, the more extensive lesions were associated with increased risk of arthritis, stiffness, and ongoing pain. Failure to return to sport at the preinjury level is quite common, occurring 10% to 20% of the time in the best case series.

SPECIAL CONSIDERATIONS

The elite female gymnast/competitive cheerleader represents a special population. Although osteochondrosis (Panner's disease) is more common in this age range (under 10), the lesions in these athletes behave more like a severe osteochondritis. It may often occur bilaterally and should be managed in an aggressive but nonoperative manner. In these patients, evaluation of the opposite elbow by radiographs and MRI is recommended.

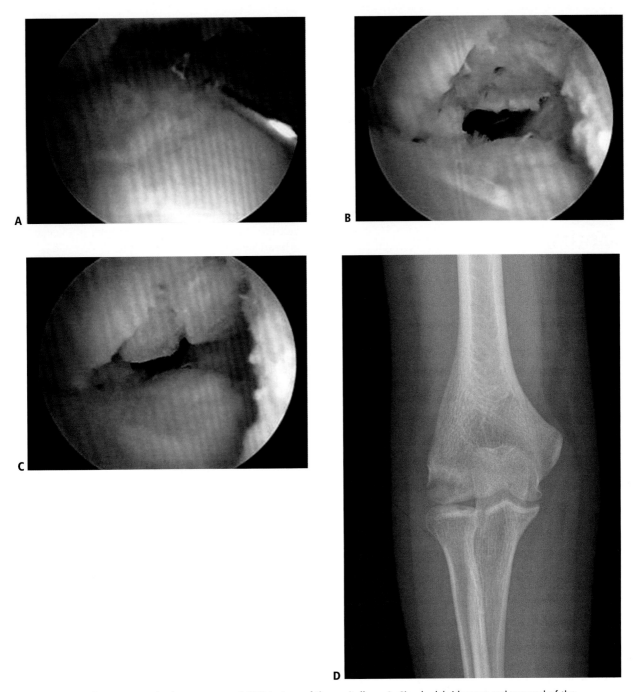

FIGURE 33.6. The sequences in the treatment of OCD lesions of the capitellum. **A:** Simple debridement and removal of the loose fragment. The arthroscope is in the posterolateral superior portal, and the instruments are through the distal soft spot portal. **B:** Drilling and/or microfracture of the residual defect to stimulate cartilage formation. The capitellar defect is above and the radial head below in this view from the superior soft spot portal. **C:** In rare late-stage OCD or when the lateral aspect of the capitellum has been compromised, arthroscopic osteochondral grafting may be indicated to bolster the lateral joint and possibly prevent instability and progressive arthritis. Note the two plugs within the center of the defect. **D:** Radiograph of the patient in **(C)** 6 weeks postosteochondral grafting, revealing reconstitution of the lateral cortex or "shoulder" of the capitellum.

Jackson et al. presented the classic article on elite female gymnasts with osteochondritis and found only 1 of 10 was able to continue her career. Surgery in these patients will often end their career, so early detection and management by bracing and protection are essential. Surgery should be undertaken with great reluctance and with full knowledge of the possibility of a good objective patient outcome but poor subjective athletic result.

PEARLS AND PITFALLS

1. Lateral elbow pain in a repetitive athlete should signal a warning sign of OCD.
2. Presenting symptoms are loss of motion and swelling on the lateral aspect of the elbow.
3. Radiographs may be equivocal, but, MRI is diagnostic.
4. Early detection and treatment give the best results.
5. Gymnasts/competitive cheerleaders look bilaterally.
6. Bracing assists nonoperative management.
7. Arthroscopic surgery is typically successful but results in <90% return to sport.

REHABILITATION

In most cases of debridement, the patient is started on a CPM machine on the day of surgery. The elbow is placed in a brace to off-load the capitellum. Physical therapy for gentle stretching, compressive pumping out of edema, and hand and wrist exercises are initiated as early as possible, usually within 1 week of surgery. The patient is started on general conditioning within the first 3 weeks of surgery. The elbow is followed clinically and with serial radiographs. Once pain-free range of motion and satisfactory strength are obtained, return to sports is allowed. This is variable and can be expected to occur between 6 and 16 weeks.

DISCUSSION

There is no level-one study available on OCD of the elbow. Most long-term studies are case series identified retrospectively.

Takahara followed 24 patients with OCD of the capitellum nonoperatively for an average of 5.2 years and found the results correlated directly with the severity of the lesion on presentation, with 6 of 11 "early" lesions healing or improving. In the same year, he presented a comparison study of 53 patients with 14 managed nonoperatively and 39 managed by surgery. The end results correlated mostly with the size of the lesion rather than type of treatment; however, this was not a randomized study.

Surgery in athletes has been reported through several case series with mixed results. Baumgarten et al. and Ruch et al. have reported relatively good results with short-term follow-up after arthroscopic debridement. In both series, more extensive lesions at the time of treatment had less successful results.

In contrast to the above work, Byrd and Jones presented a retrospective cohort series of ten baseball players treated arthroscopically. In their series, only four patients returned to unrestricted play and five patients developed arthrofibrosis. Other series have echoed the findings of the above authors with results related to the size of the lesion rather than treatment.

FUTURE DIRECTIONS

Future treatment may involve osteochondral grafting for more severe defects. El Attreche and Savoie have presented (but not published) cases of osteochondral grafts placed for loss of the structural integrity of the capitellum with satisfactory short-term results.

SUGGESTED READINGS

Konig F. Ueber freie Korper in den Gelenken. *Deutsche Zeitschr Chir* 1887;27:90–109.

Panner HJ. A peculiar affection of the capitulum humeri, resembling Calve Perthes' disease of the hip. *Acta Radiol.* 1927;10:234–242.

Haraldsson S. The vascular pattern of a growing and fullgrown human epiphysis. *Acta Anat (Basel).* 1962;48:156–167.

Minami M, Nakashita K, Ishii S. Twenty-five cases of osteochondritis dissecans of the elbow. *Rinsho Seikei Geka.* 1979;14:805–810.

Bradley JP, Petrie RS. Osteochondritis dissecans of the humeral capitellum: diagnosis and treatment. *Clin Sports Med.* 2001;20:565–590.

Baumgarten TE, Andrews JR, Satterwhite YE. The arthroscopic classification and treatment of osteochondritis dissecans of the capitellum. *Am J Sports Med.* 1998;26:520–523.

Jackson DW, Silvino N, Reiman P. Osteochondritis in the female gymnast's elbow. *Arthroscopy.* 1989;5:129–136.

Oka Y, Ikeda M. Treatment of severe osteochondritis dissecans of the elbow using osteochondral grafts from a rib. *J Bone Joint Surg Br.* 2001;83:738–739.

Takahara M, Ogino T, Fukushima S, et al. Nonoperative treatment of osteochondritis dissecans of the humeral capitellum. *Am J Sports Med.* 1999;27:728–732.

Takahara M, Ogino T, Sasaki I, et al. Long term outcome of osteochondritis dissecans of the humeral capitellum. *Clin Orthop.* 1999;363:108–115.

Ruch DS, Cory JW, Poehling GG. The arthroscopic management of osteochondritis dissecans of the adolescent elbow. *Arthroscopy.* 1998;14:797–803.

Byrd JW, Jones KS. Arthroscopic surgery for isolated capitellar osteochondritis dissecans in adolescent baseball players: minimum three-year follow-up. *Am J Sports Med.* 2002; 30:474–478.

The Stiff Elbow: Degenerative Joint Disease and Arthrofibrosis

Steven A. Giuseffi • Scott P. Steinmann

The operative treatment of the stiff and/or arthritic elbow has traditionally included open joint debridement or joint replacement. These open procedures were met with reasonable success, but results were tempered by relatively long recovery periods and high complication rates. As arthroscopic techniques have evolved, orthopedic surgeons have grown more interested in a more minimally invasive approach to elbow stiffness. Arthroscopic debridement of the stiff elbow offers the potential advantages of improved intraoperative articular visualization, decreased postoperative pain, and more rapid patient recovery in comparison with open procedures. Furthermore, several recent series have documented equivalent outcomes between open and arthroscopic techniques for elbow arthritis.

The articular anatomy of the elbow is complex, and the relatively small elbow capsule is surrounded by important neurovascular structures. The combination of a small working space and proximity to vital nerves and arteries initially deterred many surgeons from pursuing complex arthroscopic elbow procedures. Elbow arthroscopy was initially performed primarily for joint evaluation and loose body removal. However, an increased understanding of local neurovascular anatomy as well as increased experience with elbow arthroscopy has led to an expansion of potential surgical indications.

Elbow arthroscopy can be used for resection of symptomatic plicae, synovectomy for inflammatory arthritis, lateral epicondylitis debridement, treatment of osteochondritis dissecans, and fixation of simple elbow fractures. In addition to these indications, elbow arthroscopy may be especially useful in the setting of arthrofibrosis and/or elbow arthritis. The results of arthroscopic capsular release as well as joint debridement and osteophyte resection have been promising. The focus of this chapter will be the application of arthroscopic techniques for patients with stiff and/or arthritic elbows.

CLINICAL EVALUATION

History

Osteoarthritis, rheumatoid arthritis, and posttraumatic contractures may all lead to a stiff elbow joint. Osteoarthritis patients often have pain and stiffness, especially at the extremes of elbow motion. These patients often have relatively pain-free elbow motion in the midmotion arc. Loss of terminal extension is classically observed (1). Patients may also note weakness, cosmetic deformity, and instability. The patient should be questioned about mechanical symptoms such as locking or catching. Inflammatory arthritis often presents with elbow effusion and synovitis, polyarthropathy, morning stiffness, and systemic symptoms. Patients with this presentation warrant rheumatologic workup.

It is important to get an adequate history regarding the timeline of elbow pain and stiffness as well as any inciting events or exacerbating factors. In particular, it is crucial to ask the patient regarding any past traumatic episodes. Distal humerus fractures with resultant articular deformity can cause posttraumatic arthritis. Stiffness may also develop in the absence of bony deformity, with hemarthrosis leading to capsular contraction and fibrosis.

Any treatment received by the patient prior to presentation should also be noted. In particular, patients should be questioned regarding any physical therapy and/or splinting that they have undergone. If they have received physical therapy or undergone splinting, it is pertinent to know what type of therapy exercises were performed, the duration of therapy and/or splinting, and the patient's results from these interventions.

The patient's handedness as well as vocational and avocational activities are also pertinent. Osteoarthritis of the elbow is most frequently seen in the dominant arms of men with a history of heavy labor. Patients who are avid weight lifters or who are throwing athletes are also predisposed to elbow arthritis.

Physical Examination

The physical examination begins with inspection of the extremities for effusion or synovitis that may suggest inflammatory arthropathy. The elbow joint is evaluated for visual deformity as well as effusions. The elbow carrying angle is noted. The skin is inspected for rashes and prior surgical or traumatic scars. A complete neurovascular exam is essential prior to elbow arthroscopy to document preoperative function and sensation.

Examination of elbow range of motion is particularly valuable, and it is important to note both the passive and the active elbow motion arc and compare it with the contralateral side. Range of motion testing will help determine severity of functional impairment as well as provide a baseline for subsequent evaluation. Flexion contractures are commonly observed in the setting of osteoarthritis as well as arthrofibrosis. The experienced clinician may be able to distinguish between a "soft" and a "hard" endpoint that will suggest extrinsic versus intrinsic articular pathology.

Patients with osteoarthritis often have pain at the endpoints of the elbow motion arc. Crepitus may be noted. The examiner may note that the elbow locks or catches in certain positions. Testing of elbow stability is also critical and completes the physical examination.

Imaging

Imaging studies are obtained and correlated with the history and physical examination. Standard radiographic views of the elbow should include anteroposterior, lateral, and oblique projections. These are closely inspected for signs of posttraumatic deformity as well as loose bodies, which are indicative of underlying osteoarthritis. The clinician should particularly pay close attention to the olecranon and coronoid processes as well as the olecranon and coronoid fossae of the humerus, as these areas are prone to osteophytic degeneration.

CT is a valuable preoperative examination that helps characterize the size and location of osteophytes. These images are very useful for preoperative planning, particularly if three-dimensional reconstructions are obtained. CT is also indicated in the setting of malunion and posttraumatic deformity.

OPERATIVE PLANNING AND TECHNIQUE

Indications

Elbow arthroscopy is a reasonable option in the patient with symptomatic osteoarthritis and/or arthrofibrosis with loss of functional range of motion. A trial of nonoperative measures such as activity modification, nonsteroidal anti-inflammatory medications, and physical therapy and splinting are warranted prior to surgical intervention. The patient should be appropriately informed regarding the potential risks to neurovascular structures inherent in elbow arthroscopy. The patient must be willing and able to participate in any anticipated postoperative therapy or splinting regimen. Open procedures are preferred over arthroscopy in patients who have undergone significant prior elbow surgery (particularly on the lateral aspect of the elbow as this may lead to scarring near radial nerve) or who have severe bony deformity or capsular retraction.

Anesthesia and Patient Positioning

The first decision in performing elbow arthroscopy is to determine the type of anesthesia to be used. The authors recommend general anesthesia for various reasons, though axillary blocks may also be used. Elbow arthroscopy requires that the patient assume a prone or lateral decubitus position, which can be uncomfortable and awkward for the patient. In a complex arthroscopic case with duration exceeding 1 hour, the patient may experience significant discomfort that can be difficult to control and may jeopardize the success of the procedure. In addition, the use of a nerve block precludes an accurate postoperative neurologic examination. As there is a very real risk of neurovascular injury during elbow arthroscopy, an accurate postoperative examination is critical. In the setting of an axillary nerve block, it may be several days before a postoperative neurologic complication is discovered. Therefore, general anesthesia is recommended as long as the patient's overall medical health does not preclude it.

Patient positioning for elbow arthroscopy is dependent on surgeon preference. Poehling and colleagues (2) first described prone positioning, and many orthopedic surgeons have modified this to a lateral decubitus position. The lateral decubitus position allows the elbow to be positioned, so that it is highest in the operative field, which improves access to the joint and allows the surgeon to maneuver arthroscopic equipment around the elbow without impinging against the side of the patient's body (3).

It is best to obtain an elbow arm support made specifically for elbow arthroscopy (3). The use of a knee holder impedes access to the elbow. The patient can be tilted 10° to 20° toward the operating surgeon to prevent rollback of the patient and to maintain proper positioning within the arm holder. This helps avoid compression on the antecubital fossa.

A pillow is placed between the patient's legs and the proximal fibulae are well padded. A back support brace is applied to maintain torso positioning, and a strap is placed over the patient's waist. A nonsterile tourniquet is applied as proximally as possible on the operative arm at the level of the arm holder (Figs. 34.1 to 34.4).

Starting Portal Placement

The potential for neurovascular injury with elbow arthroscopy is relatively high as compared with arthroscopy of the knee and shoulder, and much attention has been given to safe portal placement. It is essential to understand the local anatomy and know the safe zones for portal placement.

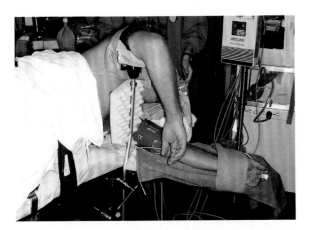

FIGURE 34.1. Patient positioned for elbow arthroscopy. Lateral decubitus position with the unaffected elbow on an arm board. (From Steinmann SP. Elbow arthroscopy. *J Am Soc Surg Hand.* 2003;3:199–207; Figure 1, with permission.)

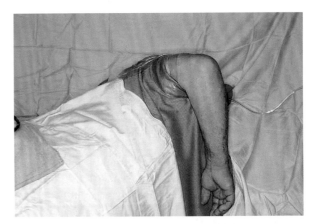

FIGURE 34.3. Patient positioned for elbow arthroscopy. The elbow is elevated to allow 360° of access. (From Steinmann SP. Elbow arthroscopy. *J Am Soc Surg Hand.* 2003;3:199–207; Figure 3, with permission.)

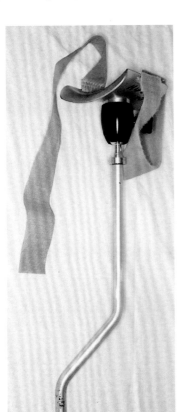

FIGURE 34.2. Elbow arthroscopy arm holder attaches to the side of the operating table. (From Steinmann SP. Elbow arthroscopy. *J Am Soc Surg Hand.* 2003;3:199–207; Figure 2, with permission.)

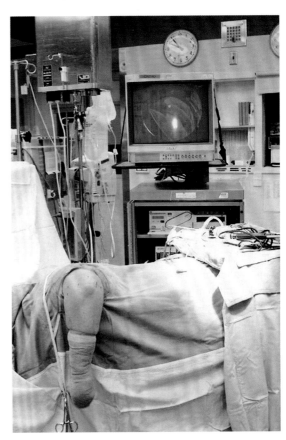

FIGURE 34.4. The surgeon's view during elbow arthroscopy. Monitor positioned on opposite side of the table. (From Steinmann SP. Elbow arthroscopy. *J Am Soc Surg Hand.* 2003;3:199–207; Figure 4, with permission.)

The order of portal placement is not as critical as a solid understanding of relevant elbow anatomy.

All portal sites should be marked prior to surgery. This allows the surgeon to determine bony landmarks before the joint is distended or the soft tissues edematous. The lateral epicondyle, medial epicondyle, radial head, capitellum, and olecranon should all be marked out. The elbow is then distended with 20 to 30 cc of saline, using a syringe and 18G needle. The needle is usually placed through the "soft spot" that lies in the middle of the triangle bordered by the olecranon, radial head, and lateral epicondyle. Alternatively, the joint can be distended with an injection directly posterior just proximal to the olecranon tip. Distending the elbow prior to establishing the starting portal is an important step, as distending the joint positions the major neurovascular structures further from the starting portal and facilitates initial portal insertion. In a nondistended elbow, inserting the trocar for the starting portal is considerably more difficult and more dangerous.

After the joint is distended, it is time to establish a starting portal. The choice of starting portal is a matter of surgeon preference. The surgeon's experience and anatomic knowledge is more important in preventing neurovascular injury than the order of portal placement. Portal sites should be made with a no. 11 blade. The knife scalpel should be drawn across the skin only without penetration into the deeper soft tissues. Once the skin is divided, a small hemostat can be used to spread down to the joint capsule and enter the joint. Joint entry is confirmed by release of the previously injected saline from the capsule. The blunt trocar is then used to enter the joint. Using a sharp trocar is avoided during elbow arthroscopy as this can damage neurovascular structures.

The trocar is then exchanged for the arthroscope, and evaluation of the joint commences. A 4-mm, 30° arthroscope is the workhorse for elbow arthroscopy. Some advocate the use of a 70° scope, but as this is seldom used in general arthroscopic practice, it may be disorienting. A 2.7-mm arthroscope can be used in a contracted joint but is not needed in most patients. However, in certain spots such as the direct lateral (soft spot) portal, the smaller scope may be easier to manipulate.

Once the arthroscope has entered the joint, the surgeon must then obtain visualization and create a space in which to work. This can be performed through pressure distention or mechanical retraction. Both methods function well, but pressure distention will eventually cause fluid to extravasate into the tissues during the course of the procedure. Kelly and colleagues (4) recommended using retractors as a means of mechanical retraction to avoid this complication. Simple lever retractors such a Howarth or large, blunt Steinmann pins are effective. Retractors are typically placed into the elbow joint through an accessory portal that is 2 to 3 cm proximal to the viewing portal (Fig. 34.5).

Again, the choice of starting portal is a matter of surgeon preference as safe entry into the joint can occur from either the medial or the lateral approach. The radial nerve is the structure at greatest risk during portal placement. There are two methods of minimizing risk of radial nerve injury. The first technique is to establish the anterolateral portal first when bony landmarks are clearly palpable. The anteromedial portal can then be established from a direct inside-out approach.

Alternatively, the surgeon can choose to establish the anteromedial portal first and then create an anterolateral portal under direct arthroscopic visualization. The anteromedial portal is relatively distant from the medial and ulnar nerves, and it is fairly safe to start with this portal. Arthroscopic observation of the lateral capsule during anterolateral portal placement, however, is not fail proof.

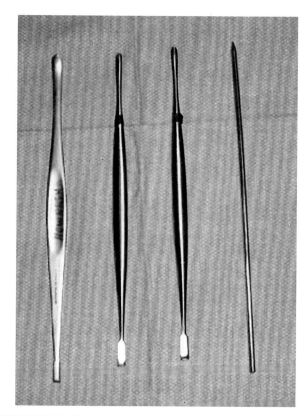

FIGURE 34.5. Elbow arthroscopy retractors. Three Howarth retractors and one blunt Steinmann pin. (From Steinmann SP. Elbow arthroscopy. *J Am Soc Surg Hand.* 2003;3:199–207; Figure 8, with permission.)

A misdirected needle or trocar could damage the radial nerve despite intra-articular visualization.

SPECIFIC PORTALS

Anterolateral

The anterolateral portal was originally described by Andrews and Carson (5). Anatomic studies have shown that the posterior antebrachial nerve and radial nerve are quite close to the anterolateral portal (6). A safe approach is to place the portal in the sulcus between the radial head and the capitellum. This area is fairly easy to locate prior to the onset of fluid extravasation and soft tissue edema. The skin is incised, a hemostat is used to spread to the joint and aimed toward the joint center. To minimize risk of radial nerve injury, it is advisable to place a cannula in the anterolateral portal and then pass all instruments through the cannula. This eliminates blind passes into the joint.

Once in the joint, the surgeon should be able to visualize the medial radial head, coronoid process, trochlea, and coronoid fossa from the anterolateral portal. The anteromedial portal can then be started through an inside-out technique. The arthroscope is removed from the sheath, and a blunt trocar is passed through the sheath straight across the joint until it tents the medial elbow skin. The skin is then incised over this trocar, and the sheath is pushed out of the skin. A cannula is then placed over the tip of the sheath, and the arthroscope is inserted into this cannula while gently retracting the trocar. In this manner, the cannula and trocar are pulled back into the joint together, with the arthroscope inside the cannula and following the trocar down into the elbow joint. Because the interval between the median and the ulnar nerves is relatively wide on the medial elbow, this inside-out technique of establishing the anteromedial portal is quite safe (Figs. 34.6 to 34.8).

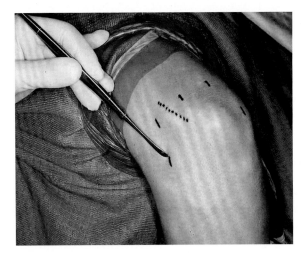

FIGURE 34.8. Anteromedial portal. Dotted line represents ulnar nerve. (From Steinmann SP. Elbow arthroscopy. *J Am Soc Surg Hand.* 2003;3:199–207; Figure 7, with permission.)

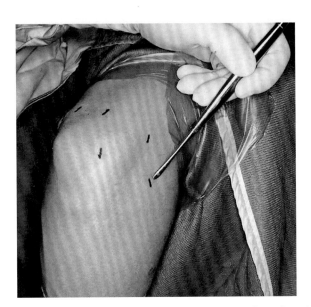

FIGURE 34.6. Anterolateral portal located anterior to the radiocapitellar joint. (From Steinmann SP. Elbow arthroscopy. *J Am Soc Surg Hand.* 2003;3:199–207; Figure 5, with permission.)

Proximal Anterolateral

The proximal anterolateral portal is used mainly as a retractor portal. It should be placed 2 cm proximal to the lateral epicondyle, with care taken not to place it too close to the standard anterolateral portal as instruments could interfere with each other. The proximal anterolateral portal is a suboptimal viewing portal, as visualization of the medial trochlea and coronoid fossa is difficult. It is a relatively safe portal, however, with the radial nerve on average 9.9 mm away and the posterior antebrachial cutaneous nerve 6.1 mm away (6). Therefore, it can be used as a starting portal in patients with very stiff elbows. In typical cases, though, the proximal anterolateral is most useful as a retracting portal. Howarth retractors or Steinmann pins can be used through this portal to elevate the anterior capsule off the humerus and establish a working space for the anterolateral portal instruments.

Direct Lateral or Midlateral Portal

The direct (midlateral) portal is placed at the "soft spot" in the center of the triangle formed by the olecranon, lateral epicondyle, and radial head. This portal is not routinely used, as it does not afford adequate visualization of the anterior joint. It can be particularly useful in a patient with osteochondritis dissecans, however, as it provides the best view of the posterior capitellum, radial head, and radioulnar articulation. Because of the small and shallow dimensions of this portal, a 2.7 arthroscope may be useful in this area.

Anteromedial Portal

Prior to establishing any medial portals, it is crucial to palpate the ulnar nerve and evaluate for any tendency to subluxate anteriorly out of the cubital tunnel. The anteromedial portal is typically placed 2 cm distal and 2 cm anterior to the medial epicondyle (5). Instruments placed

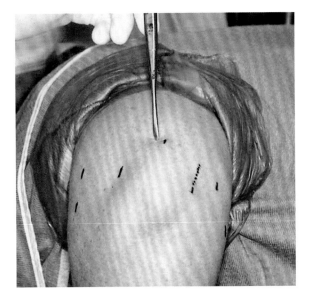

FIGURE 34.7. Direct posterior portal. (From Steinmann SP. Elbow arthroscopy. *J Am Soc Surg Hand.* 2003;3:199–207; Figure 6, with permission.)

II. The Elbow

through this entry point tend to penetrate the common flexor origin and the brachialis prior to entering the joint. The medial antebrachial cutaneous nerve is most at risk from anteromedial portal placement, as it is on average only 1 mm away from the portal site (6). The median nerve is on average 7 mm away. Lindenfeld (7) described the establishment of the anteromedial portal 1 cm proximal and 1 cm anterior to the medial epicondyle and reported an average distance of 22 mm away from the median nerve using this approach. The anteromedial portal can be established as the initial portal, or it can be placed through inside-out technique from the lateral side as described above. Surgeon preference dictates the order of portal placement.

Proximal Anteromedial Portal

The proximal anteromedial portal was first described by Poehling et al. (2), who placed this portal 2 cm proximal to the medial epicondyle and directly anterior to the intermuscular septum. This portal placement is a safe distance away from both the median and the ulnar nerves. The medial antebrachial cutaneous nerve is most at risk from this portal with an average distance of 2.3 mm away (6). The median nerve averages 12.4 mm away and the ulnar nerve 12 mm away from this portal. This portal is the safest of the medial portal locations, but it offers limited visualization of the radiocapitellar joint or the radial fossa of the humerus. Therefore, it is probably best to use this portal as a retractor portal and use the standard anteromedial portal as the viewing or working portal.

Posterolateral Portal

The posterolateral portal is an excellent viewing portal for the posterior elbow. It is important to confirm the location of the ulnar nerve prior to placing any posterior portals. Fortunately, the ulnar nerve (unlike the median and radial nerves) is palpable, and posterior portal placement is safe once the location of the ulnar nerve is confirmed. With the elbow flexed 90°, the posterolateral portal is placed at the lateral joint line level with the olecranon tip. The trocar tip is aimed toward the center of the olecranon fossa. Viewing through the posterolateral portal is nearly always difficult initially, as the fat pad occupies a large volume of the potential working space. A second portal is usually established in simultaneous fashion to debride the fat pad in order to facilitate visualization and develop adequate working space.

Direct Posterior Portal

The direct posterior portal is a good initial working portal. While viewing through the posterolateral portal, the direct posterior portal can be used to debride osteophytes and remove loose bodies. This portal is placed 2 to 3 cm proximal to the tip of the olecranon at the proximal margin of the olecranon fossa. As the triceps is quite thick at this level, a knife is needed to penetrate directly into the elbow joint. After creation of the portal, an arthroscopic

shaver or radiofrequency probe can be used for joint debridement. The arthroscope and shaver may need to be frequently switched back and forth between the direct posterior and the posterolateral portals to facilitate complete posterior debridement. As the posterior portals are relatively safe, a cannula is not needed in the posterior elbow, and the instruments can be alternated directly. It is advisable to maintain an outflow cannula in the anterior elbow, however, to limit fluid extravasation into the soft tissues while working posteriorly.

Posterior Retractor Portal

Given that the portal location is sufficiently distant from the ulnar nerve, a posterior retractor portal can be placed at any location needed to increase arthroscopic viewing. One should avoid placing the retractor portal too near other portals, however, to impingement of instruments. A useful retractor portal position is 2 cm proximal to the direct posterior portal, with orientation slightly medial or lateral as needed. A Howarth or similar retractor can be used from this position to elevate the joint capsule without impinging on working instruments.

ARTHROSCOPIC TREATMENT OF DEGENERATIVE ELBOW ARTHRITIS

Degenerative arthritis of the elbow is characterized by loose body formation, osteophyte development, and capsular contraction (8, 9). It naturally follows that arthroscopic treatment of degenerative elbow arthritis consists of loose body removal, osteophyte resection, and release of capsular contractures. Where anatomically the surgeon decides to initiate debridement depends on the patient's clinical examination. As a general rule, it is safest and easiest to release capsular contractures prior to fluid extravasation and soft tissue edema. Therefore, in a patient who predominantly lacks flexion (tight posterior capsule), arthroscopic debridement often starts in the posterior elbow so that the ulnar nerve can be identified and protected during posteromedial capsular release. In contrast, arthroscopic debridement of a patient who primarily lacks elbow extension would usually begin in the anterior aspect of the elbow (Fig. 34.9A,B).

The posterior elbow compartment is visualized well from the posterolateral portal. The direct posterior portal functions well as a working portal, and a proximal retractor portal can also be used. Posterior osteophytes usually develop on the tip of the olecranon as well as along the medial and lateral ulna. The olecranon tip osteophytes are more easily visualized, and attention is often focused on debridement of these. However, it is equally as important to fully visualize both the medial and the lateral olecranon, as osteophytes in these locations could go otherwise undetected. In addition to the olecranon, it is also essential to evaluate and debride the olecranon fossa of the humerus. Osteophytes on the posterior humerus often match

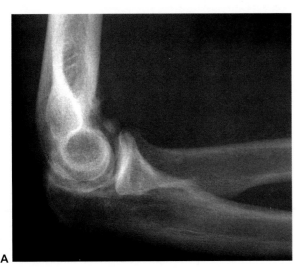 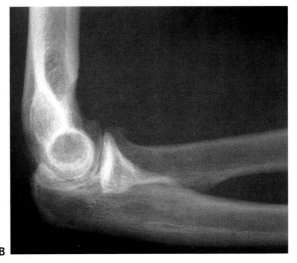

A   B

FIGURE 34.9. A: Preoperative radiograph demonstrating anterior and posterior osteophytes. **B:** Postoperative radiograph made after removal of anterior and posterior osteophytes. (From Steinmann SP, King GJ, Savoie FH. Arthroscopic treatment of the arthritic elbow. *J Bone Joint Surg.* 2005;87:2114–2121; Figure 4A,B, with permission.)

those on the olecranon, and care must be taken to debride osteophytes in both locations (Table 34.1).

Patients who lack elbow flexion preoperatively should undergo posterolateral and posteromedial capsular release. As mentioned above, particular care should be taken when performing posteromedial gutter release to identify and protect the ulnar nerve. It is reasonable to address the posteromedial capsule through a mini-open incision to allow identification and retraction of the ulnar nerve prior to capsular release. As greater experience is gained, it is possible to release the tight posteromedial capsule arthroscopically while identifying and protecting the area of the ulnar nerve. In patients with preoperative elbow flexion of less

than 90°, preoperative ulnar nerve symptoms, and/or large expected postoperative elbow flexion gains one should consider ulnar nerve decompression or transposition.

Similar steps are taken for debridement of the anterior compartment. Initial inspection is carried out and loose bodies are removed. The surgeon's attention is then turned toward any necessary bony work, as performing bony work prior to capsular release helps to limit soft tissue edema. The anterior elbow often has prominent osteophytes on the coronoid process, and these should be removed with a shaver or burr. There are often also osteophytes in the radial and coronoid fossae of the humerus, and care must be taken not to overlook these. The medial coronoid should

Table 34.1

Surgical steps

1. Mark all portal sites and surface anatomy
2. Elbow distention
3. Establish portals
4. Begin work in posterior compartment
5. Capsular release (posterior capsule first if patient lacks flexion)
6. Remove osteophytes along olecranon and olecranon fossa
7. Move to anterior compartment
8. Remove all obvious loose bodies; remove radial and coronoid osteophytes
9. Anterior capsulectomy off of humerus (lateral viewing portal)
10. Viewing from the medial portal, perform capsulectomy from radial head and capitellum

From Strickland JP, Steinmann SP. Elbow arthroscopy for the arthritic elbow. In: Cole BJ, Sekiya JK, eds. *Surgical Techniques of the Shoulder, Elbow, and Knee in Sports Medicine.* Philadelphia, PA: Elsevier/Saunders; 2008:345–353, with permission.

also be inspected for osteophytes, as they may be missed if not deliberately sought. The use of motorized burrs and shavers without attached suction devices avoids the inadvertent damage of neurovascular structures (Fig. 34.10).

After all the anterior osteophytes have been removed, the surgeon can turn his/her attention to the anterior capsule. It is often easiest to first take the capsule off the humerus, as this will increase the anterior working space. The surgeon then uses a lateral viewing portal while excising the anterior capsule with a shaver or punch. The median nerve is the closest important structure but is protected behind the brachialis. After the anterior capsule has been excised to the joint midline, the viewing portal is then changed to the medial side and the shaver inserted through the lateral portal. Great care must be taken when excising the capsule anterior to the radial head and capitellum, as the radial nerve is at risk of injury in this location. The radial nerve lies just anterior to a small fat pad that can be visualized by the arthroscopist. This fat pad warns the surgeon of the radial nerve's proximity (Table 34.2).

After completion of osteophyte resection and capsular release, the patient's range of motion is evaluated. If satisfactory, the portals are closed in standard fashion with 3 to 0 nylon or prolene sutures. The arm is held in an extended position, and a sterile compressive dressing is placed in circumferential fashion. It is important to place the arm in extended position, as this limits the accumulation of intra-articular fluid and elbow swelling. As soon as the patient is awake, the operative arm should be evaluated to confirm intact neurovascular status.

Postoperative Care

The patient's arm is elevated overnight in "Statue of Liberty" position to limit postoperative swelling. Motion can be delayed for 24 hours postoperatively to allow the resolution of edema. Splinting or continuous passive range of motion can then be initiated to maintain range of motion achieved in the operating room. Continuous passive motion (CPM) is often reserved for those patients who have significant preoperative motion limitations.

Continuous passive motion is often reserved for those patients who have significant preoperative motion limitations. It is usually not necessary in those patients with modest joint contractures. There is little evidence showing that patients who use continuous passive motion machines postoperatively have greater restoration of motion than those who receive physical therapy or splints.

Postoperative continuous passive motion protocols typically consist of 23-hour range of motion, with small breaks for eating, cleaning, and activities of daily living. The range of motion is usually set at the maximum motion achieved in the operating room. We do not often use passive range of motion regimens that start with a small motion arc and gradually increase up to the operating room range of motion. Continuous passive motion machines can be used with axillary nerve blocks or intravenous narcotics for pain control. The passive range of motion protocol is usually used for 3 to 4 weeks after surgery.

Splinting is also an effective method of maintaining postoperative elbow range of motion in patients with mild to moderate preoperative motion loss. Static splints are typically used, and regimens alternate between maximal elbow flexion and extension. For example, the patient may be splinted in full extension for an hour, and then change to a splint that maintains full flexion for an hour. The patient alternates between flexion and extension splints at periodic intervals.

Regardless of whether the postoperative regimen consists of splinting or continuous passive motion, it is crucial to regularly check the patient's neurovascular status. Particular attention should be paid to the status of the ulnar nerve, as ulnar neuropathy has been noted to occur following arthroscopic or open capsular release of patients who had less than 90° of flexion preoperatively or in whom surgery restores a large amount of elbow flexion (4, 10). Because of this potential complication, the surgeon may consider intraoperative ulnar nerve transposition in patients who achieve significant restoration of the flexion arc after anterior osteophyte removal and capsular release.

Complications

As with any surgery, there are various complications that may ensue during or after elbow arthroscopy. The most common of these is prolonged portal drainage. Septic arthritis and compartment syndrome have been reported. Persistent or new-onset elbow joint contracture may also been seen. Much of the literature has focused on the risk of neurovascular injury, which is higher in elbow arthroscopy than with knee and shoulder arthroscopy.

Patient risk factors for iatrogenic neurovascular injury include previous elbow operations, rheumatoid arthritis, and joint contractures requiring capsular release.

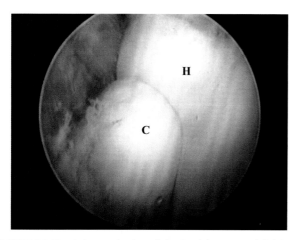

FIGURE 34.10. Arthroscopic view of the tip of the coronoid *(C)* distal humerus *(H)*. (From Strickland JP, Steinmann SP. Elbow arthroscopy for the arthritic elbow. In: Cole BJ, Sekiya JK, eds. *Surgical Techniques of the Shoulder, Elbow, and Knee in Sports Medicine.* Philadelphia, PA: Elsevier/Saunders; 2008:345–353, with permission.)

Table 34.2

Pearls and pitfalls

- Although plain radiographs are adequate for preoperative planning, three-dimensional CT scanning is helpful for fully evaluating areas of osteophyte formation
- Block anesthesia can be used for elbow arthroscopy, however, if the lateral or prone position is used, it can be difficult for the patient. In addition, if block anesthesia is used, the surgeon will be unable to evaluate for a potential nerve injury until many hours postoperatively
- An arm holder made specifically for elbow arthroscopy makes positioning easier and helps eliminate instrument impingement
- If the lateral decubitus position is used, the elbow should be positioned high in the operative field. This helps eliminate impingement of the arthroscope and instruments against the patient's body or surgeon drapes
- If the patient is tilted slightly to the surgeon this helps prevent the arm holder from impinging on the antecubital fossa. This area must be kept free to allow saline distention of the anterior joint
- Any portal can be used as an initial starting portal. However, the anterolateral portal is closest to a major nerve (radial nerve) and should be established either first before any swelling has begun and bone landmarks can be palpated, or early in the procedure
- Do not use suction on the shaver in the anterior aspect of the joint. This may inadvertently put a nerve or vital structure into the shaver or burr
- Attempt to do all bone work first in the elbow joint before removing capsule. This helps limit edema and potentially protects vital structures
- Heterotopic bone can form even after an arthroscopic procedure on the elbow. To potentially limit this process, use the shaver after the burr to remove as many bone fragments as possible
- Elevation of the patient's arm overhead in a fully extended "Statue of Liberty" position overnight can help quickly remove postoperative swelling to allow early active motion

From Strickland JP, Steinmann SP. Elbow arthroscopy for the arthritic elbow. In: Cole BJ, Sekiya JK, eds. *Surgical Techniques of the Shoulder, Elbow, and Knee in Sports Medicine.* Philadelphia, PA: Elsevier/Saunders; 2008:345–353, with permission.

Kelly et al. (4) reported on 473 elbow arthroscopies and noted several transient nerve palsies but no permanent nerve injuries. Prolonged wound drainage, infection, and elbow contracture were other complications noted, with 50 patients in total suffering complications. Savoie and Field (11) reviewed the results of 465 elbow arthroscopies presented in the literature and found a 3% prevalence of neurologic complications. Severe injuries to the ulnar, median, and radial nerve have all been reported with elbow arthroscopy. The appropriate use of retractors for improved visualization is essential in decreasing this risk.

Results

Various reports of patient results after arthroscopic debridement of elbow osteoarthritis have shown satisfactory results. Cohen et al. (12) reported excellent pain relief and no major complications in 26 patients treated with a modification of the Outerbridge–Kashiwagi procedure (fenestration of the olecranon fossa to allow greater olecranon and coronoid excursion). Savoie et al. (13) reviewed the results of 24 patients who underwent an arthroscopic

modification of the Outerbridge–Kashiwagi procedure. All patients noted a decrease in their pain and an average elbow range of motion improvement of 81° was obtained. Philips and Strasburger (14) reported satisfactory results in 25 patients, with a 41° average increase in elbow motion arc. In a study of 30 patients with elbow degenerative arthritis, Kim and Shin (15) reported that 92% had improved range of motion. In their study, preoperative motion arcs averaged 81° and improved to an average of 121° postoperatively. Adams and Steinmann (8) reviewed the results of 41 patients and noted 81% good to excellent results with average postoperative motion arcs of 8.4° to 131.6°. Krishnan et al. (16) recently reported on the results of arthroscopic treatment of elbow degenerative arthritis in 11 patients less than 50 years of age. They reported a total arc of motion increase from 60° preoperatively to 133° postoperatively. Mean subjective pain decreased from 9.2 to 1.7 on a 10-point scale after surgery. The literature supports good to excellent results in regard to range of motion improvement and pain relief for patients who undergo arthroscopic treatment of elbow arthritis (Table 34.3).

Author	Results
Cohen et al. (12)	Twenty-six patients with excellent pain relief, no major complications
Savoie et al. (13)	Twenty-four patients; all had decrease in pain, 81° increase in arc of motion
Phillips and Strasburger (14)	Satisfactory results in 25 patients with an increase in 41° in total arc of motion
Kim and Shin (15)	Thirty patients with 92% improvement in the range of motion, from a mean of 81° preoperatively to a mean of 121° postoperatively
Adams and Steinmann (8)	Forty-one patients with 81% good-excellent results; postoperative range of motion, 8.4° to 131.6°
Krishnan et al. (16)	—

From Strickland JP, Steinmann SP. Elbow arthroscopy for the arthritic elbow. In: Cole BJ, Sekiya JK, eds. *Surgical Techniques of the Shoulder, Elbow, and Knee in Sports Medicine.* Philadelphia, PA: Elsevier/Saunders; 2008:345–353, with permission.

ARTHROSCOPIC MANAGEMENT OF ARTHROFIBROSIS

Elbow stiffness may stem from various etiologies related to the joint capsule and the underlying elbow articulation. Range of motion loss may be extrinsic, with stiffness secondary to posttraumatic capsular contraction. Capsular fibrosis can form as a result of hemarthrosis after fractures, dislocations, or other elbow trauma. Elbow stiffness can also occur from intrinsic bony pathology, with loose bodies, degenerative osteophytes, or articular incongruity limiting motion.

History and physical examination are useful in determining the etiology of elbow stiffness. Patient with mechanical symptoms such as locking as catching of their elbow often have intrinsic articular pathology or loose bodies. When evaluating patient range of motion, the experienced clinician may be able to distinguish between the "hard" endpoint of degenerative arthritis and the "soft" endpoint of capsular fibrosis. Radiographs and three-dimensional CT are invaluable in the evaluation of degenerative osteophytes or articular incongruity that may cause bony impingement.

Indications for operative management for posttraumatic capsular contracture include functional loss of motion and failure of nonoperative management. Most activities of daily living require an elbow flexion arc of 100° (from 30° to 130°) (17). Nonoperative treatment options include physical therapy, static splinting, and sometimes manipulation under local or regional anesthesia. Extensive postoperative physical therapy is essential to a successful outcome, and surgical intervention is contraindicated in patients who are unable or unwilling to participate in an involved postoperative physical therapy program.

The arthrofibrotic elbow can be treated surgically through either an open or an arthroscopic approach. Open surgical release is an established treatment option for the stiff elbow and may include anterior capsulectomy as well as partial release of collateral ligaments and biceps and/or brachialis lengthening. As an open surgical approach causes significant soft tissue trauma, postoperative inflammation and scarring can lead to recurrent elbow contracture. Significant postoperative pain and swelling may delay initiation of postoperative physical therapy regimens in patients who undergo open surgical intervention. Furthermore, open surgical release does not allow complete examination of the elbow joint and often precludes treatment of intra-articular pathology. An arthroscopic approach allows the surgeon to treat both intrinsic and extrinsic elbow pathology while minimizing soft tissue trauma and allowing the early initiation of postoperative physical therapy programs.

Surgical Technique for Release of Arthrofibrotic Elbow Contractures

The operative setup for arthroscopic treatment of the arthrofibrotic elbow is as described above in the degenerative arthritis section of the text. However, unlike the posterior capsular stiffness seen in degenerative arthritis, arthrofibrosis is characterized by contracture of the anterior capsule. Therefore, the operative procedure usually begins with the anterior compartment. Anteromedial and anterolateral portals are established. The contracted anterior capsule is readily visualized and should be released and resected with a similar technique as that described above. A blunt trocar can be used to release adhesions and lift the capsule off the anterior humerus. An oscillating shaver can then be used to debride synovium and residual adhesions, with care taken not to use suction or direct the shaver toward the capsule.

When capsular adhesions have been thoroughly released, sharp anterior capsulotomy is then performed. Vital structures are protected by the brachialis, which lies deep to the neurovascular bundle but superficial to the capsule. A plane between the capsule and the brachialis is established, and a basket resector is used to incise the capsule under direct arthroscopic visualization. Care must be taken to avoid damage to neurovascular structures, with particular attention paid to the small fat pad anterior to the radial neck, which marks the position of the radial nerve.

After anterior capsule resection, the anterior aspect of the elbow joint can be further evaluated. The coronoid fossa and radial head fossa are examined and deepened if necessary to improve elbow flexion. The radiocapitellar joint as well as the proximal radioulnar joints should be evaluated. Damage to these joints may warrant radial head excision in the patient without signs of valgus instability. After the entire anterior compartment has been inspected and the capsule resected, attention is turned to the posterior compartment.

Work in the posterior compartment commences with debridement of the olecranon fossa. In patients with posttraumatic contracture, the olecranon fossa is often filled with scar tissue and adhesions that need to be resected to obtain visualization. In most elbows with arthrofibrosis, the triceps is attached to the posterior humerus through scar tissue and needs to be elevated to allow full elbow flexion. After management of the contracted soft tissues posteriorly, attention is then directed at the olecranon tip. Resection of the olecranon tip may be necessary for full elbow range of motion. The medial and lateral gutters should be inspected and debrided, with careful attention to protect the ulnar nerve when debriding medially. If resection of the medial capsule is required, identification and careful protection of the ulnar nerve should be performed (Fig. 34.11).

Postoperative care

After surgery, continuous-passive-range-of-motion machines are often used for 3 weeks. Alternatively, splinting

regimens as described above can be initiated. Patients are encouraged to use their arms for activities of daily living right after surgery. If loss of motion recurs within 3 weeks postoperatively, sedation and gentle manual manipulation can be used to break up adhesions.

Results

Savoie and colleagues reported their results after arthroscopic release of 388 arthrofibrotic elbows. They noted an average increase in elbow extension from –40 to –5 and an overall increase in elbow motion arc of 65° postoperatively. Ninety-three percent of patients reported satisfactory results (18). Ball and associates (19) reported on 14 consecutive patients who underwent arthroscopic treatment of posttraumatic elbow arthrofibrosis. The mean patient-elbow-motion arc improved from 69° to 119° after operative intervention. All patients reported improved function after their surgery. Timmerman and Andrews (20) published their results from arthroscopic treatment of 19 patients with elbow arthrofibrosis. Patients in their study had improvement in extension from –29° to –11° and flexion from 123° to 134°. Good-to-excellent results were achieved in 79% of patients.

CONCLUSION

Arthroscopy has improved the surgeon's ability to treat patients with degenerative arthritis and arthrofibrosis of the elbow. Elbow arthroscopy remains technically challenging and carries an associated risk of neurovascular injury. Thorough knowledge of the regional elbow anatomy and careful surgical technique are essential. When performed safely, elbow arthroscopy can significantly improve patient pain and elbow range of motion with results similar to those obtained with open surgical intervention.

REFERENCES

1. O'Driscoll SW. Elbow arthritis. *J Am Acad Orthop Surg.* 1993;1:106–116.
2. Poehling GG, Whipple TL, Sisco L, et al. Elbow arthroscopy: a new technique. *Arthroscopy.* 1989;5:222–224.
3. Steinmann SP. Elbow arthroscopy: where are we now? *Arthroscopy.* 2008;23:1231–1236.
4. Kelly EW, Morrey BF, O'Driscoll SW. Complications of elbow arthroscopy. *J Bone Joint Surg.* 2001;83A:25–34.
5. Andrews JR, Carson WG. Arthroscopy of the elbow. *Arthroscopy.* 1985;1:97–107.
6. Strothers K, Day B, Regan WR. Arthroscopy of the elbow: anatomy, portal sites, and a description of the proximal lateral portal. *Arthroscopy.* 1995;11:449–457.
7. Lindenfeld TN. Medial approach in elbow arthroscopy. *Am J Sports Med.* 1990;18:413–417.
8. Adams JE, Steinmann SP. Arthroscopy for elbow arthritis. *Tech Shoulder Elbow Surg.* 2007;8:120–125.
9. Steinmann SP, King GJ, Savoie FH. Arthroscopic treatment of the arthritic elbow. *J Bone Joint Surg.* 2005;87:2114–2121.

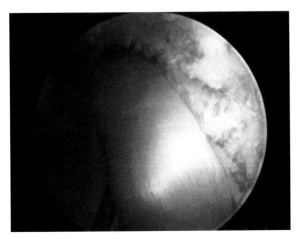

FIGURE 34.11. The ulnar nerve is seen after posterior medial capsular release. (From Steinmann SP, King GJ, Savoie FH III. Arthroscopic treatment of the arthritic elbow. *J Bone Joint Surg.* 2005;87:2114–2121; Figure 5, with permission.)

10. Wright TW, Glowczewskie F Jr, Cowin D, et al. Ulnar nerve excursion and strain at the elbow and wrist associated with upper extremity motion. *J Hand Surg.* 2001;26A:655–662.

11. Savoie F, Field LD. Complications of elbow arthroscopy. In: Savoie F, Field LD, eds. *Arthroscopy of the Elbow.* New York, NY: Churchill Livingstone; 1996:151–156.

12. Cohen AP, Redden JF, Stanley D. Treatment of osteoarthritis of the elbow: a comparison of open and arthroscopic debridement. *Arthroscopy.* 2000;16:701–706.

13. Savoie FH III, Nunley PD, Field LD. Arthroscopic management of the arthritic elbow: indications, technique, and results. *J Shoulder Elbow Surg.* 1999;8:214–219.

14. Philips BB, Strasburger S. Arthroscopic treatment of arthrofibrosis of the elbow joint. *Arthroscopy.* 1998;14:38–44.

15. Kim SJ, Shin SJ. Arthroscopic treatment for limitation of motion of the elbow. *Clin Orthop Relat Res.* 2000;375:140–148.

16. Krishnan SG, Harkings DC, Pennington SD, et al. Arthroscopic ulnohumeral arthroplasty for degenerative arthritis of the elbow in patients under fifty years of age. *J Shoulder Elbow Surg.* 2007;16:443–448.

17. Morrey BF, Askew LJ, Chao EY. A biomechanical study of normal functional elbow motion. *J Bone Joint Surg.* 1981;63A:872–877.

18. Geib TM, Savoie FH III. Elbow arthroscopy for posttraumatic arthrosis. *Instr Course Lect.* 2009;58:473–480.

19. Ball CM, Meunier M, Galatz LM, et al. Arthroscopic treatment of post-traumatic elbow contracture. *J Shoulder Elbow Surg.* 2002;11:624–629.

20. Timmerman LA, Andrews JR. Arthroscopic treatment of posttraumatic elbow pain and stiffness. *Am J Sports Med.* 1994;22:230–235.

21. Strickland JP, Steinmann SP. Elbow arthroscopy for the arthritic elbow. In: Cole BJ, Sekiya JK, eds. *Surgical Techniques of the Shoulder, Elbow, and Knee in Sports Medicine.* Philadelphia, PA: Elsevier/Saunders; 2008:345–353.

Arthroscopic Radial Head Resection: Indications and Technique

Darryl K. Young • Graham J. W. King

Deformity of the radial head is usually the result of a post-traumatic or inflammatory process. It is also seen in the setting of congenital radial head dislocation. This deformity can lead to pain and stiffness referable to the radiocapitellar or proximal radioulnar joint incongruency and arthrosis. In this setting, radial head resection may be an effective treatment for appropriately selected patients. Radial head excision reduces impingement between the deformed radial head and the corresponding articulation with the capitellum or proximal ulna, thus improving forearm rotation and decreasing pain.

Radial head resection has been classically performed through an open arthrotomy (1). Arthroscopic radial head resection has only been described more recently (2–4) but is gaining popularity. Although there is little evidence to support arthroscopic over open techniques, there are theoretical advantages. One of the primary advantages is less soft-tissue disruption, theoretically reducing the severity and duration of postoperative pain and stiffness. Another advantage is the improved intra-articular visualization, thus allowing the surgeon to address concomitant pathologies, such as synovitis, capsular contracture, osteophytes, or loose bodies.

It is worth emphasizing that radial head resection has very narrow indications. Surgeons treating patients with symptomatic radial head deformity should be well aware of the contraindications of radial head resection. In this chapter, we will outline the patients we feel are the ideal candidates for arthroscopic radial head resection. We will emphasize the appropriate preoperative evaluation, treatment alternatives, surgical technique, and "pearls and pitfalls" of managing these patients.

BIOMECHANICS AND PATHOANATOMY

The role of the radial head as a stabilizer of the elbow has been well established. Biomechanical studies have investigated the effect of radial head resection and replacement on the kinematics and stability of the elbow. The radial head has been demonstrated to be an important stabilizer in the setting of valgus instability due to medial collateral ligament (MCL) insufficiency (5–7). Posterolateral rotatory instability (PLRI) (5, 8–10) due to loss of tensioning of the lateral collateral ligament and proximal migration of the radius (11) due to deficiency of the interosseous membrane have also been reported following radial head excision. In addition, radial head excision results in increased loading of the ulnohumeral (UH) articulation due to altered elbow kinematics and the loss of load sharing by the radiocapitellar articulation. This may explain the high incidence of osteoarthritis, which is commonly reported after radial head excision (12–14). Likewise, biomechanical evidence reveals that prosthetic replacement of the radial head offers beneficial stabilizing effects (5–7, 15, 16).

The sum of these findings leads us to believe that, in most circumstances, the radial head should be preserved where possible and replaced after it is resected. This is particularly true in the setting of acute trauma where occult ligament injuries are common.

Arthroscopic radial head resection is usually performed in the setting of rheumatoid arthritis or posttraumatic arthritis. The posttraumatic arthritis often is associated with a previous radial head fracture. Although less common, radial head resection is occasionally performed for other conditions such as hemophilic arthropathy of the elbow and both congenital and acquired radial head dislocations. A fractured radial head can result in deformity of the radial head secondary to fracture malunion or osteophyte formation and joint derangement associated with progression of posttraumatic arthritis. Chronic inflammatory or hemophilic synovitis of the elbow can lead to enlargement and irregularity of the radial head. A hypertrophic or irregular radial head can impinge against the proximal ulnar facet acting as a mechanical block to forearm rotation. Likewise, there may be a mechanical block at the radiocapitellar joint affecting elbow flexion and extension.

CLINICAL EVALUATION

History

Patients with symptomatic radiocapitellar deformity often complain of pain and stiffness that is more pronounced with pronosupination rather than elbow flexion and extension. Mechanical symptoms such as clicking, catching, or locking may be present as well. A history of prior elbow trauma or surgery and other treatment to date is essential to guide diagnosis and treatment. The past medical history can reveal the underlying disease process (inflammatory arthritis, posttraumatic arthritis, primary osteoarthritis, hemophilia, etc.).

Physical Examination

The physical examination starts with inspection of the elbow carrying angle, bony contours, and evidence of surgical scars. The range of motion of the elbow and forearm should be measured accurately with the use of a goniometer. Any motion deficits should be distinguished as having either a "soft" or a "firm" endpoint, which correlate with a soft-tissue cause or osseous impingement, respectively. In the setting of rotational stiffness, one should confirm that the proximal radius articular deformity is the impediment, since the distal radioulnar joint (DRUJ) may be contributing in some cases. For this reason, physical examination and imaging of the wrist are important.

The patient population that are candidates for radial head resection are prone to instability, particularly due to prior trauma or ligament attenuation secondary to chronic inflammation. It is important to evaluate for elbow and forearm instability since valgus, posterolateral rotational, and axial instability are contraindications to radial head resection. The examination for valgus instability includes the valgus stress testing, the "milking maneuver," and the moving valgus stress test. The examination for PLRI includes the lateral pivot shift test, the posterolateral drawer test, and the supine and seated push-up tests. Although axial radioulnar instability is more difficult to detect on clinical examination, the presence of tenderness or dorsal prominence of the ulna at the DRUJ should raise the suspicion for this condition.

The location and function of the ulnar nerve should be assessed whenever elbow arthroscopy is planned. A previous ulnar nerve transposition will make standard percutaneous placement of medial portals risky. In this setting, open placement of the medial portals should be used to prevent iatrogenic nerve injury.

Imaging

Plain radiographs usually confirm the diagnosis of radiocapitellar joint derangement (Fig. 35.1). In addition to the standard AP and lateral views, a radiocapitellar view is often helpful to bring the radial head into profile. Radiographs of the wrist should be performed to ensure that there is no other cause of painful or limited forearm rotation, such as DRUJ pathology or radioulnar synostosis. Longitudinal radioulnar dissociation is best detected by bilateral wrist views to compare the ulnar variance with the contralateral normal side. If the diagnosis of instability is uncertain based on the physical

exam, live fluoroscopic examination, and stress views should be performed to evaluate for valgus, varus, and axial instability.

CT with sagittal, coronal, and three-dimensional (3D) reconstructions will provide the best detail of the bony anatomy (Fig. 35.2). CT often provides important additional information about the UH, radiocapitellar, and proximal radioulnar joint spaces. Cartilage loss, articular incongruity, loose bodies, osteophytes, and heterotopic ossification will be seen in more detail. If these other osseous deformities are contributing to symptoms, they will also need to be addressed as an isolated radial head resection will be of limited value in this setting.

TREATMENT

Nonoperative

Surgical intervention should be reserved for patients with symptoms refractory to routine nonoperative treatment. Activity modification and anti-inflammatories are the mainstay of nonoperative treatment for both conditions. Patients with rheumatoid arthritis should undergo an adequate trial of disease-modifying medications as directed by a rheumatologist.

Operative Indications and Contraindications

Arthroscopic radial head resection is indicated for radial head articular deformity or arthritis causing pain or impeding motion in a stable elbow and forearm. The radial head deformity can cause a mechanical block at either the radiocapitellar or the proximal radioulnar articulations or both. The goal of this procedure is to remove the mechanical block and thus increase motion and decrease pain. It is particularly useful in addressing limited and painful forearm rotation.

Radial head excision is contraindicated in patients with valgus, posterolateral rotatory, or axial instability. Such preexisting instability can be exacerbated if the stabilizing effects of the radial head are removed. Advanced UH arthritis is a relative contraindication. In this setting, an isolated radial head excision will not address symptoms originating from the arthritic UH articulation. Furthermore, radial head excision will increase the load across the remaining UH articulation, which may further exacerbate UH joint pain. Arthroscopic radial head excision is not generally recommended for acute radial head fractures. This is due to the high incidence of concomitant ligament injuries associated with acute fractures and the concern that the torn capsule in the acute fracture setting can result in significant extravasation of fluid making it higher risk and more technically challenging. A final word of caution would be that arthroscopic radial head resection for a rheumatoid elbow should only be performed by surgeons with considerable elbow arthroscopy experience. Arthroscopy of synovitic elbows is technically demanding since synovial proliferation, stiffness, and deformity all result in diminished capsular

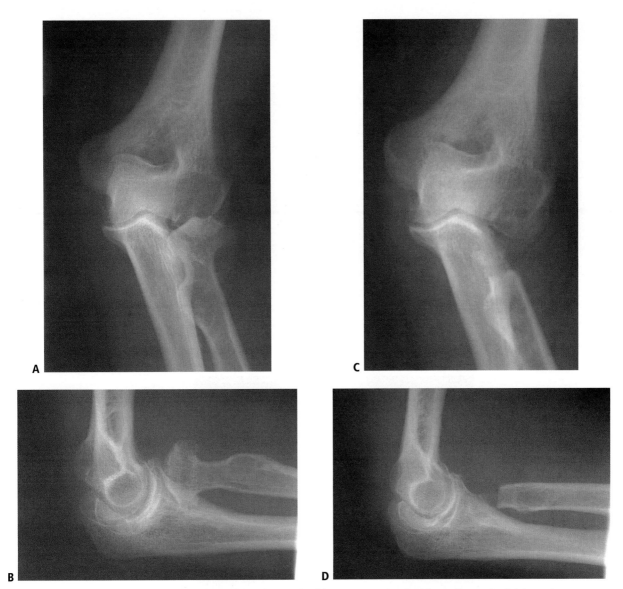

FIGURE 35.1. Imaging of a patient with congenital radial head subluxation associated with crepitus and painful rotation referable to the radiocapitellar joint and significant radial head deformity. Preoperative AP (**A**) and lateral (**B**) radiographs. Postoperative AP (**C**) and lateral (**D**) radiograph after arthroscopic radial head resection. Preoperative range of motion was 20° to 130° of flexion with full pronation and 50° of supination. Postoperative range of motion was 15° to 140° of flexion with full rotation and no pain.

volume reducing the available working room and visibility in the elbow. There is an increased risk of nerve injuries with elbow arthroscopy in the setting of inflammatory arthritis. A surgeon with less arthroscopy experience should manage these patients with open surgery.

If the capitellum is well preserved, radial head excision with prosthetic replacement may be preferred due to the favorable stabilizing and load transfer effects of the prosthetic replacement. Alternatively, if the capitellum is diseased, replacement of both the radial head and the capitellum can be considered. Although there is limited experience with radiocapitellar replacement, it may be a useful alternative in the setting of instability where isolated radial head excision is contraindicated. Older and low-demand patients with concomitant advanced UH

articular destruction and deformity may be better treated with a total elbow arthroplasty.

SURGICAL TECHNIQUE

The procedure is typically performed under general anesthesia. A continuous brachial plexus block can be useful for postoperative analgesia and to facilitate early mobilization in patients with severe stiffness. Standard elbow arthroscopic positioning, equipment, and portals are used. The senior author prefers a lateral decubitus position. The arm is positioned over a well-padded bolster. Gravity inflow is used to maintain low inflow pressures to avoid excessive joint swelling. A 4.0-mm arthroscope is used. The initial view after scope insertion is often poor due to extensive

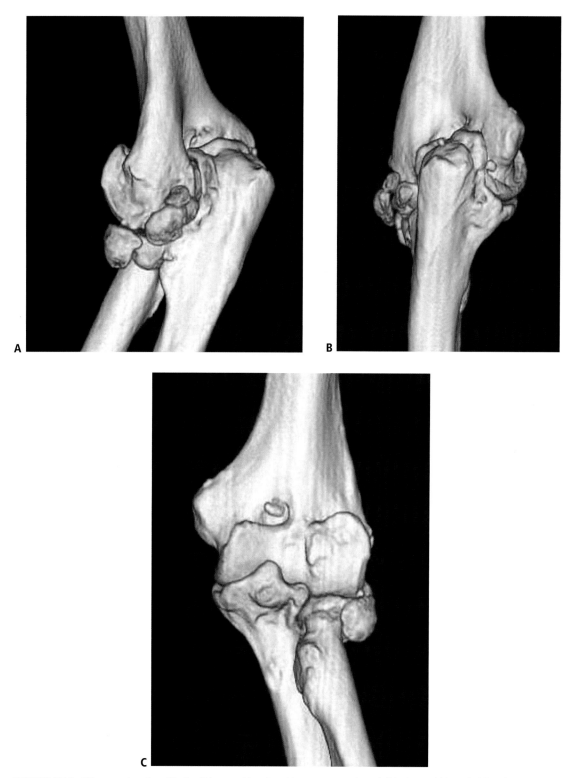

FIGURE 35.2. 3D reconstruction CT of a 76-year-old male with posttraumatic arthritis. Part of his radial head was resected years prior for a fracture. He presented with locking, impingement pain, and grinding localized to the radiocapitellar joint.

synovitis. A full radius resector is used for synovectomy as needed for visualization. A diagnostic arthroscopy of the entire elbow should be performed to identify any associated abnormalities such as cartilage defects of the capitellum, synovitis, loose bodies, and capsular contracture.

The radial head resection is initiated with the arthroscope viewing from a proximal anteromedial portal (Fig. 35.3). After achieving an adequate view, a motorized burr is introduced through a cannula placed in a midanterolateral portal placed at the level of the radial

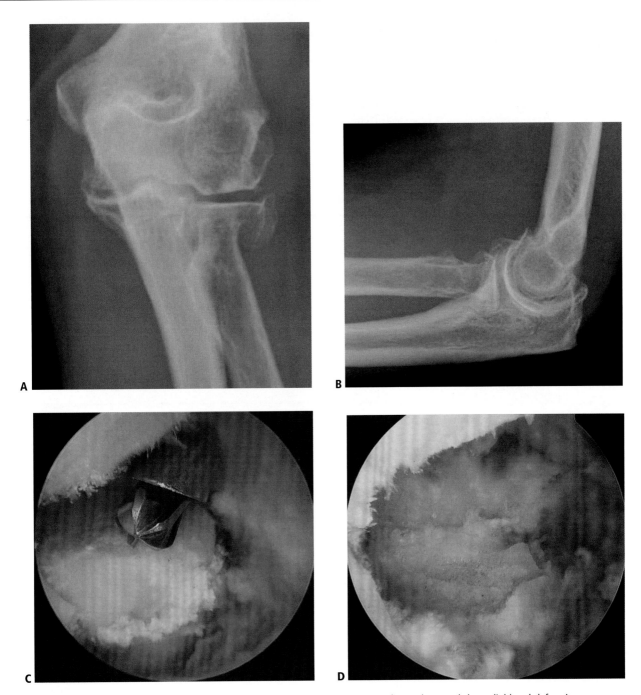

FIGURE 35.3. The same patient described in Fig. 35.2. **A** and **B**: Preoperative radiographs reveal the radial head deformity. **C**: The radial head deformity viewed from an anteromedial portal with a burr introduced in the proximal anterolateral portal. **D**: The appearance after resection of the radial head viewed from the proximal anterolateral portal. **E** and **F**: Postoperative radiographs. Preoperative range of motion was 30° to 130° of flexion with 40° pronation and 50° of supination. Postoperative range of motion was 10° to 140° of flexion with 70° pronation and 60° of supination.

head. If necessary to improve visualization and to protect the posterior interosseous nerve (PIN), a retractor can be placed in a proximal anterolateral portal. A drainage cannula is placed in the posterior central portal for outflow. Starting anterior and working posteriorly with the motorized burr, the radial head is resected in a piecemeal fashion. The cutting surface of the burr should be kept facing in a posterior direction to avoid injury to the PIN, which lies adjacent to the anterior capsule at this level. Resection is continued distally to the radial neck just past the level of the sigmoid notch of the ulna. The annular ligament should be preserved since it contributes to varus and posterolateral rotatory stability of the elbow. While continuing to view from the proximal anteromedial portal, the burr

II. The Elbow

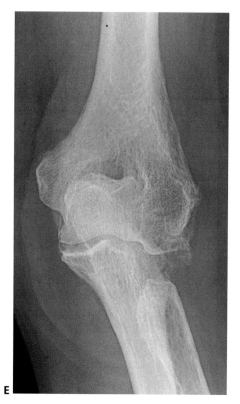
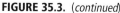
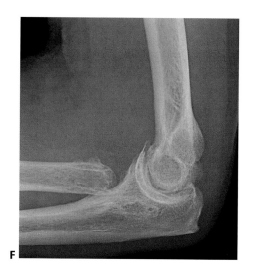

FIGURE 35.3. *(continued)*

is then transferred to a posterolateral "soft spot" portal to complete the posterior resection of the radial head. A full-radius resector or a pituitary rongeur can be used to remove the remaining cartilage and bony debris from the joint.

The goal is to resect the head just distal to the sigmoid notch of the ulna, so there is no impingement with rotation. Once the resection is complete, the elbow should be supinated and pronated under arthroscopic vision to ensure that there is no remaining mechanical impingement or block to rotation. A final check is to use an image intensifier to confirm that an adequate amount of bone has been resected from the radial neck and to evaluate for valgus, varus, posterolateral, and axial instability.

Once the procedure is completed, the portal sites are sutured to prevent formation of synovial fistulas. A bulky dressing is applied to control swelling while allowing early elbow range of motion.

AUTHORS' PREFERRED TREATMENT

Radial head resection is uncommonly indicated. It should be avoided if other options are available. Alternative treatment options include synovectomy alone with retention of the radial head, radial head debridement, radial head replacement, radiocapitellar interposition, or replacement arthroplasty and total elbow arthroplasty.

Retention of the radial head should be considered in most patients undergoing synovectomy and debridement for rheumatoid and osteoarthritis. Radial head resection should be considered only in cases where there is severe deformity interfering with rotation or symptoms specifically referable to the radial head. Rather than excising the radial head, debriding and contouring of the retained radial head have been used by some in the setting of rheumatoid arthritis with aims to improve forearm rotation (16).

If radial head resection is deemed necessary, there are a number of options for replacement. A radial head prosthesis will preserve the stabilizing effect of the radial head (5–7, 15, 16). However, radial head replacement is not ideal if there is anticipated maltracking of a prosthetic radial head. This is often the case in the setting of chronic subluxation or dislocation of the proximal radioulnar joint. Likewise, a deformed native capitellum may become a pain generator if it articulates with a radial head hemi-arthroplasty, making excision without replacement more ideal in this setting. More recently, radiocapitellar prostheses have become available to address such cases where there is deformity on both articulations of the radiocapitellar joint. However, these have not been extensively studied to date. Radiocapitellar interposition arthroplasty with fascia or dermal grafts is another option in the setting of radiocapitellar arthritis where radial head excision is not an option and the patient is too young or their demands are too great to consider a replacement-type radiocapitellar arthroplasty. Total elbow arthroplasty UH remains the procedure of choice for patients with more advanced arthritis of both the radiocapitellar and the UH joints.

REHABILITATION

The patient is usually discharged from hospital the same day. Immediate active range of motion as tolerated is initiated. If a concomitant contracture release is performed, the patient is admitted for a continuous regional block for the first few days combined with immediate continuous passive motion device. Indomethacin 25 mg three times daily for 3 weeks should be considered to reduce the incidence of heterotopic ossification, postoperative swelling, and pain in patients who do not have a contraindication.

COMPLICATIONS, CONTROVERSIES, AND SPECIAL CONSIDERATIONS

Complications

The published reports of arthroscopic radial head resection are limited in number and duration of follow-up (2–4). There are no published clinical trials comparing the outcomes of open versus arthroscopic radial head resection. Thus, our understanding of the outcomes of arthroscopic radial head resection is based largely on our experience with open radial head resection. Arthroscopic radial head excision will likely have similar complications as have been reported following open resection, including cubitus valgus, proximal radial migration, DRUJ symptoms, PLRI, residual radiocapitellar, or proximal radioulnar impingement due to inadequate resection, loss of strength, degenerative OA, heterotopic ossification, and nerve injury (9, 17–19).

Complications reported specifically during arthroscopic radial head resection in one series of 12 patients include a moderate loss of strength in three patients (25%) that did not interfere with activities of daily living and proximal migration of the radius measuring 2 and 3 mm in two patients (17%) (3). There was no objective or subjective evidence of elbow instability, cubitus valgus, heterotopic ossification, infection, nerve injury, or vascular injury. Another series in which the radial head was excised arthroscopically in 18 of the 24 patients undergoing arthroscopic elbow debridement reported a 13% complication rate, which included a superficial infection in one patient, heterotopic ossification in one patient, and recurrent effusions in two patients (4). There was no report of late instability.

Controversies and Special Considerations

In the appropriately selected patient, one must consider whether the radial head resection should be performed open or arthroscopically. As previously mentioned, there are no published clinical trials comparing the outcomes of open versus arthroscopic radial head resection. However, open radial head resection should be considered in the hands of surgeons who are not experienced with elbow arthroscopy due to the technical difficulty and theoretical increased risk of nerve injury associated with elbow arthroscopy.

PEARLS AND PITFALLS

There are a number of technical pearls to remember during arthroscopic radial head resection. As with any elbow arthroscopy, there are important principles such as low inflow pressures, gravity suction on the motorized resectors, and keeping the motorized resectors directed away from the capsule to prevent inadvertent nerve injury. Technical pearls specific to arthroscopic radial head resection include ensuring there is adequate resection by rotating the forearm under direct visualization to assess for any residual mechanical block and by using intraoperative fluoroscopy. The use of a retractor to improve visualization and to move the anterior capsule and PIN away from the burr improves the safety of the procedure.

The most significant pitfall is poor patient selection. The treating surgeon must be certain that the radial head deformity is the source of symptomatology. There is often a component of UH arthrosis present, which may be contributing to the patient's symptoms. Not only is an isolated radial head resection in this setting less likely to offer any benefit, but what is worse is that the radial head resection may exacerbate a symptomatic UH joint by increasing the load across the UH articulation.

The other significant pitfall related to patient selection is performing a radial head resection in the setting of elbow or forearm instability. The instability may worsen after radial head resection. Alternative treatments must be considered in this setting, which include radial head debridement, prosthetic radial head replacement, radiocapitellar interposition arthroplasty, replacement radiocapitellar arthroplasty, or total elbow arthroplasty.

CONCLUSIONS AND FUTURE DIRECTIONS

Resection of the radial head is an effective treatment in appropriately selected patients with a radial head articular deformity or arthritis causing pain and impeding motion. However, radial head resection is uncommonly indicated and one should aim to preserve or replace the radial head when possible. This will help to maintain the stability of the elbow and forearm and prevent late complications.

Arthroscopic radial head resection offers theoretical benefits over open resection such as less injury to the annular and lateral collateral ligament, earlier return of function, and less stiffness due to the less invasive surgical approach. However, there is currently insufficient evidence in the literature to support these theoretical advantages. Also, one must consider the increased risk of nerve injury associated with elbow arthroscopy. Regardless, arthroscopic radial head resection is a proven technique that will likely continue to become more popular as surgeons gain more experience with elbow arthroscopy.

II. The Elbow

REFERENCES

1. Lee BPH, Morrey BF. Synovectomy of the elbow. In: Morrey BF, ed. *The Elbow and Its Disorders*. 3rd ed. Philadelphia, PA: WB Saunders; 2000:708–717.

2. Lo IK, King GJ. Arthroscopic radial head excision. *Arthroscopy*. 1994;10(6):689–692.

3. Menth-Chiari WA, Ruch DS, Poehling GG. Arthroscopic excision of the radial head: clinical outcome in 12 patients with post-traumatic arthritis after fracture of the radial head or rheumatoid arthritis. *Arthroscopy*. 2001;17:918–923.

4. Savoie FH III, Nunley PD, Field LD. Arthroscopic management of the arthritic elbow: indications, technique, and results. *J Shoulder Elbow Surg*. 1999;8(3):214–219.

5. Beingessner DM, Dunning CE, Gordon KE, et al. The effect of radial head excision and arthroplasty on elbow kinematics and stability. *J Bone Joint Surg Am*. 2004;86:1730–1739.

6. Johnson JA, Beingessner DM, Gordon KD, et al. Kinematics and stability of the fractured and implant-reconstructed radial head. *J Shoulder Elbow Surg*. 2005;14:195S–201S.

7. King GJ, Zarzour ZD, Rath DA, et al. Metallic radial head arthroplasty improves valgus stability of the elbow. *Clin Orthop Relat Res*. 1999;368:114–125.

8. Jensen SL, Olsen BS, Søjbjerg JO. Elbow joint kinematics after excision of the radial head. *J Shoulder Elbow Surg*. 1999;8:238–241.

9. Hall JA, McKee MD. Posterolateral rotatory instability of the elbow following radial head resection. *J Bone Joint Surg Am*. 2005;87-A(7):1571–1579.

10. O'Driscoll SW, Bell DF, Morrey BF. Posterolateral rotatory instability of the elbow. *J Bone Joint Surg Am*. 73:440–446.

11. Morrey BF, Chao EY, Hui FC. Biomechanical study of the elbow following excision of the radial head. *J Bone Joint Surg Am*. 1979;61: 63–68.

12. Ikeda M, Oka Y. Function after early radial head resection for fracture: a retrospective evaluation of 15 patients followed for 3–18 years. *Acta Orthop Scand*. 2000;71:191–194.

13. Janssen RP, Vegter J. Resection of the radial head after Mason type-III fractures of the elbow: follow-up at 16 to 30 years. *J Bone Joint Surg Br*. 1998;80:231–233.

14. Leppilahti J, Jalovaara P. Early excision of the radial head for fracture. *Int Orthop*. 2000;24:160–162.

15. Pomianowski S, Morrey BF, Neale PG, et al. Contribution of monoblock and bipolar radial head prostheses to valgus stability of the elbow. *J Bone Joint Surg*. 2001;A83:1829–1834.

16. Schneeberger AG, Sadowski MM, Jacob HA. Coronoid process and radial head as posterolateral rotatory stabilizers of the elbow. *J Bone Joint Surg*. 2004;86-A(5):975–982.

17. Kauffman JI, Chen AL, Stuchin S, et al. Surgical management of the rheumatoid elbow. *J Am Acad Orthop Surg*. 2003;11(2):100–108.

18. Morrey BF. Radial head fracture. In: Morrey BF, ed. *The Elbow and Its Disorders*. 3rd ed. Philadelphia, PA: WB Saunders; 2000:341–364.

19. Morrey BF, Schneeberger AG. Anconeus arthroplasty: a new technique for reconstruction of the radiocapitellar and/or proximal radioulnar joint. *J Bone Joint Surg Am*. 2002;84:1960–1969.

Arthroscopic Management of Lateral Epicondylitis

Champ L. Baker III • Champ L. Baker Jr

In 1873, Runge first described the pathologic entity of lateral humeral epicondylitis. Ten years later, Morris noted an association between lawn tennis and lateral epicondylitis, leading to its common designation as tennis elbow. Since these original descriptions, various etiologies regarding the pathogenesis of lateral epicondylitis have been proposed. Advancing the works of Cyriax (1), Goldie (2), and Coonrad and Hooper (3), Nirschl and associates (4, 5) noted the basic underlying lesion is in the origin of the extensor carpi radialis brevis (ECRB) tendon. Repetitive overuse leads to microtears in the ECRB origin. Subsequent failed tendon healing and replacement with immature reparative tissue follows. Histologic examination of the essential lesion reveals a degenerative, noninflammatory process characterized with fibroblasts, disorganized collagen, and vascular hyperplasia. These findings have been termed angiofibroblastic hyperplasia with later modification to angiofibroblastic tendinosis. Despite advances in our understanding of the pathoanatomy of lateral epicondylitis, controversy remains regarding its optimal treatment. Various nonoperative and operative interventions have been proposed with most yielding short-term success. For patients who require surgery for recalcitrant symptoms, the authors have had high rates of clinical success with arthroscopic resection of pathologic tissue at both short- and long-term follow-up (6, 7).

CLINICAL EVALUATION

The most common presenting complaint is pain about the lateral aspect of the elbow. The pain may extend distally into the dorsal forearm or radiate proximally. Typically, the pain is of insidious onset with a history of repetitive activity. Patients often report a decrease in grip strength and difficulty holding or lifting objects, especially away from their body with their arms extended. On clinical examination, the patient may give minimal effort or wince with a handshake. Evaluation of the elbow reveals characteristic point tenderness to palpation at

an area just anterior and distal to the lateral epicondyle. Reproducible pain localized to the lateral epicondyle is found with resisted wrist extension with the elbow fully extended. Passive wrist flexion, again with the elbow extended, places the ECRB on stretch and can reproduce pain. Evaluation of the cervical spine and upper extremity can help to differentiate lateral epicondylitis from other causes of lateral elbow pain, such as cervical radiculopathy, radial tunnel syndrome, osteochondritis dissecans of the capitellum, radiocapitellar arthrosis, posterolateral rotatory instability of the elbow, and posterolateral elbow plica.

Although lateral epicondylitis is a clinical diagnosis, we routinely obtain plain anteroposterior, lateral, and axial elbow radiographs as part of the initial evaluation in the patient presenting with elbow pain. Radiographs may demonstrate soft tissue calcification adjacent to the lateral epicondyle, which is present in approximately 25% of patients, especially if the patient has had previous steroid injections. MRI can provide additional information regarding suspected intra-articular disorders, the extent of extensor tendon involvement, the presence of associated tendon tears, and the integrity of the lateral collateral ligamentous complex.

TREATMENT

Currently, no consensus exists regarding the optimal treatment for lateral epicondylitis. Various nonoperative measures have been recommended, including activity modification, physical therapy, nonsteroidal anti-inflammatory medications, counterforce bracing, and corticosteroid injections. More recent approaches include injections of botulinum toxin, buffered platelet-rich plasma, and application of extracorporeal shock-wave therapy. Most patients respond successfully to various conservative methods. In the reported studies of Coonrad and Hooper (3), Nirschl and Pettrone (4), and Boyd and McLeod (8), only 4% to 11% of patients required operative intervention for recalcitrant symptoms.

Indications for surgical treatment include persistent lateral elbow pain and dysfunction that interferes with the patient's activities despite appropriate nonoperative treatment. We recommend a minimum of 6 months of nonoperative treatment before considering surgery. Although rare, we consider earlier surgical intervention in the patient who sustained a direct trauma, resulting in a partial tear of the ECRB. Many different operative procedures have been reported: percutaneous, endoscopic, or open extensor tendon release; open techniques for excision of abnormal degenerative tissue with either simple suture repair or formal repair of the extensor tendons back to the lateral epicondyle; and arthroscopic release or resection of degenerative tissue.

We prefer arthroscopic management of lateral epicondylitis because we have found it to be safe and reproducible with proven high rates of clinical success at long-term follow-up. In addition, it affords the opportunity to evaluate and treat for coexistent intra-articular pathoanatomy and offers a potentially shorter postoperative rehabilitation with expedited return to work and unrestricted activities. Relative contraindications to the arthroscopic technique include previous medial elbow surgery with ulnar nerve transposition or with a subluxating ulnar nerve.

AUTHORS' PREFERRED TREATMENT

For the arthroscopic procedure, patients can be placed in the supine, lateral, or prone position. We prefer the prone position with the use of a general anesthetic (Fig. 36.1). This position allows for an accurate postoperative neurovascular assessment. A well-padded tourniquet is placed about the upper arm. For larger individuals, a sterile tourniquet can be used. The arm is placed into a commercially available arm holder and is prepared and draped in the standard sterile fashion. The following anatomic landmarks are identified and outlined on the skin to safely create the arthroscopic portals: medial epicondyle and intermuscular septum, ulnar nerve, olecranon tip, lateral

epicondyle, and radial head (Figs. 36.2 and 36.3). Next, we mark the lateral soft spot in the center of the triangle created by the radial head, olecranon, and lateral epicondyle. We wrap the forearm with a compressive dressing to prevent leakage of fluid into the distal soft tissues. The limb is exsanguinated, and the tourniquet insufflated to approximately 250 mm Hg.

Before we create the portals, the elbow joint is distended with approximately 20 to 25 mL of normal saline through the lateral soft spot (Fig. 36.4). Joint distention displaces the neurovascular structures anteriorly to help protect against iatrogenic injury during portal creation and introduction of the instruments. In particular, the ulnar nerve should be identified and protected. First, we establish the proximal medial portal approximately 2 cm proximal and 1 cm anterior to the palpable medial epicondyle (Fig. 36.5). For larger individuals, we place this portal slightly more proximal and anterior. After incising the skin, we utilize a straight hemostat to spread the subcutaneous tissues (Fig. 36.6). This "nick-and-spread" technique helps prevent injury to the sensory nerves. A blunt trocar and cannula without side portals is inserted through this portal aiming toward the center of the joint while maintaining contact with the anterior humeral

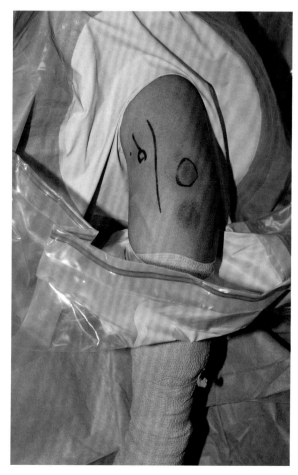

FIGURE 36.2. Landmarks outlined include medial epicondyle and intermuscular septum, ulnar nerve, and olecranon tip.

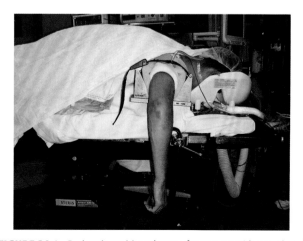

FIGURE 36.1. Patient is positioned prone for surgery with arm placed in arm holder.

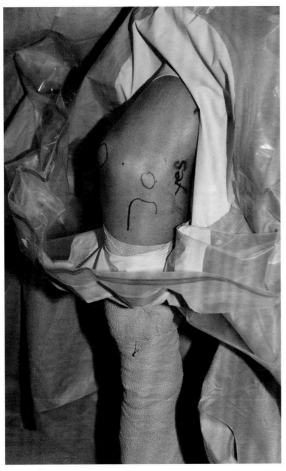

FIGURE 36.3. Landmarks outlined include the lateral epicondyle and radial head.

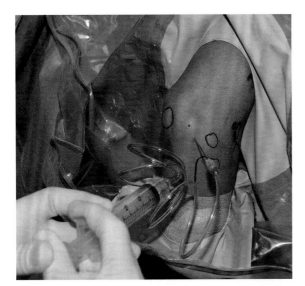

FIGURE 36.4. To distend the joint and displace the neurovascular structures anteriorly, 20 to 25 mL of saline are injected through the lateral soft spot.

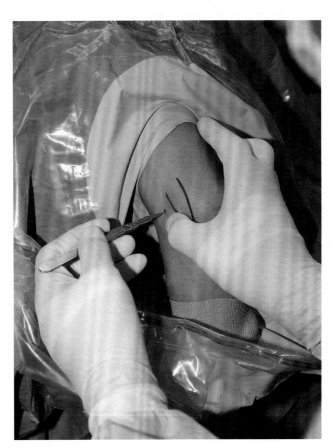

FIGURE 36.5. Location of the proximal medial portal.

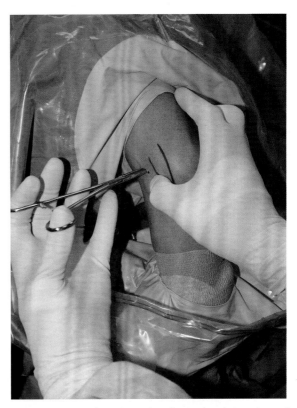

FIGURE 36.6. For safety, the nick-and-spread technique is used to spread the subcutaneous tissues.

II. The Elbow

border. Backflow of fluid confirms intra-articular placement (Fig. 36.7). Stothers et al. (9) found the ulnar nerve to be located, on average, 12 mm away from this proximal medial portal posterior to and protected by the medial intermuscular septum. This portal is also an average of 2.3 mm from the medial antebrachial cutaneous nerve, 7.6 mm from the median nerve, and 18 mm from the brachial artery with the elbow in flexion (Fig. 36.8).

A 4-mm, 30° arthroscope is inserted, and a careful, systematic evaluation is performed. Initially, the radiocapitellar articulation is visualized (Fig. 36.9). Pronation and supination of the arm allows for a complete examination of the radial head. Chondromalacia of the radiocapitellar joint is occasionally present. Irregular extension of the annular ligament overlying the radial head, or synovial fringe, can sometimes be appreciated. We believe this structure can be a source of lateral elbow symptoms often mimicking lateral epicondylitis and should be removed concomitant with the ECRB resection (10). The undersurface of the lateral capsule is inspected and classified. We classify the condition of the capsule as type I (intact capsule), type II (linear capsular tears), or type III (capsular rupture) (6). The arthroscope is carefully retracted medially to visualize the coronoid.

Next, we establish a proximal lateral portal using an outside-in technique. This portal is typically located 1 to 2 cm proximal to the lateral epicondyle along the anterior humeral surface. We localize this portal by pressing with a finger over the lateral aspect of the elbow proximal to the lateral epicondyle and visualize the capsule moving underneath. An 18G needle is inserted at this location to ensure proper positioning in the joint (Fig. 36.10).

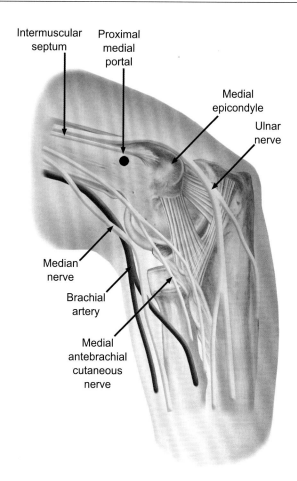

FIGURE 36.8. Relationship of the proximal medial portal to surrounding neurovascular structures.

We use a knife to incise the skin and capsule percutaneously. We have found that creating a hole in the capsule with the knife allows easier introduction of the blunt trocar into the joint. Stothers et al. (9) noted the radial nerve and the posterior branch of the antebrachial cutaneous nerve to be located at an average of 9.9 and 6. 6 mm,

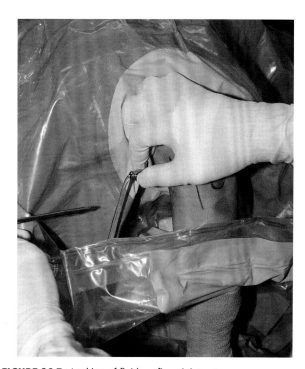

FIGURE 36.7. Leaking of fluid confirms joint entry.

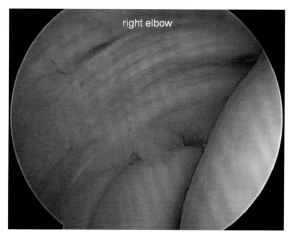

FIGURE 36.9. The radiocapitellar articulation can be seen and examined from the proximal medial portal.

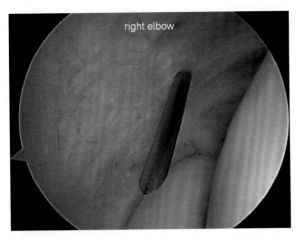

FIGURE 36.10. The proximal lateral portal is established using an outside-in technique. A needle is inserted for proper positioning.

respectively, from the proximal lateral portal with the elbow flexed (Fig. 36.11).

A small, motorized shaver is inserted through the cannula into the joint (Fig. 36.12). A portion of the lateral capsule is removed to expose the confluent ECRB

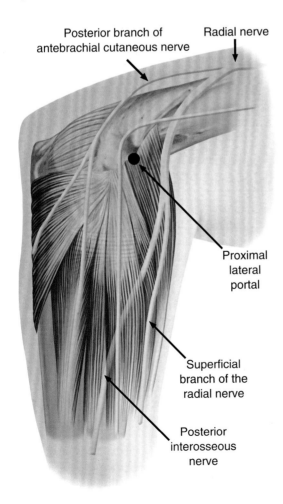

FIGURE 36.11. Relationship of the proximal lateral portal to surrounding neurovascular structures.

Posterior branch of antebrachial cutaneous nerve

Radial nerve

Proximal lateral portal

Superficial branch of the radial nerve

Posterior interosseous nerve

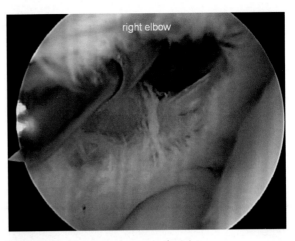

FIGURE 36.12. The shaver is seen in the joint.

(Fig. 36.13). The ECRB lies between the capsule and the common extensor origin. Using a radiofrequency probe, we resect the ECRB tendon origin from its insertion and ablate the tendinosis tissue (Figs. 36.14 and 36.15). Resection begins proximally and progresses distally. Anatomic studies have demonstrated safe, complete resection of the ECRB origin as long as dissection does not extend posterior to a line bisecting the radial head (11–13). The lateral ligamentous structures are thus protected without iatrogenic creation of posterolateral rotatory instability. Early in our experience, we routinely decorticated the lateral epicondyle; however, several patients developed a postoperative bony tenderness not present preoperatively. For this reason, we no longer decorticate the lateral epicondyle. If, on preoperative evaluation, the patient had concurrent posterior or posterolateral pain on terminal elbow extension, we then inspect the posterior compartment through either the posterolateral or direct lateral portal. There can be a posterolateral synovial reaction that can be a pain generator. If found, this area is gently debrided with a shaver. The portal sites are then closed with simple nylon ligature, and a sterile dressing is applied.

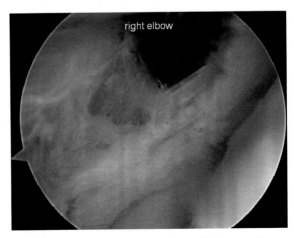

FIGURE 36.13. A portion of the lateral capsule is removed to reveal the underlying ECRB tendon.

II. The Elbow

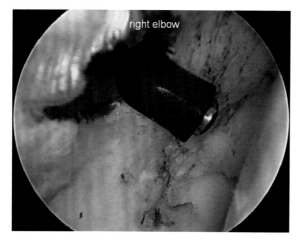

FIGURE 36.14. We prefer to use a radiofrequency device to resect the ECRB origin from its insertion.

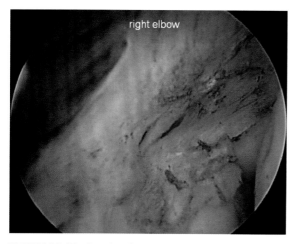

FIGURE 36.15. Completed resection.

COMPLICATIONS, CONTROVERSIES, AND SPECIAL CONSIDERATIONS

With any elbow arthroscopic procedure, there is always concern for injury to the neurovascular structures. Using the nick-and-spread technique to create the proximal medial portal can minimize potential injury to the medial antebrachial cutaneous nerves and painful neuroma formation. The surgeon should always be cognizant with previous surgery on the medial aspect of the elbow, such as ulnar nerve transposition or with a subluxating ulnar nerve. Location and protection of the nerve prior to creation of the proximal medial portal anterior to the medial intermuscular septum is critical. Although it has not been our personal experience, posterior interosseous nerve injury can occur. Danger to the nerve increases the more distal the proximal lateral portal is placed. Distention of the elbow joint before creating the portals also increases the distance from the instrumentation to the anterior neurovascular structures.

Cohen et al. (12) recently characterized the anatomical ECRB footprint as between the most proximal aspect of the capitellum and the midline of the radiocapitellar joint. The lateral ulnar collateral ligament lies posterior to the ECRB origin. The lateral collateral ligamentous complex is not disrupted during arthroscopy as long as resection of the ECRB and elbow capsule is kept anterior to a line bisecting the radial head. Posterolateral rotatory instability of the elbow has been reported after open procedures for lateral epicondylitis, but this complication can be prevented with careful attention to surgical landmarks and to extent of resection.

Persistent pain after arthroscopy can usually be attributed to an improper or incomplete preoperative diagnosis or an inadequate resection of tendinosis tissue. Cummins (14) recently described the results of arthroscopic debridement of the pathologic tissue followed by a traditional open exposure to assess the effectiveness of the arthroscopic removal. Gross and histologic analysis was done on 18 elbows at the time of the open procedure. The first six patients' elbows had residual gross tendinopathy present at open inspection. Of the next 12 elbows, no patient had residual gross tendinopathy present, but four elbows had residual tendinopathy on histologic analysis only. This study confirms that although a learning curve exists, arthroscopic debridement can effectively remove all of the gross pathologic tissue seen during an open exposure.

Another complication is postoperative loss of motion, particularly in extension. This is an infrequent occurrence due to immediate institution of range-of-motion exercises. The assistance of a physical therapist is employed if motion loss is noted at the first postoperative visit.

PEARLS AND PITFALLS

1. If a concurrent open procedure is planned, a sideboard can be affixed to the table.
2. The tourniquet and arm holder should be placed as proximal as possible to allow easy joint access with instrumentation. A sterile tourniquet may be required for larger arms.
3. For patients with larger arms, we place our proximal medial portal slightly more anteriorly and proximally than usual.
4. The "nick-and-spread" technique decreases potential injury to the medial sensory nerves during the creation of the proximal medial portal.
5. Preoperatively, the surgeon must identify with a previous ulnar nerve transfer or a subluxating ulnar nerve. If the patient has had a subcutaneous ulnar nerve transfer previously, we first make a medial incision, identify and protect the ulnar nerve, and then create the proximal medial portal under direct visualization. For a subluxating ulnar nerve, we hold the nerve posterior to the medial intermuscular septum with our thumb as we create the portal as described by O'Driscoll.

6. We use cannulas without sideports to decrease fluid extravasation into the soft tissues.

7. A second more proximal lateral portal can be created to insert a retractor if visualization becomes difficult.

8. Annular ligament extension with synovial tissue can become entrapped between the radial head and the capitellum, becoming a source of lateral elbow pain. It should be excised concurrently with the tendinosis resection.

REHABILITATION

All procedures are performed on an outpatient basis. Initially, the arm is placed into a sling for comfort only. The patient is encouraged to begin active and passive range-of-motion exercises of the elbow. Sutures are removed at the first postoperative visit, which is within 7 days from surgery. If the patient has difficulty regaining full extension or if potential motion loss is a concern, formal physical therapy is prescribed. Home exercises that include simple stretching and strengthening are initiated as the patient's symptoms allow. Return to light activities is typically at 2 weeks after surgery and to sports at approximately 6 weeks after surgery.

CONCLUSIONS AND FUTURE DIRECTIONS

We recently reviewed the long-term outcomes in a series of patients treated with arthroscopic debridement of the ECRB origin (7). Thirty elbows in 30 patients were evaluated at a mean of 130 months after surgery (range, 106 to 173 months). At final follow-up examinations, patients were asked to rate their pain on a visual analog scale from 0 (no pain) to 10 (severe pain). Patients were also asked to rate their elbows according to the functional portion of the Mayo Clinic Elbow Performance Index. The mean pain score at rest was 0, for activities of daily living 1.0, and for work or sports 1.9 out of 10. The mean functional score was 11.7 out of a possible 12 points on the Mayo Clinic Elbow Performance Index. No patient required repeat injections or surgeries. One patient continued to wear a counterforce brace with heavy activities. Eighty-seven percent of patients were satisfied, and 97% of patients stated they were "much better" or "better" at final follow-up. Twenty-two of 30 patients (73%) were still employed at the time of final follow-up, with 14 patients performing office or desk-type work and eight patients involved in heavy labor. Six patients had retired, and the remaining two patients were not working for reasons unrelated to their elbow. Only one patient had changed jobs due to the condition of her elbow at the time of her operation.

Other authors have noted similar high rates of clinical success in patients managed arthroscopically for lateral epicondylitis with results comparable to traditional open methods. In a retrospective study, Szabo et al. (15) compared 23 percutaneous, 38 open, and 41 arthroscopic procedures at a mean follow-up of 48 months. There were no statistically significant differences among the three surgical groups with regard to recurrences, complications, failures, preoperative, or postoperative Andrews-Carson scores or visual analog pain scores. The authors were unable to determine the rate at which the patients returned to work and activities of daily living without discomfort, but they concluded each method is a highly effective way to treat recalcitrant lateral epicondylitis.

We believe arthroscopic resection of pathologic tendinosis tissue is a safe, effective procedure for the management of lateral epicondylitis refractory to nonoperative treatment. High rates of clinical success are maintained at long-term follow-up. Results are comparable with open and percutaneous techniques. In addition, arthroscopy affords the ability to perform a complete intra-articular assessment with evaluation of the anterior and posterior compartments of the elbow. Associated pathoanatomy can be diagnosed and treated. Regardless of the operative technique chosen, successful operative management of lateral epicondylitis is dependent on proper patient selection, identification of pathology, and complete resection of the ECRB tendinosis.

REFERENCES

1. Cyriax JH. The pathology and treatment of tennis elbow. *J Bone Joint Surg Am.* 1936;18:921–940.
2. Goldie I. Epicondylitis lateralis humeri (epicondylalgia or tennis elbow): a pathogenetical study. *Acta Chir Scand Suppl.* 1964;57:339.
3. Coonrad RW, Hooper WR. Tennis elbow: its course, natural history, conservative, and surgical management. *J Bone Joint Surg Am.* 1973;55:1183–1187.
4. Nirschl RP, Pettrone FA. Tennis elbow: the surgical treatment of lateral epicondylitis. *J Bone Joint Surg Am.* 1979;61:832–839.
5. Kraushaar BS, Nirschl RP. Tendinosis of the elbow (tennis elbow): clinical features and findings of histological, immuno-histochemical, and electron microscopy studies. *J Bone Joint Surg Am.* 1999;81:259–278.
6. Baker CL Jr, Murphy KP, Gottlob CA, et al. Arthroscopic classification and treatment of lateral epicondylitis: two-year clinical results. *J Shoulder Elbow Surg.* 2000;9:475–482.
7. Baker CL Jr, Baker CL III. Long-term follow-up of arthroscopic treatment of lateral epicondylitis. *Am J Sports Med.* 2008;36:254–260.
8. Boyd HB, McLeod AC Jr. Tennis elbow. *J Bone Joint Surg Am.* 1973;55:1177–1182.
9. Stothers K, Day B, Regan WR. Arthroscopy of the elbow: anatomy, portal sites, and a description of the proximal lateral portal. *Arthroscopy.* 1995;11:449–457.
10. Mullett H, Sprague M, Brown G, et al. Arthroscopic treatment of lateral epicondylitis: clinical and cadaveric studies. *Clin Orthop Relat Res.* 2005;439:123–128.
11. Smith AM, Castle JA, Ruch DS. Arthroscopic resection of the common extensor origin: anatomic considerations. *J Shoulder Elbow Surg.* 2003;12:375–379.

12. Cohen MS, Romeo AA, Hennigan SP, et al. Lateral epicondylitis: anatomic relationships of the extensor tendon origins and implications for arthroscopic treatment. *J Shoulder Elbow Surg.* 2008;17:954–960.

13. Kuklo TR, Taylor KF, Murphy KP, et al. Arthroscopic release for lateral epicondylitis: a cadaveric model. *Arthroscopy.* 1999;15:259–264.

14. Cummins CA. Lateral epicondylitis: in vivo assessment of arthroscopic debridement and correlation with patient outcomes. *Am J Sports Med.* 2006;34:1486–1491.

15. Szabo SJ, Savoie FH III, Field LD, et al. Tendinosis of the extensor carpi radialis brevis: an evaluation of three methods of operative treatment. *J Shoulder Elbow Surg.* 2006;15:721–727.

Elbow Instability: Arthroscopic Management Options and Medial Collateral Ligament Reconstruction

Christopher C. Dodson • David W. Altchek

Excessive valgus and extension forces are generated during the throwing motion in several sports, most notably baseball, tennis, football, and certain track and field events (1). The repetition required to excel in these sports can ultimately lead to fatigue and even failure of key stabilizing structures in the elbow. The medial ulnar collateral ligament (MUCL) is the primary restraint to valgus load during the throwing motion and is most susceptible to injury after repetitive throwing. MUCL insufficiency leads to valgus instability, a condition that is only significant in overhead athletes. Overtime, chronic valgus instability can result in a unique constellation of elbow pathologies that are indicative of repetitive overhead throwing.

The most common injuries seen in the elbow of the throwing athlete are MUCL injuries, ulnar neuritis, postero-medial impingement/osteophyte formation, flexor-pronator strain, ulnar stress fractures, osteochondritis dissecans of the capitellum, and capsular contracture (2–5). Although not all pathology in the thrower's elbow is amenable to arthroscopic management, it is essential that any clinician who cares for throwing athletes be familiar with all pathologic conditions and comfortable with both open and arthroscopic treatments.

Over the past decade, clinicians have gained a better understanding of the complex interplay between the dynamic and static stabilizers of the elbow. Furthermore, the desire for minimally invasive treatment of these conditions has led to the development of advanced techniques and instrumentation for elbow arthroscopy. This discussion will be limited to the arthroscopic treatment of common elbow injuries in throwing athletes, including those that can be managed entirely arthroscopically as well as in conjunction with a common open procedure for valgus instability (i.e., MUCL reconstruction).

ANATOMY/PATHOANATOMY

The elbow is a hinge joint with the bony ulnohumeral articulation providing stability at the extremes of motion,

from 0° to 20° of flexion and beyond 120° of flexion (2). The intervening 100°, which is the primary arc of motion used in overhead throwing, relies progressively on the static and dynamic soft tissue restraints to provide stability. The anatomy of MUCL has been well described; it is actually not a single ligament but rather a complex consisting of an anterior bundle, a posterior bundle, and a transverse component (Fig. 37.1). The anterior bundle is the most well-defined structure and originates on the medial epicondyle and inserts on the sublime tubercle. The anterior bundle is subdivided into three components: an anterior band, a central band, and a posterior band. The anterior and posterior bands tighten in a reciprocal manner during flexion and extension, respectively. The posterior bundle is a less distinct fan-shaped structure, and the transverse ligament is the least distinct anatomic structure and provides very little stability to the elbow, because it does not cross the joint. Biomechanical studies have demonstrated that the anterior bundle is the primary constraint to valgus stress about the elbow; the anterior band of the anterior bundle provides most of the stability from 30° to 90° of flexion, whereas the posterior bundle becomes functionally significant between 60° and maximum flexion (6, 7).

The mechanics of overhead throwing, particularly pitching, accounts for the various pathologies seen in overhead athletes. Valgus forces have been estimated to reach 64 N during the late cocking and early acceleration phases of throwing (3–5). After the early and late cocking phases, the elbow goes from rapid flexion to extension, and the tangentially directed forces produce a valgus and extension moment, with resulting tensile forces across the medial side of the elbow, compressive forces across the lateral aspect of the joint, and shear forces in the posterior compartment (3–5). The repetitive stress on the MUCL eventually leads to attenuation and ultimately rupture, resulting in an insufficient ligament complex, abnormal valgus rotation of the elbow, and

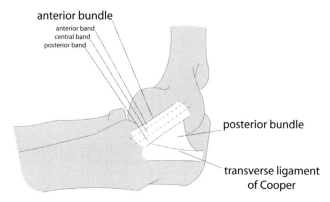

FIGURE 37.1. Schematic drawing of the MCL complex. Note that the anterior bundle is composed of three bands. The anterior band of the anterior bundle is the primary restraint to valgus stress.

instability. The term valgus extension overload describes this phenomenon (8). As the athlete continues to throw with instability, the valgus overload is accentuated and excessive valgus moments lead to stretch of other medial structures, resulting in ulnar neuritis, flexor-pronator tendonopathy, or medial epicondyle apophysitis in the skeletally immature patient. Corresponding overload on the lateral side of the elbow may lead to radiocapitellar chondromalacia, osteophyte formation, and loose bodies. Finally, during extension, posterior shear forces can produce olecranon osteophytes at the posteromedial tip with a corresponding "kissing lesion" on the posteromedial trochlea (3). It is imperative that the clinician who treats throwing athletes be familiar with these various pathologies and possess a high index of suspicion for underlying MUCL insufficiency as the etiology for many of these disorders because treating the pathology alone, without ligament reconstruction, will often fail to relieve the athletes' symptoms and to allow them to return to sport.

CLINICAL EVALUATION

History

A comprehensive patient history is crucial to developing a differential diagnosis for recalcitrant elbow pain and disability in the throwing athlete. The nature, mechanism, acuity of onset, and symptoms associated with the pain or injury are important factors to elucidate, as with any chief complaint. In addition, the phase of throwing and any change in accuracy, velocity, stamina, or strength can help provide information about the specific diagnosis. Pain during the late cocking phase on the medial side of the elbow can indicate MUCL insufficiency. Young throwing athletes with OCD lesions often report progressive lateral elbow pain during the late acceleration and follow-through phases, with the loss of extension and episodes of locking. A history of mechanical symptoms, such as locking or catching, and posterior pain exacerbated by forced extension are also important as these symptoms

may be caused by loose bodies, chondral flaps, or posteromedial impingement.

It is of utmost importance to inquire about ulnar nerve symptoms not only because this can be a source of elbow pain in the throwing athlete, but also because it is vulnerable to arthroscopic injury. Sharp pain radiating down the medial portion of the forearm with paresthesias in the fifth digit and in the ulnar-innervated half of the fourth digit can indicate ulnar neuritis. When these symptoms are associated with a snapping or popping sensation, ulnar nerve subluxation may be the cause. It is critical to make the diagnosis of a subluxating ulnar nerve because it is a risk factor for injury when making and utilizing medial portals during elbow arthroscopy.

Physical Examination

The physical examination of the elbow begins with cervical spine and includes the ipsilateral shoulder and the contralateral elbow, followed by examination of the involved elbow. Neurovascular assessment of the involved extremity, including motor and sensory testing and reflexes, is equally important.

Inspection of the elbow begins with an assessment of the resting position of the elbow and its carrying angle. A normal carrying angle is approximately 11° of valgus for men and 13° of valgus for women (2). An increase in the carrying angle of further valgus may indicate an adaptation to the repetitive stress of valgus instability. Angles of greater than 15° in professional pitchers have been documented in the literature (9). Next the lateral, posterior, medial, and anterior regions of the involved elbow should be examined for any swelling, obvious deformity, scars, or signs of previous trauma.

Following careful inspection, the four regions of the elbow should be palpated in an orderly fashion. The patients' history generally guides the examiner toward a specific location, but palpating all four anatomic regions ensures that concomitant pathology is not missed. The medial region of the elbow is often a focus when examining throwing athletes. Tenderness on the medial epicondyle and flexor-pronator mass can suggest an avulsion fracture (adolescents) or flexor-pronator tendonosis (adults). The patient with tendonosis will exhibit local tenderness and pain with resisted flexion and forearm pronation. The MUCL can be palpated under the mass of the flexor-pronator origin when the elbow is flexed greater than 90° at its insertion at the sublime tubercle; tenderness to palpation at this location can be indicative of MUCL insufficiency. In the posteromedial region of the elbow, the ulnar nerve is easily palpable in the groove, which is located between the medial epicondyle and the olecranon. The examiner should test not only for a Tinel's sign but also for hypermobility. This is done by palpating the nerve as the elbow is brought from extension to terminal flexion to determine whether the nerve subluxates or completely dislocates over the medial epicondyle. Palpation of the posteromedial region of the elbow should also focus on the olecranon, which can reveal osteophytes or swelling, which are present in the throwing athlete with valgus extension overload syndrome. The medial subcutaneous border of the olecranon should also be palpated for tenderness, which in the throwing athlete, can be caused by a stress fracture (10). Lastly, examination of the lateral region of the elbow begins with palpation of the lateral epicondyle. Tenderness directly over the epicondyle is consistent with lateral epicondylitis; tenderness directly-over the anconeus soft spot can indicate a symptomatic lateral plica, a condition that is commonly found in throwing athletes. In a recent study, this was the most reproducible finding in a group of patients who were treated for this condition (11).

Range of motion should be assessed for elbow flexion/extension and forearm supination/pronation, as well as the nature of the extension and flexion end points. Normal extension terminates in the firm sensation of the posterior bony articulation making contact in the olecranon fossa, and normal flexion terminates in the abutment of the soft tissues of the distal humerus and the proximal forearm. Variations in the normal end points particularly a bony end-feel in extension can be indicative of pathology such as posterior osteophytes. The examiner should focus on the end-feel at extension and not necessarily on motion itself; elbow flexion contractures can be a normal physical examination finding in high-level throwers and is not necessarily indicative of injury.

Evaluation of medial stability is the cornerstone of the assessment of the overhead athlete with valgus extension overload. Multiple techniques have been described in the literature for the optimal assessment of medial elbow stability. We typically find the valgus stress test and the moving valgus stress test to be the most specific and do both provocative maneuvers when examining throwing athletes. To perform the valgus stress test, the examiner places the patient's distal forearm under the axilla and applies a valgus load to the elbow in 30° of flexion (Fig. 37.2). The absence of a distinct endpoint combined with pain and/or tenderness indicates a positive test and insufficiency of the anterior band of the anterior bundle of the MCL. The moving valgus stress test, as described by O'Driscoll et al. (12), is performed with the patient in an upright position and the shoulder abducted 90° (Fig. 37.3). Starting with the elbow in full flexion and the shoulder in maximal external rotation, the elbow is quickly extended while a constant valgus torque is maintained. For an examination to be positive, the pain generated by the maneuver must reproduce the medial elbow pain that the patient has with activities, and the pain should be maximal between the position of late cocking (120°) and early acceleration (70°) as the elbow is extended. Other relevant tests in the throwing athlete include the radiocapitellar compression test for osteochondritis dissecans of the radiocapitellar joint, the clunk test for posterior olecranon impingement, and the

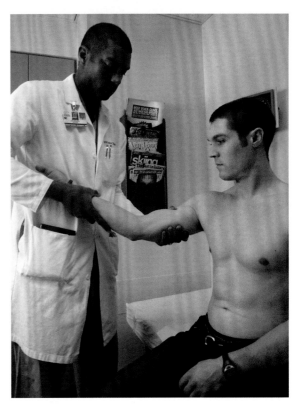

FIGURE 37.2. The valgus stress test is performed with the elbow at approximately 30°. It is important to place the distal forearm under the axilla to control rotation.

flexion-pronation test to detect a symptomatic snapping lateral plica. The radiocapitellar compression test is performed by placing the elbow in full extension and loading the joint with supination and pronation to produce mechanical symptoms. The clunk test for posterior olecranon impingement is simply stabilizing the upper arm and bringing the elbow into extension to produce posterior elbow pain (Fig. 37.4). The flexion pronation test is performed by placing the arm in maximum pronation and then passively flexing the elbow to approximately 90°, which will cause snapping in a positive test (11). Lastly, we reemphasize the importance of examining the ulnar nerve for subluxation, as many patients will be unaware of this "normal" variant.

Diagnostic Imaging

The routine preoperative radiographic evaluation of the elbow include AP, lateral, and oblique views. Stress views may be helpful in assessing ligamentous laxity and olecranon axial views at 110° of flexion may reveal posteromedial osteophytes in valgus extension overload syndrome. However, it has been our experience that a true lateral of the elbow in hyperflexion is adequate to diagnose posteromedial osteophytes. Contralateral comparison imaging studies of the elbow are helpful when evaluating elbow joint laxity and when trying to distinguish true growth disturbances from variant ossification centers in the pediatric

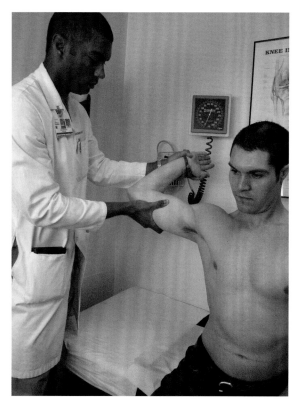

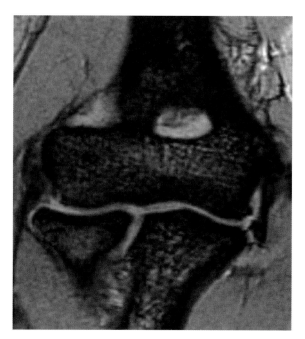

FIGURE 37.5. Coronal fat-suppression MRI demonstrating a "T-sign," which is indicative of a complete tear of the MCL complex at its humeral origin.

FIGURE 37.3. The moving valgus stress test. Starting with the arm in full flexion and the shoulder in maximal external rotation, the examiner then applies a constant valgus force and quickly extends the elbow. A positive test occurs when the patient experiences pain, reproduction of symptoms, or apprehension from 120° of flexion to 70° of extension.

population. CT scans can be helpful when trying to assess suspected bony pathology including stress fractures and avulsion fractures.

MRI remains the gold standard for the evaluation of the soft tissues about the elbow, including ligamentous injury, tendinopathy, and lesions of the articular cartilage. The accuracy of MRI in the evaluation of subtle MCL

injuries and the role of arthrography and contrast remain controversial. At our institution, we use a noncontrast MRI with specially designed sequences (Fig. 37.5). Potter et al. (13) have demonstrated a high sensitivity and specificity in detecting ligamentous, soft-tissue, and cartilaginous injuries using this technique. This technique maintains the minimally invasive nature of the test and limits cost. A major additional advantage is excellent visualization of the articular cartilage in a highly specific and sensitive manner.

TREATMENT

Nonoperative Treatment

Initially, a nonoperative treatment regimen is initiated consisting of a period of rest and anti-inflammatory medication to reduce pain and inflammation. Throwing athletes with partial MCL tears or those with overlapping symptoms secondary to medial epicondylitis or ulnar nerve symptoms are treated with activity modification and a shoulder-and-elbow-strengthening program. It is important that cortisone injections be avoided to prevent further tendon or ligament injury.

Athletes who fail conservative management are candidates for surgery. It is not uncommon for throwing athletes to have a myriad of pathologies that require arthroscopic treatment as well as open MCL reconstruction. In addition to our aforementioned criteria for arthroscopic management of valgus extension overload, we will perform an MCL reconstruction concomitantly based on the following criteria: (1) MRI evidence of MCL injury, (2) a history

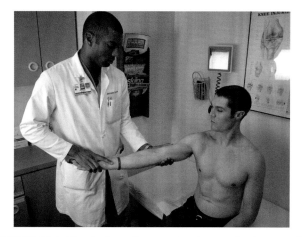

FIGURE 37.4. The clunk test for posterior olecranon impingement is simply performed by stabilizing the upper arm and bringing the elbow into extension to produce posterior elbow pain.

of medial elbow pain in the region of the MCL, which develops during the late cocking and early acceleration phase, and (3) pain that is severe enough to prevent the athlete from an acceptable level of competition.

Operative Indications/Contraindications

Arthroscopy is an important method utilized for the diagnosis and treatment of many of the pathologies of valgus extension overload with careful consideration given to choosing the appropriate indications. When valgus overload injury results in disabling symptoms for the athlete, surgical reconstruction of the anterior band of the ulnar collateral ligament may be indicated. Further indications for elbow arthroscopy in the throwing athlete include removal of loose bodies, excision of olecranon osteophytes, synovectomy, capsular release, capsular contracture, debridement of impinging osteophytes, articular cartilage lesions addressed, and the assessment and treatment of OCD of the capitellum (14).

The primary contraindication to elbow arthroscopy is any change in the normal bony or soft-tissue anatomy that precludes safe entry of the arthroscope into the elbow joint. In addition, we do not recommend performing arthroscopy when there has been a previous ulnar nerve transposition or when adequate distension of the joint cannot occur. Furthermore, arthroscopy should not be done in the presence of local soft tissue infection in the area of the portal sites, and the surgeon should have a comprehensive understanding of the surrounding anatomy, as well as advanced technical experience of arthroscopic technique. Lastly, attention to detail is essential to prevent compromise of the surrounding neurovascular structures or damage to the delicate articular cartilage.

AUTHORS' PREFERRED TECHNIQUE

Anesthesia

Regional or general anesthesia may be used for elbow arthroscopy. Regional anesthesia, with or without intravenous sedation, includes interscalene block, axillary block, and Bier block. In general, the advantage of regional anesthesia is that it optimizes postoperative pain control, minimizes postoperative nausea associated with general anesthesia, and facilitates positioning in cooperation with the patient. Disadvantages to regional anesthesia include limitations in patient tolerance of certain positions and the inability to perform a thorough postoperative neurological examination of the involved extremity to determine if nerve injury has occurred. In our work with experienced regional anesthesiologist, we have not had any cases of nerve damage after regional anesthesia; therefore, we typically use axillary block anesthesia with intravenous sedation, because we find it maximizes patient tolerance and allows for supine positioning while also maximizing postoperative comfort.

The advantages of general anesthesia include more options for patient positioning (prone and lateral decubitus positions) as well as total muscle relaxation. Disadvantages include postoperative pain tolerance and the potential for a longer postanesthesia recovery.

Patient Positioning

Patient positions routinely utilized for arthroscopic evaluation of the elbow include the prone position, lateral decubitus position, standard supine position, and supine-suspended position.

The prone position places the patient prone on chest rolls with the arm stabilized by an arm holder and allowed to hang off the table. The shoulder is abducted to 90°, and the elbow is flexed to 90°. Some surgeons prefer this position, because it eliminates the need for traction, places the elbow in a more stable position, and allows easier access to the posterior aspect of the joint. If necessary, this position may also allow for conversion from arthroscopy to an open surgical procedure, but we have found this to be very difficult. Disadvantages of the prone position include general anesthesia and poor access to the airway by the anesthesiologist.

The lateral decubitus position has advantages similar to those of the prone position including improved arm stability and posterior joint access. However, in the lateral decubitus position, the anesthesiologist's access to the airway is not compromised. The main disadvantage is that access to the anterior compartment may require repositioning by placing the patient in a lateral position with the shoulder flexed forward at 90° over a padded bolster.

The supine-suspended position positions the shoulder in 90° of abduction, with the elbow flexed 90° and the forearm, wrist, and hand suspended by a mechanical traction device. We prefer a modification of this position with the shoulder flexed 90° such that the forearm and humerus are suspended over the patient's chest for arthroscopic evaluation of the elbow. This position requires a mechanical arm holder as it securely positions the arm in space and eliminates the need for an additional assistant. Several options are available including the McConnell arm holder (McConnell Orthopedic Manufacturing, Greenville, TX) and the Spider hydraulic arm holder (Spider Limb Positioner, Tenet Medical Engineering, Calgary, Alberta, Canada). We prefer the Spider hydraulic arm holder because it more rigidly suspends the arm in space and can be easily adjusted to allow for any desired changes in position (Fig. 37.6). This allows for easy access to both the anterior and posterior compartments when facilitating arthroscopic work. With the forearm and humerus flexed over the chest, the anterior neurovascular structures effectively drop away from the anterior capsule, allowing for easier and safer work to be done on the anterior compartment. This supine position also provides clear access to the posterior compartment when performing osteophyte debridement or microfracture to address posteromedial impingement in the throwing athlete. In addition, the supine position affords the anesthesiologist excellent

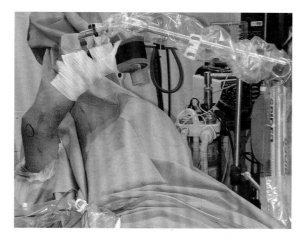

FIGURE 37.6. The modified supine position for elbow arthroscopy. This position, with the arm suspended over the chest, helps to facilitate patient positioning and allows for easy conversion to an open procedure when necessary.

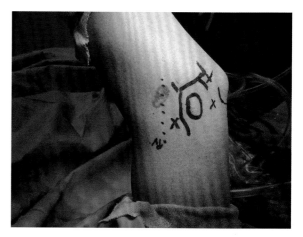

FIGURE 37.7. Lateral view of the elbow demonstrating our typically used portals, which are marked with an "X." The midlateral or "soft spot" portal is at the upper right, the posterolateral portal is at the lower right, and the proximal lateral portal is at the lower left. The radial nerve *(dotted line)* is carried away from the proximal lateral portal in flexion when the joint is distended.

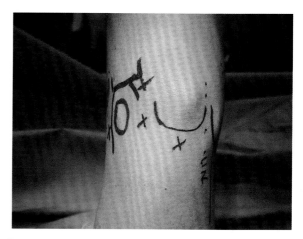

FIGURE 37.8. Posterior view of the elbow demonstrating the posterolateral portal *(left)* and the transtriceps portal *(center)*.

access to the airway. Furthermore, the conversion to an open procedure can be easily performed by removing the arm from the holder and placing it across the arm board where the seated surgeon can proceed with an open surgical procedure.

We have found this technique to be very successful and have not experienced the disadvantages historically reported in the literature such as arm instability, difficult orientation, and poor access to the posterior compartment. A tourniquet should be placed around the proximal aspect of the arm but should only be inflated when blood loss impairs arthroscopic visualization.

Portal Placement

The most common portals utilized for elbow arthroscopy include the anterolateral, midlateral, anteromedial, proximal medial, proximal lateral, and straight posterior. We most commonly use the midlateral, proximal lateral, posterolateral, and transtriceps portals (14) (Figs. 37.7 to 37.9).

The midlateral portal, also known as the soft-spot portal or direct lateral portal, is located in the center of the triangle formed by the lateral epicondyle, the tip of the olecranon and the radial head. The anconeus is penetrated in this portal and the nearest neurovascular structure is the posterior antebrachial cutaneous nerve (14). This portal is often used to inject fluid to distend the capsule but can also be utilized to remove loose bodies stuck in the lateral gutter (14).

The proximal lateral portal is located 2 cm proximal to the epicondyle and lies directly on the anterior surface of the humerus. The capsular attachments are such that, in flexion, the radial nerve is carried away from the nerve when the joint is distended. This allows for clear visualization of the medial and lateral sides of the joint, the anterior and lateral aspect of the radial head and capitellum as well as the lateral gutter.

The posterolateral portal is located 3 cm proximal to the tip of the olecranon and immediately lateral to the triceps tendon. The nearest neurovascular structures are the posterior brachial cutaneous and posterior antebrachial cutaneous nerves. This portal provides unobstructed visualization of the entire posterior compartment.

The transtriceps portal is a straight posterior portal located in the midline, 3 cm proximal to the tip of the olecranon. It is mostly used to debride the posteromedial olecranon of osteophytes and the olecranon fossa of chondral lesions as well as for the removal of loose bodies.

Operative Technique

Following anesthesia administration and proper patient positioning, the elbow joint is insufflated with 20 to 30 ml of saline, which is injected through the soft spot in the midlateral portal. Distending the joint in this manner

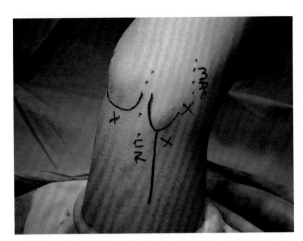

FIGURE 37.9. Medial view of the elbow demonstrating the proximal medial portal *(proximal)* and the anteromedial portal *(distal)*. These portals are made after the scope is in the elbow joint under direct spinal needle localization. When making the proximal medial portal, it is important to stay above the intermuscular septum *(straight line)* to avoid injury to the ulnar nerve *(dotted line)*. The anteromedial portal is close to the medial antebrachial cutaneous nerve *(MAC)*, which should also be avoided.

shifts the neurovascular structures away from the penetrating instruments and allows for the safe entry of the instruments. Avoiding overdistension of the capsule is important, as it can lead to capsular rupture and an inability to effectively maintain adequate fluid pressure for the ensuing arthroscopy.

Anterior Arthroscopy

The arthroscope is introduced through the proximal lateral portal into the anterior compartment (Fig. 37.10). A diagnostic arthroscopy is then performed anteriorly to evaluate the articular cartilage and synovium, as well as to look for loose bodies. The coronoid process is examined for the presence of bone spurs, and the anterior trochlea

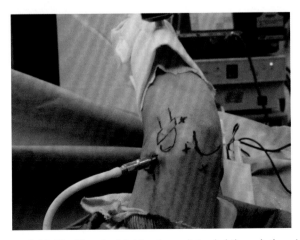

FIGURE 37.10. After the joint has been distended through the midlateral portal, the arthroscope is introduced into the anterior compartment by the proximal lateral portal.

and coronoid fossa are examined for cartilage lesions. The anterior radiocapitellar joint is evaluated for osteochondral lesions of the capitellum and any matching pathology of the radial head. The radial nerve lies on, or at least within a few millimeters of, the anterolateral joint capsule. Therefore, debridement in this area requires considerable caution. The anterior capsule is then evaluated for thickening or contracture in the context of a loss of passive extension.

To confirm the diagnosis of medial collateral ligament insufficiency, the arthroscopic valgus stress test is performed during assessment of the anterior compartment. With the arthroscope in the proximal lateral portal visualizing the medial compartment, valgus stress is applied manually to the elbow. A gap between the ulna and humerus greater than 3 mm is consistent with ulnar collateral ligament insufficiency (Fig. 37.11A, B). A probe of known dimensions can then be inserted through the proximal medial portal to aid in the measurement of the ulnohumeral opening. If such a portal is not necessary, then valgus opening can be visualized and appropriately estimated. If work needs to be performed in the anterior

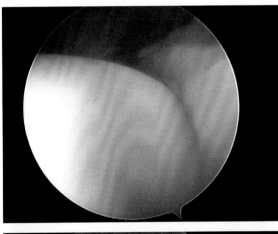

A

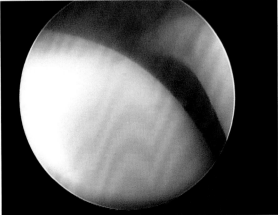

B

FIGURES 37.11. A, B. In cases of suspected MCL insufficiency, we perform the arthroscopic valgus stress test. When a valgus stress is applied in this setting, a gap between the ulna and the humerus greater than 3 mm will occur.

compartment such as debridement, synovectomy, capsular release, or removal of loose bodies, a proximal medial portal is established under direct visualization.

Posterior Arthroscopy

Following completion of the anterior arthroscopy, the cannula and its camera is retained with fluid inflow attached to maintain distention of the joint (Fig. 37.12). A posterolateral portal is then established, and the camera is removed from the anterior cannula and inserted through this portal. We typically maintain the anterior cannula to facilitate reentry into the anterior compartment if necessary and to ultimately drain the elbow of fluid at the conclusion of the case.

If work needs to be performed posteriorly, a transtriceps portal is established (Fig. 37.13). The medial,

lateral, and central olecranon are then evaluated for the presence of osteophytes. The corresponding olecranon fossa and posteromedial aspect of the humeral condyle are evaluated for matching chondral defects. The posterior radiocapitellar joint is evaluated by advancing the arthroscope down the lateral gutter. One of the most common errors made in elbow arthroscopy is to miss a loose body that is caught in the posterior radiocapitellar joint. When such a loose body is present, an accessory midlateral portal through the soft spot will often be necessary for removal.

In the throwing athlete, the most common problem encountered is a fragmented spur on the posteromedial olecranon as a result of posterior shear stresses seen in valgus extension overload (15, 16) (Fig. 37.14). These spurs should be anticipated as they can be seen in the preoperative radiographs and MRI. With the camera in the posterolateral portal and the shaver in the transtriceps portal, the extent and dimensions of the osteophyte should be evaluated. Excess soft tissue, including synovial reflections, are removed from the olecranon tip by carefully using a radiofrequency device (15, 16). The osteophyte is removed from the posteromedial olecranon using a gentle medial-to-lateral movement (Fig. 37.15). The optimal amount of olecranon to be debrided has been a matter of debate. Common surgical practice involves debridement of the osteophyte along with a variable amount of native olecranon bone. Biomechanical studies have demonstrated that excessive olecranon resection can lead to elbow instability and MCL strain in the throwing athlete (17). Therefore, it is recommended that resections be limited to approximately 3 mm because resections greater than this may jeopardize the

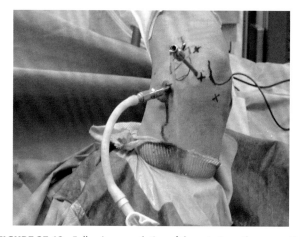

FIGURE 37.12. Following completion of the anterior arthroscopy, the posterolateral portal is established. The camera is switched from the anterior cannula to this portal, but we maintain the anterior cannula to facilitate reentry into the anterior compartment if necessary.

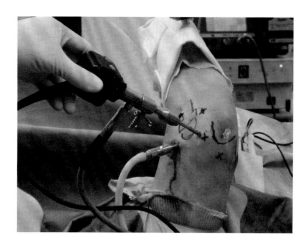

FIGURE 37.13. After the posterolateral has been established, the transtriceps portal is established by spinal needle localization. The transtriceps portal is the working portal in the posterior compartment.

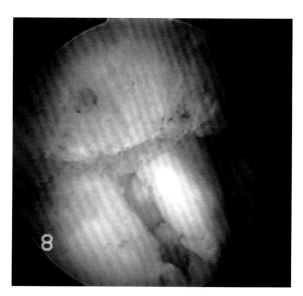

FIGURE 37.14. In throwing athletes, it is not uncommon to encounter posteromedial osteophytes *(top)* with a concomitant "kissing lesion" indicative of chondral abrasion *(bottom)* opposite the osteophyte.

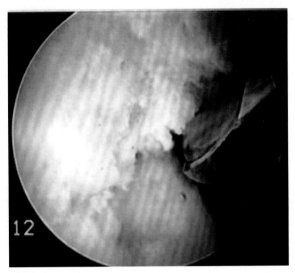

FIGURE 37.15. A shaver is introduced into the posterior compartment through the transtriceps portal and is used to resect the osteophyte. It is important to try to preserve as much native bone as possible but remove the offending pathology at the same time.

native or the reconstructed MCL. Practically speaking, our goal of arthroscopic debridement is to remove the osteophyte only and preserve as much native bone as possible. Once the osteophyte is removed, the humeral chondral surface can be visualized more completely and the "kissing lesion" of chondral abrasion opposite the osteophyte will be in direct view. Loose chondral flaps are debrided and if necessary a microfacture is performed (Fig. 37.16). Upon completion of the posterior arthroscopy, the portals are briefly irrigated and closed with interrupted nylon sutures.

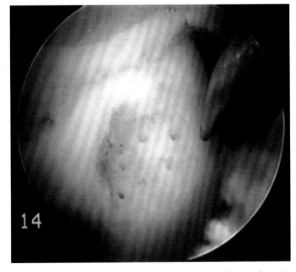

FIGURE 37.16. Once the osteophyte has been adequately excised, any loose chondral flaps can be debrided and microfractured when necessary.

OPEN MEDIAL ULNAR COLLATERAL LIGAMENT RECONSTRUCTION

If medial collateral ligament reconstruction is needed, the forearm is easily removed from the arm holder and is placed onto the table extension. In cases where the palmaris longus tendon is absent, the gracilis tendon is harvested at this time. Otherwise, the ipsilateral palmaris longus tendon is harvested through a 1-cm incision in the volar wrist flexion crease over the tendon. The visible portion of the tendon is then tagged with locking Krakow sutures, and the remaining tendon is then harvested using a tendon stripper. The incision is then irrigated and closed using interrupted nylon sutures.

Once the arm is exsanguinated to the level of the tourniquet, an 8- to 10-cm incision is made starting 2 cm proximal to the medial epicondyle in line with the intermuscular septum. The incision is carried distally, approximately 2 cm beyond the sublime tubercle. When exposing the flexor-pronator mass, the median antebrachial cutaneous nerve is often observed and should be identified and protected. A muscle splitting approach is then used through the posterior one-third of the common flexor-pronator mass within the most anterior fibers of the flexor carpi ulnaris muscle. This is located at the raphe between the flexor carpi and ulnaris muscle and the anterior portion of the flexor bundle. The advantage of this particular approach is that it utilizes a true internervous plane (18). The anterior bundle of the MCL is now excised to expose the joint.

The ulna tunnel sites are exposed first. The anterior and posterior portions of the sublime tubercle are exposed subperiosteally as care is taken to protect the ulnar nerve. A 3-mm bur is then used to create tunnels anterior and posterior to the sublime tubercle. A curette is used to connect two tunnels while preserving the body bridge.

To expose the humeral tunnel position, the incision within the native MCL is extended proximally to the level of the epicondyle. A longitudinal tunnel is created along the axis of the medial epicondyle using a 4-mm bur. Careful consideration is taken not to violate the posterior cortex of the proximal epicondyle. Using a 1.5-mm bur, two small exit punctures are created on the anterior surface of the epicondyle anterior to the intermuscular septum. This allows the sutures on each end of the graft to be passed from the humeral tunnel.

With the forearm supinated and a mild varus stress applied to the elbow, the graft is passed through the ulnar tunnel from anterior to posterior. The posterior limb of the graft with sutures is then docked into the humeral tunnel, with the sutures exiting through one of two exit holes in the anterior portion of the epicondyle. With sutures exiting the second puncture hole in the anterior portion of the epicondyle. A graft that is too long cannot be properly tensioned, therefore, it is extremely important that the final the elbow reduced, the graft is tensioned in flexion

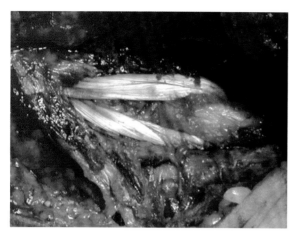

FIGURE 37.17. In cases of MCL insufficiency, an MCL reconstruction is performed after the arthroscopic component of the procedure has been completed. We have had excellent results using the docking technique for MCL reconstruction.

and extension to determine the optimal length by placing the graft adjacent to the humeral tunnel. Final length is determined by referencing the graft to the exit hole in the humeral tunnel. This point is then marked on the graft, and another Krakow stitch is placed. The excess graft is then excised above this point, and the end of the graft is securely "docked" in the anterior humeral tunnel, with the second set of graft length being short of where the graft suture will exit the epicondyle.

The final tensioning is then performed by taking the elbow through a complete range of motion while a varus stress is applied. Once the surgeon is satisfied, the two suture ends are tied over the medial epicondyle, with the elbow in approximately 20° of flexion and full supination (Fig. 37.17). This position is chosen because it reduces excessive tension or laxity in either of the two limbs. After the tourniquet is deflated and hemostasis achieved, an ulnar nerve transposition is performed if indicated. Otherwise, the fascia over the flexor-pronator mass is reapproximated, and the remaining wound is closed in layers. The elbow is placed in a plaster splint at 45° flexion to reduce excessive laxity or tension on either limb and forearm supination to keep the joint reduced.

COMPLICATIONS, CONTROVERSIES, AND SPECIAL CONSIDERATIONS

The safety of elbow arthroscopy, both as clinical and cadaveric studies, has dramatically increased our understanding of portal placement and the relative positions of surrounding neurovascular structures. Most complications of elbow arthroscopy are neurovascular in nature (19). Injury can be caused by direct laceration from a knife penetrated deep into the skin or from a trocar. In addition, compression from a cannula, from fluid extravasation, or from the use of local anesthetics has also been reported (19). Fortunately, most of the reported neurovascular injuries are transient; however, extreme care need to be taken to avoid potential disastrous complications. Probably one of the most important ways to avoid such complications is to distend the capsule with saline prior to trocar penetration.

Other complications of elbow arthroscopy are similar to those reported for arthroscopy in general. These include infection, articular cartilage injury, synovial fistula formation, instrument breakage, and tourniquet-related complications (14).

Many of the complications associated with elbow arthroscopy are the result of poor technique or a lack of knowledge regarding the surrounding bony anatomy about the elbow. Therefore, we recommend drawing the bony anatomy directly on the patients elbow in each case, using an 18G spinal needle to confirm the correct portal location before introducing larger arthroscopic instruments and, again, making sure that the elbow is maximally distended at all times to displace the neurovascular structures away from the entering instruments.

PEARLS AND PITFALLS

Positioning Pearls

1. We prefer the supine-suspended position with the arm flexed over the chest (Figs. 37.5 and 37.6). In this position, the anterior neurovascular structures effectively drop away from the anterior capsule.
2. The anterior and posterior compartments can be easily accessed.
3. This position also facilitates conversion to an open surgical procedure when necessary (e.g., MCL reconstruction).

Portals/Exposures Pitfalls

1. Identify and mark bony landmarks before the capsule is distended, which can make palpation of landmarks more difficult.
2. The joint should be distended with 20 to 40 cc of fluid through midlateral portal *before* establishing the initial viewing portal. This significantly increases the distance between the joint surfaces and neurovascular structures.
3. When creating portals, avoid penetrating the subcutaneous tissues. A hemostat or clamp should be used to spread the tissue down to capsule.
4. Avoid using any local anesthetic, which can prevent appropriate postoperative assessment of the neurologic status.
5. Avoid multiple penetrations of the capsule to prevent excessive fluid extravasation, which can lead to excessive swelling and potential risk of injury to neurovascular structures.

Surgical Procedure Pearl—Removal of Loose Body

1. One of the most common errors is to miss a loose body that is caught in the posterior radiocapitellar joint. If present, use an accessory midlateral portal through the soft spot to aid in removal.

Surgical Procedure Pitfall—Olecranon Resection

1. When removing osteophyte from the olecranon, limit the resection to the osteophyte only; excessive postero-medial resection of the olecranon can lead to valgus instability particularly in the throwing athlete.

REHABILITATION

Specific physical therapy regimens vary depending on the procedure performed, especially if the arthroscopy is followed by reconstruction the MCL. The following description is designed to serve as a general guideline for rehabilitation following only elbow arthroscopy.

Postoperatively, we prefer a compressive dressing for 48 hours, cryotherapy, and routine wound care. Sling immobilization is minimal and is for comfort only. We then proceed in a triphasic rehabilitation program that focuses on the restoration of joint range of motion and flexibility within the healing parameters of the structures involved in the surgery. Rehabilitation progresses through each phase only after the major goals of the previous phase have been successfully achieved. Generally speaking, we recommend the athlete achieve the following criteria to safely return to play: painless and full range of motion, no elbow pain or tenderness, satisfactory isokinetic muscular strength testing, and a satisfactory clinical examination. Overall, rehabilitation following elbow arthroscopy can be somewhat aggressive because the procedure causes minimal postoperative morbidity. For a more comprehensive review of non- and postoperative rehabilitation of the athlete's elbow, we recommend the text by Wilk and Levinson (20). The authors outline the three-phase approach to rehabilitation in detail and explain how such a program allows the surgeon and therapist to tailor the program to the individual patient's needs. A summary of our postoperative protocol is depicted schematically in Table 37.1.

CONCLUSIONS AND FUTURE DIRECTIONS

Elbow arthroscopy is a powerful tool in the diagnosis and treatment of the various pathologies seen in the throwing athlete's elbow. The preoperative evaluation should consist of a complete history and physical examination and as the use of appropriate imaging modalities in order to make a prompt diagnosis and facilitate a rapid return to play for the athlete. The arthroscopic recognition and treatment of related pathology is directly correlated with appropriate

Table 37.1

Postoperative Rehabilitation Program

Phase I (0–6 weeks)
Sling immobilization-MD directed
Codmans/pendulum exercises
Wrist/elbow ROM exercises
Gripping exercises
FF-AAROM (supine)-limit to 90°
Passive ER to neutral
Passive elbow abduction to 30°
Scapula tightening
Modalities PRN
Patient has begun above program as directed by MD starting on first post-op day
Discontinue sling-MD directed
Continue FF-AAROM (wand/pulleys)
ER-AAROM to 30°
Manual scapular stabilization exercise-sidelying
Begin pain-free IR/ER isometrics in modified neutral-Modalities PRN

Phase II (6–10 weeks)
Begin biceps/triceps strengthening
Progress scapular strengthening in protective arcs (emphasis on closed-chain activities)
Begin isotonic IR/ER strengthening in modified neutral
Begin latissimus strengthening-below 90° elevation
Begin FF in plane of scapula/add weights as tolerated (emphasis on scapulohumeral rhythm)
Continue to increase AAROM for ER/FF
Begin upper body ergometer below 90° elevation
Begin humeral head stabilization exercises (if adequate strength and ROM exists)
Continue aggressive scapula strengthening
Advance strengthening for deltoid, biceps, triceps, and latissimus as tolerated
Begin PNF patterns
Continue humeral head stabilization exercises
Advance IR/ER to elevated position in overhead athletes (must be pain free and have good proximal strength)
Continue UBE for endurance training
Begin general flexibility exercises

Phase III (10–24 weeks)
Continue full upper extremity strengthening
Restore normal shoulder flexibility
Begin activity specific polymeric program
Continue endurance training
Continue flexibility exercises
Continue full strengthening program
Begin return to interval throwing-MD directed

II. The Elbow

surgical technique, most notably proper portal placement and adequate surgical instrumentation. Therefore, it is crucial that the clinician who wishes to utilize arthroscopy as a tool for the treatment of the thrower's elbow be proficient in basic arthroscopic techniques, coupled with a thorough understanding of elbow anatomy and biomechanics.

The role of elbow arthroscopy in the athlete who suffers from valgus instability is most beneficial in the removal of loose bodies, plica excision, spur debridment/excision, and the treatment of intra-articular cartilage lesions. Futures advances may allow surgeons to treat ulnar neuritis and perform MCL ligament reconstruction with the aid of the arthroscope, but such procedures are currently limited to open techniques.

REFERENCES

1. O'Holleran JD, Altchek DW. Elbow arthroscopy: treatment of the thrower's elbow. *Instr Course Lect.* 2006;55:95–107.
2. Chen AL, Youm T, Ong BC, et al. Imaging of the elbow in the overhead throwing athlete. *Am J Sports Med.* 2003;31:466–473.
3. Cain EL Jr, Dugas JR, Wolf RS, et al. Elbow injuries in throwing athletes: a current concepts review. *Am J Sports Med.* 2003;31:621–635.
4. Ball CM, Galatz LM, Yamaguchi K. Elbow instability: treatment strategies and emerging concepts. *Instr Course Lect.* 2002;51:53–61.
5. Chen FS, Rokito AS, Jobe FW. Medial elbow problems in the overhead throwing athlete. *J Am Acad Orthop.* 2001;9(2):99–113.
6. Morrey BF, An KN. Articular and ligamentous contributions to the stability of the elbow joint. *Am J Sports Med.* 1983;11:315–319.
7. Callaway GH, Field LD, Deng XH, et al. Biomechanical evaluation of the medial collateral ligament of the elbow. *J Bone Joint Surg Am.* 1997;79:1223–1231.
8. Wilson FD, Andrews JR, Blackburn TA, et al. Valgus extension overload in the pitching elbow. *Am J Sports Med.* 1983;11:83–88.
9. King JW, Brelsford HJ, Tullos HS. Analysis of the pitching arm of the professional baseball pitcher. *Clin Orthop Relat Res.* 1969;67:116–123.
10. Schickendantz MS, Ho CP, Koh J. Stress injury of the proximal ulna in professional baseball players. *Am J Sports Med.* 2002;30:737–741.
11. Antuna SA, O'Driscoll SW. Snapping plicae associated with radiocapitellar chondromalacia. *Arthroscopy.* 2001;17:491–495.
12. O'Driscoll SW, Lawton RL, Smith AM. The "moving valgus stress test" for medial collateral ligament tears of the elbow. *Am J Sports Med.* 2005;33(2):231–239.
13. Gaary EA, Potter HG, Altchek DW. Medial elbow pain in the throwing athlete: MR imaging evaluation. *AJR Am J Roentgenol.* 1997;168:795–800.
14. Dodson CC, Nho SJ, Williams RJ III, et al. Elbow arthroscopy. *J Am Acad Orthop Surg.* 2008;16:574–585.
15. O'Holleran JD, Altchek DW. Throwers elbow: arthroscopic treatment of valgus extension overload syndrome. *HSS J.* 2006;2:83–93.
16. Kamineni S, Hirahara H, Pomianowski S, et al. Partial posteromedial olecranon resection: a kinematic study. *J Bone Joint Surg Am.* 2005;85-A:1005–1011.
17. Kamineni S, ElAttrache NS, O'Driscoll SW, et al. Medial collateral ligament strain with partial posteromedial olecranon resection: a biomechanical study. *J Bone Joint Surg Am.* 2004;86-A:2424–2430.
18. Smith GR, Altchek DW, Pagnani MJ, et al. A muscle-splitting approach to the ulnar collateral ligament of the elbow. Neuroanatomy and operative technique. *Am J Sports Med.* 1996;24:575–580.
19. O'Driscoll SW, Morrey BF. Arthroscopy of the elbow: diagnostic and therapeutic benefits and hazards. *J Bone Joint Surg Am.* 1992;74:84–94.
20. Wilk KE, Levinson M. Rehabilitation of the athlete's elbow. In: Altchek DW, Andrews JR, eds. *The Athlete's Elbow.* Philadelphia, PA: Lippincott Williams & Wilkins; 2001:249–273.

Distal Biceps Tendon Tears: Surgical Indications and Techniques

Cory Edgar • Augustus D. Mazzocca

The surgical treatment of distal biceps ruptures is becoming a more commonly performed procedure. It is unclear if the incidence, reported in 2002 to be approximately 1.2 patients per 100,000 in the general population (1), has changed much in the last 10 years. However, the increasing demands of a middle-aged population, along with multiple advances in the fixation technology and a renewed focus on the local anatomy, have allowed for less invasive exposures and decreased complications and permit a more aggressive postoperative rehabilitation.

The injury is most commonly observed in males, within the dominant extremity, and in a middle-aged population 40 to 50 years old (1–4). Reported risk factors include smoking or nicotine exposure (1, 5) and anabolic steroid use (5, 6). The mechanism is most commonly attributed to eccentrically loaded arm under tension while the elbow is flexed at about 90° and pulled into extension.

The etiology of the distal biceps ruptures is still unclear as many patients report no pain prior to the moment of rupture, whereas others report an insidious deep elbow pain for weeks to months leading up to the rupture. Utilizing a cadaver injection study in 27 elbows, a consistent vascular pattern was identified and supported the theory of a hypovascular zone within the tendon approximately 2.14 cm in length within the central zone 2 of the tendon (7). This may lead to degenerative tendon associated with repeated microtrauma to the tendon (7). Morrey and others (8–10) have suggested that an abnormal boney prominence or irregularities at the radial tuberosity are associated with tendon degeneration and lead to ruptures; however, boney abnormalities at this location may simply be normal anatomic variant (11). Some combination of anatomic factors and local tendon degeneration probably contribute to failure of the distal biceps tendon, but the precise mechanism has yet to be demonstrated.

ANATOMY/OSTEOLOGY

An understanding of the anatomy of the biceps origin and the osteology of the bicipital tuberosity is an essential aspect to getting an anatomic repair and better postoperative function. The biceps tendon inserts like a ribbon at the ulnar side of the lesser tuberosity, rather than as a cylinder on the center of the tuberosity (Fig. 38.1). The distal insertion of the short head positions it to be a more powerful flexor of the elbow, and the insertion of the long head on the tuberosity farther from the axis of rotation of the forearm increases leverage for supination. The average length of the biceps tendon insertion on the tuberosity is 21 mm, with an average width of 7 mm, indicating that the tendon insertion does not occupy the entire bicipital tuberosity (11, 12). The tuberosity does demonstrate some anatomic variability but has a mean length of 22 to 24 mm, a mean width of 15 to 19 mm, and it is located on the ulnar, posterior aspect of the proximal radius on average 25 mm from the radial head (11). The tendon insertion footprint is a ribbon-shaped configuration on the most ulnar aspect of the tuberosity, and it occupies 63% of the length and 13% of the width of the entire boney tuberosity (11).

The lacertus fibrosus (bicipital aponeurosis) typically originates from the distal short head of the biceps tendon, passes anterior to the elbow joint, and expands ulnarly blending with the fascia of the forearm (Fig. 38.2). It is composed of three layers that originate from the short head of the tendon and assists in stabilizing the tendon distally. As the forearm flexors contract, they tense the lacertus, subsequently causing a medial pull on the biceps tendon and perhaps contributing to its rupture, and can commonly mask a complete rupture during clinical examination.

CLINICAL EVALUATION AND WORKUP

Patients with complete distal biceps tendon ruptures usually report feeling a sudden, sharp, painful tearing sensation in the antecubital region of the elbow when an unexpected extension force was applied to the flexed/supinated arm. Occasionally, pain is also present in the posterolateral aspect of the elbow. The acute pain subsides

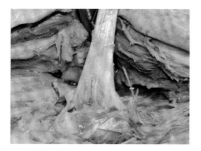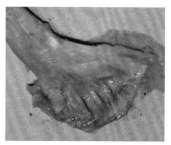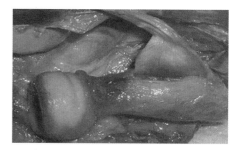

FIGURE 38.1. Cadaver dissections of distal biceps origin demonstrating the ulnar and posterior attachment and the ribbon footprint at the tendon entheses.

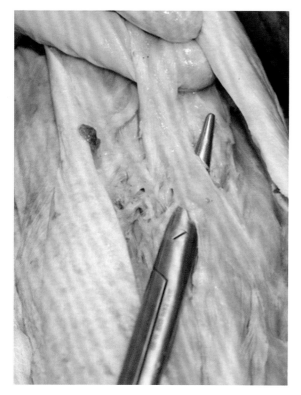

FIGURE 38.2. Cadaver dissection demonstrating the lacertus fibrosus (bicipital aponeurosis).

in a few hours and is replaced by a dull ache. Elbow range of motion is typically not affected, but symptoms of weakness and fatigue can occur with repetitive flexion and supination activities. Examination reveals tenderness in the antecubital fossa in the acute setting, and a defect can usually be palpated there. The "hook test," as described by O'Driscoll et al. (13), is a means of palpating the tendon under resisted elbow flexion at about 70°; the biceps tendon can be "hooked" with a deep probing digit working lateral to medial just proximal to the crease.

The biceps is the main supinator of the arm and secondary flexor. Active flexion and supination of the elbow causes the biceps muscle belly to retract proximally, accentuating the defect in the antecubital fossa. If the biceps tendon can be palpated in the antecubital fossa, a partial rupture of the distal biceps tendon should be considered. Ecchymosis and swelling are usually evident in the antecubital fossa and along the medial aspect of the arm and proximal forearm. Plain radiographs generally do not show any bony changes, although irregularity and enlargement of the radial tuberosity and avulsion of a portion of the radial tuberosity have been reported with complete ruptures of the distal biceps tendon. We feel this is important to obtain for complete evaluation of the patient. MRI can be helpful to distinguish complete from partial ruptures and to differentiate partial rupture from tendinosis, tenosynovitis hematoma, and brachialis contusion. More importantly, in the rare but potentially difficult situation of a more proximal rupture of the distal biceps approaching the myotendinous junction, an MRI may aid in diagnosis (Fig. 38.3). In this setting, an allograft Achilles tendon should be made available to augment the length of the shortened tendon.

TREATMENT

Nonoperative Versus Operative Repair

There is a small role for nonsurgical management of distal biceps ruptures in the patient with low demand work and recreational activity function, older age or within a medically high-risk patient. There have been a few studies demonstrating some success with nonoperative treatment of distal biceps ruptures, stating patients had minimal functional loss and could lead to a full return to work as early as 4 weeks after injury (14, 15). However, more recent studies clearly show that unrepaired avulsion of the distal biceps tendon frequently leaves the patient with substantial weakness of supination and elbow flexion (16–19). Excellent subjective and objective results of surgical repair have been reported (4, 10, 19–22). Results with surgical repair have been superior to nonsurgical treatment in terms of restoring elbow flexion strength (30% improved), supination strength (40% improved), and upper extremity endurance (14). This statement is supported by the study by Baker and Bierwagen (16) in which cybex strength testing was performed on 13 patients treated with and without distal biceps reattachment. They reported 40% loss of supination strength, 79% loss of supination endurance,

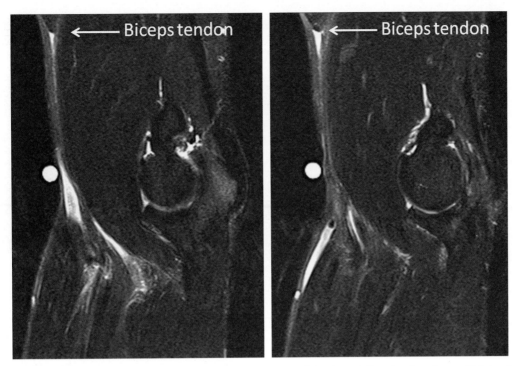

FIGURE 38.3. MRI right elbow, two cuts 9 mm apart moving medial to lateral. Note the ulnar–humeral joint and the very proximal, barely in the scanned field proximal biceps tendon tear and edema within the antecubital fossa.

30% loss of flexion strength, and 30% loss of flexion endurance in those patients treated nonoperatively (16). In a similar study, Morrey and coworkers (19) also showed a 40% loss of supination and 30% loss of flexion strength following nonoperative treatment for distal biceps ruptures.

Partial Rupture

Partial rupture of the distal biceps tendon is a less commonly reported injury, and a limited number of case reports exist in the literature regarding its management. Diagnosis can be difficult and subtle symptoms usually lend themselves to conservative treatment for a period. Typically, partial ruptures can present with pain in the antecubital fossa without a palpable defect or positive "hook test," but may have complaints of weakness during elbow flexion and more commonly in repetitive supination activity. Other causes of antecubital fossa pain should be ruled out, including biceps tendinitis, bicipital bursitis, and pronator syndrome. Lack of a specific traumatic event and subtle clinical findings make MRI a more important diagnostic tool for diagnosis. MRI is capable of quantifying the extent of the tear, as well as tenosynovitis, tendinitis, or bursitis, which may accompany the tear. Initial treatment consists of nonoperative management, including nonsteroidal anti-inflammatory medication and rest, with progression to a physical therapy program for stretching and strengthening. Should surgical intervention be necessary, most investigators advocate conversion of the partial tear into a complete tear, followed by reinsertion onto the radial tuberosity (23–26).

SURGICAL TECHNIQUE

Complications

Injury to the superficial lateral antebrachial cutaneous nerve is the most common complication of distal biceps repair. Paresthesia can occur for a variable amount of time, and in our experience it is usually the consequence of aggressive retraction or can be the result of aggressive dissection during a chronic biceps tendon repair. Injury to the PIN and radial nerve paresthesias have also been reported and are best avoided by careful treatment of the lateral soft tissue and minimal to no retraction lateral on the radial neck during bicipital tuberosity exposure. Also, it is very important to maintain the arm in hypersupination to maintain the posterior interosseous nerve as far lateral and away as possible from surgical exposure.

Most of the complications reported for both the one- and the two-incision techniques can be stratified into heterotopic ossification (synostosis formation between the proximal ulna and the radius) or nerve injuries. Synostosis presents in the earlier stages with pain and swelling, leading to loss of rotation, primarily supination. Earlier studies reported associated nerve injuries following repair using the one-incision technique (14, 27). The original Boyd–Anderson (28) two-incision technique resulted in less nerve injury, but higher rates of heterotopic ossification (29). The modified Boyd–Anderson technique attempted to decrease the rate of heterotopic ossification by using a muscle-splitting approach. The two largest series looking at complications following a two-incision repair show that abnormal bone formation can still occur despite a muscle splitting approach, but it rarely results in functional limitations (30, 31). Other less common complications include infection, re-rupture, complex regional pain syndrome, and a proximal radius fracture (1, 2, 4, 30–32).

Ideally, surgical treatment should occur within a few weeks from the date of injury; further delay may preclude a straightforward, primary repair. A more extensile approach or a secondary incision at the level of the retracted tendon may be required in a chronic rupture to capture the retracted and scarred distal biceps tendon.

AUTHORS' PREFERRED METHOD OF REPAIR

Anatomic Repair of Distal Biceps Tendon Ruptures Using a Combined Anatomic Interference Screw and Cortical Button

Volar Single-Incision Approach

The patient is positioned supine on the operating room table with a hand table extension and mini C-arm present. A nonsterile tourniquet is placed as close to the axilla as possible. It is important to allow room for a secondary incision if necessary to localize a proximally retracted tendon. If this is impossible secondary to patient habitus, a sterile tourniquet is preferred. We typically insufflate the tourniquet and have had no problems with proximal biceps muscle belly entrapment preventing tendon mobility distal to the footprint, postoperative arm pain, or with arm deep vein thrombosis.

The approach is made through a volar forearm incision, centered over the biceps tuberosity, which is usually three finger breadths from the flexion crease or approximately 3 to 4 cm distal to the skin crease at the antecubital fossa (Fig. 38.4). The subcuticular tissue is carefully dissected to avoid injury to the lateral antebrachial cutaneous nerve. As this is a commonly injured nerve during dissection and retraction, we routinely localize the nerve under direct visualization. The interval above the deep fascia is located and with blunt finger dissection proximally dissection is carried out until the proximally retracted tendon is localized (Fig. 38.5). It is important not to get too deep and stay above the brachialis fascia in the arm, and in the forearm the fascia overlying the pronator and brachioradialis. It is important to develop the interval between fascia and overlying skin for a large radius to allow for a very mobile window that allows the small incision to be centered over the proximal tendon or the tuberosity footprint.

Preparation of the Distal Bicep Tendon

Depending on the chronicity of the tear, the biceps tendon is usually retracted from the tuberosity and forms a

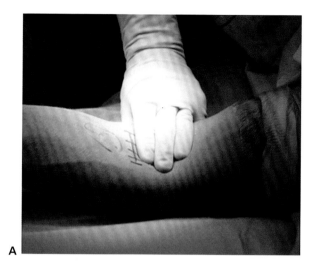

A

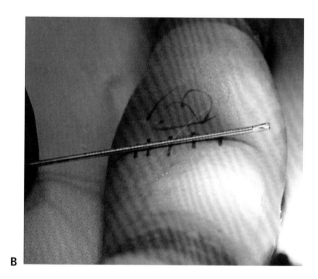

B

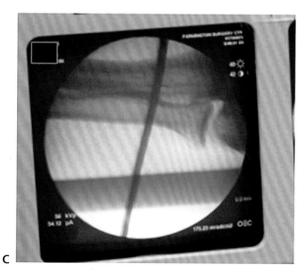

C

FIGURE 38.4. Right elbow incision location, approximately three finger breadths from flexion crease (**A**). This position coincides with biceps tuberosity position (**B**), which can be checked on mini-C arm, which should be present in the room (**C**).

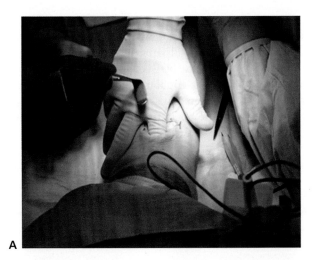

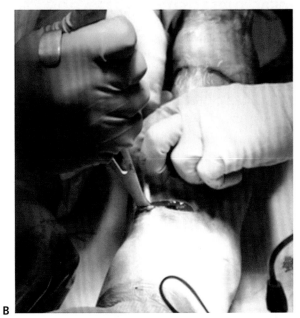

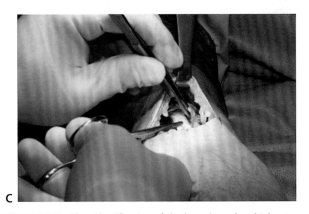

scarred bulbous end. The isolated tendon end should be isolated and carefully dissected free of soft tissue, and the pseudocapsule scar around the injured tendon incised. Often the tendon is folded back upon itself. The degenerative and abnormal tendon should be debrided and trimmed to an 8-mm thickness. If the tendon end is frayed with degenerated collagen, up to 1 cm can be resected from the end without compromising the ability to reattach it to the tuberosity. Two no. 2 fiberwire (Arthrex Inc., Naples, FL) sutures are then placed in the distal tendon (Krackow or whipstitch fashion) (Fig. 38.6A). It is very important to use high-strength suture during preparation of the remnant tendon as the suture strength is directly related to the pull-out strength of the endobutton construct. Also, the way in which the suture is placed through the tendon is important for fixation (Fig. 38.6). The first suture is started distal and then baseball stich, is brought proximal up the tendon for a

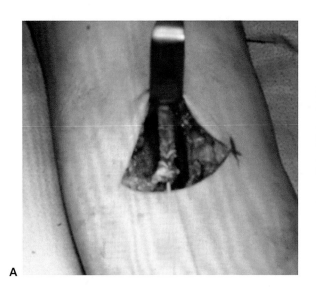

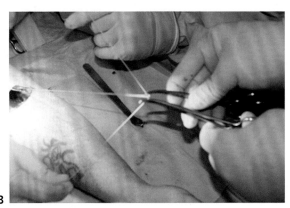

FIGURE 38.5. After identification of the lateral antebrachial cutaneous nerve, the dissection is carried bluntly proximal over the biceps. **A:** Often the proximal extent of the biceps is found within a wad of scar tissue and needs to be dissected free or the tendon is folded upon its self and more length of the tendon can be used. **B, C:** Using the "mobile window" of the incision that can be flexed to aid elbow with exposure of the tendon stump proximal.

FIGURE 38.6. Preparation of the proximal portion of the tendon for reattachment to the tuberosity. **A:** Tendon is isolated, debrided of scar to healthy tissue, and then fiberwire or another high-tension suture is placed from proximal to distal in the tendon for a minimum of 1 cm. **B:** Suture limbs are brought through a cortical button in opposite directions to allow the suture to slide and use the cortical button as a fulcrum for reduction of the tendon into the bone tunnel.

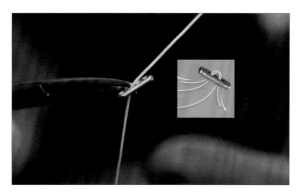

FIGURE 38.7. Suspension fixation with a "Tension-slide" technique. An Arthrex BicepsButton or a regular cortical button can be used. Two limbs of high-strength suture are brought through the central holes around a metal post in *opposite* directions to allow for friction slide of the suture around a fixed point—the cortical button.

length of 10 to 12 mm, then brought distal down the other half of the tendon and then looped through the center holes of a cortical button in opposite directions to create a tension slide orientation (Figs. 38.6 and 38.7). An alternative method is to start the suture proximal on the tendon, bring it distal, loop the cortical button center holes, and

then baseball stitch the tendon proximally until the level of the suture and then tied down (Fig. 38.8). It should be noted that the suture will typically loosen a few millimeters, and it is a balance between having enough slack in the suture to allow the endobutton to be flipped on the far cortex and having minimal slack so that the most tendon is present within the bone tunnel for healing. The tails of this suture are cut. The second suture begins distally, captures the endobutton, travels proximally 12 mm, and ends distally (Fig. 38.8). One end of this suture should be left long and the other short. The long "tail" of the suture is paned through the cannulated of the tendon screw driver in looped wire (Fig. 39.9 B). These will be used to pass the endobutton through the distal cortex.

BICEPS TUBEROSITY PREPARATION

It should be restated that anatomic dissections demonstrate that the distal biceps tendon attaches on the ulnar side of the tuberosity in a 2 × 14 mm ribbonlike configuration after rotating 90° from the musculotendinous junction (Fig. 38.1). Once the tendon has been isolated, deep dissection toward the tuberosity is carried within muscular

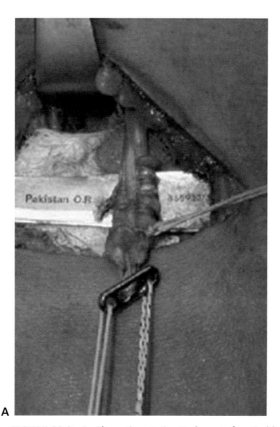
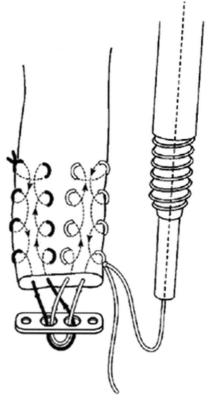

A B

FIGURE 38.8. A: Alternative, static attachment of cortical button to the biceps tendon for passage through the far cortex of radius with the use of a Beath pin and standard endobutton technique, flipping the button with end-passing suture. **B:** Cartoon explaining the suture configuration—Black suture for cortical button only ant passed proximal to distal. White suture also passed through cortical button but distal to proximal to allow attachment to tenodesis screw. (Reproduced with permission from (11) *Tech Should Elbow Surg.* 2005;6:108–115.)

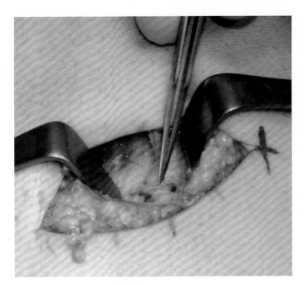

FIGURE 38.9. As the dissection is carried between the pronator and the brachioradialis, a sling of vessels should be identified and coagulated with the bipolar cautery. This allows deeper exposure toward the ulnar side of the radius where the tuberosity is found.

interval between the pronator teres and the brachioradialis is developed to the level of the lacertus fibrosis and surrounding hematoma or scar. Directly in the plane of the dissection is a series of veins (leash of Henry) (Fig. 38.9) and the recurrent branch of the radial artery that must be addressed by suture ligature, coagulation, or retraction. The frayed edge of the tendon is usually found at this level or proximal to it.

Arm positioning during exposure of the tuberosity is critical, maximal supination and extension to adequately visualize the tuberosity and protects the posterior interosseous nerve from injury (Fig. 38.10). It is important to visualize the entire tuberosity. It is possible for the tunnel to be placed too proximal if using the two-incision approach and looking for the ridge. Care should be taken while retracting the deep tissues for exposure not to retract too vigorously on the radial side of the proximal radius, as this may damage the posterior interosseous nerve. The tuberosity is frequently covered with a fibrous layer of immature scar. This should be removed, enabling complete visualization. A 2.7- or 3.2-mm drill tip guide pin with an eyelet to allow passage of suture is placed into the center of the tuberosity and drilled through both cortices. These are present in the Arthrex distal biceps set, or a 2.7 drill can be used bicortical and then a Beath pin used to pass the suture through the bone tunnel and out the dorsal side with the elbow flexed to 90°. It should be noted that the direction of pin placement should be in the center of the footprint and then directed more ulnar by 20°. Once the drill bit or pin is within the far cortex, it is used as a guide pin to ream a unicortical, 8-mm bone tunnel with a cannulated reamer (Arthrex Inc.). Again, this is critical that the 8-mm tunnel is through the proximal cortex only (Fig. 38.11). Care must be used to not continue reaming after penetrating the cortex, as the endobutton fixation is dependent on the far cortex for suspension fixation. The tuberosity should be irrigated and any reamings or soft tissue obscuring the cortical bone tunnel entrance should be debrided to clearly visualize and allow for easy passage of the tendon. The second "free" suture is attached to the biotenodesis screwdriver; a single limb is brought up through the driver and snapped on the handle.

II. The Elbow

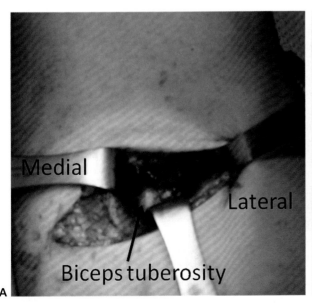

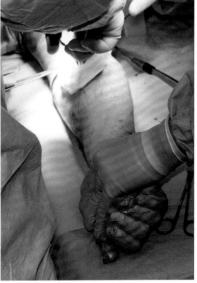

FIGURE 38.10. A: Placement of retractors and exposure of the biceps tuberosity deep, ulnar side of the proximal radius. **B:** For exposure and protection of the posterior interosseous nerve, the arm should be kept in extreme, maximal supination.

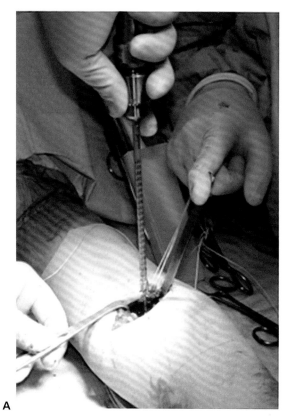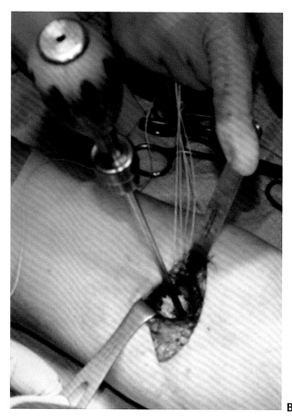

A   B

FIGURE 38.11. A: The near cortex is reamed with an 8-mm reamer on power, but removed by hand "chucked off" the drill to limit any widening of the proximal cortical bone tunnel. **B:** The bone tunnel is "tapped" with an 8-mm tap prior to placement of the tendon. Tapping the hard bone in the patient allows for improved fixation of the tenodesis screw.

Reduction of the Tendon

The remaining outside two holes in the endobutton are then loaded with two different color no. 2 fiberwire sutures to allow the endobutton to be passed on the end through the far cortex with the use of a Beath pin, and then by pulling the counter suture, the button is toggled and flipped on the far side of the cortex, completing the suspensory fixation. The two sutures placed onto the lateral holes of the endobutton (traction sutures) are then placed into the eyelet of the Beath pin (Fig. 38.8). The arm is flexed, and the Beath pin is pushed through the soft tissue penetrating the dorsal skin. This pin is placed as ulnarly as possible to avoid damage to the neurovascular structures. One of the sutures is pulled until the endobutton passes the distal cortex; the second suture is then toggled, and the endobutton is deployed (Figs. 38.12 and 38.13). A portable radiographic image is obtained (mini c-arm) to confirm that the endobutton is deployed and that there is close apposition to bone (Fig. 38.14).

Tenodesis

The Tenodesis driver consists of a cannulated handle and post. Sutures from the end of the prepared tendon can be passed through the driver after the chosen screw has been placed onto the driver. The post is used to insert the tendon to the bottom of the prepared socket and hold the tendon in place while the interference screw is advanced over it. To perform the tenodesis, one limb of the fiberwire suture is then placed through the tenodesis driver with the 8-mm × 12-mm screw attached (Fig. 38.11). The driver is then inserted into the 8-mm hole, making sure that the tendon is on the ulnar side of the tuberosity (Fig. 38.12). While the tendon is stabilized with an Adson forceps, the screw is advanced through the tenodesis driver as described above (Fig. 38.13). After the screw is inserted and the tenodesis driver is removed, the suture passing through the cannulated screw is then tied to the outside of the interference screw. Thus, there is both an interference fit of the tendon to bone as well as a suture anchor effect. Three modes of fixation now exist (interference fit, endobutton, and suture anchor-like fixation), which allows this method to have superior strength and cyclic load characteristics.

Prior to closure of the wound, the tourniquet can also be released and all venous bleeding stopped to minimize postoperative hematoma. We have had a few patients notice a "defect" within the antecubital fossa, and currently, we put in a few deep 3-0 undyed absorbable suture to close the fascia within the interval. The skin is closed with a running subcuticular 3-0 monocryl or polydioxanone (PDS) suture. Steri-strips are applied and a soft dressing

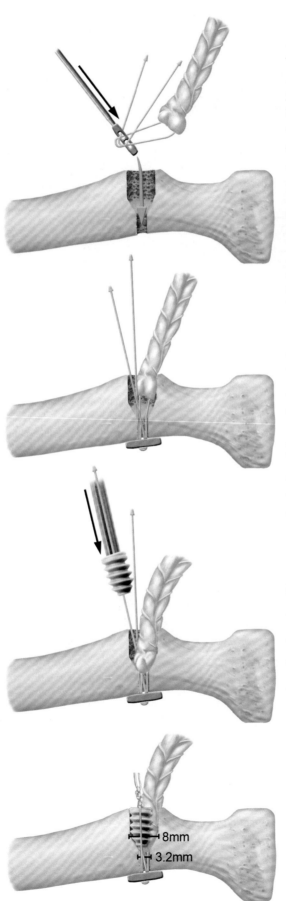

FIGURE 38.12. A: Cartoon representation of a reduced tension slide construct and reduction of the tendon into the bone tunnel. **B:** Cartoon of reduced tendon fixed with bio-tenodesis screw providing improved pullout strength and better native biceps footprint re-creation.

II. The Elbow

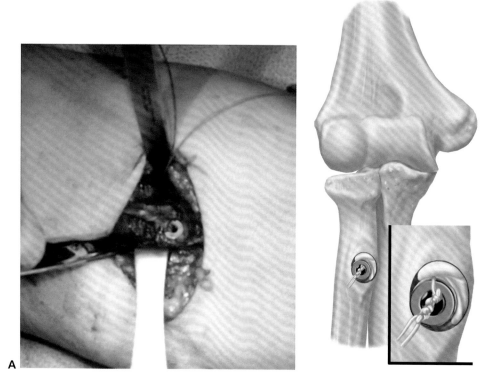

A   B

FIGURE 38.13. A: Clinical picture of reduced biceps tendon within bone tunnel at tuberosity and secondary fixation with an 8-mm tenodesis screw. **B:** Cartoon of the footprint and placement of tenodesis screw on the radial side of the footprint to improve placement of the tendon more ulnar for more native function and improved biomechanical function during supination.

is used. We use accelerated postoperative rehabilitation program that allows full active-assisted range of motion immediately, and the patient is encouraged to achieve full extension/flexion by the time the sutures are removed at 7 to 10 days. This is followed by active range of motion, with strengthening beginning at 12 weeks. To date, all of our re-ruptures have failed after 6 weeks and were associated with a traumatic event.

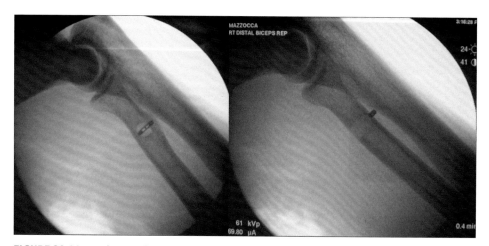

FIGURE 38.14. Final C-arm shots intraoperative taken with 90° of radial rotation through supination and pronation. Note the position of the cortical button, unicortical 8-mm bone tunnel, and placement of the tunnel in relation to the tuberosity.

REFERENCES

1. Safran MR, Graham SM. Distal biceps tendon ruptures: incidence, demographics, and the effect of smoking. *Clin Orthop Relat Res.* 2002;(404):275–283.

2. Sutton KM, Dodds SD, Ahmad CS, et al. Surgical treatment of distal biceps rupture. *J Am Acad Orthop Surg.* 2010;18:139–148.

3. Mazzocca AD, Spang JT, Arciero RA. Distal biceps rupture. *Orthop Clin North Am.* 2008;39(2):237–249.

4. Miyamoto RG, Elser F, Millett PJ. Distal biceps tendon injuries. *J Bone Joint Surg Am.* 2010;92(11):2128–2138.

5. Schneider A, Bennett JM, O'Connor DP, et al. Bilateral ruptures of the distal biceps brachii tendon. *J Shoulder Elbow Surg.* 2009;18(5):804–807.

6. Visuri T, Lindholm H. Bilateral distal biceps tendon avulsions with use of anabolic steroids. *Med Sci Sports Exerc.* 1994;26(8):941–944.

7. Seiler JG III, Parker LM, Chamberland PD, et al. The distal biceps tendon. Two potential mechanisms involved in its rupture: arterial supply and mechanical impingement. *J Shoulder Elbow Surg.* 1995;4(3):149–156.

8. Davis WM, Yassine Z. An etiological factor in tear of the distal tendon of the biceps brachii; report of two cases. *J Bone Joint Surg Am.* 1956;38-A(6):1365–1368.

9. Morrey BF. Injury of the flexors of the elbow: biceps in tendon injury. In: Morrey BF, ed. *The Elbow and Its Disorders.* 3rd ed. Philadelphia, PA: W.B. Saunders; 2000:468–478.

10. Morrey BF. Chapter 34: biceps tendon injury. In: Warner JP, ed. *Instructional Course Lectures: Shoulder and Elbow.* Rosemont, IL; American Academy of Orthopedic Surgeons: 2005:369–374.

11. Mazzocca AD, Cohen M, Berkson E, et al. The anatomy of the bicipital tuberosity and distal biceps tendon. *J shoulder Elbow Surg.* 2007;16(1):122–127.

12. Hutchinson HL, Gloystein D, Gillespie M. Distal biceps tendon insertion: an anatomic study. *J Shoulder Elbow Surg.* 2008;17:342–346.

13. O'Driscoll SW, Goncalves LB, Dietz P. The hook test for distal biceps tendon avulsion. *Am J Sports Med.* 2007;35:1865–1869.

14. Dobbie RP. Avulsion of the lower biceps brachii tendon: analysis of fifty-one previously unreported cases. *Am J Surg.* 1941;51:662–683.

15. Carroll RE, Hamilton LR. Rupture of the biceps brachii: a conservative method of treatment. *J Bone Joint Surg.* 1967;49:1016.

16. Baker BE, Bierwagen D. Rupture of the distal tendon of the biceps brachii. Operative versus non-operative treatment. *J Bone Joint Surg.* 1985;67(3):414–417.

17. Meherin JM, Kilgore ES Jr. The treatment of ruptures of the distal biceps brachii tendon. *Am J Surg.* 1960;99:636–640.

18. Norman WH. Repair of avulsion of insertion of biceps brachii tendon. *Clin Orthop.* 1985;193:189–194.

19. Morrey BF, Askew LJ, An KN, et al. Rupture of the distal tendon of the biceps brachii. A biomechanical study. *J Bone Joint Surg Am.* 1985;67:418–421.

20. Agins HJ, Chess JL, Hoekstra DV, et al. Rupture of the distal insertion of the biceps brachii tendon. *Clin Orthop.* 1988;234:34–38.

21. D'Alessandro DF, Shields CL Jr, Tibone JE, et al. Repair of distal biceps tendon ruptures in athletes. *Am J Sports Med.* 1993;21:114–119.

22. Leighton MM, Bush-Joseph CA, Bach BR Jr. Distal biceps brachii repair. Results in dominant and nondominant extremities. *Clin Orthop.* 1995;317:114–121.

23. Bourne MH, Morrey BF. Partial rupture of the distal biceps tendon. *Clin Orthop Relat Res.* 1991;(271):143–148.

24. Rokito AS, McLaughlin JA, Gallagher MA, et al. Partial rupture of the distal biceps tendon. *J Shoulder Elbow Surg.* 1996;5(1):73–75.

25. Vardakas DG, Musgrave DS, Varitimidis SE, et al. Partial rupture of the distal biceps tendon. *J Shoulder Elbow Surg.* 2001;10(4):377–379.

26. Kelly EW, Steinmann S, O'Driscoll SW. Surgical treatment of partial distal biceps tendon ruptures through a single posterior incision. *J Shoulder Elbow Surg.* 2003;12(5):456–461.

27. Meherin JM, Kilgore ES. The treatment of ruptures of the distal biceps brachii tendon. *Am J Surg.* 1954;88:657–659.

28. Boyd HB, Anderson LD. A method for reinsertion of the distal biceps brachii tendon. *J Bone Joint Surg Am.* 1961;43:1041–1043.

29. Failla JM, Amadio PC, Morrey BF, et al. Proximal radioulnar synostosis after repair of distal biceps brachii rupture by the two-incision technique. Report of four cases. *Clin Orthop Relat Res.* 1990;(253):133–136.

30. Kelly EW, Morrey BF, O'Driscoll SW. Complications of repair of the distal biceps tendon with the modified two-incision technique. *J Bone Joint Surg Am.* 2000;82-A(11):1575–1581.

31. Bisson LJ, de Perio JG, Weber AE, et al. Is it safe to perform aggressive rehabilitation after distal biceps tendon repair using the modified 2-incision approach? A biomechanical study. *Am J Sports Med.* 2007;35(12):2045–2050.

32. Duncan SF, Sperling JW, Steinmann SP. Infected distal biceps tendon repairs: three case reports. *Clin Orthop Relat Res.* 2007;(461):14–16.

II. The Elbow

39

Avoiding Complications in Elbow Arthroscopy

E. Rhett Hobgood • Larry D. Field

Elbow arthroscopy is a useful technique in the management of various pathologic conditions. It has demonstrated utility in the treatment of loose bodies, plicae, osteoarthritis, rheumatoid arthritis, osteochondritis dissecans, contracture, fractures, and even some causes of elbow instability. However, it is a technically demanding procedure due to the remarkable congruity of the articular surfaces as well as the close proximity of neurovascular structures. Because of these factors, complications can often occur.

Complications include superficial infection, persistent drainage from portal sites, postoperative contracture, compartment syndrome, septic arthritis, and, most commonly, nerve injury. Some authors have shown the rate of complications after elbow arthroscopy to be much higher (approximately 10%) than that reported after knee or shoulder arthroscopy (1% and 2%). Although permanent neurologic injuries are uncommon, when they do occur, they can be devastating.

Avoiding complications requires a thorough knowledge of both intra-articular and extra-articular anatomy of the elbow combined with a systematic operative technique. The aim of this chapter is to help surgeons avoid complications by reviewing anatomic considerations, proper positioning, and use of instruments. Specific complications and associated risk factors are also discussed. Finally, we present the authors' preferred method of treatment and situations that deserve special consideration.

ANATOMIC CONSIDERATIONS

Neurovascular injury is the primary concern during elbow arthroscopy. Understanding several important anatomic considerations can help decrease the likelihood of injuring these vital structures. These considerations influence our surgical technique in the following ways: (1) marking anatomic landmarks prior to initiating the procedure, (2) positioning the elbow in 90° of flexion, (3) understanding the effect of joint distention on the relationship between the joint capsule, the bone, and the neurovascular

structures, (4) incising only the skin to protect cutaneous nerves, and (5) utilizing proximal portals in the anterior compartment.

The bony landmarks of the elbow, the ulnar nerve, and the portal sites are marked on the skin prior to joint distention (Fig. 39.1). This is important because anatomic landmarks may become obscured secondary to swelling once the procedure is initiated. The important bony landmarks to outline include the medial and lateral epicondyles, radial head, and olecranon. It is especially important to mark the position of the ulnar nerve, as subluxation and anterior dislocation can occur in approximately 16% of the population. This can place it at risk during the placement of the anteromedial portal.

Positioning the elbow in 90° of flexion is recommended. In this position, the neural structures are further away from both the bone and the capsule than in the extended position. Miller et al. demonstrated in a cadaveric study that the capsule-to-nerve and the bone-to-nerve

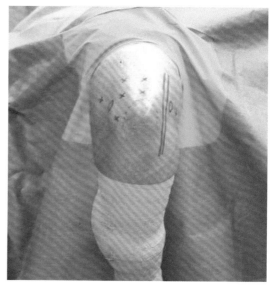

FIGURE 39.1. Anatomic landmarks are outlined on the skin.

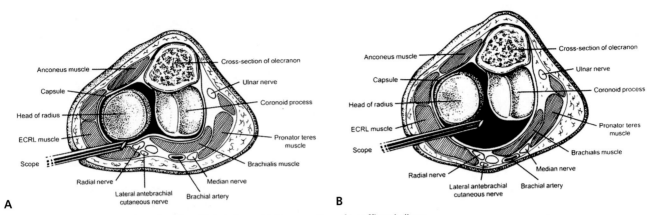

FIGURE 39.2. **A:** Cross-section of noninsufflated elbow. **B:** Cross-section of insufflated elbow.

distances increased for both the radial and the median nerves in flexed elbows when compared with matched extended elbows. However, they found that the distance between the ulnar nerve and the capsule did not vary with elbow flexion and extension, remaining essentially on the capsule in most specimens. Most importantly, elbow extension eliminates the protective effect of insufflation.

Joint insufflation with 20 mL of sterile saline should always be performed prior to portal placement. Insufflation increases the distance between the bone and the radial and median nerves. However, the bone-to-ulnar nerve distance does not change significantly with insufflation. Importantly, joint distention does not increase the distance between the joint capsule and the adjacent neurovascular structures (Fig. 39.2A, B). Therefore, it does not protect these structures from work performed against the joint capsule. An additional benefit is that joint distention makes capsule penetration easier and more reliable.

However, distention of the joint with more than 25 mL of saline risks capsular rupture. This may result in poor visualization and fluid extravasation during the procedure. In addition, exercise caution when insufflating degenerative or posttraumatic elbows as they may not have the capacity to hold more than 10 mL.

Cutaneous nerves should be protected during portal placement (Fig. 39.3A, B). When establishing portals, we advise only incising the skin to protect the subcutaneous nerves. Blunt dissection through the subcutaneous tissues is then performed prior to cannula insertion. Stab incisions should always be avoided.

When performing arthroscopy in the anterior compartment, utilize proximal portals, as they are safer than distal portals. Field et al. showed that a proximal anterolateral portal is located farther away from the radial nerve than the standard anterolateral portal (Fig. 39.4A, B). In addition, they found that the more

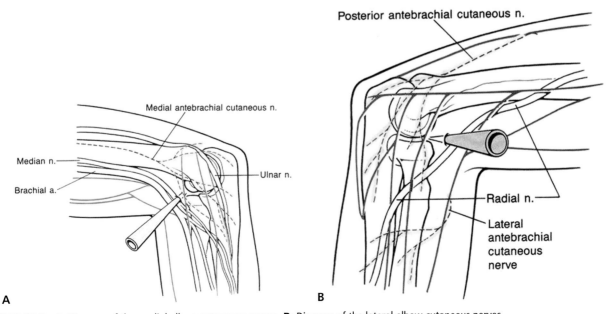

FIGURE 39.3. **A:** Diagram of the medial elbow cutaneous nerves. **B:** Diagram of the lateral elbow cutaneous nerves.

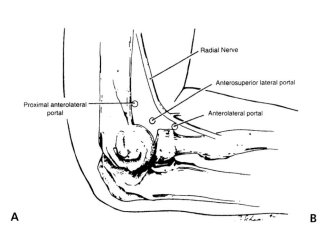

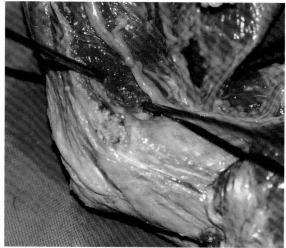

FIGURE 39.4. A: Diagram depicting the proximal anterolateral and standard anterolateral portals in relation to the radial nerve. **B:** Anatomic dissection of the lateral side of the elbow demonstrating the proximity of the radial nerve to the proximal antero-lateral *(left)* and standard anterolateral *(right)* portals.

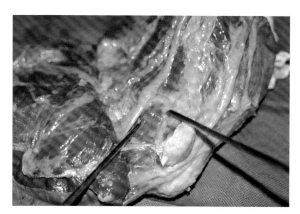

FIGURE 39.5. Anatomic dissection of the medial side of the elbow demonstrating the proximity of the median nerve to the proximal an-teromedial *(right)* and standard anteromedial *(left)* portals.

proximal portal provided equivalent visualization. The proximal anteromedial portal popularized by Poehling et al. has also been shown to be safer than the antero-medial portal. As Figure 39.5 demonstrates, the median nerve is significantly further from a more proximally placed anteromedial portal than a standard anterome-dial portal. In addition, the more proximal position al-lows the arthroscope to be directed distally, resulting in the arthroscope being almost parallel to the median nerve in the coronal plane.

PATIENT POSITIONING AND INSTRUMENTS

Proper patient positioning and equipment are integral components of a successful arthroscopy. The position of the elbow and the specific types of trocars and cannulas

are reviewed in this section. We also discuss the use of small osteotomes and retractors to aid in visualization while protecting neurovascular structures.

As discussed previously, placing the elbow in 90° of flexion helps ensure that neural structures are farther away from both the bone and the capsule than in the ex-tended position. Patients may be positioned in one of four ways to accomplish this: supine, supine suspended, prone, and lateral decubitus. Each position has specific advan-tages and disadvantages, which are described in more de-tail elsewhere.

The surgeon should be familiar with the type of can-nulas and trocars used, as there are important differences. Side-vented inflow cannulas should be avoided because the distance between the skin and the joint capsule is often very small (Fig. 39.6). This can result in the can-nula being intra-articular, whereas the side vents remain extra-articular. This can result in fluid extravasation into the surrounding soft tissues. In addition, trocars should be conical and blunt tipped to decrease the possibility of neurovascular and articular injury during cannula placement.

Small osteotomes are a valuable tool for removal of bony spurs and prominences (Fig. 39.7). They are eas-ily introduced through a cannula and can be used to re-move spurs in a more controlled manner compared with a burr. The loose fragments are then removed with an arthroscopic grasper. This technique is especially use-ful when bony spurs are adhered to the adjacent capsule where an arthroscopic burr with suction would increase the potential for neurovascular injury.

Retractors should also be utilized to decrease the like-lihood of nerve injury. As shown in Figure 39.8, retrac-tors improve visualization and physically protect specific structures during at-risk procedures. Both capsular release

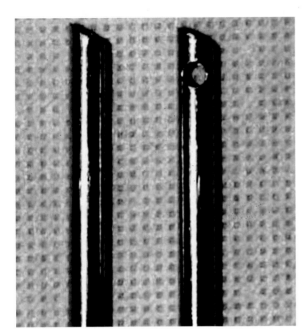

FIGURE 39.6. Side-vented inflow cannulas *(right)* should be avoided because the side vents may lie outside of the elbow joint, resulting in fluid extravasation into the surrounding soft tissues. Fluid flow should occur from the end of the cannula *(left)*.

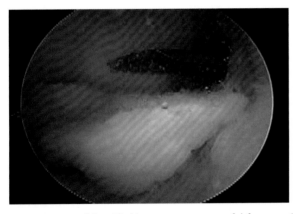

FIGURE 39.7. Small hand-held osteotomes are useful for removing bony spurs and prominences.

and radial head excision are examples of procedures in which retractors can be utilized to protect neurovascular structures.

Finally, as with any arthroscopic technique, it is imperative that the surgeon maintains visualization of instruments and articular surfaces at all times. The risk of inadvertent injury is increased exponentially when the tips of burrs, shavers, or other instruments cannot be visualized.

COMPLICATIONS

The complications associated with elbow arthroscopy include superficial infection, persistent drainage from portal

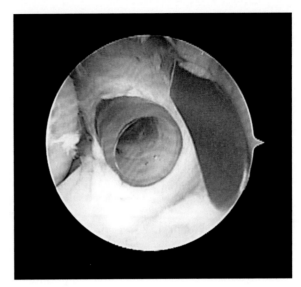

FIGURE 39.8. Arthroscopic view from the proximal anterolateral portal showing a retractor utilized to improve visualization and protect neurovascular structures.

sites, heterotopic ossification, postoperative contracture, compartment syndrome, septic arthritis, and nerve injuries. This section reviews the incidence and treatment of each complication and any risk factors identified in the literature. This knowledge may assist the treating surgeon in avoiding the complication.

Superficial Infection

Superficial infection is an uncommon complication when performing elbow arthroscopy. Two of the largest series (Thomas et al. and Kelly et al.) found an incidence of 2% in 334 and 473 cases of elbow arthroscopy, respectively. All infections resolved with a course of oral antibiotics and no particular risk factors were identified in either study. Attention to sterile technique and use of perioperative antibiotics may help reduce the incidence of this complication.

Persistent Drainage

Drainage from portal sites has been noted in 3% to 5% of elbow arthroscopies. The lateral portal sites appear to be most susceptible because the subcutaneous tissues are thin and are often unable to provide a barrier between the joint and the skin. We recommend suture closure of portal sites, particularly lateral ones, to help prevent this complication.

Heterotopic Ossification

This is a rare complication occurring in only 0.9% of patients in one of the largest series of patients evaluated. One case report involved a young throwing athlete undergoing arthroscopic debridement for posterior impingement. It was also reported in patients who underwent ulnohumeral

II. The Elbow

arthroplasty for degenerative arthritis. Treatment involved a combination of physical therapy and open excision of the heterotopic bone. No particular risk factors have been identified; however, this complication should be considered in patients who are unable to recover full range of motion after elbow arthroscopy.

Postoperative Contracture

Contracture occurred in 3% of elbows undergoing elbow arthroscopy in the largest series in the literature. Motion loss occurred in the flexion–extension plane and was <20° in all patients. Most cases were associated with conditions that predispose the elbow to stiffness (e.g., inflammatory arthritis and osteochondritis dissecans). The explanation for loss of motion after arthroscopy is uncertain; however, immediate postoperative motion with the assistance of an occupational therapist may prevent this complication.

Septic Arthritis

This serious complication has been reported in 0.6% to 0.8% of elbow arthroscopies. It may have an association with intra-articular steroid injection at the end of the procedure. Patients require irrigation and debridement combined with a prolonged course of intravenous antibiotics. Routine administration of preoperative intravenous prophylactic antibiotics as well as avoiding corticosteroid injections may help prevent this potentially devastating complication.

Neurologic Injury

Neurologic complications after elbow arthroscopy range from 0% to 14%. Injuries to the radial, median, ulnar, posterior interosseous, and anterior interosseous nerves (AINs) have all been reported. Several case reports detail permanent neurologic injury; however, most injuries are transient. Risk factors associated with the development of a transient nerve palsy include rheumatoid arthritis, contracture, and performance of a capsular release. Nerve injury may be secondary to portal placement, local anesthetic, prolonged tourniquet compression, indwelling catheters, compression due to swelling, and direct injury from instruments.

The posterior interosseous nerve (PIN) is at risk for injury near the inferior aspect of the anterolateral capsule. This complication was reported in two case series in which an anterior capsular release was performed. Both authors recommend stopping the debridement once the fibers of the brachioradialis or brachialis are visualized. Thus, caution must be exercised when working near the anterolateral capsule just distal to the radiocapitellar joint. As previously discussed, retractors can be utilized to protect the anterolateral capsule in this area.

AIN injury is a rare complication. One case report involved a rheumatoid patient who underwent extensive arthroscopic synovectomy with removal of multiple loose bodies. Subsequent surgical exploration revealed diffuse scarring involving the anterior capsule with complete transection of the anterior interosseous branch of the median nerve. Other authors have noted that patients with rheumatoid arthritis have a thin anterior capsule and atrophic brachialis muscle. We recommend that surgeons maintain extreme caution when performing arthroscopic synovectomy or capsular release in rheumatoid patients as anterior structures, including the median nerve and AIN, are at increased risk for injury.

Ulnar nerve injury can occur for various reasons. Anteromedial portal placed too far posteriorly risks direct injury to the nerve, and posterior portals should never be placed medial to the midline of the arm. Also, intra-articular work performed near the posteromedial gutter risks injury due to the close proximity of the nerve to the capsule. Stretch-induced ulnar neuropathy is a documented complication after arthroscopic capsular release, where flexion is greatly increased. In fact, a decreased flexion–extension arc has been identified as a risk factor for neuropathy in one retrospective review of 191 consecutive arthroscopies. Therefore, we recommend routine decompression of the ulnar nerve in patients undergoing capsular release when <95° of elbow flexion is present preoperatively.

Complete transection of nerves is an exceedingly rare complication; however, transection of both the median and the radial nerves has been reported. Haapaniemi et al. describe this devastating complication after arthroscopic release of a posttraumatic elbow contracture. They note that elbow trauma may change anatomy, making correct portal placement difficult. In addition, the capsule has reduced compliance and capacity leading to markedly reduced fluid distension. This consequently reduces the working distance between the articular surface and the neurovascular structures.

SPECIAL CONSIDERATIONS

There are several situations that require unique technical consideration. These are synovectomy in rheumatoid patients, radial head resection, capsular release, and posttraumatic contractures. These should be considered "at-risk" procedures and almost all cases of severe nerve injury have been associated with them. Each situation presents unique challenges and specific recommendations to prevent complications.

Synovectomy in Rheumatoid Patients

Rheumatoid arthritis is a significant risk factor for the development of nerve injury. Patients with rheumatoid arthritis have a thin and filmy anterior capsule. The brachialis muscle, which normally provides a stout barrier to injury of anterior structures, is typically thin and atrophic. Surgeons need to bear in mind the thickness of the anterior capsule and overlying brachialis when performing synovectomy in rheumatoid patients.

Radial Head Resection

The PIN is at risk for injury, as this procedure places instruments adjacent to the inferior capsule (Fig. 39.9). In addition, prior trauma may cause the PIN to adhere or scar down to the capsule increasing the risk.

Capsular Release

Prevention of neurologic injury during arthroscopic anterior capsular release is aided by several measures. The release must be performed on the anterior aspect of the distal humerus and stopped once the muscular layer of the brachialis or brachioradialis is identified (Fig. 39.10). In addition, care must be taken not to direct the shaver blade toward the anterolateral capsule just distal to the radiocapitellar joint where the PIN is located. Some

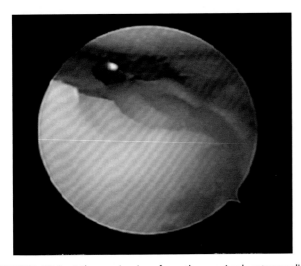

FIGURE 39.9. Arthroscopic view from the proximal anteromedial portal demonstrating radial head resection.

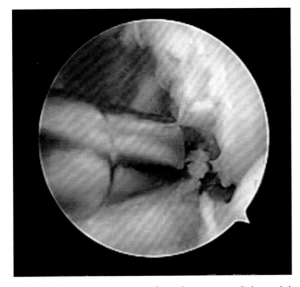

FIGURE 39.10. Arthroscopic view from the anteromedial portal demonstrating fibers of the brachialis seen during anterior capsular release.

experienced elbow arthroscopists consider trauma that produces excessive scarring in the vicinity of the PIN, a contraindication to arthroscopic capsular release.

Posttraumatic Contractures

Trauma may change the anatomy making correct placement of portals difficult. The joint capsule has a reduced compliance and capacity leading to reduced fluid distension and consequently a reduced working distance between the articular surface and the neurovascular structures.

CONCLUSIONS/KEY POINTS

Elbow arthroscopy is a valuable tool that can be utilized for various pathologic conditions. However, it is a technically challenging procedure due to the anatomic constraints of the joint and the proximity of neurovascular structures. Avoiding complications requires a thorough understanding of elbow anatomy and a methodical surgical technique. The following key points highlight how to perform a safe and successful arthroscopy.

- Define landmarks and palpate ulnar nerve.
- Distend joint prior to portal placement.
- Incise skin only to protect cutaneous nerves.
- Keep elbow flexed 90° when possible.
- Utilize proximal anterior portals.
- Always maintain visualization of arthroscopic instruments.
- Avoid inferior aspect of anterolateral capsule (PIN) and posteromedial gutter (ulnar nerve) when possible.
- Consider exploring and protecting nerves during complex "at-risk" arthroscopic procedures.
- Abandon procedure if visualization/orientation compromised, as prevention of nerve injury in elbow arthroscopy is EVERYTHING!

REFERENCES

1. Abboud JA, Ricchetti ET, Tjoumakaris F, et al. Elbow arthroscopy: basic setup and portal placement. *J Am Acad Orthop Surg.* 2006;14(5):312–318.
2. Dumonski ML, Arciero RA, Mazzocca AD. Ulnar nerve palsy after elbow arthroscopy. *Arthroscopy.* 2006;22(5):577.
3. Field LD, Altchek DW, Warren RF, et al. Arthroscopic anatomy of the lateral elbow: a comparison of three portals. *Arthroscopy.* 1994;10:602–607.
4. Haapaniemi T, Berggren M, Adolfsson L. Complete transection of the median and radial nerves during arthroscopic release of post-traumatic elbow contracture. *Arthroscopy.* 1999;15(7):784–787.
5. Jones GS, Savoie FH III. Arthroscopic capsular release of flexion contractures (arthrofibrosis) of the elbow. *Arthroscopy.* 1993;9(3):277–283.
6. Kelly EW, Morrey BF, O'Driscoll SW. Complications of elbow arthroscopy. *J Bone Joint Surg Am.* 2001;83-A(1):25–34.
7. Miller CD, Jobe CM, Wright MH. Neuroanatomy in elbow arthroscopy. *J Shoulder Elbow Surg.* 1995;4(3):168–174.

II. The Elbow

8. Morrey BF. Complications of elbow arthroscopy. *Instr Course Lect.* 2000;49:255–258.

9. O'Driscoll SW, Savoie FH. Arthroscopy of the elbow. In: Morrey BF, ed. *Master Techniques in Orthopaedic Surgery: The Elbow.* Philadelphia, PA: Lippincott Williams & Wilkins; 2002:27–45.

10. Park JY, Cho CH, Choi JH, et al. Radial nerve palsy after arthroscopic anterior capsular release for degenerative elbow contracture. *Arthroscopy.* 2007;23(12):1360.

11. Ramsey ML, Naranja RJ. Diagnostic arthroscopy of the elbow. In: Baker CL Jr, Plancher KD, eds. *Operative Treatment of Elbow Injuries.* New York, NY: Springer-Verlag; 2002:163–169.

12. Ruch DS, Poehling GG. Anterior interosseus nerve injury following elbow arthroscopy. *Arthroscopy.* 1997;13(6):756–758.

13. Sodha S, Nagda SH, Sennett BJ. Heterotopic ossification in a throwing athlete after elbow arthroscopy. *Arthroscopy.* 2006;22(7):802.

14. Thomas R, Savoie FH, Field LD. Complications of elbow arthroscopy (SS-67). *Arthroscopy.* 2007;23(6):e34.

15. Huffman GR, O'Driscoll SW. Delayed onset ulnar neuropathy after arthroscopic elbow contracture release (SS-63). *Arthroscopy.* 2006;22(6):e32.

Wrist Arthroscopy Basics: Anatomy, Portals, and Diagnostic Arthroscopy

Mark Morishige • Robert C. Dews • Larry D. Field • Felix H. Savoie III

Wrist arthroscopy has been utilized for the past 30 years since it was first described by Chen in 1979 (1). Then it provided only a partial evaluation of the articular surfaces and few investigators routinely utilized it. Not until 1986 when Whipple et al. (2) advocated distraction techniques and precise portal placement did an extensive evaluation of the wrist joint become an option. Still, diagnosis was the primary function and therapeutic indications were minimal.

Since that time, arthroscopy of the wrist has evolved into one of the most reliable and productive means of diagnosing, qualifying, and treating wrist pathology, and it has rapidly obtained widespread acceptance. Diagnostic and therapeutic arthroscopy have advanced our knowledge of the wrist by increasing understanding of both anatomy and function, thus facilitating anatomic repair of previously unrecognized pathology. Continued advances in instrumentation and technology will improve the ability to perform challenging and innovative procedures as the principles of open surgery become adapted to arthroscopy (3).

CLINICAL EVALUATION

Pertinent History

A meticulous history is essential prior to arthroscopic evaluation of the wrist. The history helps the examiner focus the physical examination toward the suspected pathology. It should include duration of symptoms, location, intensity, aggravating or relieving factors, and the effects of treatment modalities already utilized as well as the past medical and surgical history, medications, allergies, and family history. Sports and repetitive activities should also be identified. The mechanism of injury including the position of the hand, direction of force, and resultant area of pain must be fully detailed during the evaluation. The patient's age and sex should also be considered. Young patients (<40 years) are more prone to posttraumatic carpal injuries, whereas older patients are more susceptible to systemic and degenerative processes. The medical and family history are helpful for diagnosing patients with systemic and hereditary disorders that can present in the

wrist. Laboratory values are often helpful in this situation. The effect of the wrist pain on the patient's work and leisure activities is also important.

Physical Examination

Physical examination is the most accurate method to diagnose wrist pathology (4). It begins with a systematic inspection of swelling, erythema, warmth, nodules, skin lesions, and deformities or prior surgical incisions. If possible, tenderness is localized to a specific anatomic structure. Wrist range of motion should be noted, paying careful attention to any snapping or clicking. "Clicks," which may indicate carpal instability, can sometimes be felt throughout the wrist range of motion but are usually not significant unless they reproduce the patient's clinical symptoms.

All joints must be palpated and evaluated with the appropriate use of provocative tests. Radially, the grind test can assess carpal metacarpal (CMC) thumb arthritis. Arthritis of the scaphotrapeziotrapezoid joint should also be evaluated. Anatomic snuffbox tenderness may indicate scaphoid or scapholunate ligament pathology. This ligament can be further assessed with Watson's (5) "scaphoid shift test." Ulnarly, the shear or ballottement test can indicate lunotriquetral instability by manipulating the two bones relative to each other. Ulnocarpal abutment and triangular fibrocartilage complex (TFCC) tears are considered with pain just distal to the ulnar styloid and reproduction of symptoms after axial loading and ulnar wrist deviation. Instability of the midcarpal joint is suggested by the "catch-up" clunk produced when the wrist is moved from radial to ulnar deviation during axial loading. Pain or crepitation during compression of the distal radioulnar joint (DRUJ) suggests instability or arthritic changes there. Volarly, tenderness with palpation of the pisiform or hook of the hamate may represent pisotriquetral arthritis or a hamate fracture.

To complete the wrist examination, the tendons are examined to exclude tenosynovitis. Evaluation of motor and sensory nerves may indicate compressive neuropathies.

Finally, the vascular status is assessed using capillary refill and Allen's test to exclude insufficiency or thrombosis.

Diagnostic Imaging

The initial radiographic evaluation should consist of three views of the wrist: standard posteroanterior (PA), oblique, and lateral views. They should be examined for fractures, alignment, and congruence of joint spaces, as well as evidence of arthritic changes and mineralization. The lateral view is important for assessment of the carpal alignment. A scapholunate angle of greater than 60° suggests possible scapholunate instability, and an angle of less than 30° suggests ulnar-sided wrist instability. Additional radiographs may be needed depending on the clinical scenario. The "clenched fist" view improves visualization of scapholunate pathology, and the "carpal tunnel view" can better elucidate the bony structures of the carpal tunnel.

Musculoskeletal ultrasound may prove useful for the evaluation of soft-tissue abnormalities such as tendinopathy, ganglia, and synovial cysts but is highly operator dependent.

Arthrography is helpful to evaluate the integrity of capsular structures and interosseous ligaments, especially the scapholunate, lunotriquetral, and TFCC (6). It may show localized synovitis or abnormal leaks between normally "compartmentalized" spaces.

CT provides the best assessment of osseous and articular morphology. It can provide images in any plane (such as the oblique axis of the scaphoid) and gives clear detail to fractures that are difficult to visualize with plain radiographs, such as the hook of the hamate.

MRI provides important detail about the soft tissues of the wrist and bony vascularity. Avascular necrosis of carpal bones, such as the lunate and scaphoid, as well as occult ganglions, soft-tissue tumors, tendinitis, and joint effusions, are well visualized. MRI has been shown to have a 90% sensitivity when evaluating tears of the TFCC. Accuracy also approaches 90% when evaluating the scapholunate ligament but drops to 50% for lunotriquetral tears (7). The most definitive study seems to be the MR arthrogram that begin with a radiocarpal injection following by a DRUJ injection (8).

TREATMENT

Nonoperative

Prior to arthroscopy, nonoperative measures should usually be exhausted. Temporarily immobilization of the wrist in a splint or brace and anti-inflammatory medication may be helpful. Diagnostic and therapeutic injections can frequently provide some benefit. A physical therapy regimen for wrist range of motion and strengthening may prove definitive for some wrist pathology.

Operative Indications

Wrist arthroscopy has been a useful tool for diagnosis in patients with wrist pain, motion loss, and weakness where noninvasive diagnostic and treatment protocols have failed. It is also useful in patients with well-defined pathology such as nonunions, Kienbock disease, scapholunate or lunotriquetral dissociations where evaluation of the articular surfaces are of prognostic and therapeutic importance. Many definitive treatments can be performed at the time of arthroscopy such as loose body removal, synovectomy, intra-articular adhesion release, lavage of septic wrist, and debridement of chondral lesions as well as hypertrophic or torn ligaments and tears of the TFCC. It provides a useful adjunct in the reduction of distal radius and scaphoid fractures and has been used for dorsal ganglion excision. More recently, midcarpal, DRUJ, and volar portals have expanded the arthroscope's use for evaluation and treatment of midcarpal chondral lesions of the hamate, articular damage to the ulnar head or extensive synovitis. These portals also improve visualization of volar articular surfaces and dorsal capsular structures (9). Bone excision procedures such as radial styloidectomy and partial resection of distal ulna (wafer procedures) have been performed. Arthroscopy has even been described for advanced procedures such as proximal row carpectomy, excision of proximal pole of the scaphoid, excision of Kienbock disease, and capitolunate arthrodesis (10, 11).

Contraindications to wrist arthroscopy are mainly limited to conditions of trauma or swelling, which distorts the normal anatomy or significantly damages capsular integrity leading to fluid extravasation.

TECHNIQUE—SURFACE ANATOMY

The wrist is made up of the eight carpal bones each with multiple articular surfaces as well as the intrinsic and extrinsic ligaments, and TFCC surrounded by tendons and neurovascular structures (10, 11). A thorough understanding of the relationship between the surface anatomy of the wrist and these underlying structures is essential for accurate arthroscopic portal placement and adequate arthroscopy. Understanding these relationships will help to prevent injury to the cutaneous nerves, tendons, and vascular structures as well as minimize the risk to the articular surfaces in the wrist. It will also help to perform increasingly complicated arthroscopic wrist procedures.

The surface anatomy should be mapped and labeled prior to making the first portal incision. Bony landmarks that should be familiar include Lister's tubercle, the radius and ulna with their styloids, the radiocarpal joint level, the radial border of third ray, and central portion of the forth ray. In addition, the capitate sulcus or "soft spot" should be palpated.

The extensor retinaculum is an oblique structure spanning the dorsal distal radius and ulna. It compartmentalizes the 12 extensor tendons into 6 compartments and prevents bowstringing (Fig. 40.1). The extensor pollicis longus (EPL) is the only tendon in the third compartment and is easily palpated especially after application of traction. The EPL should be marked as it passes just ulnar to Lister's tubercle. The area bordered by the EPL and

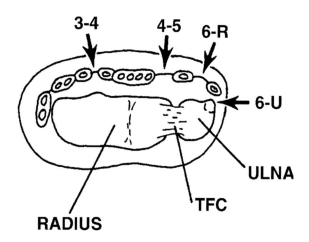

FIGURE 40.1. Cross-sectional anatomy of the dorsal compartments. (From Geissler WB, Freeland AE, Weiss AP, et al. Techniques of wrist arthroscopy. *Instr Course Lect.* 2000;49:225–237, used with permission.)

extensor pollicis brevis (EPB) together and the extensor carpi radialis longus (ECRL) define the margins of the anatomic snuffbox. The extensor digitorum communis (EDC) is just ulnar to EPL. The extensor carpi ulnaris (ECU), and the ECRL and extensor carpi radialis brevis (ECRB) tendons are easily palpated and should be drawn as well. The intersection of these tendons and the bony structures allows accurate placement of arthroscopic portals.

AUTHORS' PREFERRED TREATMENT

Arthroscopic Technique: Setup

Regional or general anesthesia may be used. The patient is positioned supine with the operative extremity on an arm table. The OR table is angled so that the surgeon is positioned above the arm table near the patient's head, and the assistant is positioned directly across the arm table within the patient's axilla (Fig. 40.2). A nonsterile tourniquet is applied and the arm and hand is prepped and draped with the forearm in a vertical position (Fig. 40.3).

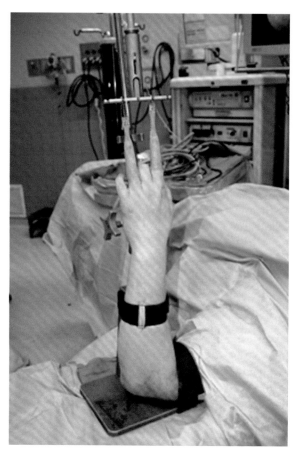

FIGURE 40.3. Draping and tower placement.

Distraction is essential to improve visualization and provide adequate space for maneuverability during wrist arthroscopy. Several distraction options currently exist. A dedicated sterile or nonsterile traction tower is a popular choice (Fig. 40.4). Alternatives include the use of horizontal traction with a pulley and weight system as well as nonsterile traction boom devices.

We prefer a sterile traction tower with nylon finger traps. This provides convenient application of wrist

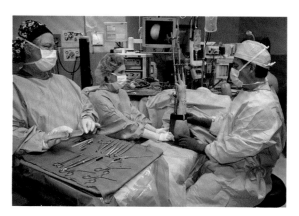

FIGURE 40.2. OR setup with position of assistant and surgical assistant.

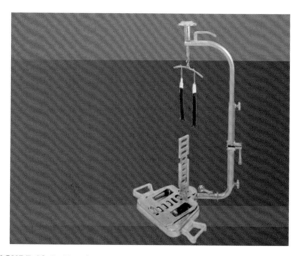

FIGURE 40.4. Traction tower.

distraction in flexion, extention, and radial and ulnar deviation. This system allows adjustability to both the distraction force and the position of the wrist. In addition, it permits easy conversion to open procedures if necessary.

The prepped arm is then placed in an abducted position, and the upper arm is secured to the traction tower. Soft nylon finger traps are used to secure the index and long finger to the tower for most procedures (Fig. 40.5). Soft traps have increased surface area and distribute the force better than wire devices. In the case of poor or fragile skin, additional fingers in the traps can decrease the force to the skin (4). To improve visualization for ulnar-sided pathology, we will frequently use the index and ring fingers. Generally, 5 to 10 pounds of traction is adequate for most procedures.

Arthroscopic Equipment

Proper equipment is essential to perform a quality wrist arthroscopy. This begins with basic equipment such as video arthroscope and monitor with printer and video recorder to document the intra-articular findings. In addition to adequate visualization, a major improvement came with the development of instruments specifically designed for use in small joints. Larger instrumentation used for knee and shoulder arthroscopy is not adequate for procedures in the wrist. A small 2- to 3-mm diameter arthroscope is required to allow adequate mobilization while minimizing the risk

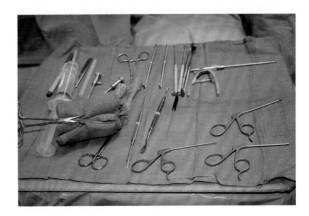

FIGURE 40.6. Mayo setup.

of injury to surrounding structures and articular surfaces. In addition to the standard 30° arthroscope, a 70° scope is occasionally useful.

Other small joint arthroscopy equipment is available and necessary for mastery of wrist arthroscopy (Fig. 40.6). This includes a small joint shaver (2.7 or 2.9 mm) with multiple tips, a wrist probe (1.7 or 2.0 mm), and many smaller versions of large joint arthroscopic instruments (11, 12). As arthroscopy has advanced, more specialized equipment has become available, allowing for advanced surgical procedures. These including TFCC repair kits, retrograde retrievers, ablation shrinkage devices, and fracture fixation devices. Spinal needles and passing sutures are also helpful tools that have been adapted from other arthroscopic repair techniques.

Clear physiologic crystalloid solution such as lactated ringers is preferable because it can be rapidly absorbed into the tissues and prevent excessive distention. Irrigant can be introduced through the sheath of the arthroscope or by separate inflow and outflow portals. Gravity inflow has proven adequate in our practice. Pinch chambers can introduce small boluses of irrigant to clear the visual field (4). Fluid pumps that can precisely control the pressure in the joint are available. However, pressurized injection increases the risk of fluid extravasation into subcutaneous tissues and is usually unnecessary.

Portals

Wrist arthroscopy portals can be organized into radiocarpal, midcarpal, distal radioulnar, and volar portals. Traditionally, arthroscopic viewing portals are described by their relationship to the six extensor compartments of the wrist (Fig. 40.7). There are 11 historical access portals typically used. These include five radiocarpal, four midcarpal, and two distal radioulnar. There are also two additional volar portals that have become increasingly popular.

Precise portal placement allows complete wrist arthroscopy while minimizing iatrogenic injury to the wrist joint and surrounding structures. Incorrect portal placement can result in the damage to neurovascular structures

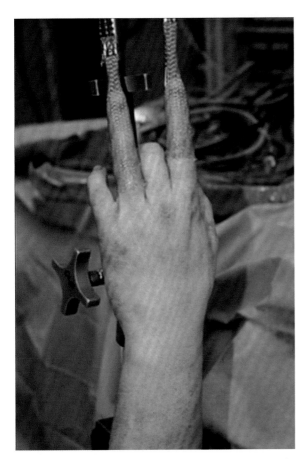

FIGURE 40.5. Soft finger trap placement for ulnar-sided procedure.

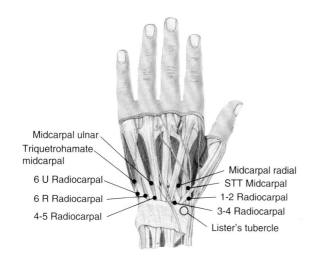

FIGURE 40.7. Dorsal wrist anatomy and portal locations.

and the articular cartilage. Marking portals after the application of traction helps prevent distortion and improper portal sites (Fig. 40.8).

Radiocarpal portals include the 3-4, 4-5, 6-R, 6-U, and 1-2 portals. Radiocarpal portals show smooth carpal articulations, whereas the midcarpal portals will show more irregular articulations (12). Portals are named according to the interspace between extensor compartments. The 3-4 portal divides the third and fourth extensor compartments.

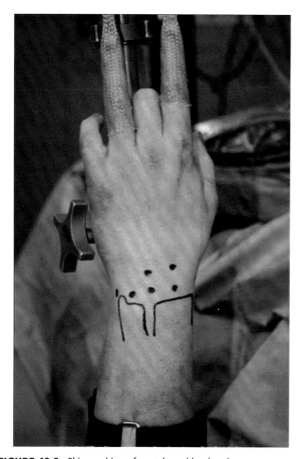

FIGURE 40.8. Skin marking of portals and landmarks.

The 6-R and 6-U portals are named by their relationship to the ECU, with the 6-R on the radial aspect and the 6-U ulnar (11). Palpation between these compartments will show soft spots of the wrist, which provide the least traumatic entry points into the joint.

3-4 Portal

The 3-4 portal is usually the first portal established and is the primary viewing portal. It is bordered on the radial side by the EPL and ECRB, on the ulnar side by the EDC, on the proximal side by the distal radius, and on the distal side by the scapholunate ligament. The 3-4 portal is placed 1 cm distal to Lister's tubercle and is located by palpating the distal edge of the radius between the ulnar border of the ECRB and the radial margin of EDC in line with the radial border of the long finger. This is the soft spot between the third and the fourth compartments. A spinal needle can then be inserted at an angle parallel to the radial articular surface. This portal is the workhorse of standard wrist arthroscopy and provides a broad view of most of the radiocarpal joint on the volar side. This portal is relatively safe with branches of the sensory branch of the radial nerve (SBRN) radial, a mean distance of 16 mm and a mean of 26.3 mm from the radial artery (13).

4-5 Portal

The 4-5 portal is bordered on the radial side by EDC, on the ulnar side by the extensor digiti quinti (EDQ), proximally by the attachment of the radius and the TFCC, and distally by the lunate. It is established 1 cm ulnar and slightly more proximal to the 3-4 portal due to the inclination of the radius (11). It can be found by palpating the soft spot directly ulnar to the EDC. A spinal needle should then be placed just proximal to the lunate. Entry through this portal places instruments directly adjacent to the midportion of the TFCC (14). The 4-5 portal is typically the main working portal for instrumentation on the ulnar side of the wrist. It may also be used as a viewing portal for ulnar-sided structures. This portal has minimal neurovascular risk unless there is an aberrant branch of the SBRN (13).

6-R Portal

Frequently used as an alternative to the 4-5 portal, the 6R portal is bordered radially by the EDQ, ulnarly by the ECU, proximally by the TFCC, and distally by the lunotriquetral joint. It enters the wrist joint just distal to the ulnar attachment of the TFCC. This portal is found by using the proximal border of the triquetrum rather than distal ulna as a surface landmark to avoid damaging the TFCC. It is established under arthroscopic visualization by introducing a needle just radial to the ECU. The 6-R portal is typically used for instrumentation or for outflow. It also provides visualization of the TFCC and the ulnolunate, ulnotriquetral, and interosseous LT ligaments. The 6-R has a mean distance of 8.2 mm from the dorsal sensory branch of the ulnar nerve (DBUN) (13).

6-U Portal

The 6-U portal is established volar to the ECU tendon because of its proximity to the DBUN it is not routinely used. The skin incision may be placed as far volar as the dorsal border of the ECU tendon. The portal enters the wrist joint through the prestyloid recess between the ECU tendon and the ulnar styloid. The portal is distal to the TFCC and dorsal ulnar to the ulnotriquetral ligament. The 6-U is typically used for the inflow/outflow cannula. It may be used as an accessory portal for viewing ulnar-sided structures or instrumentation during TFCC repairs. The mean distance of the DBUN is 4.5 mm, but there can be multiple branches in some patients (13).

1-2 Portal

The 1-2 portal is not used frequently. It is established between the first and the second extensor compartments 1 to 2 mm distal to the radial styloid. This portal is placed by finding the soft spot between the first extensor compartment containing the abductor pollicis longus (APL) and EPB and the second compartment with ECRL and ECRB tendons along the far ulnar part of the anatomic snuffbox. It is located just proximal to the waist of the scaphoid. The radial artery is located at the volar and radial aspect of the snuffbox. This necessitates placement of this portal as far dorsal as possible to avoid injury to the artery (14). The 1-2 portal provides access to the radial styloid, scaphoid, and articular surface of the distal radius but allows only a limited view of the lunate (3). There is significant risk with the placement of this portal. Two branches of the SBRN are a mean of 3 mm radial and 5 mm ulnar to the portal, and the radial artery was a mean of 3 mm radial to the portal (13).

Midcarpal Portals

Midcarpal evaluation should be done as a routine part of wrist arthroscopy. The four midcarpal portals include the midcarpal radial, midcarpal ulnar, triquetrohamate, and triscaphe portals (STTs). The most commonly used are the radial and ulnar midcarpal portals. The very limited room in the midcarpal space requires extra care when entering the joint. Once established, these portals should be maintained to minimize the difficulty reestablishing them due to fluid extravasation (11). Normally, there is no communication between the radiocarpal and the midcarpal spaces.

Evaluation of wrist instability with midcarpal arthroscopy is better than with radiocarpal arthroscopy alone. Studies show instability of scapholunate or lunotriquetral ligament diagnosed with radiocarpal arthroscopy was always seen on midcarpal arthroscopy but that seen by midcarpal arthroscopy was not always noted when performing radiocarpal arthroscopy alone. Grading of instability was also equal to or greater on the midcarpal examination (15).

Visualization of the scaphoid–trapezoid–trapezium (STT) joint, midcarpal extrinsic ligaments, the capitohamate joint, and the articular surfaces of the midcarpal bones is improved with midcarpal arthroscopy. Midcarpal arthroscopy can be mastered quickly and adds little time to wrist arthroscopy. It has a low morbidity rate and should routinely be used for a thorough evaluation of the wrist (15).

Midcarpal Radial Portal

The midcarpal radial (RMC) portal is the most commonly used midcarpal portal. It is bordered radially by the ECRB, ulnarly by the EDC, proximally by the scapholunate ligament, and distally by the capitate. It should be established in line with the radial border of the third metacarpal, 1 cm distal to the 3-4 portal. A soft spot may be palpated on the radial side of the proximal capitate between the base of the third metacarpal and the dorsal margin of the distal radius. The arthroscope enters between the capitate and the scaphoid. This allows evaluation of the midcarpal space, as well as the SL, LT, and STT articulations. This portal is relatively safe with branches of the SBRN found radially at a mean distance of 15.8 mm (13).

Midcarpal Ulnar Portal

The midcarpal ulnar portal (UMC) is bordered radially by the EDC, ulnarly by the EDQ, proximally by the lunotriquetral joint, and distally by the capitate hamate joint. It is in line with the center of the fourth metacarpal. As with the RMC portal, it is placed approximately 1 cm distal to the 4-5 portal, at about the same level as the RMC portal. This portal enters through capitate–hamate–triquetral–iunate interval. It is used primarily for instrumentation within the midcarpal joint. There is minimal risk when making this portal as the SBRN branches are usually remote to this portal (13).

Triquetrohumate Portal

The triquetrohumate (TH) portal is established on the ulnar side of the wrist distal to the triquetrum and ulnar to the midcarpal ulnar portal. The EDQ borders it on the radial side and the end of the ECU on its ulnar side. It enters the TH joint, just ulnar to the ECU tendon. It provides excellent access for an inflow or outflow cannula and can also be used for instrumentation in the TH joint.

Triscaphe Portal

The STT is on the radial side of the midcarpal space. It is established ulnar to EPL or more recently radial to APL in line with the radial margin of the second metacarpal at the level of the distal pole of the scaphoid. The more recent STT-R provides additional view and access to the STT joint (16). Staying ulnar to EPL will help to avoid the radial artery. The ulnar aspect of the ECRL tendon can also be used to check the location of this portal because the EPL is quite mobile at the level of the STT joint. Care must be taken to prevent displacing the tendon radially while establishing the STT portal to protect the radial artery. The STT joint can be entered directly through this portal, and it is used primarily for instrumentation in this

III. The Wrist

joint (14). Care should be taken to avoid the small terminal branches of the SBRN.

Volar portals have become increasingly popular to complete the view of diagnostic wrist arthroscopy as well as provide access for procedures that are not feasible from the dorsal entry sites. Bain suggests the concept of the box approach to wrist arthroscopy (Fig. 40.9). By utilizing portals around the circumference of the wrist, adequate visualization and access to all surfaces within the wrist is improved (17). The viewing and working portals can then be adjusted for the specific diagnostic or therapeutic procedure (3). The volar portals allow improved treatment for dorsal pathology such as dorsal rim fractures of the distal radius, dorsal rheumatoid synovial proliferation, and volar segment tears of the SL and LT interosseous ligaments (17).

Volar Radial Portal

To place the volar radial (VR) portal, a mini-open technique is utilized over the FCR on radial side of volar proximal wrist crease. In an anatomic study, there was a safe zone that included the width of the FCR and at least 3 mm in all directions at this level from the palmar cutaneous branch of median nerve (ulnarly) and radial artery (radially) (18). Because of this safe zone, a 2-cm transverse incision can then be made over the FCR tendon. The transverse incision provides superior cosmesis while maintaining minimal risk for the volar structures. The tendon sheath is divided and the radial artery is retracted radially and the FCR and median nerve are retracted ulnarly. The radiocarpal joint is identified with a spinal needle, and the portal is opened with a blunt instrument. This portal is used to assess the dorsal aspect of the scapholunte interosseous ligament (SLIL) and the dorsal radiocarpal ligament (DRCL) (18).

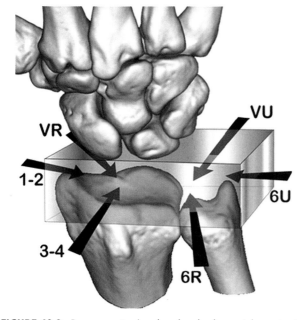

FIGURE 40.9. Box concept using dorsal and volar portals as viewing and working portals to encircle the wrist. (From Bain GI, Munt J, Turner PC. New advances in wrist arthroscopy. *Arthroscopy.* 2008;24:355–367, used with permission.)

Volar Ulnar Portal

The volar ulnar (VU) portal also utilizes a mini-open technique. A 2-cm longitudinal incision is centered over the proximal wrist crease along the ulnar edge of the common flexors. The interval between FCU and common flexor tendons is then used. The common flexors are retracted radially and FCU and the ulnar nerve are retracted ulnarly. The joint space is identified with a spinal needle, and the capsule is again opened bluntly. There is no true safe zone for the VU portal so this portal requires a careful dissection and spread technique (19). This portal provides access for reduction of distal radius fracture and a view of the dorsal articular surfaces and dorsal ligaments.

Distal Radioulnar Portals

The DRUJ is difficult to examine and arthroscopy is not frequently used here. Portals include the proximal and the distal DRUJ portals named by their location proximal or distal to the ulnar head. The DRUJ portals are bordered radially by the EDC and ulnarly by the ECU. The joint is entered from at the base of the DRUJ bordered by the radius and ulna. The proximal portal is placed in this line just proximal to the DRUJ. The forearm is supinated to relax dorsal capsule and arthroscope is then introduced between radius and ulna underneath the TFCC and proximal to the articular surface. The radioulnar articular surfaces can then be seen. Examination during pronation and supination will increase the available surface area.

The distal portal is not always accessible. Use of this portal allows the surgeon to examine the distal articular surface of the ulna and the undersurface of the TFCC. The DRUJ portal uses a mini-open approach. It is located just proximal to the TFCC and care must be taken to stay below the TFCC and prevent injury to this structure. In addition, there is some risk to the posterior interosseous nerve (10). There is minimal risk to sensory nerves with the closest 17.5 mm distally (13).

DIAGNOSTIC ARTHROSCOPY

To perform an adequate diagnostic arthroscopy requires familiarity with the normal appearing structures and the ability to differentiate them from pathologic structures. The normal white smooth articular cartilage should be easily differentiated from the more yellow fibrocartilage. In addition, the surgeon should be able to identify and note cracked and fibrillated tissue as well as eburnated bone. Ligaments should have a white or yellow appearance and should be taught when probed especially under traction. Pathologic ligaments may become attenuated with fraying due to injury or degeneration. Inflammation may cause the synovium to become hypertrophic and reddish. A discolored or brown tinge to synovial fluid likely represents a pathologic problem. Joints should be congruous without step-offs, and ligaments should be tight without the ability to pass a probe from the radiocarpal joint (14).

Radiocarpal Evaluation

Diagnostic wrist arthroscopy begins with the 3-4 portal. This is the primary viewing portal. A spinal needle is inserted and the joint may be distended with 5 to 7 mL of saline (Fig. 40.10). The skin is incised and a small, blunt hemostat is used to spread the soft tissues (Fig. 40.11). Next, a blunt trocar should be inserted at approximately a 20° proximal angle to match the distal radius articular slope. This angle will help avoid damaging the dorsal articular surface (6, 11, 20). The inflow and outflow are interchangeable and can be maintained through the arthroscopic cannula or a separate 6-U portal established under direct arthroscopic visualization. We prefer the inflow through the arthroscope to push debris away instead of pulling it toward the camera. Once a 3-4 portal is established, a diagnostic radiocarpal arthroscopy is performed.

The radial styloid and radial capsule are examined first. The scaphoid superiorly and the radial styloid inferiorly can be evaluated for signs of arthritic change or articular injury (Fig. 40.12). The proximal border of the radial facet is then evaluated as are the volar extrinsic ligaments, the radioscaphocapitate ligament, and long radiolunate ligament (Fig. 40.13). The long radiolunate ligament is a wide structure usually two to three times the width of the radioscaphocapitate ligament (11, 14). They should be taut on probing because of the traction applied to the wrist. Ulnar to these is the radioscapholunate ligament, also called the ligament of Testut, which is a vascularized tuft of tissue without any significant structural integrity. This tuft marks the scapholunate interval and sagittal ridge (14, 21, 22). Blood vessels are frequently noted along this ligament, which has a natural redundancy that should not be mistaken for a tear.

Following the scaphoid ulnarly, the slightly concave-shaped scapholunate interosseous ligament can be examined for tears or scapholunate diastasis (Fig. 40.14). An intact ligament may not be immediately obvious because it mimics the appearance of cartilage. Complete injury to this ligament, however, will allow the arthroscope to pass between the scaphoid and the lunate (drive-through sign) (6).

Next, the proximal surface of the lunate and the distal surface of the radius can be evaluated. The two fossae of the distal radius, the scaphoid and the lunate fossae, are separated by a sagittal ridge. Fraying or fissuring of this area, suggestive of chondromalacia, should be documented. Normally, in the neutral wrist position, half of the lunate will articulate with the lunate facet and half will articulate with the TFCC (14).

The radial attachment of the TFCC is evaluated as is the volar and dorsal radioulnar ligaments. The lunotriquetral interosseous ligament is evaluated by identifying a sulcus or concavity in the otherwise convex articular surfaces of the lunate and triquetrum (23). A probe can be inserted through the 4-5 or 6-R portal to evaluate the integrity of the lunotriquetral ligament. Next, the peripheral attachment of the TFC and the ulnar prestyloid recess should be examined. The TFCC is "wedge-shaped" in the coronal plane with a thickened periphery and a thin radial attachment (22). A probe can be used to evaluate the tension of the TFCC by ballottement (the trampoline test) (21, 23) (Fig. 40.15). The triangular fibrocartilage is also known as the articular disc and should be taut. Lack of tension raises suspicion of a central or peripheral TFCC tear. The peripheral 15% to 20% of the TFCC is vascularized and therefore has healing potential if torn (6). The prestyloid ulnar recess is a normal anatomical finding approximately 3 to 4 mm wide and should not be mistaken for a peripheral tear (14). The ulnolunate and ulnotriquetral ligaments may be more easily evaluated by placing the arthroscope in the 4-5 or 6-R portals. These ligaments are identified as capsular thickenings in the volar aspect of the ulnar capsule.

Midcarpal Evaluation

Once a complete examination of the radiocarpal joint has been performed, the arthroscope can be used to evaluate the midcarpal space. The RMC portal, located approximately 1 cm distal to the 3-4 radiocarpal portal, is typically used to establish a diagnostic arthroscopy portal. The midcarpal joint can be distended with 3 to 5 mL fluid through any of the portals. This will allow easier access into the joint and minimize the risk of damaging the articular

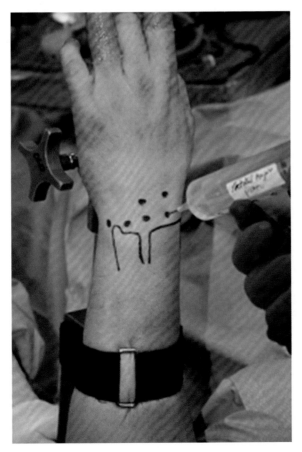

FIGURE 40.10. Injection of 3-4 portal.

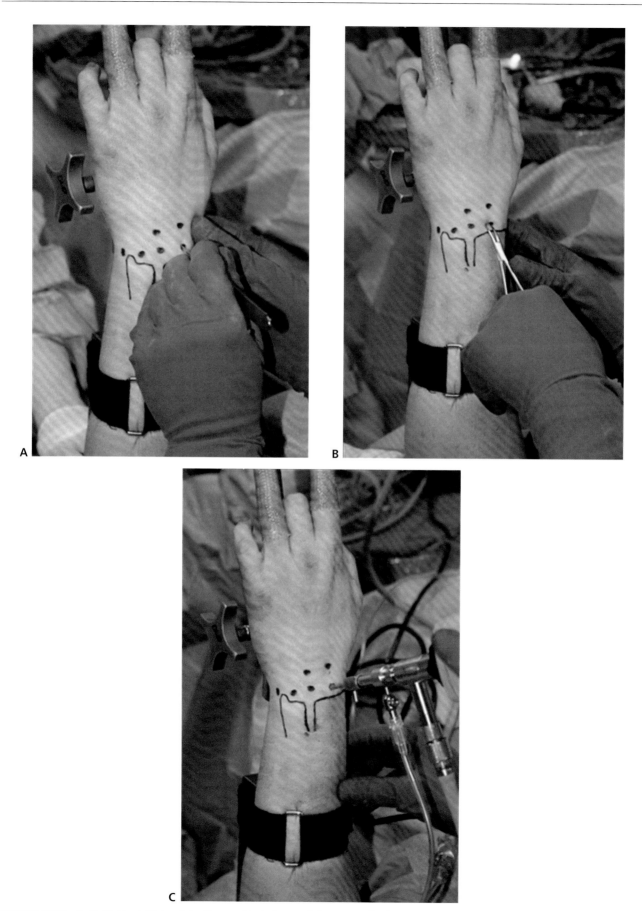

FIGURE 40.11. A–C: Making initial portal with spread technique and placement of arthroscope.

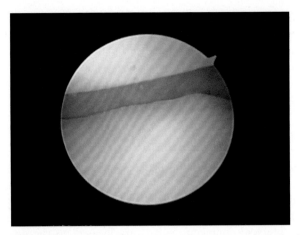

FIGURE 40.12. Radiocarpal joint viewing from the 3-4 portal. Scaphoid superiorly and distal radius inferiorly.

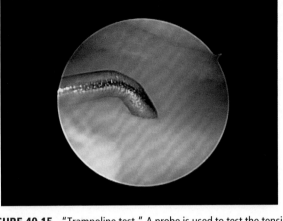

FIGURE 40.15. "Trampoline test." A probe is used to test the tension of the TFC.

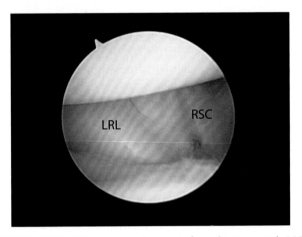

FIGURE 40.13. Volar extrinsic ligaments from the 3-4 portal. RSC, radioscaphocapitate ligament; LRL, long radiolunate ligament.

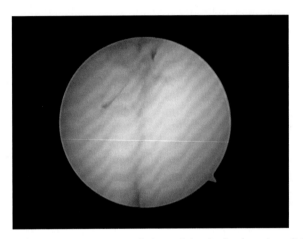

FIGURE 40.16. Congruent scapholunate joint viewing from the radial midcarpal (RMC) portal.

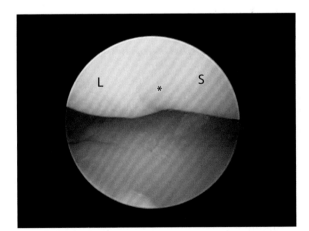

FIGURE 40.14. Convexity of the scapholunate interosseous ligament *(asterisk). S*, scaphoid; *L*, lunate.

cartilage (14). Normally, there is no communication between the radiocarpal and the midcarpal spaces. Care must be taken when entering the radial midcarpal space as it is less than half the depth of the radiocarpal space (6).

The UMC portal is created for instrumentation as well as visualization of the ulnar portion of the midcarpal joint. The arthroscopic evaluation in this area begins with visualization of the convexity of the capitate (superiorly) and the scapholunate joint (inferiorly). The scapholunate joint should be perfectly congruous (Fig. 40.16). The scapholunate ligament is not present on the distal edge of the scapholunate joint and therefore, the joint is best viewed from this perspective. Intraoperatively, the stability of the joint may be assessed by performing Watson's "scaphoid shift test (15, 24)."

The distal surface of the lunate and the triquetrum are then evaluated, as is the concave proximal surface of the hamate (Fig. 40.17). The lunotriquetral joint is also well visualized from this view and a ballottement test can be performed to assess stability. Within the distal row, the capitate and capitohamate articulation can also be examined from this portal. Further ulnarly, the triquetrohamate joint may be used to establish an accessory portal. The triquetrohamate joint is a saddle-shaped joint, which is

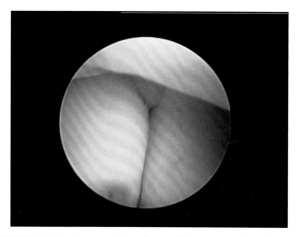

FIGURE 40.17. Congruent lunotriquetral joint viewing form the radial midcarpal (RMC) portal.

normally quite tight and difficult to view across unless pathologic laxity is present (24).

The scaphotrapeziotrapezoid joint can be seen by passing the arthroscope radially, and early osteoarthritic changes, common in this area, should be noted (25). In the STT joint, the trapezoid is in the foreground and the trapezium is in the background (Fig. 40.18). Bubbles frequently collect here and may impair visualization of the joint. These bubbles may be evacuated with a 21G needle, and debridement can be performed with a small motorized shaver through an accessory STT portal (24).

DRUJ Evaluation

Upon completion of the diagnostic midcarpal arthroscopy, a proximal distal radial ulnar joint portal can be established and the ulnar surface of the radius, the radial surface of the ulna, and the distal surface of the ulnar head, as well as the proximal surface of the TFCC can be evaluated. DRUJ arthroscopy is performed with the forearm in supination suspended in the wrist traction device but without any traction applied. A blunt trocar is angled slightly distal

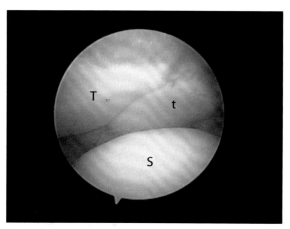

FIGURE 40.18. View from the RMC portal of the scaphotrapeziotrapezoid joint. S, scaphoid; T, trapezoid; t, trapezium.

and placed in the joint. If required, outflow can be created by placing an 18G needle into the distal portion of the joint. Through pronation and supination of the wrist, the articular margin of the ulna can be visualized. Evaluation is useful for lysis of adhesions, debridement, exostectomy, or capsulotomy of the DRUJ (4, 6).

COMPLICATIONS

Because of the absence of major neurovascular structures, most wrist arthroscopy utilizes the dorsum of the wrist. Only the deep branch of the radial artery and the superficial dorsal sensory branches of the radial, ulnar, and lateral antebrachial cutaneous nerves are located on the dorsal side of the wrist (10). Injury to these structures can cause numbness and at the worst extreme, a painful neuroma and complex regional pain syndrome. Certain portals have increased risk of iatrogenic neurovascular injury. The greatest risk to the radial artery and dorsal radial and ulnar sensory nerve branches occur with the 1-2, 6R, and 6U portals. The midcarpal, 3-4, 4-5, and DRUJ portals are relatively safe. Risk does exists even in safe portals because aberrant sensory nerve branches can be dangerously close (13).

In general, complications during and after wrist arthroscopy are quite rare. Most authors report rates less than 2% (3, 12). The most common complication was dorsal ulnar sensory neuropraxia and was associated with open procedures (26). Complications can be the result of traction and arm positioning or related to establishment of portals. They can also be procedure-specific complications or general arthroscopic complications. Major complications include compartment syndrome, permanent nerve injury, postsurgical joint infection, vascular injury, complex regional pain syndrome, permanent stiffness, and tendon rupture (26).

Most of these complications can be prevented with a prior knowledge of the risks and simple precautions used when performing the surgery. Large instrumentation within a small joint space predisposes iatrogenic injuries to nerves, the radial artery, and extensor tendons. The EPL and EDQ are the tendons most at risk during wrist arthroscopy. Flexible nylon finger traps help prevent skin damage for patients with friable skin (3). Using a spinal needle ensures adequate pathway. Incisions should be longitudinal and made by pulling only the skin over a blade and bluntly spreading through the subcutaneous tissue. When piercing the capsule, only a blunt trochar should be used to minimize risk to the articular surfaces.

Excessive extravasation of fluid may occur in recently injured patients with torn capsules or if the inflow cannula is placed extra-articularly. If extravasation does occurs, the causative factor should be addressed or the arthroscopic portion should be stopped. Pressure diminishes quickly when the inflow is halted and elevating the extremity is usually all that is necessary for correction. Physiologic solutions allow better fluid absorption in the soft tissues and further decreases risk with extravasation (11). Whipple reports the risk of compartment syndromes is minimal to none because even in the case of intra-articular fractures, extravasated fluid is rapidly absorbed by clysis and does not increase compartment pressures long enough to compromise circulation. Caution is advised if pressure pumps are used (27).

Postoperative infection is extremely uncommon. With any evidence of superficial infection, oral antibiotics are usually sufficient. If a deep intra-articular infection develops, irrigation, arthroscopic debridement, and intravenous antibiotic therapy are usually required.

CONTROVERSIES

Dry Wrist Arthroscopy

A new technique that utilizes wrist arthroscopy without irrigation has some been tried in some instances. Proponents claim that there is a theoretical benefit to arthroscopy without water. Suggested benefits include limiting loss of vision and compartment syndrome. Another possible advantage includes the ability to do open procedures without soft-tissue infiltration of the tissue. The authors also suggest the possibility of less pain and swelling after surgery (28). No prospective studies have evaluated these reported benefits and this technique is still in its early stages.

PEARLS AND PITFALLS

1. Skin.
   a. Use only soft finger traps. If poor skin quality, minimize traction and limit duration of procedure.
2. Neurovascular structures.
   a. Draw portals and landmarks AFTER applying traction to the wrist as anatomic structures may change.
   b. Incise only the dermis by pulling the skin against a scalpel.
   c. Bluntly spread before cannula placement.
   d. Use care with all portals but use extreme caution with high-risk portals.
   e. Place the 1-2 portal in the most dorsal portion of the snuffbox to protect the radial artery.
3. Protect the articular surfaces.
   a. Know the precise portal location and anatomy.
   b. Localize the joint space with a spinal needle before establishing a portal.
   c. Insert with the angle of radial inclination and volar tilt.
   d. Use only blunt instruments and cannulas.
4. See what you are doing.
   a. Use volar and dorsal portals to see the area required.
   b. Maintain a clear visual field.
   c. Prevent or remove bubbles.
   d. Place inflow on camera to push debris away from scope.
   e. Have assistant maintain fluid flow with finger pressure pump.

5. Probe articular surfaces, ligaments, and the TFCC for tears and pathology.
6. Evaluate the midcarpal joint space.
7. Prevent fluid extravasation. Use adequate outflow. Use gravity inflow if possible.

POSTOPERATIVE TREATMENT AND REHABILITATION

For debridement and resection procedures, a compressive wrap is used in the postoperative phase. Range of motion is started immediately and exercises are initiated 1 week postoperative. If necessary, formal physical therapy is started 3 to 4 weeks postoperatively. Normal use is allowed as pain and strength dictate.

In repair procedures, we favor the use of a müenster cast for approximately 6 weeks. The wrist is placed in slight dorsiflexion and neutral pronation/supination. This cast prevents pronation/supination of the forearm. Approximately 4 weeks post-op, a removable müenster splint is used and gentle range of motion is initiated. The splint is discontinued and exercises begin 6 to 8 weeks postoperative. Full recovery takes 3 to 9 months.

CONCLUSIONS

Arthroscopy of the wrist has become a common technique for the evaluation and treatment of intra-articular wrist disorders. It provides excellent visualization under bright, magnified conditions with less morbidity than arthrotomy (11). Although once used as a tool for diagnosis only this is no longer the case. As technology advances, our ability to master new and advanced procedures will continue to improve. Although simple to learn and relatively easy to master, it requires a thorough understanding of principles and anatomy to perform successfully. With adherence to standard precautions, wrist arthroscopy will continue to prove increasingly beneficial in the management of disorders of the wrist.

REFERENCES

1. Chen YC. Arthroscopy of the wrist and finger joints. *Orthop Clin North Am.* 1979;10:723–733.
2. Whipple TL, Marotta JJ, Powell JH III. Techniques of wrist arthroscopy. *Arthroscopy.* 1986;2:244–252.
3. Bain GI, Munt J, Turner PC. New advances in wrist arthroscopy. *Arthroscopy.* 2008;24:355–367.
4. Whipple TL, Cooney WP III, Osterman AL, et al. Wrist arthroscopy. *Instr Course Lect.* 1995;44:139–145.
5. Watson HK, Ashmead D IV, Makhlouf MV. Examination of the scaphoid. *J Hand Surg Am.* 1988;13:657–660.
6. Geissler W. *Wrist Arthroscopy.* New York, NY: Springer; 2005:xiv, 201.
7. Nagle DJ. Evaluation of chronic wrist pain. *J Am Acad Orthop Surg.* 2000;8:45–55.
8. Maizlin ZV, Brown JA, Clement JJ, et al. MR arthrography of the wrist: controversies and concepts. *Hand (N Y).* 2009;4:66–73.

III. The Wrist

9. Trumble TE, Budoff JE. *Wrist and Elbow Reconstruction and Arthorscopy*. Rosemont, IL: Publisher is American Society for Surgery of the Hand. 2006.

10. Gupta R, Bozentka DJ, Osterman AL. Wrist arthroscopy: principles and clinical applications. *J Am Acad Orthop Surg*. 2001;9:200–209.

11. Geissler WB, Freeland AE, Weiss AP, et al. Techniques of wrist arthroscopy. *Instr Course Lect*. 2000;49:225–237.

12. Haisman JM, Matthew B, Scott W. Wrist arthroscopy: standard portals and arthroscopic anatomy. *J Am Soc Surg Hand*. 2005;5:175–181.

13. Abrams RA, Petersen M, Botte MJ. Arthroscopic portals of the wrist: an anatomic study. *J Hand Surg Am*. 1994;19:940–944.

14. Bettinger PC, Cooney WP III, Berger RA. Arthroscopic anatomy of the wrist. *Orthop Clin North Am*. 1995;26:707–719.

15. Hofmeister EP, Dao KD, Glowacki KA, et al. The role of midcarpal arthroscopy in the diagnosis of disorders of the wrist. *J Hand Surg Am*. 2001;26:407–414.

16. Carro LP, Golano P, Farinas O, et al. The radial portal for scaphotrapeziotrapezoid arthroscopy. *Arthroscopy*. 2003;19:547–553.

17. Abe Y, Doi K, Hattori Y, et al. A benefit of the volar approach for wrist arthroscopy. *Arthroscopy*. 2003;19:440–445.

18. Slutsky DJ. Wrist arthroscopy through a volar radial portal. *Arthroscopy*. 2002;18:624–630.

19. Slutsky DJ, Nagle DJ. Wrist arthroscopy: current concepts. *J Hand Surg Am*. 2008;33:1228–1244.

20. Roth JH. Radiocarpal arthroscopy. *Orthopedics*. 1988;11:1309–1312.

21. North ER, Thomas S. An anatomic guide for arthroscopic visualization of the wrist capsular ligaments. *J Hand Surg Am*. 1988;13:815–822.

22. Roth JH, Poehling GG, Whipple TL. Arthroscopic surgery of the wrist. *Instr Course Lect*. 1988;37:183–194.

23. Berger RA. Arthroscopic anatomy of the wrist and distal radioulnar joint. *Hand Clin*. 1999;15:393–413, vii.

24. Viegas SF. Midcarpal arthroscopy: anatomy and portals. *Hand Clin*. 1994;10:577–587.

25. Viegas SF. Advances in the skeletal anatomy of the wrist. *Hand Clin*. 2001;17:1–11, v.

26. Beredjiklian PK, Bozentka DJ, Leung YL, et al. Complications of wrist arthroscopy. *J Hand Surg Am*. 2004;29:406–411.

27. Whipple TL. Precautions for arthroscopy of the wrist. *Arthroscopy*. 1990;6:3–4.

28. del Piñal F, Garcia-Bernal FJ, Pisani D, et al. Dry arthroscopy of the wrist: surgical technique. *J Hand Surg Am*. 2007;32:119–123.

Arthroscopic Treatment of Dorsal and Volar Ganglions

Scott G. Edwards • Evan Argintar

DORSAL WRIST GANGLION CYSTS

Introduction

Arthroscopic wrist ganglion resection offers several theoretical advantages over open techniques, including improved recovery, better joint visualization, lower complication and recurrence rates, and more satisfying cosmetic results. Initial outcomes of dorsal wrist ganglia resected arthroscopically have been favorable (1–3). Although arthroscopic resection of dorsal wrist ganglion cysts is a procedure that is becoming more accepted, several questions still remain unanswered. Based on a critical review of the sparse literature on the subject and on clinical observations, this chapter attempts to clarify the ambiguity surrounding arthroscopic dorsal wrist ganglion resection and determine whether this is a useful technique to add to the arsenal or a triumph of technology over reason.

Anatomy and Pathoanatomy

Intra-articular Cystic Stalks

Cystic stalks, which may appear to be pedunculated or sessile protuberances, may be viewed in the radiocarpal joint at the interval between the dorsal scapholunate ligament and the capsule inflection that separates the radiocarpal and midcarpal joints (Fig. 41.1). In reviewing the current literature, the exact roles of intra-articular cystic stalks are somewhat ambiguous. According to previous reports, although not specifically stated, it has been implied that the identification and surgical excision of the stalk is paramount when using standard arthroscopic technique for ganglion excision. However, the presence of this important structure has been variable in the literature. Osterman and Raphael (1) identified a stalk in two-thirds of their patients undergoing arthroscopic ganglion excision. Despite the fact that one-third of their patients had no identifiable stalk, ganglions were successfully excised with no recurrences. Other studies have reported a stalk incidence as low as 10% (2–4). Despite vastly different reports on stalk identification, the importance of such pathology must be questioned. Rather than a cystic

stalk, Edwards and Johansen (4) described intra-articular cystic material and redundant capsular tissue in the vast majority of their patients with ganglion cysts (Fig. 41.2). This finding, which was more consistently evident, was the focus of their resection, rather than the stalk.

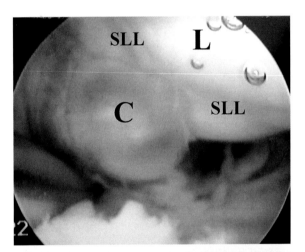

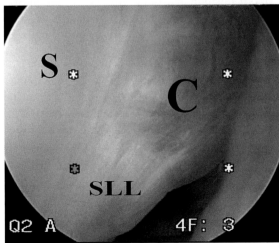

FIGURE 41.1. Intra-articular cystic stalk as viewed from the radiocarpal joint compartment. Cysts may be **(A)** pedunculated or **(B)** sessile in appearance. C, cyst; S, scaphoid; L, lunate; SLL, scapholunate ligament.

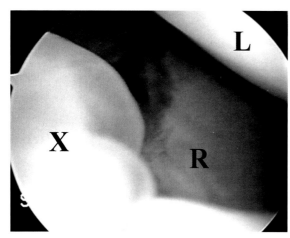

FIGURE 41.2. Diffuse cystic material and redundant capsule often occur more commonly than a discreet cystic stalk. X, cystic material and redundant capsule; R, radius; L, lunate.

The intra-articular limitations of arthroscopic viewing may explain the paucity of stalk identification. The radiocarpal and midcarpal joints are separated by the extrinsic capsular ligaments. At this separation, the dorsal capsular reflection is adherent to the interosseous scapholunate ligament. It is possible that a ganglion stalk travels toward the scapholunate ligament within the substance of the dorsal capsular reflection, rather than through the radiocarpal or midcarpal spaces, and the stalk may never be visualized by arthroscopy. Certain observations during arthroscopic resections may support this theory. On several occasions, extravasations of cystic fluid can be noted during the debridement of the dorsal capsular reflection between the radiocarpal and the midcarpal joints when stalks had not been visualized in either compartment. In other words, the stalk may have been hidden within the dorsal capsular extrinsic ligaments.

Intra-articular Associations

The dorsal ganglion may be an overt sign of intra-articular pathology. Povlsen and Puckett (5) found intra-articular abnormalities in 75% of patients with painful ganglia. They concluded that, like popliteal cysts in the knee, the dorsal ganglion was a marker of joint abnormality. Osterman and Raphael (1) found abnormalities in 42% predominated by findings at the scapholunate ligament (24%), triangular fibrocartilage (8%), lunatotriquetral ligament (3%), and significant chondromalacia. Despite only the ganglion being treated, wrist pain resolved in all cases. Edwards and Johansen (4) elaborated on this notion by showing that most ganglia are associated with type II and III scapholunate and type III lunatotriquetral laxities, as determined by the Geissler grading system (Table 41.1). Although it is reasonable to propose that increased intercarpal laxity may contribute to ganglion formation, the actual significance is unclear given that the natural incidence of these ligamentous laxities in the general population is not known. Cadaveric studies have suggested that type II and III laxities are actually within normal physiologic ranges (7).

Table 41.1.

Arthroscopic classification of interosseous ligament tears (6)

Grade	Description
1	Attenuation and/or hemorrhage of interosseous ligament as observed from the radiocarpal joint. No incongruence of carpal alignment in midcarpal space
2	Attenuation and/or hemorrhage of interosseous ligament as observed from the radiocarpal joint. Incongruence and/or step-off as observed from midcarpal space. A slight gap (less than the width of a 2-mm probe) between carpals may be present
3	Incongruence and/or step-off of carpal alignment are observed in both the radiocarpal and the midcarpal space. The width of a 2-mm probe may be passed through gap between carpals
4	Incongruence and/or step-off of carpal alignment are observed in both the radiocarpal and the midcarpal space. Gross instability with manipulation is noted. A 2.7-mm arthroscope may be passed through the gap between carpals

Clinical Evaluation

History and Physical Examination

The first question to answer when a patient presents with a mass is whether it is a cyst or a tumor. Many elements of the history and physical are not conclusive. Occurrence, progression, size, shape, texture, the presence or absence of pain, and association with traumatic or repetitive activities provide little more than suggestions either way. One element of history, however, can be quite helpful in determining whether the lesion is cystic. Both cysts and tumors get larger, but only cysts get smaller. There are rare exceptions to this rule, such as some vascular tumors that involute over a period of months to years. Cysts, on the other hand, may decrease in size as quickly as overnight. On physical exam, transillumination can be helpful in differentiating a cyst from a tumor. This is performed by holding a penlight up against the lesion. A cystic lesion will allow the light to transmit through its fluid medium. The solid tissue of a tumor, however, will prevent any propagation of light.

Occasionally, cysts may herald a more dubious underlying pathology, such as a scapholunate ligament injury. The history and physical should focus on any recent or remote trauma. Oftentimes, patients may have incompetent scapholunate ligaments that remain clinically unapparent until the manifestation of an associated ganglion cyst. Palpation of the dorsal portion of the scapholunate ligament, a positive Watson scaphoid shift test, or positive straight finger resistance test may be suggestive of scapholunate ligament pathology. Cysts may resemble other pathologies such as gouty tophus, tenosynovitis, and rheumatoid pannus. A careful history and physical should be able to differentiate these conditions.

Diagnostic Imaging

MRI and ultrasound remain the most commonly used imagery to differentiate fluid-filled cysts from solid tumors. Although both differentiate with equal reliability, MRI may suggest an etiology of a solid tumor, whereas ultrasound cannot. Even given this difference, there has been more of a shift toward using ultrasound as the preferred technique given its lesser comparable cost. Very small ganglions, though clinically significant, may be readily overlooked by both ultrasound and MRI. Surgeons should keep a high index of suspicion for these lesions despite a negative reading.

Treatment Options

Nonoperative Treatments

Although there is no consensus about the best nonoperative treatment for ganglion cysts, restriction of wrist activity seems to be well accepted. The efficacy of anti-inflammatory medications is more controversial. Some believe that reducing inflammation help painful cysts, whereas others believe that the medications may make the cystic fluid less viscous and possibly more likely to spontaneously decompress. Neither belief has been substantiated in the literature. Needle aspiration seems to be relatively safe for dorsal ganglion cysts, but volar ganglions place neurovascular structures at particular risk with blind aspiration. Patients need to understand that recurrences after aspiration can be high. In summary, nonoperative treatments for dorsal ganglion cysts are unpredictable and the evidence to support such measures is largely anecdotal. Most surgeons, however, will attempt a trial of nonoperative treatment for some duration before committing the patient to surgical excision.

Surgical Indications and Contraindications

Indications and contraindications for arthroscopic dorsal wrist ganglion resection are still evolving. Ho et al. (2) reported two recurrences following resection of ganglia originating from the midcarpal joint. They concluded that arthroscopic resection was not indicated for cysts originating from the midcarpal joint. Many would agree that most dorsal wrist ganglia originate from the scapholunate interval. Given the capsular limitation in the wrist, however, this interval is only partially visualized from the radiocarpal joint. One study (4) observed that cysts communicated with the midcarpal joint in 75% of cases. In the same report, 25% of cysts were accessed exclusively through the midcarpal joint, which suggests that evaluation of the midcarpal

joint is not only indicated, but also mandatory for successful resection. Although most cysts may be resected successfully through an isolated radiocarpal portal, some cysts may need supplemental debridement from the midcarpal joint.

Regarding recurrent cysts, one group of investigators has suggested that recurrent cysts following previous open surgical excision should be considered a contraindication for arthroscopic resection (8). Appropriate concerns are the risk of extensor tendon injury due to their potential displacement by the scar from the previous surgery. Thus, most previous studies have used recurrence as an exclusion criterion. One significant exception was a series in which 15% of the patients included recurrent ganglia (4). Patients with recurrent cysts had comparable outcomes with primary cyst resections. Therefore, the authors believe that arthroscopic resection of recurrent cysts is not contraindicated. In fact, arthroscopic resection may be helpful in identifying a potential cause of the recurrence. Previous studies have identified intra-articular abnormalities such as ligament tears, excessive intercarpal laxities, chondromalacia, and triangular fibrocartilage tears as being associated with ganglion cysts (1, 4). It is unclear whether these findings contribute to cystic development, but to the degree they have a role, arthroscopy is more effective at identifying and addressing these abnormalities compared with open excision. Given a recurrent cyst, an arthroscopic evaluation may identify a partial scapholunate ligament tear, which could be debrided, thus lowering the probability of further recurrence. An open technique may not identify the cause as easily and thus doom the recurrent excision to another recurrence.

Cosmetic reasons sometime drive decisions to pursue any endoscopic technique. Although an open incision across the dorsum of the wrist may not seem excessive to a surgeon, the patient may have another perspective. One study reported a very high postoperative satisfaction rate despite having 17% of patients be asymptomatic preoperatively and only opting for surgery for cosmetic reasons (4). There is no similar report for open resections. This implies that it would be reasonable to offer arthroscopic ganglion resections for patients primarily interested in the cosmetic appearance of their hands.

Surgical Technique for Arthroscopic Resection of Dorsal Wrist Ganglions

A tourniquet was placed on every patient as a precaution, and inflated in the event that intra-articular bleeding obscured visualization. While suspending the patient's arm in a traction tower with 5 to 10 lb of traction applied, a 6R or 6U portal is created as a visualization portal. The more radial 3-4 or 4-5 portals are avoided at this time to prevent inadvertently decompressing the cyst (Fig. 41.3). Once the 2.7-mm arthroscopic camera is directed toward the dorsal compartment of the wrist, the capsule adjacent to the scapholunate ligament is visualized. Occasionally, either a sessile or pedunculated protrusion into the joint

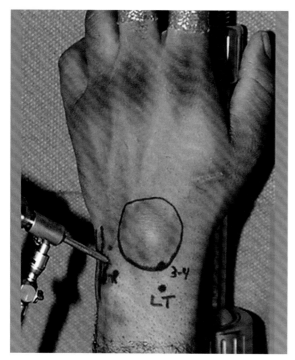

FIGURE 41.3. The arthroscopic setup for ganglion resection. Note that the 3-4 arthroscopic portal is modified slightly to avoid penetrating the cyst directly.

can be seen in the area where the extrinsic capsule joins the distal portion of the dorsal scapholunate ligament. This capsular reflection serves as part of the barrier between the radiocarpal and the midcarpal joints, and the protrusion located here has been termed the cystic stalk (Fig. 41.1). More often, however, one may be impressed with the amount of synovitis and redundant capsule in this area instead of an actual cystic stalk (Fig. 41.2).

A common technique for arthroscopic ganglionectomy is to place the shaver through the cystic sac, since it often resides directly over the usual 3-4 portal. This action will consequently decompress the cyst and may obscure any presence of an intra-articular stalk. Some feel that this is of some therapeutic benefit while critics of the procedure will argue that arthroscopic excisions are nothing more than "glorified aspirations." The authors recommend a method that attempts to avoid decompressing the cyst with the shaver prior to actual excision in order to observe the possibility of an undisturbed cystic stalk and its path elsewhere outside the radiocarpal joint. The working portal is created adjacent to the immediate area of the cyst, rather than directly over the 3-4 portal. Consequently, this "modified" working portal is usually just distal and sometimes slightly radial to the actual 3-4 portal. A 2.9-mm full-radius shaver is introduced through this "modified" portal with every attempt not to decompress the cyst with simple introduction of the shaver. If the cyst were decompressed too soon, the surgeon would not be able to confirm by palpation whether the cyst was adequately resected or simply decompressed with a "glorified aspiration."

Although the procedure implies that the cyst is removed by the arthroscope, this is often not the case. In actuality, the arthroscopy procedure disrupts the communication between the cyst and the joint, leaving a deflated sac behind that cannot reinflate. Eventually, the empty sac is resorbed. Recurrences would only happen if another cyst were generated.

The focus of the resection begins at the site of ganglion stalk or redundant capsular material, if identified. Cystic stalk seems to be present variably, and their presence appears to have no effect on the outcomes of the resection. Redundant capsular material has been described and reported to serve as a more reliable landmark for resection. This billowing, redundant material appears different from typical reactive synovitis. Although its exact significance is unclear, it seems to be continuous with the capsule that lies adjacent to the cyst. With this landmark, surgeons may confidently begin their capsulotomy. If neither is identified, the debridement begins adjacent to the dorsal scapholunate ligament and distal capsular reflection. Commonly, the cyst travels within the capsular reflection as it communicates with the scapholunate joint. Care should be taken to keep the blade of the shaver away from the scapholunate ligament at all times. Upon initial debridement of the capsular reflection, occasionally a flash of viscous cystic fluid may be visualized escaping into the joint.

The debridement continues until approximately 1 cm of capsule has been removed. It is important to be constantly aware of what the shaver is actually cutting. Since it takes some pressure to cut into the extrinsic ligaments of the wrist, which is necessary for a complete capsulotomy, that same pressure may easily cut inadvertently into an extensor tendon lying on the other side of the capsule. Even the most experienced arthroscopists should stop frequently and reassess the terrain.

A common mistake is to make the capsulotomy too small, which is quite easy to do under magnification. Using the 2.9-mm shaver as a reference is helpful in gauging the size of the capsulotomy. Another common mistake is to create an incomplete capsulotomy, which fails to communicate with the extra-articular space. The authors advise direct visualization of the extensor tendons to verify that complete capsulotomy has been performed (Fig. 41.4). Removing the cystic sac is not necessary since it often resorbs over time once detached from its origin at the joint. If the cyst is particularly large, resorption may take some time and patients may complain about the residual prominence on the dorsum of the hand. Removal of the truncated sac may be performed by pulling it out of the 3-4 portal with a hemostat. Because this is a blind maneuver and the risk of neuroma formation is relatively high, the authors believe that if removal of the cystic sac is elected, it should be done from inside the joint arthroscopically, provided the surgeon is comfortable with the technique. Careful extensor tenosynovectomy may be performed at the same time with the shaver, if desired. When performing this,

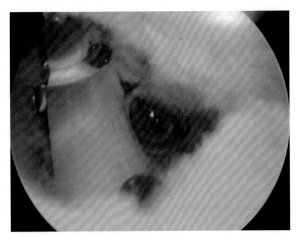

FIGURE 41.4. Radiocarpal joint after capsulotomy. Viewing the extensor tendons confirmed complete capsulotomy and communication with the extra-articular space.

however, shaver suction should be paused to reduce the chances of inadvertently pulling the tendon into the blade of the shaver.

Once the capsulotomy and cyst excision have been completed from the radiocarpal joint, the camera is removed and the dorsal wrist is palpated to determine the efficacy of the debridement. If a portion of the cyst remains, there is some degree of communication between the cyst and the midcarpal joint that has not yet been addressed. To remedy this, the arthroscopic camera is introduced through an ulnar midcarpal portal and a similar capsulotomy is performed adjacent to the scapholunate interval through the radial midcarpal portal. During debridement from the midcarpal joint, often a fenestration is created between the midcarpal and the radiocarpal joints through the capsular reflection. Upon removing the arthroscopic equipment, the wrist is palpated again to ensure that the cyst has been completely excised. This may be difficult especially given the possibility of fluid extravasation, substantial amounts of adipose tissue obscuring the cyst, or having a very small cyst prior to resection.

Some surgeons close each arthroscopic portal with one simple nonabsorbable suture, but other surgeons leave them open with no cosmetic detriment. Open arthroscopic wounds can rarely form sinus tracts reported in other joints, so the authors prefer to close their wounds. A sterile wrist dressing is used in all. Some authors recommend postoperative splinting for 1 week, whereas others believe splinting is unnecessary.

Recurrences and Complications

Recurrence rates have been low in virtually every report (0% to 10%) (1–3), which would imply that the recurrence rate for arthroscopic resection may be less than that for open excision, which have typically showed slightly higher recurrence rates. However, most previously reported studies had small cohort sizes, selection bias, and poorly defined follow-up, all of which could potentially distort the actual recurrence rates. In four separate studies (3, 4, 9, 10) with a combined cohort of 233 patients undergoing arthroscopic ganglion resection with an average follow-up of 2 years, only seven recurrences were reported. One prospective series (10) comparing arthroscopic with open resection found no statistical differences between recurrence rates, 10.7% arthroscopic versus 8.7% open. Based on a critical review of the relevant literature, recurrence rates between open and arthroscopic techniques are similar and should not be the sole determining factor in selecting either technique.

Complications for open ganglion resections have been reported and include neuroma formation and scapholunate ligament laceration. Similar complications for arthroscopic resections have not been reported. Although arthroscopy may prove to be a safer method of excision, there may be other reasons to explain the discrepancy in the literature. First, there are more overall reports on open ganglion resections and, consequently, will have more complications reported from a statistical standpoint. Second, much of the literature on open ganglion resections is older. The more recent studies do not report on the same variety and extent of complications. We may surmise with some degree of reasonability that recent techniques have improved, making these previously reported complications not as prevalent.

Reactive tenosynovitis may occur after any arthroscopy although not commonly. Reports of this complication following any wrist arthroscopy techniques are rare. One study evaluating the complications of wrist arthroscopy not limited to ganglionectomy reviewed 210 cases and found "extensor tendon irritation" in only four cases (11). There has been only one report of extensor tenosynovitis following arthroscopic ganglion resection, and in this series it occurred in 6% of patients. The authors contributed the discrepancy to the extensive capsulotomy required during ganglion excision that does not occur during other arthroscopic procedures. In any case, the risk of extensor synovitis should be part of the preoperative discussion with patients.

VOLAR WRIST GANGLION CYSTS

Introduction

The volar wrist ganglion is the second most common mass in the wrist (20%) (12). As with dorsal cysts, arthroscopic volar wrist ganglion resection offers the theoretical advantages previously discussed, including improved recovery, better joint visualization, better joint visualization, lower complication and recurrence rates, and more satisfying cosmetic results. Reports on outcomes are more limited compared with the literature available for dorsal arthroscopic ganglion cyst resection. Arthroscopic volar ganglion cyst resection, in certain situations, appears to be similarly favorable, also conferring a greater degree of protection from complications that are present with open volar surgery. This chapter attempts to define the indications and contraindications, clarify surgical technique, and describe and, more importantly, navigate how to avoid complications found with arthroscopic volar wrist ganglion resection.

Anatomy and Pathoanatomy

As with dorsal cysts, volar ganglions arise from mucinous degeneration of the capsular and ligamentous structures around the radiocarpal joint. Visible most commonly at the level of the volar wrist crease on the radial side of the palmaris longus tendon, most volar ganglion cysts arise from the radiocarpal joint (35% to 80%) (12, 13). Here, intra-articular inspection often reveals a capsular defect between the radioscaphocapitate (RSC) and the long radiolunate ligament (LRL) intervals (12) (Fig. 41.5). Uncommonly, volar cysts may arise from the midcarpal joint (10% to 25%) (14). Regardless of joint, tumefaction, by means of long stalks, may place the visible ganglion mass in approximation to its articular origination. The superficial radial nerve and artery found volar to these cysts makes open approached particularly challenging. As a result, common complications from open resections include hematoma, digital cold sensitivity, paresthesias, and painful neuroma formation.

Treatment Options

Traditional conservative treatment of volar ganglion cysts by means of puncture, aspiration, and/or steroid injection has shown to have high reoccurrence rates. Although these treatments avoid the risks inherent with operative inventions, often, persistent pain, anxiety regarding mass identity, and/or cosmetic concern lead to surgical treatment.

Before the advent of arthroscopy, open excision was considered the standard of care for operative treatment of volar ganglion cysts. Retrospective review clearly has

shown that open surgical excision carries risks not present with dorsal cyst removal. Jacobs et al. (14) reviewed 71 open volar cyst excisions and found a reoccurrence rate of 28%, occurring on an average, 4 months postoperatively. Furthermore, the palmar cutaneous branch of the median nerve was damaged 28% of the time. Gündeş et al. (15) retrospectively evaluated 16 volar cysts treated with open excision and found a complication rate of 56%. Of this group, two patients sustained neuropraxia injuries to the palmar cutaneous branch of the median nerve, and two patients sustained lacerations to branches of the radial artery. Other complications cited included decreased wrist motion greater than 20° compared with the contralateral side and persistent wrist pain. The reoccurrence rate was 31%, and of those that underwent revision open excision, all volar cysts were found to originate from the scaphotrapezium (ST) joint. Certainly, given these complications, a less invasive method would be a welcomed alternative.

Arthroscopic decompression of radiocarpal volar ganglion cysts been shown to be safer and more successful compared with open procedures. Ho et al. (16) first achieved arthroscopic success with no complications or reoccurrences in his five patient series. Mathoulin et al. (9) reviewed 32 patients who underwent arthroscopic decompression at an average 13 months after needle aspiration. With average follow-up at 26 months, all patients had normal mobility, were pain free, without any complications. One patient was reported to have developed a moderate hematoma that spontaneously resolved at 3 days. Rocchi et al. (17) found 1 reoccurrence in 17 volar ganglion cysts treated with arthroscopic decompression. The remaining 16 (94%) had normal motion, without persistent pain or complication development (14). In the only prospective randomized trial conducted to date, Rocchi et al. (17) compared open excision with arthroscopic decompression of volar ganglion cysts. The 20 radiocarpal volar ganglion cysts treated by open surgical incision collectively sustained four injuries to a branch of the radial artery, two cases of a stiff wrist associated with a painful scar, one case of neuropraxia, and one reoccurrence. Arthroscopically treated cysts developed one case of neuropraxia and one injury to branch of the radial artery. All other patients treated had no visible mass, full range of active wrist motion, full grip strength, asymptomatic, with a cosmetically appealing scar. Furthermore, mean functional recovery time following open volar ganglion resection was 9 days longer and mean time lost from work was 13 days longer compared with volar ganglion cysts treated with arthroscopic decompression (9).

The success seen with radiocarpal volar ganglion cysts, unfortunately, has not been matched with similar treatment of cysts originating from the Scapho-trapezio-trapezoid (STT) joint. Of six patients treated, Ho et al. (16) converted one case to an open procedure when faced with his lone STT-originating volar ganglion cyst. Of the four STT volar ganglion cysts treated by Rocchi et al. (17) in his initial study, three were considered failures, with

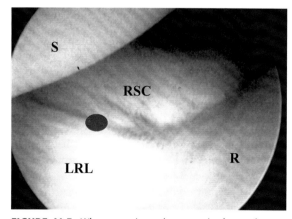

FIGURE 41.5. When resecting volar cysts, the focus of attention for performing a capsulotomy should be between the RSC and the LRL ligaments (note *red mark*). RSC, radioscaphocapitate ligament; LRL, long radiolunate ligament; S, scaphoid; R, radius.

the development of one injury to a branch of the radial artery and one neuropraxia to the radial nerve. Of these two complications, the arterial injury, along with an additional case, was, respectively, converted to open procedures due to hemostasis control and poor visibility (13). Lastly, in Rocchi's (17) more recent prospective review, his only three recurrences from the group treated arthroscopically all originated from the STT joint. For these reasons, it would seem that STT volar ganglion cysts should be treated by open excision, with specific care to avoid injury to the radial nerve and artery. The problem is that sometimes it is difficult to know preoperatively whether a volar cyst is arising from the radiocarpal or STT joint.

Surgical Technique for Arthroscopic Resection of Volar Ganglion Cysts

Radiocarpal ganglion cysts

A supine patient should be placed in wrist traction of 5 lb with any standard wrist arthroscopy tower. General and/or local anesthesia should be selected, with a sterile tourniquet application, but not inflated. This allows for both intraoperative radial pulse palpation and avoidance of muscle ache associated with prolonged tourniquet time (16). General, regional, and/or local anesthesia may be utilized. Portal sites are identified and marked, and local anesthetic may be injected into the subcutaneous tissues.

In planning which arthroscopic portal to utilize, the 3-4 dorsal portal typically allows direct access to the volar radial capsule. As previously mentioned, volar ganglion cysts commonly can be localized between the RSC and the LRL intervals (Fig. 41.5). The 3-4 portal also is optimal for instrumentation (4). Additional 4-5 or 1-2 portals should be utilized for visualization once instrumentation has begun through the initial portal site. Ho et al. (16) reported improved visualization through the 1-2 portal; however, he found this location was associated with a higher complication rate. Alternatively, the arthroscope may remain in the 3-4 portal, with instrumentation placed through the 1-2 portal (13).

The radiocarpal joint should initially be distended with 2 to 5 mL of normal saline. Portal sites should be incised by sharp skin incision followed by blunt hemostat dissection and arthrotomy. This maneuver is particularly important for the 1-2 portal in order to protect radial artery and nerve (16). A 2.7-mm 30° arthroscope should be inserted into the 3-4 portal, with standard radiocarpal and midcarpal articular exploration and evaluation. The 6U portal or needle arthrotomy may be utilized for outflow.

After inspection, the volar cyst stalk should be localized and decompressed. Location confirmation can be confirmed by external manual palpation, which may reveal capsular bulging (15, 16). With difficulty in cyst localization, alternatively, the midcarpal joint must be suspected as the source for the ganglion.

A 2.0- to 2.9-mm arthroscopic shaver should next be inserted intra-articularly into the surgeon's preferred portal. The shaver is focused at the interval between the radioscaphocapitate ligaments and long radiolunate ligaments. Successful resection can be confirmed with a sudden gush of mucinous material into the radiocarpal joint. Visualizing a sudden gush is not necessary for successful resection, but the cyst should no longer be palpable. If it is, consider evaluating the midcarpal joint and/or the STT joint and proceeding with a capsulotomy in a similar manner. The tendon synovitis and ganglion may be resected once decompression is complete. Upon completion of capsulotomy, the flexor tendons may be visible in the operative field. The radial artery may be routinely palpated to confirm avoidance of iatrogenic injury (16), provided the tourniquet is not inflated. Excessive anterior debridement must be avoided in an effort to protect the important volar neurovascular structures at risk.

After successful resection and decompression, portal sites may be closed with suture and/or steri-strips and covered with a soft sterile bandage. Patients may be instructed to begin immediate active and passive range of motion with avoidance of heavy lifting.

STT ganglion cysts

In situations where radiocarpal pathology cannot be conclusively identified, the midcarpal joint must be suspected as a potential cyst source. Although not recommended by some authors (12, 13, 16), decompression may be accomplished arthroscopically.

The arthroscope may be inserted in the metacarpophalangeal portal, where the ganglion cyst stalk may be identified at the STT joint. Due to the anatomical limitations of this small joint, a 1.9-mm scope is recommended. Additional thumb-based traction should be applied. Carefully, with sequential sharp and blunt arthrotomy technique as previously described, a 2.0-mm shaver may be placed in the STT portal. Caution must be exercised in order to protect the dorsal branches of the radial artery and terminal branches of the radial nerve.

As with volar radiocarpal ganglion cysts, successful resection and decompression can be verified with intra-articular visualization of a rush of mucinous fluid, as well as confirming the disappearance of the ganglion cyst with visualization and palpation externally. If a tourniquet is used, it must be deflated before ending the operation in order to identify possible iatrogenic arterial injuries.

Similarly, portal sites may be closed with suture and/or steri-strips and covered with a soft sterile bandage. Patients may be instructed to begin immediate active and passive range of motion with avoidance of heavy lifting.

Postoperative Rehabilitation Protocol

Following dorsal or volar arthroscopic cyst resections, immediately postoperative digital motion is encouraged and sutures are removed in 7 to 10 days. Very seldom is any supervised therapy required. If there is residual fullness over the ganglion or its portal, the use of an elastomer as a pressure scar modulator may be helpful. Activity is resumed as tolerated, and the patient is advised against forceful loading of the wrist for 4 weeks. The theoretical advantages of a minimally invasive procedure to reliably remove wrist ganglion cysts seem intuitive, but strangely have not been validated until recently. Reduced recovery times, less postoperative pain, and quicker returns to work and athletics have been reported (4, 8).

Patients can expect decreased pain and increased function within 6 weeks following surgery. Outcome surveys, often regarded as the most important assessment of patients, showed considerable improvements in both the short term and the long term (4). Unfortunately, the positive short-term outcomes cannot be referenced to open excisions since there have not been comparable reports dealing with open excisions.

Although more and more studies are demonstrating that arthroscopic ganglion resection is a safe and effective technique with a predictable and easy recovery, there have been only two prospectives, randomized study comparing arthroscopic resection with more traditional open techniques (10, 17). One study could not demonstrate compelling differences in outcomes at 1 year postoperatively. The other study, however, suggested that the short-term outcomes favored the arthroscopic technique. This is consistent with most perceptions that the true benefits of a minimally invasive arthroscopy would be most profound within the first 4 weeks. However, neither study can be considered definitive given their small cohorts. Until an adequately powered study evaluating both the short-term and the long-term outcomes of arthroscopic and open ganglion resections, it is difficult to make any meaningful comparisons between the two techniques.

CONCLUSIONS

A summation of the literature and clinical experience on arthroscopic dorsal wrist ganglion resection has quieted the debate on several issues, but still leaves some issues open. First, patients can experience significant increases in function and decreases in pain within 6 weeks, following arthroscopic dorsal wrist ganglion resection, and these initial benefits can be expected to be maintained for at least 2 years. Second, the recurrence and complication rates for arthroscopic ganglion resection appear to be comparable with, if not less than, that those reported for open resections. Third, ganglion cysts have a high association with intra-articular abnormalities, but the significance of this is unclear. Fourth, despite previous reports, recurrent ganglia and ganglia originating from the midcarpal joint are not contraindications for arthroscopic resection. In fact, assessment of the midcarpal joint is necessary for complete resection of most ganglia. Finally, identification of a discrete stalk is not always necessary for successful resection. Rather, attention should be focused on any cystic material or

redundant capsular thickening within the joints as well as performing an adequate capsulotomy.

Although occurring less commonly their dorsal counterpart, volar ganglion cysts originating from the radiocarpal joint can safely and effectively be treated with arthroscopic decompression. In this situation, arthroscopy not only is a reasonable alternative to open excision, but there is evidence to suggest that open excision should be avoided due to potential injuries to the palmar cutaneous branch of the median nerve. Volar ganglion cysts originating from the STT joint, however, should be treated with careful open excision, as the arthroscopic technique seems to be complicated by radial artery and nerve injury and higher rates of reoccurrence.

Regardless of whether dorsal or volar cysts are concerned, the debate of whether arthroscopic wrist ganglion resection is a preferable technique to open resection has shifted issues. Concerns of recurrence and long-term efficacy seem to have been put to rest and determined to be equivalent. Currently, the debate has turned to whether arthroscopic resection offers patients any benefits in terms of decreased pain and increased motion over open resection in the initial postoperative course. Further comparative investigation specifically focusing on the immediate short term is required to answer this question. At the very least, for the most part, arthroscopic ganglion resection remains a safe and effective technique to offer patients.

REFERENCES

1. Osterman AL, Raphael J. Arthroscopic resection of dorsal wrist ganglion of the wrist. *Hand Clin*. 1995;11(1):7–12.
2. Ho PC, Griffiths J, Lo WN, et al. Current treatment of ganglion at the wrist. *Hand Surg*. 2001;6(1):49–58.
3. Rizzo M, Berger RA, Steinman SP, et al. Arthroscopic resection in the management of dorsal wrist ganglion: results with a minimum 2-year follow-up period. *J Hand Surg [Am]*. 2004;29(1):59–62.
4. Edwards SG, Johansen JA. Prospective outcomes and associations of wrist ganglion cysts resected arthroscopically. *J Hand Surg [Am]*. 2009;34(3):395–400.
5. Povlsen B, Peckett WR. Arthroscopic findings in patients with painful wrist ganglia. *Scand J Plast Reconstr Surg Hand Surg*. 2001;35(3):323–328.
6. Geissler WB, Freeland AE, Savoie FH, et al. Intracarpal soft-tissue lesions associated with an intra-articular fracture of the distal end of the radius. *J Bone Joint Surg [Am]*. 1996;78(3):357–365.
7. Rimington TR, Edwards SG, Lynch TS, et al. Intercarpal ligamentous laxity in cadaveric wrists. *J Bone Joint Surg Br*. 2010;92(11):1600–1605.
8. Singh D, Culp R. Arthroscopic ganglion excisions. Paper presented at ASSH, 2002.
9. Mathoulin C, Hoyos A, Pelaez J. Arthroscopic resection of wrist ganglia. *Hand Surg*. 2004;9(2):159–164.
10. Kang L, Akelman E, Weiss AP. Arthroscopic versus open dorsal ganglion excision: a prospective, randomized comparison

of rate of recurrence and of residual pain. *J Hand Surg [Am]*. 2008;33(4):471–475.

11. Beredjiklian PK, Bozenka DJ, Leung YL, et al. Complications of wrist arthroscopy. *J Hand Surg [Am]*. 2004;29(3):406–411.

12. Angelides AC, Wallace PF. The dorsal ganglion of the wrist: its pathogenesis, gross and microscopic anatomy, and surgical treatment. *J Hand Surg [Am]*. 1976;1(3):228–235.

13. Rocchi L, Canal A, Pelaez J, Fanfani F, Catalano F. Results and complications in dorsal and volar wrist Ganglia arthroscopic resection. *Hand Surg*. 2006;11(1–2):21–26.

14. Jacobs LG, Govaers KJ. The volar wrist ganglion: just a simple cyst? *J Hand Surg [Br]*. 1990;15(3):342–346.

15. Gündeş H, Cirpici Y, Sarlak A, et al. Prognosis of wrist ganglion operations. *Acta Orthop Belg*. 2000;66(4):363–367.

16. Ho PC, Lo WN, Hung LK. Arthroscopic resection of volar ganglion of the wrist: a new technique. *Arthroscopy*. 2003;19(2):218–221.

17. Rocchi L, Canal A, Fanfani F, et al. Articular ganglia of the volar aspect of the wrist: arthroscopic resection compared with open excision. A prospective randomized study. *Scand J Plast Reconstr Surg Hand Surg*. 2008;42(5):253–259.

Triangular Fibrocartilage Complex Tears: Arthroscopic Management Options

Kevin D. Plancher • Sheryl L. Lipnick

CLINICAL EVALUATION

Pertinent History

The functions of the distal radial ulnar joint (DRUJ) as well as its major structure, the triangular fibrocartilage complex (TFCC), have been reported extensively. The TFCC acts as a cushion between the distal end of the ulna and the radial ulnocarpal joint. It is a ligamentous connection between the distal radius and the ulnar side of the carpus. Loss of TFCC support may result in subluxation or dislocation of the DRUJ. Complete excision of the TFCC, a previously recommended treatment for the painful DRUJ, has been shown to lead to an increase in ulnar lunate abutment and erosion of the cartilage, causing increasing wrist pain.

The TFCC consists of various parts including the triangular fibrocartilage, the articular disk, the dorsal and palmar ligamentous attachments, the meniscus homologue, and the extensor carpi ulnaris (ECU) subsheath (Fig. 42.1A, B).

TFCC injuries are a common cause of ulnar-sided wrist pain, especially in athletes. There are multiple pathologies that can result in ulnar-sided wrist pain. The differential diagnosis includes ligamentous/tendinous, osseous, vascular, neurologic, and other etiologies. Ligamentous/tendinous injuries include TFCC tears, intrinsic or extrinsic ligamentous damage, tendinitis of the flexor carpi ulnaris or ECU tendons, and ECU tendon subluxation. Osseous sources such as fracture, nonunion, malunion, and arthritis can also cause ulnar-sided wrist pain. Ulnar artery thrombosis, hemangiomas, ulnar nerve entrapment, neuritis and complex regional pain syndrome represent vascular and neurologic sources of pain. Tumors and avascular necrosis of the lunate (Kienbock's disease) are additional causes of ulnar-sided wrist pain.

The majority of the blood supply to the TFCC has been shown to be along the peripheral edge of the TFCC (Fig. 42.2). The primary vascular supply comes from the anterior interosseous artery and the ulnar artery. The dorsal branch of the interosseous artery supplies most of the dorsal periphery, and the palmar branch supplies the volar

periphery near the radial attachment. The ulnar artery supplies the styloid region and ulnar portion of the volar periphery. Vascular penetration extends to only the peripheral 15%, leaving the central portion of the disk relatively avascular. There has also been a concern over the healing potential of radial-sided TFCC lesions. However, Cooney et al., Plancher et al., and others have showed adequate healing of radial-sided TFCC repairs. The neural supply, similar to the vascular supply, excludes the central portion of the disk. The ulnar nerve supplies the volar and ulnar portions of the TFCC, while the posterior interosseous nerve supplies the dorsal portion. There is a variable contribution of the dorsal sensory branch to all portions of the TFCC.

One main function of the TFCC is load transmission, which is dependent upon forearm rotation. The TFCC has been shown in biomechanical studies to distribute up to 20% of the load across the ulnar wrist. The ulna assumes a relatively shortened position in supination and a relatively lengthened position in pronation. The primary stabilizers of the DRUJ are the dorsal and volar radial ulnar ligaments. The TFCC has a number of primary functions. It extends over the articular surface of the distal radius to cover the ulnar head. It partially absorbs the load while it transmits an axial force across the ulnocarpal joint. The TFCC provides a strong but flexible connection between the distal ulna and the radius, allowing for forearm rotation. Lastly, the TFCC supports the ulnar portion of the carpus through the connections established to both the ulna and the radius.

The history of a patient with a TFCC tear may include ulnar-sided wrist pain with pronation or supination, especially with weight-bearing. The patient may also report a sense of clicking or popping with forearm rotation, such as turning a doorknob or swinging a racquet or golf club. Activity usually exacerbates the symptoms, where rest can relieve them. Traumatic TFCC injuries are usually the result of a fall on an outstretched hand, where there is an extension-pronation force on an axially loaded wrist. Other mechanisms include either a dorsal rotation injury or a distraction force applied to the volar forearm or wrist. In addition, patients with distal radius fractures have been found to have tears of the TFCC.

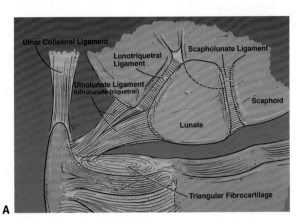 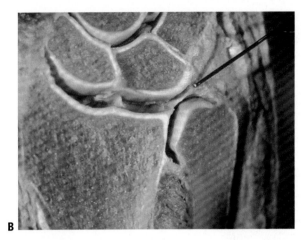

FIGURE 42.1. A: Artist's rendering of normal triangular fibrocartilage complex (TFCC) anatomy. **B:** Anatomical cross-section of the wrist revealing normal TFCC anatomy. (© Kevin D. Plancher.)

Physical Examination

The physical examination of a patient with a suspected TFCC tear begins with adequate inspection of both the affected and the unaffected sides. The wrist, forearm, and DRUJ should be assessed for swelling. The extremity should be palpated for tenderness, specifically over the TFCC in the soft spot between the flexor carpi ulnaris, the ulnar styloid, and the triquetrum (Fig. 42.3). Range of motion of the wrist and DRUJ, both active and passive, should be evaluated and compared with the opposite extremity. The examiner should be aware of other wrist pathologies that may mimic TFCC tears, such as DRUJ arthritis, ECU tendinitis/subluxation, and lunotriquetral ligament tears. Supination and ulnar deviation should exacerbate subluxation of the ECU. The shear or ballottement test can aid in the evaluation of lunotriquetral ligament tears.

DRUJ instability is assessed with passive manipulation of the ulna and radius. Increased translation in the anteroposterior plane is evident and should be evaluated in a neutral, supinated, and pronated forearm position. The ulnocarpal stress test may reproduce the symptoms caused by disk tears or ulnocarpal degeneration. The forearm is placed in a vertical position on the examiner's table. An axial load is then placed through the wrist while the wrist is moved through radial and ulnar deviation with

simultaneous pronation and supination. The press test is another way to dynamically load the ulnocarpal joint. The patient grasps the arms of a chair and pushes up to a standing position. The press test, although not particularly specific, is positive if symptomatic ulnar wrist pain is elicited with this maneuver.

Imaging

Radiographs, including a zero-rotation posteroanterior (PA) and lateral views of the wrist, should be obtained. Ulnar variance measurements can be obtained on the PA view, which is taken with the shoulder abducted to 90° and the elbow flexed to 90° with the hand flat on an X-ray cassette. DRUJ instability can be accentuated through a lateral stress view in which the patient holds a 5-lb (2.26 kg) weight with the forearm pronated and the X-beam directed "cross-table."

Arthrography, while once having a key role in assessing for TFCC tears, has slowly fallen out of favor due to poor clinical correlation and increased use of MRI and arthroscopy. Not only has a high incidence of perforations been detected in asymptomatic wrists of various ages but studies have also shown low sensitivity of arthrography compared with arthroscopy. Nonetheless, a negative arthrogram can be a useful screening tool. After arthrogram,

FIGURE 42.2. Blood supply to the TFCC (From Bednar MS, Arnoczky SP, Weiland AJ. The microvasculature of the triangular fibrocartilage complex: its clinical significance. *J Hand Surg.* 1991;16A(6):1101–1105, with permission).

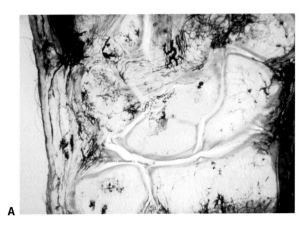 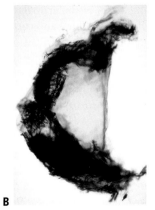

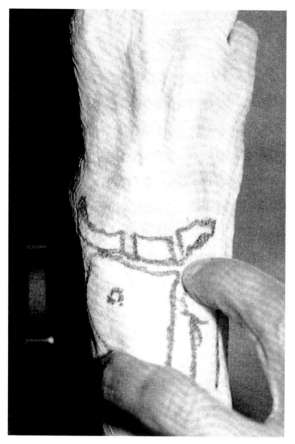

FIGURE 42.3. Palpation of the TCFF for tenderness in the soft spot between the flexor carpi ulnaris, the ulnar styloid, and the triquetrum. (From Whipple T, *The Wrist* Philadelphia, PA: Lippincott Williams & Wilkins with permission)

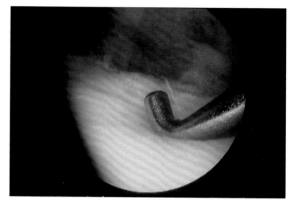

FIGURE 42.4. The "trampoline" effect is shown by directly probing a lax or hypermobile TFCC. The increased laxity represents a tear of the TFCC. (© Kevin D. Plancher.)

Decision-Making Algorithms

Classification

Palmer's classification is the most recognized system. There are two categories described: traumatic and degenerative. Traumatic TFCC tears are further subdivided based on location of the tear. Degenerative tears are usually a result of chronic, excessive loading of the ulnocarpal joint from ulnar impaction syndrome (UIS). Degenerative lesions are further classified by the location and severity of degeneration of the TFCC, ulnar head, and carpus. Treatment generally involved debridement of the joint and reduction of load across the ulnocarpal joint.

Palmer's classification of TFCC lesions

Class I: Traumatic lesions
A. Central rupture
B. Ulnar avulsion
   With styloid fracture
   Without styloid fracture
C. Distal avulsion (from carpus)
D. Radial avulsion
   With sigmoid notch fracture
   Without sigmoid notch fracture

Class II: Degenerative lesions
A. Superficial
B. Degenerative tear with chondral changes on the lunate or ulna
C. Degenerative perforation with chondral lesion of the lunate or ulna
D. Degenerative perforation with chondral lesion of the lunate or ulna and lunotriquetral instability
E. Degenerative perforation with lunotriquetral instability and ulnocarpal arthritis

if dye is present within the substance of the TFCC, a partial thickness tear is suspected. A full thickness tear should be suspected if the dye passes from the wrist joint into the radioulnar joint.

CT can evaluate for fractures, degenerative arthritis, and possibly DRUJ instability. To adequately assess for DRUJ instability, both forearms need to be evaluated in identical forearm positions. MRI, which is noninvasive, is commonly used to assess injuries of the TFCC. The sensitivity, specificity, and accuracy, however, vary widely. MRI can also be used to evaluate for bony edema, the thickness of the articular cartilage, the subchondral bone of the distal ulna and carpal bones, and the integrity of the lunotriquetral ligament.

Arthroscopy can be used as a diagnostic and therapeutic modality and is considered to be the gold standard for diagnosing injuries of the TFCC. A number of other wrist injuries or carpal pathologies can also be treated with arthroscopy. A lax or hypermobile TFCC can be determined with direct probing. This "trampoline" effect is indicative of an unstable TFCC (Fig. 42.4). Evidence of TFCC injury may also include scarring or vascular invasion seen along the periphery and tears of the lunotriquetral interosseous ligament or ECU sheath.

Class IA tears are located in the central portion of the triangular fibrocartilage. These are relatively common injuries and generally produce pain and clicking, usually due to an unstable flap. There is no DRUJ instability. These usually do not require acute treatment and should be treated with rest, immobilization, anti-inflammatory medications, and corticosteroid injections. Arthroscopic treatment is reserved for persistent symptoms. Tears should be debrided to a stable edge, making sure to leave an intact peripheral border.

Class IB tears are avulsions formfrom the ulnar attachment, with and without an ulnar styloid fracture. Concomitant ECU sheath disruption may occur with subluxation of the tendon. The DRUJ usually, but not always, remains stable. The chance of DRUJ instability increases if the fracture is at the base as opposed to the more common shaft or tip. Physical findings may include tenderness over the fovea region and pain with dorsal and volar translation. These injuries are less likely to produce a click. Initial treatment includes 4 to 6 weeks of immobilization. Surgical indications include persistent symptoms or DRUJ instability. These tears can be treated by suturing the tear to the capsule arthroscopically or by open repair, which may be preferred in cases of chronic instability with ulnar styloid nonunion.

Class IC injuries are defined as having complete or partial tears of the ulnocarpal ligaments. The tears are located at their attachments to the lunate and triquetrum or in their midsubstance. There is a higher probability of healing potential due the good peripheral vascular supply. The volar "sag" of the carpus relative to the ulnar head is classic for this injury pattern. Conservative management is the mainstay of treatment unless mechanical instability is present. Arthroscopic or open procedures have been described in limited cases.

Class ID tears are partial or complete avulsions of the TFCC from the sigmoid notch of the radius. A bony fragment may or may not be present. Many class ID injuries are associated with distal radius fractures and can be treated with adequate fracture reduction. Instability of the DRUJ is rare for these types of tears. Repair of the tear back to the radius can be accomplished by both open and arthroscopic procedures.

Class II tears are degenerative TFCC lesions caused by ulnocarpal impaction syndrome. Many of the symptomatic degenerative tears are the result of chronic overloading of the ulnocarpal joint and generally progressive.

TREATMENT

Nonoperative

Initial treatment of ulnar-sided wrist pain with localized tenderness over the ulnar fovea region with a stable DRUJ consists of rest, anti-inflammatory medication, and immobilization. The patient can be splinted or placed in a short-arm cast for 3 to 4 weeks. Cortisone injections, administered into the wrist joint through area of the 6 R portal site, may also be beneficial in aiding to alleviate discomfort.

Operative Indication

Persistent symptoms highly suggestive of a TFCC tear require wrist arthroscopy and TFCC repair. Indications for operative treatment for class I tears include tears associated with neutral or negative ulnar variance, suspected or proven injury with ulnar wrist symptoms, which significantly interfere with activities and failure of nonoperative treatment.

TECHNIQUE–ULNA SIDED TFCC REPAIR

Standard wrist arthroscopy is performed with the extremity suspended by finger traps with 5 to 15 lb (2.26 to 6.80 kg) of countertraction (Fig. 42.5). A wrist traction tower may be used. An upper arm tourniquet is applied but is not initially inflated. TFCC tears are identified by direct visualization of the tear or by finding a loss of tension of the TFCC. The "trampoline effect," as described by Hermansdorfer and Kleinman, reveals a loss of resiliency in the central portion of the TFCC upon probing. Inflamed synovium, most notably seen in ulnar-sided tears, is another indication of a tear.

Several arthroscopic methods have been described for TFCC repair based on the direction of suture passage. Techniques can be classified as "inside-out," "outside-in," or "all-inside." The "inside-out" technique has been described using a Tuohy (Becton Dickson, Franklin Lakes, NJ) needle. The needle is introduced into the wrist joint from the radial side, passing it through the TFCC tear and out through the palmar skin over the ulnar carpal region. A second area of the TFCC tear is punctured in a similar fashion and both ends of the suture are retrieved. 2-0 PDS is used to make this horizontal mattress repair. "Outside-in" repairs can vary in technique depending on instrumentation and slight surgical modifications. A small incision is made adjacent to the TFCC tear, and arthroscopic needles are passed through the capsule and TFCC. A 2-0 PDS or 3-0 Fiberwire suture is passed through the needle, and a grasper is used to retrieve the suture, which is then tied

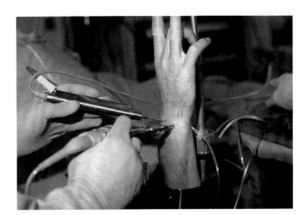

FIGURE 42.5. Arthroscopic setup of the right wrist using a wrist traction tower. (© Kevin D. Plancher.)

over the dorsal wrist capsule. Two to four sutures are generally required for adequate repair.

AUTHORS' PREFERRED TREATMENT

Class IA tears: Standard wrist arthroscopy is performed as previously described. A 2.3-mm arthroscope is established through the 3-4 portal. The 4-5 and the 6-R portals are used for instrumentation, usually starting with a mini 3.5-mm full-radius motorized suction shaver. The associated synovitis is debrided and a probe is then used to assess for additional flap stability, TFCC tension, and other ligament integrity. A shaver or banana blade is used to resect the unstable flap. The peripheral attachments must remain undisturbed. Portal sites are closed with monocryl suture in a subcuticular fashion. Caution is taken to avoid injury to the dorsal ulnar sensory nerve.

Class IB tears: Standard wrist arthroscopy is performed as previously described. Carpal portals are established between the 3-4, 4-5 and the 6-R intervals. The 3-4 and the 4-5 portals are used for viewing using a 2.3-mm arthroscope. The 6-R portal, and possibly the 4-5 portal, if needed, are used for instrumentation. The tear edges are debrided with a full-radius shaver to aid in the healing process. A 1.5 to 2.0 cm longitudinal incision is made adjacent to the tear, which is usually located ulnar to the 6-R portal. Blunt dissection is carried out to identify the dorsal ulnar sensory branch and the transverse branch. Take care not to violate the wrist capsule. A curved meniscal needle is then introduced through the ulnar capsule then piercing the TFCC, which is done under arthroscopic visualization. The straight meniscal needle is placed just above the curved needle. A suture retrieval instrument or wire basket loop is then employed to bring the 2-0 PDS or 3-0 Fiberwire suture, which is advanced through the curved needle, out through the capsule through the straight needle. The needles are removed and the suture is tied down to the wrist capsule in a vertical mattress fashion. Additional sutures can be placed in a similar fashion.

The proximity of the dorsal sensory branch of the ulnar nerve to the suture may cause impingement of the nerve leading to pain and/or parasthesias. In this situation, it is possible to exteriorize the suture using Bunnell needles to bring the suture limbs out through the dorsal skin. The sutures are advanced through a button and tied down to the back of the wrist. This procedure, however, is rarely performed.

Unstable peripheral tears with an associated nonunion of the ulnar styloid fragment must be treated with an open procedure. The ulnar styloid fragment should either be reattached or be excised with reattachment of the TFCC to the distal ulna.

Class IC tears: A small 1-cm incision is made volar to the ECU tendon. Caution is taken to avoid the dorsal sensory branch of the ulnar nerve and the volar ulnar

neurovascular structures. Needles are passed in an "outside-in" fashion through the capsule over the tear similar to class IB repairs. The dorsal ulnar portion of the TFCC can be reefed to obtain adequate tissue for repair.

Class ID tears: Standard wrist arthroscopy is performed as described above. Carpal portals are established between the 3-4 interval and the 6-R and 6-U intervals. The 3-4 portal is used for viewing, and the 6-R and 6-U portals are used for instrumentation. After completion of the diagnostic arthroscopy and identification of the radial-sided tear (Fig. 42.6), a small diameter burr is used to debride and decorticate the radial site of the TFCC detachment. Once a rough and bleeding surface has been established along the dorsal or volar aspect of the radio-sigmoid notch, a suture passer is used to place sutures through the torn free edge of the TFCC. The suture ends are retrieved through the 6-R or 6-U portal. Alternatively, a drill guide may be used to place a meniscal needle from the ulnar to the radial side of the wrist by using a soft tissue sleeve.

A 1- to 1.5-cm longitudinal incision is placed over the interval between the second and the third extensor compartments. Using blunt dissection, the dorsal cortex of the distal radius is identified. Identification of the Kirschner wire and protection of the superficial radial nerve is performed (Fig. 42.7). A 2-0 PDS or 3-0 Fiberwire suture is passed with the use of a suture passer and is tied with a mulberry knot drawn into the joint to suture the radial-sided tear. A suture is then tied on the dorsal cortex of the radius. Alternatively, prethreaded meniscal needles may be used to tie a horizontal mattress suture (Fig. 42.8).

An alternative placement of the Kirschner wires by free hand can be done by using a targeting drill guide placed into the radiocarpal joint through the 6-R or 6-U portal, with the barrel of the guide seated on the radius between the second and the third extensor compartments. Confirmation of drill guide placement is made

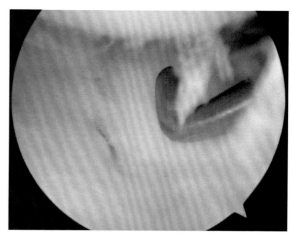

FIGURE 42.6. Radial avulsion of the triangular fibrocartilage complex. (© Kevin D. Plancher.)

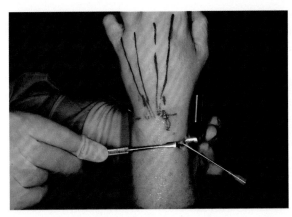

FIGURE 42.7. Longitudinal incision with Kirschner wire protruding from the ulnar side of the radius. (© Kevin D. Plancher.)

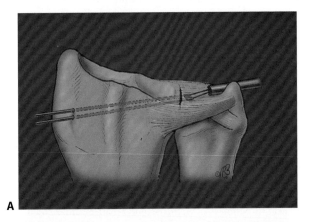

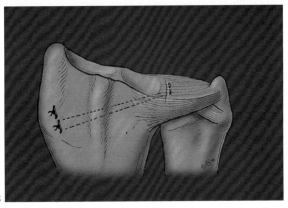

FIGURE 42.8. A: Suture placed in the triangular fibrocartilage complex through drill holes with a prethreaded meniscal needle. **B:** Suture tied over a bony bridge between the second and the third extensor compartments. (© Kevin D. Plancher.)

arthroscopically and fluoroscopically. After the drill guide has been seated, a 2-mm drill hole is established. Care is taken to avoid the articular surface of the lunate facet of the distal radius. A second drill hole converges to the same site within the sigmoid notch of the radius. A Hewson suture passer is then advanced through the drill hole and used to retrieve one suture limb that had been previously placed within the TFCC. The Hewson passer is

then used to retrieve the second suture limb through the second drill hole. The TFCC is then visualized, and the forearm position that most accurately reduces the TFCC is determined while tension is applied to the suture. The sutures are tied over the bony bridge, between the second and the third extensor compartments, with the forearm in this position. Up to three sutures can be passed through each drill hole.

More recent, innovative techniques have also been described. Fellinger et al. described the technique for repair of radial avulsion of the TFCC with a T-fix suture anchoring device. In this technique, a Kirschner wire is passed from the sigmoid notch through the radial cortex of the distal radius. The Kirschner wire is then overreamed to 2.5 mm, followed by insertion of the suture anchor. The suture is then secured to the periosteum of the radius. Of note, previous studies have revealed irritation in the postoperative period caused by the T-fix suture anchors. With our technique, two drill holes are used, and the sutures are tied over a bony bridge or one suture is tied as a mulberry knot. We believe our technique provides a more secure fixation and accurate placement of sutures into the periosteum of the radius (two drill holes).

Class IIA and IIB injuries are treated with standard arthroscopic evaluation and synovial debridement. An open ulnar shortening osteotomy is performed after the arthroscopy. Class IIC perforations require debridement. The 3-4 portal is used as a viewing portal with an ulnar portal used to introduce a 4-mm burr. An arthroscopic wafer procedure is performed to resect between 3 and 4 mm of the radial portion of the ulna. Pronation and supination of the wrist will help to evenly resect the distal ulna. The radius can be used as a guide to help determine the amount of bone removed. An 18G needle is then placed in the DRUJ beneath the tear. An operative portal is established in the DRUJ. A burr or small 1/8 in osteotome is inserted through this portal. The ulnar portion of the distal ulna beneath the TFCC is removed to the level of the base of the ulna. Class IID and IIE injuries involve lunotriquetral ligament disruption with instability. Significant DRUJ arthritic changes require resection of the distal ulna. If no significant DRUJ arthritic changes are seen, arthroscopic debridement similar to the treatment described for class IIC injuries can be performed. The lunotriquetral interval must be evaluated through both the radiocarpal and the midcarpal joints. Fraying of the lunotriquetral ligament without instability can be treated with an arthroscopic wafer procedure, similar to the class IIC injuries. If lunotriquetral instability is present, an ulnar shortening osteotomy is needed after arthroscopic synovectomy and chondroplasty. The osteotomy with allow for secondary ulnar extrinsic ligament tightening. If instability is still present, percutaneous Kirschner wire fixation of the lunotriquetral interval is performed using two or three 0.045 in wires, which are buried in the subcutaneous tissue.

III. The Wrist

COMPLICATIONS/CONTROVERSIES/ SPECIAL CONSIDERATIONS

Complications of TFCC repair include injury to the dorsal sensory branch of the ulnar nerve, the dorsal sensory branch of the radial nerve, the radial artery, extensor tendons, and iatrogenic chondromalacia. Meticulous technique and attention to detail can prevent most of these complications. The ulnar dorsal sensory nerve is especially at risk with arthroscopic treatment of the wrist. Patients may complain of pain and/or parasthesias due to nerve damage or irritation from suture knot impingement. If symptoms persist, patients may require return to the operating room for neurolysis and suture removal.

REHABILITATION

Class IA tears should be treated with a splint for approximately 1 week for support. Over the next 3 weeks, patients should wear the splint intermittently and should avoid forceful grasping or repetitive rotatory activities. A formal therapy program may be needed in select patients.

For class IB, IC, and ID tears, the wrist and forearm are immobilized in a Muenster cast or with pinning of the distal ulna to the distal radius. Both of these methods control forearm rotation. The position of immobilization is determined intraoperatively and is based on the position that most appropriately reduces the TFCC. After 4 to 6 weeks, the forearm immobilization is exchanged for a standard forearm cast for an additional 4 weeks. After immobilization, physical therapy is initiated, with active assisted range of motion, passive range of motion, and gentle strengthening exercises.

Postoperative treatment for class IIA, IIB, and IIC injuries should involve intermittent use of a short-arm splint for 4 weeks with active range-of-motion exercises for the wrist. At that time, graduated strengthening exercises are started. Class IID and IIE injuries are treated with a short arm cast for 4 to 8 weeks. Pins are removed in the office at 6 to 8 weeks. Therapy is started with maximum improvement seen at approximately 4 months.

CONCLUSIONS/FUTURE DIRECTIONS

Wrist arthroscopy and MRI has allowed for increased recognition of tears of the TFCC as a cause of ulnar-sided wrist pain. The continued advancement in arthroscopic devices and instrumentation has allowed for successful arthroscopic repair of these injuries.

Open techniques have also been described for repair of the TFCC with satisfactory results. The arthroscopic approach minimizes the amount of dissection required for TFCC repair and has the theoretical advantage of reducing subsequent scar formation and wrist stiffness. These arthroscopic techniques are technically difficult and should be performed by surgeons experienced in wrist arthroscopy.

SUGGESTED READINGS

Adams B. Distal radioulnar joint instability. In: Green D, Hotchkiss R, Pederson W, Wolfe S, eds. *Green's Operative Hand Surgery.* 5th ed. Philadelphia, PA: Elsevier; 2005:605–644.

Culp R, Osterman A, Kaufmann R. Wrist arthroscopy: operative procedures. In: Green D, Hotchkiss R, Pederson W, Wolfe S, eds. *Green's Operative Hand Surgery.* 5th ed. Philadelphia, PA: Elsevier; 2005:784–792.

Micucci C, Schmidt C. Arthroscopic repair of ulnar-sided triangular fibrocartilage complex tears. *Oper Tech Orthop.* 2007; 17:118–124.

Nagle D. Triangular fibrocartilage complex tears in the athlete. *Clin Sports Med.* 2001;20(1):155–166.

Plancher K, Faber K. Arthroscopic repair of radial-sided triangular fibrocartilage complex lesions. *Tech Hand Up Extrem Surg.* 1999;3(1):44–51.

Tracy M, Wiesler E, Poehling G. Arthroscopic management of triangular fibrocartilage tears in the athlete. *Oper Tech Sports Med.* 2006;14:95–100.

The Role of Wrist Arthroscopy in the Management of Intra-articular Distal Radius Fractures

William B. Geissler

The use of wrist arthroscopy is a valuable adjunct in the management of displaced intra-articular distal radius fractures as it has the advantage of viewing the articular surface under bright light and magnified conditions with minimal surgical morbidity. Fracture hematoma and debris removed arthroscopically may potentially improve the patient's final range of motion. In addition, any associated soft tissue intra-articular injuries may be managed at the same sitting. Often, pathology—not readily identifiable on plain radiographs—is discovered during arthroscopic-assisted reduction of internal fixation distal radius fractures. It is much easier to manage an acute soft tissue injury that occurs with a fracture of the distal radius than a chronic injury.

Displaced intra-articular fractures of the distal radius are a unique subset of distal radius fractures. These fractures usually develop high-energy injury and are less amenable to traditional closed manipulation and casting. The prognosis for intra-articular fractures of the distal radius has been shown to depend on numerous factors. These include the amount of radial shortening, residual extra-articular angulation, articular reduction of both the radial carpal and the radial ulnar joints, and associated soft tissue injuries.

Lafontaine has described several radiographic features that signify when a fracture of the distal radius is unstable (1). These include initial dorsal angulation greater than 20°, extensive dorsal comminution, associated ulnar styloid fractures, significant intra-articular involvement, and patients above the age of 60.

Edwards et al. (2) described the advantage of viewing the articular reduction by wrist arthroscopy compared with monitoring reduction under fluoroscopy alone. In their series, 15 patients underwent arthroscopic evaluation of the articular surface of the distal radius following reduction and stabilization under fluoroscopy. They noted that 33% of the patients had articular step-off of 1 mm or more as viewed arthroscopically. Often, the fragment was rotated. Wrist arthroscopy is particularly useful in judging

the rotation of fracture fragments, which is not readily identifiable under fluoroscopic guidance alone. Edwards et al. concluded that utilizing wrist arthroscopy is a useful adjunct and may detect residual gapping not previously identified under fluoroscopy.

Two millimeters or less of articular displacement for reduction has been the well-established threshold over the past several years. Knirk and Jupiter (3), in their classic article, demonstrated the importance of articular reduction within 2 mm or less. Bradway et al. (4) further substantiated their findings in their previously published study. Fernandez and Geissler, in their series of 40 patients, noted that the critical threshold may be as low as 1 mm or even less. They found the incidence of complications was substantially lower when articular reduction was within 1 mm or less (5).

A high incidence of associated intra-articular soft tissue injuries involving the triangular fibrocartilage complex and the interosseous ligaments has been shown by several studies as displaced intra-articular fractures of the distal radius. Mohanti and Kar (6) and Fontes et al. (7), in two separate wrist arthrogram studies, noted a high incidence of tears to the triangular fibrocartilage complex in associated distal radius fractures. Mohanti and Kar (6) noted the triangular fibrocartilage complex injury in 45% of 60 patients in their study. Similarly, Fontes et al. (7) noted a 66% incidence of tears to the triangular fibrocartilage complex in 58 patients with fractures of the distal radius.

Several arthroscopic studies have documented the incidence of associated intracarpal soft tissue injuries associated with fractures of the distal radius. In three recent studies, tears to the triangular fibrocartilage complex are the most commonly associated intra-articular soft tissue injury (8–10). Geissler et al. (8) reported their experience with 60 patients with displaced intra-articular fractures of the distal radius undergoing arthroscopic-assisted reduction. In Geissler et al. series, 49% of the patients had a tear of the triangular fibrocartilage complex. However, tears to the interosseous ligament were less common. Injuries to the scapholunate interosseous ligament and the lunotriquetral interosseous ligament were identified in 32% and 15% of the patients, respectively.

Hanker (9), in a study of 65 patients, noted that tears of the triangular fibrocartilage complex were present in 55% of the patients in his series of arthroscopic-assisted reduction of distal radius fractures. Lindau (10), in an arthroscopic study of 50 patients, noted that injury to the triangular fibrocartilage complex was identified in 78% of patients, injury to the scapholunate interosseous ligament was identified in 54% of patients, whereas tears of the lunotriquetral interosseous ligament were far less common and were seen in only 16% of patients.

Geissler et al. (8) noted that there was a spectrum of injuries that occurred to the interosseous ligaments, based on his findings of associated soft tissue injuries with fractures of the distal radius (8). An arthroscopic classification of interosseous ligament injuries was described. He noted that the ligament attenuates and eventually tears usually in a volar to dorsal direction. This arthroscopic classification of carpal instability is based on observations of the interosseous ligaments from both the radiocarpal and the midcarpal spaces (Table 43.1).

The normal scapholunate and lunotriquetral interosseous ligaments have a concave appearance between the carpal bones when viewed from the radiocarpal space. The scapholunate interosseous ligament is best seen with the arthroscope in the 3-4 portal, and the lunotriquetral interosseous ligament is best observed with the arthroscope in either the 4-5 or 6-- portal. In the midcarpal space, the scapholunate interval should be tight and congruent without any articular gap or step-off. Similarly, the lunotriquetral interval may

be congruent, but usually a 1-mm step-off or increased play may normally be seen between the lunate and the triquetrum when viewed from the radial midcarpal space.

In Geissler grade 1 injuries, there is a loss of the normal concave appearance between the carpal bones as the interosseous ligament attenuates to become convex as seen with the arthroscope in the radiocarpal space. Hemorrhage may be seen within the interosseous ligament itself. However, in the midcarpal space, there is no rotation between the carpal bones, and the carpal interval is tight and congruent.

In Geissler grade 2 injuries, the interosseous ligament continues to stretch and becomes attenuated with a convex appearance as seen with the arthroscope in the radiocarpal space. In the midcarpal space, the carpal bones are no longer congruent, and a step-off is present. With scapholunate instability, there is slight palmar flexion of the dorsal edge of the scaphoid in relation to the lunate. With lunotriquetral instability, increased play will be seen between the triquetrum and the lunate when palpated with a probe in the ulnar midcarpal portal.

In Geissler grade 3 injuries, the interosseous ligament starts to tear usually in a volar to dorsal direction as seen with the arthroscope in the radiocarpal space. A gap is seen between the carpal bones. In the midcarpal space, a probe may be inserted between the carpal bones. A portion of the interosseous ligament is still intact, and a complete separation of the carpal bones is not seen.

In Geissler grade 4 injuries, the interosseous ligament is completely detached and the arthroscope may be passed freely between the radiocarpal and the midcarpal spaces. (This is the so-called drive-through sign.)

Table 43.1

Geissler arthroscopic classification of carpal instability

Grade	Description	Management
1	Attenuation/hemorrhage of interosseous ligament as seen from the radiocarpal joint. No incongruency of carpal alignment in the midcarpal space	Immobilization
2	Attenuation/hemorrhage of interosseous ligament as seen from the radiocarpal joint. Incongruency/step-off as seen from midcarpal space. A slight gap (less than the width of a probe) between the carpal bones may be present	Arthroscopic reduction and pinning
3	Incongruency/step-off of carpal alignment is seen in both the radiocarpal and the midcarpal spaces. The probe may be passed through gap between the carpal bones	Arthroscopic/open reduction and pinning
4	Incongruency/step-off of carpal alignment is seen in both the radiocarpal and the midcarpal spaces. Gross instability with manipulation is noted. A 2.7-mm arthroscope may be passed through the gap between the carpal bones	Open reduction and repair

Large joint instrumentation is not appropriate for arthroscopic-assisted reduction of distal radius fractures. Smaller joint instrumentation is essential. A smaller joint arthroscope of 2.7 mm or less is recommended. When the arthroscope is initially placed in the wrist, fracture debris and hematoma often obscure vision. It is important to irrigate out the fracture debris to improve utilization. A 3.5-mm or smaller shaver is used to help clear fracture hematoma and debris.

A traction tower is quite useful in the management of arthroscopic-assisted reduction of distal radius fractures. The tower allows continuous traction to the fracture fragments. It also allows the surgeon to flex, extend, and ulnar and radial deviate the wrist to help reduce the fracture fragments while maintaining constant traction. It is generally easier to insert the arthroscope with the wrist in slight flexion. The tower allows for slight flexion of the wrist during initial introduction of the arthroscope and cannulae.

A new traction tower is designed to allow the surgeon to simultaneously evaluate the wrist arthroscopically to manipulate the articular reduction and monitor the reduction under fluoroscopy (Fig. 43.1). The traction bar is uniquely placed at the side of the forearm and wrist so that it does not block fluoroscopic evaluation and the surgeon does not need to work around a central bar. In addition, the new traction tower allows the surgeon to perform arthroscopic-assisted fixation in the vertical or horizontal position, depending on the surgeon's preference. If a traction tower is not available, the wrist may be suspended with a finger trap attached to weights suspended over the end of a horizontal hand table or suspended with a shoulder holder in the vertical position. A small bump placed under the wrist is useful if weights are being utilized over the end of the table to maintain the wrist in slight flexion to ease entry on reduction of instrumentation.

Patients who present with a fracture of the distal radius often have a swollen wrist. Because of this, it may be difficult to palpate the traditional extensor tendon landmarks for wrist arthroscopy. However, the bony landmarks are usually still palpable. These bony landmarks include the bases of the metacarpals, the dorsal lip of the radius, and the ulnar head. The 3-4 portal is made in line with the radial border of the long finger. The 4-5 portal is made at the mid-axial line to the ring finger. Precise portal placement is mandatory for arthroscopic-assisted reduction of distal radius fractures. If the portals are placed too proximally, the arthroscope may be placed within the fracture itself, or if placed too distally can injure the articular cartilage of the carpus. It is very important to place an 18G needle into the proposed location of a portal before making a skin incision. The needle should enter into the joint easily without interference. The portals are made upon the skin with the surgeon's thumb against the tip of a no. 11 blade to avoid injury to the cutaneous nerves.

Blunt dissection is continued with the hemostat to the level of the joint capsule, and the arthroscope with a blunt trocar is introduced into the 3-4 portal. The 3-4 portal is the primary viewing portal in wrist arthroscopy. Fracture hematoma and debris are washed out to improve visualization through the 6-U portal. It is helpful to have a separate inflow provided with a 14G needle through the 6-U portal. Outflow is provided through the arthroscopic cannula. It is felt that a separate inflow and outflow are important to improve irrigation of the joint rather than inflow through the arthroscopic cannula alone. The small joint cannula in wrist arthroscopy does not allow much space between the cannula and the arthroscope itself and limits the amount of fluid irrigation into the joint. In addition, a separate outflow limits fluid extravasation into the soft tissues of the forearm and hand.

The ideal timing for arthroscopic-assisted reduction of intra-articular distal radius fractures appears to be between 3 and 10 days. Earlier attempts at arthroscopic fixation may result in troublesome bleeding obscuring visualization. Fractures that are stabilized after 10 days postinjury may be difficult to disimpact and elevate with arthroscopic techniques and manipulation.

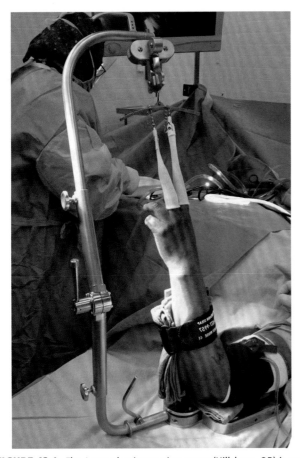

FIGURE 43.1. The Acumed wrist traction tower (Hillsboro, OR) is very useful for arthroscopic management of distal radius fractures. The suspending arm is located at the side and does not block fluoroscopic visualization while performing arthroscopy.

III. The Wrist

Fractures without extensive comminution are most ideal for arthroscopic-assisted management. Radial styloid fractures, die-punch fractures, three-part T fractures, and four-part fractures are all amenable to arthroscopic-assisted reduction and internal fixation. Radial styloid fractures are particularly amenable to arthroscopic reduction and are an ideal fracture pattern to gain experience in arthroscopic management of these fractures.

Three-part and four-part fractures with metaphyseal comminution are managed with a combination of open reduction and arthroscopic-assisted fixation. In these instances, the fracture is stabilized by a volar plate inserted through a volar approach, and the joint capsule is not opened. The articular reduction is provisionally pinned as viewed under fluoroscopy. The wrist is then suspended in traction, and articular reduction may be fine-tuned arthroscopically. Distal screws are then used to stabilize the fracture. Any associated soft tissue injuries are detected and managed in the same sitting.

RADIAL STYLOID FRACTURES

Radial styloid fractures are an ideal fracture pattern to manage arthroscopically, particularly if one is beginning to gain experience in arthroscopic management of wrist fractures (11). In addition, radial styloid fractures are often associated with injury to the scapholunate interosseous ligament (12). Arthroscopic management allows for management of the fracture as well as observation and possible treatment for any associated interosseous ligament injuries. There are several options to manage this fracture arthroscopically.

A closed reduction and percutaneous fixation of the radial styloid may be performed under fluoroscopy. The fractured fragment is reduced as anatomically as possible under fluoroscopy in the AP and lateral planes. The fracture may then be placed in traction and the wrist arthroscopically evaluated. The arthroscope is initially placed in the 3-4 portal and a shaver is brought in through the 6-R portal to clear the joint of debris and hematoma. The 4-5 or 6-R portal is best to evaluate the fracture reduction and in particular to judge rotation of the radial styloid fragment. Often, the articular reduction will look anatomic under fluoroscopy but may be rotated as viewed arthroscopically. If this is the case, the provisional fixation may be backed out, leaving the guidewires alone in the radial styloid fragment where they can then be used as joysticks and the fracture is rereduced and provisionally pinned. In addition, a trocar may be introduced through the 3-4 portal to provide additional control of the displaced radial styloid fragment as it is being manipulated with the guidewire joysticks. The position of the guidewires is then checked under fluoroscopy. If the guidewires are appropriate, a cannulated screw may be placed over the guidewire through the radial styloid fragment into the radial shaft to stabilize the fracture fragment.

Initially, the author only placed Kirschner wires to stabilize the radial styloid fragment. This provided good provisional fixation, but delayed any type of early range of motion as the patient had to be splinted. Often, patients complained of pin track infections and pain over the protruding Kirschner wires. Currently, the author prefers headless cannulated screws that are placed over the guidewires. In this manner, the screws are flush with the bone and do not cause any soft tissue or skin irritation. As the fixation is more stable, early range of motion can be performed as well.

It is vital that when the initial guidewires are placed, they are placed in oscillation mode with the drill to avoid injury to the dorsal sensory branch of the radial nerve. Similarly, if a headless screw is placed, a small incision is made and a trocar and cannula are placed. All drilling and placement of the screws are done through a cannula to prevent injury to the dorsal sensory branch of the radial nerve.

An alternative technique is to advance the Kirschner wire under fluoroscopy into the radial styloid fragment alone and not across the fracture site (Figs. 43.2 and 43.3). The ideal position of the guidewire in relation to the fracture and to its starting point is viewed directly under fluoroscopy. The wrist is then suspended in the traction tower, and the standard arthroscopy portals are made. As previously described, the wrist is debrided with the arthroscope in the 3-4 portal and the shaver in the 6-R portal. The arthroscope is then switched to the 6-R portal to best judge rotation of the radial styloid fragment. The Kirschner wire is then used as a joystick and the fracture is manipulated

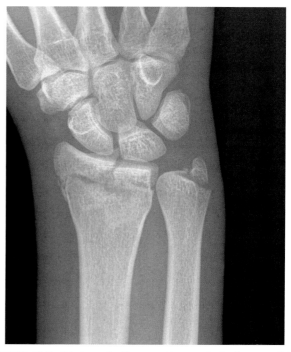

FIGURE 43.2. AP view of a three-part intra-articular fracture of the distal radius with an associated ulnar styloid fragment.

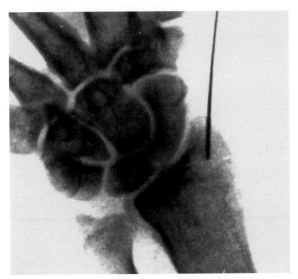

FIGURE 43.3. Under oscillation, a guidewire is placed only in the radial styloid fragment to be utilized as a joystick for reduction.

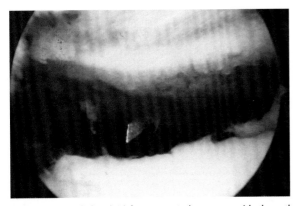

FIGURE 43.4. Radial styloid fractures are best seen with the arthroscope in the 6-R portal by looking across the wrist. The joystick guidewire can be seen in the radial styloid fragment to help reduce the fragment back through the lunate facet.

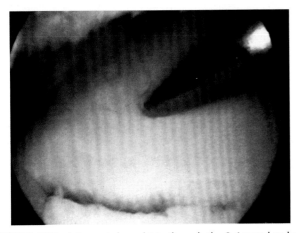

FIGURE 43.5. A trocar is brought in through the 3-4 portal to help control rotation of the fragment as a guidewire is then placed across the fracture.

under direct observation and anatomically reduced (Figs. 43.4 and 43.5). At that point, the guidewire is advanced across the fracture site. Once the fracture has been judged to be anatomic as viewed both arthroscopically and under fluoroscopy, headless cannulated screws are placed (Figs. 43.6 to 43.8).

It is important to remember that the zone of injury may pass through the fracture of the radial styloid and continue distally into the scapholunate interosseous ligament. For this reason, radial styloid fractures are associated with a high incidence of injury to the scapholunate

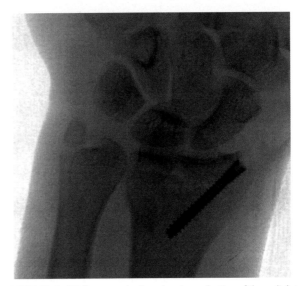

FIGURE 43.6. PA fluoroscopic view showing reduction of the radial styloid fragment. This can then be used as a landmark to reduce the lunate facet.

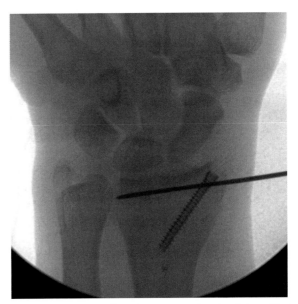

FIGURE 43.7. The lunate facet fragment is reduced and the guidewire is placed in oscillation mode for the radial styloid and lunate facet. It is important to pronate and supinate the forearm to ensure the guidewire is not penetrating the distal radial ulnar joint.

III. The Wrist

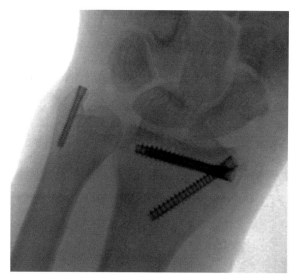

FIGURE 43.8. Headless cannulated screws are then placed in a subchondral fashion to secure the lunate facet fragment. Using headless screws decreases soft tissue irritation to promote earlier range of motion.

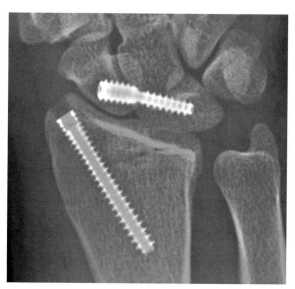

FIGURE 43.10. The radial styloid fragment was arthroscopically reduced and stabilized. Arthroscopic evaluation of the scapholunate interval showed a Geissler grade 3 tear to the scapholunate interosseous ligament. An Acumed SLIC screw was placed across the interval of this acute injury to stabilize the interval as the interosseous ligament healed.

interosseous ligament (Figs. 43.9 and 43.10). Following reduction to the radial styloid fracture, the arthroscope is placed back in the 3-4 portal to evaluate the integrity of the scapholunate interosseous ligament. The scapholunate interosseous ligament can also be evaluated with the arthroscope in the radial midcarpal portal to evaluate the scapholunate interval in the midcarpal space. Carpal instability should be evaluated from both the radial carpal and the midcarpal spaces (Figs. 43.11 to 43.13). In addition, articular cartilage damage may be identified in the

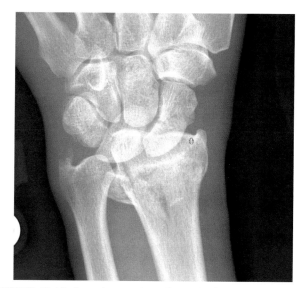

FIGURE 43.11. Posterior anterior radiograph of a displaced fracture of the distal radius and scaphoid.

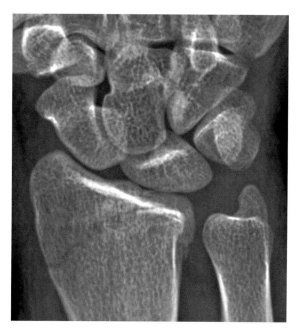

FIGURE 43.9. AP radiograph of a fracture of a patient with a fracture of the radial styloid with concern of scapholunate instability.

midcarpal space with cartilaginous loose bodies that are not normally detected on plain radiographs. Any associated injuries are then managed arthroscopically.

THREE-PART FRACTURES

Three-part fractures involve a fracture of the radial styloid and the lunate facet. Often, the radial styloid fragment may reduce under closed manipulation. The radial styloid fragment is closed reduced and percutaneously pinned

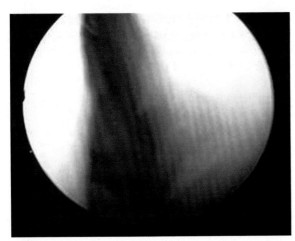

FIGURE 43.12. Following reduction of the distal radius and arthroscopic fixation of the scaphoid fracture, a Geissler grade 4 tear to the scapholunate interosseous ligament was identified. This is not readily apparent on the prereduction radiographs.

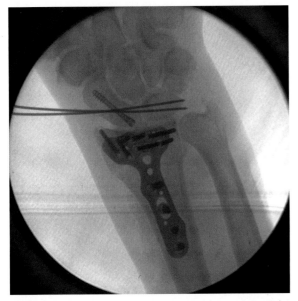

FIGURE 43.13. PA radiograph showing stabilization of the distal radius, scaphoid, and stabilization of the scapholunate interval.

under fluoroscopic control. It is important to protect the dorsal sensory branch of the radial nerve when inserting the guidewires. Once the radial styloid fragment is anatomically reduced, it may be used as a landmark for the reduction of the depressed lunate facet fragment.

Following reduction of the radial styloid fragment under fluoroscopy, the wrist is suspended in the wrist traction tower. Debris and hematoma are then evacuated, and the depressed lunate fragment is evaluated. The depressed lunate facet fragment is best seen with the arthroscope in the 3-4 portal. An 18G needle may be placed percutaneously directly over the depressed fragment as viewed arthroscopically. This can then be used as a landmark, and a large Steinmann pin is placed approximately

2 cm proximal to the 18G needle into the depressed lunate facet fragment. The Steinmann pin is then used to gently elevate the lunate facet fragment back in line with the previously reduced radial styloid fragment. A bone tenaculum may be very useful to further reduce any fracture gap that exists between the radial styloid fragment and the depressed lunate facet fracture. The bone tenaculum provides provisional fixation. Once the fracture fragment is found to be anatomic as viewed arthroscopically with the arthroscope both in the 3-4 and in the 6-R portals, guidewires are placed transversely from the radial styloid fragment subchondrally into the lunate facet fragment. If the lunate facet fragment is primarily dorsal, it is vital to aim the guidewires dorsally to capture this fracture fragment. In addition, it is easy to violate the distal radioulnar joint with the transverse guidewires. It is important to pronate and supinate the wrist to ensure that the transverse pins have not violated the distal radioulnar joint. The reason is that owing to the concave nature of the distal radioulnar joint, the pins that may appear under fluoroscopy do not penetrate the joint when in fact they have mechanically protruded into the space. For this reason, it is important to pronate and supinate the wrist to ensure there is no mechanical block to forearm rotation.

In the author's earlier experience, Kirschner wires alone were used to stabilize the fracture fragments. Now, headless cannulated screws are utilized if at all possible. One screw is placed to stabilize the radial styloid fragment, and one or two are then placed transversely to stabilize the lunate facet fragment. The use of headless cannulated screws increases soft tissue irritation, which enhances rehabilitation and promotes earlier range of motion. Bone grafting may be placed into a small dorsal incision between the fourth and the fifth dorsal compartments to avoid late settling of the fracture fragment if extensive metaphyseal comminution is present.

THREE- AND FOUR-PART FRACTURES WITH METAPHYSEAL COMMINUTION

A combination of open surgery and wrist arthroscopy is used for three- and four-part fractures with metaphyseal comminution. In patients who have a four-part fracture, the lunate facet is split into volar and dorsal fragments (Figs. 43.14 and 43.15). The volar fragment cannot be reduced with closed manipulation. Traction on the volar fragment causes rotation if it does not allow for a closed reduction. For this reason, an open approach is utilized to stabilize the volar ulnar fragment.

A standard volar approach is made to the distal radius centered over the radial side of the flexor carpi radialis tendon. The incision is placed on the radial side of the flexor carpi radialis tendon to protect the palmar cutaneous branch of the median nerve. The flexor carpi radialis tendon is identified and retracted radially to protect the radial artery. Next, the flexor pollicis longus tendon is identified and retracted ulnarly to protect the median nerve. The pronator quadratus is released from the radial border of the distal radius. It is quite helpful to release the brachioradialis from the radial styloid to facilitate reduction of this fracture fragment. However, it is important to release the brachioradialis from a proximal to distal direction. In this manner, there is decreased risk of injury to the tendons of the first dorsal compartment. The brachial radialis performs as a floor to the first dorsal compartment.

The joint capsule is not opened (Fig. 43.16). A volar plate is placed on the volar aspect of the distal radius.

The fracture is provisionally stabilized and pinned with Kirschner wires (Fig. 43.17). As always, the Kirschner wires are placed in oscillation mode to limit injury to the dorsal sensory branch of the radial nerve. The first screw is placed in the volar plate as in the offset hole so that the plate may be shifted proximally or distally. Under fluoroscopy, the fracture is reduced as anatomically as possible. Kirschner wires are placed through the plate to provide provisional stabilization.

The wrist is then suspended in the traction tower, and articular reduction is arthroscopically evaluated. The arthroscope is introduced into the standard 3-4 portal, working portal is made in the 6-R portal, and

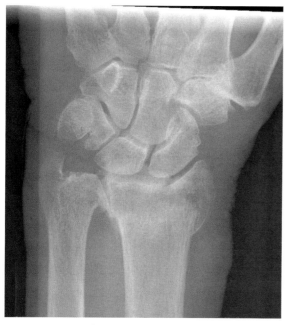

FIGURE 43.14. PA radiograph of a displaced four-part fracture to the distal radius.

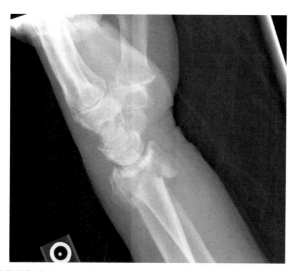

FIGURE 43.15. Lateral radiograph showing the lunate facet to be fractured in the anterior and posterior fragments.

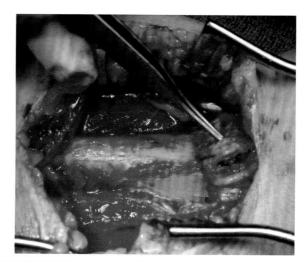

FIGURE 43.16. A standard volar approach centered over the flexor carpi radialis tendon is made. The fracture is reduced on the volar aspect.

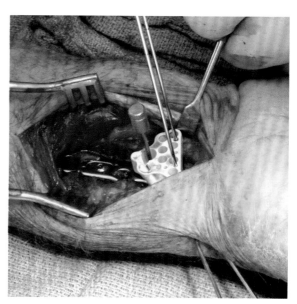

FIGURE 43.17. An Acumed Acu-Loc (Hillsboro, OR) plate is placed on the volar aspect of the distal radius. The intra-articular fracture is provisionally pinned under fluoroscopic visualization.

inflow in the 6-U portal. Locking and nonlocking screws are placed in the distal portion of the plate if the fracture reduction is deemed anatomic as viewed arthroscopically. If the reduction is not anatomic, the provisional Kirschner wires are removed from the plate, and reduction is fine tuned under arthroscopic visualization (Figs. 43.18 and 43.19). The plate is used as a fulcrum to further reduce the articular fragments with the wrist in traction in slight flexion manipulating the fracture fragment against the plate. It is important to ensure that there is no gap between the plate and the distal radius. Flexion of the wrist helps prevent any gaps between the plate and the fracture fragments. This will help decrease irritation to the flexor tendons and particularly to the flexor pollicis longus.

In four-part fractures, the lunate facet is divided into volar and dorsal fragments. Through a volar approach, the radial styloid fragment and the volar ulnar fragment are anatomically reduced back to the shaft of the distal radius. Furthermore, the joint capsule is not open and the reduction is performed extra-articularly utilizing the metaphyseal fracture pattern for the reduction. The volar distal radius plate is used to provisionally stabilize the radial styloid and the volar ulnar fragment. Ideally, a single distal fitting plate is utilized to stabilize both the radial styloid and the volar ulnar fragment. If the volar ulnar fragment is quite small and distal, then potentially a separate plate may be utilized to stabilize the radial styloid and the volar ulnar fragment. In this instance, the volar ulnar plate is placed. Sutures are then placed through the capsule and thus potentially through the fracture fragment and passed through the plate itself. The volar fracture fragments are provisionally stabilized

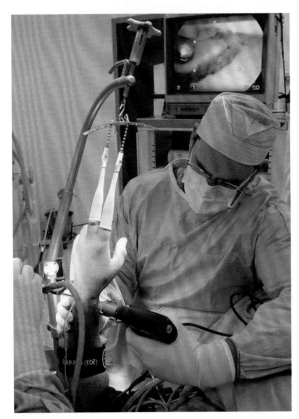

FIGURE 43.19. Under arthroscopic control, the fracture line will be anatomically reduced with percutaneous manipulation.

as previously described with either a single plate or dual plates.

The volar ulnar fragment is best visualized with the arthroscope in the 3-4 portal. The reduction of this fragment to the radial styloid is directly observed and any fine tuning will be performed at this point. Any rotation of the radial styloid fragment and the dorsal lunate fragment is best visualized with the arthroscope in the 6-R portal. The dorsal lunate fragment is visualized and percutaneously elevated up to the radial styloid and the previously reduced volar ulnar fragment (Figs. 43.20 and 43.21). The volar ulnar fragment has been previously reduced through the volar approach. This is used as a landmark to reduce the dorsal lunate fragment as viewed arthroscopically. Once anatomic reduction of the fracture fragments has been viewed arthroscopically, distal locking and nonlocking screws are then placed through the volar plate to stabilize the articular surface (Fig. 43.22).

Dorsal lip fracture fragments are best seen with the arthroscope in the 6-R portal. Alternatively, the arthroscope may be placed through the volar radial portal. This portal is made between the radial scaphocapitate ligament and the long radial lunate ligament. The portal is made by placing the arthroscope between the interval of the radial scaphocapitate and long radial lunate ligament. The arthroscope is then removed, and a trocar is placed into the cannula and advanced from an inside-to-outside technique tinting the skin volarly. The skin is incised on

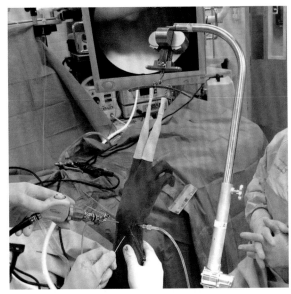

FIGURE 43.18. Arthroscopic visualization shows the fracture line still to be displaced. The lunate facet dorsal fragment is then percutaneously elevated as viewed arthroscopically.

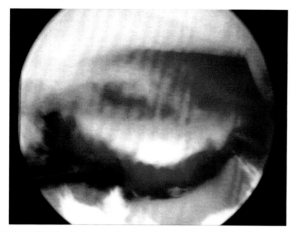

FIGURE 43.20. Arthroscopic view showing the displaced lunate facet fragment with the arthroscope in the 6-R portal.

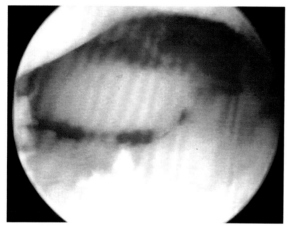

FIGURE 43.21. Following percutaneous elevation, the fracture line is now anatomic as viewed arthroscopically with the arthroscope in the 6-R portal.

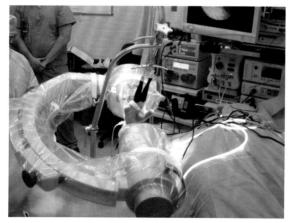

FIGURE 43.22. The reduction is confirmed with the C-arm following arthroscopic-assisted reduction.

the volar aspect of the wrist, and a cannula is then placed over a joystick placed between a dorsal cannula and entering the volar aspect of the incision. The cannula is placed over the joystick and advanced back into the wrist to form

a volar portal. It is the author's experience that usually the dorsal lip can be easily visualized from the 6-R portal. However, if difficulty is experienced, a volar radial portal can easily be made.

Volar plate stabilization using wrist arthroscopy as an adjunct to view the articular reduction is preferred if metaphyseal comminution is present (Figs. 43.23 and 43.24). Utilizing a strong volar plate allows a very stable construct, which enables early range of motion and rehabilitation compared with the use of Kirschner screws or headless screw alone. Potentially, this would avoid late settling of the fracture fragments when percutaneous Kirschner wires or cannulated screws are used alone. Patients also prefer the use of a plate compared with percutaneous Kirschner wires to avoid skin irritation and allow early range of motion.

ULNAR STYLOID FRAGMENT

There is considerable controversy over management of an associated ulnar styloid fragment. Information gained from arthroscopic evaluation of the wrist following stabilization of a distal radius fracture provides some rationale about when to stabilize an associated ulnar styloid fracture. Following reduction of a distal radius fracture, the patient's articular disk is palpated with a probe. The arthroscope is placed in the 3-4 portal, the probe is inserted through the 6-R portal, and the tension of the disk is evaluated. When there is good tension to the articular disk as it is palpated, the majority of the fibers of the triangular fibrocartilage complex are still attached to the base

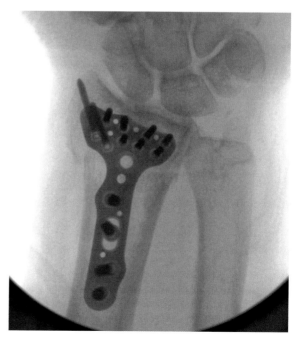

FIGURE 43.23. PA fluoroscopic view showing anatomic restoration to the joint surface.

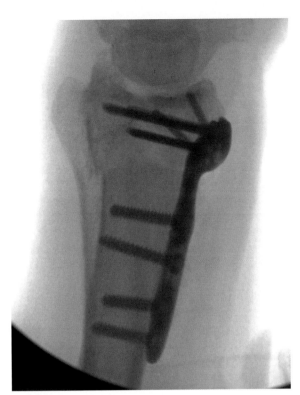

FIGURE 43.24. Lateral radiograph showing arthroscopic reduction to the volar and dorsal fragments of the four-part fracture to the distal radius.

of the ulna. A peripheral tear of the triangular fibrocartilage complex is suspected when there is loss of tension to the articular disk. Often, a peripheral tear is covered with hematoma (Fig. 43.25). The hematoma must be debrided with the shaver in the 6-R portal to allow direct visualization to the articular disk. The articular disk is best visualized with the arthroscope in the 3-4 portal.

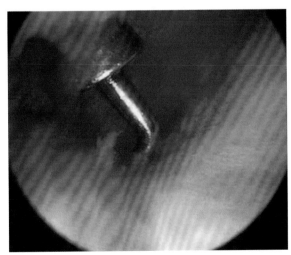

FIGURE 43.25. Following reduction to the distal radius, the distal radial ulnar joint is evaluated. Clinically, there is gross instability. Arthroscopic evaluation confirmed a peripheral tear to the articular disk of the triangular fibrocartilage complex with instability.

A peripheral tear of the triangular fibrocartilage complex is repaired arthroscopically when associated with the fracture to the distal radius (Figs. 43.26 and 43.27).

Stabilization of a large ulnar styloid fragment is considered when there is considerable tension to the articular disk and no peripheral ulnar tear of the articular disk is identified. In this instance, the majority of the fibers of the articular disk are attached to the ulnar styloid fragment alone. A small incision is made between the extensor carpi ulnaris and the flexor carpi ulnaris, and blunt dissection is carried down to protect the dorsal sensory branch of the ulnar nerve, which runs along the volar aspect of the incision. The ulnar styloid fragment is then anatomically reduced and stabilized by a tension band configuration, Kirschner wire, or preferably with a small headless cannulated screw to decrease soft tissue irritation.

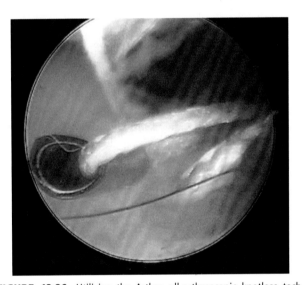

FIGURE 43.26. Utilizing the Arthex all-arthroscopic knotless technique, a horizontal stitch of 2.0 fiber wire is placed to the articular disk with the suture lasso.

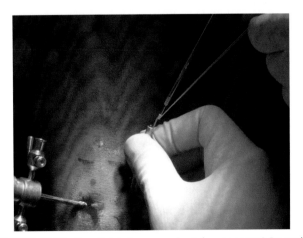

FIGURE 43.27. The stitch is then passed out the accessory 6-R portal, placed into a mini push lock anchor (Arthex, Naples, FL), and impacted into the distal ulna at the base of the fovea for all arthroscopic knotless repair of the disk back to bone.

III. The Wrist

DISCUSSION

The literature is relatively sparse regarding results of arthroscopic-assisted fixation of intra-articular displaced fractures of the distal radius. Stewart and Berger (13) presented a comparative study of 12 open and 12 arthroscopic-assisted reductions of comminuted intra-articular fractures of the distal radius. In the arthroscopic group, they noted five excellent, six good, and one fair result. The open group had no excellent results. The authors concluded that the arthroscopic group had significantly increased range of motion compared with the group that underwent open stabilization.

Similarly, Doi et al. (14) reported their results in a comparative study of 38 patients who underwent arthroscopic-assisted fixation as against patients who underwent open reduction. They found that the arthroscopic group had a significantly improved range of motion in comparison with the open group.

Ruch et al. (15) reported their results in a comparison study of 15 patients who underwent arthroscopic-assisted reduction as against 15 others who underwent closed reduction and were stabilized by external fixation. This study focused on the importance of associated soft tissue lesions. In the 15 patients who underwent arthroscopic reduction, 10 patients presented with an associated tear of the triangular fibrocartilage complex. Seven of these tears were peripheral and underwent arthroscopic repair. No patient in the arthroscopic group had any signs of instability of the distal radioulnar joint at final follow-up visit. Among the 15 patients who underwent closed reduction external fixation, 4 presented with chronic instability to the distal radioulnar joint. Potentially, these patients had an associated peripheral tear of the triangular fibrocartilage complex, which could be detected and managed at the same sitting as the fracture reduction.

Geissler and Freeland (16) reviewed their results of 33 patients who underwent arthroscopic-assisted reduction of comminuted intra-articular fractures of the distal radius. In their series, 25 patients had anatomic reduction and 8 had a 1-mm or less step-off. Utilizing the modified Mayo wrist score, there were 20 excellent, 10 good, and 3 fair results in their series. Simple articular fractures had a better result compared with complex articular fractures.

The authors particularly reviewed the results based on associated intra-articular soft tissue injuries. They noted that when a Geissler grade 2 scapholunate interosseous ligament was present, it did not affect the final prognosis. However, when a Geissler grade 3 or 4 tear was present in AO Type C fractures, it significantly affected the results. In the five patients with an AO Type C fracture without an interosseous ligament tear, all patients presented excellent results. However, in comparison, among the five patients with AO Type C fracture with a Geissler grade 3 or 4 interosseous ligament tear, there were four good results and one fair result. It appeared that the presence of a significant Geissler grade 3 or 4 interosseous ligament injury affected the final prognosis in their study.

Wrist arthroscopy is a valuable adjunct in the management of displaced intra-articular fractures of the distal radius (17, 18). It allows for evaluation of the joint surface under bright light and magnified conditions. As noted by the studies of Knirk and Jupiter (3) and substantially by others, restoration of the articular surface is significantly important for the patient's final prognosis. Arthroscopy, in particular, allows for detection of malrotation of fracture fragments, which is very difficult to judge under fluoroscopy. Arthroscopy allows for derotation of these fracture fragments and allows for potentially anatomic reduction as possible. In addition, washing the joint out of fracture debris and hematoma may allow for improved range of motion as noted by the studies of Stewart and Berger (13) and Doi et al. (14).

Wrist arthroscopy also allows for detection and management of associated intra-articular soft tissue injuries shown to occur with a high incidence with intra-articular fractures to the distal radius. Management of an acute soft tissue injury certainly has a better prognosis compared with a chronic reconstruction.

Tears of the triangular fibrocartilage complex have been shown to be often associated with fractures of the distal radius (19). This has been confirmed by several arthroscopic and arthrogram studies (6–10). This may be an explanation for why some patients continue to complain of ulnar-sided wrist pain for several months despite post anatomic restoration of the joint surface. As noted by Ruch et al. (15), repair of peripheral tears of the TFC resulted in no signs of instability of the distal radioulnar joint at final follow-up visit. Chondral defects or loose bodies that would normally not be seen on plain radiographs can be identified arthroscopically and removed from the radiocarpal and midcarpal spaces.

Finally, wrist arthroscopy provides some rationale for when or when not to stabilize the displaced large ulnar styloid fragment when associated with a fracture of the distal radius.

REFERENCES

1. Lafontaine M, Hardy D, Delince P. Stability assessment of distal radius fractures. *Injury.* 1989;20:208–210.
2. Edwards CC III, Harasztic J, McGillivary GR, et al. Intraarticular distal radius fractures: arthroscopic assessment of radiographically assisted reduction. *J Hand Surg.* 2001;26:A1036–A1041.
3. Knirk JL, Jupiter JB. Intraarticular fractures of the distal end of the radius in young adults. *J Bone Joint Surg.* 1986;68A:647–658.
4. Bradway JK, Amadio PC, Cooney WP. Open reduction and internal fixation of displaced comminuted intraarticular fractures of the distal end of the radius. *J Bone Joint Surg.* 1989;71A:839–847.
5. Fernandez DL, Geissler WB. Treatment of displaced articular fractures of the radius. *J Hand Surg.* 1991;16:375–384.

6. Mohanti RC, Kar N. Study of triangular fibrocartilage of the wrist joint in Colles' fracture. *Injury*. 1979;11:311–324.
7. Fontes D, Lenoble E, DeSomer B, et al. Lesions ligamentaires associus aux fractures distales du radius. *Ann Chir Main*. 1992;11:119–125.
8. Geissler WB, Freeland AE, Savoie FH, et al. Carpal instability associated with intraarticular distal radius fractures. In: Proceedings, American Academy Orthopedic Surgeons Annual Meeting; 1993; San Francisco, CA.
9. Hanker GJ. Wrist arthroscopy in distal radius fractures. In: Proceedings, Arthroscopy Association North America Annual Meeting; 1993; Albuquerque, NM.
10. Lindau T. Treatment of injuries to the ulnar side of the wrist occurring with distal radial fractures. *Hand Clin*. 2005;21:417–425.
11. Geissler WB. Arthroscopically assisted reduction of intraarticular fractures of the distal radius. *Hand Clin*. 1995;11:19–29.
12. Mudgal CS, Jones WA. Scapholunate diastasis: a component of fractures of the distal radius. *J Hand Surg*. 1990;15B:503–505.
13. Stewart NJ, Berger RA. Comparison study of arthroscopic as open reduction of comminuted distal radius fractures.

Presented at: 53rd Annual Meeting of the American Society for Surgery of the Hand (Programs and Abstracts); January 11, 1998; Scottsdale, AZ.
14. Doi K, Hatturi T, Otsuka K, et al. Intraarticular fractures of the distal aspect of the radius arthroscopically assisted reduction compared with open reduction and internal fixation. *J Bone Joint Surg*. 1999;81A:1093–1110.
15. Ruch DS, Vallee J, Poehling GG, et al. Arthroscopic reduction versus fluoroscopic reduction of intraarticular distal radius fractures. *Arthroscopy*. 2004;20:225–230.
16. Geissler WB, Freeland AE. Arthroscopically assisted reduction of intraarticular distal radial fractures. *Clin Orthop*. 1996;327:125–134.
17. Geissler WB, Savoie FH. Arthroscopic techniques of the wrist. *Mediguide Orthop*. 1992;11:1–8.
18. Geissler WB. Intraarticular distal radius fractures: the role of arthroscopy? *Hand Clin*. 2005;21:407–416.
19. Hollingworth R, Morris J. The importance of the ulnar side of the wrist in fractures of the distal end of the radius. *Injury*. 1976;7:263.

Endoscopic Carpal Tunnel Release: Chow Technique

James C. Y. Chow • James Campbell Chow • Athanasios A. Papachristos

INTRODUCTION

Historical Note

Sir James Paget first described a median nerve compression following a distal radius fracture in 1854 (1). Subsequently in 1880, James Putman, a neurologist from Boston, reported similar symptoms in a group of his patients. The first formal description of a surgical decompression for the treatment of this condition was reported in 1933 followed by Phalen's classic article in 1950. Since then, open carpal tunnel release has been established as the gold standard for the surgical treatment of carpal tunnel syndrome.

Dr. James C.Y. Chow began working on an endoscopic release of the transverse carpal ligament in 1985, unaware that Dr. Ichiro Okutsu in Japan as well as Dr. John Agee in California were concurrently and separately working toward similar goals. The primary motivation of Dr. Chow's concept was to create a method for the surgical treatment of carpal tunnel syndrome that would be able to preserve the unaffected surrounding normal anatomic structures of the wrist and hand. Through these pursuits, Dr. Chow developed the slotted cannula late in 1986. After a thorough cadaveric trial period, the procedure was completed in May 1987, and it was performed in a patient for the first time in September of the same year.

The first two reports in the literature on endoscopic carpal tunnel release (ECTR) Chow et al. (2). In the next year, Chow presented a conference paper based on his clinical results after ECTR in 149 cases at the 1990 AANA Annual Meeting in Orlando, Florida. In the fall of the same year, another conference paper by Agee et al. (3) was presented at the 1990 American Society for Surgery of the Hand Annual Meeting in Toronto, Canada, regarding the clinical results of a multicenter study with the use of the Agee technique for the endoscopic release of the carpal ligament. Since the publishing of the three original endoscopic carpal ligament release techniques, there has been an increasingly continuous interest and much debate among surgeons regarding the safety and efficacy of the endoscopic procedure versus that of the open one. Several modifications and variations to the three original ideas have been made since their initial demonstration.

Anatomy/Pathoanatomy

The carpal tunnel is bounded deeply by the volar surface of the distal radius, ulnarly by the hook of hamate, radially by the scaphoid, and superficially by the confluence of the rather stout transverse carpal ligament, palmar aponeurosis, and antebrachial fascia. The carpal tunnel contains nine tendons (the flexor digitorum sublimus and profundus to all four fingers and the flexor pollicus longus) as well as the median nerve.

Carpal tunnel syndrome is a compressive neuropathy of the median nerve at the wrist. As such, it can result from any etiology that increases intracarpal tunnel pressure. This can include irritation and swelling of any of the nine flexor tendons and their tenosynovium, edema of the median nerve itself, anatomical abnormality or scarring of any of the bordering structures of the carpal tunnel, anomalous lumbrical anatomy, an intracarpal tunnel mass (such as a deep ganglion cyst), or stiffening and contracture of the transverse carpal ligament itself.

Over the past 25 years of endoscopic carpal ligament release surgery, an otherwise undescribed soft tissue structure has become evident. Further cadaver dissection has revealed an additional soft-tissue band, volar to the resected carpal ligament. This soft tissue band courses between the thenar and the hypothenar musculatures (Fig. 44.1). Microscopic examination shows this band to be a distinct structure when compared with the transverse carpal ligament. While the carpal ligament is formed solely by compact collagen fibers, this soft tissue band contains small nerves and vessels (Fig. 44.2). In reference to its location, the authorship has named this structure the "intramuscular soft-tissue band." Because of its location and histology, the authorship believes that the preservation of this anatomy is paramount for the rapid recovery seen in ECTR compared with open carpal tunnel release. Theoretically, this can be attributed to (1) prevention of bowstringing of the flexor tendon, (2) decreased pain (possibly pillar pain),

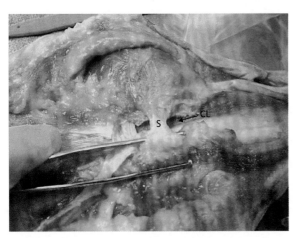

FIGURE 44.1. Anatomical study. S, soft tissue band; CL, carpal ligament.

and family history. Congenital diseases or anomalies, connective tissue diseases, systemic and metabolic disorders, and a previous sustained injury to the distal forearm and wrist should be taken into consideration.

Physical examination is critical for accurate diagnosis. In an acute case, there is tenderness along the carpal canal area. Light percussion over the median nerve at the wrist area produces an "electric current" sensation that radiates to the median nerve distribution known as Tinel sign. Phalen sign is evoked by holding the wrists at maximum flexion and the dorsal aspects of the hands in full contact such as a "reverse praying" position. This position narrows the carpal canal and if it reproduces the paresthesias in the fingers within 60 seconds, the sign is considered positive. As the pathologic condition advances, less time is necessary to evoke a response. Other examinations include

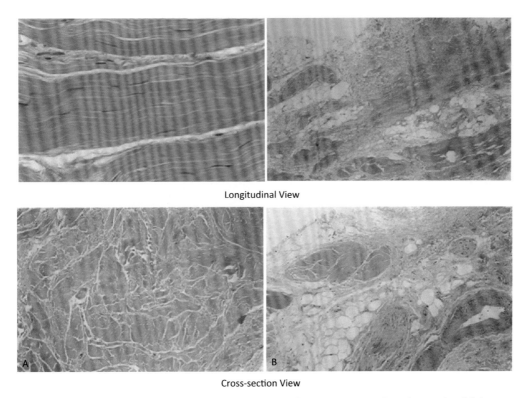

Longitudinal View

Cross-section View

FIGURE 44.2. Microscopic examination of carpal ligament **(A)** versus intramuscular soft tissue band **(B)**.

(3) decreased bleeding, and (4) increased muscle strength of the thenar and hypothenar muscles.

CLINICAL EVALUATION

Carpal tunnel syndrome accounts for approximately 463,673 carpal tunnel releases performed annually in the United States (4). Patients who have developed this syndrome usually present with a history of characteristic symptoms such as nocturnal pain and paresthesias, numbness in the median nerve distribution distal to the wrist, and thenar muscular weakness. In addition, the physician should be aware of the patient's general health condition

the monofilament test, two-point discrimination, reverse Phalen's test, and tourniquet test. In the late stages, with thenar muscle atrophy, one can observe the muscle waste in the thenar area. Muscle weakness is tested subjectively by resisted palmar abduction of the thumb against the examiner's index finger and comparison of one hand with the other.

A carefully performed history and physical examination can help the physician distinguish between an isolated compression neuropathy at the wrist and a double crush syndrome (5). Clinical correlation of the double crush phenomenon has been demonstrated by the high incidence of concurrent carpal syndrome in patients with

III. The Wrist

cervical radiculopathy. An equally high incidence of associated carpal tunnel syndrome with a more proximal entrapment of the median nerve has also been reported (6). Therefore, the physician must concomitantly exclude thoracic outlet syndrome, pronator compression syndrome in the forearm, and CNS disease.

Electromyography and nerve conduction velocity (NCV) tests aid in the detection of carpal tunnel syndrome. Indications for surgery should not be decided or altered according to the results of NCV tests, especially when the results are normal but the patient has the clinical signs and symptoms of the syndrome. A delay of the distal latency of the median nerve of 7.0 milliseconds or longer represents significant compression of the median nerve; if present, surgery should be considered without further delay. The most important aspects in diagnosing carpal tunnel syndrome are the history and physical examination. Electrodiagnostic studies of the median nerve are an adjunct used to confirm the diagnosis and perhaps suggest how the patient will respond to surgery.

Wrist radiography can rule out the possibility of congenital or acquired bone and joint deformity, abnormality, or pathology. Previously sustained fractures of the distal forearm and wrist should be taken into consideration. A malunited fracture of the distal radius, previously performed surgery in the wrist area, and a hypoplastic or aplastic hook of the hamate (7) can produce difficulties for the surgeon while placing and operating through the slotted cannula. Therefore, standard anteroposterior and lateral views of the distal forearm-wrist and a tunnel view of the wrist are required. If a more extensive study is indicated, MRI, CT scan, ultrasound, bone scan, or arthrogram of the wrist may be necessary.

TREATMENT

Conservative Management

Conservative management includes daily or nightly wrist splinting, alteration of daily activities, physical therapy, and nonsteroidal anti-inflammatory oral medication. Intracarpal tunnel steroid injections have been used with varying reported success.

Open versus Arthroscopic Management

The indications for the open surgical release of transverse carpal tunnel ligament have been well established and, in most cases, they apply to ECTR.

The advantages of endoscopic over open carpal tunnel release include the following: no hypertrophic scar or scar tenderness, no pillar pain, less compromise to pinch or grip strength, and an earlier return to work and daily activities. However, ECTR has the potential to become a dangerous procedure if performed by an inexperienced surgeon (8). Considerable intraoperative complications have been reported throughout the United States by surgeons using this technique (9, 10). This situation has raised a

controversy among surgeons regarding the value of endoscopic carpal tunnel surgery. However, it has also been shown that ECTR can be performed safely by experienced surgeons. Despite its steep learning curve, ECTR can give both the patient and the surgeon a great deal of satisfaction (11). As the knowledge, technique, and instrumentation have evolved, the safety of ECTR has improved.

AUTHORS' PREFERRED TREATMENT: TWO-PORTAL ENDOSCOPIC TECHNIQUE

The original technique was described by Chow as a transbursal approach to the carpal tunnel requiring penetration of the ulnar bursa. Based on the results of a multicenter study, the original technique has been modified in an attempt to decrease the complications and the learning curve. The conversion to an extrabursal technique has made the surgical procedure much easier and safer, thus offering a better visualization of the proximal transverse carpal ligament. The following is a description of the extrabursal, dual-portal technique.

Operating Room Setup

The patient is placed in a supine position and a hand table is used. Two video monitors are preferred, although some surgeons can manage the procedure with only one. One of the two monitors should face the surgeon and the other should face the assistant. The surgeon sits on the ulnar side of the patient and the assistant faces the surgeon (Fig. 44.3). The arthroscopic equipment consists of a short 4.0 mm × 30° video endoscope that prevents light guide from interfering with the patient's forearm by having the light post on the same side as the direction of view, a camera apparatus, a light cord, a camera input device, and a light source device. Optional equipment includes a DVD video recorder and a video printer for the printing of any captured images. Water pump and shaver equipment are not used.

A standard handset should be available. Specific instrumentation for the procedure, designed by Dr. Chow,

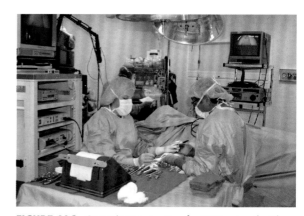

FIGURE 44.3. Operating room setup for ECTR using the Chow dual-portal technique.

comprises an ECTRA System Kit and an ECTRA Disposable Kit (Smith & Nephew Endoscopy, Andover, MA). The ECTRA System Kit includes the video endoscope, slotted cannula, dissecting obturator, curved blunt dissector, palmar arch suppressor, probe, retractors, and hand holder. The dissecting obturator is attached with a detachable handle that can also take some other types of obturators included in the kit (conical or boat-nose obturator), although the latter is not being used routinely. The ECTRA Disposable Kit includes a probe knife, a triangle knife, a retrograde knife, a hand pad, and swabs. These knives allow the surgeon to determine both the direction and the depth of cut. Standard preparations and draping are performed as usual without the application of a tourniquet. Before the introduction of local anesthesia, a skin marker is used to map landmarks for the entry and exit portals.

Anesthesia

Local anesthesia combined with intravenous medication is recommended for the procedure because it allows the patient and the surgeon to communicate. An alert patient can inform the surgeon, during the procedure, about any abnormal sensation in the hand, indicating a potential problem from any variance of nerve structure in the wrist and palm region (12–14). Usually, when the patient first comes into the operating room, fentanyl citrate (Sublimaze) (Baxter Healthcare Corporation, Westlake Village, CA) 100 µg is given intravenously. This is a narcotic analgesic type of medication with an onset period of 7 to 8 minutes and a peak action of approximately 30 minutes. Normally, the surgical time does not exceed 10 minutes. Xylocaine 1% (Astra, Westboro, MA) without epinephrine is injected at the entry and exit portals, approximately 2 to 3 cc at the entry portal and 6 to 7 cc at the exit portal owing to the higher degree of sensitivity of the skin on the palmar region. Special care is taken to limit the injection to the skin and subcutaneous tissue and to avoid affecting the nerve by penetrating deeply.

Positioning the Entry Portal

The proximal end of the pisiform bone is palpated on the volar surface of the wrist within the flexor carpi ulnaris tendon at the distal wrist flexor crease and is marked with a small circle. A line from the proximal pole of the pisiform is drawn radially, approximately 1.0 to 1.5 cm in length. From this point, a second 0.5-cm line is drawn proximally. A third dotted line, approximately 1.0 cm in length, is drawn radially from the proximal end of the second line to create the entry portal (Fig. 44.4A). The average dimensions of these lines will vary slightly, depending on the overall size of the hand.

Positioning the Exit Portal

The patient's thumb is placed in full abduction. A line is drawn across the palm from the distal border of the thumb to the approximate center of the palm, perpendicular to the long axis of the forearm. A second line is drawn from

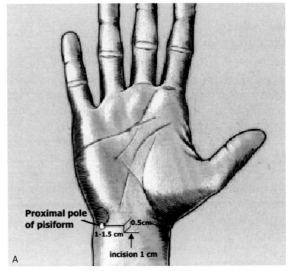

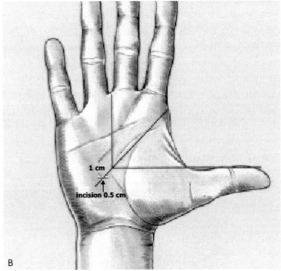

FIGURE 44.4. **A:** The entry portal is located by drawing a line 1 to 1.5 cm radially from the proximal pole of the pisiform bone, then drawing an approximately one-third length from the end of the first one, and finally, drawing an approximately 1-cm third line radially from the proximal end of the second line to create the entry portal. **B:** The exit portal is located by drawing a line from the distal border of the fully abducted thumb perpendicular to the long axis of the forearm. A second line is drawn from the third web space parallel to the long axis of the forearm. These two lines form a right angle. A third line is drawn, bisecting this angle and extending approximately 1.0 cm from its vertex to determine the exit portal.

the third web space, parallel to the long axis of the forearm, to meet the first line. These two lines should form a right angle. A third line is drawn, bisecting this angle and extending approximately 1.0 cm proximally from its vertex, which serves to establish the site of incision for the exit portal (Fig. 44.4B). The surgeon should be able to palpate the hook of hamate. The exit portal should fall into the soft spot at the center of the palm and line up with the ring finger, just slightly radial to the hook of hamate.

Creation of Portals and Placement of the Cannula

The procedure begins with the creation of the entry portal. A transverse incision of approximately 1.0 cm length (Fig. 44.5A) is made at the marked entry portal site extending just through the skin. Subcutaneous tissue is bluntly dissected off the volar forearm fascia with the use of a hemostat and is retracted with the retractors. Care must be taken to avoid damage to the small subcutaneous blood vessels. A knife is used to make a small longitudinal opening of the antebrachial fascia that is extended distally with the use of a Stephen's tenotomy scissors (Fig. 44.5B, C). If the palmaris longus is present, the longitudinal cut should be along the ulnar border of the palmaris longus tendon. Care should be taken, as sometimes there are two layers of fascia that must both be cut. Retractors are passed just beneath the fascia with one of them lifting the skin distally to create a vacuum that will separate the transverse carpal ligament from the ulnar bursa. A blunt curved dissector is gently slipped into the carpal tunnel just under the transverse carpal ligament. Maneuvering the dissector back and forth should result in a type of "washboard" feeling owing to the rough undersurface of the carpal ligament. The curved dissector is then removed. A dissecting obturator/slotted cannula assembly unit can now be guided into the space vacated by the curved dissector. The slotted cannula assembly is advanced into the carpal tunnel on the underside of the transverse carpal ligament to the level of the hook of hamate, staying to the ulnar side of the carpal tunnel (Fig. 44.5D). With the tip of this unit touching the hook of the hamate, the surgeon gently picks up and hyperextends the hand. The hand and cannula assembly are now moved as a unit (Fig. 44.5E) and placed on the hand holder with the wrist and fingers in full hyperextension. The cannula assembly is advanced along the under surface of the carpal ligament, while the assistant keeps the hand onto the hand holder, until the tip of the cannula assembly can be easily palpated in the palm area where the mark for the exit portal was previously made. A small transverse or oblique incision is made just over the palpable cannula assembly tip cutting only the skin (Fig. 44.5F). The palmar skin and soft tissue are depressed using the palmar arch suppressor, and the cannula assembly is then pushed into the receptacle of the palmar arch suppressor to exit through the distal portal (Fig. 44.5G). The obturator is then removed from the cannula, which should lie just below the transverse carpal ligament, and the hyperextended hand is strapped onto the hand holder (Fig. 44.5H). Hyperextension of the wrist brings the superficial palmar arch to a level lower than the exiting point of the slotted cannula assembly, thereby protecting it from injury. The creation of two portals is very essential, because they serve to stabilize the slotted cannula while it passes through both of them and thus ensure the reproducibility of the technique.

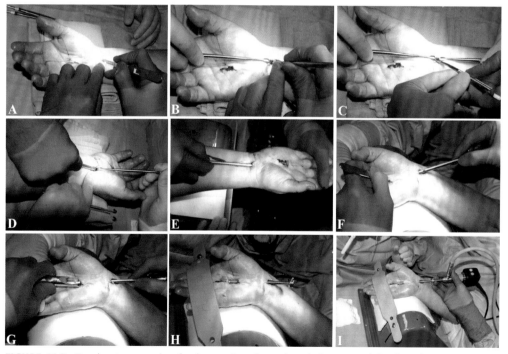

FIGURE 44.5. Step-by-step procedure for the creation of portals and placement of the slotted cannula. **A:** Skin incision. **B, C:** A small longitudinal opening of the antebrachial fascia is created and is extended distally using a tenotomy scissors. **D:** Insertion of the dissecting obturator/slotted cannula assembly into the carpal canal. **E:** Placement of the hand onto the hand holder. **F, G:** Skin incision, and use of the arch suppressor in order for the cannula assembly to exit through the distal portal. **H:** The dissecting obturator has been removed leaving the slotted cannula into the carpal canal. **I:** The scope is inserted into the carpal canal through the proximal portal.

The slotted portion of the cannula allows a safe cutting zone, while delicate structures such as the median nerve and flexor tendons are protected by the walls of the cannula.

Endoscopic Examination

The video endoscope is inserted into the slotted cannula at the proximal portal (Fig. 44.5I). The camera and scope should rest comfortably in the first web space of the surgeon's hand. A cotton swab can be inserted into the tube from the distal portal to clean the lens while the focus is adjusted to the best visualization (Fig. 44.6A). A blunt probe is inserted to palpate the undersurface of the transverse carpal ligament (Fig. 44.6B) proximally to distally, and in case a thin bursal membrane is seen above the cannula's slotted opening, this is carefully dissected with the probe to gain access to the ligament, which has an "ivory type" white appearance with its fibers running transversely. If the median nerve is present (Fig. 44.7A), the patient will feel sharp pain radiating to the fingers when the nerve is probed and this should alert the surgeon. If abundant soft tissue is noted in the opening of the cannula, the procedure should not be performed. The slotted cannula may need to be reinserted to ensure a better visualization; however, to avoid irreversible damage, surgery should not be carried out if tendons (Fig. 44.7B) or other important structures are entrapped between the slotted cannula and the undersurface of the carpal ligament.

If there is only a minimal amount of synovium obstructing the view, the obturator is replaced into the slotted cannula. The slotted cannula assembly unit can then be rotated radially about 355° to 360° to provide the visualization and protection required. It has to be emphasized that surgeons should not hesitate to convert an endoscopic procedure to an open one if they are not able to obtain adequate visualization.

Technique for the Release of the Transverse Carpal Ligament

With the scope in the proximal portal and the probe in the distal portal, the distal border of the transverse carpal ligament is identified. The probe knife, which permits forward cutting only, is inserted into the distal portal. The blunt edge of the knife can be used to probe proximally to distally along the ligament. The cutting edge is then used to release the distal border of the ligament by drawing the knife distally to proximally (Fig. 44.8A). Anything beyond the distal border of the carpal ligament should not be excised. The scope is withdrawn proximally about 1 cm, and the triangle knife is used to make a small upward cut in the midsection of the ligament (Fig. 44.8B). The retrograde knife is now inserted through the distal portal, and its blunt tip is gently positioned at the incision made by the triangle knife (Fig. 44.9B.1, B.2). The proximal cutting edge of the retrograde knife is drawn distally, making an incision that joins the previous two cuts, thereby completing the release of the distal portion of the transverse carpal ligament (Fig. 44.9B.3, B.4).

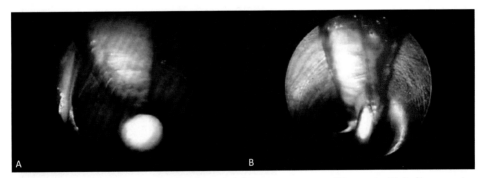

FIGURE 44.6. A: Endoscopic normal appearance of the transverse carpal ligament with its fibers running transversely. **B:** The thicker bursal membrane that sheathes the undersurface of the proximal portion of the carpal ligament has been probed proximally depicting the fibers of ligament.

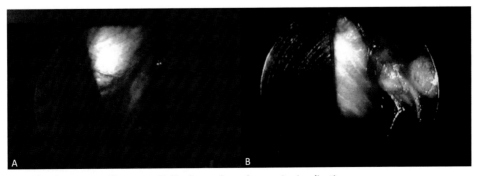

FIGURE 44.7. A: Median nerve. **B:** Tendon under arthroscopic visualization.

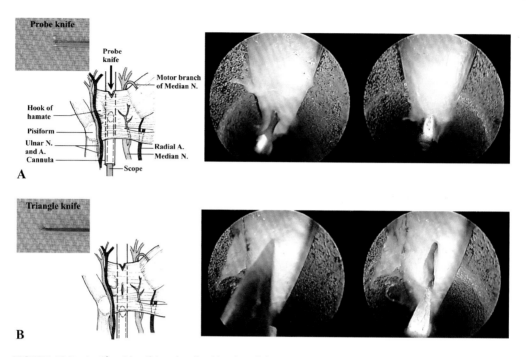

FIGURE 44.8. A: After identifying the distal border of the transverse carpal ligament, the probe knife is used to make the first cut distally to proximally. **B:** The scope is withdrawn proximally and the triangle knife is used to make a small cut in the midsection of the transverse carpal ligament. A, artery; N, nerve.

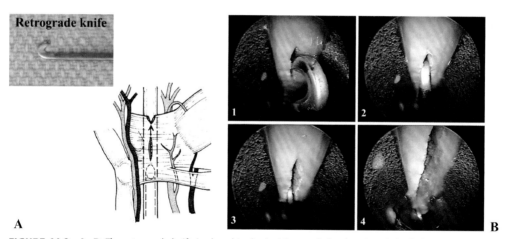

FIGURE 44.9. A, B: The retrograde knife is placed in the incision made by the triangle knife **(B1, B2),** and it is drawn distally to make an incision that joins the previous two cuts **(B3, B4).**

The scope is removed from the proximal portion and inserted into the distal opening of the slotted cannula. The camera view on the screen now forms a mirror effect. The surgeon should realize that the previous ulnar side is now the radial side. By moving the scope proximally and distally, the previous distal cut is identified. The probe knife is inserted into the proximal portal and is drawn toward the level of the previous distal cut with its blunt tip touching the underside of the transverse carpal ligament, just before the beginning of the distal cut (Fig. 44.10B1). From this point, the blunt edge of the knife is used to retract the thick

bursal membrane, which sheathes the proximal portion of the carpal ligament, distally to proximally along the ligament's undersurface (Fig. 44.10B.2). When the cutting edge of the knife has engaged to the proximal border of the ligament, the knife is advanced distally to make an incision that joins the previous cut and thus to accomplish the release of the transverse carpal ligament (Fig. 44.10B.3, B.4). This is a slight modification of the technique that was described in previous textbooks, (15, 16) where the retrograde knife was used to complete the release of the ligament. The thick bursal membrane contains small vessels, and it should be

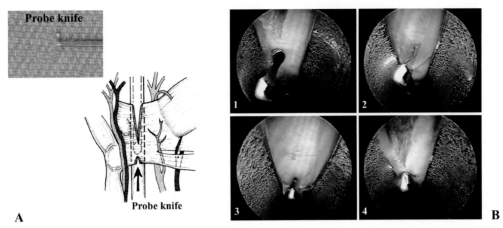

FIGURE 44.10. A, B: Once the scope has been switched from the proximal to the distal opening of the slotted cannula, the tip of the probe knife is placed just before the beginning of the distal cut **(B1)**. From this point, the knife's blunt edge is used to retract the thick bursal membrane distally to proximally **(B2)**. When the knife has engaged to the proximal border of the transverse carpal ligament, it is advanced distally to complete the release of the ligament **(B3, B4)**.

preserved to avoid bleeding into the carpal canal. Finally, the slotted cannula is gently rotated about a few degrees, clockwise and counterclockwise sequentially, enabling the surgeon to view the edges of the transected carpal ligament. If there are any additional fibers remaining, the triangle knife, or any other knife that feels appropriate, can be used to release these fibers until the surgeon is satisfied.

Owing to the position of the patient's hand, the cut edges of the transverse carpal ligament should spring apart and disappear from the slotted opening of the cannula. If the edges can still be seen through the opening, the release is incomplete. Although the assistant fully abducts the patient's thumb, the uncut portion of the ligament can be identified and the surgeon is able to complete the transection. There is a soft tissue band that bridges the thenar and hypothenar musculatures lying volar to the transverse carpal ligament that has to be preserved as well as the palmaris brevis muscle, if present. This soft tissue band prevents bowstringing of the flexor tendons after surgery, thereby maintaining their strength during contraction. Only one suture is required for the closure of each portal. Immediately after the procedure, the surgeon should clinically examine the patient while still in a sterilized environment. If there is any dysfunction indicating intraoperative damage to the median nerve or tendons, exposure and exploration of the carpal tunnel can be performed at the same time.

COMPLICATIONS, CONTROVERSIES, AND SPECIAL CONSIDERATIONS

Several complications after ECTR with the use of the Chow technique have been reported in the literature. Nagle et al. (17) performed a multicenter prospective review study on 640 cases. The initial transbursal technique was used in 110 cases and the modified extrabursal technique was used in the remaining 530 cases. An overall (perioperative and late) complication rate of 11% was found in the cases that were done with the transbursal technique compared with 2.2% in the cases that were done with the extrabursal technique. Perioperative complications occurred in 21 of the total 640 cases (3.3%). Fourteen of these 21 cases involved neurapraxia, all of which resolved without sequelae, and no nerves were lacerated or transected. There was one laceration of the superficial flexor tendon of the ring and small fingers, four incomplete releases, and two cases with hematoma and laceration of the superior palmar arch. Late complications included three cases of reflex sympathetic dystrophy (0.5%). This complication resolved in all cases without the use of sympathetic nerve blocks. The authors of this study concluded that ECTR using the dual-portal extrabursal technique reliably decompresses the carpal tunnel and can be effectively performed with low perioperative and late complication rates.

Malek and Chow (10) in a national study of the complications of 10,246 cases in 9,562 patients using the dual-portal Chow technique found a complication rate of 2.3% (240 cases with complications were reported). Of these, there were 154 nerve-related complications (median or ulnar nerve neurapraxias, lacerations, and transections), 38 complications related to blood vessels, 15 tendon injuries, 18 incomplete releases of the transverse carpal ligament, and 6 reflex sympathetic dystrophy complications. The remaining nine were listed as miscellaneous complications, including hematoma or superficial wound infection. The majority of intraoperative nerve injuries occurred in cases where general or regional anesthesia was used.

The complication rates of ECTR that have been reported compare favorably with published series of open carpal tunnel release. Complications of the latter include incomplete ligament release, nerve injuries, palmar hematomas, bowstringing of the flexor tendons, adhesions between nerve and tendons, reflex sympathetic dystrophy, deep wound infections, scar tenderness, pillar pain, tendon lacerations, and vascular injuries. Most of the damage to the surrounding anatomical structures that occur during carpal tunnel surgery, either open or endoscopic, usually requires a second surgical procedure to be repaired.

PEARLS AND PITFALLS

Pearls

1. When administering local anesthetic, preference is given to the subcutaneous regions proximally at the entry portal and distally at the exit portal. These are the areas of greatest pressure from the slotted cannula.
2. To best visualize the fibers of the transverse carpal ligament, the light source must often be dimmed. The senior author routinely turns off the "auto" function on his light source and dims it according to the available picture. This can markedly improve visualization, and thus safety, during the procedure.
3. Because of the symmetric nature of the visual field, it is easy to lose orientation when operating through the slotted cannula. To avoid this, the senior author always introduces instrumentation into the cannula with the blade facing ulnarly.
4. It is safest not to use a tourniquet. This allows palpation of the ulnar artery before making the skin incision for the entry portal, thus protecting the ulnar neurovascular bundle.
5. If necessary, your assistant can provide direct pressure to the palm between the two portals over the slotted cannula to control bleeding while operating.

Pitfalls

As with any endoscopic procedure, visualization is paramount. Regardless of the circumstance, if the surgeon is unable to obtain a clear view of the undersurface of the carpal ligament, the endoscopic procedure should be abandoned.

A common pitfall is the ulnar placement of the entry portal. To avoid this situation, the following steps should be taken:

1. Watch the entire width of the wrist to ensure the central location of the entry portal.
2. Make sure that the landmarks of both the entry and the exit portals are aligned along the long axis of the forearm.
3. Palpate and mark the hook of hamate. Both portals should be located radially to the hook of hamate.
4. During the entire procedure, surgical instruments that are introduced in the wrist and hand should follow the long axis of the forearm.

REHABILITATION

Active range of motion is encouraged immediately after the effects of local anesthesia have subsided. The patient is advised to avoid heavy lifting or pressure on the palm region until the discomfort disappears, usually within 2 to 3 weeks. Active movement of the fingers decreases the formation of scar tissue in the wrist region and therefore prevents adhesions on the tendons or nerve at the surgical site. Sutures are removed in 1 week. If the patient engages in hard occupational activities, such as heavy lifting, too soon after surgery, there might be swelling and prolonged pain in the palm region. If these occur, myofascial release and fluidotherapy treatment will help to decrease the condition.

CONCLUSIONS AND FUTURE DIRECTIONS

The advantages of endoscopic over open carpal tunnel release include absence of hypertrophic scar or scar tenderness, no pillar pain, less compromise to the pinch or grip strength, and an earlier return to work and daily activities. However, the surgeon can be in front of unexpected difficulties (e.g., ganglion, neurofibroma, neurilemmoma) that limit visualization into the carpal canal. As in any surgical procedure, safety and success are dependent upon a thorough knowledge of the anatomy of the area, adequate training, and familiarity with the uses and capabilities of the instrumentation. Surgeons who are not familiarized with endoscopes and arthroscopic techniques may give rise to major iatrogenic complications.

In addition, recognition of the intramuscular soft tissue band is both new and important. Common awareness of this structure may change the fundamental understanding of compressive neuropathies at the wrist and the associated carpal ligament release. The Chow dual-portal technique may be the most favorable method to preserve this valuable anatomic structure.

Data gathered from the experience of the past 25 years strongly indicate that, owing to the preservation of normal anatomical structures of the hand (specifically the intramuscular soft-tissue band), clinical results of ECTR are better than those of the standard open procedure. ECTR with the Chow dual-portal technique is a reliable method of treating carpal tunnel syndrome and can be performed safely by a well-trained surgeon. Although a debate among surgeons still exists, the endoscopic release of the transverse carpal ligament has established its position as an accepted minimally invasive surgical technique.

REFERENCES

1. Pfeffer GB, Gelberman RH, Boyes JH, et al. The history of carpal tunnel syndrome. *J Hand Surg [Br]*. 1988;13:28.
2. Chow JCY. Endoscopic release of the carpal ligament: a new technique for carpal tunnel syndrome. *Arthroscopy* 1989; 5:19–24.; Okutsu I, Nonomiya S, Takatori Y, Ugawa Y. Endoscopic management of carpal tunnel syndrome. *Arthroscopy* 1989; 5:11

3. Agee JM, Tortsua RD, Palmer CA, Berry C. Endoscopic release of the carpal tunnel: a prospective randomized multicenter study. Presented at: 45th Annual Meeting of the American Society for Surgery of the Hand; September 24–27, 1990; Toronto, Canada.

4. Duncan KH, Lewis RC, Foreman KA, et al. Treatment of carpal tunnel syndrome by members of the American Society for Surgery of the Hand: results of a questionnaire. *J Hand Surg [Am]*. 1987;12:384–391.

5. Upton A, McComas A. The double crush in nerve entrapment syndromes. *Lancet*. 1973;2:359.

6. Hurst L, Weissberg D, Carroll R. The relationship of the double crush to carpal tunnel syndrome (an analysis of 1000 cases of carpal tunnel syndrome). *J Hand Surg [Br]*. 1985;10:202–204.

7. Chow JC, Weiss MA, Gu Y. Anatomic variations of the hook of hamate and the relationship to carpal tunnel syndrome. *J Hand Surg [Am]*. 2005;30:1242–1247.

8. Chow JCY, Malek M, Nagle D. Complications of endoscopic release of the carpal ligament using the Chow technique. Presented at: 47th Annual Meeting of the American Society for Surgery of the Hand; November 11–14, 1992; Phoenix, AZ.

9. Chow JCY, Malek MM. Complications of endoscopic release of the carpal ligament using the Chow technique. Presented at: 60th Annual Meeting of the American Academy of Orthopaedic Surgeons; February 18–23, 1993; San Francisco, CA.

10. Malek MM, Chow JCY. National study of the complications of over 10,000 cases of endoscopic carpal tunnel release. Presented at: 61st Annual Meeting of the American Academy of Orthopaedic Surgeons; February 24–March 1, 1994; New Orleans, LA.

11. Chow JC, Hantes ME. Endoscopic carpal tunnel release: thirteen years' experience with the Chow technique. *J Hand Surg [Am]*. 2002;27:1011–1018.

12. Mannerfelt L, Hybbinette CH. Important anomaly of the thenar motor branch of the median nerve. *Bull Hosp Jt Dis*. 1972;33:15.

13. Lanz U. Anatomical variations of the median nerve in the carpal tunnel. *J Hand Surg [Am]*. 1977;2:44.

14. Seradge H, Seradge E. Median innervated hypothenar muscle: anomalous branch of median nerve in the carpal tunnel. *J Hand Surg [Am]*. 1990;15:356–359.

15. Chow JCY. Endoscopic carpal tunnel release. In: Chow JCY, ed. *Advanced Arthroscopy*. New York, NY: Springer-Verlag; 2001:271–286.

16. Chow JCY. Carpal tunnel release. In: McGinty JB, ed. *Operative Arthroscopy*. 3rd ed. Philadelphia, PA: Lippincott Williams & Wilkins; 2003:798–818.

17. Nagle D, Fischer T, Harris G, et al. A multi-center prospective review of 640 endoscopic carpal tunnel releases using the Chow technique. *Arthroscopy*. 1996;12:139–143.

III. The Wrist

Clinical Assessment and Patient Selection for Hip Arthroscopy

Olusanjo Adeoye • Marc R. Safran

There has been a recent increase in interest and awareness of nonarthritic hip injuries in the active population. As our understanding of hip pathology progresses, noninvasive imaging techniques improve, and arthroscopic and other minimally invasive operative techniques continue to evolve, the focus is shifting toward earlier identification and treatment of hip pathology. Emerging treatment options may address some of these conditions in the early stages and prevent or slow the progression of hip degeneration.

The differential diagnosis of hip pain is quite broad in the active population. Hip pain can be caused by intra-articular or surrounding extra-articular pathology or be referred to the hip from a variety of truncal sources. Intra-articular sources of hip pain include labral tears, chondral damage, ligamentum teres tears, loose bodies, femoroacetabular impingement, hip dysplasia, and hip instability (15). Periarticular sources include greater trochanteric bursitis, snapping hip syndrome, hip flexor strains and tendinopathy, hamstring strain and tendinopathy, piriformis syndrome, and gluteus medius tendinopathy and tears. Furthermore, the hip is commonly a location of referred pain from the lumbar spine and sacrum as well as the abdomen and pelvis. It is important to examine the spine, pelvis, and abdomen to rule out referred pain from those areas. Details of those examinations are beyond the scope of this chapter.

Making a correct diagnosis is imperative to appropriate management of hip injuries. A careful history, physical examination, and standard radiographs may provide important clues, with advanced imaging, such as MRI arthrography, helping confirm the diagnosis. Arthroscopy has also been advocated as a diagnostic tool for intra-articular hip pathology, although this is necessary in only a small minority of patients. As we begin to understand hip anatomy, mechanics, and pathomechanics better, improvements and refinements in examination and imaging will also advance, along with management options.

CLINICAL EVALUATION

Pertinent History

The first step in evaluating the hip is to obtain a thorough history from the patient. The presence or absence of trauma (including mechanism of injury), as well as the location of the pain, onset, duration, and severity of symptoms should be determined. Exacerbating and alleviating factors along with specific limited activities of daily living should be identified. The examiner should inquire about prior hip consultations, past surgeries, old injuries, and prior treatments including activity modifications, oral medications, physical therapy, injections, and assistive devices. Recreational history and athletic participation should also be probed. It is important to discern a history of ligamentous laxity or treatment for acetabular dysplasia as an infant. It is also important to obtain a history of hip pain as an adolescent that may be a clue to previous hip problems such as slipped capital femoral epiphysis (SCFE) and Legg–Calve–Perthes (15).

A thorough history will help delineate intra-articular versus extra-articular sources of pain. Patients with symptomatic intra-articular problems, such as chondral flaps and labral tears, will often complain of pain and mechanical symptoms (17). Typically, the pain is deep and localized in the anterior groin or inguinal region, although this pain may be referred to the medial thigh, the region proximal to the greater trochanter laterally, or in the buttocks. Frequently, patients will note the pain is deep within the joint, grabbing their hip with the thumb in the inguinal region and the long finger posterolaterally, stating the pain is at the junction of the fingers—known as the C-sign (Fig. 45.1) (1–3). This can be misinterpreted as lateral soft tissue pathology; however, the patient often describes deep interior hip pain. Posterior-superior pain requires a thorough evaluation in differentiating hip and back pain.

Other characteristics of intra-articular sources of mechanical hip pain include discreet episodes of sharp pain

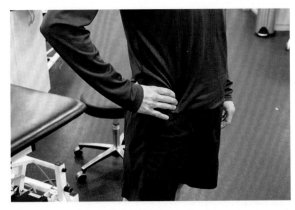

FIGURE 45.1. Depicting the "C-sign," a characteristic sign, patients with intra-articular hip pain will often demonstrate.

with weightbearing that may be exacerbated by pivoting or twisting, discomfort with sitting with the hip flexed, and pain or catching on arising from a seated position. Patients may also complain of catching, clicking, popping, or locking within the joint with ambulation or other hip motion, although this is less specific for intra-articular sources of symptoms.

Patients with extra-articular sources or referred pain will have varying complaints. Pain located in the thigh or buttocks, or pain that radiates distally below the knee, is likely to originate from the lumbar spine or buttock and proximal thigh musculature. Pain located in the lower abdomen and/or at the adductor tubercle can indicate athletic pubalgia or osteitis pubis. Pain located around the greater trochanter and associated with snapping can be external snapping hip syndrome. External snapping hip is often visible, or seen by the patient and others, and sometimes is described as the hip dislocating by the patient. Internal snapping hip is usually audible or palpable and felt deep inside or in the groin. Identification of associated symptoms such as weakness or numbness, back pain, and exacerbation with coughing or sneezing, may indicate thoracolumbar pathology. Individuals with athletic pubalgia may also note pain with sit-ups. Furthermore, one must remember that hip problems may present as pain in the knee.

A general medical and surgical history, as well as any developmental problems, should be explored. Patients should specifically be asked about systemic illnesses such as malignancy, coagulopathies, and inflammatory disorders. Various coagulation and metabolic disorders such as abnormality of lipids, thyroid, homocysteine, and clotting mechanisms have been shown to impede vascular supply to the femoral head. Social history should be reviewed to determine current or prior use of alcohol, steroids, and tobacco, or altitude issues, which might place the patient at risk for osteonecrosis.

The report of present illness, surgical and medical history, and family history should provide the clinician with enough information to develop a preliminary differential diagnosis. This differential diagnosis will allow the clinician to pay special attention to specific areas of the complete hip examination.

Physical Examination

Physical examination of the hip follows the same basic principles of any other area of the body. However, the hip is difficult to examine due to it being a deep structure, surrounded by a thick envelope of muscles and other soft tissues, that is also well constrained. Furthermore, examination of the hip is difficult because hip pain may be a result of intra-articular hip pathology as well as a myriad of extra-articular and referred sources of pain. It is crucial to perform a consistent, comprehensive physical examination to best identify the underlying diagnosis. A systematic approach includes inspection, palpation, range of motion, strength, and special or provocative tests (4, 16, 17). A complete examination of the hip must be performed, even if the differential diagnosis appears very narrow, to help reduce the likelihood of an incorrect diagnosis. The order of the examination should be easy on the patient and flow for the physician. An efficient order of patient positioning for the examination begins with standing tests followed by seated, supine, lateral, and ending with prone tests (2).

Inspection

Observe the patient as they walk into the room, how they are sitting, how they get up from the interview chair, and how they transfer to the examination table—these may be essential initial clues in the examination of the hip. Notation is made with regard to favoring, splinting, or compensating for the injured limb. Patients with piriformis syndrome may lean off the affected hip, whereas some patients with femoroacetabular impingement or anterior labral tear may slouch in the chair to reduce hip flexion. Antalgic gait, with decreased stance phase, shortened swing phase, or avoidance of hip extension is noted. Also, Trendelenburg gait may be seen because of abductor weakness or as the patient tries to place their center of gravity over the hip, reducing the forces on the joint. Abductor weakness is present if the pelvis drops contralateral to the stance leg or the patient shifts his/her entire body over the stance leg to compensate for the deficient abductors. As this weakness progresses, a compensatory shift of weight toward the affected side may occur. Known as an abductor lurch, this gait pattern places the center of gravity closer to the hip and thus decreases the force required from the abductors.

Observation for swelling and bruising at the greater trochanter for bursitis or at the iliac crest for hip pointers or avulsion fractures, for example, may also provide a clue to the diagnosis. Observation of the pelvic region and spine for asymmetry, deformity, masses, redness, atrophy, malalignment, and pelvic obliquity is also made. Leg lengths are measured standing (assessing from the back for pelvic tilt) and laying supine (measured from the anterosuperior iliac spine [ASIS] to the medial malleolus bilaterally).

Palpation

Intra-articular pathologies usually do not have palpable areas of tenderness, although compensation for longstanding intra-articular problems may result in tenderness of muscles or bursae. Palpating bony prominences around the hip is an essential part of the physical examination and is very useful in delineating extra-articular causes of pain. Common areas of tenderness include the greater trochanter with trochanteric bursitis and snapping hip from the iliotibial band (Fig. 45.2). Tenderness posterior to the greater trochanter is suggestive of piriformis tendonitis, whereas tenderness just superior to the greater trochanter may be because of gluteus medius tendonitis. The ASIS is the origin of the sartorius, a common location of apophyseal avulsion fractures in adolescent athletes. Just medial to the ASIS, the lateral femoral cutaneous nerve crosses under the inguinal ligament. Compression of the nerve at this site, known as meralgia paresthetica, may produce dysesthesias over the proximal anterolateral aspect of the thigh. Reproduction of symptoms with deep palpation just medial to the ASIS is diagnostic for this condition. Tenderness and swelling at the iliac crest following direct trauma is commonly known as a "hip pointer" or in the skeletally immature athlete may be related to iliac crest avulsion injury. The anterior inferior iliac spine (AIIS) is the origin of the rectus femoris. Tenderness at this location in a skeletally immature athlete suggests an apophyseal avulsion injury.

Tenderness at the pubic symphysis or ramus may occur as the result of recurrent stress created by powerful adductors. This condition, termed pubic symphysitis or osteitis pubis, is most frequently seen in soccer and hockey players. The ischial tuberosity may be palpated with the patient either in the prone or in the supine position with the hip flexed. Acute tenderness at this site is found in hamstring avulsion injuries, but tenderness may also be seen with hamstring tendinopathy. Tenderness in the absence of acute injury may be attributable to inflammation of the overlying bursa. Ischiogluteal bursitis, or weaver's bottom, is most commonly found in seated athletes such as rowers, bikers, and equestrian athletes.

Other areas of pain, as located by the patient, should be palpated. It is important not to forget to palpate other potential areas of referred pain to the hip, including the lumbar spine, sacrum, and sacroiliac (SI) joint. Palpation of the femoral artery should be included in the general hip examination as well as the neurovascular evaluation because an aneurysm of this artery may uncommonly cause swelling and pain about the hip.

Range of Motion

Range of motion is assessed checking the normal, unaffected limb first (Table 45.1). It is important to evaluate hip range of motion with the patient in the seated, supine, and prone positions. Excessive femoral anteversion will present with increased internal rotation and decreased external rotation. It is important to distinguish motion from the hip joint itself from compensatory motion occurring in the pelvis and lumbar spine. Flexion contracture is measured with the contralateral hip flexed and the lumbar spine stabilized with the examination table using the Thomas test (Fig. 45.3). This is performed properly by having the subject flex hip to the chest. If there is no

Table 45.1	
Active normal range of motions of the hip	
Flexion	110°–120°
Extension	10°–15°
Abduction in extension	30°–50°
Adduction in extension	30°
External rotation in flexion	40°–60°
Internal rotation in flexion	30°–40°

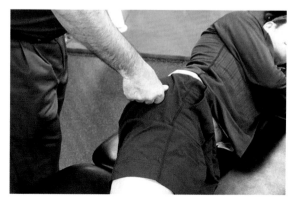

FIGURE 45.2. Palpating the greater trochanter to elicit tenderness on physical examination.

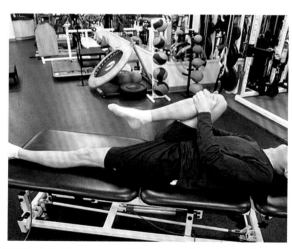

FIGURE 45.3. Thomas test. Utilized to evaluate for hip flexion contractures. If there is no flexion contracture, the extended hip and extremity will be flat on the examination table.

flexion contracture, the hip being tested remains on the examining table. If a flexion contracture is present, the patient's contralateral leg will rise off the table.

Hamstring tightness is also evaluated by measuring the popliteal angle. With the subject supine, the hip is flexed 90° with the knee flexed. The knee is then passively extended. The degree of knee extension is indicative of hamstring tightness, with full extension indicative of hamstring flexibility.

Hip abductor tightness or tensor fascia lata contracture is measured using the Ober test (Fig. 45.4) (2, 4, 5). In the lateral decubitus position, the lower hip and knee is flexed for stability. The examiner then passively flexes the hip being examined to 90° and then abducts the hip fully and extends the hip past neutral with the knee in 90° of flexion. At this point, the hip and knee are allowed to adduct while the hip is held in neutral rotation. If the knee does not reach to midline, then the hip abductors are tight.

Rectus femoris tightness can be assessed in the prone position. The patient's knee is passively flexed. If on flexion of the knee the ipsilateral hip also flexes, then the rectus femoris is tight and the test is positive. This test is also known as Ely's test (2, 4, 5). The degree of knee flexion should also be compared between the two sides to assess for rectus femoris tightness (Fig. 45.5).

With chondral flaps or labral tears, usually there is only a mild decrease in hip range of motion. More often there is pain or discomfort at the extremes of motion. For those with SCFE and femoroacetabular impingement, it is common for the individual's hip to abduct and externally rotate as the hip is being flexed. With femoroacetabular impingement (FAI), there is usually loss of internal rotation. Those with arthritis will have diffuse loss of range of motion. However, the first ranges to be lost are internal rotation and abduction (4).

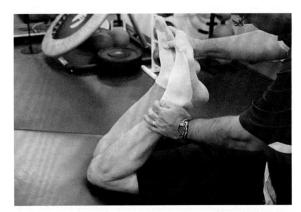

FIGURE 45.5. Examination for rectus femoris tightness or contracture. The degree of knee flexion is evaluated and compared with contralateral side. Here the patient's left quadriceps are tighter than the right.

Strength

Strength testing may elicit weakness as a cause of pain or compensatory loss from hip pathology. This is performed in all directions of hip motion. Pain with strength testing may guide the diagnosis as to whether the etiology of hip pain is musculotendinous in origin because resisted contraction may reproduce localized symptoms of the muscle being tested. Hip abductor weakness is assessed with the Trendelenburg test in single leg stance as described previously. Pain at the proximal tendon of the adductor longus may be provoked by resisted adduction of the hip (Fig. 45.6). Iliopsoas bursitis symptoms may be exacerbated by testing hip flexion strength while the patient is seated.

Provocative or Special Tests
Intra-articular pathology

The dynamic external rotatory impingement test (DEXRIT) and the dynamic internal rotatory impingement test (DIRI) are both performed with the patient lying supine with the contralateral hip maximally flexed to eliminate lumbar lordosis. The affected hip is then brought to 90° of flexion.

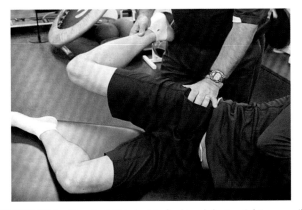

FIGURE 45.4. Ober test. This test is for hip abductor tightness or iliotibial band contracture. It is performed with the patient in the lateral decubitus position. The hip and knee are first flexed, then the hip abducted, then extended and let fall into adduction. Inability of the knee to drop below neutral is considered positive, or tightness of the iliotibial band.

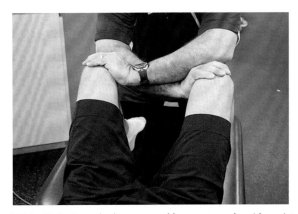

FIGURE 45.6. A method to test adductor strength with resisted adduction—this test is performed in hip flexion as well as in extension.

In the DIRI, the hip is passively ranged through a wide arc of adduction and internal rotation while extending the hip. In the DEXRIT, the hip is passively ranged through a wide arc of abduction and external rotation with hip extension. For both maneuvers, a positive test will recreate the patient's pain. Both tests may also be performed during arthroscopy to provide direct visualization of femoral neck and acetabular congruence.

The flexion/adduction/internal rotation (FADDIR) test may be performed in either the supine or lateral positions (Fig. 45.7). The examined hip is passively brought into 90° of flexion, adducted, then internally rotated. Reproduction of the patient's pain indicates a positive test. The degree of flexion and internal rotation achieved at the onset of pain should be documented. Although this test has been called the impingement test, it is very sensitive for intra-articular hip pathology, not necessarily just FAI. However, this test has also been shown to yield a high percentage of false-positive results. Groin pain provoked by the dynamic impingement test described by McCarthy indicates intra-articular pathology as well (6). It is performed by having the supine patient start with maximum hip flexion, adduction, and internal rotation moving to full extension, then immediately moving into maximum flexion, abduction, and external rotation moving to full extension.

Having the patient perform a straight leg raise against resistance, known as the Stinchfield test, is an effective screening tool for intra-articular hip pathology (2, 4). The patient is asked to perform an active straight leg raise to 45°, and then the examiner directs a downward force (Fig. 45.8). A positive test produces either pain or weakness. This maneuver is designed to simulate normal walking and creates a force double the patient's body weight across the hip joint. With active resistance, the psoas places pressure on the labrum, and thus helps detect intraarticular pathology. Extra-articular pathologies, including hip flexor tendonitis, a hip flexor avulsion fracture, or a psoas abscess, will also produce a positive result.

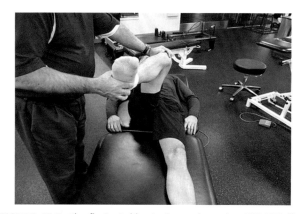

FIGURE 45.7. The flexion/adduction/internal rotation (FADDIR) "impingement" test. Here the hip is flexed to 90°, then adducted, and then internally rotated. Although this test is called the impingement test, it is not pathognomonic for femoroacetabular impingement but is sensitive for other sources of intra-articular hip pathology.

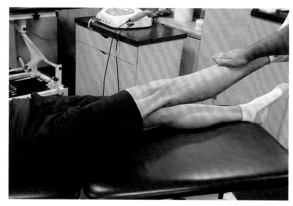

FIGURE 45.8. Stinchfield test. This test is performed with a straight leg raise against resistance. This can be an effective screening tool for intra-articular hip pathology or hip flexor inflammation or injury.

The foveal distraction test is performed with the patient in the supine position. The leg is abducted 30° and axial traction is placed on the leg. This maneuver reduces intra-articular pressure, and relief of pain is indicative of an intra-articular source of hip pain.

The log roll test is a sensitive maneuver to evaluate for intra-articular pain.

The hop test is an effective test to diagnose a stress fracture. The patient performs a single leg hop on the affected leg. Pain in the groin, hip, or anterior thigh is considered a positive test.

Extra-articular pathology

SI joint—The flexion/abduction/external rotation test (FABER), also known as the Patrick test, is helpful to detect SI pain (2, 4). The patient is placed supine on the edge of examining table with the buttock of the extremity to be examined partly off the table, and the examined extremity is place in the figure-of-4 position with the knee flexed and the ipsilateral ankle resting on the contralateral thigh. The examiner directs a downward force of the flexed knee with one hand while stabilizing the pelvis at the contralateral ASIS with the other hand (Fig. 45.9). This test stresses the SI joint. If this maneuver produces posterior hip pain, SI joint pathology should be suspected. The FABER test can also elicit pain with true intra-articular hip pathology; however, the pain will typically be localized to the anterior groin.

Gaenslen's test is another test that places stress on the SI joint (2, 4, 5). The patient is positioned supine with the examined hip shifted toward the side of the table. Both knees are flexed up toward the patient's chest. The examiner stabilizes the pelvis with one hand while extending the examined thigh over the edge of the table. This maneuver stresses the SI joint and is positive if the patient experiences pain on the provoked side.

Pubic symphysis—The pubic symphysis stress test is useful for identifying pathology at that site. The test is performed in the supine position. One of the examiner's hands

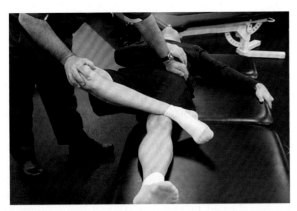

FIGURE 45.9. FABER test/Patrick's test. In this test, the patient's buttock is off the edge of the table, and then the ipsilateral leg is brought into a "figure-of-4" position. While stabilizing the contralateral pelvic brim, downward force is applied to the knee. Posterior pain is often elicited as a result of sacroiliac pathology, whereas anterior pain may be the result of pubic symphysis pain or anterior labral damage.

is placed at the superior border at one side of the pubis, and the other is placed at the inferior border of the pubis on the contralateral side. The two hands are then pressed together, creating a shearing force at the pubic symphysis. A positive test will reproduce the patient's pain at this location. The pelvic compression test may be performed in the supine or lateral positions (Fig. 45.10). These maneuvers produce a compression force at the pubic symphysis, which, in a positive test, will cause pain at that site.

Snapping hip—With external snapping hip (coxa sultans externa), the iliotibial band produces tenderness over the greater trochanter, and the pain can be reproduced with repetitive flexion and extension. External snapping hip is usually visually identified, though may be heard occasionally. Most patients can voluntarily produce this snapping while standing and shifting their hip laterally. The bicycle test may also be helpful in diagnosing external snapping hip syndrome. This test is performed with the patient laying in the lateral position. A bicycle pedaling motion is

simulated with the extremity away from the table, and a positive test will reproduce snapping of the iliotibial band.

Internal causes of snapping hip produce pain along the inguinal crease and medial thigh. The snapping occurs when the iliopsoas is suddenly forced under tension over the iliopectineal eminence or the femoral head. Internal snapping hip is generally audible, and occasionally palpable. The snap can be made more obvious or reproduced with one of a series of active motions performed by the supine patient. One test, described by Byrd (7), begins with the hip in flexion, then abducted, externally rotated, and extended. The senior author has found this to be the most sensitive test to evaluate for internal snapping hip. Another maneuver that we have found useful is ranging the hip a flexed, abducted, and externally rotated position to an adducted, internally rotated, and extended position. A last provocative test used to reproduce internal snapping of the hip from the iliopsoas is to have the supine patient lift the leg to be examined 24 in off the table and move the leg from an abducted and externally rotated position to an adducted and internally rotated position. The common theme to each of these tests is to move the contracted iliopsoas muscle–tendon unit from a position lateral to the femoral head to a position medial to the femoral head and is associated with a very loud clunk. Gentle pressure over the femoral head may prohibit the snap from occurring.

The piriformis test is used to confirm or rule out piriformis syndrome. To test for this clinical syndrome, the patient is examined in the lateral decubitus position. The patient flexes the test hip to 60° of flexion with the knee also flexed. The examiner stabilizes the hip with one hand and applies a downward (adducting/internally rotating) force to the knee. If the piriformis is tight, pain is elicited in the muscle. If the piriformis is compressing the sciatic nerve, the pain may be in the buttocks and radiate distally to the back of the thigh to the knee. Additionally, while the patient is in this position, the piriformis is palpated to elicit tenderness (as compared with the contralateral side), which may be seen with piriformis syndrome (Fig. 45.11).

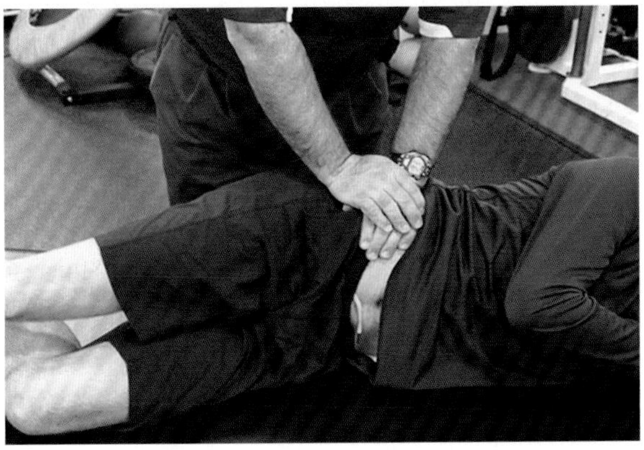

FIGURE 45.10. Lateral compression test. With the patient in a lateral position, downward force on the pelvis may produces pain anteriorly at the pubic symphysis or posteriorly for the SI joint.

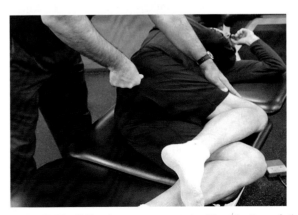

FIGURE 45.11. Piriformis test augmented with palpation of the sciatic nerve to assess for piriformis syndrome.

Sports hernia—The resisted sit-up test is helpful in diagnosing a sports hernia (8). With the patient in the supine position, legs extended, the examiner places a hand on the patient's chest and provides resistance. A positive test produces pain at the rectus abdominus insertion or in the groin. Another test we have found useful to detect a sports hernia is reproduction of pain when the patient does a sit-up while the clinician palpates the edge of the rectus abdominus near its insertion into the pubis (Fig. 45.12).

Imaging and Procedures

Plain Radiographs

Routine radiographs should be obtained in all patients with hip pain. Plain hip radiographic series includes an anteroposterior (AP) view of the pelvis, an AP view of the affected hip, and a lateral view of the hip. The AP of the pelvis is imperative because most of the radiographic lines and relationships have been validated with the AP pelvis view. As radiographs are a series of divergent beams (only one perpendicular beam), there will be a difference in the relationship of the various radiographic lines between the AP pelvis and the AP hip—the single perpendicular beam is centered on the center of the pelvis in an AP pelvis view, whereas it is on the center of the femoral head in an AP hip view (where it would be angled on an AP pelvis). Additionally, the AP pelvis radiograph allows visualization of closely related areas that may present with hip pain, such as the pubic symphysis, sacrum, SI joints, ilium, and ischium (Fig. 45.13).

It is important to obtain an orthogonal view to the AP radiograph. There are several lateral views that may be obtained, including a cross-table lateral, a Dunn view, modified Dunn view, frog table lateral, and false profile view,

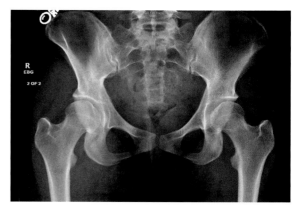

FIGURE 45.13. Routine appropriate AP pelvis radiograph. An appropriate AP pelvis radiograph is confirmed by the tip of the coccyx being centered 1 to 3 cm above the pubic symphysis. An AP pelvis can be helpful because it allows comparison with the asymptomatic side to evaluate subtle variations in bony architecture as well as allowing visualization of closely related areas that may present with hip pain. Furthermore, measurements and relationships of pelvic bony structures have been validated with AP pelvis radiographs and not just AP of the hip.

to name a few (3, 9). Of the lateral views used, the senior author prefers a cross-table lateral radiograph, as it is easy to obtain a reproducible lateral view and is a lateral of the proximal femur and acetabulum (Fig. 45.14). The frog leg lateral is often obtained; however, it is not a true lateral of the hip, it is a good lateral of the femoral head and neck and provides more information about the proximal femur, but is still an AP view of the acetabulum.

Plain radiographs may help identify degenerative joint changes, osteonecrosis, loose bodies, stress fractures, and osseous pathology. One should assess for subtle acetabular dysplasia, using center-to-edge (CE) angle and other appropriate measurements such as the crossover sign or the posterior wall sign, indicators acetabular retroversion (3, 9). The CE angle should be at least 20° and preferably 25°

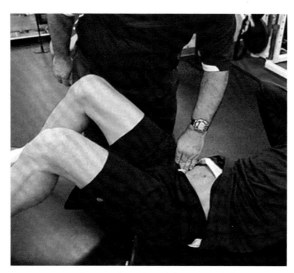

FIGURE 45.12. Palpating the edge of the rectus abdominus near its insertion while the patient does a sit-up is a test that is helpful to evaluate for a sports hernia. Exacerbation of symptoms with this provocative maneuver is consist with athletic pubalgia/sports hernia.

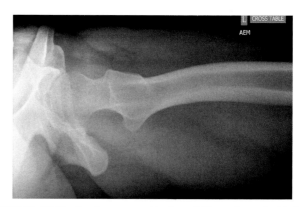

FIGURE 45.14. Routine cross-table lateral hip radiograph. Notice how this is a true lateral of the proximal femur (femoral head and neck) and the acetabulum. Care should be taken to not have the greater trochanter posterior to the shaft of the femur, which is an externally rotated view of the proximal femur.

to ensure normal seating of the femoral head and ideally equal distribution of forces on the bony acetabulum. The AP pelvic radiograph should be evaluated for protrusion, as well as coxa profunda, where the floor of the cotyloid fossa reaches the ilioischial line and the center edge angle is greater than 35°. Plain radiographs are also evaluated for a prominent femoral neck or femoral head–neck asymmetry indicative of femoroacetabular cam impingement. Both of these problems may result in labral tears and/or articular cartilage damage.

Although labral tears are usually not seen on plain radiographs (other than calcification or ossification of the labrum), Wenger et al. (10), found that most patients with labral tears have associated bony abnormalities. Certainly, plain radiographs also are useful in diagnosing associated pathology and in excluding other sources of hip symptoms.

Magnetic Resonance Imaging

MRI has traditionally been used to evaluate soft-tissue injury, such as labral tears, bursitis, and tendinous injuries. MRI has also been found to be useful in the early detection of stress fractures of the femoral neck and osteonecrosis. The routine use of MRI in assessing labral injuries has been questioned by some because of the relatively low sensitivity and specificity of MRI (3, 4, 11, 12). MRI of the pelvis has a less than 10% sensitivity to detect labral tears, whereas MRI of the hip (a smaller field of view) is significantly more sensitive (13). False-positive results may also occur with MRI. Several studies have shown morphologic variants, degeneration, and increased signal within the labrum in asymptomatic controls (1, 3, 4, 11, 12). MRI has proved important in identifying sources of hip pain other than labral tears including loose bodies, pigmented villonodular synovitis, synovial chondromatosis, and other intra-articular pathology. Newer techniques and more powerful magnets have increased the ability to detect labral tears as well as isolated chondral defects of the femoral head and acetabulum.

MRI Arthrography

MRI combined with arthrography appears to increase the utility of this imaging modality in the diagnosis and description of labral pathology and articular cartilage loss (Fig. 45.15A, B). Magnetic resonance arthrography is a minimally invasive means of improving the ability to diagnose labral and cartilage problems with a higher sensitivity and specificity than MRI (1, 11, 12, 14). Magnetic resonance arthrography has a 90% sensitivity and a 91% specificity (1, 11, 12, 14).An intra-articular local anesthetic can be used in conjunction with Gadolinium to assess pain relief in addition identification of anatomic evidence of intra-articular pathology.

Intra-articular Anesthetic Injection

An intra-articular local anesthetic can be used to assist in the diagnosis of intra-articular hip pain and to help

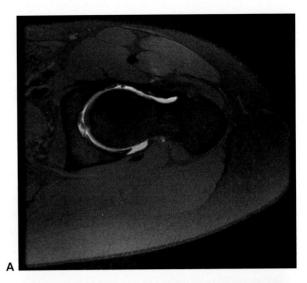

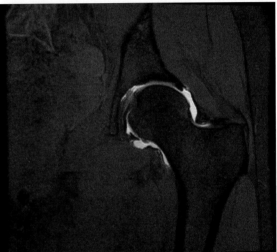

FIGURE 45.15. MRI arthrogram with intra-articular gadolinium enhances the sensitivity of the MRI study in the evaluation of the painful hip. Notice the improved visibility of the labrum and other intra-articular structures. **A:** An axial cut from routine MRI arthrogram study. **B:** A coronal cut from routine MRI arthrogram.

determine whether intra-articular pathology seen on MR is producing the patients pain (Fig. 45.16). Because labral tears may be asymptomatic and because MRIs may be falsely negative, pain relief with the local anesthetic is considered important in determining the true intra-articular nature of symptoms and if hip arthroscopy may be of benefit. If there is no relief with the intra-articular injection, one must consider other sources of pain. Extravasation of anesthetic and traumatic injections precludes this from being 100% specific for intra-articular etiology of pain. Corticosteroids are only added when a patient has degenerative arthritis. The intra-articular local anesthetic can be used independently (under ultrasound or fluoroscopic guidance) or in conjunction with contrast as part of an MRI arthrographic study.

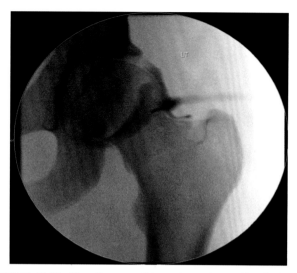

FIGURE 45.16. Hip arthrogram. This can be used to confirm the intra-articular placement of contrast, anesthetic solution, or corticosteroid.

Decision Making

Successful hip arthroscopy is most clearly dependent on proper patient selection. A well-executed procedure will fail when performed for the wrong reasons. Hip pain, particularly in the young adult, may arise from several soft tissue structures in and around the hip joint. Patient expectation is also paramount. The patient should have reasonable goals and knows what can be accomplished with arthroscopy, which is only partially dictated by the nature of the pathology. The pathomechanics, pathoanatomy, and natural history of many of these lesions being surgically addressed are still being studied and not fully understood. However, an increasing amount of clinical experience exists upon which patients can be offered reasonable expectations on outcomes.

Hip arthroscopy offers a less invasive alternative to hip procedures that would otherwise require an open procedure, including surgical dislocation of the hip. In addition, this procedure allows surgeons to address a wide range of intra-articular derangements that were previously undiagnosed and untreated. With the exception of loose bodies, no literature exists to suggest that recommending nonsurgical interventions first is harmful for most of the problems that are now being recognized and addressed. Most disorders will declare themselves over time through failure of response to conservative measures. As such, most patients should have a committed trial of nonoperative treatment before recommending hip arthroscopy.

Hip arthroscopy has been very effective for the treatment of numerous injuries including labral tears, capsular laxity with iliofemoral ligament deficiency, femoroacetabular impingement and decreased femoral head–neck junction offset, lateral impact injury and chondral injuries, injuries to the ligamentum teres, extra-articular conditions

(internal and external snapping hip), and loose bodies. Other less common indications for hip arthroscopy include management of osteonecrosis of the femoral head, synovial chondromatosis and other synovial abnormalities, crystalline hip arthropathy (gout and pseudogout), infection, management of posttraumatic intra-articular debris, and management of mild to moderate hip osteoarthritis with mechanical symptoms. In addition, patients with long-standing, unresolved hip joint pain and positive physical findings may benefit from arthroscopic evaluation. Our indications for hip arthroscopy include the actual or suspected diagnoses above in patients (and thus not extra-articular cause of pain) who get pain relief with an intra-articular injection and have failed nonoperative management.

Hip arthroscopy is contraindicated in patients with hip fusions, advanced arthritis, open wounds or cellulitis, obesity, stress fractures in the femoral neck, severe dysplasia, osteonecrosis with collapse of the femoral head, and stable avascular necrosis.

CONCLUSIONS AND FUTURE DIRECTIONS

Interest in nonarthritic hip problems in patients has recently grown as a result of newer understanding of hip joint problems, easier and more reproducible diagnostic modalities, and less invasive treatment options, especially the technical advances of hip arthroscopy. In conjunction with this increased interest, has been an increased effort and emphasis on clinical evaluation of the hip, as outlined in this chapter.

The application of arthroscopic techniques to the hip joint appears to be the last frontier for the minimally invasive management of intra-articular injuries in athletes. Until the recent advent of improved surgical techniques, advanced imaging modalities, and more versatile instrumentation, the hip joint was largely inaccessible because of numerous anatomic and technical constraints. With these improvements, however, hip arthroscopy can now be performed safely and effectively as an outpatient procedure. Patients with reproducible symptoms and physical findings that reveal limited functioning and who have failed an adequate trial of conservative treatment and had pain relief with an injection of an intra-articular anesthetic will have the greatest likelihood of success after surgical intervention. Strict attention to thorough diagnostic examination, detailed imaging, and adherence to safe and reproducible surgical techniques are essential for the success of this procedure.

REFERENCES

1. Burnett RS, Della Rocca GJ, Prather H, et al. Clinical presentation of patients with tears of the acetabular labrum. *J Bone Joint Surg Am.* 2006;88(7):1448–1457.

2. Martin HD, Shears SA, Palmer IJ. Evaluation of the hip. *Sports Med Arthrosc.* 2010;18(2):63–75.

3. Nepple JJ, Carlisle JC, Nunley RM, et al. Clinical and radiographic predictors of intra-articular hip disease in arthroscopy. *Am J Sports Med.* 2011;39(2):296–303.

4. Safran MR. Evaluation of the hip: history, physical examination, and imaging. *Oper Tech Sports Med.* 2005;13(1):2–12.

5. Plante M, Wallace R, Busconi BD. Clinical diagnosis of hip pain. *Clin Sports Med.* 2011;30(2):225–238.

6. McCarthy JC, Noble PC, Schuck MR, et al. The Otto E. Aufranc Award: the role of labral lesions to development of early degenerative hip disease. *Clin Orthop Relat Res.* 2001;393(393):25–37.

7. Byrd JW. Evaluation and management of the snapping iliopsoas tendon. *Instr Course Lect.* 2006;55:347–355.

8. Swan KG Jr, Wolcott M. The athletic hernia: a systematic review. *Clin Orthop Relat Res.* 2007;455:78–87.

9. Clohisy JC, Carlisle JC, Beaule PE, et al. A systematic approach to the plain radiographic evaluation of the young adult hip. *J Bone Joint Surg Am.* 2008;90(suppl 4):47–66.

10. Wenger DE, Kendell KR, Miner MR, et al. Acetabular labral tears rarely occur in the absence of bony abnormalities. *Clin Orthop Relat Res.* 2004;426(426):145–150.

11. Byrd JW, Jones KS. Diagnostic accuracy of clinical assessment, magnetic resonance imaging, magnetic resonance arthrography, and intra-articular injection in hip arthroscopy patients. *Am J Sports Med.* 2004;32(7):1668–1674.

12. Chan YS, Lien LC, Hsu HL, et al. Evaluating hip labral tears using magnetic resonance arthrography: a prospective study comparing hip arthroscopy and magnetic resonance arthrography diagnosis. *Arthroscopy.* 2005;21(10):1250.e1–1250.e8.

13. Toomayan GA, Holman WR, Major NM, et al. Sensitivity of MR arthrography in the evaluation of acetabular labral tears. *AJR Am J Roentgenol.* 2006;186(2):449–453

14. Leunig M, Werlen S, Ungersbock A, et al. Evaluation of the acetabular labrum by MR Arthrography. *J Bone Joint Surg Br.* 1997;79-B(2):230–234.

15. Clohisy JC, Beaulé PE, O'Malley A, et al. AOA symposium. Hip disease in the young adult: current concepts of etiology and surgical treatment. *J Bone Joint Surg Am.* 2008;90(10):2267–2281.

16. Martin HD, Kelly BT, Leunig M, et al. The pattern and technique in the clinical evaluation of the adult hip: the common physical examination tests of hip specialists. *Arthroscopy.* 2010;26(2):161–172.

17. Martin R, Kelly B, Leunig M, et al. Reliability of clinical diagnosis in intraarticular hip diseases. *Knee Surg Sports Traumatol Arthrosc.* 2010;18(5):685–690.

Hip Arthroscopy: The Supine Position

Christopher M. Larson • Corey A. Wulf

There has been increased interest in the area of hip arthroscopy over the past decade. Increasing numbers of surgeons are performing or considering incorporating hip arthroscopy into their practice. There is a steep learning curve when performing hip arthroscopy that even the most experienced hip arthroscopists continue to climb. It is imperative to develop consistent and predictable techniques that allow for safe and effective management of hip disorders through the central and peripheral compartment. Patient positioning is the starting point when optimizing various techniques for hip arthroscopy. Hip arthroscopy can be performed in either the supine or the lateral position. This chapter will describe hip arthroscopy in the supine position with a focus on patient position, portal placement, techniques to improve visualization, and the use of intraoperative fluoroscopy in an attempt to optimize surgical techniques and ultimately patient outcomes.

ANESTHESIA

In order to achieve appropriate distraction for work in the central compartment, an adequate motor block is necessary when performing hip arthroscopy. General anesthesia is the most common anesthetic approach and reliably allows for adequate distraction and muscle paralysis if necessary. Most patients undergoing hip arthroscopy are relatively young and general anesthesia is safe and efficient. Spinal anesthesia can also be utilized as long as an adequate motor blockade is achieved. Infrequently, if traction is difficult with spinal anesthesia, a general anesthetic may need to be administered during the case. There are no studies evaluating other regional blocks (i.e., lumbar plexus blocks, sacral plexus blocks, obturator blocks, and lumbar paravertebral blocks) as the sole form of anesthesia during hip arthroscopy.

There is a variable level of postoperative pain seen after hip arthroscopy and the most patients are discharged on an outpatient basis with the use of a local anesthetic at the conclusion of the procedure. Occasionally, there may be patients who have a history of poor pain tolerance or

who experience severe postoperative pain in the recovery room after hip arthroscopy. In these patients, a regional block can be considered. Regional blocks that may be helpful in these situations include lumbar plexus blocks, combined lumber plexus and sacral plexus blocks, L1 and L2 paravertebral blocks, and obturator and psoas compartment blocks (1–3). There are, however, no large series evaluating the efficacy of these regional blocks for pain after hip arthroscopy.

EXAMINATION UNDER ANESTHESIA

Patient positioning in the supine position does have some advantages when compared with the lateral position. The supine position simplifies positioning at the beginning of the procedure and is user friendly for the anesthesia team (4–6). The supine position may also decrease the rarely reported risk of intra-abdominal fluid extravasation when compared with the lateral position. Ultimately, the choice of position to be used during hip arthroscopy is based on surgeon preference, experience, and neither the supine nor the lateral position has proven to be superior to the other.

Basic Setup

Hip arthroscopy requires traction, which can be achieved with the use of a standard fracture table or with commercially available distraction devices designed for hip arthroscopy. We prefer to use a standard fracture table. We believe that the operating room staff's familiarity with the fracture table aids in efficient setup and eases their ability to adjust the table throughout the case if needed.

The patient is placed in the supine position with care taken to pad all bony prominences. Initially an examination under anesthesia is performed to assess range of motion (ROM). This is particularly useful in cases of femoroacetabular impingement (FAI) and adhesive capsulitis. For these specific cases, ROM, in particular internal rotation and flexion/abduction/external rotation deficits, can be assessed preoperatively and improvements assessed at the completion of the procedure. The patient is then moved distally on the table until contact is made between the medial thigh of the operative leg and the perineal post. The peroneal post should be adequately padded to decrease the risk for local neural and cutaneous injuries. The feet are placed in a well-padded boot or wrapped in cast padding after applying an ABD pad to the dorsomedial aspect of the forefoot. Padding protects the foot from skin and nerve pressure injuries as the feet need to be secure to avoid inadvertent slippage and loss of traction during the case. The feet are placed in the traction boots and further secured with cloth tape. The nonoperative leg is then maximally abducted and externally rotated with the knee in extension. The operative leg is positioned in neutral abduction, neutral to 15° of hip flexion, maximal internal rotation, and full knee extension. The pelvis is leveled by rotating the bed (typically toward the operative side) until the anterior superior iliac spines (ASIS) are at the same height and parallel to the floor/ceiling. A mayo stand is brought in from the contralateral side of the patient and placed over the upper torso and head. This acts as a working platform where instruments are easily accessed by the surgeon or assistant while allowing a working space under the surgical drape for the anesthesiologist. Finally, the video monitor is placed at the patient's head, next to fluoroscopic monitor (Fig. 46.1).

Intraoperative Fluoroscopic Evaluation

Although some surgeons routinely perform hip arthroscopy without intraoperative imaging, we find fluoroscopic guidance to be very useful. Intraoperative fluoroscopy aids in safe portal placement, maintenance of correct orientation throughout the surgical procedure, and evaluation of bony resections when indicated.

The fluoroscopy machine (C-arm) is brought in between the patients' lower extremities at an angle of 45° to the neutrally abducted operative leg (Fig. 46.2). The base can be locked in place and the arm telescoped in and out, so as not to interfere with the manipulation of instruments while allowing the surgeon to efficiently obtain imaging when necessary.

We perform a fluoroscopic evaluation of the hip prior to draping or distraction. An anteroposterior (AP) view of the hip is initially obtained to verify neutral abduction of the leg and correct rotation of the pelvis. Variable degrees of abduction or adduction of the operative leg may be required based on trochanteric height and acetabular inclination. The pelvic rotation can be estimated as noted in the previous section and verified radiographically by aligning the coccyx and pubic symphysis. There should be approximately 0 to 3 cm between the tip of the coccyx and symphysis in the cranial to caudal plane for neutral pelvic tilt. The goal is to obtain an intraoperative fluoroscopic view identical to a well-aligned preoperative AP radiograph of the patient's pelvis. The anterior and posterior walls are identified, allowing the surgeon to identify any area of rim resection (RR) that has been planned or templated on preoperative radiographs. Next, the femoral head–neck junction (FHNJ) is evaluated with an "around-the-world" inspection (7). With the hip in extension, fluoroscopic images are obtained in maximal hip internal rotation, neutral rotation, and maximal external rotation (Fig. 46.3). This provides assessment of the superior and inferior head–neck junction corresponding to the preoperative AP radiograph. Next, the hip is evaluated in 45° of hip and knee flexion. This is performed with the foot in the traction boot and allowing the entire bracket to slide proximally. Fluoroscopic images are obtained in maximal hip internal, neutral, and maximal external rotation (Fig. 46.4). This allows for inspection of the anterior and posterior head–neck junction corresponding to preoperative lateral radiographs. The neutral image (greater trochanter in line with the femoral neck (FN)) with the hip in flexion is similar to a modified Dunn view. We also obtain a cross-table lateral to assess femoral version

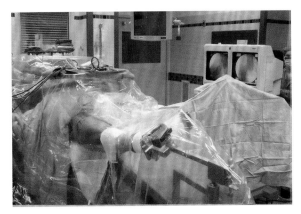

FIGURE 46.1. Hip arthroscopy setup in the supine position (*right hip*).

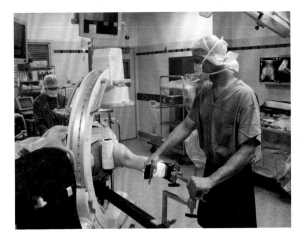

FIGURE 46.2. Fluoroscopy machine brought in between the legs during the supine approach (*left hip*).

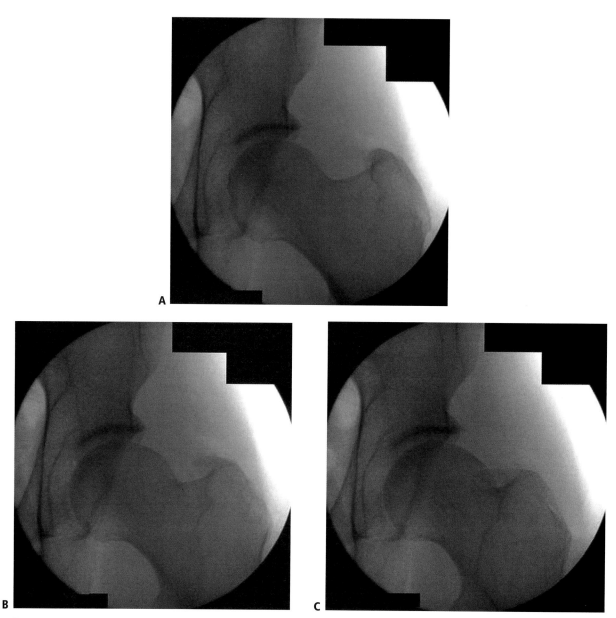

FIGURE 46.3. Fluoroscopic images intraoperatively with the hip in extension and **(A)** internal rotation, **(B)** neutral rotation, and **(C)** external rotation (left hip).

and complete the evaluation of the head–neck junction (Fig. 46.5). Finally, the operative leg is brought back to the "starting position" (neutral abduction, hip flexion of 15° to 20°, full-knee extension, and maximal internal rotation) and traction is applied until adequate distraction of the FH is achieved (Fig. 46.6). In some cases, breaking the seal may be difficult to achieve and gently shaking the hip along with IR and ER of the foot typically achieves atraumatic release of the intra-articular seal in these cases. If the seal is still difficult to release, excessive traction should be avoided and the use of a spinal needle at the beginning of the case will allow for an atraumatic release of the seal. The traction is then released while the leg is prepped and draped to minimize traction time.

Draping

The thigh and groin are prepped from the ASIS proximally to the knee distally. The entire posterior and lateral aspect of the thigh is also prepped medially to the perineal post. A sterile down drape is placed over the nonoperative leg. A second sterile down drape is placed over the mayo stand and extended just proximal to the ASIS. The surgical landmarks (ASIS and greater trochanter) are identified and marked with a surgical marker. A hip fracture drape is then adhered to the thigh and pulled over the operative leg and abdomen (Fig. 46.1). This transparent hip fracture drape is invaluable for hip arthroscopy, allowing for visualization of the traction apparatus and ease of manipulation of the leg during the procedure.

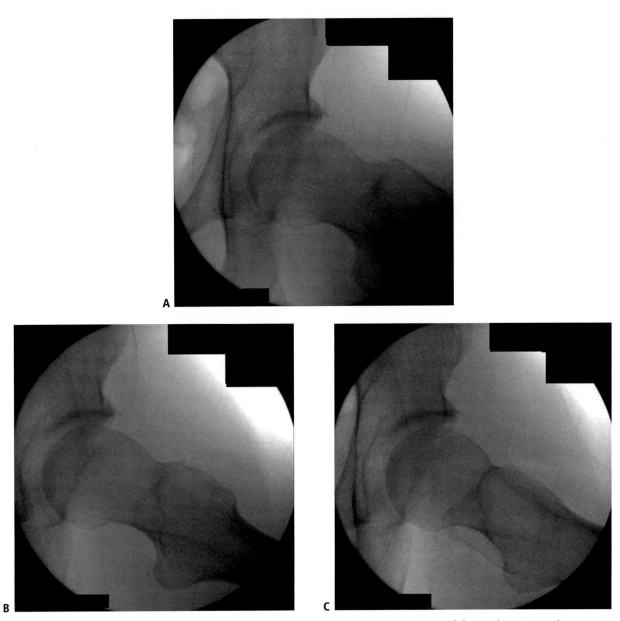

FIGURE 46.4. Fluoroscopic images intraoperatively with the hip in flexion and **(A)** internal rotation, **(B)** neutral rotation, and **(C)** external rotation *(left hip)*.

Specialized Instrumentation

Instruments specifically designed for hip arthroscopy are available through multiple vendors. Specifically designed instrumentation (baskets, punches, curettes, microfractures awls, suture passers, and graspers) improves the ease and safety with which hip arthroscopy is performed. In addition to an arthroscopic hip set, our standard instrumentation includes a slotted cannula, an extended length burr and curved shaver, a flexible tissue ablation probe, and a long-handled, curved beaver blade (BB).

PORTAL PLACEMENT AND ANATOMY

Exposure is essential to the success of any surgical procedure. Portal placement is the equivalent of exposure for arthroscopic surgery. Correct portal placement allows maximal visualization, reduced risk for iatrogenic injuries to intra-articular or neurovascular structures, and effective manipulation of instrumentation. The placement of arthroscopic portals about the hip poses unique challenges. The relatively thick soft tissue envelope restricts palpation of the osseous articular structures and joint space commonly used in portal placement for other joints. The highly constrained three-dimensional structure of the hip restricts intra-articular placement without significant distraction. Finally, the reduced volume of the capsule in a distracted hip provides a very little working space in the peripheral greater than central compartments. Despite these challenges, techniques for portal placement have evolved to allow for

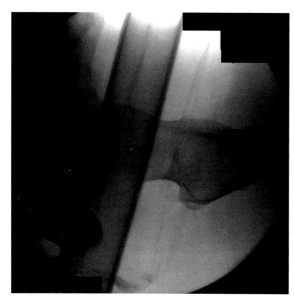

FIGURE 46.5. Cross-table lateral fluoroscopic image of the hip intraoperatively *(left hip)*.

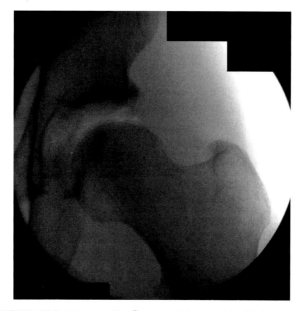

FIGURE 46.6. Intraoperative fluoroscopic image of the hip in traction verifying adequate distractibility *(left hip)*.

safe placement and adequate visualization of the central, peripheral, and peritrochanteric compartments of the hip.

There have been multiple portals described for treatment of both intra-articular and extra-articular pathologies about the hip (8–10) (Tables 46.1 and 46.2). The knowledge and use of multiple portals allow the surgeon to address a vast array of pathology. In the author's experience, two to three standard portals provide adequate access for most cases, with accessory portals used when necessary. A clear understanding of the anatomic relationships between portals and important structures reduces the risk of injury. All described portals are placed

in reference to key superficial anatomical structures: the anterior superior iliac spine and greater trochanter. Both structures are palpated and marked with a surgical marker for easy referencing during the procedure. It is important to acknowledge the variability from patient to patient with respect to neck-shaft angle, the height of the greater trochanter, FN version, and acetabular inclination. The individual variations may require the surgeon to adjust portal placement and/or leg position in order to maintain maximal visualization.

Anterolateral Portal

The anterolateral (AL) portal (anterior paratrochanteric portal) is placed approximately 1 cm anterior and 1 cm superior to the tip of the greater trochanter (9) (Fig. 46.7). The typical trajectory is 15° cephalad and 15° posterior (10). This portal takes advantage of the interval between the tensor fascia lata (TFL) anteriorly and the gluteus maximus posteriorly (10), before piercing the gluteus medius muscle belly and entering the lateral aspect of the joint capsule. The AL portal is a relatively safe portal. The superior gluteal nerve poses the biggest risk of neurologic injury, but lies safely 4 to 6 cm superior. The nerve passes posterior to anterior, deep to the gluteus medius muscle after exiting the greater sciatic notch. Iatrogenic injuries to the FH or labrum pose the largest overall risk.

Posterolateral Portal

The posterolateral (PL) portal (posterior paratrochanteric portal) is established in a similar manner to the AL portal, but on the posterior aspect of the trochanter. The portal is placed 1 cm posterior and 1 cm superior to the tip of the greater trochanter (Fig. 46.7) (9). A spinal needle is directed medially with a trajectory of 5° cephalad and 5° anterior (10). The portal pierces the gluteal fascia, gluteus medius, and gluteus minimus muscle bellies

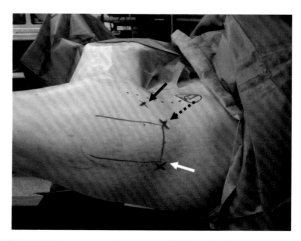

FIGURE 46.7. Intraoperative image of the left hip depicting the typical anterior *(black solid arrow)*, AL *(black dashed arrow)*, and PL *(white arrow)* portals. A circle outlines the ASIS, and the greater trochanter is outlined with a surgical marker.

Table 46.1

Distance from portal to anatomic structures

Portal	Anatomic Structure	Average (cm)	Range (cm)
Anterior	Anterior superior iliac spine	6.3	6.0–7.0
	LFCN[a]	0.3	0.2–1.0
	Femoral nerve		
	Level of sartorius[b]	4.3	3.8–5.0
	Level of rectus femoris	3.8	2.7–5.0
	Level of capsule	3.7	2.9–5.0
	Ascending branch of lateral circumflex femoral artery	3.7	1.0–6.0
	Terminal branch[c]	0.3	0.2–0.4
Anterolateral	Superior gluteal nerve	4.4	3.2–5.5
Posterolateral	Sciatic nerve	2.9	2.0–4.3

[a]Nerve had divided into three or more branches and measurement was made to closest branch.
[b]Measurement made at superficial surface of sartorius, rectus femoris, and capsule.
[c]Small terminal branch of ascending branch of lateral circumflex femoral artery identified in three specimens.

From Byrd JW, Pappas JN, Pedley MJ. Hip arthroscopy: an anatomic study of portal placement and relationship to the extra-articular structures. *Arthroscopy*. 1995;11:418–423, with permission.

before entering the lateral aspect of the posterosuperior capsule. Byrd (11) described the portal as coursing superior and anterior to the piriformis muscle tendon prior to entering the capsule. However, Robertson and Kelly (10) found that the PL portal passed through the piriformis tendon. This discrepancy may be due to the slight variation in the two authors' portal placement.

The PL portal is also a relatively safe portal. Injury to the sciatic nerve represents a potentially catastrophic complication. Fortunately, the nerve is located approximately 2 to 3 cm posterior to this portal (8,10). Placing the leg in maximal internal rotation will move the greater trochanter more anterior and facilitate a safe distance. Another potentially catastrophic complication involves injury to medial femoral circumflex artery. The artery courses superiorly and laterally as it runs between the quadratus femoris and the obturator externus (12). It crosses the tendon of the obturator externus and enters the posterior capsule at the femoral attachment becoming the lateral retinacular vessels. Sussmann et al (13). found that the medial femoral circumflex artery is on average 10.1 mm from the PL portal when the portal passes through the piriformis tendon. The authors felt that the greater trochanter protects the medial circumflex artery from injury. Anecdotally, this is verified by the rarity of avascular necrosis (AVN) associated with hip arthroscopy.

Anterior Portal

The anterior portal has been described with several variations. Byrd et al (8). described placement of the anterior portal at the intersection of a sagittal line drawn distally from the anterior superior iliac spine and a transverse line drawn across the superior edge of the greater trochanter. The trajectory of the portal courses 45° cephalad and 30° posterior, penetrating the muscle belly of the sartorius and the rectus femoris before entering through the anterior capsule. Robertson and Kelly (10) described an anterior portal that was placed 1 cm lateral to the ASIS and in line with the AL portal. The portal is directed medially with the trajectory being 35° cephalad and 35° posterior. The portal penetrated the muscle belly of the TFL and then passed through an interval between the gluteus minimus and the rectus femoris before entering the joint through the anterior capsule. We prefer to make the anterior portal approximately one-finger breath (1 cm) lateral to the ASIS and two finger breaths (2 cm) distal to the level of the AL portal (Fig. 46.7).

Injury to the lateral femoral cutaneous nerve (LFCN) is a potential complication associated with the anterior portal and likely underreported. The LFCN has variable branching as it courses underneath the inguinal ligament and distally down the leg. Byrd et al (8). found the average distance of the LFCN to be 3 mm from their described anterior portal. Robertson and Kelly, having moved the portal more laterally in an effort to avoid the LFCN, found the average distance to be 15.4 mm. However, the range was 1 to 28 mm, emphasizing the high variability of the LFCN. Moving the portal more distal than the described portals and off the ASIS line laterally will further minimize risk to the LFCN. As the portal is moved more distal, you do

Table 46.2

Results of central and peripheral compartment portals

Portal	Approximate Portal Insertion Angle	Anatomic Structure	Distance (mm)		
			Mean	SD	Range
Central compartment					
AP	35° cephalad, 35° posterior	LFCN	15.4	9.7	1–28
		Femoral nerve at sartorius	54.3	10.5	40–73
		Femoral nerve at rectus femoris	45.4	11.7	34–71
		Femoral nerve at capsule	35.4	10.2	18–52
		Ascending LCFA	31.0	13.1	13–53
		Terminal branch of ascending LCFA	14.7	11.1	2–33
AL	15° cephalad, 15° posterior	Superior gluteal nerve	64.1	13.1	39–81
		Sciatic nerve	40.2	8.0	31–51
MAP	35° cephalad, 25° posterior	LFCN	25.2	9.3	9–38
		Femoral nerve at sartorius	63.8	13.8	46–87
		Femoral nerve at rectus femoris	53.0	15.1	35–85
		Femoral nerve at capsule	39.9	9.2	26–54
		Ascending LCFA	19.2	11.2	5–42
		Terminal branch of ascending LCFA	10.1	8.2	1–23
PL	5° cephalad, 5° anterior	Sciatic nerve	21.8	8.9	11–38
Peripheral compartment					
AL	15° Caudad, 5° posterior	Superior gluteal nerve	69.4	11.0	52–85
		Sciatic nerve	57.7	12.2	38–66
MAP	15° cephalad, 20° posterior	LFCN	30.2	11.1	7–47
		Femoral nerve at sartorius	70.0	14.3	51–93
		Femoral nerve at rectus femoris	57.0	15.8	35–85
		Femoral nerve at capsule	39.4	11.5	18–57
		Ascending LCFA	21.0	12.3	5–41
		Terminal branch of ascending LCFA	14.7	10.8	1–30
PMAP	40° caudad, 25° posterior	Superior gluteal nerve	50.3	7.4	35–59
		Sciatic nerve	58.4	9.3	49–83
PL	25° caudad, 15° anterior	Sciatic nerve	33.6	9.7	17–50

From Robertson WJ, Kelly BT. The safe zone for hip arthroscopy: a cadaveric assessment of central, peripheral, and lateral compartment portal placement. *Arthroscopy.* 2008;24:1019–1026, with permission.

increase the risk of injuring the ascending branch of lateral femoral circumflex artery (LFCA). The ascending branch of the LFCA was found to terminate 31 mm distal to the anterior portal described by Robertson and Kelly (10). To further reduce risk to the LFCN, the skin incision should not pass deeper than the dermis. A deeper "stab" incision should be avoided.

Mid lateral Portal

The mid lateral (mid anterior) portal is utilized as an accessory portal and facilitates central compartment procedures such as suture anchor placement for labral repairs of the anterosuperior acetabulum and microfracture of the acetabulum. The portal is typically placed an equal distance between distal to the AL and anterior portals (10). The portal is established under direct visualization with the spinal needle directed medially with a trajectory of 15° cephalad and 20° posterior. The portal passes through the TFL and then passes between the gluteus minimus and the rectus femoris entering the anterior capsule. We typically use a position that is distal and further lateral to the anterior portal, but strictly based on the ability to directly visualize the proper trajectory for the purpose of the needed accessory portal (i.e., improved angle for microfracture of the acetabulum).

The mid lateral portal carries the same risk as the anterior portal. Moving more distal not only reduces risk to the LFCN but also increase the risk of injury to the ascending branch of the LFCA. The LFCA was on average 19.2 mm from the mid lateral portal (10). The LFCN was on average 25.2 mm from the portal.

Superior and Inferior Trochanteric Portals

The superior trochanteric and inferior trochanteric portals are utilized to access the peritrochanteric space in cases of trochanteric pain syndrome and external coxa saltans. The portals are established 3 cm above and 3 cm below the tip of the GT, in line with the axis of the femur (14). The portals are developed superficial to the iliotibial band (ITB) initially. A thermal ablation device is then used to develop a window through the ITB, allowing access to the peritrochanteric space.

The portals have no associated anatomic studies to correlate their relationships to neurovascular structures. There are no structures at risk with these portals as they are more superficial and only penetrate the skin and subcutaneous fat prior to reaching the ITB. Ilizaliturri et al (14). noted no complications with this technique. We have utilized the portals on numerous occasions with no associated complications.

Additional/Alternative Peritrochanteric Portals

The anterior portal, as previously described (10), can also be used to access the peritrochanteric space by directing the cannula lateral and posteriorly between the ITB and the greater trochanter (15). The leg is placed in full extension, 0° of abduction, and 10° to 15° of internal rotation to allow the cannula to be easily redirected. Two addition peritrochanteric portals, proximal anterolateral accessory (PALA) portal and peritrochanteric space portal (PSP), have been described in conjunction with the anterior portal for repair of gluteus medius tendon tears, bursectomy, and treatment of external coxa saltans. These portals have been found to be safe with very little risk to neurovascular structures (10).

BASIC ARTHROSCOPIC EXAMINATION

Central Compartment

We routinely establish portals into the central compartment first. The AL portal is typically the first portal established as it lies most centrally in the "safe zone." With fluoroscopic guidance, a spinal needle is directed medially into the hip joint between the acetabulum and the distracted FH (Fig. 46.8). We recommend placing the bevel of the spinal needle toward the FH to decrease the risk of iatrogenic cartilage damage. It is helpful to initially direct the spinal needle inferiorly toward the FH in order to place it under the labrum. Once the capsule is penetrated, the needle is directed cephalad in order to avoid the FH articular cartilage. If the surgeon is unable to place the spinal needle under the labrum, the spinal needle can be introduced into the joint and the stylet is then removed releasing the intra-articular pressure. The joint can then be further distended with saline and the spinal needle repositioned prior to placement of the obturator-cannula assembly. Adjusting the location of the AL portal may facilitate the ease with which specific procedures are performed. The appropriate angle for placement of suture anchors can be obtained by adjusting the AL portal slightly distal/caudal (1 cm). Adjusting the portal more proximal/cephalad improves the angle for accessing the fovea for treatment of injuries to the ligamentum teres (LT) or loose body removal from the fovea.

Once appropriate placement of the spinal needle is achieved, the stylet is removed and a guide wire is passed through the needle. The needle is withdrawn and the obturator-cannula assembly is placed over the guide wire and into the joint (Fig. 46.8). This should be done carefully and if excessive resistance is felt, additional traction or repositioning of the portal should be performed. The 70° arthroscope is then introduced into the joint. A combination of 30° and 70° arthroscopes allows for maximum visualization of the central and peripheral compartments. We routinely use a 70° arthroscope and reserve the 30° arthroscope for better visualization of the fovea and/or peripheral compartment when necessary. The AL portal is the only portal made without direct arthroscopic visualization. At this point the anterior labrum, anterior acetabulum, anterior capsule, and anterior FH should be well visualized (Fig. 46.8). If visualization is poor, this

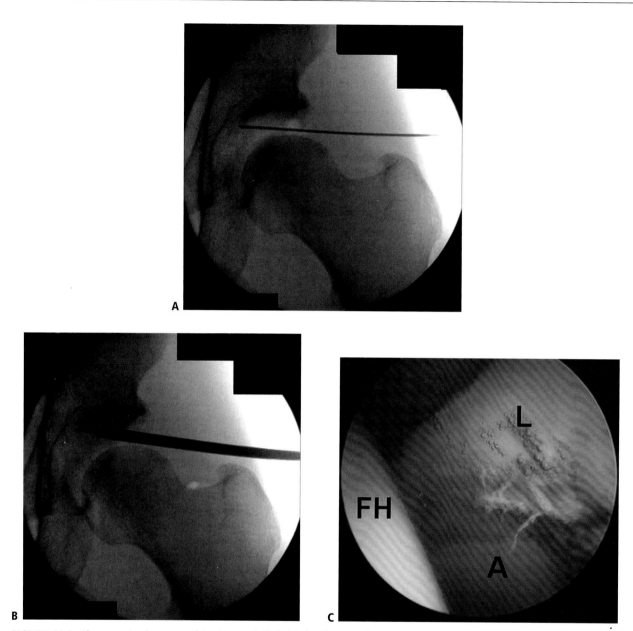

FIGURE 46.8. Fluoroscopic placement of the AL portal *(left hip)* with a spinal needle **(A)** and obturator cannula assembly **(B)**. Arthroscopic view of the anterior labrum (L), femoral head (FH), and acetabulum (A) through the AL portal **(C)**.

can be secondary to a prominent anterior bony acetabular lip (pincer) or inadvertent penetration of the acetabular labrum.

The anterior portal is next established under direct arthroscopic visualization. We adjust the portal relative to the size of the patient's leg. The portal is moved more medial in smaller diameter legs and more lateral in larger diameter legs in relation to a line dropped distally from the ASIS. This maintains appropriate distance (approximately 3 to 4 cm) between the AL and anterior portals for ease of triangulation and manipulation of instruments while a more distal site improves the angle for suture anchor placement. A spinal needle is introduced through the anterior capsule between the labrum and the FH through triangulation and with fluoroscopic assistance if

necessary (Fig. 46.9). A guide wire is then passed through the spinal needle followed by the obturator-cannula assembly (Fig. 46.9). We find it helpful to perform capsulotomies early to improve maneuverability during hip arthroscopy (Fig. 46.9). The degree of capsulotomy is based on the procedure to be performed with an extended capsulotomy performed when femoral resection osteoplasty is planned.

At this point, the camera is turned posterior to view the posterosuperior labrum, capsule, and femur. A spinal needle is introduced through the PL portal position (Fig. 46.10). Although this portal can be formally established at this point, we typically remove the stylet and use this for outflow. We find that most pathology can be adequately addressed with the anterior and AL portals and

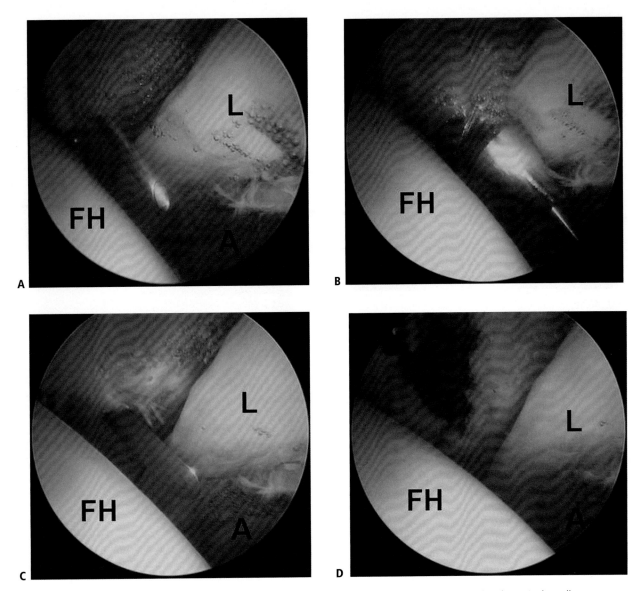

FIGURE 46.9. Arthroscopic view through the AL portal *(left hip)*. Establishment of the anterior portal with a spinal needle **(A)**, obturator cannula assembly **(B)**, introduction of a BB **(C)**, and performing a capsulotomy **(D)**. L, labrum; A, acetabulum; FH, femoral head.

reserve establishment of the PL portal for posterior labral and rim pathology, and posteriorly located loose bodies and synovial disorders.

The arthroscope is then placed into the anterior portal and a switching stick is placed in the AL cannula. Viewing from the anterior portal allows visualization of the superior/lateral labrum, acetabulum, FH, and both the AL and the PL portal placements (Fig. 46.11). If the AL portal has penetrated the lateral labrum, this portal is repositioned outside the labrum prior to making any capsular incisions. A BB is then introduced and a capsulotomy is performed through the AL portal (Fig. 46.11). Closed cannula systems should be utilized during placement of suture anchors and knot tying. Open or slotted cannulas can be utilized when exchanging instruments and cannulas,

which may help to minimize the amount of fluid extravasation within the extra-articular hip structures while still maintaining enough pressure to displace the capsule for visualization.

After placement of portals and performing capsulotomies, the central compartment of the hip is systematically evaluated. A descriptive arthroscopic evaluation of the hip joint has been published (6) and this can be done in any order as long as the examination is thorough. We typically begin our evaluation with the arthroscope in the anterior portal. The lateral/superior labrum, acetabulum, FH, and lunate fossa with its associated LT, pulvinar, and transverse acetabular ligament are inspected and probed (Fig. 46.12). The arthroscope is then placed into the AL portal. Looking anteriorly reveals the anterior labrum, acetabulum, lunate

IV. The Hip

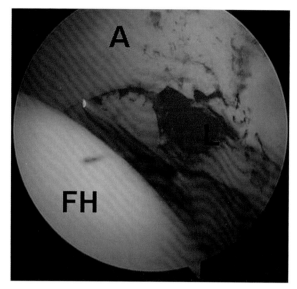

FIGURE 46.10. Arthroscopic view *(left hip)* through the AL portal and placement of a spinal needle in the PL portal. L, labrum; A, acetabulum; FH, femoral head.

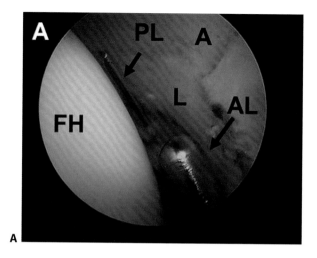

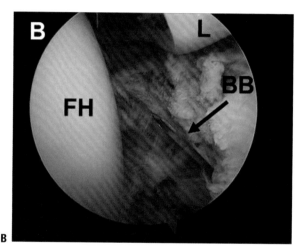

FIGURE 46.11. View through the anterior portal *(left hip)* reveals **(A)** a spinal needle in the PL portal and switching stick in the AL portal. **B:** A BB is used to create a capsulotomy through the AL portal. L, labrum; A, acetabulum; FH, femoral head.

fossa, and FH, and looking posteriorly reveals the supero-posterior labrum, acetabulum, lunate fossa, and FH. The location of pathology can be defined by the clock system or the zones system (16). Orientation is of paramount importance when evaluating pathology and its associated location. When capsular incisions are made, the psoas tendon (3:00 R hip) and the reflected head of the rectus tendon (12:00 R hip) can be helpful with respect to orientation. At this point, central compartment pathology should be well defined and the appropriate definitive procedures begin. Typically 50 lb of traction is adequate and traction time of greater than 2 hours should be avoided in order to minimize complications secondary to prolonged traction (4,5).

Peripheral Compartment

After management of central compartment pathology, attention is paid to the peripheral compartment. The peripheral compartment can be accessed by removal of instruments, flexion of the hip, and placement of a spinal needle through the AL incision and onto the anterior FN. Alternatively, when larger capsular incisions are made, we find it most efficient to back the arthroscope and instruments just outside the central compartment while still visualizing the FH and acetabulum, followed by release of traction. The hip is then flexed 30° to 40°. We typically keep the arthroscope in the anterior portal and use the AL portal as our working portal although alternating between portals may be helpful to improve visualization and working angles in some situations. The posterior spinal needle should be removed prior to release of traction. The anatomy of the peripheral compartment has been described in detail (6,17). At this point, the anterior FH, FHNJ, and acetabular rim/labrum are well visualized (Fig. 46.13).

When extended transverse capsulotomies have been performed, the arthroscope can be driven under the anterior inferior capsular limb revealing the inferomedial synovial fold (MSF), zona orbicularis (ZO), anteroinferior FH, acetabulum, and labrum (Fig. 46.14). This is rarely a site for pathology with the exception of an occasional loose body, synovial disorders (pigmented villonodular synovitis (PVNS), synovial chondromatosis), or inferior extension of some cam and pincer lesions. Driving the arthroscope superior/lateral will reveal and AL head–neck junction and labrum (Fig. 46.15). The arthroscope can then be driven under the superolateral capsular limb to reveal the lateral synovial fold (LSF), which is the site of the lateral retinacular vessels (Fig. 46.15). With respect to location, the MSF is generally located at about the 5:30 position (R hip) and the LSF is located at the 12:00 position. This initial evaluation is performed with the hip in flexion. To visualize the more superoposterior FHNJ, the hip can be extended and internally rotated.

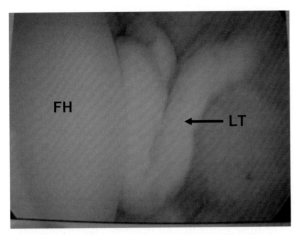

FIGURE 46.12. View of the lunate fossa and LT through the anterior portal. LT, ligamentum teres; FH, femoral head.

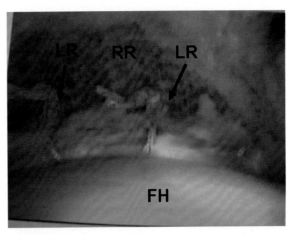

FIGURE 46.13. Release of traction *(left hip)* and viewing through the anterior portal reveals the anterior FH, labral refixation (LR), and RR.

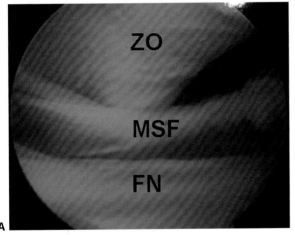

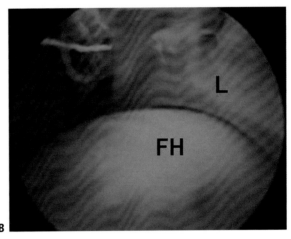

FIGURE 46.14. Driving the arthroscope anterioinferior *(left hip)* reveals the ZO, MSF, FN, FH, and inferior labrum (L).

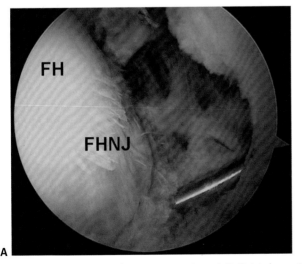

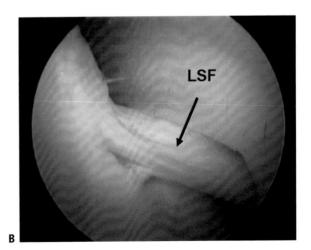

FIGURE 46.15. Driving the arthroscope superolateral *(left hip)* reveals the superolateral FH, FHNJ, and LSF.

INDICATIONS FOR HIP ARTHROSCOPY

Indications and contraindications for hip arthroscopy continue to evolve based on our understanding of hip pathology and the results of outcomes studies. Indications include labral tears, FAI, articular cartilage injury, hip subluxation/dislocation, LT disorders, loose bodies, recalcitrant internal and external snapping hip, psoas impingement, recalcitrant greater trochanteric pain syndrome, synovial disorders, septic hip, and some cases of mild to mod dysplasia. Contraindications include extensive heterotopic bone formation limiting access to the hip joint, advanced degenerative arthritis, and significant dysplasia with structural instability. Some common indications for hip arthroscopy and some technical PEARLS for performing these procedures are listed below:

Labral Tears

Labral tears are typically located anterosuperior and are often associated with other disorders such as FAI, dysplasia, and hip subluxation/dislocation. Placement of portals further distal/caudad may allow for better angles for suture anchor placement. When performing labral repairs/refixation, it is imperative then any associated pathology such as FAI be addressed to decrease the risk for recurrent labral damage. Emerging data suggest that labral preservation is preferable to indiscriminate labral debridement/excision (18).

Femoroacetabular Impingement

FAI has become one of the most common indications for hip arthroscopy. There is a steep learning curve for understanding and treating this entity. Generous capsulotomies allow for improved maneuverability and the ability to more easily perform labral takedown, pincer, and cam resection procedures. Intraoperative fluoroscopic in addition to direct arthroscopic evaluation can help to optimize bony resections and decrease the risk for bony underresection, overresection, or both. Symptomatic posterior femoral lesions are difficult to access arthroscopically and may be better addressed with open surgical dislocation. Heterotopic bone formation after bony resections can be minimized with meticulous removal of bony debris and prophylaxis with nonsteroidal anti-inflammatory drugs (NSAIDs) postoperatively.

Articular Cartilage Pathology

Some degree of articular cartilage pathology is found during the majority of hip arthroscopies. Lesions are typically located anterosuperiorly about the acetabulum and are frequently associated with other disorders such as FAI and dysplasia. Microfracture is the most common treatment method, and underlying disorders should ideally be addressed concomitantly. Accessory portals placed further distally/caudad may allow for better angles for the microfracture technique. Preoperative radiographic joint space narrowing will underestimate the true degree of articular cartilage damage and may have a significant negative impact on outcomes.

Ligamentum Teres Pathology

Ligamentum teres disorders can present similar to labral tears and are often missed on MRI. Use of multiple portals and a more proximal/cranial portal location can improve access to these disorders within the lunate fossae.

Dysplasia

Dysplasia should be approached arthroscopically with caution. Moderate to severe dysplastic forces can only be corrected with open procedures and FH lateralization should be considered a relative contraindication to hip arthroscopy. Every attempt to preserve the labrum, avoid RR, and close extensive capsular incisions should be considered in these situations. Acetabular retroversion in the setting of acetabular dysplasia should not be treated with anterior RR as this can lead to catastrophic structural instability.

Synovial Disorders

Although focal synovial disorders such as pigmented villous nodular synovitis and synovial chondromatosis can be managed arthroscopically, diffuse and posterior-based lesions are more definitively managed with open and combined arthroscopic and limited open approaches. The posterior aspect of the hip joint is difficult and in some cases impossible to fully address with hip arthroscopy.

Internal Snapping/Psoas Impingement

Psoas tenotomies can be performed at the level of the lesser trochanter, peripheral compartment, or central compartment. Psoas impingement is characterized by labral bruising/maceration anteroinferior as opposed to the typical labral pathology noted anterosuperior seen in association with other disorders. There is a significant risk for postoperative heterotopic bone formation after psoas tenotomy, and prophylaxis should be considered for 3 weeks with NSAIDs.

COMPLICATIONS

The reported complication rates after hip arthroscopy range from 1.34% to 3.8% (19–22). Neuropraxias of the perineal, LFCN, pudendal, sciatic, and femoral nerves are reported complications and are related to positioning and traction. Other traction injuries include pressure ulcers to the perineum, labia, scrotum, or dorsum of the foot. Positioning and traction injuries may be prevented by adequately padding the perineal post and minimizing the time spent in traction. Laceration of the LFCN, or a branch of the LFCN, is associated with establishment of portals, in particular the anterior portal. Skin incisions for the portals should be made no deeper than the dermis to avoid penetrating the subcutaneous tissue and injuring the LFCN. Other reported complications after hip arthroscopy include intra-abdominal fluid extravasation, iatrogenic cartilage and labral damage, instrument breakage, and FH AVN. Disease-specific complications related to FAI include inadequate RR or femoral resection osteoplasty. The rate of inadequate femoral resection osteoplasty has been reported to range from 72% to 92% in the setting of revision hip arthroscopy (9,22). Overresection of the acetabular rim may result in iatrogenic hip instability, whereas aggressive head and neck resection or inadequate protection postoperatively may result in FN fractures. Protected weight bearing for 2 to 6 weeks and avoidance of high-impact activity for 6 to 10 weeks even after an appropriate head/neck resection are recommended to minimize risk of postoperative FN fracture.

CONCLUSIONS

Hip arthroscopy in the supine position has been established as an effective and safe method for managing hip disorders. It is important to understand the appropriate setup, anatomical considerations, and basic and advanced surgical techniques in order to optimize outcomes for individuals with hip disorders amenable to hip arthroscopy.

REFERENCES

1. De Visme V, Picart F, Le Jouan R, et al. Legrand A, Savry C, et al. Combined lumbar and sacral plexus block compared with plain bupivacaine spinal anesthesia for hip fractures in the elderly. *Reg Anesth Pain Med.* 2000;25:158–162.

2. Touray ST, de Leeuw MA, Zuurmond WW, et al. Psoas compartment block for lower extremity surgery: a meta-analysis. *Br J Anaesth.* 2009;101;750–760.

3. Lee EM, Murphy KP, Ben-David B. Postoperative analgesia for hip arthroscopy: combined L1 and L2 paravertebral blocks. *J Clin Anesth.* 2008;20:462–465.

4. Byrd JW. The supine approach. In: Byrd JW, ed. *Operative Hip Arthroscopy.* 2nd ed. New York, NY: Springer; 2005:145–169.

5. Byrd JW. Hip arthroscopy by the supine approach. *Instr Course Lect.* 2006;55:325–336.

6. Bond JL, Knutson ZA, Ebert A, et al. The 23-point arthroscopic examination of the hip: basic set up, portal placement, and surgical technique. *Arthroscopy.* 2009;25(4):416–429.

7. Larson CM, Giveans MR. Arthroscopic management of femoroacetabular impingement: early outcomes measures. *Arthroscopy.* 2008;24:540–546.

8. Byrd JW, Pappas JN, Pedley MJ. Hip arthroscopy: an anatomic study of portal placement and relationship to the extraarticular structures. *Arthroscopy.* 1995;11:418–423.

9. Philippon MJ, Stubbs AJ, Schenker ML, et al. Arthroscopic management of femoroacetabular impingement: osteoplasty technique and literature review. *Am J Sports Med.* 2007;35:1571–1580.

10. Robertson WJ, Kelly BT. The safe zone for hip arthroscopy: a cadaveric assessment of central, peripheral, and lateral compartment portal placement. *Arthroscopy.* 2008;24;1019–1026.

11. Byrd JW. *Operative Hip Arthroscopy.* 2nd ed. New York, NY: Springer; 2005:113.

12. Kalhor M, Beck M, Huff TW, et al. Capsular and pericapsular contributions to acetabular and femoral head perfusion. *J Bone Joint Surg Am.* 2009;91:409–418.

13. Sussmann PS, Zumstein M, Hahn F, et al. The risk of vascular injury to the femoral head when using the posterolateral arthroscopy portal: cadaveric investigation. *Arthroscopy.* 2007;23:1112–1115.

14. Ilizaliturri VM, Martinez-Escalante FA, Chaidez PA, et al. Endoscopic iliotibial band release for external snapping hip syndrome. *Arthroscopy.* 2006:22: 505–510.

15. Voos JE, Rudzki JR, Shindle MK, et al. Arthroscopic anatomy and surgical techniques for peritrochanteric space disorders in the hip. *Arthroscopy.* 2007:23:1246.e1–1246.e5.

16. Ilizaliturri VM Jr, Byrd JW, Sampson TG, et al. A geographic zone method to describe intra-articular pathology in hip arthroscopy: cadaveric study and preliminary report. *Arthroscopy.* 2008;24(5):534–539.

17. Dienst M, Gödde S, Seil R, et al. Hip arthroscopy without traction: in vivo anatomy of the peripheral hip joint cavity. *Arthroscopy.* 2001;17(9):924–931.

18. Larson CM, Giveans MR. Arthroscopic debridement versus refixation of the acetabular labrum associated with femoroacetabular impingement. *Arthroscopy.* 2009;25(4):369–376.

19. Byrd JW. Complications associated with hip arthroscopy. In: Byrd JW, ed. *Operative Hip Arthroscopy.* New York, NY: Thieme; 1998:171–176.

20. Sampson TG. Arthroscopic treatment of femoroacetabular impingement. *Tech Orthop.* 2005;20:56–62.

21. Clarke MT, Villar RN. Hip arthroscopy: complications in 1054 cases. *Clin Orthop Relat Res.* 2003;406:84–88.

22. Heyworth BE, Shindle MK, Voos JE, et al. Radiologic and intraoperative findings in revision hip arthroscopy. *Arthroscopy.* 2007;23:1295–1302.

Hip Arthroscopy: The Lateral Position

Victor M. Ilizaliturri Jr • Alberto N. Evia-Ramirez

After adequate patient selection, patient positioning is the first and most important step in hip arthroscopy. Modern hip arthroscopy requires a dynamic technique of patient positioning. Traction is used to access the central compartment of the hip, which is the articular portion of the joint (1, 2). Structures in the central compartment are the acetabular articular surface, the acetabular labrum, the acetabular fossa and its contents, and most of the femoral head. The hip periphery (3), which is the intracapsular nonarticular portion of the hip joint, is usually accessed without traction. The hip periphery is considered to begin lateral to the free margin of the labrum. The structures inside the hip periphery are a small portion of the femoral head, the femoral neck, and the hip capsule with its synovial folds and zona orbicularis. Furthermore, hip mobility is frequently evaluated dynamically to assess clearance or improve access to different parts of the hip periphery. Therefore, effective patient positioning implies effective traction to separate the femoral head from the acetabulum and versatility to provide range of motion to the hip joint without traction to perform an adequate evaluation of the hip periphery.

Two techniques for patient positioning have been described for hip arthroscopy: the supine position (1) and the lateral position (4, 5). Both have evolved from only static traction techniques to a dynamic hip evaluation technique.

TECHNIQUE FOR LATERAL PATIENT POSITIONING

The lateral positioning technique for hip arthroscopy was developed by Glick and Sampson (4) in San Francisco. It was first used successfully in a case where the patient presented morbid obesity and the developers failed to gain arthroscopic access into the hip using the supine approach. They decided to try the technique with the patient in lateral decubitus, expecting to produce the fatty tissue to "fall away" from the trochanteric region, thus providing access through the less soft tissue between the portal sites and the inside of the joint. The lateral position was also adopted and further developed by McCarthy et al. (6) in Boston.

The operating room setup for the lateral position is different from the setup for the supine position. When the patient is supine, both the surgeon and the assistant are on the operative side of the patient and monitors are on the opposite side. When the lateral position is used, the surgeon stands in front of the patient because most of the pathology inside the hip is in the front. The surgical assistant stands at the back side of the patient and in front of the surgeon. It is more comfortable to have access to an endoscopy suite that has monitors in every side of the room. If there is access to an arthroscopy cart with only a single monitor, we position it on the back side of the patient and proximal to the patient's head; this will give a very adequate view both to the surgeon standing in the front side and to the assistant standing at the back side of the patient. The monitors of the image intensifier are positioned at the back side of the patient distal to the patient's feet; these will provide a very adequate view to the surgeon and to the surgical assistant (Fig. 47.1).

When the lateral position is used, only the operative side foot is fixed to the traction device; pelvic tilt from the application of traction is avoided by the patient's body weight and the length of the nonoperative leg resting free on the operative table.

In the supine position, pelvic tilt is avoided by fixing both feet to traction devices. Countertraction is applied on the foot in the nonoperative side.

Both the lateral and the supine positions use a perineal post to fix the pelvis and upper body in position on the surgical table while traction is applied. The position of the perineal post in both cases is lateralized relative to the patient's body, with the perineal post resting on the medial upper thigh. This protects the pudendal nerve from direct compression and lateralizes the vector of force from traction, aligning it closer to the direction of the femoral neck than to the direction of the femoral shaft (Fig. 47.2A and B). For both the lateral and the supine techniques, an oversized perineal post of at least 10-cm diameter is used (4). The position of the patient's genitalia should be verified before traction is established to protect them from compression injury.

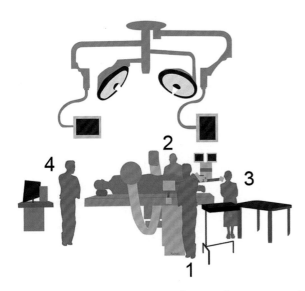

FIGURE 47.1. The drawing represents the operating room setup for hip arthroscopy in the lateral position. The patient is in right lateral decubitus, and only the left foot is fixed to the traction device. The arch of the image intensifier is horizontal under the operating table. In position number 1 is the surgeon, 2 is the surgical assistant, 3 is the scrub nurse, and 4 is the anesthesiologist.

When using the lateral position, lateralization of the perineal post is obtained by raising the position of the post relative to the operating table, and the surgeon should be careful not to over-raise the post, producing a "hanging patient" situation.

The arch of the image intensifier is positioned horizontally to obtain an antero posterior view of the affected side hip. Our preference is to position the arch under the surgical table (Fig. 47.3). In some patients the size of the arch may not be large enough to reach the operative side hip from under the table (because the patient is in lateral decubitus, the operative hip is on the upper side of the patient opposite to the operating table). If this is the case, the arch can be brought into the operating field in an over-the-top position and tilted in the direction of the patient's head to prevent it from obstructing the surgical team.

Foot fixation is a very important step in patient positioning. As mentioned above, when the lateral position is used, only the operative side foot is fixed to the traction device. Fracture tables and dedicated hip distractors have a foot platform, which is connected to the traction device. The way the foot is fixed to the platform varies and depends on the design of the table or distractor and surgeons' preference. The objective is to provide adequate and stable foot fixation to the traction device so that the traction force is effectively applied to the foot and transmitted through the lower extremity onto the hip joint, producing effective separation of the femoral head from the acetabulum. Separation occurs at the hip because the pelvis is stabilized with the perineal post. Adequate padding of the foot should always be performed to prevent

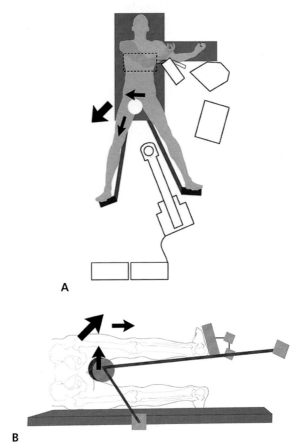

A

B

FIGURE 47.2. A: The drawing represents a patient in supine position for arthroscopy of the right hip. Both feet are fixed to traction devices. The perineal post is lateralized resting on the medial upper thigh. The *small arrows* represent the traction vector, lateral from lateralization of the post and longitudinal from the direction of force from the traction device. The *bigger arrow* represents the resultant direction of traction. **B:** The drawing represents a patient in left lateral decubitus; the right foot is fixed to the traction device. The *small arrows* represent the vectors of force created from traction lateralization (by raising the perineal post) and by longitudinal pull from the traction device. The *bigger arrow* represents the resulting traction vector of the combined forces.

compression injury. There are different methods of foot fixation to the traction platform:

1. *Elastic bandage and taping.* We have found this method to be effective and inexpensive. A cotton wrap is used around the foot for padding, the foot is fixed to the traction platform using an AC-bandage, and finally it is stabilized using adhesive tape to prevent foot separation from the platform. The result is like a boxer's bandage.

2. *Traction booties.* Most of the fracture tables provide traction booties as fixation devices to the platform. Belt buckles or Velcro straps are available for fixation of the booties over the feet. In our experience, Velcro straps seem to be more stable. It is also important to provide adequate padding to the foot inside the bootie. Fixation may be complemented with an elastic bandage around the bootie.

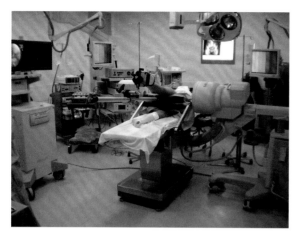

FIGURE 47.3. The photograph demonstrates a panoramic view of the operating room. A patient is positioned in left lateral decubitus for hip arthroscopy. The arch of image intensifier is horizontal under the operating table. Multiple roof mounted arthroscopy monitors provide an unobstructed view from either side of the patient. The fluoroscopy monitors are on the back side of the patient to provide an unobstructed view to the surgeon (who stands in front) and an adequate view to the assistant (who stands at the back side).

3. *Ski boots.* McCarthy introduced the concept of a ski boot-like design for the Inomed lateral distractor (Savannah, GA). This is the most effective fixation device. It provides a stable fixation between the foot and the boot and between the boot and the traction platform. Care must be taken to ensure adequate padding of the foot within the ski boot. It is the most expensive of the foot fixation systems and may not be available for every traction table or distractor.

FRACTURE TABLES

Fracture tables are the option of choice when hip arthroscopy is performed in the supine approach, because the positioning technique is very similar to the position used for fracture fixation. Fracture tables may also be used with the lateral position but special accessories are necessary, and they may not be available at every hospital (Fig. 47.4A–C). Because most of the cases of hip arthroscopy today require dynamic hip positioning, the surgeon and the operating room team should be very familiar with the design of the fracture table to operate it adequately to provide traction, traction release, and hip range of motion during the case. It is very important that the unscrubbed surgical team understand the operation of the fracture table because the surgeon will be in the sterile field and the table will be operated at the request of the surgeon by unsterile operating room staff.

DEDICATED HIP ARTHROSCOPY DISTRACTORS

Dedicated hip arthroscopy distractors were originally designed for the lateral approach because many of the fracture

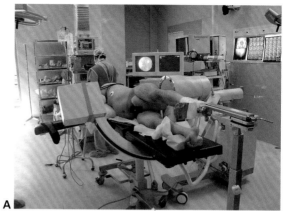
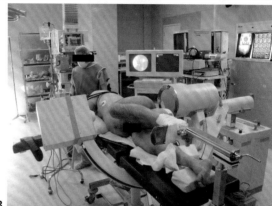
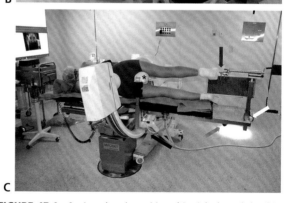

FIGURE 47.4. A: A patient is positioned in right lateral decubitus for arthroscopy of the left hip. An oversized perineal post is resting on the upper medial thigh. Only the left foot is fixed to a traction device, the right lower limb is resting free on the table. Bone prominences are protected to avoid compression. The arch of the image intensifier is horizontal under the table. **B:** A patient is positioned in right lateral decubitus for arthroscopy of the left hip. The hip is in flexion of about 90° neutral rotations and abduction/adduction to demonstrate hip mobility using the fracture table system. **C:** The photograph demonstrates the special accessories needed to position a patient lateral with traction on a Maquet fracture table (Rasttat, Germany). A model is resting in left lateral decubitus positioned for arthroscopy of the right hip. The *black arrow* indicates the crank used to elevate the traction post, *(asterisk)* indicates the oversized perineal post. The *orange arrow* points to a blue screw used to slide the traction bar away or in the direction of the table. The *white arrow* points to a white screw used to elevate to position of the traction device. The *green arrow* points to the traction device. The *blue arrow* points to the device that allows rotations and foot flexion of extension.

table designs had no accessories for the lateral position. The main advantage of dedicated distractors is that they can be used in combination with a standard surgical table. The first generation of hip distractors was designed to provide only traction to obtain separation of the femoral head from the acetabulum and perform surgery of the central compartment. In these early designs, dynamic examination of the hip periphery was not considered.

More recent distractors have been designed for providing traction and range of motion without traction for arthroscopic access of both the central and the peripheral compartments. Ease of operation is also a design feature of modern hip distractors to facilitate their operation by unsterile operating room personnel under the sterile drapes (Fig. 47.5A and B).

Dedicated supine distractors for hip arthroscopy are also available today. They are a good option for surgical centers where fracture tables are not available and have a very competitive cost compared with the cost of a fracture table system.

OTHER POSITIONING SYSTEMS

Positioning system technology such as the Spider (Tenet Medical, Calgary, Canada) has been a very popular option in shoulder and ankle surgeries. The system consists of a multiple joint "arm" that uses pneumatic pressure. When the system is pressurized, the joints are stable, and the arm holds a position. When pressure is released, the joints are loose, and range of motion can be reproduced. To apply the spider in hip arthroscopy, a perineal post and the Spider are attached to the surgical table; a traction device and a fixation boot are attached to the end of the Spider; the system is used to bring the lower extremity to a pre-traction position; and the system is stabilized and traction is applied with the traction device (Fig. 47.6). When the traction time is completed, the system pressure is released, allowing range of motion to be applied to the hip joint. The system can be pressurized again at any position of the hip the surgeon decides. The system is the most versatile for range of motion and gives full control of pressure release to the surgeon, making it very easy to operate. The disadvantages of the system are that it may be insufficient for very heavy or muscular patients and that a lateral rail extension is necessary to mount the Spider distally.

TRACTION POSITION AND TRACTION TEST

The position of the hip for traction has been a matter of debate among different authors. Our preference is to position the patient with neutral hip rotations. Internal rotation may place the sciatic nerve closer to the posterior margin of the greater trochanter, increasing the risk of puncture while introducing a needle through the posterolateral portal (at the posterior superior corner of the greater trochanter). The hip is positioned in slight flexion,

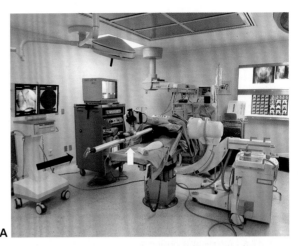

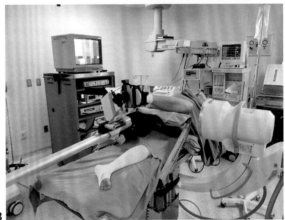

FIGURE 47.5. A: A patient is in left lateral decubitus positioned for arthroscopy of the right hip on a lateral hip distractor (Smith and Nephew Endoscopy, Andover, MA). Only the right foot is fixed to the traction device, the contralateral limb rests free on the table. The image intensifier is horizontal under the table. The *black arrow* points to the orange "T Handle" at the end of the traction bar; this releases a ball joint located at the connection between the perineal post and the traction bar (not visible) to provide mobility of the bar, allowing to extend, flex, adduct or abduct the hip. The *white arrow* points to an orange screw under the traction sled, which is used to lock or unlock the sled on the traction bar. If the sled is pulled away from the perineal post, the hip is in tension and preliminary traction is established. If the sled is pushed in the direction of the perineal post, hip flexion occurs. The *red arrow* points to a black crank, which is used to adjust final traction. **B:** A patient is in left lateral decubitus positioned for arthroscopy of the right hip on a lateral hip distractor (Smith and Nephew Endoscopy, Andover, MA). Only the right foot is fixed to the traction device; the contralateral limb rests free on the table. The hip is in flexion provided by sliding the traction sled in the direction of the perineal post. The *black arrow* points to a black screw in the base of the foot plate, which is used to provide foot rotations and foot flexion and extension.

of 15° to 20° to relax the anterior hip capsule. More flexion may increase tension on the sciatic nerve (7). Slight adduction of about 3° to 5° is applied to take mechanical advantage of the perineal post, using it to slightly lever the hip laterally with the proximal femur.

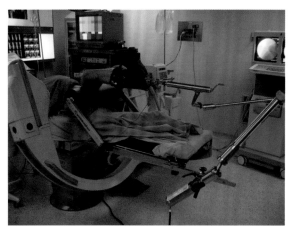

FIGURE 47.6. A patient is positioned in left lateral decubitus for arthroscopy of the right hip. A perineal post from the Smith and Nephew Lateral distractor is used. A spider positioning device (Tenet Medical, Calgary, Canada) is used for traction and limb positioning. In the photograph, the hip is flexed 30° and slightly abducted. This position is used to access the hip periphery. The foot is fixed to a specially designed traction device for the Spider using a ski boot. At the right side of the photograph, the Spider is attached to an extension side bar on the table; this is necessary to distance the Spider from the perineal post to provide traction.

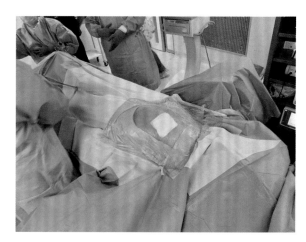

FIGURE 47.7. A patient positioned in left lateral decubitus for arthroscopy of the right hip. Sterile drapes are in position covering the patient and the image intensifier. A transparent adhesive drape is over the surgical field. A gauze is under the transparent drape on the area where the portals will be established.

Once the patient is in position with the anesthetic procedure installed and the arch of the image intensifier has been placed optimally to provide an antero posterior view of the operative hip, a traction test is performed before draping. Separation of at least 10 mm from the acetabular rim and the superior femoral head should be documented with the image intensifier (6). With the traction test applied, the surgeon must do a final examination of contact areas from the perineal post, make sure the patient's genitalia are free of compression, verify there are no compression points or lift off of the foot from the traction plate, and confirm padding is adequate. If the traction test was successful, traction is released and the patient is prepared and draped. In the case of an unsuccessful traction test, the surgeon should verify every step of patient positioning and look for the problem.

PREPARING AND DRAPING THE PATIENT

After a successful traction test we proceed to prepare the patient using an iodine solution.

When applying sterile drapes we start by covering both ends of the C arm using sterile bags. Then waterproof adhesive sterile drapes are placed in a standard fashion. The surgeon should be careful not to cover the landmarks or the portal sites with the drapes. The medial drape should be slightly medial to the anterior superior iliac spine. The posterior drape should be behind the posterior edge of the greater trochanter. The superior drape should be at the level of the anterior superior iliac spine,

and the distal drape should be 10 to 15 cm below the tip of the greater trochanter. After drapes are in position, we place sterile gauze over the area where the portals will be established and an adhesive transparent surgical drape is placed over the surgical area (over the gauze). This will seal the operative area to the adhesive drapes and prevent fluid from leaking under the drapes to the patient when the procedure starts (Fig. 47.7).

After cables and tubes for arthroscopy are ready, traction is applied (traction starting time should be recorded to monitor its duration). With the traction established, the gauze is removed from the surgical area with the adhesive drape that covers it. The plastic adhesive material is removed from the surgical area to prevent fragments of plastic from being introduced into the joint with the needles or the cannulas.

Landmarks are identified and marked on the skin with a skin marker (we prefer to mark the skin after traction is applied to avoid migration of the marks).

GENERAL TECHNIQUE

Portal Establishment: Central Compartment and Management of Hip Arthroscopy Cannulas

Traditionally, three portals have been described to access the central compartment in hip arthroscopy: the anterolateral, posterolateral, and direct anterior (Fig. 47.8) (8). There is variation among different authors about the situation of the portals and the order in which they are established. In general, one or two lateral portals (in the greater trochanteric region) are used and an anterior portal always lateral to a vertical line coming down from the anterior superior iliac spine. The anterior portal may be at the same height as the tip of the greater trochanter or more distal.

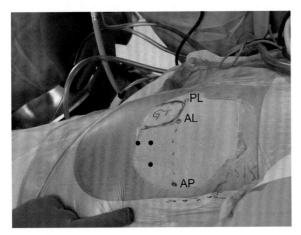

FIGURE 47.8. A patient positioned in left lateral decubitus for arthroscopy of the right hip. The sterile gauze and part of the transparent adhesive drape have been removed. The greater trochanter *(GT)* and the anterior superior iliac spine *(ASIS)* have been outlined on the skin. The situation of the anterolateral *(AL)*, posterolateral *(PL)*, and anterior *(AP)* portals is also indicated (these are typically used for the central compartment). The *black dots* demonstrate the site of different accessory portals (these are typically used for the hip periphery).

A description of our preferred technique follows:

We start by using a skin marker for topographical landmarks in the skin. The anterior superior iliac spine and the greater trochanter are the main landmarks for hip arthroscopy.

The anterolateral portal, located at the anterior superior corner of the greater trochanter, is always established first because it lies in the middle of the safety zone, which is limited posteriorly by the posterior edge of the greater trochanter (the sciatic nerve lies approximately 1.5 cm posterior to the femur) and anteriorly by a vertical line descending from the anterior superior iliac spine (the femoral neurovascular bundle lies medial to this line) (8).

With traction established, the patient prepared, and landmarks marked on the skin, we start by introducing a 17G spinal needle at the site of the anterolateral portal. The needle is navigated into the joint using fluoroscopy. Even though the anterolateral portal is at the center of the safe zone, it has the highest risk of iatrogenic injury to the intra-articular structures because it is done blindly without direct arthroscopic vision and guided only by fluoroscopy. Good separation of the femoral head and

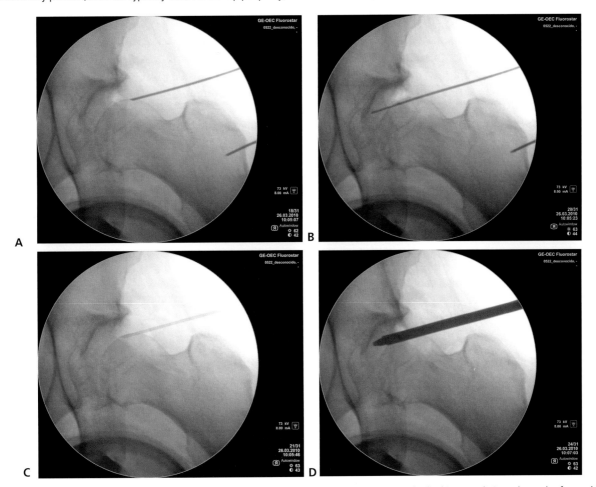

FIGURE 47.9. A: Fluoroscopy image of a left hip with distraction. A needle is in position inside the hip capsule just above the femoral head as far away as possible from the labrum. **B:** A guidewire has been introduced through the needle and is used to palpate the medial aspect of the acetabulum. It is directed toward the acetabular fossa (an osteophyte at the fossa is right in front of the guidewire). **C:** The capsule has been distended with fluid (note the increase in the separation between the acetabulum and the femoral head compared with **(A and B)**. The needle is in position on top of the femoral head, indicating it is not through the labrum. **D:** A cannula and cannulated obturator in position inside the hip joint.

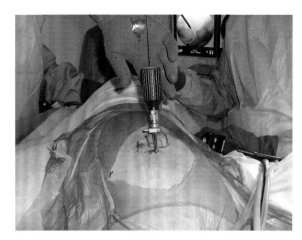

FIGURE 47.10. A modular cannula is introduced at the anterolateral portal using a guidewire (note the cannulated obturator).

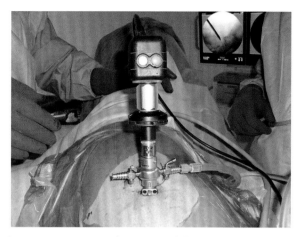

FIGURE 47.11. A 70° arthroscope-modular bridge-modular cannula assembly in position at the anterolateral portal. Inflow has been connected to one of the valves.

acetabulum is the first step to avoid iatrogenic injury. At this point, the separation depends on adequate traction. The spinal needle is introduced following the direction of the femoral neck as close as possible to the femoral head to avoid labrum penetration, with the tip of the needle in the opposite direction of the femoral head to contact the femoral head cartilage with the blunt side of the needle. Access into the joint is confirmed by feeling the penetration of the hip capsule and not by "landing" the needle on the acetabulum to avoid injury to the acetabular cartilage. Once the capsule has been penetrated, the stylus can be removed from the needle and a Nitinol (flexible metal alloy) guidewire can be passed though the needle to "palpate" the medial acetabulum with its blunt tip and confirm the intra-articular position of the needle. The guidewire must be directed to the acetabular fossa. The guidewire is removed and 40 cc of saline is injected into the joint for distension. Distension increases separation of the acetabulum and the femoral head (2, 8). Once the joint has been distended, a Nitinol guidewire is reintroduced through the needle and the needle is removed. At this point the cannulated hip arthroscopy instruments are used. A modular cannula with a cannulated obturator is passed into the joint using the guidewire as a monorail (Fig. 47.9A–D). The intra-articular placement of the modular cannula is confirmed with fluoroscopy (at this point it is better to use a small-diameter cannula to protect cartilage from damage as the cannula is introduced) (Fig. 47.10). The cannulated obturator is removed from the cannula, and a modular bridge with fluid management valves and a distal and proximal locking mechanism is attached to the cannula. The distal locking mechanism attaches the bridge to the cannula and the proximal one to the arthroscope (Arthrogarde Cannulas, Smith & Nephew Endoscopy, Andover, MA). A 70°, 4-mm arthroscope is positioned inside the cannula and attached to the modular bridge (Dyonics, Smith & Nephew Endoscopy, Andover, MA). One valve is used for inflow, which is set at 70 mm Hg using a hi-flow pump, and suction is placed at the second valve (Fig. 47.11). Next, the direct anterior portal is

established. The anterior triangle is identified arthroscopically (the anterior triangle is formed by the free margin of the anterior labrum superiorly, the superior anterior femoral head inferiorly, and the limit of the arthroscopic field of view laterally). The area inside the triangle is the anterior hip capsule. A needle is introduced at the site of the anterior portal and triangulated toward the center of the anterior triangle. The intra-articular position of the needle is confirmed arthroscopically as it pierces the anterior hip capsule at the center of the anterior triangle (Fig. 47.12). With the needle in position, the stylus is removed, a Nitinol guidewire introduced, and the needle removed. At this point two different techniques may be used: (1) The portal may be established using a second modular cannula, which will function as a working portal (Fig. 47.13), or (2) a switching stick can be introduced over the guidewire and then used to slide a slotted cannula into the joint (Fig. 47.14) (9, 10). With the slotted cannula in position, the switching stick and guidewire are removed, and the open side of the slotted cannula is ready for instrument introduction. After the instrument has been introduced, the slotted cannula is removed and the instrument is used "freehanded" inside the joint.

Slotted cannulas are not a good option for suture management, which is better though a closed cannula (Fig. 47.15A–D). The main advantage of a slotted cannula is that it allows curved or angled instruments to be introduced into the hip joint through its open side (Figs. 47.16A and B and 47.17A and B) (9).

To establish posterolateral portal or other accessory portals when necessary, the same technique of spinal needle, guidewire, and cannulated instruments is performed.

The posterolateral portal located at the posterior superior corner of the greater trochanter is frequently used as an outflow portal and may be necessary to access the posterior labrum, cartilage lesions on the posterior femoral head, or loose bodies located posteriorly within the hip.

For surgeons who use a classic anterior portal (located slightly literal to the vertical line descending from

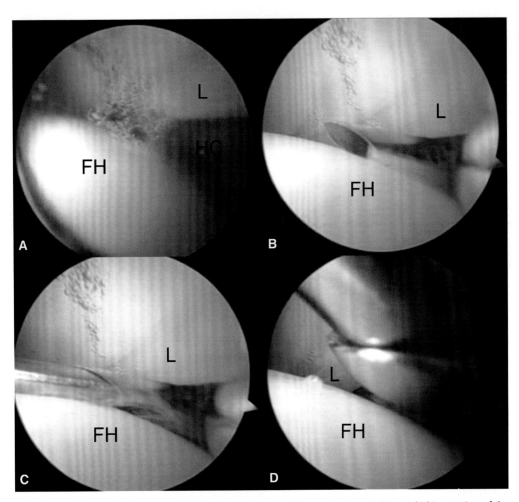

FIGURE 47.12. Arthroscopic photographs demonstrating the sequence to establish an anterior portal in a right hip. **A:** View of the anterior triangle. The upper limit is the labrum *(L)* at the top. The inferior limit is the femoral head *(FH)* at the bottom. The lateral limit is the limit of the arthroscopic field of view. The hip capsule *(HC)* is at the center of the triangle. The vision is slightly distorted because there is no outflow. **B:** A needle is in position at the anterior triangle between the labrum *(L)* and the femoral head *(FH)*. Note the vision is clear because of outflow. **C:** A flexible guidewire is introduced through the needle. **D:** A switching stick is in position through the anterior portal. A slotted cannula is being inserted using the switching stick as a guide.

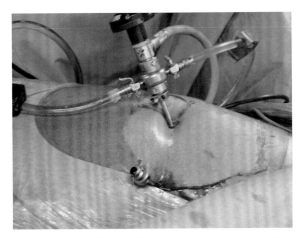

FIGURE 47.13. The photograph demonstrates an arthroscope in position at the anterolateral portal and a second modular cannula inside the anterior portal in a right hip.

the anterior superior iliac spine at the level of the tip of the greater trochanter), anchor placement at the anterior acetabular rim may require a lower accessory anterior portal (Fig. 47.18A and B).

INSTRUMENT EXCHANGE

The basic difference between the modular cannula technique and the slotted cannulas is that modular cannulas are full pipes; they typically remain in position in the portals, and instruments are driven into the joint through them. Instrument exchange is just a matter of taking out an instrument, leaving the modular cannula in place and then using it to introduce the new instrument.

The slotted cannula has an open side and is inside the portal only while instruments are introduced or exchanged. When using a slotted cannula for instrument

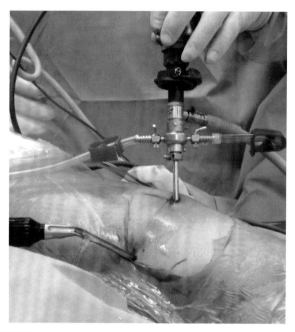

FIGURE 47.14. The photograph demonstrates an arthroscope in position at the anterolateral portal and a slotted cannula inside the anterior portal in a right hip.

exchange, the surgeon should remember that there should always be an instrument or the slotted cannula itself inside the joint to avoid losing the portal. For instrument exchange, the instrument inside the portal is used as a guide to slide the slotted cannula into the joint. With the slotted cannula in position, the instrument is removed and the new instrument brought in. When the new instrument is in position, the slotted cannula is removed from the portal.

PORTAL INTERCHANGING

Portal interchange with a modular cannula system is only a matter of closing the fluid valve, unlocking the bridge from the cannula that is in use as a viewing cannula, removing the arthroscope from the cannula, and reinserting it and locking it in the modular cannula that was originally used as a working cannula. The fluid is restarted and arthroscopic examination begins from the new position.

Portal interchange with a slotted cannula is slightly more complex and can be achieved using a slotted cannula only technique or combining the slotted cannula with modular cannulas: (1) *Slotted cannula only technique.* The slotted cannula is brought into the working portal

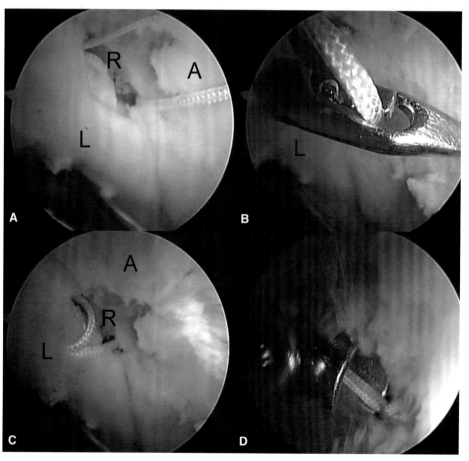

FIGURE 47.15. Arthroscopic sequence presenting a labral repair in a left hip. Suture management is done through a closed cannula. A: A loop is created with one of the limbs of the suture and passed into the joint between the labrum (L) and the acetabular rim (R). Medial to the exposed subchondral bone is the acetabular cartilage (A). B: The labrum (L) is pierced with a Bird Peak and the suture loop is caught. C: One suture limb is passed through the labral tissue as the Bird Peak is pulled out. D: Arthroscopic knots tied on the articular side of the labrum. Note how the suture is managed though a close cannula (5.5 mm).

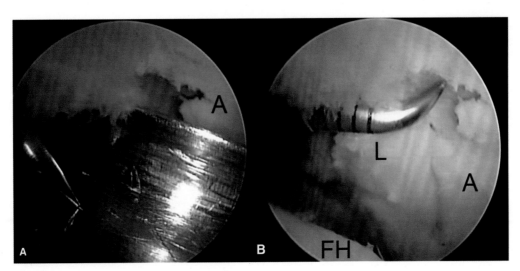

FIGURE 47.16. This arthroscopic sequence follows the sequence presented in Figure 47.15. **A:** A 60° microfracture awl is introduced using a slotted cannula. **B:** The labrum *(L)* has been fixed to the acetabular rim using a suture anchor. A 60° microfracture awl is used to do microfractures at an area of exposed subchondral bone on the anterior acetabulum *(A)*. The femoral head *(FH)* is below.

using the previous instrument in the portal as a guide, the instrument is removed, and a switching stick is introduced through the slotted cannula. The slotted cannula is removed, leaving the switching stick in position inside the original working portal, and reintroduced around the cannula in the viewing portal (the modular cannula inside the viewing portal is used as a guide for the slotted cannula) until the intra-articular position of the slotted

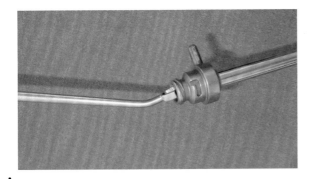

A

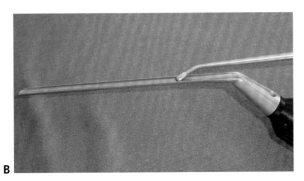

B

FIGURE 47.17. A: The photograph demonstrates how an angled curette cannot go through a closed 5.5-mm hip arthroscopy modular cannula. **B:** The photograph demonstrates how an angled curette is slid over a slotted cannula.

cannula is confirmed with direct arthroscopic vision. The fluid inflow is closed and the arthroscope-bridge-modular cannula assembly is removed from the inside of the joint, leaving the slotted cannula in position inside the original viewing portal. In the outside the arthroscope is removed from the bridge-modular cannula assembly. The assembly is then introduced over the switching stick positioned at the original working portal. The switching stick is removed and the arthroscope introduced and locked in the assembly and the fluid restarted; the slotted cannula is already in position for instrument introduction (2). *Hybrid technique using a slotted cannula and multiple modular cannulas.* A slotted cannula is brought into the working portal using the instrument in the portal as a guide. The instrument is taken out of the portal, leaving the slotted cannula in position inside the portal. A second modular cannula and obturator are introduced through the slotted cannula into the working portal. When the tip of the modular cannula is confirmed inside the joint with arthroscopic vision, the obturator from inside the modular cannula and the slotted cannula are removed. The inflow is closed, the modular bridge and arthroscope are removed from the first modular cannula (used as a cannula for the arthroscope) and introduced in the second modular cannula, and inflow is restarted. At this point the original working cannula is the new viewing cannula. A switching stick is introduced through the first modular cannula (now the working portal), the modular cannula is removed, and a slotted cannula is slid over the switching stick into the joint.

CAPSULOTOMY

The capsulotomy technique was introduced by Glick (11), who originally enlarged the portal entry site on the hip capsule using an arthroscopic knife. The result was a slot rather than a hole at the entry site of the portal on the

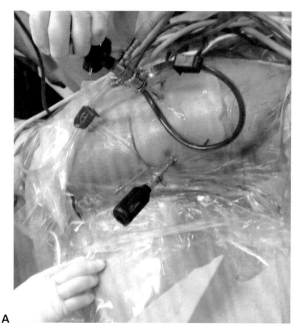
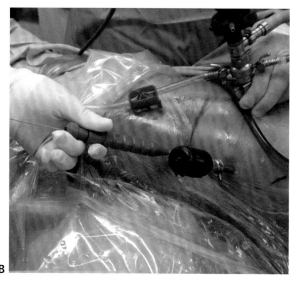

FIGURE 47.18. A: The photograph demonstrates establishment of an accessory portal in a right hip. The arthroscope is inside the anterolateral portal. A modular cannula and obturator are in position at the anterior portal. The needle is in position at an anterior inferior accessory portal. **B:** The anchor delivery instruments are in position at the anterior inferior accessory portal. A percutaneous technique using a flexible guidewire was used.

hip capsule. This slot improved instrument mobility and access to pathology within the central compartment. The technique evolved into a complete capsulotomy, in some cases joining the entry sites of the anterolateral portal and the anterior portal from inside the hip capsule (Fig. 47.19A and B). The capsular cut is also frequently prolonged in the direction of the femoral neck, creating a T-shaped capsulotomy on the anterior hip capsule, often used to expose the anterior femoral head and neck junction.

AIMING DEVICES

Aiming devices were introduced to facilitate portal establishment of the anterior portal while minimizing the amount of radiation used during hip arthroscopy (12). The anterior portal is out of the plane that can be ideally navigated by the image intensifier and is established by the surgeon using a triangulation technique (8). The first generation of aiming devices was inspired on an anterior

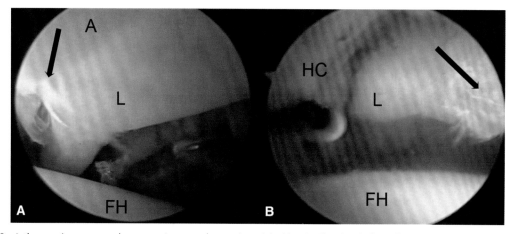

FIGURE 47.19. Arthroscopic sequence demonstrating capsulotomy in a right hip. **A:** The view is from the anterolateral portal. A radiofrequency hook is used to perform a retrograde cut on the anterior hip capsule *(HC)*. The anterior labrum *(L)* is at the center, the anterior acetabulum *(A)* at the top and the anterosuperior femoral head *(FH)* at the bottom. The *black arrow* points to an anterior labral detachment. **B:** The view is from the anterior portal. A radiofrequency hook probe is used to perform a retrograde cut on the lateral hip capsule *(HC)* (the goal is to connect this cut to the anterior capsular cut, presented in Fig. 47.17A). The lateral labrum *(L)* is at the top and the femoral head *(FH)* at the bottom. The *black arrow* points to a lesion of the free margin of the anterolateral labrum.

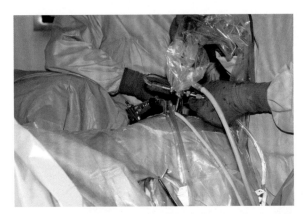

FIGURE 47.20. The photograph demonstrates a patient in left lateral decubitus; arthroscopy of the right hip is performed. The arthroscope is in position at the posterolateral portal. The tip of the aiming device is in position through the anterolateral portal. The aiming arch is attached to the aiming tip. The bullet and the needle have been introduced through the anterior portal.

cruciate ligament tibial tunnel guide using an intra-articular reference to guide the needle into the hip joint. For this, two lateral portals were necessary: the anterolateral and posterolateral portals, which were established with the aid of fluoroscopic navigation. The posterolateral portal was used as the viewing portal and an intra-articular aimer was introduced through the anterolateral portal using a slotted cannula. The tip of the aimer was directed to the selected entry point on the anterior hip capsule. The aiming device was assembled outside of the joint and the aiming bullet fully introduced at the site of the anterior portal based on the arthroscopic landmarks. With the bullet in position, a spinal needle was introduced through the bullet and observed inside the joint as it pierced through the selected spot (Fig. 47.20). A more recent evolution of the aiming devices uses the arthroscope itself as a reference point for the aimer. With the arthroscope in position inside the joint, the anterior triangle (formed by the free margin of the anterior labrum as the upper limit, the anterosuperior femoral head as the lower limit and laterally the limit of the arthroscopic field of view) is identified, and the center of the hip capsule inside the triangle is positioned at the center of the screen. The arch of the aiming device is attached to the arthroscope, the aiming bullet introduced through the selected site of the anterior portal based on skin landmarks, and a needle introduced though the bullet (Fig. 47.21). The tip of the needle is observed arthroscopically as it pierces the selected spot on the anterior hip capsule. Both techniques can be used to establish other accessory portals.

TRACTION TIME

We think about traction as we think about tourniquet time. Traction time should never exceed 1.5 hours and is best limited to 1 hour. Usually, most of the central compartment work can be achieved in less than 1 hour of traction

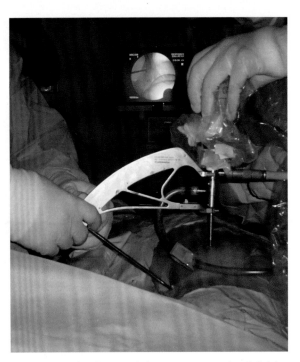

FIGURE 47.21. The photograph demonstrates a patient in left lateral decubitus; arthroscopy of the right hip is being performed. The arthroscope is in the anterolateral portal. The aiming arch is attached to the arthroscope. The aiming bullet is inserted through the anterior portal to guide the needle to the anterior hip capsule.

time. If more time is necessary for the central compartment, the surgeon can release traction and work at the hip periphery to allow the patient to rest from traction for 20 to 30 minutes. Then traction may be reestablished and the central compartment procedure completed.

PORTAL ESTABLISHMENT: PERIPHERAL COMPARTMENT

There are two ways to access the hip periphery after central compartment arthroscopy is completed:

1. *Using the same portals established for the central compartment.* Instruments are pulled out of the articular portion of the hip joint but remain inside the capsule, taking advantage of the capsulotomy as traction is released. To perform this, we prefer to have the arthroscope positioned at the anterolateral portal and a slotted cannula at the anterior portal. The femoral head is observed as it comes into the acetabulum when traction is released; evaluation of the labral seal on the femoral head can be done at this point. After the head is completely inside the acetabulum, the femoral head-neck junction comes into view, and, if necessary, an arthroscopic knife or a radiofrequency device can be used to extend the capsulotomy distally in the direction of the femoral neck. The result is a "T-shaped" capsulotomy. The capsulotomy is useful to further expose the anterior femoral head-neck

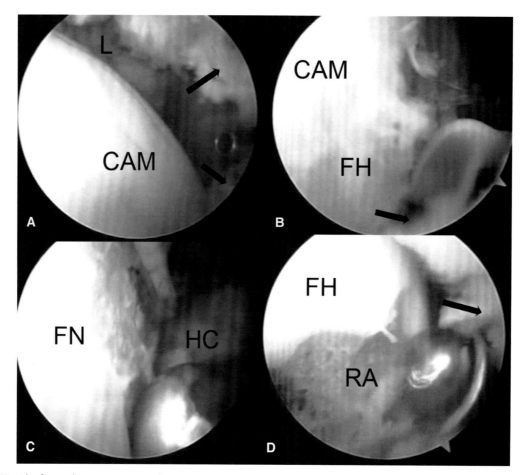

FIGURE 47.22. The figure demonstrates an arthroscopy sequence accessing the femoral head-neck junction by pulling back the instruments. **A:** The arthroscope is in the anterolateral portal; it was pulled back and traction was released. A cam deformity *(CAM)* at the femoral head-neck junction is at the center of the photograph. The labrum *(L)* is at the top. The *arrows* point to the limits of a capsulotomy that was performed when accessing the central compartment. A switching stick is in position at the anterior portal. **B:** The capsulotomy is extended distally using a radiofrequency hook *(black arrow)* in the direction of the femoral neck *(FN)*. The distal portion of the cam *(CAM)* deformity is at the top. **C:** A shaver is used to resect synovial tissue from the hip capsule *(HC)* to further expose the femoral neck *(FN)* area. **D:** A burr is used to remodel the cam deformity. The femoral head *(FH)* is at the top, the resected area *(RA)* is below the head. The *arrow* points to one of the capsular flaps created by the "T capsulotomy."

junction and the adjacent femoral neck (Fig. 47.22). Dynamic examination is used at this point to evaluate clearance of hip motion. If necessary, the portals may be interchanged to access different areas of the hip periphery. The 70° arthroscope may also be exchanged for a 30° arthroscope in the hip periphery. This technique is very useful for femoroacetabular impingement surgery. Accessory portals may also be necessary for this technique at the hip periphery, and they are established under direct arthroscopic vision using spinal needles, guidewires, and cannulated instruments, as described for the central compartment.

2. *Instrument pullout, traction release, and reestablishing portals for the hip periphery.* We use this technique to access the lower part of the femoral neck or the iliopsoas bursa, transcapsular or at the level of the lesser trochanter (13, 14). Instruments are removed from the joint and traction is released. A new portal for the hip periphery is established using a spinal needle introduced through the portal incision of the anterolateral portal, but this time directed anteriorly to the inferior femoral head-neck junction roughly perpendicular to the direction of the femoral neck. Once in position, the stylus is removed from the needle; fluid escape through the needle confirms its intracapsular position. A guidewire is introduced through the needle, the needle removed, and a modular cannula with cannulated obturator is introduced, using the guidewire as a monorail. The obturator is removed and a 30° 4-mm arthroscope and modular bridge assembly are introduced and locked into position in the modular cannula. Examination of the hip periphery begins at this point. A working portal is established using an accessory portal entry site. A triangulation technique using a spinal needle, guidewire, and cannulated hip arthroscopy access instruments is used (Fig. 47.23).

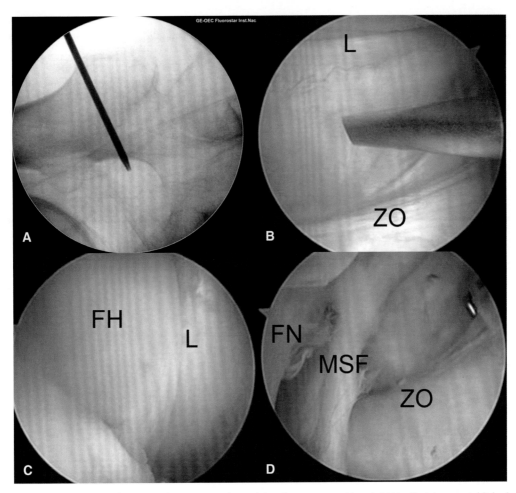

FIGURE 47.23. Arthroscopy sequence demonstrating access to the peripheral compartment in a right hip. Portals are established after removal of instruments from the central compartment. **A:** A switching stick guided to position at the anterior inferior hip capsule using fluoroscopy. **B:** Once in the hip periphery an accessory working portal is triangulated using a spinal needle. The labrum *(L)* is at the top and the zona orbicularis *(ZO)* at the bottom. **C:** View of the anterior labrum *(L)* and the anterior femoral head *(FH)*. **D:** Detail of the inferior hip capsule showing the femoral neck *(FN)* to the left, the medial synovial fold *(MSF)* and its relation to the zona orbicularis *(ZO)*.

SUMMARY

Both the supine and the lateral patient position techniques are effective in providing safe and reproducible access to the central and peripheral compartments of the hip. Today hip arthroscopy is performed mode dynamically, and patient positioning should be designed to provide not only adequate traction for effective separation of the femoral head from the acetabulum but also hip range of motion after traction has been released to access the hip periphery and evaluate clearance of hip motion. All of these requirements have made hip arthroscopy a very technical and technologic procedure. For the surgeon interested in hip arthroscopy, infrastructure as well as dedicated hip instruments must be available to ensure a safe and reproducible surgical procedure with good results. The learning curve of hip arthroscopy has been described as complicated; surgeon visits and attending to cadaver training laboratories are effective educational tools.

REFERENCES

1. Byrd JW. Hip arthroscopy utilizing the supine position. *Arthroscopy.* 1994;10:275–280.
2. Byrd JW. Avoiding the labrum in hip arthroscopy. *Arthroscopy.* 2000;16:770–773.
3. Dienst M, Godde S, Seil R, et al. Hip arthroscopy without traction in vivo anatomy of the peripheral joint cavity. *Arthroscopy.* 2001;17:924–931.
4. Glick JM, Sampson TG, Gordon RB, et al. Hip arthroscopy by the lateral approach. *Arthroscopy.* 1987;3:4–12.
5. Ilizaliturri VM Jr, Mangino G, Valero FS, et al. Hip arthroscopy of the central and peripheral compartment by the lateral approach. *Tech Orthop.* 2005;20:32–36.
6. McCarthy JC, Day B, Busconi B. Hip arthroscopy: applications and technique. *J Am Acad Orthop Surg.* 1995;3:115–122.
7. Dienst M, Seil R, Godde S, et al. Effects of traction, distension and joint position on distraction of the hip joint: an experimental study in cadavers. *Arthroscopy.* 2002;18:865–871.

IV. The Hip

8. Byrd JW, Pappas JN, Pedley MJ. Hip arthroscopy: an anatomic study of portal placement and relationship to the extraarticular structures. *Arthroscopy*. 1995;11:418–423.

9. Ilizaliturri VM Jr, Acosta-Rodriguez E, Camacho-Galindo J. A minimalist approach to hip arthroscopy: the slotted cannula. *Arthroscopy*. 2007;23:560, e1–e3.

10. Ilizaliturri VM Jr, Mangino G, Valero FS, et al. Special instruments and technique for hip arthroscopy. *Tech Orthop*. 2005;20:9–16.

11. Glick JM. Hip arthroscopy: the lateral approach. *Clin Sports Med*. 2001;20:733–747.

12. Ilizaliturri VM Jr, Valero FS, Chaidez PA, et al. An aiming guide for anterior portal placement in hip arthroscopy. *Arthroscopy*. 2003;19:E125–E127.

13. Ilizaliturri VM Jr, Villalobos FE Jr, Chaidez PA, et al. Internal snapping hip syndrome: treatment by endoscopic release of the iliopsoas tendon. *Arthroscopy*. 2005;21:1375–1380.

14. Ilizaliturri VM Jr, Chaidez C, Villegas P, et al. Prospective randomized study of 2 different techniques for endoscopic iliopsoas tendon release in the treatment of internal snapping hip syndrome. *Arthroscopy*. 2009;25:159–163.

Management of Labral and Articular Lesions

Carlos A. Guanche

Our understanding of the pathology causing hip pain is evolving. The exact prevalence of acetabular labral tears and cartilage injuries in the general population is unknown. Injuries to the acetabular labrum are the most consistent pathologic findings identified at the time of hip arthroscopy (1). In one review of 300 cases, labral tears were present in 90% of patients. These tears are most frequently found in the anterior aspect and often are associated with sudden twisting or pivoting motions. The incidence of cartilage injuries is as not as well documented, however.

Current surgical options as well as the indications for surgery are being developed. The ideal indication for labral repair is a tear from a recent traumatic injury. The common presentation, however, has no inciting event and is caused by chronic repetitive injury, leading to an attritional tear. Likewise with cartilage injuries, there is typically a long history of chronic pain with no obvious etiological event. It is therefore important to understand that treatment of the underlying pathology is as important as treating the problem, or the long-term results will be poor.

The hip labrum is a fibrocartilaginous structure that surrounds the rim of the acetabulum in a nearly circumferential manner. The labrum is widest in the anterior half, thickest in the superior half, and merges with the articular hyaline cartilage of the acetabulum through a transition zone (2) of 1 to 2 mm. The labrum is firmly attached to the rim of the acetabulum. Its junction with the osseous margin is irregular, and there may be extension of bone into the substance of the labrum. A group of three or four vessels are located in the substance of the labrum on the capsular side of this bony extension and penetrate into the peripheral one-third of the labrum. The labrum is separated from the hip capsule by a narrow synovial-lined recess (Fig. 48.1). Extrapolating from our understanding of the healing capacity of the meniscus, repair strategies should be considered in tears involving only the peripheral labrum.

We are only beginning to understand the function of the labrum. It functions as a secondary stabilizer by extending the acetabular congruity as well as helping to maintain the negative intra-articular pressure within the joint. This

has been confirmed through a poroelastic finite model that showed the labrum functions to provide structural resistance to lateral motion of the femoral head within the acetabulum (3) and decreases the contact pressures within the hip probably as a result of its effect on maintaining the articular fluid in contact with the weight-bearing cartilage (4).

CLINICAL EVALUATION

History and Physical Examination

Since the differential diagnosis of hip pain is so broad, the examiner must detail the patient's history with regard to their medical history, any hip surgery/trauma, or pediatric hip disease, as well as any social or occupational hazards. The clinical presentation of patients with a tear of the labrum or chondral injury is variable, and, as a result, the diagnosis is often missed initially. One study has shown that in a series in which the diagnosis of a labral tear had been made by arthroscopy, the mean time from onset of symptoms to diagnosis was 21 months (3). An average of 3.3 health care providers had seen each patient prior to diagnosis. Groin pain was the most common complaint (92%) with the onset of symptoms most often insidious. The most common exam finding was a positive "impingement sign," which occurred in 95% of patients in this series.

Although most patients do not specifically report loss of hip range of motion, this finding is almost universally seen. Hips with structural abnormalities, such as acetabular retroversion, coxa profunda, or pistol grip deformities, may have decreased range of motion(ROM) from anatomic limitations, but may also be limited by pain. Patients with pathologic hip conditions also commonly develop late capsulitis, synovitis, and/or trochanteric bursitis. Differential diagnosis of the classic mechanical symptoms (painful catching or clicking) of labral tears and/or chondral injury includes snapping iliotibial tendon or a hypermobile psoas tendon (1). The differential diagnosis should include sacroilitis, degenerative disk disease, abductor muscle problems, osteonecrosis, psoas tendinitis, pubic rami fractures,

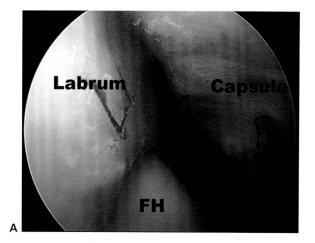

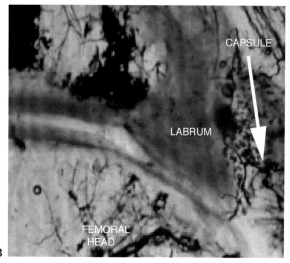

FIGURE 48.1. Hip labral vascularity. **A:** Clinical picture of the inter-section of the hip capsule. Labrum and acetabulum **B:** Cross-sectional image at the same level depicting that areas of vascularity of the labrum. Note the extensive plexus at the capsulolabral junction.

and stress fractures of the proximal femur. More chronic problems are usually associated with trochanteric bursitis.

Clinical examination of the affected hip should begin with an evaluation of the patient's gait, foot progression angle, and measurement of leg length. The antalgic gait pattern should be differentiated from the Trendelenburg gait (seen in patients with hip dysplasia who have weak abductors). Patients with deformities secondary to slipped capital femoral epiphysis may ambulate with an externally rotated extremity and an open foot progression angle (>10°). Hip pathology may be detected on inspection of the lower extremity rotation with the legs at rest. Typically, both feet rest symmetrically at approximately 10° to 30° of external rotation. Asymmetric external rotation of the legs may indicate acetabular retroversion, femoral retrotorsion, or femoral head–neck abnormalities, which can be a source of primary pathology.

The hip is then carried through a range of motion, with one hand placed over the spinous process during

flexion to allow immediate detection of pelvic flexion once the proximal femur contacts the acetabulum. Rotation is then measured with the hip flexed at 90°. The patient with retroversion and femoroacetabular impingement (FAI) has limited flexion and/or internal rotation.

Findings on physical examination can include a positive McCarthy sign (with both hips fully flexed, the patient's pain is reproduced by extending the affected leg, first in external rotation, then in internal rotation). Also common is inguinal pain with flexion, adduction, and internal rotation of the hip as well as anterior inguinal pain with ipsilateral resisted straight leg raising (5).

The impingement test was first described for patients with femoroacetabular impingement but is equally useful for labral injuries. With the hip at 90° of flexion, maximum internal rotation and adduction is performed. Contact between the anterosuperior acetabular rim and the femoral neck elicits pain. Although there is no specific examination to assess for chondral injuries, this same maneuver is also highly sensitive for intra-articular patholog (6). The hip can also be tested at varying degrees of flexion. Posterior labral tears should be tested with the leg externally rotated and in hyperextension.

Diagnostic Imaging

Weight-bearing AP pelvis and frog lateral radiographs are critical in the initial assessment to evaluate the patient for arthritis and FAI, as well as dysplasia.

Multiple studies have demonstrated the superior accuracy of magnetic resonance arthrography (MRA) over standard MRI in diagnosing labral tears. Intra-articular gadolinium has been shown to improve the sensitivity of diagnosing labral pathology from 25% to 92% using a small field of view (7). Therefore, when clinical suspicion of a hip labral tear or chondral articular disruption exists, MRA using a small field of view is the study of choice.

An intra-articular bupivacaine injection may be useful in situations where the diagnosis of labral or chondral pathology is equivocal or if a tear has been diagnosed by MRA, but it is uncertain whether symptoms are related. Similar to its use in diagnosing external impingement of the shoulder, if patients experience relief from their symptoms following the injection, the diagnosis of pain secondary to hip intra-articular pathology is more certain (8). However, intra-articular pathology could still be present without pain relief from the injection (9).

Research utilizing delayed gadolinium-enhanced MRI of cartilage (dGEMRIC), which measures loss of glycosaminoglycans in early stages of arthritis, has demonstrated that dGEMRIC has the ability to detect early stages of osteoarthritis due to hip dysplasia and femoroacetabular impingement (10). In addition, this technique has shown promise with regard to staging of cartilage lesions before and following surgical interventions.

TREATMENT

Nonoperative

Once the diagnosis of a labral tear has been made, conservative treatment options include avoiding activities that cause symptoms and a supervised therapy program emphasizing hip range of motion and core strengthening. Although it is unlikely that the tear will heal over time, it is possible that symptoms may stabilize to the point that the patient no longer experiences symptoms. If conservative management is elected, the patient should understand the need to avoid activities that produce symptoms and the possibility that the tear may progress and potentially predispose to arthritic changes in the hip. There are no published series detailing the long-term results of this treatment regimen.

Likewise, the mainstay of treatment for cartilage injuries consists of prompt diagnosis and activity modification. If these fail to ameliorate symptoms, surgical treatment is recommended. There are numerous accepted surgical options most of which are based on the historical treatment of these injuries in the knee. The procedure depends on the underlying etiology, overall alignment of the joint, the extent of involvement, and size of the lesion. For more advanced processes, treatment options include acetabular and femoral osteoplasties, redirectional osteotomies, trap-door procedures, hip resurfacing, and total joint replacement. For well-circumscribed lesions in a prearthritic well-aligned joint, options include debridement, microfracture, and isolated cartilage restoration as well as resurfacing procedures. Although open surgery is still the gold standard, these procedures are increasingly being performed arthroscopically.

Operative Debridement of Lesions

Most labral tears and chondral injuries are treated with debridement. However, some labral tears are amenable to arthroscopic repair. As discussed, the blood supply to the labrum enters from the adjacent joint capsule, with vascularity detected in the peripheral one-third of the labrum while the inner two-thirds were avascular. Thus peripheral tears have healing potential, and repairs should be considered if this is observed at the time of surgery. However, McCarthy et al. (6) reported 436 consecutive hip arthroscopies including 261 labral tears, with all of the tears located at the relatively avascular articular junction.

It is the author's preference to use a general anesthetic supplemented with a lumbar plexus block for postoperative analgesia as well as relaxation (11). The procedure can be performed in either the supine or the lateral position and should use both a 30° and a 70° arthroscope for a thorough assessment of the joint. Modified arthroscopic flexible instruments, extended shavers, and hip-specific instrumentation should be available.

A diagnostic arthroscopic examination of the central compartment can be done systematically not only to evaluate the labrum from anterior to posterior but also to locate possible cartilage lesions on both the acetabular and the femoral side (5). The typical cartilage lesions are adjacent to injured labrum. The acetabular notch should be evaluated and the integrity of the ligamentum teres should be assessed. This can be a source of pain as a result of impingement of the soft tissues between the femoral head and the acetabulum. In addition, severe synovitis can be found in this area. If encountered, it should be debulked or removed(Fig. 48.2). Any loose bodies should be noted and their source identified. Finally, an assessment should be made of any obvious capsular redundancy or laxity.

Many patients will have a significant synovitis associated with the labral tearing and an effort should be made to resect some of the inflamed tissue, not only for visualization of the joint but also to decrease the associated pain. It is the author's preference to use a radio frequency (RF) probe in order to decrease the potential for bleeding and subsequent compromise of the surgical field.

The goal of the procedure should be to preserve as much tissue as is technically feasible, while resecting the degenerative or damaged portions. This is important in order to maintain the labrum's role as a secondary joint stabilizer and to minimize the potential for arthrosis. Frayed labral tears should be debrided with the use of either motorized shavers or RF probes (Fig. 48.3). Placing absorbable suture through the defect and tying the suture through the capsule can stabilize intrasubstance labral tears. It is important to delineate the areas of abnormal tissue that are identified both on radiographs (in the form of perilabral calcifications) and on MRI/A (abnormal signal intensity) in order to thoroughly address the labral pathology. Occasionally, perilabral calcifications can be in the formative stage and these should be sought out and decompressed (Fig. 48.4).

An outcome correlated classification system of labral injuries and chondral damage has been created by Wardell et al., stage 0, as compared with normal

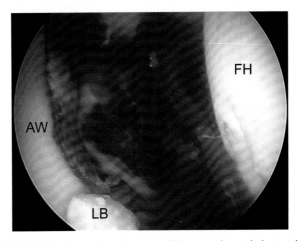

FIGURE 48.2. Synovitis in the area of the central acetabular notch. Note the loose body (LB) in the notch, also. AW, Acetabular wall; FH, Femoral head.

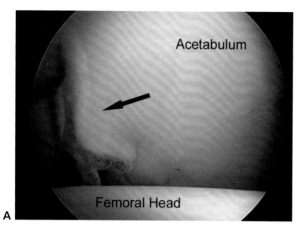

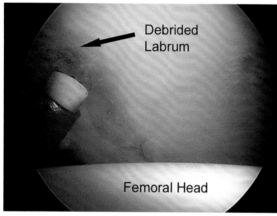

FIGURE 48.3. Labral debridement with the use of an RF probe. View is of a right hip, visualized from the anterior portal. **A:** Initial view of labral fraying *(arrow)*. **B:** Final view after debridement and stabilization of edges.

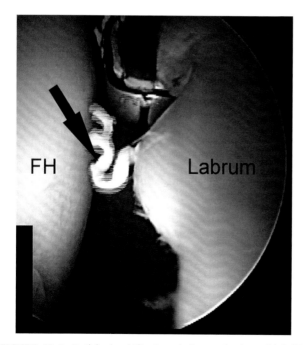

FIGURE 48.4. Perilabral calcification. Arthroscopic view of left hip from the anterolateral portal showing decompression of calcified material *(arrow)*. FH, Femoral Head.

acetabular labrum, constitutes a contusion of the labrum with adjacent synovitis; stage I is a discrete labral free margin tear with intact articular cartilage of the acetabulum and femoral head; stage II is a labral tear with focal articular damage to the subjacent femoral head but with intact acetabular articular cartilage; stage III is a labral tear with an adjacent focal acetabular articular cartilage lesion with or without femoral head articular cartilage chondromalacia (12). In the author's experience, this is the most common type of tear seen in those patients with cam impingement.(Fig. 48.5). Stage IV constitutes an extensive acetabular labral tear with associated diffuse arthritic articular cartilage changes in the joint. Ninety-five percent of the time the labral injury involved the anterior half of the joint. All patients who had combined anterior and lateral labral injuries had associated degenerative arthritis in the joint. This classification is loosely used to establish a general algorithm for treatment of these complex patients.

Adjacent cartilage damage should be searched for and thoroughly assessed. Superficial lesions can be gently debrided with mechanical shavers and perhaps stabilized with the use of RF probes. Grade 4 Outerbridge lesions may be managed with a thorough debridement down to a bleeding bed and preparation with microfracture awls (discussed below).

OPERATIVE TECHNIQUE FOR ARTHROSCOPIC LABRAL REPAIR

The decision to perform a labral repair is still evolving (Table 48.1). The current indications are symptomatic tears that have either obvious vascularity within their substance or are repairable to the acetabular bony wall (or the adjacent capsule). In general, a tear less than 1 cm in length does not require repair because there is minimal associated instability and mechanical symptomatology. Expert arthroscopic skills and appropriate instrumentation are also required.

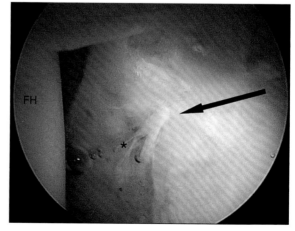

FIGURE 48.5. Stage III tear—Labral tear *(arrow)* with adjacent focal acetabular cartilage lesion *(asterisk)*. FH, Femoral head.

Table 48.1

Indications for labral repair

Mechanical symptoms with rotational activities
Unremitting pain in groin with weight-bearing
  activities
Concomitant femoroacetabular impingement with
  healthy, repairable tissue
Traumatic dislocation or subluxation with ongoing
  mechanical symptoms
Subluxation episodes in high performance athletes
Tissue with obvious vascularity in proper
  (capsular) anatomic zone
Tears >1 cm

The arthroscopic technique uses routine anterior and anterolateral portals. The anterior portal is started approximately 3 cm distal and 3 cm lateral to the intersection of line from the anterior, superior iliac spine and the top of the greater trochanter (Fig. 48.6). This accessory portal allows for a more appropriate angle for suture anchor placement. In addition, it avoids damage to the lateral femoral cutaneous nerve branches as well as the psoas tendon sheath. However, caution should be taken in creating this portal since excessively distal placement places the ascending lateral circumflex artery at risk with the possibility of bleeding and compromise of the surgical field (13).

As with labral debridements, the procedure includes a diagnostic arthroscopy with treatment of any associated pathology. Any degenerative tissue is debrided, and the labrum is elevated from the bone. The bony bed is prepared by decorticating with a curette or shaver to stimulate healing (Fig. 48.7).

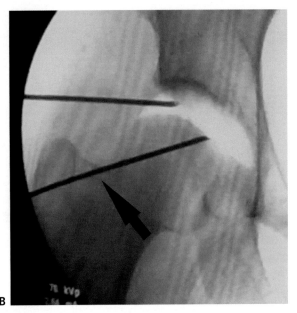

FIGURE 48.6. Modified anterior portal. **A:** The portal *(arrow)* is created approximately 3 cm distal and lateral to the intersection of the two lines *(dotted)* drawn across the top of the greater trochanter (GT) and parallel to the femoral shaft, beginning at the anterior, superior iliac spine *(asterisk)*. **B:** Fluoroscopic view of portal positions. Note the angle formed by the lower needle *(arrow)*.

Mobility within the joint to insert instruments, manipulate sutures, and insert anchors is critical to a successful outcome. Unlike the shoulder, the hip capsule is significantly thicker and less forgiving. A generous capsulotomy should be considered in many cases so that instruments can be moved within the joint and to limit the amount of iatrogenic damage. The capsulotomy can be performed with either an arthroscopic knife or a radiofrequency probe (Fig. 48.8). Slotted cannulas can also make delivery of curved instruments significantly easier (Fig. 48.9).

Similar to arthroscopic labral repair in the shoulder, suture anchors are used. The position of the anchor is critical in reestablishing the normal anatomy of the labrum. It should be placed on the acetabular rim, with care to avoid penetrating into the articular cartilage. In contrast to the shoulder, the acetabular cavity is concave. This makes the angle of anchor insertion significantly more acute. Avoiding chondral injury, both to the head (delivery of the anchor) and with respect to acetabular penetration is important, as it can become a factor in joint degeneration. Both endoscopic and fluoroscopic visualization are essential (Fig. 48.10). There are many options for suture anchors, some requiring traditional arthroscopic knot tying, and recently knotless anchors (Fig. 48.11). Once the anchor is placed, a suture-passing device is used to penetrate the labrum and standard knot-tying techniques may be used. Most available instruments have been adapted from those employed in shoulder arthroscopy.

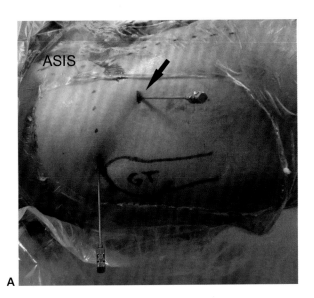

ASIS

GT

A

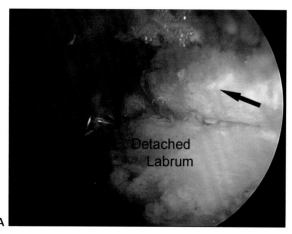
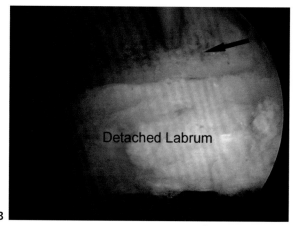

FIGURE 48.7. Preparation of labral bony bed for adequate healing. View is of right hip from anterolateral portal. **A:** Initial view of labral detachment and bony wall *(arrow)* without obvious vascularity. **B:** Final prepared bony site *(arrow)*. Note the punch for the anchor in the upper, central section.

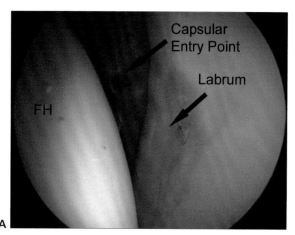
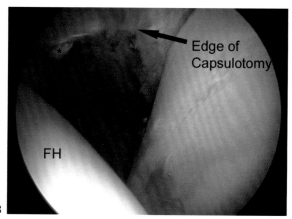

FIGURE 48.8. Capsulotomy with the use of a radiofrequency probe. FH, femoral head. **A:** Initial view prior to capsular incision. **B:** Final capsulotomy with device *(asterisk)* in place.

With a tear in the labrocapsular junction, the repair can be performed attaching the labrum to the adjacent capsular tissue. Intrasubstance tears may be addressed in a similar manner. The cleavage plane in the labrum should be defined and debrided of nonviable tissue. A suture shuttle device can be used to deliver a looped monofilament suture between the junction of the articular cartilage and the labrum. A suture penetrator is then employed through the capsule to grasp the loop of monofilament. The looped shuttle is then used to pass a monofilament suture around the labral tear and through the capsule. The suture is then tied in an extra-articular position (Fig. 48.12).

OPERATIVE TECHNIQUE FOR ARTHROSCOPIC MICROFRACTURE

Since microfracture of the knee has been shown a safe and effective procedure, many arthroscopists have applied the same principles to the hip (14). Microfracture provides an enriched environment for tissue regeneration by taking

advantage of the body's own healing abilities. After the procedure, a marrow clot is established within the treated area. This clot provides an environment for pluripotential and mesenchymal stem cells to differentiate into fibrocartilaginous tissue. The indications for microfracture of the hip include focal and contained lesions, typically less than 2 to 4 cm in size. Some authors have noted that lesions less than 400 mm (2) tend to respond better to microfracture than lesions 400 mm (2) or greater (15). As in the knee, intact subchondral bone is critical. The cartilage loss can either be full thickness in weight-bearing areas or be unstable partial lesions. Patients benefiting from microfracture include those with impingement, trauma, pediatric hip disease, or early degenerative disease. Other considerations for performing the procedure include patient age, activity level, and the ability to comply with postoperative rehabilitation.

Contraindications to the procedure include stable partial thickness defects, subchondral bony disease or defects associated with the chondral lesions and extensive degenerative disease. Other specific contraindications

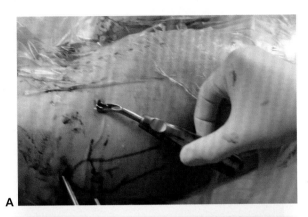

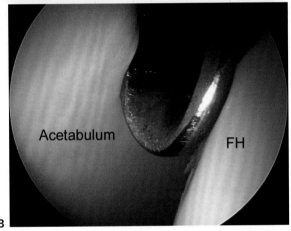

FIGURE 48.9. Use of a slotted cannula for insertion of instruments. **A:** Internal view of device. **B:** External view of device.

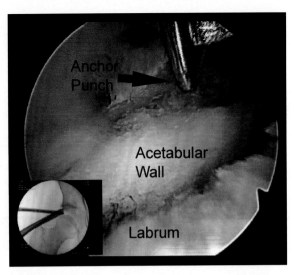

FIGURE 48.10. Endoscopic and fluoroscopic visualization of anchor insertion angle. Note the corresponding fluoroscopic view in the lower left hand corner of the image, assuring divergence from the joint.

include inflammatory arthritides, immune-mediated disease, or other systemic diseases.

Once the chondral defect is identified, the extent of the lesion is documented. Debridement of all remaining unstable cartilage from the exposed bone is completed using a full-radius resector and curettes. A ring curette is particularly useful for preparation of the defect and creating a smooth, perpendicular border. Particular attention must be paid while resecting the surrounding rim of the defect. Debridement should be deep enough to remove the calcified cartilage layer while maintaining the integrity of the subchondral plate (16). The edges of the lesion should be perpendicular to the adjacent, unaffected cartilage to allow for the marrow clot to form effectively. Arthroscopic awls are used to make multiple penetrations (microfractures) in the exposed subchondral plate. The penetrations are separated by about 3 to 4 mm. A depth of approximately 2 to 4 mm is enough to visualize bleeding once the fluid pressure is decreased (Fig. 48.13).

Other techniques have also been attempted in order to repair cartilage flaps. First, a microfracture is performed as previously described. Then using arthroscopic techniques and absorbable sutures, the cartilage flap is repaired. This technique is employed in select patients with a much high healing potential (i.e., younger patients).

PEARLS AND PITFALLS

Perform a Capsulotomy (Enlarge Your Portals for Better Mobility)

A beaver blade can be inserted under direct visualization in the joint. The blade can be used to enlarge the portals by opening the capsule. Any portal can be extended in this fashion to gain more mobility. This is especially important for the novice hip arthroscopist as establishment of the portals in the ideal location takes some experience. Alternatively, the portal can also be enlarged with the use of a radiofrequency probe.

Slotted Cannulas

The use of slotted cannulas, instead of disposable plastic devices, makes the insertion of longer and curved tools easier. The hip capsule is very restricting, and insertion of plastic cannulas is fraught with difficulties including articular cartilage damage upon insertion. With the use of a slotted cannula, the capsular entry point is preserved and maneuverability enhanced compared with a closed cannula.

Treat the Underlying Pathology (Look for Subtle Indicators of Impingement)

In the broadest sense, there are two types of impingement, cam and pincer. When conducting the diagnostic arthroscopy of the central compartment, the type of labral pathology and the presence or absence of chondral delamination can serve as a subtle clue with any impingement pathology.

Use Fluoroscopic and Endoscopic Visualization for Anchor Placement

The liberal use of fluoroscopy while anchor insertion points are chosen will allow for anchors to be placed in a safe location that will have a minimal likelihood of penetrating the articular cartilage and causing iatrogenic

IV. The Hip

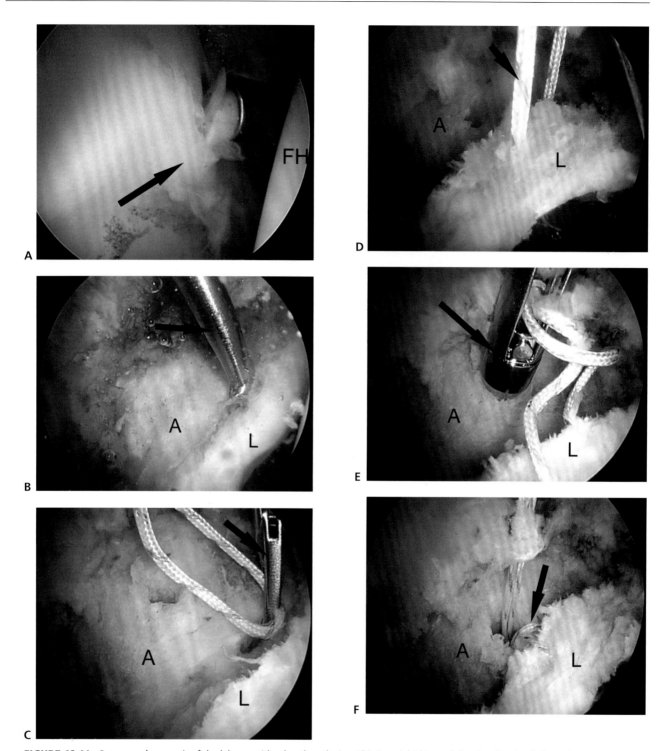

FIGURE 48.11. Suture anchor repair of the labrum with a knotless device. This is a right hip and the visualization is from the anterolateral portal with all of the tools inserted via the modified anterior portal. FH, femoral head; A, Acetabulum; L, Labrum. **A:** Initial view of tear *(arrow)*. Note the ablator tool in place. **B:** Mobilization of labral tear with an elevator tool *(arrow)*. **C:** Suture penetrator in place *(arrow)*. Note the suture that is being passed at the labral–acetabular interface. **D:** Suture in place *(arrow)*. **E:** Anchor *(arrow)* in position prior to implantation. Note the loose suture material that is now positioned in the anchor device. **F:** Final anchor position with loose suture *(arrow)*. **G:** Final suture advancement. Note the increased tension and approximation of labrum to acetabulum. **H:** Intra-articular view of completed repair. The *arrow* is showing the suture material in place.

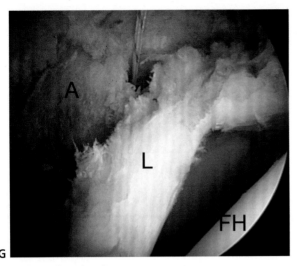

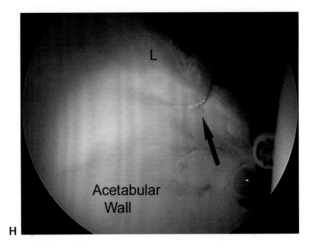

FIGURE 48.11. (*Continued*)

damage. Unlike the glenoid cavity, the acetabulum is concave, making the safe angle of approach completely different. The distortion that accompanies the use of the 70° arthroscope further confuses the situation and makes the use of fluoroscopy even more important.

LOOK FOR ANATOMIC VARIANTS

In the acetabular fossa, several normal variants have been noted. These are confusion and may appear like cartilage lesions. One is the stellate crease, which is located superior

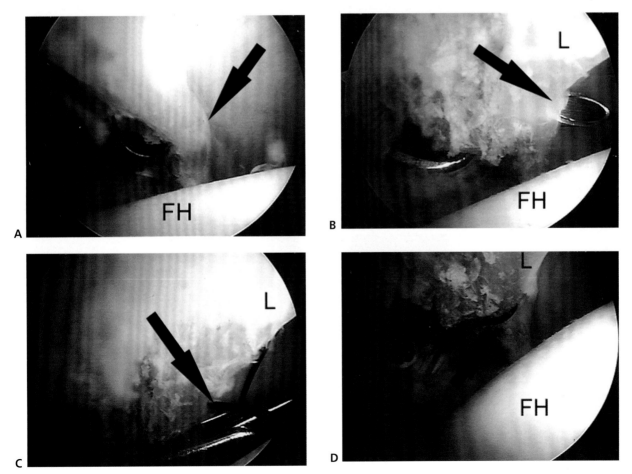

FIGURE 48.12. Intrasubstance labral repair in a right hip viewed from the anterior portal. **A:** Initial view of unstable labral flap (*arrow*) laterally. **B:** Suture passer (*arrow*) in place through labral tear. **C:** Passed suture (*arrow*) in place with grasping tool at the lower margin of the photo. **D:** Final labral repair (*arrow*).

IV. The Hip

and has a star like appearance. Another is the physeal scar, a remnant of the triradiate cartilage, which can be anterior or posterior in the fossa (Fig. 48.14). One other common variant is the keyhole complex. This is an extension of the acetabular notch and has been especially noted in younger patients (Fig. 48.15).

COMPLICATIONS

Hip arthroscopy has been shown to be relatively safe in several studies documenting its effectiveness as well as several complications. In one large series, there was a 1.6% complication rate with problems including transient palsy of either the sciatic or the femoral nerves, paresthesias secondary to lateral femoral cutaneous nerve palsy, perineal injury, and instrument breakage (17). While this study was not specific to the repair of the hip labrum, certainly specific problems may be associated with this procedure. As a result of the tight confines and the multiple instruments that are inserted into the joint, the possibility of serious articular cartilage damage exists. Care should

be taken while working within the joint to limit cartilage damage. In addition, with the insertion of suture anchors, there is a possibility of joint penetration. The liberal use of fluoroscopy to document the position of anchor insertion angles prior to committing to a specific position is critical. In addition, limiting the amount of traction time also minimizes the risk of neurological injury.

REHABILITATION

After Debridement (Labrum and Cartilage)

Formal therapy for range of motion and strengthening of the operative hip is begun 7 to 10 days following surgery. Weight-bearing following an isolated arthroscopic debridement should be unrestricted with the use of crutches limited to the early postoperative period only (3 to 5 days). The standard protocol includes a gradual progression from increasing the range of motion, to unrestricted strengthening. Strengthening is only begun once the patient attains approximately 75% of normal motion. Aggressive hip flexor strengthening should be limited until full range of

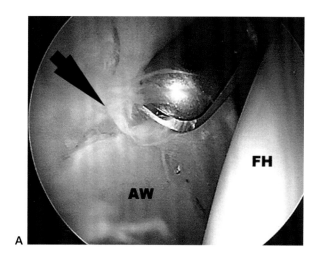
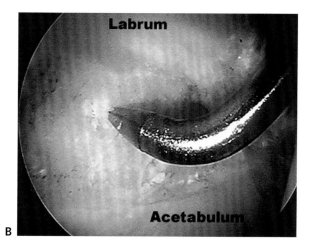
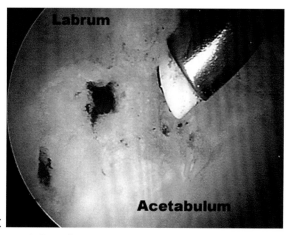

FIGURE 48.13. Chondroplasty of the acetabular wall. **A:** Initial view of chondral injury *(arrow)* prior to bony bed preparation. FH, femoral head; AW, acetabular wall. **B:** Lesion following curetting and preparation of the base. The awl is in place and the lesion is well-demarcated along the lower margin of the picture. **C:** Final area of chondroplasty. Note the punctate bleeding from two of the perforations.

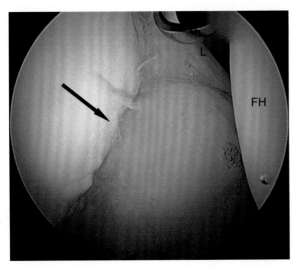

FIGURE 48.14. Anatomic variant *(arrow)*, which is a remnant of the triradiate epiphyseal fusion in a 19-year-old patient with a labral tear. FH, femoral head; L, Labrum. View is of a right hip viewed from the anterolateral portal.

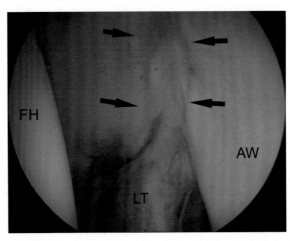

FIGURE 48.15. Keyhole complex. Arthroscopic view of the complex in a left hip viewed from the anterolateral portal. Note the area outlined by the arrows which appears to be an extension of the acetabular notch. AW, acetabular wall; FH, femoral head.

motion is obtained and hip mechanics are normalized. In cases where patients develop abnormal mechanics to assist the recovering psoas and/or hip flexors, a significant tendonitis can occur. This entity is difficult to treat and slows the patient's recovery. Explosive and rotational activities should also be limited for at least 6 weeks. The return to unrestricted activity is predicated on a full, painless range of motion and normal strength of the pelvic, abdominal, and lower extremity musculature.

After Labral Repair

Formal therapy for range of motion and strengthening of the operative hip is also begun early following surgery. Early initiation is important in order to limit the scarring in the joint associated with the surgical trauma. Weight-bearing following repair should be restricted to foot-flat (20% of body weight) ambulation for the first 4 weeks. The most important principle is to limit the rotational stresses that the repaired labrum experiences in the first few weeks. The range that puts the repair at risk includes flexion past 90°, abduction past 25°, and internal or external rotation past 25° (18). Limitations are placed on flexion past 90° for 10 days, while abduction and adduction are limited to 25° for 4 weeks. Beginning at 4 weeks, a gradual progression from increasing the range of motion to unrestricted strengthening is begun. The use of stationary bicycling is encouraged and instituted in the first 10 days. Aggressive hip flexor strengthening should also be limited until full range of motion is obtained and hip mechanics are normalized. As mentioned previously, a significant tendinitis can develop, thus slowing recovery. Explosive and rotational activities should be limited for at least 12 weeks. The return to unrestricted activity is also predicated on a full, painless range of motion, and normal strength of the pelvic, abdominal, and lower extremity musculature. This typically occurs at approximately 6 months postoperatively.

After Microfracture

The most important principle in postoperative management is to maintain the marrow clot and thus the ideal environment for healing, while regaining range of motion and strength. Crutch-assisted 30 lb (13.6 kg) flat-foot weight bearing is allowed for 4 weeks with advancement to full weight bearing at 6 weeks. A continuous passive motion (CPM) machine is utilized throughout the 4-week period in some situations. Initial physical therapy consists of passive motion progressing to active-assisted motion and eventually active motion with particular emphasis on regaining internal rotation of hip. Specific limitations also depend on associated procedures performed. Stationary bicycle exercises without resistance are useful and can be started immediately. Impact sports are delayed until at least 4 to 6 months postoperatively and only after range of motion, strength, and functional agility have returned to normal.

CONCLUSIONS AND FUTURE DIRECTIONS

The mechanical effects of the labrum appear to substantiate the need to preserve as much tissue as possible. With resection of the labrum, synovial fluid may not be maintained in the central joint, which is probably detrimental on a long-term basis. Therefore, the labrum should be preserved as much as possible in patients who have mechanical symptoms from labral pathology.

IV. The Hip

The available literature supports the concept that the labrum is important both for stability and for cartilage homeostasis. More research needs to be done to evaluate the long-term effects of labral repair or excision. Intuitively, it would appear that the preservation of as much relatively normal labral tissue with any surgical procedure is critical to the long-term preservation of the native hip joint.

Likewise, the ideal treatment for cartilage defects has yet to be delineated. While some semblance of cartilaginous tissue is generated with the current microfracture techniques, the outcomes are variable even in contained lesions. Similarly, the outcome of repair of cartilage flaps is highly variable with very little, if any, support in the literature. The next phases of treatment likely will involve genetic engineering with the development of more predictably cartilage-like tissue.

REFERENCES

1. Kelly BT, Weiland DE, Schenker ML, et al. Arthroscopic labral repair in the hip: surgical technique and review of the literature. *Arthroscopy*. 2005;21:1496–1504.
2. Seldes RM, Tan V, Hunt J, et al. Anatomy, histologic features, and vascularity of the adult acetabular labrum. *Clin Orthop Relat Res*. 2001;382:232–240.
3. Burnett RS, Della Rocca GJ, Prather H, et al. Clinical presentation of patients with tears of the acetabular labrum. *J Bone Joint Surg Am*. 2006;88:1448–1457.
4. Ferguson SJ, Bryant JT, Ganz R, et al. The influence of the acetabular labrum on hip joint cartilage consolidation: a poroelastic finite element model. *J Biomech*. 2000;33:953–960.
5. Bond JL, Knutson ZA, Ebert A, et al. The 23-point arthroscopic examination of the hip: basic set-up, portal placement and surgical technique. *Arthroscopy*. 2009;25:416–429.
6. McCarthy J, Noble P, Aluisio FV, et al. Anatomy, pathologic features, and treatment of acetabular labral tears. *Clin Orthop Relat Res*. 2003;406:38–47.
7. Toomayan GA, Holman WR, Major NM, et al. Sensitivity of MR arthrography in the evaluation of acetabular labral tears. *Am J Roentgenol*. 2006;186:449–453.
8. Byrd JW, Jones KS. Diagnostic accuracy of clinical assessment, magnetic resonance imaging, magnetic resonance arthrography, and intra-articular injection in hip arthroscopy patients. *Am J Sports Med*. 2004;32:1668–1674.
9. Martin RL, Irrgang JJ, Sekiya JK. The diagnostic accuracy of a clinical examination in determining intra-articular hip pain for potential hip arthroscopy candidates. *Arthroscopy*. 2008;24:1013–1018.
10. Kim YJ, Jaramillo D, Millis MB, et al. Assessment of early osteoarthritis in hip dysplasia with delayed gadolinium-enhanced magnetic resonance imaging of cartilage. *J Bone and Joint Surg*. 2003;85-A:1987–1992.
11. Marino J, Russo J, Kenny M, et al. Continuous lumbar plexus block for postoperative pain control after total hip arthroplasty. A randomized controlled trial. *J Bone Joint Surg Am*. 2009;91:29–37.
12. McCarthy J, Wardell S, Mason J, et al. Injuries to the acetabular labrum: classification, outcome, and relationship to degenerative arthritis. Paper presented at the Annual Meeting of the American Academy of Orthopaedic Surgeons; 1997; San Francisco, CA.
13. Robertson WJ, Kelly BT. The safe zone for hip arthroscopy: a cadaveric assessment of central, peripheral, and lateral compartment portal placement. *Arthroscopy*. 2008;24:1019–1026.
14. Crawford K. Microfracture of the hip in athletes. *Clin Sports Med*. 2006;25:327–335.
15. Steadman JR, Outcomes of microfracture for traumatic chondral defects of the knee: average 11-year follow-up. *Arthroscopy*. 2003;19:477–484.
16. Steadman JR, Rodkey WG, Rodrigo JJ. Microfracture: surgical technique and rehabilitation to treat chondral defects. *Clin Orthop Relat Res*. 2001;391(suppl):S362–S369.
17. Griffin DR, Villar RN. Complications of arthroscopy of the hip. *J Bone Joint Surg Br*. 1999;81:604–606.
18. Ikeda T, Awaya G, Suzuki S, et al. Torn acetabular labrum in young patients. Arthroscopic diagnosis and management. *J Bone Joint Surg Br*. 1988;70:13–16.

Snapping Hip Syndromes and Peritrochanter Disorders

Craig S. Mauro • James E. Voos • Bryan T. Kelly

Snapping hip syndromes and peritrochanter disorders, including internal and external coxa saltans, trochanteric bursitis, and gluteus medius and minimus tears, have been well documented (1–9). Since numerous intra-articular lesions that may cause hip pain and, occasionally, popping or snapping have been identified, the term internal coxa saltans is best reserved for iliopsoas tendon snapping and external coxa saltans for iliotibial band snapping (9). For this chapter, these entities will be the focus of the snapping hip syndromes. The peritrochanteric disorders have previously been grouped into the "greater trochanteric pain syndrome" (4,6,7). Conservative treatment is the primary therapeutic modality for these disorders and includes local corticosteroid and anesthetic injections combined with a structured physical therapy program (10). However, patients who fail conservative treatment may require surgery. While open surgical treatment for snapping hip syndromes and peritrochanter disorders has been utilized for many years, (11–17) endoscopic treatment has more recently been described (18–28). This chapter reviews the clinical evaluation, treatment (including the authors' preferred technique), complications of treatment, and rehabilitation of snapping hip syndromes and peritrochanter disorders.

CLINICAL EVALUATION

An in-depth patient history is one of the most effective tools for evaluating a complaint of hip snapping or pain. A historical description of hip pain can help to differentiate intra-articular from extra-articular pathology. Patients with intra-articular pathology often localize the pain to the groin and state that it is exacerbated with prolonged sitting or strenuous activity. Those patients with pathology involving the peritrochanteric compartment more often localize the symptoms to the lateral hip surrounding the greater trochanter. They may note lateral hip pain during strenuous activity or with activities as simple as lying on the affected side. However, intra-articular pathology can certainly present as isolated lateral hip pain, so a heightened suspicion and appropriate evaluation are always necessary. In addition, it is important to consider the lumbar spine, sacroiliac joint, and intrapelvic pathology in the differential diagnosis. The diagnostic differential can be narrowed with descriptive characteristics and physical examination findings specific to each snapping hip syndrome and peritrochanter disorder.

Internal coxa saltans occurs as the iliopsoas tendon subluxates from lateral to medial across the iliopectineal eminence or the anterior aspect of the femoral head and capsule when the hip is brought from a flexed, abducted, externally rotated position into extension and internal rotation. (1) Patients typically describe, and may be able to reproduce, a painful clicking or popping sensation coming from the anterior groin. However, they may also describe flank, buttock, or sacroiliac pain.

External coxa saltans has been attributed to an excessively thick, taut posterior border of iliotibial band or anterior gluteus maximus tendon moving over the greater trochanter (1). Anatomically, with the hip extended, the iliotibial band lies posterior to the greater trochanter and slips anteriorly over the greater trochanter during hip flexion. The tight anterior attachments of the tensor fascia latae, the presence of the gluteus maximus posteriorly, and the association with gluteus medius aponeurosis restricts the iliotibial band over the greater trochanter throughout hip range of motion (1). The slipping motion produces the snapping sensation and resultant lateral hip pain. Patients with external coxa saltans may describe a palpable or audible lateral snapping as the hip moves from flexion to extension. It most often occurs with athletic activity but may be symptomatic with activities of daily living.

Trochanteric bursitis and greater trochanteric pain syndrome have been described as overuse injuries occurring most commonly in older females. It has also been associated with long distance running, low back pain, coxa saltans, iliotibial band syndrome, and hip arthroplasty and osteotomy (2,12,29–31). Symptoms are characterized by chronic, intermittent aching pain over the lateral aspect of the hip.

Tears at the insertions of the gluteus medius and minimus at the greater trochanter have been described synonymously with tears of the rotator cuff tendons (3,5). Descriptions of calcific tendonitis of the hip have also included relationships with gluteus medius and minimus tears, thus further substantiating the rotator cuff similarity (32–34). Tears were initially identified in the setting of open debridement for recalcitrant trochanteric bursitis, total hip arthroplasty, and treatment of femoral neck fractures (5,7,35). However, tears of the gluteus medius and minimus tendons at the greater trochanter may also occur with trauma in otherwise normal hips or in the setting of hip abductor tendinopathy (36,37). Symptoms are characterized by lateral hip pain and an ambulatory limp, likely related to hip abductor weakness.

After obtaining the patient history, the physician should perform thorough examination of the entire hip joint. Diagnosis of internal coxa saltans begins by placing the patient supine. The examiner moves the hip from flexed, abducted, externally rotated position into extension with internal rotation. This motion may elicit an audible popping sound that corresponds to the sensation experienced by the patient. However, the popping may be difficult to reproduce passively and sometimes the patient may be able to better actively demonstrate it. The diagnosis of external coxa saltans may be distinguished from internal coxa saltans on physical examination by demonstrating a lateral palpable or audible snapping as the hip is moved from flexion to extension. This examination maneuver should be performed with the patient lying on his or her side and while standing.

A more focused evaluation of the lateral aspect of the hip should then be used to further define an offending peritrochanter disorder. Lateral hip pain can arise from pathology in the peritrochanteric space or be referred pain from intra-articular pathology. Palpation of the lateral hip aids in this differential as referred pain may be reproduced with passive and active joint motion but should not produce tenderness with direct palpation. In this vein, palpation should begin with the origin of the gluteus maximus at the inferior-posterior aspect of the ileum and sacrum. The insertion can then be examined in two locations: the lateral base of the linea aspera on the proximal femur and the tensor fascia latae. Next, the gluteus medius should be palpated from its origin on the anterior and middle aspect of the ileum to its two insertions on the middle and superoposterior facet of the greater trochanter. The gluteus minimus can be examined from its origin deep to the gluteus medius to its insertion at the greater trochanter anterior facet. The greater trochanteric bursa should also be appreciated overlying the greater trochanter at the mid posterior proximal aspect of the femur. Patients with trochanteric bursitis demonstrate point tenderness over the greater trochanter with occasional warmth and/or swelling.

Physical examination of muscle strength should be conducted with the hip in flexion to assess the tensor fascia latae, in neutral to evaluate the gluteus medius, and in extension to evaluate the gluteus maximus. This examination should be performed with the knee both flexed and extended to allow tension and relaxation of the iliotibial band, respectively. Weakness may be seen with all entities because of pain, but significant weakness may be suggestive of a gluteus medius and/or minimus tendon tear. Also, the 30-second single-leg stance and resisted external derotation tests have been shown to have very good sensitivity and specificity for identifying tendinous lesions in patients with peritrochanteric pain (38).

Ober's test may be used during the physical examination to evaluate for contractures of the abductor muscles. This test should also be conducted with the hip in flexion, neutral, and extension. Classically, Ober's test is performed in hip extension to assess tension across the tensor fascia latae. The knee should then be flexed to relax the iliotibial band and allow effective evaluation of possible gluteus medius contracture. In this position, the knee should be able to internally rotate such that it can touch the table in the absence of pathologic tension.

All patients presenting with hip pain are evaluated with an anteroposterior (AP) radiograph of the pelvis as well as a Dunn lateral radiograph (90° of hip flexion with 20° of abduction and the beam centered on and perpendicular to the hip) to assess for avulsions of the greater trochanter, cam and pincer lesions, loss of joint space, cross-over sign, acetabular dysplasia, and sacroiliac joint pathology. Our AP pelvis radiographs are performed according to Siebenrock et al. (39) who recommended taking radiographs of the pelvis in neutral rotation and in a standardized position of pelvic inclination, which is indicated by the distance between the symphysis and the sacrococcygeal joint (approximately 32 mm in men and 47 mm in women).

MRI provides the most information regarding the soft tissues surrounding the hip (40). At our institution, we utilize noncontrast MRI to evaluate the hip joint (41). Every MRI study of the hip performed at our institution includes a screening examination of the whole pelvis, acquired with use of coronal inversion recovery and axial proton density sequences. Detailed hip imaging is obtained with use of a surface coil over the hip joint, with high-resolution cartilage-sensitive images acquired in three planes (sagittal, coronal, and oblique axial) with use of a fast-spin-echo pulse sequence and an intermediate echo time (42). Other authors have advocated the use of magnetic resonance arthrography of the hip for evaluation of hip pathology (43–45). Cvitanic et al. concluded MRI showed good accuracy for the diagnosis of tears of the gluteus medius and gluteus minimus tendons. The identification of an area of T2 hyperintensity superior to the greater trochanter had the highest sensitivity and specificity for tears at 73% and 95%, respectively (46). Suspected gluteus medius tendon tears in patients with trochanteric bursitis may be confirmed with MRI (47). This modality aids to confirm the clinical suspicion in patients with refractory trochanteric bursitis with lateral hip pain and an ambulatory limp likely related to hip abductor weakness (48).

Ultrasound may be used to confirm placement of injections into the trochanteric space or into the iliopsoas bursa for diagnostic and therapeutic purposes (49). Dynamic ultrasound has also been used to evaluate internal and external coxa saltans, especially when surgical treatment is being considered (49–51). It provides real-time images of sudden abnormal displacement of the iliopsoas tendon or the iliotibial band or gluteus maximus muscle overlying the greater trochanter, which can be correlated with a painful snap during hip motion (49–51). In addition, Connell et al. (52) concluded that sonography can identify gluteus medius and minimus tendinopathy and provides information about the severity of the disease.

TREATMENT

In the vast majority of cases of internal or external coxa saltans, the patient is either asymptomatic or can be treated conservatively with rest, activity modification, stretching, anti-inflammatory medications, corticosteroid injections, and physical therapy (1,8,19). Conservative management for trochanteric bursitis, in the form of local corticosteroid and anesthetic injections performed at the area of maximal tenderness combined with physical therapy, is the cornerstone of diagnosis and treatment (10). The predictable diagnostic and therapeutic results produced by history, physical exam, and relief of symptoms with anesthetic injection have obviated the need for routine MRI except in recalcitrant cases where other concomitant pathology may exist. Conservative therapy is not always benign, however. Multiple or inappropriately placed corticosteroid injections have been associated with gluteus medius injury (48). MRI may be used to confirm potential gluteus medius and minimus tears and further guide surgical treatment. While conservative treatment is often successful with these snapping hip syndromes and peritrochanter disorders, some patients are persistently symptomatic and surgical treatment is indicated.

Open lengthening of the iliopsoas tendon has been described for treatment of the internal coxa saltans (14–17). These techniques involve either an open medial, ilioinguinal, or iliofemoral approach and fractional lengthening of the iliopsoas tendon. Endoscopic iliopsoas tendon release has been described more recently (20,26–28). With the endoscopic approaches, the iliopsoas tendon may be released either at the insertion of the tendon on the lesser trochanter (8,19,26) or through the central or peripheral compartments of the hip joint through an anterior hip capsulotomy (25,28). Ilizaliturri et al. (27) prospectively evaluated endoscopic iliopsoas tendon release at the lesser trochanter with endoscopic transcapsular release from the peripheral compartment and found no clinical difference in the outcomes.

Zoltan et al. (13) described an open surgical technique for treatment of recalcitrant external coxa saltans that involved excision of an ellipsoid-shaped portion of the iliotibial band overlying the greater trochanter and removal of the trochanteric bursa. A minimally invasive technique using transverse step cuts in the fascia along a longitudinal facial incision has also been described (53).

While these open techniques have shown positive results in treating external coxa saltans, treatment of external coxa saltans with endoscopic iliotibial band release has been described with promising results (19). The iliotibial band may be released through an "outside-in" or an "inside-out" approach (19,24). Ilizaliturri et al. treated 11 patients endoscopically and all patients experienced no postoperative complaints and full return to previous activity level (19). In his series, the iliotibial band was released with an "outside-in" approach by first making a vertical cut in the iliotibial band a radiofrequency hook probe. A transverse cut was then made at the middle of the vertical release, creating a cross-shape. The four resulting flaps were resected to make a diamond-shaped defect.

Open trochanteric bursectomy has been described for refractory cases of trochanteric bursitis (2,12). Trends toward arthroscopic treatment have also produced descriptions of endoscopic bursectomy in the literature (11,18,23). Baker et al. (18) recently published a prospective follow-up in 25 patients treated with endoscopic bursectomy at a mean follow-up of 26.1 months. Significant improvement was found in visual analog scores, Harris Hip Score, and SF-36. Improvements in a patient's status are usually evident by 1 to 3 months after surgery and appear to be lasting.

Open surgical techniques have been also described for treatment of gluteus medius and minimus tendon tears (3,5,36). Endoscopic treatment of calcific tendonitis of the gluteus medius and minimus has been reported by Kandemir et al., (21) whereas Voos et al. (22) reported the technique for endoscopic repair of gluteus medius and minimus tendon tears. More recently, Voos et al. (54) reported the outcomes of 10 patients with gluteus medius tears who had failed conservative management and were treated with endoscopic repair. At an average of 25-month follow-up, they found endoscopic repair provided pain relief and return of strength in all 10 patients.

AUTHORS' PREFERRED TECHNIQUE

Diagnostic Arthroscopy

The importance of proper portal placement is critical in hip arthroscopy. For arthroscopy of peritrochanteric space, a technique has been described using both traditional and unique portals (22,42,55). The technique begins with accurate identification of the trochanter and marking of the arthroscopic portals. The case begins with routine central compartment hip arthroscopy to rule out associated intra-articular pathologies. Labral tears may occur in association with internal coxa saltans in a directly anterior location, adjacent to the iliopsoas tendon, and without any associated osseous abnormalities. Central compartment arthroscopy is performed in all cases of peritrochanter disorders to document and treat any associated labral or chondral pathology that may coexist with the lateral-based pathology.

The anterolateral portal is established first using the standard Seldinger technique. A cannulated trochar is inserted over a guide wire into the central compartment under fluoroscopic guidance. In order to minimize trauma to the lateral femoral cutaneous nerve, a mid anterior portal is then established. This portal is made slightly more lateral and distal than the traditional anterior portal (56). The portal is critical for entry into the peritrochanteric space, as it is the primary initial viewing portal. Thus, fluoroscopy is used to assist with optimal placement of the mid-anterior portal over the lateral prominence of the greater trochanter.

Iliopsoas Tendon Release

In the case of internal coxa saltans, the iliopsoas tendon is addressed through the central compartment. If there is a labral tear associated with the snapping iliopsoas tendon, labral debridement or repair is performed first. Then, with the camera in the anterolateral portal, the capsule overlying the iliopsoas identified. The capsule and synovium overlying the psoas tendon may be hyperemic as a result of the snapping psoas tendon. A shaver is introduced through the mid anterior portal and is used to remove the capsule and expose the iliopsoas tendon (Fig. 49.1). The tendinous portion of the iliopsoas is then released with an electrocautery device. Care is taken to leave the overlying muscle belly intact. Prior to entry into the peritrochanteric

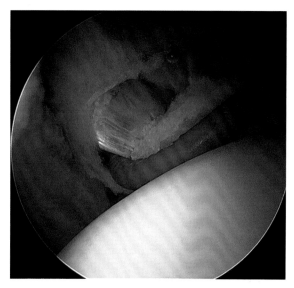

FIGURE 49.1. A shaver has been used to remove the capsule and expose the iliopsoas tendon. The tendinous portion of the iliopsoas is then released with an electrocautery device.

space and after completion of the central compartment evaluation, the peripheral compartment should be entered if there is any concern for peripheral compartment pathology. Rarely, if the iliopsoas tendon is noted to snap over and cause a groove in the femoral head, the tendon is released through the peripheral compartment at the site of contact instead of through the central compartment.

Trochanteric Bursectomy

Diagnostic arthroscopy of the peritrochanteric space then begins with the placement of blunt trochar in the mid-anterior portal. This trochar is then used to swipe between the IT band and the vastus ridge, in a manner similar to that which is performed in the subacromial space of the shoulder. The trochar is aimed directly toward the lateral prominence of the greater trochanter. This position is the safest starting position for blunt trochar placement. If the trochar is placed too proximally initially, violation of the gluteus medius musculature may occur; if it is placed too distally, the trochar may disrupt the fibers of the vastus lateralis. The use of fluoroscopy helps to precisely identify the starting position and to avoid iatrogenic injury to the surrounding soft tissue. Unlike arthroscopy of the central compartment, traction is not necessary for visualization of the peritrochanteric space. The perineal post is removed and the hip is placed in an extended position with the leg abducted slightly. However, minimal traction may be used to maintain tension on the abductors.

Once the space has been defined, a 70° scope is placed in the mid anterior portal. The camera is oriented so that both the light source and the camera base are pointed distally. The first structure that is visualized is the gluteus maximus tendon inserting on the femur just below the vastus lateralis. This insertion is a reproducible landmark that provides good orientation within the space. It is typically unnecessary to work distal to the gluteus maximus tendon, and one should avoid exploration posterior to the tendon, as the sciatic nerve lies within close proximity (2 to 4 cm). The camera light source is then directed to the lateral aspect of the femur where the longitudinal fibers of the vastus lateralis can be visualized and followed proximally to the vastus ridge. Proximal to the vastus ridge, the insertion and muscle belly of the gluteus medius is identified. The gluteus medius has two separate bony attachment sites on the greater trochanter. The posterior muscle fibers attach to the superoposterior portion or facet of the greater trochanter, whereas most of the central and all of the anterior muscle fibers attach to the lateral facet (57). The gluteus minimus insertion is located more anteriorly and is mostly covered. Finally, with the camera looking proximally and laterally, the IT band is identified (Fig. 49.2).

After performing a diagnostic arthroscopy, a spinal needle is placed under direct arthroscopic visualization 4 to 5 cm distal to the anterolateral portal. This portal is the distal anterolateral accessory portal, which is

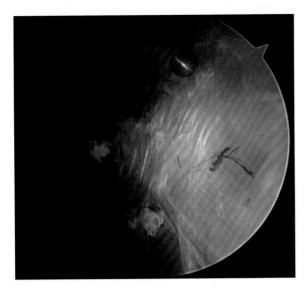

FIGURE 49.2. The iliotibial band, as visualized with the 70° arthroscope in the mid anterior portal with the camera looking proximally and laterally.

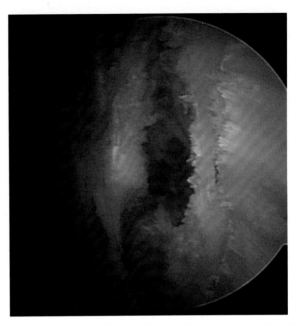

FIGURE 49.3. The iliotibial band, after being released within the peritrochanteric space through the "inside-out" approach.

roughly in line with anterolateral portal. An arthroscopic shaver is then placed in the distal anterolateral accessory portal, and a thorough trochanteric bursectomy is performed over the distal portion of the space. Initially, distended bursal tissue and fibrinous bands are cleared off the gluteus maximus tendinous insertion distally. The bursectomy is then performed from distal to proximal. An additional portal can be made 2 to 3 cm proximal to the anterolateral portal (proximal anterolateral accessory portal) to access the most proximal portions of the in-flamed bursal tissue. This portal can also be used as a viewing portal to get a more complete perspective on the underlying pathology.

Iliotibial Band Release/Lengthening

After a thorough bursectomy has been performed, attention is turned to the IT band. The pathologic entity is the thickened posterior one-third of the IT band that snaps over the greater trochanter. Often a "kissing lesion" can be seen on the lateral prominence of the trochanter where a bruised or erythematous zone of injury corresponds to the site of impact. With the 70° scope in the mid-anterior portal, the proximal anterolateral accessory portal is made under direct visualization. A beaver blade is then placed in this portal and a controlled transverse or cruciate style lengthening is performed. When this release is performed within the peritrochanteric space through this "inside-out" approach, it is fairly easy to confirm adequate release as direct visualization of the region of injury on the trochanter is possible (Fig. 49.3).

Gluteus Medius and Minimus Repair

If there is evidence of significant gluteus medius or minimus pathology, an arthroscopic repair is performed.

Occasionally, gentle distraction of the hip is needed to place the gluteus medius muscle fibers on tension to more clearly delineate proximal bursal tissue from gluteus medius muscle fibers. The 70° arthroscope is then placed in the proximal anterolateral accessory portal to get a more global view of the abductors. The working instruments can then be placed in the mid anterior and distal antero-lateral accessory portals.

Most commonly, the gluteus medius is degenerated and torn off its distal insertion on the lateral facet of the greater trochanter (Fig. 49.4). Often, the tear is predomi-nantly an undersurface tear, analogous to an articular-sided rotator cuff tear, which extends posteriorly and becomes a full-thickness tear. These tears may be visualized by

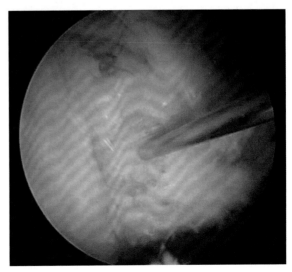

FIGURE 49.4. Gluteus medius tendon tear.

developing the plane at the anterior margin of the gluteus medius, between the gluteus minimus and the medius, and visualizing the undersurface of the tendon. Close scrutiny of the MRI is critical to correlate intraoperative findings with the preoperative imaging. Sometimes the initial intraoperative evaluation demonstrates significant thinning of the tendon insertion and completion of the tear with facet bone preparation and reattachment is necessary (Fig. 49.5).

The technique for fixing these tears is quite similar to the techniques for rotator cuff repair. First, a probe or grasper is used to manually reduce the tear to its anatomic position in the footprint (Fig. 49.6) (57). The lateral facet is then burred to a bleeding edge of bone. Due to the hard nature of bone in the trochanter, two metallic anchors are usually placed. These anchors can be placed percutaneously to achieve the optimal angle into the bone (Fig. 49.7). A spinal needle is used to find

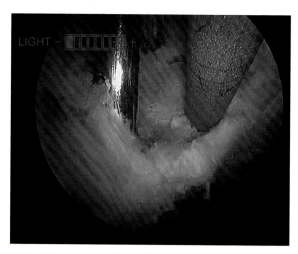

FIGURE 49.7. Two metallic anchors are usually placed percutaneously to achieve the optimal angle into the bone.

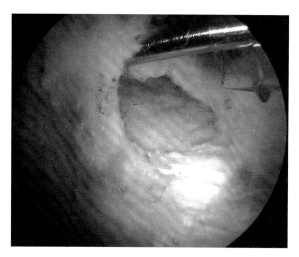

FIGURE 49.5. A completed gluteus medius tendon tear.

the proper position and angle for anchor placement. Fluoroscopy is useful at this stage of the procedure to confirm proper positioning of the anchors. A suture-passing device is then used to sequentially pass the sutures through the tendon from posterior to anterior (Fig. 49.8). Proper suture management is critical. Extra long cannulas are used to help manage the sutures and to aid with arthroscopic knot tying. After all the sutures have been passed, arthroscopic sliding, locking knots are placed with a knot pusher to secure the medius back to its native footprint on the trochanter (Fig. 49.9).

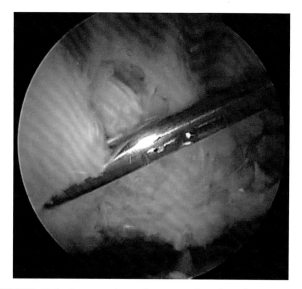

FIGURE 49.6. A grasper is used to manually reduce the tear to its anatomic position in the footprint.

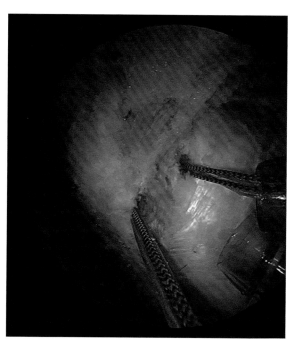

FIGURE 49.8. A suture-passing device is used to sequentially pass the sutures through the tendon from posterior to anterior.

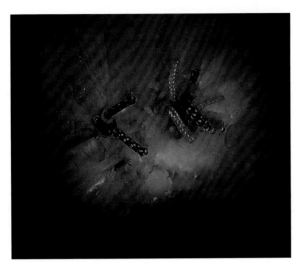

FIGURE 49.9. Arthroscopic sliding, locking knots secure the gluteus medius tendon back to its native footprint on the trochanter.

COMPLICATIONS, CONTROVERSIES, AND SPECIAL CONSIDERATIONS

There are few complications inherent to surgical procedures for snapping hip syndromes and peritrochanter disorders. Symptomatic heterotopic bone formation and hip flexion weakness in the early postoperative period may occur as a result of the iliopsoas tendon release. Heterotopic bone formation has been an issue primarily with iliopsoas tendon release off the lesser trochanter. A postoperative course of anti-inflammatory medications may decrease this risk. Other potential complications include fluid extravasations into the soft tissues and hematoma. There have been no formal reports in the literature reporting the incidence of these complications.

Recurrence of internal coxa saltans has been reported although this recurrence has primarily been identified with open techniques. (15,16) Recurrence of trochanteric bursitis, painful external coxa saltans, and retear of gluteus medius tendon repairs can all occur. However, the incidence of these complications has not been reported either.

The senior author has identified one deep venous thrombosis postoperatively after addressing peritrochanteric space pathology. Patients may be at a higher risk for deep venous thrombosis after surgery involving the peritrochanter space because the patient population is generally older, the cases may be longer, and the postoperative rehabilitation often requires a period of limited weight bearing.

PEARLS AND PITFALLS

Placement of the initial mid-anterior portal should be performed under fluoroscopic guidance to confirm placement over the lateral prominence of the greater trochanter to avoid entry into vastus lateralis distally and gluteus medius muscle proximally.

The initial view in the space should be directed toward identifying the gluteus maximus tendon insertion into the linea aspera. This allows the surgeon to gain proper orientation in the space and provides a boundary to protect the sciatic nerve 2 to 4 cm posterior to its insertion.

A complete bursectomy should be performed prior to tendon evaluation.

Slight axial traction on the limb will help to tension the gluteus medius fibers to allow for easy distinction between the inflamed bursa and the normal gluteus medius muscle tissue.

Place anchors perpendicular to the trochanter with fluoroscopic assistance.

A small stab incision at level of posterolateral peritrochanteric portal is an ideal location for anchor placement.

Plastic, extra long-threaded cannulas should be used during suture passage to provide optimal suture management.

REHABILITATION

Postoperative rehabilitation for patients undergoing iliopsoas tendon release, iliotibial band release, or bursectomy consists of 20 lb foot-flat weight bearing as tolerated with crutches for the two postoperative weeks. Full weight bearing is advanced without crutches as the patient's pain tolerates. Range of motion and hip strengthening without restrictions begin as soon as the patient's pain allows. It is important to avoid aggravating the lateral hip with aggressive therapy immediately after surgery.

In patients undergoing repair of the gluteus medius and minimus tears, physical therapy consists of 6 weeks of 20 lb foot-flat weight bearing with crutches. The patient is fitted with a hip abduction brace that blocks active abduction. No limitation of hip flexion or extension is required. Isometric strengthening of the hip abductors should begin at 6 weeks. At 12 weeks, more aggressive strengthening and activity is introduced. Running is not allowed until the patient displays equal abductor strength bilaterally to support the pelvis.

At the first preoperative visit and at the 3-, 6-, and 12-month follow-up visits, patients are asked to complete the Modified Harris Hip Score and Hip Outcomes Score Surveys as validated by Martin et al. (58,59)

CONCLUSIONS AND FUTURE DIRECTIONS

With greater surgeon experience in arthroscopic techniques and improved imaging modalities, instrumentation and diagnostic understanding, the treatment of snapping hip syndromes, and peritrochanter disorders will continue to develop. Although conservative management should still be the mainstay of treatment, endoscopic treatment of trochanteric bursitis, internal and external coxa saltans, and gluteus medius and minimus tears provides an additional treatment option for refractory cases. A thorough understanding of each disease entity, arthroscopic hip anatomy, and proper placement of portals is crucial for successful outcomes. Continued improvements through basic and clinical science studies with longer follow-up will expand the viable treatment options and allow more effective management of these disorders.

REFERENCES

1. Allen WC, Cope R. Coxa saltans: the snapping hip revisited. *J Am Acad Orthop Surg.* 1995;3:303–308.
2. Brooker AF Jr. The surgical approach to refractory trochanteric bursitis. *Johns Hopkins Med J.* 1979;145:98–100.
3. Bunker TD, Esler CN, Leach WJ. Rotator-cuff tear of the hip. *J Bone Joint Surg Br.* 1997;79:618–620.
4. Collee G, Dijkmans BA, Vandenbroucke JP, et al. Greater trochanteric pain syndrome (trochanteric bursitis) in low back pain. *Scand J Rheumatol.* 1991;20:262–266.
5. Kagan A II. Rotator cuff tears of the hip. *Clin Orthop Relat Res.* 1999;(368):135–140.
6. Karpinski MR, Piggott H. Greater trochanteric pain syndrome. A report of 15 cases. *J Bone Joint Surg Br.* 1985;67:762–763.
7. Tortolani PJ, Carbone JJ, Quartararo LG. Greater trochanteric pain syndrome in patients referred to orthopedic spine specialists. *Spine J.* 2002;2:251–254.
8. Byrd JW. Evaluation and management of the snapping iliopsoas tendon. *Instr Course Lect.* 2006;55:347–355.
9. Schaberg JE, Harper MC, Allen WC. The snapping hip syndrome. *Am J Sports Med.* 1984;12:361–365.
10. Ege Rasmussen KJ, Fanø N. Trochanteric bursitis. Treatment by corticosteroid injection. *Scand J Rheumatol.* 1985;14:417–420.
11. Fox JL. The role of arthroscopic bursectomy in the treatment of trochanteric bursitis. *Arthroscopy.* 2002;18:E34.
12. Govaert LH, van der Vis HM, Marti RK, et al. Trochanteric reduction osteotomy as a treatment for refractory trochanteric bursitis. *J Bone Joint Surg Br.* 2003;85:199–203.
13. Zoltan DJ, Clancy WG Jr, Keene JS. A new operative approach to snapping hip and refractory trochanteric bursitis in athletes. *Am J Sports Med.* 1986;14:201–204.
14. Gruen GS, Scioscia TN, Lowenstein JE. The surgical treatment of internal snapping hip. *Am J Sports Med.* 2002;30:607–613.
15. Jacobson T, Allen WC. Surgical correction of the snapping iliopsoas tendon. *Am J Sports Med.* 1990;18:470–474.
16. Taylor GR, Clarke NM. Surgical release of the 'snapping iliopsoas tendon'. *J Bone Joint Surg Br.* 1995;77:881–883.
17. Dobbs MB, Gordon JE, Luhmann SJ, et al. Surgical correction of the snapping iliopsoas tendon in adolescents. *J Bone Joint Surg Am.* 2002;84-A:420–424.
18. Baker CL Jr, Massie RV, Hurt WG, et al. Arthroscopic bursectomy for recalcitrant trochanteric bursitis. *Arthroscopy.* 2007;23:827–832.
19. Ilizaliturri VM Jr, Martinez-Escalante FA, Chaidez PA, et al. Endoscopic iliotibial band release for external snapping hip syndrome. *Arthroscopy.* 2006;22:505–510.
20. Ilizaliturri VM Jr, Villalobos FE Jr, Chaidez PA, et al. Internal snapping hip syndrome: treatment by endoscopic release of the iliopsoas tendon. *Arthroscopy.* 2005;21:1375–1380.
21. Kandemir U, Bharam S, Philippon MJ, et al. Endoscopic treatment of calcific tendinitis of gluteus medius and minimus. *Arthroscopy.* 2003;19:E4.
22. Voos JE, Rudzki JR, Shindle MK, et al. Arthroscopic anatomy and surgical techniques for peritrochanteric space disorders in the hip. *Arthroscopy.* 2007;23:1246.e1–1246.e5.
23. Wiese M, Rubenthaler F, Willburger RE, et al. Early results of endoscopic trochanter bursectomy. *Int Orthop.* 2004;28:218–221.
24. Voos JE, Ranawat AS, Kelly BT. The peritrochanteric space of the hip. *Instr Course Lect.* 2009;58:193–201.
25. Larson CM, Guanche CA, Kelly BT, et al. Advanced techniques in hip arthroscopy. *Instr Course Lect.* 2009;58:423–436.
26. Flanum ME, Keene JS, Blankenbaker DG, et al. Arthroscopic treatment of the painful "internal" snapping hip: results of a new endoscopic technique and imaging protocol. *Am J Sports Med.* 2007;35:770–779.
27. Ilizaliturri VM Jr, Chaidez C, Villegas P, et al. Prospective randomized study of 2 different techniques for endoscopic iliopsoas tendon release in the treatment of internal snapping hip syndrome. *Arthroscopy.* 2009;25:159–163.
28. Wettstein M, Jung J, Dienst M. Arthroscopic psoas tenotomy. *Arthroscopy.* 2006;22:907.e1–907.e4.
29. Clancy WG. Runners' injuries. Part two. Evaluation and treatment of specific injuries. *Am J Sports Med.* 1980;8:287–289.
30. Collee G, Dijkmans BA, Vandenbroucke JP, et al. A clinical epidemiological study in low back pain. Description of two clinical syndromes. *Br J Rheumatol.* 1990;29:354–357.
31. Robertson WJ, Kadrmas WR, Kelly BT. Arthroscopic management of labral tears in the hip: a systematic review of the literature. *Clin Orthop Relat Res.* 2007;455:88–92.
32. Callaghan BD. Unusual calcification in the region of the gluteus medius and minimus muscles. *Australas Radiol.* 1977;21:362–366.
33. Gordon EJ. Trochanteric bursitis and tendinitis. *Clin Orthop.* 1961;20:193–202.
34. Leonard MH. Trochanteric syndrome; calcareous and non-calcareous tendonitis and bursitis about the trochanter major. *J Am Med Assoc.* 1958;168:175–177.
35. Howell GE, Biggs RE, Bourne RB. Prevalence of abductor mechanism tears of the hips in patients with osteoarthritis. *J Arthroplasty.* 2001;16:121–123.
36. Lonner JH, Van Kleunen JP. Spontaneous rupture of the gluteus medius and minimus tendons. *Am J Orthop.* 2002;31:579–581.
37. Ozcakar L, Erol O, Kaymak B, et al. An underdiagnosed hip pathology: apropos of two cases with gluteus medius tendon tears. *Clin Rheumatol.* 2004;23:464–466.
38. Lequesne M, Mathieu P, Vuillemin-Bodaghi V, et al. Gluteal tendinopathy in refractory greater trochanter pain syndrome: diagnostic value of two clinical tests. *Arthritis Rheum.* 2008;59:241–246.
39. Siebenrock KA, Kalbermatten DF, Ganz R. Effect of pelvic tilt on acetabular retroversion: a study of pelves from cadavers. *Clin Orthop Relat Res.* 2003;(407):241–248.
40. Kingzett-Taylor A, Tirman PF, Feller J, et al. Tendinosis and tears of gluteus medius and minimus muscles as a cause of hip pain: MR imaging findings. *AJR Am J Roentgenol.* 1999;173:1123–1126.
41. Mintz DN, Hooper T, Connell D, et al. Magnetic resonance imaging of the hip: detection of labral and chondral

abnormalities using noncontrast imaging. *Arthroscopy*. 2005;21:385–393.

42. Shindle MK, Voos JE, Heyworth BE, et al. Hip arthroscopy in the athletic patient: current techniques and spectrum of disease. *J Bone Joint Surg Am*. 2007;89(suppl 3):29–43.

43. Kassarjian A, Yoon LS, Belzile E, et al. Triad of MR arthrographic findings in patients with cam-type femoroacetabular impingement. *Radiology*. 2005;236:588–592.

44. Kramer J, Recht MP. MR arthrography of the lower extremity. *Radiol Clin North Am*. 2002;40:1121–1132.

45. Schmid MR, Notzli HP, Zanetti M, et al. Cartilage lesions in the hip: diagnostic effectiveness of MR arthrography. *Radiology*. 2003;226:382–386.

46. Cvitanic O, Henzie G, Skezas N, et al. MRI diagnosis of tears of the hip abductor tendons (gluteus medius and gluteus minimus). *AJR Am J Roentgenol*. 2004;182:137–143.

47. Lequesne M, Djian P, Vuillemin V, et al. Prospective study of refractory greater trochanter pain syndrome. MRI findings of gluteal tendon tears seen at surgery. Clinical and MRI results of tendon repair. *Joint Bone Spine*. 2008;75:458–464.

48. LaBan MM, Weir SK, Taylor RS. 'Bald trochanter' spontaneous rupture of the conjoined tendons of the gluteus medius and minimus presenting as a trochanteric bursitis. *Am J Phys Med Rehabil*. 2004;83:806–809.

49. Blankenbaker DG, De Smet AA, Keene JS. Sonography of the iliopsoas tendon and injection of the iliopsoas bursa for diagnosis and management of the painful snapping hip. *Skeletal Radiol*. 2006;35:565–571.

50. Choi YS, Lee SM, Song BY, et al. Dynamic sonography of external snapping hip syndrome. *J Ultrasound Med*. 2002;21:753–758.

51. Pelsser V, Cardinal E, Hobden R, et al. Extraarticular snapping hip: sonographic findings. *AJR Am J Roentgenol*. 2001;176:67–73.

52. Connell DA, Bass C, Sykes CA, et al. Sonographic evaluation of gluteus medius and minimus tendinopathy. *Eur Radiol*. 2003;13:1339–1347.

53. White RA, Hughes MS, Burd T, et al. A new operative approach in the correction of external coxa saltans: the snapping hip. *Am J Sports Med*. 2004;32:1504–1508.

54. Voos JE, Shindle MK, Pruett A, et al. Endoscopic repair of gluteus medius tendon tears of the hip. *Am J Sports Med*. 2009;37:743–747.

55. Robertson WJ, Kelly BT. The safe zone for hip arthroscopy: a cadaveric assessment of central, peripheral, and lateral compartment portal placement. *Arthroscopy*. 2008;24:1019–1026.

56. Byrd JW, Pappas JN, Pedley MJ. Hip arthroscopy: an anatomic study of portal placement and relationship to the extra-articular structures. *Arthroscopy*. 1995;11:418–423.

57. Robertson WJ, Gardner MJ, Barker JU, et al. Anatomy and dimensions of the gluteus medius tendon insertion. *Arthroscopy*. 2008;24:130–136.

58. Martin RL, Kelly BT, Philippon MJ. Evidence of validity for the hip outcome score. *Arthroscopy*. 2006;22:1304–1311.

59. Martin RL, Philippon MJ. Evidence of validity for the hip outcome score in hip arthroscopy. *Arthroscopy*. 2007;23:822–826.

Femoroacetabular Impingement

J.W. Thomas Byrd

Surgical correction of various hip impingement problems was described even early in the last century (1, 2). In 1975, Harris and coauthors (3) described the "pistol grip" deformity of the femoral head observed in association with early age-onset osteoarthritis. In 1998, we described arthroscopic correction of impingement due to posttraumatic osteophytes and have also reported an arthroscopic technique of cheilectomy for femoral protuberances associated with Perthes disease (4, 5). However, it was Ganz and colleagues who formulated the concept of femoroacetabular impingement (FAI) describing pincer, cam, and combined types (6–8). Subsequently, we and other authors have reported arthroscopic methods for correcting this disorder (9–13).

FAI is not a cause of hip pain. It is simply a morphologic variant that predisposes the joint to intra-articular pathology that then becomes symptomatic. The arthroscope can be instrumental in assessing this associated intra-articular damage, which aids in establishing the correct treatment algorithm and can include arthroscopic correction of the impingement when necessary.

PATHOMECHANICS

Pincer impingement is caused by an excessive prominence of the anterolateral rim of the acetabulum. This can occur simply from overgrowth of the anterior edge or retroversion of the acetabulum. Sometimes there is a separate piece of bone along the anterolateral rim, referred to as an os acetabulum. The origin of this separate bone fragment is variable and may include a rim fracture secondary to cam impingement, an unfused physis, a traction injury from the enthesis of the rectus femoris, or ossification of a portion of the labrum. With hip flexion, the prominent rim of the acetabulum crushes the labrum against the femoral neck (Fig. 50.1). This cyclical submaximal repetitive microtrauma leads to breakdown and failure of the acetabular labrum. Secondarily, over time, a variable amount of articular failure within the adjacent acetabulum will occur. Pincer impingement occurs just about equally in males and females and more commonly starts to cause symptoms in middle age (9). More severe examples of pincer

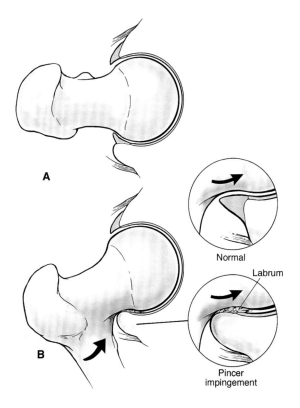

FIGURE 50.1. Pincer impingement occurs from a bony prominence of the anterior acetabulum crushing the labrum against the neck of the femur. Secondary articular failure occurs over time. (Reprinted with permission from J.W. Thomas Byrd.)

impingement occur with profunda or protrusio disorders of the acetabulum. These should be carefully assessed as some may be better corrected by open surgical procedures.

Cam-type FAI refers to the cam effect created by a non-spherical femoral head. During flexion, the prominence of the out-of-round portion rotates into the acetabulum, engaging against its surface, resulting in delamination and failure of the acetabular articular cartilage (Fig. 50.2). Early in the disease process, the labrum is relatively preserved, but, with time, it begins to sustain secondary damage. Cam impingement is classically attributed to a slipped

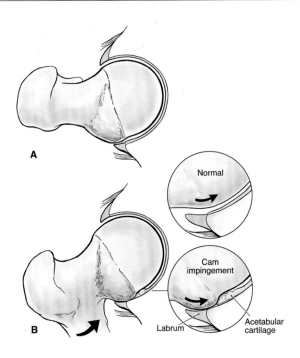

FIGURE 50.2. Cam impingement occurs with hip flexion as the bony prominence of the nonspherical portion of the femoral head (cam lesion) glides under the labrum engaging the edge of the articular cartilage and results in progressive delamination. Initially, the labrum is relatively preserved, but secondary failure occurs over time. (Reprinted with permission from J.W. Thomas Byrd.)

capital femoral epiphysis, resulting in a bony prominence of the anterior and anterolateral head–neck junction. However, the most common cause is the pistol grip deformity, attributed to a developmental abnormality of the capital physis during growth. The exact etiology of this growth disturbance is unclear; it may represent premature asymmetric closure of the physis, and it has been postulated that this could be due to late separation of the common proximal femoral growth plate that forms the physis of the greater trochanter and femoral head (14).

CLINICAL EVALUATION

The onset of symptoms associated with FAI is variable, but the damage results from the cumulative effect of cyclical abnormal wear associated with the altered joint morphology. The onset may be gradual, or often patients will recount an acute precipitating episode prior to which they were relatively asymptomatic. However, on close questioning, they will frequently recall previous nonspecific symptoms of a groin strain. Also, many patients will recount that they have never been very flexible in their hips.

Physical Examination

The trademark feature of FAI is diminished internal rotation caused by the altered bony architecture of the joint. However, there is much variation in the normative data

on hip range of motion. Also, although only one hip may be symptomatic, the altered morphology is usually present in both hips and there may not be much asymmetry in motion comparing the symptomatic with asymptomatic side. Be aware that many patients may demonstrate reduced internal rotation and still not suffer from pathologic impingement. Also, although uncommon, pathologic impingement is occasionally observed in individuals with normal or even increased internal rotation. Forced flexion, adduction, and internal rotation is called the impingement test in reference to eliciting symptoms associated with impingement (Fig. 50.3). However, virtually any irritable hip, regardless of the etiology, will be uncomfortable with this maneuver. Thus, although it is quite sensitive, it is not necessarily specific for impingement. This maneuver may normally be a little uncomfortable so the symptomatic side must be compared with the asymptomatic side. Most important is whether this recreates the characteristic type of pain that the patient experiences with activities.

These conditions often have a chronic component, even at the time of initial evaluation. Thus, secondary findings may be present due to compensatory mechanisms. Lateral pain may be present from trochanteric bursitis and posterior tenderness within the gluteal muscles may be present from overfiring, attempting to splint the joint. These secondary features may be more easily evident on examination and can obscure the underlying primary joint pathology. The anterior groin, lower abdominal, and adductor area must be carefully palpated to localize tenderness suggestive of athletic pubalgia (Fig. 50.4) (15). This can mimic or coexist with FAI. Tenderness with resisted sit-ups, hip flexion, or adduction should raise an index of suspicion for athletic pubalgia. Pain with passive flexion and internal rotation is more indicative of an intra-articular source.

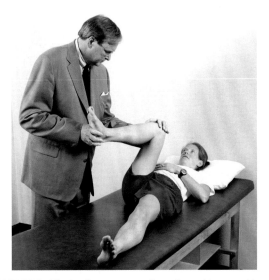

FIGURE 50.3. The impingement test is performed by provoking pain with flexion, adduction, and internal rotation of the symptomatic hip. (Reprinted with permission from J.W. Thomas Byrd.)

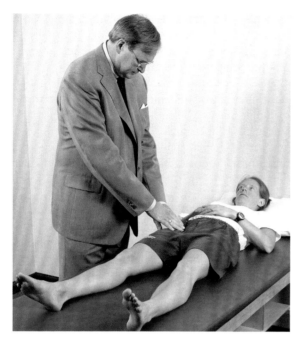

FIGURE 50.4. Careful palpation of the anterior hip, groin, lower abdominal, and adductor regions aids in assessing for the presence of soft-tissue pelvic pathology. (Reprinted with permission from J.W. Thomas Byrd.)

Imaging

Radiographs should include a well-centered anteroposterior (AP) pelvis view and a lateral view of the affected hip (Fig. 50.5) (16). These are important for assessing impingement as well as evaluating joint space preservation and other acute or chronic bony changes. Overcoverage of the anterior acetabulum, characteristic of pincer impingement, is evaluated by the presence of a crossover sign (Fig. 50.6). This can be due to acetabular retroversion, indicated by

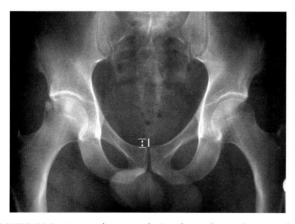

FIGURE 50.5. A properly centered AP radiograph must be controlled for rotation and tilt. Proper rotation is confirmed by alignment of the coccyx over the symphysis pubic *(vertical line)*. Proper tilt is controlled by maintaining the distance between the tip of the coccyx and the superior border of the symphysis pubis at 1 to 2 cm. (Reprinted with permission from J.W. Thomas Byrd.)

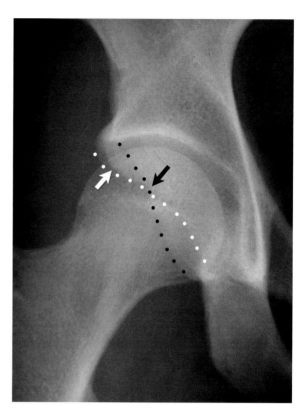

FIGURE 50.6. AP view of the right hip. The anterior *(white dots)* and posterior *(black dots)* rim of the acetabulum are marked. The superior portion of the anterior rim lies lateral to the posterior rim *(white arrow)* indicating overcoverage of the acetabulum. Anteriorly, it assumes a more normal medial position, creating the crossover sign *(black arrow)* as a positive indicator of pincer impingement. (Reprinted with permission from J.W. Thomas Byrd.)

the posterior wall sign (Fig. 50.7). The presence of an os acetabulum can also be evaluated (Fig. 50.8). The sphericity of the femoral head is assessed on both the AP and the lateral view (Fig. 50.9). There is some controversy regarding the optimal lateral radiograph. One study showed that the 40° Dunn view most predictably demonstrates the cam lesion (17). However, because of the variable shape and location of the lesion, no radiograph is consistently reliable. A frog lateral view is easy to obtain in a reproducible fashion and has demonstrated efficacy in assessing the cam lesion. Whatever lateral radiograph is chosen, the clinician must be cognizant that it can underinterpret the extent of a cam lesion. A herniation pit may be present in the region of the anterolateral femoral head–neck junction (Fig. 50.10). This has been reported with 30% prevalence in pathologic cases of FAI, but is sometimes observed in asymptomatic individuals (18). There are several caveats regarding radiographic interpretation of FAI. Indices of pincer impingement are assessed on a supine pelvis radiograph, and it is uncertain how this can be extrapolated to the orientation of the pelvis when standing. Dynamic positioning of the pelvis in real life is influenced by numerous other factors,

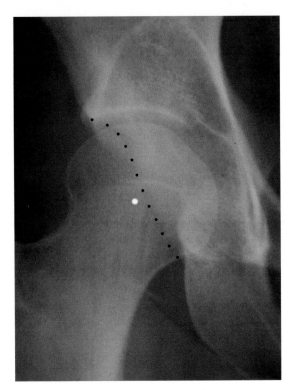

FIGURE 50.7. AP view of the right hip. Acetabular retroversion as a cause of pincer impingement is indicated by a shallow posterior wall in which the posterior rim of the acetabulum *(black dots)* lies medial to the center of rotation of the femoral head *(white dot)*. (Reprinted with permission from J.W. Thomas Byrd.)

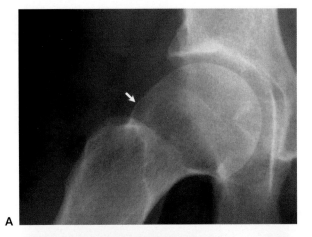

A

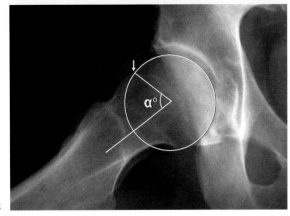

B

FIGURE 50.9. A frog lateral view of the right hip. **A:** The cam lesion *(arrow)* is evident as the convex abnormality at the head–neck junction where there should normally be a concave slope of the femoral neck. **B:** The Alpha angle is used to quantitate the severity of the cam lesion. A circle is placed over the femoral head. The Alpha angle is formed by a line along the axis of the femoral neck (1) and a line (2) from the center of the femoral head to the point where the head diverges outside of the circle *(arrow)*. (Reprinted with permission from J.W. Thomas Byrd.)

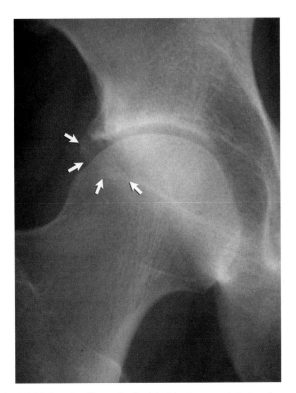

FIGURE 50.8. AP radiograph of a right hip. An os acetabulum *(arrows)* is present and, although the etiology is variable, it is often associated with FAI. (Reprinted with permission from J.W. Thomas Byrd.)

such as lumbar lordosis or kyphosis. The shape of cam lesions is variable and its epicenter may be more anterior or lateral. Thus, radiographs represent a poor two-dimensional image of the lesion's three-dimensional anatomy.

MRI and gadolinium arthrography with MRI (MRA) can both be helpful at detecting the intra-articular damage accompanying FAI. These studies are best at defining labral pathology, but are less reliable in assessing the associated articular damage (19). In the presence of a cam lesion, anticipate that the articular damage will be more extensive than the labral pathology. Also, subchondral edema in the anterior acetabulum is usually a harbinger of subjacent articular failure. With MRA's, the injection of long-acting anesthetic along with the contrast is important to substantiate whether the hip disease is the source of the patient's symptoms. This distinction may not always be clear on clinical examination alone.

IV. The Hip

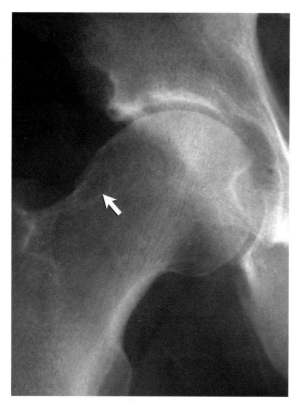

FIGURE 50.10. AP radiograph of a right hip. A herniation pit is present *(arrow)*, often associated with cam impingement. (Reprinted with permission by J.W. Thomas Byrd.)

CT is much better at showing bone architecture and structure. MRI and MRA often cannot distinguish an os acetabulum and have difficulty defining the amount of joint space narrowing. For some cases, CT provides information that complements these other studies. However, all planar two-dimensional images, whether from magnetic resonance or CT, have difficulty in quantitating cam lesions. Unless the image happens to bisect the variable apex or epicenter of the cam lesion, it often underestimates its magnitude. CT with three-dimensional reconstructions provides the clearest image of the cam lesion and its morphology. These images are especially helpful in the arthroscopic management, providing a clear interpretation of the exact shape of the abnormal bone that must be exposed and then resected.

ARTHROSCOPIC PROCEDURE

Arthroscopic management of FAI begins with arthroscopy of the central compartment. This is where the intra-articular damage, indicative of pathologic impingement, is identified. The patient is positioned supine with traction applied, and three standard portals provide optimal access for surveying and accessing intra-articular pathology (Fig. 50.11A,B) (20,21).

There are three arthroscopic parameters of pincer impingement. First is the presence of anterior labral pathology that must be present in order to have pathologic pincer impingement. Second, positioning of the anterior portal may be difficult despite adequate distraction, and this is due to the bony prominence of the anterolateral acetabulum. Third is the presence of bone overhanging the labrum where normally there would just be a capsular reflection when pincer impingement is not present. The amount of bone to be removed is determined in conjunction with the radiographic and arthroscopic findings. In determining whether to excise bone, the radiographs should be carefully assessed for evidence of dysplasia. Retroversion in a dysplastic hip can give a false sense of pincer impingement. Recontouring the acetabulum in this setting can result in iatrogenic instability.

If labral degeneration is extensive, as is often seen in middle age, then it is best managed with simple debridement. The labral damage may not be salvaged, but recontouring the acetabulum opens the joint and may substantially improve mobility and symptoms. After completely inspecting the joint, attention is turned to the labral lesion. Selective debridement of the damaged portion will reveal the overhanging lip of bone instead of the normal capsular reflection from the labrum (Fig. 50.12A–E). Once the damaged tissue has been removed, exposing the pincer lesion, the bone is then recontoured with a spherical burr. Generous capsulotomies around the portals facilitate maneuverability and access. The pincer lesion is addressed switching the arthroscope and instrumentation between the anterior and the anterolateral portals. Resection is typically carried to the articular edge of the acetabulum. The amount of bone to be removed is dictated by the severity of the pincer lesion. Proximally, the bone is resected flush with the anterior column of the acetabulum. The antero-medial and lateral extent of the bony resection is dictated by the margin of healthy labrum. The bone is recontoured to create a smooth transition with the healthy portion of the labrum, which is preserved. A variable amount of associated secondary articular damage may be present, which is addressed with a chondroplasty or microfracture for grade 4 lesions.

In the presence of good-quality labral tissue and especially in younger patients, preservation of the labrum is preferred. Sometimes the bony lesion can be exposed on the capsular side of the labrum and recontoured without compromising the labrum's structural integrity (Fig. 50.13). More often, when the labrum is failing due to pincer impingement, but maintains reasonable quality tissue, it can be mobilized to resect the pincer lesion and then refixed (Fig. 50.14). The portion of the labrum to be mobilized must be exposed at its bony attachment on the capsular side. The labrum is sharply dissected from the overlying bone to reveal the pincer lesion. The acetabulum is then recontoured with a high-speed burr, taking care to preserve the mobilized labrum. With this technique,

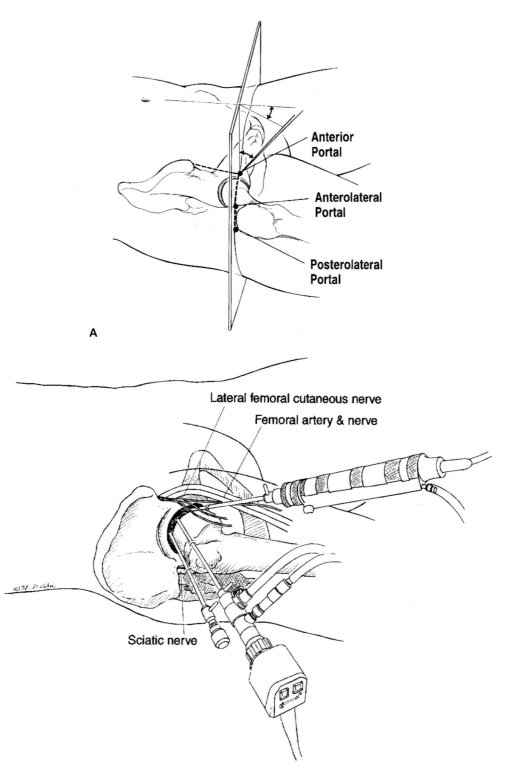

A

B

FIGURE 50.11. A: The site of the anterior portal coincides with the intersection of a sagittal line drawn distally from the anterior superior iliac spine and a transverse line across the superior margin of the greater trochanter. The direction of this portal courses approximately 45° cephalad and 30° toward the midline. The anterolateral and posterolateral portals are positioned directly over the superior aspect of the trochanter at its anterior and posterior borders. **B:** The relationship of the major neurovascular structures to the three standard portals is illustrated. The femoral artery and nerve lie well medial to the anterior portal. The sciatic nerve lies posterior to the posterolateral portal. The lateral femoral cutaneous nerve lies close to the anterior portal. Injury to this structure is avoided by using proper portal placement. The anterolateral portal is established first because it lies most centrally in the safe zone for arthroscopy. (Reprinted with permission by J.W. Thomas Byrd.)

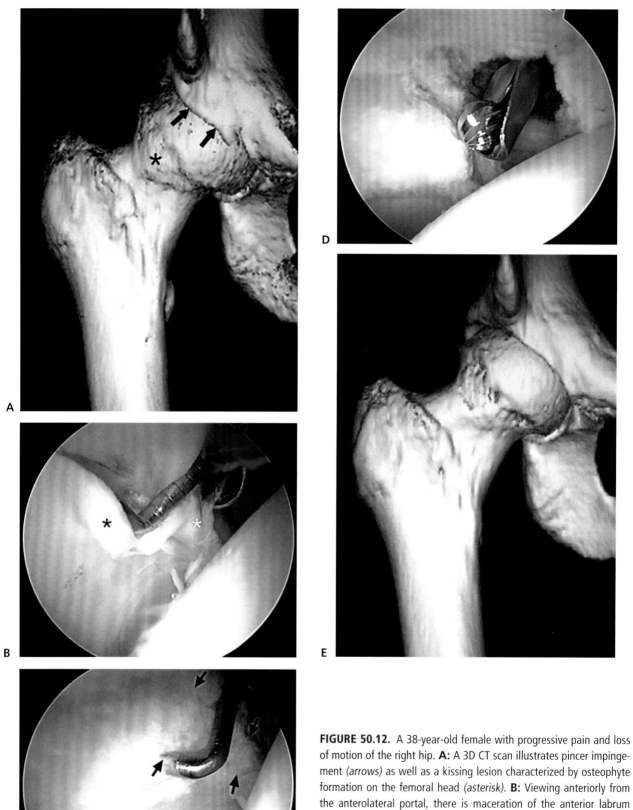

FIGURE 50.12. A 38-year-old female with progressive pain and loss of motion of the right hip. **A:** A 3D CT scan illustrates pincer impingement *(arrows)* as well as a kissing lesion characterized by osteophyte formation on the femoral head *(asterisk)*. **B:** Viewing anteriorly from the anterolateral portal, there is maceration of the anterior labrum *(white asterisk)* and some associated articular delamination *(black asterisk)*. **C:** Debridement of the degenerate labrum exposes the pincer lesion *(arrows)*. **D:** The pincer lesion is recontoured with a burr. **E:** A postoperative 3D CT scan demonstrates the extent of bony recontouring of the acetabulum and the femoral head. (Reprinted with permission by J.W. Thomas Byrd.)

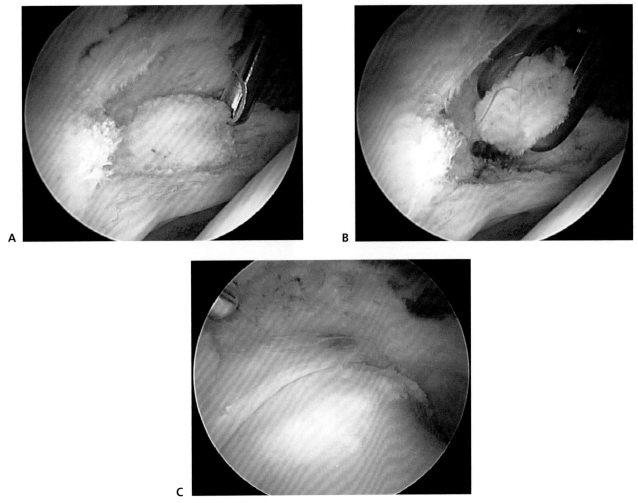

FIGURE 50.13. A pincer lesion created by an os acetabulum along the anterolateral rim of a right hip. **A:** The fragment is exposed. **B:** The fragment is being removed. **C:** The integrity of the labrum has been preserved.

adequate mobilization of the labrum is necessary to visualize the bony margins of the pincer lesion for recontouring. Inadequate exposure results in simply a small scalloped defect in the acetabular rim with incomplete correction. The depth of resection is typically 3 to 5 mm but is determined by the dimensions of the pincer lesion. After reshaping the rim, the labrum is then refixed with suture anchors. The anchors are placed in the rim of the acetabulum on the capsular side of the labrum. Anchor placement usually requires a more distal portal entry site through the skin to ensure that the anchor diverges from the joint, avoiding perforation of the articular surface. It is preferable to then pass a single limb of the suture through the main substance of the labrum to approximate it to the articular edge of the acetabulum. This technique secures the labrum, but avoids having suture interposed between the labrum and the articular surface of the femoral head. Various devices for penetrating the suture through the labrum or suture shuttle techniques can accomplish this (Fig. 50.15). Alternatively, if the quality of the tissue is marginal, the suture may simply be looped around the

labrum to secure it to the acetabulum. It is most important to ensure that the substance of the tissue sutured is sufficient to warrant the repair.

Management of cam impingement also begins with arthroscopy of the central compartment to assess for the pathology associated with cam lesion (22). The characteristic feature of pathologic cam impingement is articular failure of the anterolateral acetabulum. The femoral head remains well preserved until late in the disease course. Early stages of the disease are characterized by closed grade 1 chondral blistering, which sometimes must be distinguished from normal articular softening. Our experience has been that most already have grade 3 or 4 acetabular changes by the time of surgical intervention. The articular surface is seen to separate or peel away from its attachment to the labrum (Fig. 50.16), and this is caused by the shear effect of the cam lesion. The labrum may be relatively well preserved but, with time, progressive fragmentation occurs. Often, the damaged articular edge of the labrum can be selectively debrided, preserving the capsular margin and potentially some of its labral seal function. If there is good quality

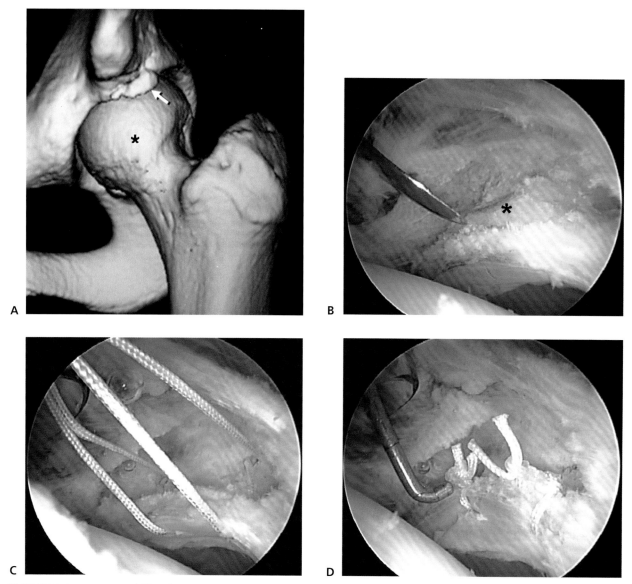

FIGURE 50.14. A 15-year-old female gymnast with pain and reduced internal rotation of the left hip. **A:** A 3D CT scan defines a pincer lesion with accompanying os acetabulum *(arrow)* and cam lesion *(asterisk)*. **B:** Viewing from the anterolateral portal, the pincer lesion, and os acetabulum *(asterisk)* are exposed with the labrum being sharply released with an arthroscopic knife. **C:** The acetabular fragment has been removed and the rim trimmed with anchors placed to repair the labrum. **D:** The labrum has been refixed. (Reprinted with permission by J.W. Thomas Byrd.)

tissue that has been detached, repair can be performed with suture anchors (Fig. 50.17). If pincer impingement is not present, the anchors can be placed adjacent to the articular surface, between the acetabulum and the labrum. The suture limbs can be grasped through the labrum with a penetrator device and tied with the knots on the capsular side of the labrum. Passing both limbs of the suture in a mattress fashion avoids suture rubbing against the femoral head, but occasionally looping the sutures may be necessary to ensure that good substance of the tissue is secured to the rim of the acetabulum. The articular pathology is addressed with chondroplasty and microfracture as dictated by its severity.

After completing arthroscopy of the central compartment, the cam lesion is addressed from the peripheral compartment. A capsulotomy is created by connecting the anterior and anterolateral portals (Fig. 50.18). The posterolateral portal can be removed and the anterior and anterolateral cannulas are simply backed out of the central compartment. The traction is released, and the hip flexed approximately 35°. As the hip is flexed under arthroscopic visualization, the line of demarcation between healthy femoral cartilage and abnormal fibrocartilage that covers the cam lesion can usually be identified. Flexing the hip too far can cause part of the cam lesion to disappear under the acetabulum.

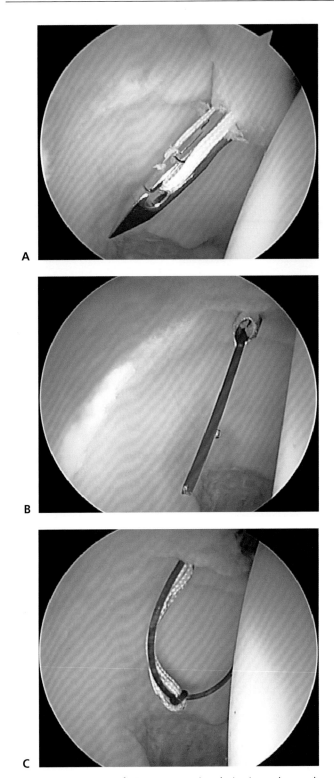

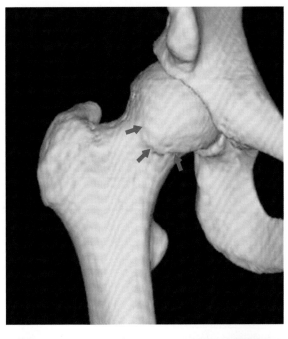

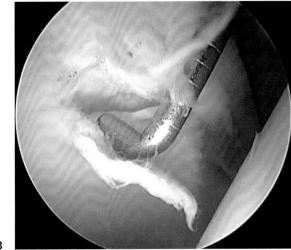

FIGURE 50.15. A: A soft tissue-penetrating device is used to push the suture limb through the labrum. **B:** A suture passing device penetrates the device to shuttle through a monofilament suture. **C:** The anchor suture is shuttled through the labrum by the monofilament secured with a single half-hitch.

A cephalad anterolateral portal is established approximately 5 cm above the anterolateral portal, entering through the capsulotomy that has already been established.

FIGURE 50.16. A 20-year-old hockey player with a 4-year history of right hip pain. **A:** A 3D CT scan defines the cam lesion *(arrows)*. **B:** Viewing from the anterolateral portal, the probe introduced anteriorly displaces an area of articular delamination from the anterolateral acetabulum characteristic of the peel-back phenomenon created by the bony lesion shearing the articular surface during hip flexion. (Reprinted with permission by J.W. Thomas Byrd.)

These proximal and distal anterolateral portals work well for accessing and addressing the cam lesion (Fig. 50.19). Removing the anterior portal provides an unobstructed image for the C-arm although the portal can be maintained if it is needed for better access to the medial side of the femoral neck.

Most of the work for performing the recontouring of the cam lesion (femoroplasty) lies in the soft tissue preparation. This includes capsular resection as necessary to ensure complete visualization of the lesion and then removal of the fibrocartilage and scar that covers the abnormal bone

IV. The Hip

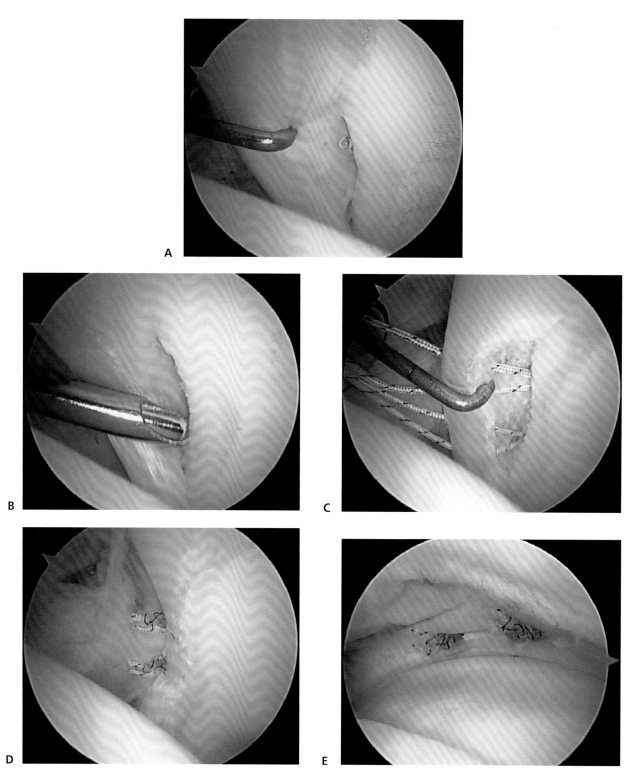

FIGURE 50.17. An anterior labral tear of a right hip is being viewed from the anterolateral portal. **A:** Pathologic detachment of the labrum from the rim of the acetabulum is being probed. **B:** Freshening the rim of the acetabulum, creating a bleeding bony surface aids in potentiating healing of the repair. **C:** Two anchors have been placed in the rim of the acetabulum with the sutures passed through the labrum in a mattress fashion. **D:** The sutures have been tied securely reapproximating the labrum to the rim of the acetabulum. **E:** Now viewing from the peripheral compartment, the repair is inspected showing approximation of the labrum against the femoral head with the sutures well removed from the articular surface.

(Fig. 50.20). With the hip flexed, the proximal portal provides better access for the lateral and posterior portion, whereas the distal portal is more anterior relative to the joint and provides best access for the anterior part of the lesion. The lateral synovial fold is identified as the arthroscopic landmark for the retinacular vessels and care is taken to preserve this structure during the recontouring (Fig. 50.21). Switching between the portals is important for full appreciation of the three-dimensional anatomy of the recontouring.

Once the bone has been fully exposed, recontouring is performed with a spherical burr. The goal is to remove the abnormal bone identified on the preoperative CT scan and recreate the normal concave relationship that should exist where the femoral neck meets the articular edge of the femoral head. It is best to begin by creating the line and depth of resection at the articular margin. The resection is then extended distally, tapering with the normal portion of the femoral head (Figs. 50.22A,B and 50.23A,B).

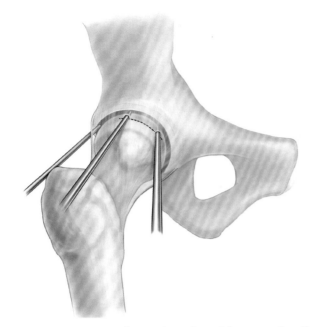

FIGURE 50.18. A capsulotomy is performed by connecting the anterior and anterolateral portals *(dotted line)*. This is geographically located adjacent to the area of the cam lesion. This capsulotomy is necessary in order for the instruments to pass freely from the central to the peripheral compartment as the traction is released and the hip flexed. (Reprinted with permission from J.W. Thomas Byrd.)

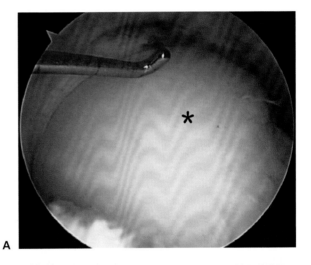

A

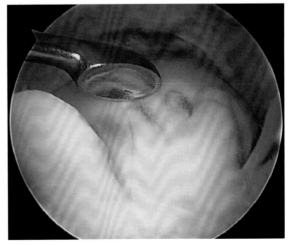

B

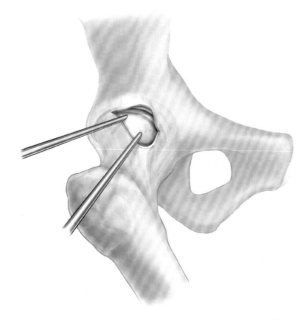

FIGURE 50.19. With the hip flexed, the anterolateral portal is now positioned along the neck of the femur. A cephalad (proximal) anterolateral portal has been placed. These two portals allow access to the entirety of the cam lesion in most cases. Their position also allows an unhindered view with the c-arm. (Reprinted with permission from J.W. Thomas Byrd.)

FIGURE 50.20. The right hip is viewed from the anterolateral portal. **A:** The cam lesion is identified, covered in fibrocartilage *(asterisk)*. **B:** An arthroscopic curette is used to denude the abnormal bone. **C:** The area to be excised has been fully exposed. The soft tissue preparation aids in precisely defining the margins to be excised. (Reprinted with permission from J.W. Thomas Byrd.)

IV. The Hip

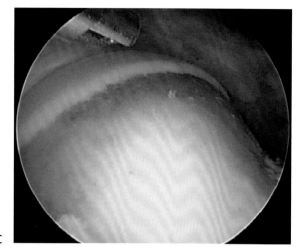

C

FIGURE 50.20. (continued)

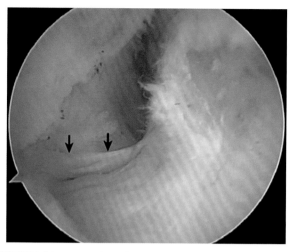

FIGURE 50.21. Viewing laterally, underneath the area of the lateral capsulotomy, the lateral synovial fold *(arrows)* is identified along the lateral base of the neck, representing the arthroscopic landmarks of the lateral retinacular vessels. (Reprinted with permission from J.W. Thomas Byrd.)

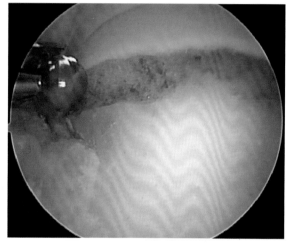

A

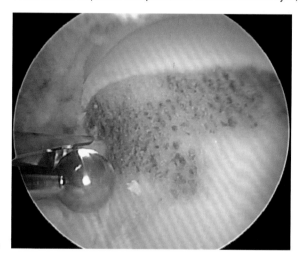

B

FIGURE 50.22. The arthroscope is in the more distal (anterolateral) portal with the instrumentation placed from the proximal portal. **A:** Bony resection is begun at the articular margin. **B:** The resection is then carried distally, recreating the normal concave relationship. (Reprinted with permission from J.W. Thomas Byrd.)

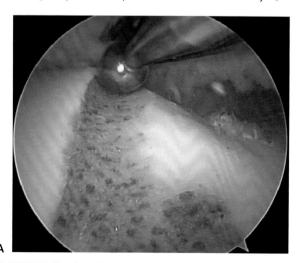

A

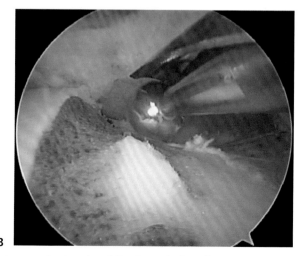

B

FIGURE 50.23. The arthroscope is now in the proximal portal with the instrumentation introduced distally. **A:** The line of resection is continued along the anterior articular border of the bump. **B:** The recontouring is completed. (Reprinted with permission from J.W. Thomas Byrd.)

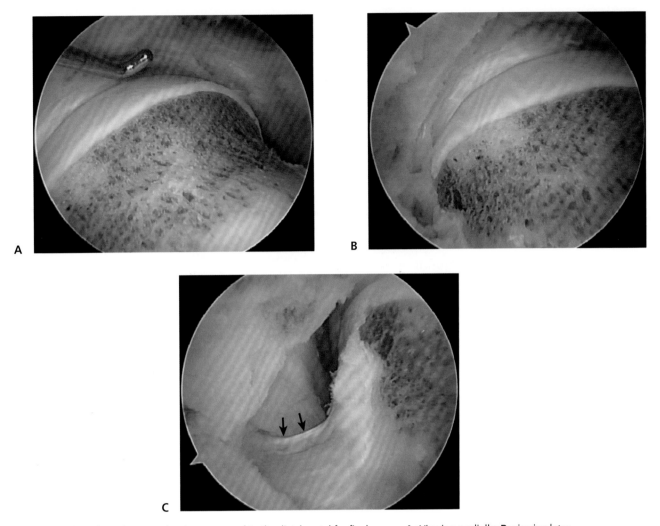

FIGURE 50.24. The arthroscope has been returned to the distal portal for final survey. **A:** Viewing medially; **B:** viewing later-ally; **C:** confirming preservation of the lateral retinacular vessels *(arrows)*. (Reprinted with permission from J.W. Thomas Byrd.)

We recommend beginning the resection at the lateral/posterior limit of the cam lesion with the arthroscope in the more distal portal and instrumentation in the more proximal portal. The posterior extent of the resection is usually the most difficult; the resection is also the most critical to avoid notching the tensile surface of the femoral neck, and particular attention must be given to avoiding and preserving the lateral retinacular vessels. Then, switching the arthroscope to the proximal portal, the burr is introduced distally and the reshaping is completed along the anterior head and neck junction. Lastly, attention is given to make sure that all bone debris is removed as thoroughly as possible to lessen the likelihood of developing heterotopic ossification. The quality of the recontouring is assessed and preservation of the lateral retinacular vessels is confirmed (Fig. 50.24A–C).

Closure of the capsulotomy is not routinely performed. In cases where instability might be a potential concern, such as dysplasia, the capsulotomy is limited and suture closure could be considered.

POSTOP REHABILITATION

The recovery strategy depends on the extent of pathology that is encountered at the time of arthroscopy and what is done to address it. For simple labral debridement and recontouring of the acetabular rim, the patient is allowed to weight bear as tolerated, with an emphasis on range of motion and joint stabilization. If the labrum is refixed, then precautions are necessary to protect the repair site during the early healing phase. This includes protected weight bearing and avoiding extremes of flexion and external rotation for the first 4 to 6 weeks.

Reshaping of the femoral head–neck junction necessitates some precautions. Fracture of the femoral neck is an unlikely, but potentially serious, complication. Full weight bearing is allowed, but crutches are used to avoid awkward twisting movements during the first 4 weeks. Once full motor control has been regained, the joint is adequately protected for light activities. Full bony remodeling takes 3 months during which time some precautions

IV. The Hip

are necessary to avoid high impact or torsional forces. If microfracture is performed, strict protected weight bearing is continued for 2 months to optimize the early maturation of the fibrocartilaginous healing response. During this time, gentle range of motion is emphasized to stimulate the healing process.

At 3 months, specific precautions are lifted and functional progression is allowed. The rate at which the individuals advance is variable and may require another 1 to 3 months for full activities. Athletes are generally advised that return to sports following surgical correction of FAI can take 4 to 6 months.

RESULTS

In 2006, Sampson (11) reported on 183 patients who underwent arthroscopic correction of impingement using the lateral position. The distribution of the types of impingement was not reported, but he described correcting the pincer and cam lesions in conjunction with labral debridement. He noted in his preliminary results that the impingement sign was eliminated in 94% and there was a high degree of satisfaction although no other specific outcome measures were reported. The results were generally noted to be poorer in the presence of more extensive articular damage.

Larson and Giveans, (12) in 2008, reported their early outcomes in 96 patients (100 hips) at an average follow-up of 10 months. There were 26 cam, 21 pincer, and 53 combined lesions. Thirty underwent labral repair or refixation and the rest debridement. Eighty-six percent had negative or only mildly positive impingement tests postoperatively. The modified Harris hip score was significantly improved with an average of 25 points (preop 60; postop 85). Three hips were converted to total hip arthroplasty during this early follow-up. There was one partial transient sciatic nerve neuropraxia and six cases of heterotopic bone formation.

In 2009, Philippon et al. (13) reported on 122 cases with minimum 2-year follow-up. Ten patients refused to participate in the follow-up, leaving 112 patients with 23 undergoing correction of cam, 3 undergoing correction of pincer, and 86 undergoing correction of combined lesions. Ten patients were converted to total hip replacement and another 12 were lost to follow-up. Excluding those, among the remaining 90, he reported an average 26-point improvement in the modified Harris hip score (preop 58; postop 84) with no specific reported complications. They found higher preoperative hip score, less joint space narrowing and labral repair to be predictors of better outcomes.

Also in 2009, we reported our initial experience in 220 patients (227 hips) with minimum 1-year follow-up (9). There were 162 cam, 21 pincer, and 44 combined lesions that were corrected. No labral repairs were performed in this early series. The median improvement was 21 points (preop 66; postop 87) with 100% follow-up. One was converted to total hip arthroplasty and six underwent repeat

arthroscopy. There were three complications including a transient neuropraxia of the pudendal nerve and one of the lateral femoral cutaneous nerve, each of which resolved uneventfully, and one mild heterotopic ossification, which did not preclude a successful outcome.

Most recently, Larson and Giveans (23) identified 39 patients who underwent labral repair in conjunction with correction of FAI and compared these with a previous matched group of 36 FAI patients in whom the labrum was debrided. They reported superior results in the labral repair group at 1-year follow-up, but noted that other variables could have influenced the outcomes. There is certainly a trend toward labral preservation, but these early results of repair versus debridement must be interpreted cautiously as there are significant methodologic biases.

Other substantial complications have also been reported in conjunction with arthroscopic correction of FAI. Several femoral neck fractures have been encountered, usually associated with poor compliance with postoperative precautions (24). Also, postoperative dislocation has been reported when rim trimming was performed in a case where dysplasia may have played a role (25). This emphasizes the importance of accurately interpreting radiographs.

SUMMARY

Many patients with FAI can be appropriately managed with arthroscopic surgery. However, the surgeon must be clinically astute in assessing the patient and interpreting the studies to be certain this is the best approach for the patient. Meticulous attention to the details of the procedure is necessary. The advantages of this less invasive approach are evident; it is performed as an outpatient with few complications and facilitates postoperative rehabilitation. The arthroscopic procedure is better suited for individuals seeking to return to an active lifestyle. Also, the imaging studies may underestimate the severity of articular loss, which may only become evident during arthroscopy.

REFERENCES

1. Vulpius O, Stoffel A. *Orthopaadische Operationslehre.* Stuttgart, Germany F. Enke; 1913.
2. Smith-Petersen MN. Treatment of malum coxae senilis, old slipped upper femoral epiphysis, intrapelvic protrusion of the acetabulum, and coxa plana by means of acetabuloplasty. *J Bone Joint Surg Am.* 1936;18:869–880.
3. Stulberg SD, Cordell LD, Harris WH, et al. Unrecognized childhood hip disease: a major cause of idiopathic osteoarthritis of the hip. In: Cordell LD, Harris WH, Ramsey PL, eds. *The Hip: Proceedings of the Third Open Scientific Meeting of the Hip Society.* St Louis, MO: CV Mosby; 1975:212–228.
4. Byrd JWT. Arthroscopy of select hip lesions. In: Byrd JWT, ed. *Operative Hip Arthroscopy.* New York, NY: Thieme; 1998:153-170.

5. Byrd JWT. Hip arthroscopy: evolving frontiers. *Oper Tech Orthop*. Special Issue: Novel Techniques in Hip Surgery, 2004;14(2):58–67.

6. Myers SR, Eijer H, Ganz R. Anterior femoroacetabular impingement after periacetabular osteotomy. *Clin Orthop*. 1999;363:81–92.

7. Ganz R, Parvizi J, Beck M, et al. Femoroacetabular impingement: a cause for osteoarthritis in the hip. *Clin Orthop*. 2003;417:112–120.

8. Lavigne M, Parvizi J, Beck M, et al. Anterior femoroacetabular impingement: part I. Techniques of joint preserving surgery. *Clin Orthop*. 2004;418:61–66.

9. Byrd JWT, Jones KS. Arthroscopic management of femoroacetabular impingement. *Instr Course Lect*. 2009;58:231–239.

10. Guanche CA, Bare AA. Arthroscopic treatment of femoroacetabular impingement. *Arthroscopy*. 2006;25(1):95–106.

11. Sampson T. Arthroscopic treatment of femoroacetabular impingement. *Instr Course Lect*. 2006;55:337–346.

12. Larson CM, Giveans MR. Arthroscopic management of femoroacetabular impingement: early outcomes measures. *Arthroscopy*. 2008;24(5):540–546.

13. Philippon MJ, Briggs KK, Yen YM, et al. Outcomes following hip arthroscopy for femoroacetabular impingement with associated chondrolabral dysfunction. Minimum two-year followup. *J Bone Joint Surg (Br)*. 2009;91-B:16–23.

14. Siebenrock KA, Wahab KHA, Werlen S, et al. Abnormal extension of the femoral head epiphysis as a cause of cam impingement. *Clin Orthop Rel Res*. 2004;418:54–60.

15. Meyers WC, Foley DP, Garrett WE, et al. Management of severe lower abdominal or inguinal pain in high-performance athletes. PAIN (Performing Athletes with Abdominal or Inguinal Neuromuscular Pain Study Group). *Am J Sports Med*. 2000;28(1):2–8.

16. Parvizi J, Leunig M, Ganz R. Femoroacetabular impingement. *J Am Acad Ortho Surg*. 2007;15(9):561–570.

17. Meyer DC, Beck M, Ellis T, et al. Comparison of six radiographic projections to assess femoral head/neck asphericity. *Clin Orthop*. 2006;445:181–185.

18. Leunig M, Beck M, Kalhor M, et al. Fibrocystic changes at anterosuperior femoral neck: prevalence in hips with femoroacetabular impingement. *Radiology*. 2005;236:237–246.

19. Byrd JWT, Jones KS. Diagnostic accuracy of clinical assessment, MRI, gadolinium MRI, and intraarticular injection in hip arthroscopy patients. *Am J Sports Med*. 2004;32(7):1668–1674.

20. Byrd JWT. The supine approach. In: Byrd JWT, ed. *Operative Hip Arthroscopy*. 2nd ed. New York, NY: Springer; 2005:145–169.

21. Byrd JWT. Hip arthroscopy by the supine approach. *Instr Course Lect*. 2006;55:325–336.

22. Byrd JWT, Jones KS. Arthroscopic "femoroplasty" in the management of cam-type femoroacetabular impingement, *Clin Orthop Relat Res*. 2009;467:739–746.

23. Larson CM, Giveans MR. Arthroscopic debridement versus refixation of the acetabular labrum associated with femoroacetabular impingement. *Arthroscopy*. 2009;25(4):369–376.

24. Sampson T. Arthroscopic treatment of femoroacetabular impingement. *Am J Orthop*. 2008;37(12):608–612.

25. Matsuda DK. Acute iatrogenic dislocation following hip impingement arthroscopic surgery. *Arthroscopy*. 2009;25(4):400–404.

Advanced Techniques and Frontiers in Hip Arthroscopy

Marc J. Philippon • Bruno G. Schroder e Souza • Karen K. Briggs

---

Hip arthroscopy is a fast evolving field in orthopedic surgery. The past decade consisted on a period in which new applications and safer techniques were developed, and more people started their experience with this procedure. In the past 10 years, the procedure has gained interest with the "rediscovery" of femoroacetabular impingement (FAI) (1), and the development of arthroscopic techniques to treat that condition (2).

Performing a fast search on Medline through PubMed using the term "hip arthroscopy," one will find that 234 papers have been published on that topic to date. Of these papers, 137 were published in the past 5 years. For the search of the "femoroacetabular impingement," which is currently the main indication for hip arthroscopy, 175 papers were found being more than half (81) were published in the past 2 years. The objective of this chapter is to present and discuss advanced techniques in hip arthroscopy that are currently in use, as well as new techniques that are on the new frontier of hip arthroscopy.

MODERN SURGICAL SETUP AND PORTAL PLACEMENT

Arthroscopy of the hip can be performed in a lateral or supine position. Our preference is the modified supine approach (2). We recommend a combination of general anesthesia with a lumbar plexus sciatic regional block, for complete muscular paralysis. After the induction of anesthesia, the patient is positioned on a standard fracture table that allows independent lower extremity traction. The perineum is positioned against a large, padded bolster with care taken to protect the genitalia. The feet are placed in padded boots that are secured with Velcro straps and reinforced with a tape wrap (Fig. 51.1). Both legs are positioned in 40° of abduction, 20° of flexion, and neutral rotation.

Gentle traction is applied through the operative hip with moderate countertraction through the nonoperative hip as needed. A lateral tilt of the table of 10° to the contralateral side is obtained to optimize traction forces. Fluoroscopy is used to obtain an anteroposterior (AP) view

of the operative hip. The fluoroscopic image should be observed for distraction of the joint space as well as the development of a "vacuum sign" or radiolucency within the joint space. Once the vacuum sign has been visualized, the operative leg is adducted to neutral. The foot is maximally internally rotated, bringing the femoral neck parallel to the floor (about 15°). Joint distraction is assessed with fluoroscopy, and additional traction is applied to restore the vacuum sign. Approximately 8 to 10 mm of distraction should be obtained between the acetabulum and femoral head to provide instrument clearance and to avoid iatrogenic damage to the labrum or chondral surfaces. The time of traction application is noted, and continuous traction time is limited to less than 2 hours.

We currently use the anterolateral and the distal lateral accessory portal in most cases. The anterolateral portal is placed approximately 1 to 2 cm superior to the tip of the greater trochanter and 1 to 2 cm anterior from this proximal point. The needle is guided slightly cephalic and posterior to converge along the direction of the femoral neck, at an angle of approximately 15° to 20° in relation to the floor. After capsular penetration, a tactile decrease in the resistance indicates the labrum has not been pierced. Fluoroscopic images may be obtained to reassure the position of the needle. The injection of 30 mL of saline helps to distend the joint and the liquid rebound confirm its intra-articular position. A 70° arthroscope is introduced into the joint with fluid pump set at 50 mm Hg of pressure and at high flow. Once within the joint, one should be able to visualize the femoral head and acetabulum. Additional traction may be applied as needed to allow improved instrument mobility within the joint.

INTRA-ARTICULAR PROCEDURES

Current Approach to FAI

The diagnosis of FAI has recently been clinically described in several publications. Patients with bony deformities causing FAI and pain should be effectively treated. Conservative measures have not shown to be effective when intra-articular lesions are present. Therefore, surgical

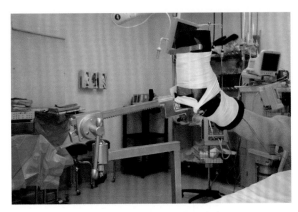

FIGURE 51.1. The feet are placed in padded boots that are secured with Velcro straps and reinforced with a tape wrap.

treatment should be considered the gold standard for those patients. We prefer the arthroscopic approach because it is effective and allows for faster recovery (3).

Acetabular Rim Trimming

In case of labral detachment at its base, which is particularly common in cases with associated cam impingement, the labrum should be separated in the watershed zone so that underling bone deformity can be corrected, and the labrum reattached with suture anchors. That is achieved by a systematic approach. First, we delineate the chondrolabral junction by controlled application of a monopolar radiofrequency chisel. This will contract the fibrocartilage and better define the tear, preventing sacrifice of healthy labral tissue as well as stabilize that adjacent acetabular cartilage. Chondral flaps are removed after demarcation with aid of the same RF device. The area between the labrum and the capsule is then dissected with a shaver, and the labrum is completely detached from the acetabular rim (Fig. 51.2). The acetabular bony overhang, responsible for the pincer deformity, is removed with a motorized burr

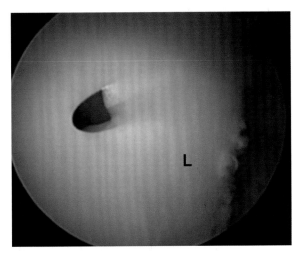

FIGURE 51.2. The labrum *(L)* is completely detached from the acetabular rim using a beaver blade. Care should be taken not to completely cut through the labrum.

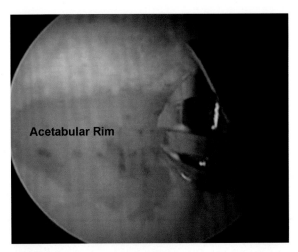

FIGURE 51.3. A motorized burr is used to remove the bony overhang responsible for the pincer deformity.

before complete labral detachment and after detachment, depending on the amount of resection required (Fig. 51.3). That amount should be estimated preoperatively by the analysis of preoperative images. There is a correlation between the center-edge angle and the amount of lateral resection in millimeters. The formula CE angle reduction = 1.8 + (0.64 × rim reduction in millimeters) was obtained in a prospective study and provides a good parameter for the resection (4). The resection should never diminish the center-edge angle to less than 25°. The working portal to perform most of the resection is the lateral portal, although switching portals is essential for the assessment of a complete work.

Femoral Osteoplasty (Cam Resection)

It is important to note that isolated pincer lesions occur in only 10.7% of the cases (5). In most cases, femoral deformities coexist and should be addressed, under risk of failure of the treatment. To approach the peripheral compartment, the traction should be released. As the traction is released and the hip is flexed, we look outside our capsulotomy and enlarge it distally to provide better visualization. In some cases, the zona orbicularis may be very tight and an additional incision starting at the medial aspect of the capsulotomy running distally in the direction of the femoral neck, may be necessary. After inspection of the femoral deformity, the femoral head–neck junction is reshaped. We resect the most prominent part of the deformity and progress until we get visual appraisal of sufficient resection (Fig. 51.4). In some cases, a thin osteotome may be necessary to remove medial osteophytes in the femoral head. The adequacy of the osteoplasty is confirmed by dynamic evaluation of the joint under direct arthroscopic visualization (Fig. 51.5). Any signs of impingement require further bone reshaping or labral contouring. The need of more anchors is commonly noted at this time of the surgery, and we proceed to provide better attachment to

IV. The Hip

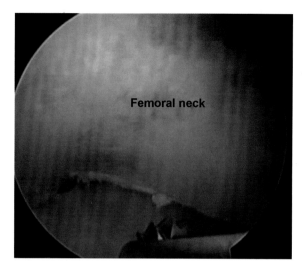

FIGURE 51.4. The femoral neck after resection of the bony prominence.

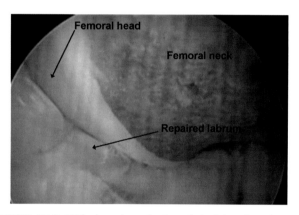

FIGURE 51.5. With dynamic evaluation of the joint, the adequacy of the osteoplasty can be assessed. Any bony prominence that causes displacement or movement of the labrum should be resected.

the labrum. In athletes, we reproduce the sports gesture to disclose any potential conflict between the femur and the labrum. Further resection is performed as deemed. The objective is to obtain maximum range of motion without impingement. Dynamic fluoroscopy may aid to determine adequacy of bone resection, but, in our opinion, it is not a substitute for direct arthroscopic inspection. The capsule is then closed, which we find important to resume rehabilitation and prevent instability and finish the procedure.

Some studies have shown that bone resection in the femur is not sufficient in some cases (6). The main reasons for revision surgery in hip arthroscopy are non-treated or insufficiently corrected bone deformities. Surgical navigation systems are being developed in an attempt to ease cam resection technique and make it more reproducible. In principle, those systems should allow more complete correction of the deformity even for less experienced surgeons. In addition, they should make the procedure safer, avoiding potential risks of excessive resection.

Labral Repair

Upon joint entry, a systematic examination should be performed of the entire acetabular labrum. The fibrocartilaginous labrum is normally adhered to the acetabular rim and transitions to the hyaline articular cartilage in a zone of approximately 1 to 2 mm. The labrum is widest anteriorly and thickest superiorly, corresponding to the weight-bearing region of the acetabulum (7). The labrum has been shown to provide approximately 5 mm of additional femoral head coverage and primarily function as a physiologic joint seal. A torn labrum is thought to alter load transmission in the joint and increase articular cartilage consolidation (5). In our practice, we observe five types of labral tears: detached, midsubstance longitudinal, flap, frayed, and degenerative. A labral tear can be a source of hip pain, but also can cause mechanical symptoms and contribute to hip instability. In the hip, labral tears have been related to joint degeneration. Patients undergoing labral repair had significantly less radiographic evidence of progression of osteoarthritis at 1 and 2 years compared with those who had their labrum resected (8).

Once the labral pathology has been characterized, correction is necessary. Most labral lesions are due to femoroacetabular impingement and these bony deformities need to be corrected to protect the repair. Tear size does not preclude arthroscopic fixation. Mechanical débridement of nonviable tissue is performed using a 4.5-mm full radius shaver. Often a previously unrecognized flap or area of gross delamination becomes more apparent. The quality of the tissue and the nature of the tear are evaluated at this point. Preserving as much of the viable acetabular labrum as possible is important to optimize joint congruence, evenly distribute force contact loads, and prevent further joint degeneration. Equally as important is recognizing an unstable construct for irreparable tissue. Generally, degenerative tears and tears that are of a frayed or flap nature in very thin labrums are not considered to be repairable. In that case, labral reconstruction might be a good option to improve stability in active patients.

Anchors are placed about 2 mm off the acetabular rim in the area of the rim trimming under direct visualization of the entry point and the adjacent articular surface (Fig. 51.6). In general, the anterolateral portal allows the insertion of anchors in the superolateral aspect of the acetabulum, where the most lesions are found. As the guide, a sleeve is directed to the trimmed acetabular margin in a divergent direction to avoid intra-articular penetration, a cranial angle of about 30° to 45° is often observed in the coronal plane. In general, the direction in the transverse plane for placement of anchors at 12-o'clock position (zone 3) in the acetabulum is parallel to the ground. As more anterior placements are necessary, a forward inclination of the guide is performed. The limits for that is usually the position corresponding to 2-o'clock position (considering the right acetabulum) where the insertion angle may be too acute. For the insertion of anterior-most (zone 1) anchors, the

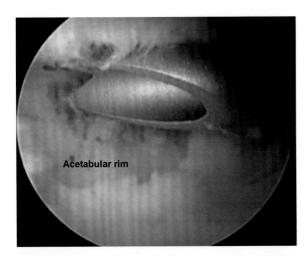

FIGURE 51.6. Anchors for labral repair are placed in the area of acetabular rim trimming. The tips of the sleeve allow you to maintain the perpendicular position during drilling and tapping of the anchor.

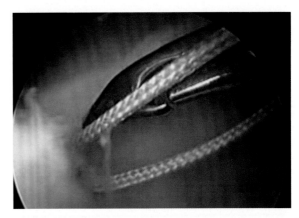

FIGURE 51.8. The arthropierce is used to move the suture under the labram and retrieve it. It can also be used to pass the suture through the labrum, if adequate labral tissue is available.

midanterior lateral portal should be used. Fluoroscopy may be used during the procedure to ensure optimal placement.

We recommend tapping the sleeve slightly into the acetabular rim and drilling the anchor path, manually drive the anchor into place using tactile sensation as guidance (Fig. 51.7). While drilling the path of the anchor, it is critical to visualize the articular surface of the acetabulum to assure that the articular surface is not being compromised. If bulging of the articular surface is noticed, the angle of the anchor must be redirected. The anchor is inserted, and once it is in place, the articular surface should again be visualized to verify that it has not been penetrated. Using an arthropierce, the suture is retrieved over the labrum (Fig. 51.8). As the suture is pulled out through the clear cannula, it is important to visualize the

anchor to assure that the correct suture limb is being retrieved. The cannula must then be pulled back slightly for improved visualization, and the suture is tied down using standard arthroscopic knot-tying techniques.

A translabral suture stitch may be performed in thick labra, on the weight-bearing zone. In that case, one limb of the suture is delivered intra-articularly between the labrum and the acetabular rim. Then the labrum is pierced with the arthropierce in its midsubstance in an outside-in direction and a loop of the intra-articular limb of the suture is pulled through it. The free end of the same suture limb is passed through the loop, retrieving it through the cannula. As both limbs of the suture are tensioned simultaneously, the labrum gets closer to the acetabular rim, allowing a suture free-margin of it to be in contact with the femoral head (Fig. 51.9). The suture is then tied down using standard arthroscopic knot-tying techniques.

Labral Reconstruction

In active young patients and on those with signs of hip instability with irreparable labral lesions, labral reconstruction

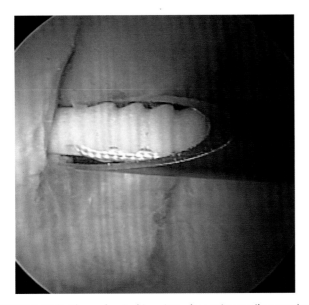

FIGURE 51.7. The anchor is driven into place using tactile sensation as guidance. The anchor is perpendicular to the acetabular rim.

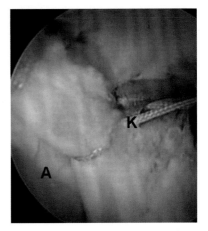

FIGURE 51.9. The suture is tied using standard arthroscopic techniques. The knot (K) is facing away from the acetabular (A) surface.

might be considered. Severely hypothrophic labrum, with complex tears or segmental deficiency are usually impossible to repair. We developed a technique for labral reconstruction using autologous illiotibial band grafts (9).

Debridement of the reminiscent labrum is performed in the area it was considered unhealthy. The objective is to obtain a stable rim for refixation of the new labrum. The need for a bleeding cancellous bed cannot be overemphasized, for the vascular in growth to the free graft must occur from this site. As soon as adequate margins for the labrum anastomosis were achieved and the acetabular rim is prepared, measurement of the gap without labrum is taken. We often use the tip of the 5.5-mm motorized burr to measure the gap (Fig. 51.10). The arthroscope is removed from the joint and traction is released.

With the leg straight and internally rotated, a longitudinal incision comprising the skin and subcutaneous is performed over the great trochanter. The illiotibial tract is exposed and a rectangle of tissue is retrieved. The longitudinal axis of the graft should correspond to 130% to 140% of the intra-articular distance measured, and the transverse axis should be approximately 1.5 in. After clearing the graft from all muscular and fatty tissue, the graft is then tubulized using absorbable sutures. A loop of the suture is left in the proximal end of the graft. The graft is then bathed in platelet-rich plasma. It should provide a tubular structure with about 5 to 7 mm width and enough length to substitute the missing labrum.

The leg is put back into traction, and a suture anchor is placed at the anterior-most part of the labrum defect on the acetabular rim. The limbs of the suture should be inside a 8.25-mm transparent cannula placed on the midanterior lateral portal. The graft is then transfixed at its distal portion with one of the suture limbs. After good fixation of the distal portion is obtained, the portals are switched and an anchor is placed at the lateral-most part of the defect in the acetabular rim (Fig. 51.11). One of

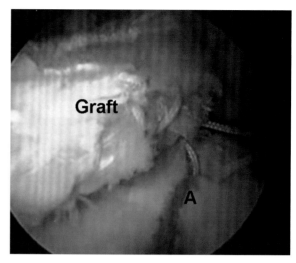

FIGURE 51.11. The anchor is placed on the rim *(A)*, and the graft is sutured down into place along the acetabular rim.

the limbs of the suture is passed through the suture loop in the proximal (posterior) end of the graft. The graft is then pushed into position by a sliding knot, and additional loop suture around the labrum is performed to grant its attachment. Further anchors should be placed in the midportion of the defect in order to provide adequate fixation and anatomical contour to the labrum as in the technique for labral refixation. Attention to the anastomosis must be taken so that no redundant tissue causes conflict with the joint (Fig. 51.12).

Management of Chondral Lesions

Chondral lesions may be cartilage softening, fraying or fissuring, subchondral cysts, chondral flaps, and total thickness abrasion with subchondral bone exposure. Peripheral chondral lesions, usually related to pincer deformities, often disappear after the resection of the underlying pathologic bone. The remaining chondral edge needs then to be

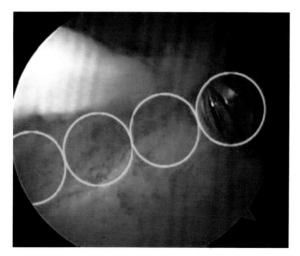

FIGURE 51.10. A 5.5-mm motorized burr is used to measure the area of labral deficiency.

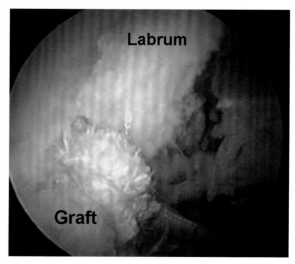

FIGURE 51.12. Attention to the anastomosis must be taken so that no redundant tissue causes conflict with the joint.

stabilized. Cam deformities are often related to more extensive articular damage. Chondral flaps usually demand debridement, and the remaining defect is usually still present after treatment of the bone deformities. When the full-thickness cartilage defect is focal and articular space is greater than 2 mm, good results can be expected with the microfracture technique. Once the chondral defect is identified, the extent of the lesion is noted. Debridement of all remaining unstable cartilage from the exposed bone is completed using a full-radius resector and curettes. A ring curette is particularly useful for preparation of the defect and creating a smooth, perpendicular border. Particular attention must be paid while debriding the surrounding rim of the defect (Fig. 51.13). Debridement should be deep enough to remove the calcified cartilage layer while maintaining the integrity of the subchondral plate. For defects of the femoral head, a chondral border is necessary to contain the clot. The edges of the lesion should be perpendicular to the adjacent, unaffected cartilage to allow for the marrow clot to form more effectively. Arthroscopic awls are used to make multiple holes (microfractures) in the exposed subchondral plate (Fig. 51.14). Place as many holes as possible, leaving about 3 to 4 mm between each. A depth of approximately 2 to 4 mm is usually enough to visualize fat droplets and blood from the holes.

Management of the Ligamentum Teres (Debridement and Reconstruction)

Lesions of the ligamentum teres are still of unclear significance and are often described in association with other conditions. Three types of tears have been described: complete tears associated with dislocation, partial tears associated with a subacute event, and degenerative tears associated with joint pathology (10). Associated pathology includes avulsed bone or cartilage fragments and labral tears. Patients describe nonspecific symptoms of catching,

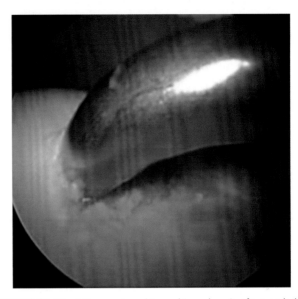

FIGURE 51.14. Arthroscopic awl is used to make microfracture holes starting at the edge of the defect.

popping, locking, or giving. Exam findings are also nonspecific, although the hip joint should be definitively identified as the source of symptoms. Patients should have pain with hip logroll and may obtain relief with an intra-articular injection.

The surgical treatment of lesions of the ligamentum teres is arthroscopic. A dynamic test for the integrity of the ligamentum is performed by having the limb rotated internally, when the ligamentum is loose and then externally with the ligamentum taut. The techniques currently used for the ligamentum teres include repair, debridement, and shrinkage. The ligamentum is approached through the anterolateral portal. Debridement of frayed, loose fibers in partially ruptured ligaments (Fig. 51.15) and of the stump in the presence of complete rupture relieves mechanical symptoms and is best performed with the hip in external

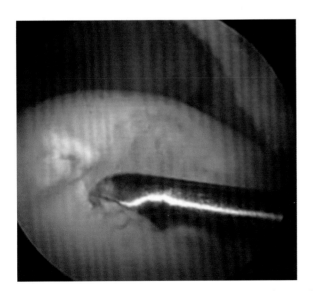

FIGURE 51.13. An curette is used to removed loose cartilage and prepare a stable surrounding rim of the defect to hold the clot.

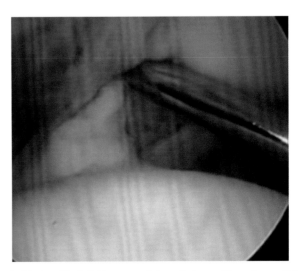

FIGURE 51.15. Debridement of frayed, loose fibers in partially ruptured ligamentum teres.

rotation, which tenses the ligamentum and delivers it anteriorly. In cases where the ruptured ligament has two distinct ends with adequate length left after debridement, a repair can be performed. The repair must be tested with motion to make sure there is enough ligament after repair to allow for full motion.

A long, thin, flexible radiofrequency ablation probe, whose tip is deflectable by up to 100°, is used to perform thermal modification. The radiofrequency probe is used to shrink the intact portion of the ligament in case of partial rupture. Shrinkage is performed with hip at neutral rotation and should not be excessive, for it could lead to restricted external rotation of the hip.

Reconstruction of the ligament teres using an autograft of fascia lata has been reported and may be an option in the treatment of complete tears in patients presenting with instability as the main symptom. Although the clinical indications and results are yet to be published, the senior author has seen promising results when the technique is used on the right patient. The reconstruction technique involves the harvest of graft from the IT band (such as in the labral reconstruction technique). Allograft may also be used. The objective is to obtain the most anatomical reconstruction. With cannulated reams, a tunnel from the lateral cortex is perforated to fovea in the femoral head. Anchors are placed at the base of the acetabular fossa, next to the acetabular notch. The graft fixed in the acetabulum with anchor and then pulled back into the tunnel into the joint through the tunnel (Fig. 51.16). Proper tensioning of the graft is obtained in maximal external rotation. The graft is then fixed in the femur with interference screws.

Management of Hip Instability (Capsular Plication and Thermal Capsulorraphy)

Hip instability is a syndrome characterized by symptoms of discomfort, giving away, popping sounds (snapping), pain, and overphysiologic hip motion in one or more directions. It can be also be defined as abnormal symptomatic motion of the hip joint that results in pain, subluxation, or dislocation (11). This syndrome may occur as consequence of failure of one or more of those stabilizing elements, but also may be a cause for intra-articular lesions. Often the capsule is elongated either primarily or as a consequence of instability due to other lesions such as labral tears. The following strategy may be used whichever cause of capsular laxity (12).

The capsule is probed in the regions of the iliofemoral and ischiofemoral ligaments and areas of redundancy are noted. A flexible monopolar TAC-S radiofrequency energy probe is used. Temperature and power settings are closely monitored at 67°C and 40 W. The probe is then moved across the redundant tissue, with minimal contact, in a striped pattern. To encourage healing in the treated tissue, sufficient healthy tissue should be left between the stripes. As the probe is moved across the tissue, the color and shrinkage of the capsular tissue is visually monitored.

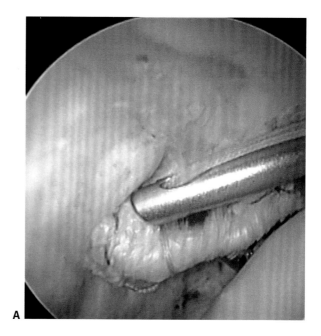

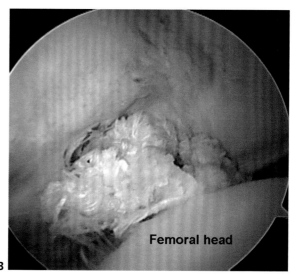

FIGURE 51.16. A: One end of the graft is secured to the cotyloid fossa with a suture anchor. **B:** The graft is then pulled back through the tunnel in the femoral head.

Overheating of the tissue must be avoided. Following focal thermal capsulorraphy, capsular plication may be performed as needed to further reduce capsular volume. Sutures are placed through the tissue and tied to reduce the capsule volume. Plication sutures are placed between the lateral arm of the iliofemoral ligament and the ischiofemoral ligament.

EXTRA-ARTICULAR PROCEDURES

Internal Snapping Hip (Transarticular Release of the Iliopsoas Tendon)

There are three types of coxa saltans or snapping hip: intra-articular snapping caused by several conditions, including loose bodies and labral pathology; internal snapping caused by the iliopsoas tendon moving over a bony prominence; and external snapping from the iliotibial (IT) band or gluteus maximus tendon snapping over the greater trochanter (13). Internal snapping of the iliopsoas tendon over the iliopectineal eminence, femoral head, or lesser trochanter may or may not be painful. Pain or discomfort associated with internal snapping is an indication of associated iliopsoas tendonitis, either as a result of acute inflammation or more chronic degeneration and tendinopathy (13). Initial management of painful iliopsoas tendonitis consists of NSAIDs and physical therapy. If pain persists, an ultrasound-guided injection with lidocaine and corticosteroid can provide relief and predict the response to surgical release. For patients who have recurrent pain after local injection, arthroscopic release at the musculotendinous junction or near the tendon insertion on the lesser trocanter have been described with good results (13).

Our current approach involves the tenotomy of the iliopsoas tendon by an intra-articular approach as described by Wettstein (14). In this approach, the tendon is visualized through an anterior capsulotomy during arthroscopy (Fig. 51.17). At this point, there is usually some muscle tissue attached to the tendon. We selectively divide the tendinous portion using an arthroscopic blade (beaver blade), leaving the muscle intact. The tenotomy can be considered complete, but some continuity between the muscle and its insertion is maintained. While this often prevents postoperative weakness, a chance for undercorrection or recurrence may be greater.

Lateral Trocantheric Syndrome (Hip Abductors Repair)

Pain at the hip trochanteric and gluteus are often blamed on bursitis. Hip abductors tendinopathy is a frequent cause of greater trochanteric pain syndrome and many cases diagnosed as bursitis are probably related to tendon lesions (15).

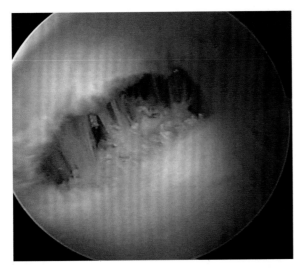

FIGURE 51.17. The iliopsoas tendon is visualized through an anterior capsulotomy during arthroscopy.

We have performed cases of arthroscopic repair of hip rotator cuff tendon lesions (16). We often perform formal hip arthroscopy to rule out and treat concomitant intra-articular problems, following our standard technique.

The hip is then abducted to about 15° and subcutaneous plane is dissected just above the fascia lata. A cruciform incision is then performed just above the trocanter, in order to decompress the underlying tissue. All the redundant bursa is debrided. The insertion of the gluteus medius and minimus tendons is identified and the tear/detachment is diagnosed. Debridement of the scar tissue over the trocanter is performed so that bleeding bone is exposed at the tendons original footprint for reinsertion. Metallic anchors are placed on those spots at an angle of at least 45° to the action line of the muscle (to prevent its avulsion). Mattress sutures are used to reattach the conjoined tendon to its original site.

Piriformis Syndrome (Arthroscopic Technique)

Piriformis syndrome is a compressive condition of the sciatic nerve by the piriformis muscle that was described by Robinson (17). The six classical findings include (1) a history of trauma to the sacroiliac and gluteal regions; (2) pain in the region of the sacroiliac joint, greater sciatic notch, and piriformis muscle that usually extends down the limb and causes difficulty with walking; (3) acute exacerbation of pain caused by stooping or lifting (and moderate relief of pain by traction on the affected extremity with the patient in the supine position); (4) a palpable sausage-shaped mass, tender to palpation, over the piriformis muscle on the affected side; (5) a positive Lasègue sign; and (6) gluteal atrophy, depending on the duration of the condition. The classical physical examination maneuver is known as Pace's sign and consists of radiated pain and weakness in association with resisted abduction and external rotation of the affected thigh. The piriformis syndrome may occur due to anatomical anomalies, trauma, and tumors. Early diagnosis can avoid prolonging ineffective empiric treatment and disability with satisfactory results achieved in most patients by conservative treatment (18,19). Patients who have a typical history and findings on physical examination with intractable pain after failure of nonoperative treatment, release of the piriformis tendon and sciatic neurolysis can give predictably good results with few complications.

CONCLUSIONS

Hip arthroscopy has been established as a safe and effective procedure to treat many condition affecting intra- and extra-articular structures. As experience in the clinical setting is gained and innovative research are published, alternatives are included in the surgeons' portfolio. Surgeons dedicated to learn and practice this minimally invasive method should take continued education for the innovations in practice are currently the rule in this specialty.

IV. The Hip

REFERENCES

1. Ganz R, Parvizi J, Beck M, et al. Femoroacetabular impingement: a cause for osteoarthritis of the hip. *Clin Orthop Relat Res.* 2003;417:112–120.

2. Kelly BT, Williams RJ III, Philippon MJ. Hip arthroscopy: current indications, treatment options, and management issues. *Am J Sports Med.* 2003;31:1020–1037.

3. Philippon MJ, Weiss DR, Kuppersmith DA, et al. Arthroscopic labral repair and treatment of femoroacetabular impingement in professional hockey players. *Am J Sports Med.* 2010;38:99–104.

4. Philippon MJ, Wolff AB, Briggs KK, et al. Acetabular rim reduction for the treatment of femoroacetabular impingement correlates with preoperative and postoperative center-edge Angle. *Arthroscopy.* 2010;26:757–761.

5. Beck M, Kalhor M, Leunig M, et al. Hip morphology influences the pattern of damage to the acetabular cartilage: femoroacetabular impingement as a cause of early osteoarthritis of the hip. *J Bone Joint Surg Br.* 2005;87:1012–1018.

6. Mardones RM, Gonzalez C, Chen Q, et al. Surgical treatment of femoroacetabular impingement: evaluation of the size of the resection. *J Bone Joint Surg Am.* 2005;87:273–279.

7. Tan V, Seldes RM, Katz MA, et al. Contribution of acetabular labrum to articulating surface area and femoral head coverage in adult hip joints: an anatomic study in cadavera. *Am J Orthop.* 2001;30:809–812.

8. Espinosa N, Rothenfluh DA, Beck M, et al. Treatment of femoroacetabular impingement: preliminary results of labral refixation. *J Bone Joint Surg Am.* 2006;88:925–935.

9. Philippon MJ, Briggs KK, Hay CJ, et al. Arthroscopic labral reconstruction in the hip using iliotibial band autograft: technique and early outcomes. *Arthroscopy.* 2010;26:750–756.

10. Rao J, Zhou YX, Villar RN. Injury to the ligamentum teres: mechanism, findings, and results of treatment. *Clin Sports Med.* 2001;20:791–799.

11. Bellabarba C, Sheinkop MB, Kuo KN. Idiopathic hip instability. an unrecognized cause of coxa saltans in the adult. *Clin Orthop Relat Res.* 1998;355:261–271.

12. Philippon MJ. New frontiers in hip arthroscopy: the role of arthroscopic hip labral repair and capsulorrhaphy in the treatment of hip disorders. *Instr Course Lect.* 2006;55:309–316.

13. Blankenbaker DG, DeSmet AA, Keene JS. Sonography of the iliopsoas tendon and injection of the iliopsoas bursa for diagnosis and management of the painful snapping hip. *Skeletal Radiol.* 2006;3:565–571.

14. Wettstein M, Jung J, Dienst M. Arthroscopic psoas tenotomy. *Arthroscopy.* 2006;22:907.e1–907.e4.

15. Kingzett-Taylor, Tirman PF, Feller J, et al. Tendinosis and tears of gluteus medius and minimus muscles as a cause of hip pain: MR imaging findings. *AJR AM J Roentgenol.* 1999;173:1123–1126.

16. Bunker TD, Esler CNA, Leach WJ. Rotator-cuff tear of the hip. *J Bone Joint Surg Br.* 1997;79:618–620.

17. Robinson, DR. Pyriformis syndrome in relation to sciatic pain. *Am J Surg.* 1947;73:355–358.

18. Benson ER, Schutzer SF. Posttraumatic piriformis syndrome: diagnosis and results of operative treatment. *J Bone Joint Surg Am.* 1999;81:941–949.

19. Foster MR. Piriformis syndrome [Comment in: *Orthopedics.* 2004;27:797–799; author reply 799].*Orthopedics.* 2002;25:821–825.

Miscellaneous Problems: Synovitis, Degenerative Joint Disease, and Tumors; Miscellaneous Conditions: Ligamentum Teres, Synovial Disease, Degenerative Joint Disease, Tumors

Thomas G. Sampson

LIGAMENTUM TERES

The ligamentum teres is located deep within the central compartment of the hip and is amenable to arthroscopic inspection. Injury to the ligament and many of the pathologic conditions involving it are associated with developmental dysplasia of the hip. Fortunately, dysplastic hips are more flexible, making it easier to distract the hip and diagnose and treat injuries and pathologies of the ligamentum teres. Patients usually present with groin pain and a limp or clicking.

Gray and Villar (1) classified pathology of the ligamentum teres using arthroscopic surgery. After looking at 472 consecutive hip arthroscopies, they identified 20 patients with ligamentum teres tears pathology. They placed them in three categories: Group 1, complete ligamentum teres rupture; group 2, partial tear of the ligamentum teres; and group 3, degenerative ligamentum teres (Fig. 52.1). All were treated with debridement. There were a few case reports of either tears or avulsion fractures involving the ligamentum teres (2, 3); however, Byrd prospectively looked at 23 patients with ligamentum teres tears and found 7 occurred from violent injuries, such as motor vehicle accidents, 3 from a fall from a height, 3 from football injuries, 1 from snow skiing, 1 from ice hockey and included 6 dislocations. The remaining 8 patients sustained twisting injury. He found a lengthy duration before diagnosis and surgery with an average of 28.5 months. All of his patients experienced groin pain, and 19 of them experienced catching, popping, locking, or giving way, as well as pain with activities. He used a variety of diagnostic

tests such as MRI, CT scan, and radionuclide bone scans. The indication for surgery was intractable hip pain.

Simpson and Villar (4) described a method for ligateres reconstruction in a 20-year-old using an artificial graft and Endo button. It appears that they are very rare indications, such as persistent hip pain and instability between the head and the acetabulum.

SYNOVIAL DISEASE

Synovitis of the hip has many causes. Five of the pathologic entities causing primary synovitis are (1) rheumatoid arthritis (RA) (2), calcium pyrophosphate dihydrate (CPPD) crystal deposition disease (3), fatty deposition disease (hyperlipoproteinemia) (4), hemochromatosis, and (5) pyarthrosis.

The role of arthroscopic synovectomy in treating synovial diseases was apparent to the earliest arthroscopists. In almost all pathology of the hip, synovitis is present. We had several undiagnosed cases of hip pain with effusions that were shown to be seronegative rheumatioid arthritis with synovial biopsy. In 1988, Ide et al. (5) performed arthroscopic synovectomy for RA on six hips in three patients using mechanical shavers through a two-portal technique with good results. With the advent of laser and radiofrequency (RF) ablation, there are now three modalities used to debride the synovium. It remains difficult to reach 100% of the joint. However, with newer, more effective medical management, debulking of the diseased synovium seems to be adequate.

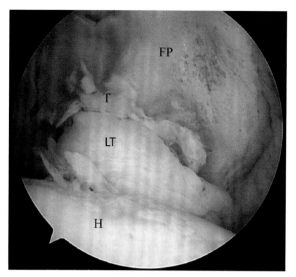

FIGURE 52.1. Degenerative tear ligamentum teres in a 48-year-old female with mild hip dysplasia. LT (ligamentum teres), T (tear), H (head), FP (fat pad).

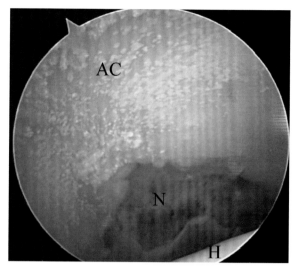

FIGURE 52.3. Lipid deposition on the articular cartilage of the acetabulum *(arrow)*, AC (acetabular cartilage), N (notch), H (femoral head.)

CPPD crystal deposition disease has not been reported as frequently in the hip as it has in the ligamentum flavum and in the knee associated with RA (6, 7). We have performed synovectomy on two patients for CPPD associated with femoroacetabular impingement (FAI). Clearly, it is an entity that should be considered in the differential diagnosis of patients with refractory synovitis (Fig. 52.2 A–B).

There are no reports in the arthroscopic literature on the treatment of hyperlipoproteinemia, hemochromatosis, or any of the metabolic arthropathies. We have performed partial synovectomy in a few patients thought to have fatty deposition and in one patient with hemochromatosis associated with arthritis (Fig. 52.3). It is presented here only to make the arthroscopic surgeon aware that metabolic arthropathies exist (8). Metabolic arthropathy appears as white or yellowish plaques on the articular cartilage associated with a mild synovitic reaction. The plaque cannot be removed without destroying the articular cartilage and therefore should be treated with synovectomy only.

Arthroscopic debridement and lavage has become the treatment of choice for septic arthritis in children, adolescents, and adults. This modality has been associated with minimal morbidity and an excellent cure rate (9–12). McCarthy et al. (13) reported on successful treatment of septic total hips in two patients using arthroscopic debridement, lavage, and intravenous antibiotics. We have successfully treated arthroscopically four patients with late hematogenous infections of their total hips. No recurrence has been noted, with the longest follow-up being

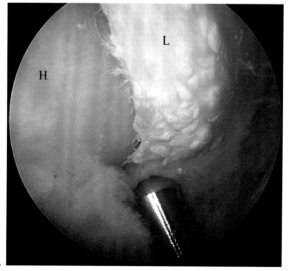

A

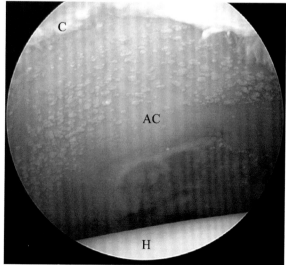

B

FIGURE 52.2. A: Calcified right anterior labrum of the hip seen from the anterolateral portal. L (labrum), H (femoral head); **B:** Calcifications of the acetabular cartilage. AC (acetabular cartilage), C (calcifications).

20 years when one patient passed away owing to natural causes at the age of 93 years.

DEGENERATIVE JOINT DISEASE

The arthroscopic treatment of degenerative joint disease (DJD) of the hip remains controversial, challenging, and difficult. Even the most experienced hip arthroscopists avoid the procedure because there are few benchmarks to predict a successful outcome. Prior to 2001, DJD was treated with arthroscopic debridement, labrectomy, synovectomy, and abrasion chondroplasty. In 28 of 290 patients who had partial labrectomies with DJD, only 21% had a good result compared with a 71% good result rate in those without DJD (14). Subsequently, with the recognition of FAI and the added correction of the abnormal morphology, the modified Harris Hip Score improved

significantly from 72 to 92 with an average of 4 years follow-up (15–17).

A residual head–neck deformity from femoral neck fractures has been a cause of FAI and DJD. Reshaping of the deformity has been done using an open surgical dislocation by Eijer et al. (18). We have treated the DJD and deformity with an arthroscopic head–neck osteoplasty and debridement, synovectomy, and abrasion chondroplasty with microfracture in three patients (Fig. 52.4 A–F).

TUMORS

Essentially all tumors that are amenable to arthroscopic treatment are benign. Pigmented villonodular synovitis (PVNS) and synovial chondromatosis may be considered synovial diseases instead of tumors, and are both difficult

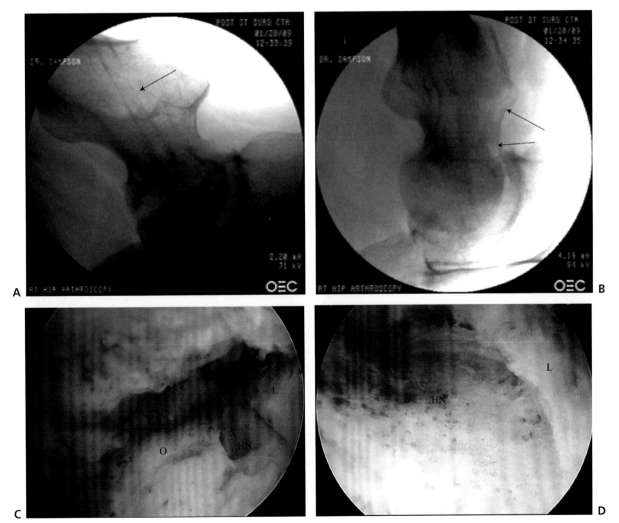

FIGURE 52.4. Osteoplasty femoral head–neck for postcervical neck fracture causing impingement and arthritis **A:** A-P and **B:** Abduction Internal Rotational lateral Radiographs, note the residual markings from the hardware bone changes, and head–neck deformity (*arrows*), **C:** Arthroscopic view anterolateral portal *(O)* osteophyte and synovitis, *(L)* labrum; **D:** After synovectomy and osteoplasty;

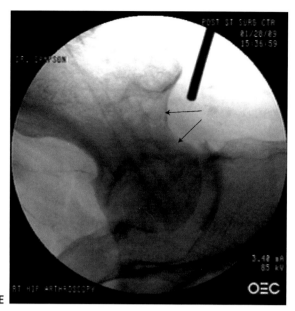
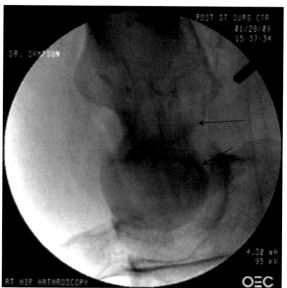

FIGURE 52.4. *(continued)* **E:** A-P and **F:** Lateral after osteoplasty.

to eradicate unless a complete synovectomy can be performed (Fig. 52.5 A–B).

Most recurrences are more often than not from either inadequate removal of the tumors or inadequate synovectomy (19–21). We advocate capsulotomy to expose *all* areas and recesses of both the central and the peripheral compartments to remove the loose and attached bodies and ablate the synovium, particularly where the lesions are forming.

Arthroscopic removal of osteoid osteoma of the hip has been described by Glick et al. in two cases in the central compartment (22). We have since removed an old,

yet active osteoid osteoma from the head–neck junction associated with a cam impingement requiring excision, synovectomy, and head–neck osteoplasty.

Heterotopic bone should be considered a pseudotumor of the hip and is most often a complication of trauma or hip surgery. There are no reports of its treatment using arthroscopic techniques; however, we favor arthroscopic excision and follow surgery with either a single dose of 700 rads of radiation or a strong dose of NSAIDs for 6 weeks. Our recurrence rate is lower with the subsequent radiation (Fig. 52.6 A–C).

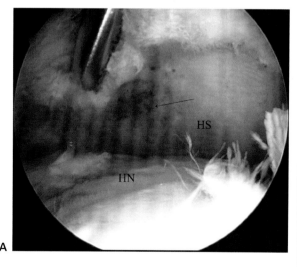
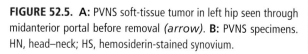
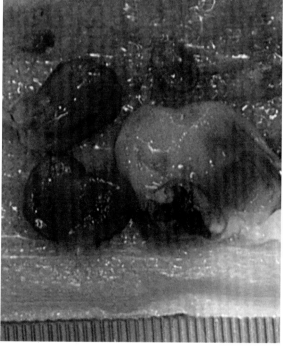

FIGURE 52.5. A: PVNS soft-tissue tumor in left hip seen through midanterior portal before removal *(arrow).* **B:** PVNS specimens. HN, head–neck; HS, hemosiderin-stained synovium.

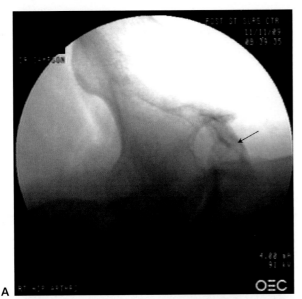

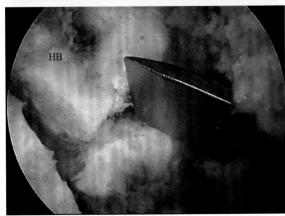

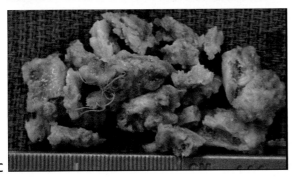

FIGURE 52.6. **A:** A-P Radiogragh of heterotopic bone right hip (*arrow*); **B:** Heterotopic bone right hip viewed through anterolateral portal being cut by an osteotome, HB (heterotopic bone) **C:** H.O. specimens after removal.

ANATOMY AND PHYSICAL EXAMINATION

Synovitis of the hip may present with pain in the groin, buttock, and trochanter. The hallmarks of the presentation and examination are associated with an irritable hip. Much like an acute abdomen that is stiff and exquisitely painful on palpation and jarring, the irritable hip is very painful on palpation and rotational movements. Synovitic hips will have pain either with all ranges of motion, or at

the extremes of motion when tested passively. Septic hips may vary on the level of pain, depending on the organism type and the tenseness of the effusion.

DJD presents with or without a limp, and difficulty walking, sitting, and putting on shoes and socks owing to restricted range of motion. With the loss of articular cartilage, a straight leg raising with the knee extended may cause pain in the groin because of the compressive forces of the opposing chondromalacic surfaces of the head and acetabulum. There may be popping and catching with rotation. Loss of internal rotation is almost always present. The Trendelenberg sign and test may be negative in milder cases. We have found if there is at least 50% range of rotational movement when tested passively compared with the normal contralateral side, and if greater than 50% of articular cartilage thickness on the AP x-ray is present, our results show a better than 80% chance of significant improvement that is durable for more than 2 years (Fig. 52.7). Radiographs showing joint space narrowing greater than 50% compared with the opposite "normal hip" are predictive of a poorer outcome, in our opinion.

Tumors present with pain and in many cases popping and catching. There may be a limp if there is an effusion. Range of motion may be restricted if catching or locking is present. Most may present with entirely normal movement. Osteoid osteomas usually cause night pain that is relieved by aspirin and other NSAIDs (22, 23).

PREOPERATIVE IMAGING AND PLANNING

Routine radiographs are mandatory for preliminary imaging of the hip in all cases of hip symptoms. This should include an AP view of the pelvis including both hips from the top of the iliac crest to below the lesser trochanters and frog-leg and cross-table lateral views. On the AP view, the tip of the coccyx should be 1 to 2 cm from the pubic symphysis to eliminate pelvic tilt. MRI and magnetic resonance arthrography with gadolinium should be done as an adjunct to the x-rays if clinically indicated.

The findings of synovitis on x-ray may be normal in the early stages to subtle erosions and cystic formation. On MRI, the findings in RA may include subchondral erosions and hypertrophic synovium (24). DJD is easily detectable on both x-rays and MRI with osteophyte formation and joint space narrowing. Since FAI may be the etiology in many osteoarthritic hips, a metaplastic bump on the head–neck junction and a rim overgrowth or prominence may be seen. In many cases, a fibro-osseous cyst of varying size appears on the neck, typically within the bump. The MRI shows capsular thickening, chondral erosions, and usually some cysts.

PVNS may only be detected on the MRI in the early stages and in late stages with periarticular erosion, effusion, and MR characteristics of hemosiderin deposition in the synovium. In these cases, it is important to thoroughly examine the entire hip, including the peripheral compartment, to assure as thorough a resection as possible.

IV. The Hip

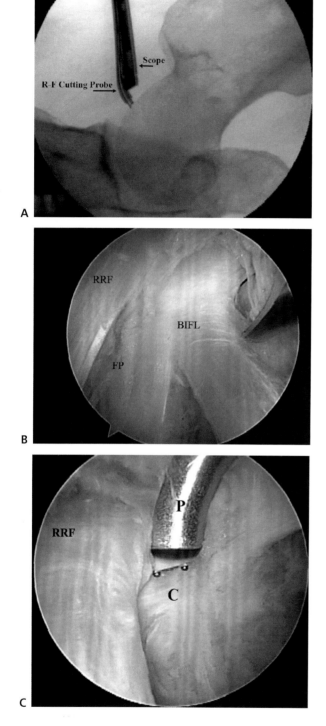

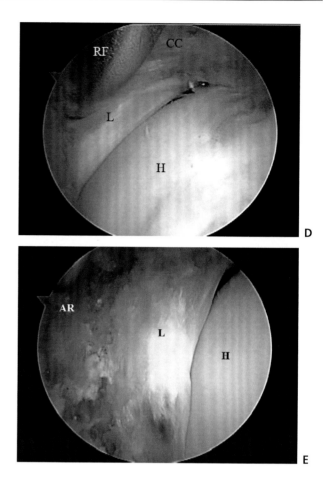

FIGURE 52.7. A: C-arm fluoroscopic view of the arthroscope and RF probe over the anterolateral capsule of a left hip before capsulotomy. **B:** Arthroscopic view external to the left anterolateral hip capsule. Note the reflected head of the rectus femoris (RRF), the fat pad over the capsule (FP), and the band of the iliofemoral ligament (BIFL). **C:** Arthroscopic view external to the left anterolateral hip capsule with the RF probe in place that matches the fluoroscopic view in (**A**) before capsulotomy. Note the reflected head rectus femoris (RRF), the capsule *(C)*, and the RF probe *(P)*. **D:** Arthroscopic view of the cut capsule (CC) with the RF probe (RF) retracting the capsule before incising it over the labrum *(L)*. Note the femoral head *(H)*. **E:** Arthroscopic view of the completed capsulotomy exposing the femoral head *(H)*, labrum *(L)*, and acetabular rim *(AR)*, much like seen in an arthrotomy.

Synovial chondromatosis presents as either cartilage type or osteocartilage type with the latter visualized on plain radiographs. MR shows the loose bodies from small uniform-sized areas attached to the synovium, to large detached multiple bodies. In some cases, large aggregates and masses are also noted.

In all cases, radiographs and MRI identify the diagnosis and the location(s) of the lesions to be addressed arthroscopically. The standard techniques of hip arthroscopy are used to confirm the diagnosis. We advise the use of a wide capsulotomy to expose the lesions. This allows for easier access of the instruments and facilitated removal of masses and loose bodies. The capsulotomy may be done either from the central compartment by connecting the portals with an arthroscopic knife, or can be done by an extracapsular method as will be described. All peripheral compartment surgery may be done without distraction.

ANESTHESIA CONSIDERATIONS

Most hip arthroscopy is done in an outpatient setting. It is difficult to predict the operative time in many of these cases, especially those with DJD and loose bodies from synovial chondromatosis. We perform the procedure with the patient in the lateral decubitus position. Awake patients under regional anesthesia may become uncomfortable lying on their side for the duration of the procedure. For this reason, as well as for relaxation and the need for paralysis, we recommend a general anesthetic.

POSITIONING

Either the supine or the lateral position may be used to treat these conditions. The preference and skill of the hip arthroscopist will determine which to use. There are multiple series documenting good outcomes with both techniques.

PORTALS

In most arthroscopic procedures for the treatment for synovitis, DJD, and tumors, the standard three portals (anterior, anterolateral, and posterolateral) are used. When more peripheral areas need to be reached, the addition of an anterior and distal portal between 5 and 8 cm from the anterior portal is useful.

PROCEDURE AND TECHNIQUE

The patient is placed in the supine or lateral decubitus position and the appropriate distractor is applied to the affected leg. A C-arm fluoroscope is brought in, and before prepping the patient, a series of four views are taken and recorded. These include AP views in neutral, internal, and external rotation as well as an AP 90° view to show the shape and interaction between the head–neck junction and the acetabulum and to appreciate any loose bodies and their change in position.

Under fluoroscopic control, the long needle is placed through the anterolateral portal directed toward the capsular area at the head–neck junction. There should be about 1 cm clearance with the greater trochanter. A Nitinol wire is placed through the needle and the skin is incised with a no. 11 blade. The arthroscope trochar sheath assembly is pushed over the wire, and the sheath is used to sweep the muscle away from the capsule. We start with a 30° arthroscope. The pump is started at 50 mm Hg pressure on low flow, allowing a view of the fat pad over the anterior hip capsule. The anterior portal is established with the same technique, and a 4-mm switching stick is used to sweep the capsule and palpate the reflected head of the rectus femoris. The key to this approach is identifying the rectus femoris, as the capsule directly beneath covers the anterolateral portion of the labrum (Fig. 52.7 A–E).

A 4-mm shaver is introduced and the fat is removed to expose the capsule. The capsulotomy is done with an RF probe beginning at the base of the neck, toward the labrum. Capsular thickening is common and in our experience may vary from a few millimeters to 2 cm. By lifting the capsule with the probe before cutting when near the articular cartilage and labrum, exposure may be done without damaging those structures. The capsulotomy is carried up and over the labrum and along the anterior and lateral acetabular rim between the labrum and the bone.

Synovitis, loose bodies, degenerative tissue, and both normal and abnormal anatomy of the head–neck region are visualized similar to an open procedure with the addition of magnification.

Once the peripheral pathology has been identified, the hip is then distracted to enter the central compartment. It may be necessary to create a posterolateral portal to work in all areas of the central compartment. The central compartment is then inspected for pathology in a methodical manner, first through the anterolateral portal using a probe from the anterior or posterolateral portals. Moving the scope to the other portals is necessary for a complete assessment of the joint.

If loose bodies are present, they are removed with a shaver and graspers. Occasionally, the fat pad hides notch bodies or is fibrotic, and is removed with the shaver. If the notch is filled with a mat of chondromata, the mass is removed with a combination of curettes, picks, and shavers. If the notch has encroaching osteophytes, we favor osteophytectomy using a long 4-mm hip burr, curettes, and picks to restore the contact forces between the head and the acetabular cartilage (25).

The rim of the acetabulum may have an anterolateral osteophytic ridge. The osteophyte is exposed behind the labrum and removed with a 4-mm hip burr. If cysts are encountered, they are curetted and saucerized with the burr.

Labral degeneration, tears, or destruction by synovitis are treated with partial labrectomy with the shaver and/ or an RF wand. In some cases, a labral repair or refixation is done. This is accomplished by abrading the base of the anticipated acetabular attachment with a 4-mm burr, followed by drilling for the anchor of choice and finally inserting the anchor. The suture is either wrapped around the labrum or sewn through with a suture passer or suture relay technique. Finally, the labrum is tied down securing it. We like to place anchors 1 cm apart, which will determine the number of anchors used.

Erosions of the articular cartilage of the head and acetabulum require excision of the delaminated tissue to stable cartilage with a shaver or curette, abrasion, and removal of the calcific layer and microfracture using awls. Most areas can be reached on the acetabular surface except for zone 6 near the transverse ligament; however, on the femoral head, we have difficulty applying instruments to zones 2m, 3m, 4m, and 6 (26).

In the peripheral compartment, the capsulotomy makes it much easier to find and remove loose bodies. The search should be performed circumferentially around the head and neck, beneath the lateral and medial synovial folds, near the transverse ligament, and the distal capsular reflection near the lesser trochanter. Once the loose bodies or PVNS lesions are removed, we recommend a synovectomy using 4-mm straight and curved shavers and RF wands. A flexible wand may be needed to reach all the areas. By doing as complete a synovectomy as possible, the recurrence rate of the disease will be reduced.

Lastly, in the case of DJD, the femoral head–neck junction may need to be reshaped in the same way it is done with FAI, and the neck may have barnacle-like osteophytes that are removed with a shaver, burr, and curettes (Fig. 52.8 A–F).

If the hip is arthritic and stiff, a generous capsulectomy is done with the 5-mm shaver, arthroscopic knife, and/or RF probe. In all other situations, we leave the capsule open, as it will heal in most cases.

The treatment of septic arthritis involves entering the central compartment first with distraction through an anterolateral portal and placing a shaver through the posterolateral portal to debride, lavage, and perform a synovectomy. The peripheral compartment may be reached by

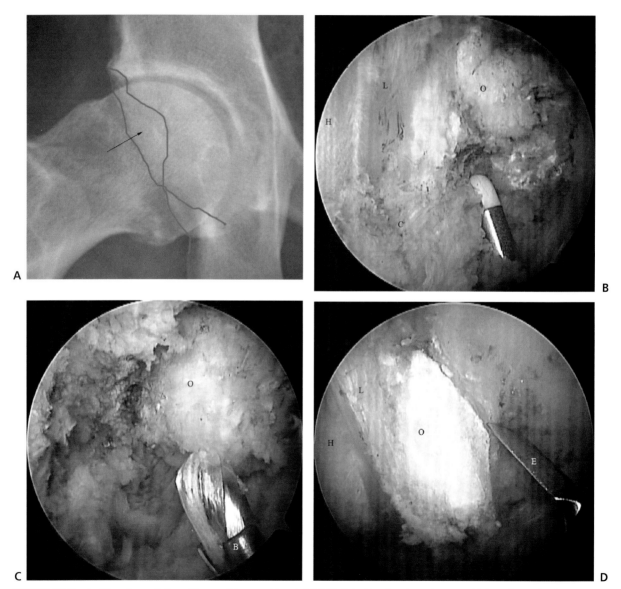

FIGURE 52.8. A: AP radiograph in a 46-year-old man with painful DJD right hip showing a large multishaped anterior impingement osteophyte (*arrow*). **B:** Arthroscopic view of the multishaped anterior rim osteophyte *(O)* with the soft tissue being dissected away by the RF wand. Note the head *(H)*, labrum *(L)* and capsule *(C)*. **C:** Arthroscopic view of the osteophyte *(O)* being excised by the 5-mm burr *(B)*. **D:** Arthroscopic view of a elevator *(E)* separating the remaining osteophyte *(O)* away from the rim.

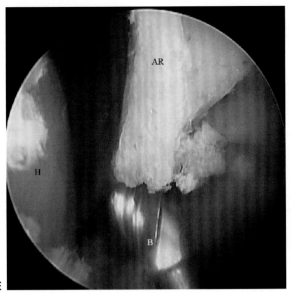
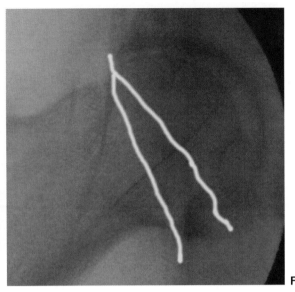

FIGURE 52.8. *(continued)* **E:** Arthroscopic view of acetabular rim *(AR)* trimming with the 5-mm burr *(B).* **F:** Postoperative fluororadiograph showing the correction and removal of the anterior rim osteophyte.

releasing traction and flexing the hip to create the space, or by the method of capsulotomy previously described. We recommend lavaging the hip with more than 3 L of saline. Drains are placed through a slotted cannula and sewn into the skin. Broad-spectrum intravenous antibiotics are started after adequate cultures are taken. The antibiotic is later changed based on the results of the culture and sensitivity. Consideration should always be given to the involvement of an Infectious Disease consultant.

POSTOPERATIVE CARE

After wound closure, 30 cc of *Ropivacaine* is administered to all patients. An NSAID such as ibuprofen, celecoxib, or diclofenac is prescribed to reduce the potential for heterotopic bone formation. On the day of surgery, weight bearing on two crutches is begun as tolerated and progressed to one crutch or a cane. When the patient is experiencing little pain on weight bearing, has no sensation of giving way, and has good hip stabilization, use of the crutches or cane can be discontinued. Beginning 1 day after surgery or when tolerated, the patient is encouraged to ride a stationary bike with little to no resistance for 20 minutes three times per day. The time is increased along with the resistance as tolerated. Sutures are removed at 1 week and elliptical and weight-training exercises are begun along with distance walking on a treadmill or outside. The patient is taught range-of-motion exercises and told not to hyperextend for 3 to 6 weeks. At 1 month, the patient is evaluated for symptoms, range of motion, and hip stability. Most of our patients continue with self-directed advancement of their exercises and activities. If the range of motion is not 80% of normal, we advise physical therapy.

We have found that symptoms may continue to some degree, even after successful surgery, for at least 1 year, and advise our patients not to be alarmed if the symptoms fluctuate in their intensity and frequency. Most symptoms improve over months. If there is a significant decline, further investigation with a simple x-ray may lead to a diagnosis of failed surgery. Surgical failure in arthritic patients is demonstrated by further loss of joint space or widening of the medial clear space and superior lateral subluxation.

COMPLICATIONS

Complications may be avoided by paying attention to the length of distraction time and the location of the neurovascular bundles, and taking great care to avoid damage to the articular cartilage.

In our series of 1,500 cases, we have found that continuous distraction lasting less than 2 hours resulted in no sciatic, femoral, or pudendal neuropraxias. We have had five cases of lateral cutaneous neuropraxia; however, all either resolved or the patient accommodated to the patch of numbness on the thigh. Approximately 1% of our cases developed heterotopic bone; in five patients, reoperation was required to alleviate symptoms. There was one nondisplaced femoral neck fracture in a patient treated for DJD and FAI, in which the treatment was placement of a single-cannulated screw. This patient had a final modified Harris Hip Score of 100 for the last 5 years. There was one case of retroperitoneal extravasation, treated with an overnight stay, diuretics, and observation, resulting in no sequelae. We have had no occurrence of deep infections.

REFERENCES

1. Gray AJ, Villar RN. The ligamentum teres of the hip: an arthroscopic classification of its pathology. *Arthroscopy.* 1997; 13(5):575–578.

2. Kashiwagi N, Suzuki S, Seto Y. Arthroscopic treatment for traumatic hip dislocation with avulsion fracture of the ligamentum teres [case reports]. *Arthroscopy.* 2001;17(1):67–69.

3. Kusma M, Jung J, Dienst M, et al. Arthroscopic treatment of an avulsion fracture of the ligamentum teres of the hip in an 18-year-old horse rider [case reports]. *Arthroscopy.* 2004;20(suppl 2):64–66.

4. Simpson JM, Field RE, Villar RN. Arthroscopic reconstruction of the ligamentum teres [case reports video-audio media]. *Arthroscopy.* 2011;27(3):436–441.

5. Ide T, Akamatsu N, Nakajima I. Arthroscopic surgery of the hip joint. *Arthroscopy.* 1991;7(2):204–211.

6. Ishida Y, Oki T, Ono Y, et al. Coffin-Lowry syndrome associated with calcium pyrophosphate crystal deposition in the ligamenta flava. *Clin Orthop Relat Res.* 1992;(275):144–151.

7. Gerster JC, Varisco PA, Kern J, et al. CPPD crystal deposition disease in patients with rheumatoid arthritis. *Clin Rheumatol.* 2006;25(4):468–469.

8. Timsit MA, Bardin T. Metabolic arthropathies. *Curr Opin Rheumatol.* 1994;6(4):448–453.

9. Broy SB, Schmid FR. A comparison of medical drainage (needle aspiration) and surgical drainage (arthrotomy or arthroscopy) in the initial treatment of infected joints. *Clin Rheum Dis.* 1986;12(2):501–522.

10. Ohl MD, Kean JR, Steensen RN. Arthroscopic treatment of septic arthritic knees in children and adolescents. *Orthop Rev.* 1991;20(10):894–896.

11. Blitzer CM. Arthroscopic management of septic arthritis of the hip. *Arthroscopy.* 1993;9(4):414–416.

12. Kim SJ, Choi NH, Ko SH, et al. Arthroscopic treatment of septic arthritis of the hip. *Clin Orthop Relat Res.* 2003;(407):211–214.

13. McCarthy JC, Jibodh SR, Lee JA. The role of arthroscopy in evaluation of painful hip arthroplasty. *Clin orthop Relat Res.* 2009;467(1):174–180.

14. Farjo LA, Glick JM, Sampson TG. Hip arthroscopy for acetabular labral tears. *Arthroscopy.* 1999;15(2):132–137.

15. Sampson T. Hip morphology and its relationship to pathology: dysplasia to impingement. *Oper Tech Sports Med.* 2005;13(1):37–45

16. Sampson T. Arthroscopic treatment of femoroacetabular impingement. *Tech Orthop.* 2005;20(1):56–62.

17. Sampson TG. Arthroscopic treatment of femoroacetabular impingement: a proposed technique with clinical experience. *Instr Course Lect.* 2006;55:337–346.

18. Eijer H, Myers SR, Ganz R. Anterior femoroacetabular impingement after femoral neck fractures. *J Orthop Trauma.* 2001;15(7):475–481.

19. Boyer T, Dorfmann H. Arthroscopy in primary synovial chondromatosis of the hip: description and outcome of treatment. *J Bone Joint Surg.* 2008;90(3):314–318.

20. Sim FH. Synovial proliferative disorders: role of synovectomy. *Arthroscopy.* 1985;1(3):198–204.

21. Yamamoto Y, Hamada Y, Ide T, et al. Arthroscopic surgery to treat intra-articular type snapping hip. *Arthroscopy.* 2005;21(9):1120–1125.

22. Khapchik V, O'Donnell RJ, Glick JM. Arthroscopically assisted excision of osteoid osteoma involving the hip. *Arthroscopy.* 2001;17(1):56–61.

23. Alvarez MS, Moneo PR, Palacios JA. Arthroscopic extirpation of an osteoid osteoma of the acetabulum. *Arthroscopy.* 2001;17(7):768–71.

24. Stoller DW, Sampson T, Bredella M. The hip. In: Stoller DW, ed. *Magnetic Resonance Imaging in Orthopaedics and Sports Medicine.* 3rd ed. Philadelphia, PA: Lippincott Williams & Wilkins; 2007:41–304.

25. Daniel M, Iglic A, Kralj-Iglic V. The shape of acetabular cartilage optimizes hip contact stress distribution. *J Anat.* 2005;207(1):85–91.

26. Ilizaliturri VM Jr, Byrd JW, Sampson TG, et al. A geographic zone method to describe intra-articular pathology in hip arthroscopy: cadaveric study and preliminary report. *Arthroscopy.* 2008;24(5):534–539.

The Knee

General

Arthroscopic Setup, Instrumentation, Portals, and Operative Pearls

Kevin W. Farmer • Gautam P. Yagnik • John W. Uribe

Knee arthroscopy is the most commonly performed orthopedic procedure (1). As surgeons add this procedure to their repertoire, it is important to develop a consistent approach to the operation. Through consistency, complications are minimized, operative time is decreased, and the potential of missed pathology is diminished. This chapter will describe the authors' approach to a basic knee arthroscopy. It is important to realize that there are several ways to approach this procedure, and surgeons should utilize their training and experience to ensure an efficient performance in the operating room.

PREOPERATIVE MARKING

Wrong-site surgery is a concern for all orthopedic surgeons. The operating surgeon should mark the operative site before the administration of any anxiolytic or narcotic medications (Fig. 53.1). An evaluation of malpractice claims found knee arthroscopy to be the most common procedure involved in a wrong-site surgery (2). Orthopedic surgeons have an estimated 25% chance of wrong-site surgery during their career (3). In 1998, the American Academy of Orthopaedic Surgeons began the "sign your site" campaign, recommending the operating surgeons initials are placed in indelible ink on the operative site such that the marking is unambiguous and will be present on the operative site after prepping and draping (see Fig. 53.1) (4). The Joint Commission on Accreditation of Healthcare Organizations further expanded the recommendations to include a time-out to verify the initials in the field, the correct patient and site, the correct procedure, correct position, and the availability of appropriate equipment (5). Recent studies have demonstrated that chloraprep was 22 times more likely to remove site markings before prepping (6), and that ink in the sterile field does not increase infection risk (7).

ANTIBIOTICS

There are no randomized controlled trials looking at the role of prophylactic antibiotics in arthroscopic surgery.

The incidence of infections with arthroscopy is extremely low, thus it would take a very large study to ensure an appropriate power (8). Nonetheless, we routinely give 2 g of cefazolin, or 600 to 900 mg of clindamycin for true penicillin allergies, within 1 hour of tourniquet use or incision.

ANESTHESIA

Local anesthetic with a mixture of lidocaine and bupivacaine both intra-articularly and at the portal sites have been used successfully in basic knee arthroscopies (9). Any bony work would have to be minimized, as this would likely elicit a pain response. Use of a tourniquet would also have to be minimized in an awake patient in this setting. It is important to confirm the maximum dose that can be safely used during the case to avoid serious complications. Given the recent findings of chondrolysis with the use of bupivacaine, this option may become less favorable with many orthopedic surgeons (10).

Regional anesthesia with sedation or spinal anesthesia are appropriate options for knee arthroscopic procedures, especially in the setting of medical comorbidities that limit general anesthesia. There is some evidence that regional anesthesia may decrease hospital admissions in an outpatient setting. A regional anesthetic is preferred to spinal due to decreased rates of urinary retention (11). Complications including femoral neuritis and hematomas have been reported. All patients with a femoral nerve block should be placed in a knee immobilizer until quadriceps function returns to minimize fall risks (12).

General anesthetic is the most commonly used modality for knee arthroscopy. It minimizes the time constraints placed by some local and regional anesthetics and allows for complete muscle relaxation if necessary. A combination of general and regional anesthetic provides effective intraoperative relaxation and postoperative pain control.

Our preferred anesthesia protocol is usually general anesthesia for simple arthroscopies. If we are expecting a more involved procedure, we will often use a regional anesthetic, if preferred by the anesthesiologist and the

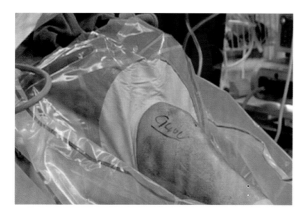

FIGURE 53.1. The surgeon's initials should be placed in the operative field and should be visible after prepping and draping.

patient, in combination with a general anesthetic. We are less likely to use a regional anesthetic in cases that have an increased risk of nerve injury, as we like to perform an adequate neurovascular examination at the end of the case.

EXAMINATION UNDER ANESTHESIA

Once the patient has appropriate muscular relaxation, an examination under anesthesia should be performed in all cases. The examination should include evaluation of effusion, range of motion, crepitance, patellar mobility, and stability. Specialized tests such as the Lachman, pivot shift, and dial test should be performed in appropriate cases (Fig. 53.2). One should always compare findings with the contralateral side.

SETUP

A well-padded tourniquet should be placed high on the thigh in all cases, even if its use is not expected (Fig. 53.3). It is important to ensure proper table positioning before draping. If fluoroscopy is needed, the table should be adjusted so all obstructing objects are out of the way. The patient should also be moved on the bed to the

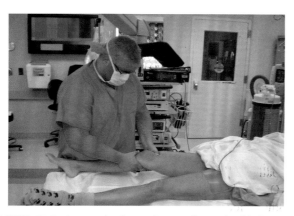

FIGURE 53.2. An examination under anesthesia should always be performed and compared with the contralateral side.

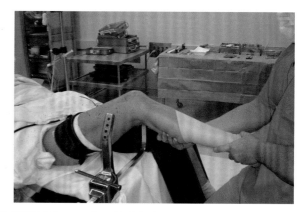

FIGURE 53.3. A well-padded thigh tourniquet should be placed high on the thigh, even if its use is not expected.

appropriate position based on surgeon's preference. This position is often distal, allowing the foot of the bed to be lowered if needed.

PATIENT POSITIONING—LEG HOLDER

The use of a leg holder is the author's preferred method for knee arthroscopy. We favor this position as it maximizes the freedom of movement of the knee and can be utilized without the need for an assistant. The leg holder is placed on the operating table at the distal break in the table. This allows the foot of the bed to be lowered during the case (Fig. 53.4). The patient should be positioned so the leg holder is four finger breadths above the superior pole of the patella (Fig. 53.5). This position provides enough room to allow varus/valgus stress without compromising portal placement, but may need to be altered based on the case (i.e., if more exposure is needed proximally for a posterolateral corner reconstruction). A pad is placed under the contralateral leg, and we let this hang off the end of the table (Fig. 53.6). A lithotomy leg positioner may also be used. Since the leg holder has a venous tourniquet effect if sufficiently tightened, we inflate the tourniquet before placing in the leg holder (see Fig. 53.3). The foam leg

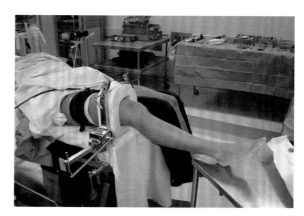

FIGURE 53.4. The operative leg holder should be placed at the distal break in the bed, so the foot of the table can be lowered.

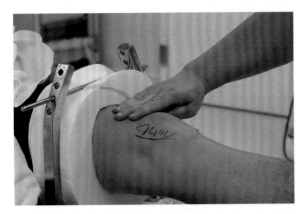

FIGURE 53.5. The leg holder should be placed approximately four finger breadths above the superior pole of the patella.

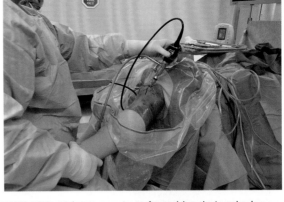

FIGURE 53.8. Valgus stress is performed by placing the leg on the surgeon's outer hip.

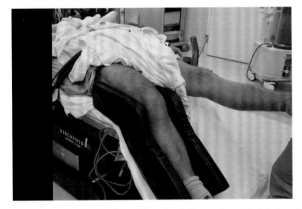

FIGURE 53.6. The contralateral leg should be well padded during the operation. Compression stockings and pneumatic compression devices are useful in longer cases.

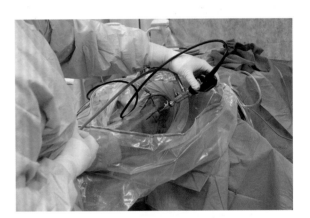

FIGURE 53.9. Varus stress is applied by placing the leg on the surgeon's inner hip.

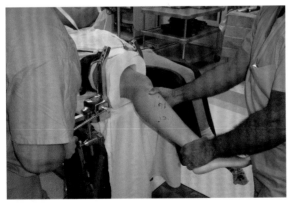

FIGURE 53.7. When tightening the operative leg holder, internally rotating the leg counteracts the natural tendency of the leg to externally rotate.

holder is then placed and tightened with the leg in internal rotation to prevent locking the leg in a naturally externally rotated position (Fig. 53.7). Examination of the medial compartment is accomplished with a valgus stress placed with the leg on the surgeon's outside hip (Fig. 53.8). Examination of the lateral compartment is accomplished by

placing a varus stress on the knee with the leg on the surgeon's inside hip (Fig. 53.9).

PATIENT POSITIONING—LATERAL POST

The lateral post is useful in conjunction with an open procedure that requires the leg in a position of extension, such as a patellar instability case. The use of a post may limit varus and valgus stresses and may require assistance with leg positioning during the case. The post should be approximately four finger breadths proximal to the superior pole of the patella (Fig. 53.10). Valgus stress is applied with the leg placed on the upper outer thigh of the surgeon (Fig. 53.11). Varus stress is applied in the figure-four position, often requiring the lateral post to be lowered and force added from an assistant (Fig. 53.12).

PREPPING AND DRAPING

The two main choices for surgical skin preparation are chlorhexidine and povidone iodine. Studies have shown that a combination of chlorhexidine with isopropyl alcohol significantly reduces bacterial counts when compared with isopropyl alcohol, chlorhexidine alone, or povidone

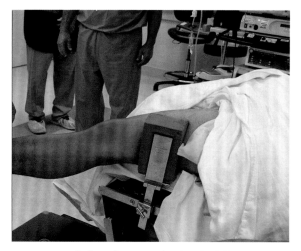

FIGURE 53.10. If a lateral post is utilized, it should be placed at least four finger breadths above the superior pole of the patella.

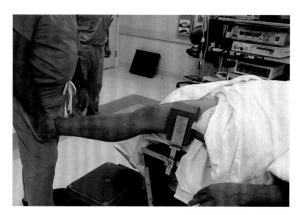

FIGURE 53.11. When using a lateral post, valgus stress is applied by placing the leg on the surgeons outer leg.

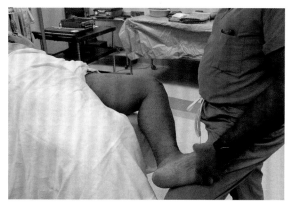

FIGURE 53.12. Varus stress is applied by placing the leg in a figure-four position when using a lateral post.

iodine. In addition, chlorhexidine has been shown to bind to proteins in the skin and mucosa, with significant antimicrobial effects up to 24 hours (13).

There are many different ways of draping a leg for arthroscopy. We prefer a sterile U-drape with adhesive placed directly on the skin. The foot is draped out with

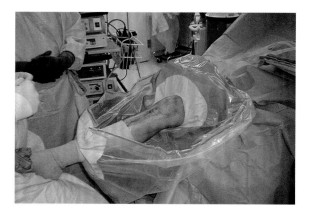

FIGURE 53.13. An arthroscopic extremity drape with collecting bag minimizes fluid collections that may prolong turnover times.

an impervious stockinette, and an arthroscopic extremity drape with collecting bag is utilized (Fig. 53.13).

INSTRUMENTATION

There are many instruments that are designed specifically for arthroscopic surgery. The 30° arthroscope is the primary tool of knee arthroscopy and is defined as a lens that is angled 30° to the long axis of the scope (Fig. 53.14). Most aspects of a knee arthroscopy can be completed with a 30° scope with adequate visualization. A 70° scope may be needed when working in the posterior compartments through the intercondylar notch (Gillquist interval), or during posterior cruciate ligament (PCL) reconstruction (14).

The choice of inflow is a matter or surgeon preference. Gravity inflow has the advantage of decreased tissue extravasation that may occur with high intra-articular pressures. A pump inflow system is the authors treatment of choice, as it allows easy adjustment of flow and intra-articular pressure. If a tourniquet is not utilized, a pump may be beneficial in improving visualization.

The first tool often used during the course of knee arthroscopy is the arthroscopic probe. The arthroscopic

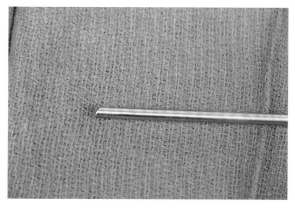

FIGURE 53.14. A 30° scope is sufficient to perform most aspects of knee arthroscopy.

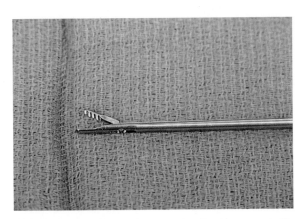

FIGURE 53.15. An arthroscopic grasper is utilized in removal of loose bodies and meniscal fragments.

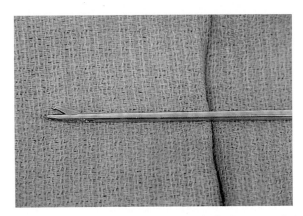

FIGURE 53.17. An arthroscopic punch is useful for fine tuning during meniscectomy.

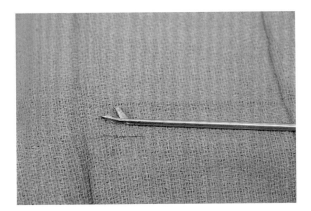

FIGURE 53.16. An up-biter is beneficial during meniscectomy, especially in the concave medial compartment.

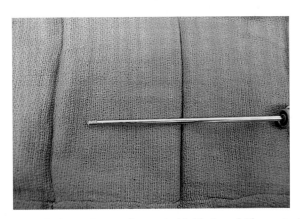

FIGURE 53.18. A 3.5-mm arthroscopic debrider is useful for most soft tissue debridements.

probe is useful in assessing the presence of meniscal tears and in determining stability. In addition, the probe is useful in evaluating chondral injuries and cruciate damage and can used in the retrieval of loose bodies. A graduated probe allows for a determination of size of pathologic lesions.

An arthroscopic grasper is useful in the retrieval of loose bodies and meniscal fragments (Fig. 53.15). Arthroscopic handheld resectors are known by various terms. "Duckbills" tend to have a larger resecting area, allowing large pieces to be removed in less time. An arthroscopic biter tends to be a midsize resector and can come in various curvatures. The most commonly used are side-biters, or curved biters, as well as an up-biter (Fig. 53.16). An arthroscopic punch is a smaller resector, allowing contouring and minimal trimming of pathology (Fig. 53.17). A pituitary rongeur is useful for taking soft tissue biopsies and in removal of loose bodies.

Arthroscopic shavers come with various cutting blades, with different sizes and shapes, as well as variations in cutting windows. For the most part, a slower oscillating speed along with suction is useful when debriding soft tissue, as more tissue is brought into the cutting zone. Faster speeds in a constant direction are utilized for bony

debridement. A debrider, or "shaver" blade come in sizes often from 2.5 up to 5.0 mm or larger. A 3.5- or 4.0-mm blade tend to be the blades we use most often. These blades have a large oval window, with a smooth cutting blade (Fig. 53.18). Debriders are most effective in synovectomy, meniscal debridement, and chondroplasty. An arthroscopic abrader, or "burr," tends to be a larger oval solid blade with a protecting sheath. This is used mainly for bony debridement. Suction can either be manually, or run through the pump system, which is our method of choice.

Bipolar radiofrequency devices have become more frequently used in arthroscopic surgery. Uses include soft tissue debridement, stabilizing chondral edges, lateral release, and meniscal debulking (Fig. 53.19) (15). Care should be taken to ensure there is adequate flow through the joint to reduce elevating intra-articular temperatures. In addition, judicious use should be utilized to minimize injury to surrounding healthy tissue.

PORTALS

Proper portal placement is the most crucial step for any arthroscopic procedure. Improper placement of portals

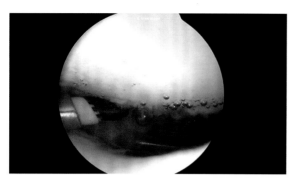

FIGURE 53.19. A bipolar radiofrequency used to stabilize chondral edges during chondroplasty of the patella.

can greatly increase the difficulty of the procedure and can lead to iatrogenic injury. If an aberrant portal is established, subsequent incisions maybe needed to allow the case to proceed. A thorough understanding of surface anatomy is the key to proper portal placement.

Inflow Portals

Superomedial or superolateral inflow portals may be established based to surgeon preference. These portals are typically made just proximal to the intersection of a line drawn from the superior pole of the patella either medially or laterally, and a line drawn proximal from the medial or lateral pole (Fig. 53.20). A small oblique incision is made in the direction of Langer's lines, and the trochar is aimed toward the superopatellar pouch, in a direction nearly parallel to the floor, with the knee in extension (Fig. 53.21). The trochar should not be aimed toward the patellar femoral joint to avoid chondral injury, nor toward the femur, as this tends to pull synovium down, leading to an extrasynovial inflow and increased swelling. The benefit of an accessory inflow portal is the increased inflow allotted through a larger cannula, and the ability to be used as an accessory portal.

Care should be taken to avoid violating the quadriceps muscle during insertion. The superomedial portal is our

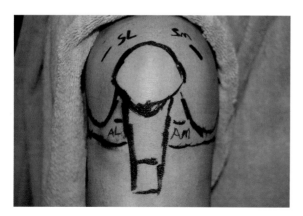

FIGURE 53.20. An anterior view of the knee with the patella, patellar tendon, femoral condyles, and tibial plateaus outlined. The anteromedial (AM), anterolateral (AL), superomedial (SM), and superolateral (SL) portals are marked.

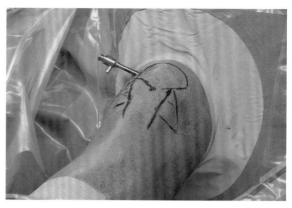

FIGURE 53.21. An inflow cannula placed in the superomedial portal with drainage from an effusion. The cannula should be placed in the superopatellar pouch in a direction that parallels the floor with the knee in extension.

preferred portal, and we pay close attention to minimizing trauma to the vastus medialis oblique muscle. The superolateral portal has less chance of injury to the quadriceps, but a slightly increased chance of chondral injury given the more proximal extension of chondral surfaces on the lateral trochlea. Inflow may become occluded during extreme flexion, and this can be minimized by a more proximal portal placement initially, or by simply switching inflow to the bridge on the camera during that part of the case.

Anterolateral Portal

The anterolateral portal is typically made after joint infiltration with saline through the superior inflow portals or may be made as the initial portal if inflow is not utilized. The arthroscope is typically placed in this portal, and most aspects of arthroscopy can be performed with this configuration. This portal is established just lateral to the patellar tendon, at the site where the lateral femoral condyle is noted to "drop-off." This is just proximal to the lateral tibial plateau, and near the level of the inferior pole of the patella (see Fig. 53.20). Placing the portal too high or too low will make access into the medial compartment or posterior compartments extremely difficult. The incision can be made either vertical or horizontal. We prefer a horizontal incision as this is better for cosmesis, but care should be taken to aim the blade away from patellar tendon to avoid iatrogenic injury. If a vertical incision is chosen, the blade should be aimed away from the tibial plateau to avoid making a radial incision in the anterior horn of the lateral meniscus. The trochar should be inserted in a direction aimed toward the intercondylar notch. This reduces the risk of chondral injury during initial and future instrument insertions and allows the surgeon an anatomic landmark to aim for, minimizing difficulty in localizing the capsulotomy.

Anteromedial Portal

The anteromedial portal is the primary instrumentation portal during most aspects of knee arthroscopy. The proper

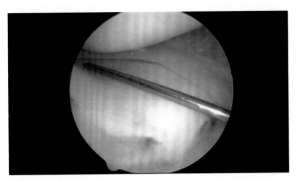

FIGURE 53.22. A needle used to localize the placement of the anteromedial portal. The portal should be placed medial to the patellar tendon, just proximal to the anterior horn of the medial meniscus.

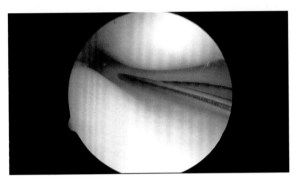

FIGURE 53.23. An arthroscopic view of the posterior horn of the medial meniscus. The anteromedial portal should be placed in a position that allows easy access to the posterior horn.

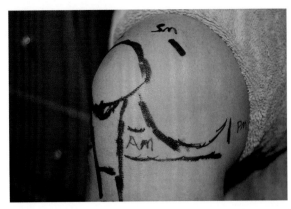

FIGURE 53.24. An medial-oblique view of the knee with the patella, patellar tendon, femoral condyles, and tibial plateaus outlined. The locations of the anteromedial (AM), posteromedial (PM), and superomedial (SM) portals are noted.

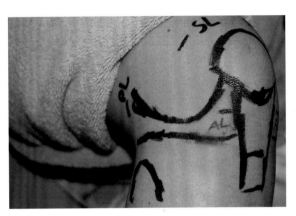

FIGURE 53.25. An lateral-oblique view of the knee with the patella, patellar tendon, femoral condyles, tibial plateaus, and fibular head outlined. The locations of the anterolateral (AL), posterolateral (PL), and superolateral (SL) portals are noted.

placement of this portal is crucial to minimizing difficulty during the case. Placement too high will lead to difficulty reaching the posterior horn of the medial meniscus due to contact with the medial femoral condyle. Placement too low will lead to a superior trajectory of the instruments over the medial tibial plateau. We always make this portal under direct visualization. We strive to make this portal just medial to the patellar tendon, and just above the anterior horn of the medial meniscus (Fig. 53.22). It is important to ensure that the trajectory of the portal allows easy access to the posterior horn of the medial meniscus (Fig. 53.23).

Posteromedial and Posterolateral Portal

These portals are accessory portals used for synovectomies, removal of loose bodies, and in PCL reconstruction. The posteromedial portal is located along the posteromedial joint-line, posterior to the medial femoral condyle (Fig. 53.24). The arthroscope is passed through the Gillquist interval, between the PCL and the medial femoral condyle (14). With the camera looking medial, a spinal needle is used to localize the correct location. A skin incision followed by blunt spreading minimizes the risk of injury to the saphenous vein and nerve.

The posterolateral portal is established at the posteromedial joint line, posterior to the lateral femoral condyle (Fig. 53.25). This portal is created under direct visualization with the arthroscope passed through the medial portal, between the anterior cruciate ligament and the lateral femoral condyle. Care should be taken to ensure the needle is located posterior to the lateral collateral ligament and anterior to the biceps femoris, and therefore, the peroneal nerve. A skin incision followed by blunt spreading should always be utilized.

OPERATIVE PEARLS

The most important aspect of knee arthroscopy is accurate portal placement. Placing a portal either inferior or superior to the ideal location can increase the difficulty of the case exponentially. If portals are misplaced, iatrogenic injury may occur, and multiple portals may need to be established. Proper portal placement will decrease tourniquet time, allow ease of access to pathology, and minimize collateral damage. With that in mind, here are a few pearls that will increase the accuracy of portal placement:

1. *Draw out anatomy.* While one is becoming more comfortable with portal placement, accurately drawing the anatomic landmarks can aid in localization. It is helpful to draw out the patella, patellar tendon, tibial tuberosity, and articular line of the femoral condyles and tibial plateaus. It is helpful to use multiple references when making portals, such as the lateral portal placed at the "drop-off" of the lateral femoral condyle, which is just proximal to the lateral tibial plateau, and often at the level of the inferior pole of the patella (Fig. 53.26).

2. *Place the knee in a position to see the posterior horn of the medial meniscus when making the medial portal.* When making the medial portal under direct visualization, it is helpful to place the knee in the position that gives the best visualization of the posterior horn of the medial meniscus. In that position, one can ensure that the portal is placed in a location that allows the best access to the posterior horn (see Fig. 53.23).

3. *In morbidly obese patients, direct visualization of both the anteromedial and the anterolateral portals may be necessary.* In the morbidly obese patients, palpation of anatomic landmarks maybe precluded by adipose tissue. Often, the patella is the only landmark palpable. In that setting, it may be helpful to establish the superomedial or superolateral inflow portal, and place the arthroscope into the portal to establish the anterolateral portal under direct visualization (16). The anteromedial portal should be established in a standard fashion, but one should realize

that this portal appears more lateral than normal due to the large amount of medial knee adipose tissue. It is critically import to establish precise portals in this population as the extra tissue is less forgiving with inaccurate placement (16).

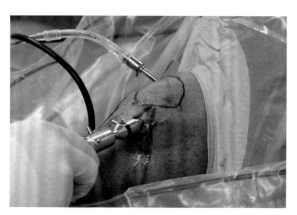

FIGURE 53.26. Anatomic marking may be beneficial for accurate portal placement during the learning curve for knee arthroscopy.

REFERENCES

1. Garrett WE Jr, Swiontkowski MF, Weinstein JN, et al. American Board of Orthopaedic Surgery Practice of the Orthopaedic Surgeon: part-II, certification examination case mix. *J Bone Joint Surg Am.* 2006;88:660–667.
2. Cowell HR. Wrong-site surgery. *J Bone Joint Surg Am.* 1998;80:463.
3. Canale ST. Wrong-site surgery: a preventable complication. *Clin Orthop Relat Res.* 2005;(433):26–29.
4. Surgeons AAoO. Information statement: wrong-site surgery 2008. http://www.aaos.org/about/papers/advistmt/1015.asp. Accessed July 19, 2009.
5. Organizations JCoAoH. Universal protocol 2004. http://www.jointcommission.org/PatientSafety/UniversalProtocol. Accessed July 19, 2009.
6. Mears SC, Dinah AF, Knight TA, et al. Visibility of surgical site marking after preoperative skin preparation. *Eplasty.* 2008;8:e35.
7. Cullan DB II, Wongworawat MD. Sterility of the surgical site marking between the ink and the epidermis. *J Am Coll Surg.* 2007;205:319–321.
8. Kurzweil PR. Antibiotic prophylaxis for arthroscopic surgery. *Arthroscopy.* 2006;22:452–454.
9. Yoshiya S, Kurosaka M, Hirohata K, et al. Knee arthroscopy using local anesthetic. *Arthroscopy.* 1988;4:86–89.
10. Dragoo JL, Korotkova T, Kanwar R, et al. The effect of local anesthetics administered via pain pump on chondrocyte viability. *Am J Sports Med.* 2008;36:1484–1488.
11. Casati A, Cappelleri G, Aldegheri G, et al. Total intravenous anesthesia, spinal anesthesia or combined sciatic-femoral nerve block for outpatient knee arthroscopy. *Minerva Anestesiol.* 2004;70:493–502.
12. Sharma S, Iorio R, Specht LM, et al. Complications of femoral nerve block for total knee arthroplasty. *Clin Orthop Relat Res.* 2009;468:135–140.
13. Lim KS, Kam PC. Chlorhexidine—pharmacology and clinical applications. *Anaesth Intensive Care.* 2008;36:502–512.
14. Gillquist J, Hagberg G. A new modification of the technique of arthroscopy of the knee joint. *Acta Chir Scand.* 1976;142:123–130.
15. Barber FA, Uribe JW, Weber SC. Current applications for arthroscopic thermal surgery. *Arthroscopy.* 2002;18:40–50.
16. Martinez A, Hechtman KS. Arthroscopic technique for the knee in morbidly obese patients. *Arthroscopy.* 2002;18:E13.

Arthroscopic Anatomy of the Knee

Jason Koh

The arthroscopic anatomy of the knee can be best described by consideration of the various parts of the knee joint that can be evaluated during a diagnostic evaluation. Familiarity with the normal anatomy and anatomical variance is important for the understanding of pathology. A complete and systematic evaluation of the knee should be performed prior to the initiation of any planned arthroscopic procedure. The precise sequence of the arthroscopic evaluation should be performed in a consistent fashion to truly assess the knee joint. We will describe the arthroscopic anatomy with regard to a standard arthroscopic evaluation (Table 54.1).

DIAGNOSTIC ARTHROSCOPY

Diagnostic arthroscopy of the knee joint typically begins with the arthroscope placed through an anterolateral portal into the knee joint. Portal creation is noted in the previous chapter; this needs to be precise and accurate both for the viewing portal and for the instrumentation portal. It is strongly recommended that the portals be created after using a spinal needle initially as a guide to the orientation of the proposed portal and instruments. If the tip of the spinal needle is able to touch the specific anatomical area of interest, this increases the likelihood that instruments will also reach those specific areas.

The scope is placed through the anterolateral portal, typically entering into the suprapatellar pouch. This should be done with care to avoid iatrogenic damage to the surrounding articular cartilage. Motions inside the joint should be done gently with regard to the tip of the scope and scope sheath.

The arthroscopic evaluation of the knee should be systematic and complete. The sequence described here is not prescriptive; rather it is meant to serve as a guide to the author's preferred technique. The precise sequence used is up to the individual surgeon; however, we recommend a thorough evaluation of all compartments.

SUPRAPATELLAR POUCH

The suprapatellar pouch is the initial location of the arthroscope. This is a normal anatomical opening above the patella separating the extensor mechanism from the anterior femur. A suprapatellar plica is a normal finding in the majority of knees (Fig. 54.1). In some cases this suprapatellar plica may be extensive enough to nearly wall off the superior portion of the suprapatellar pouch. It is important in these cases to advance the arthroscope sufficiently to view the most proximal portion of the

Table 54.1

Arthroscopic regions of the knee

Suprapatellar pouch
Patellofemoral joint
Medial gutter
Lateral gutter
Medial tibiofemoral compartment
Lateral tibiofemoral compartment
Intercondylar notch
Posteromedial compartment
Posterolateral compartment

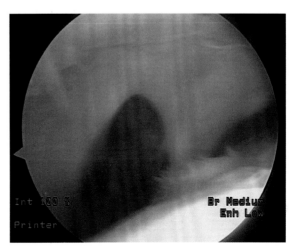

FIGURE 54.1. Normal suprapatellar plica.

suprapatellar pouch; otherwise loose bodies in this area may not be identified. The suprapatellar pouch should also be evaluated for the presence of loose bodies, synovitis, or scarring. Postsurgical or posttraumatic adhesions between the extensor mechanism and the anterior femur can decrease quadriceps mobility. The anterior femur is typically covered with a richly vascularized synovial lining and fat. Nodular or villous synovitis may also be present in this area.

MEDIAL GUTTER

The scope is then gently brought across the knee joint into the medial portion of the knee. As the scope gently sweeps across the anterior portion of the distal femur, depending on the position of the anterolateral portal and other anatomical factors such as osteophytes, it may be difficult to sweep the scope directly anteriorly without engaging the articular cartilage of the trochlea. In this situation it is recommended that the scope be gently drawn back and passed across the more distal anterior portion of the femur anterior to the border of the trochlea. Visualization can be directed anteromedially with a scope and this may demonstrate the presence of anteromedial plica (Fig. 54.2). This plica is a normal anatomical variant in many patients and is often asymptomatic. The plica itself is a normal remnant of embryonic development. About 40% of knees have medial plica originating from the medial retinaculum and inserting onto the fat pad. In some cases an anteromedial plica may become a source of pathology for the knee joint. These pathologic plica typically have significant thickening of the tissue or synovitis and may be associated with articular cartilage damage (1, 2). If a large anteromedial plica is present, it may be difficult to visualize the medial gutter directly. The knee may need to be slightly flexed or the scope placed slightly more proximally to avoid the plica. Visualization of the medial gutter should typically be performed to assess for the presence or absence of loose bodies, marginal osteophytes, and synovitis.

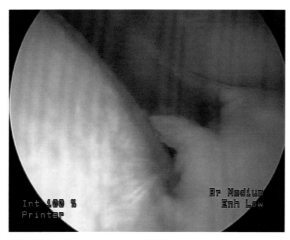

FIGURE 54.2. Normal anteromedial plica.

PATELLOFEMORAL ARTICULATION

One often takes an initial look at the distal lateral facet of the patella while inspecting the patellofemoral joint. The scope can be placed to look more proximally to inspect the more proximal portion of the patella. The more medial facet of the patella is sometimes obscured by the apex of the patella. This can sometimes be further visualized by placing the scope somewhat more distally and rotating the lens so that it looks more proximally and superiorly to visualize the medial facet (Fig. 54.3). The trochlea should also be inspected. Typically, the most proximal portion of the trochlea is seen with the knee in full extension. Visualization of the trochlea is enhanced by rotating the lens inferiorly and gently flexing the knee to expose the entire trochlea (Fig. 54.4).

Patella tracking and mobility can be assessed while placing the knee through a range of motion and also by shifting the patella medially and laterally. In some cases

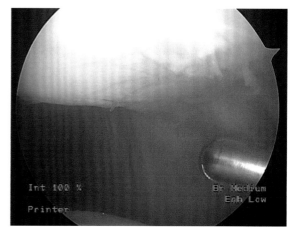

FIGURE 54.3. Medial facet of patella.

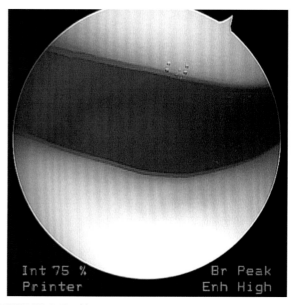

FIGURE 54.4. Trochlea.

increased patella mobility can be identified with a decrease in the amount of fluid pressure within the knee because the distended knee joint has less patella mobility than the nondistended joint. The patella should be inspected for articular cartilage damage and overhanging osteophytes. In cases of patella instability there is often evidence of trauma to the medial retinaculum. The trochlea should be inspected for evidence of trochlea dysplasia and carefully inspected for the presence or absence of articular cartilage damage. In many cases there may be minimal damage seen more proximally; however, as the knee is flexed, central trochlear damage may become more evident (Fig. 54.5). Articular cartilage lesions should be evaluated for size and depth and should be graded using a standardized grading scale such as the modified Outerbridge classification (3) or International Cartilage Research Society classification (4). It is helpful to use a probe to assess the mechanical properties of the articular cartilage resistance to compression. A

Table 54.2	
Modified outerbridge classification with Insall modification (5)	
I	Softening and swelling of cartilage
II	Fissuring to subchondral bone
III	Fibrillation of articular surface
IV	Erosion of cartilage down to exposed subchondral bone

calibrated probe can also be used to help provide a ruler for a comparison for measurement of size and also assess the stability of any articular cartilage damage.

Evaluation can also be performed by placing the scope superiorly using a suprapatellar portal. The patella tracking through a range of motion can be identified as the scope enters the trochlea in flexion and exits, going from flexion to extension (Fig. 54.6). This may also be enhanced by use of a 70° scope to evaluate the patella tracking (Table 54.2).

LATERAL GUTTER

The lateral gutter should be visualized, and again a similar inspection to the medial gutter should be performed looking for synovitis, loose bodies, and marginal osteophytes. The popliteal hiatus should be identified in this area (Fig. 54.7) and a gentle milking maneuver should be performed to assess for the presence of loose bodies that may move back and forth within the popliteal hiatus. If it is difficult to enter into the lateral gutter, it is recommended that the scope be slightly withdrawn from the joint and passed distal to the distal articular cartilage of the femur. Use of gentle suction applied to the arthroscopic sheath of the scope can help vacuum loose bodies from the popliteal hiatus. A portion of the posterior horn of the lateral meniscus can also be identified in this area.

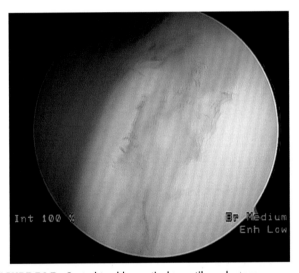

FIGURE 54.5. Central trochlear articular cartilage damage.

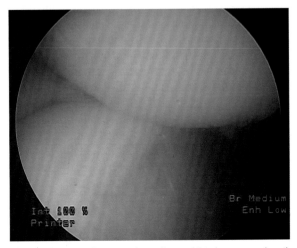

FIGURE 54.6. Identification of patella tracking by scope placed superiorly through a suprapatellar portal entering the trochlea in flexion and exiting going from flexion to extension.

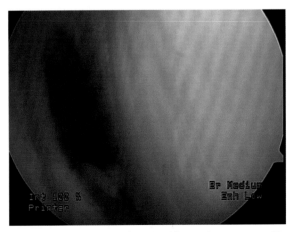

FIGURE 54.7. Assessment of popliteal hiatus for presence of loose bodies.

MEDIAL COMPARTMENT

Inspection of the medial compartment is performed with the knee slightly flexed to allow the scope to enter the compartment over the anterior horn of the medial meniscus. The knee should be placed in flexion of approximately 20° to 30° and the valgus force applied to open up the medial compartment. Typically, this is performed with use of a post or leg holder proximally to stabilize the femur. The anatomic structures evaluated in the medial compartment are the medial tibial plateau, the medial femur, and the medial meniscus. The meniscus can be initially visualized anteriorly with the scope, and then the lens of the arthroscope can be rotated so that the viewing angle is directed more posteriorly and underneath the articular cartilage of the distal femur. The meniscus should demonstrate a smooth and consistent appearance (Fig. 54.8), and it should be possible to visualize the posterior horn of the meniscus. Incomplete visualization suggests abnormal morphology or difficulties with portal placement or positioning. If necessary, the scope should be repositioned to evaluate the entire posterior horn of the medial meniscus. A diminutive posterior horn may actually be the result of a displaced fragment entrapped behind the posterior femoral condyle. The medial joint space typically opens up 3.5 to 4 mm to allow good visualization of the posterior horn of the medial meniscus. Further improvement of visualization of the posterior horn of the medial meniscus can sometimes be enhanced by gentle external rotation of the foot while the knee is flexed in the valgus position.

The meniscus should be carefully and completely evaluated. The evaluation of the arthroscopic anatomy should be performed with the assistance of a probe that is typically placed in the anteromedial portal. This author finds that a portal relatively adjacent to the patella tendon enhances palpation of the undersurface of the posteromedial aspect of the meniscus. A more medially originating portal may not allow palpation of the undersurface.

The probe should be used to evaluate the meniscus. A smooth blending into the synovial lining should be seen on the superior and inferior surfaces of the meniscus. Irregularity of the undersurface of the meniscus may be suggestive of a displaced fragment that is entrapped behind the posterior edge of the medial tibial plateau. The probe should also be used to evaluate the resistance to palpation of the meniscus. The meniscus should be smooth, firm, and creamy white. In certain cases the meniscus may appear to be yellowed, and palpation demonstrates that the central portion of the meniscus has degenerated and does not provide substantial resistance to palpation. Full or partial tears of the meniscus should also be identified and palpated.

The meniscal root should also be clearly identified. Meniscal root tears may not be visualized well with a scope in the standard femorotibial viewing location and may be potentially better visualized by withdrawing the scope slightly from the medial compartment into the

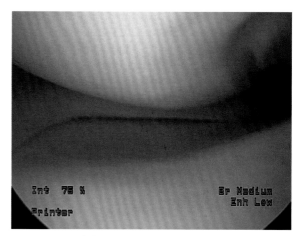

FIGURE 54.8. Medial compartment inspection.

intercondylar notch where the root can be seen more clearly. Again, abnormal morphology of the root of the meniscus, including poor visualization of the more horizontal component, suggests that there may be a tear, possibly with a displaced fragment entrapped behind the posterior femoral condyle. The articular cartilage of the knee should also be carefully inspected. Typically articular cartilage lesions in the medial compartment are often located slightly more posterior and it is important that the knee be placed through a gentle range of motion to identify the presence or absence of these hidden articular cartilage lesions. Again, the articular cartilage itself should be carefully palpated with a probe to assess the stability of any articular cartilage lesions. There is a normal distal medial femoral sulcus where the anterior horn of the medial meniscus will engage.

Occasionally, the presence of a medial collateral ligament tear or sprain can sometimes be identified by excessive medial side opening of the medial compartment. If there is significant medial side opening, the meniscus should be evaluated to find out whether it separates from the medial tibial plateau. The meniscal capsular junction can be evaluated under conditions of valgus stress and also by careful elevation of the medial meniscus. Careful palpation of the meniscus can demonstrate the stability of the meniscus or any torn attachments. In addition, careful palpation of the articular cartilage surfaces should be performed if there is concern about an osteochondritis dissecans lesion or avascular necrosis of the femoral condyle. The stability of these lesions can be assessed by careful palpation with a probe and typically the margin of the lesion can be identified with careful arthroscopic inspection.

INTERCONDYLAR NOTCH

The intercondylar notch has several structures of anatomical interest, including the anterior cruciate ligament, posterior cruciate ligament, and medial and lateral tibial eminences (Fig. 54.9). The intermeniscal ligament, the anterior insertion of the medial and lateral horns of the medial and lateral menisci, and typically a ligamentum mucosum or ligament connecting the apex of the inter-condylar notch to the fat pad can be visualized. The ligamentum mucosum (Fig. 54.10) may be very robust and if this impedes visualization, it can be resected; how-ever it does have some vascularity and can bleed. The intercondylar notch should be briefly inspected for the presence or absence of osteophytes that may be present at the margin of the intercondylar notch or in the tibial eminences. Loose bodies may also be found in the inter-condylar notch as well as synovitis. The anterior cruciate ligament should be inspected for damage (Fig. 54.11). In many patients, well-defined posterolateral and ante-rior medial bundles can be clearly identified. It is rec-ommended that the normal insertion and origin of the anterior cruciate ligament be identified as a guide to ana-tomic reconstruction in other patients. It is notable that in many patients the anterior medial bundle attaches an-terior to the posterior edge of the anterior horn of the

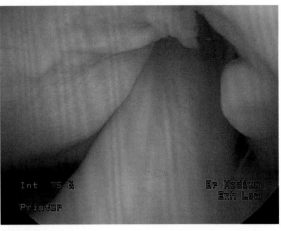

FIGURE 54.11. Anterior cruciate ligament.

lateral meniscus. The knee should be placed through a range of motion and the normal patterns of laxity of the posterolateral bundle with the knee in flexion should be observed (6). The presence or absence of synovitis or damage to the anterior cruciate ligament should be identified. If there is concern about potential damage to the ligament, a probe should be used to palpate the fibers of the ligament and determine the amount of rela-tive laxity. The ligament can undergo partial tearing or strain that can result in subsequent symptomatic insta-bility. The insertion site of the anterior cruciate ligament should be palpated. The presence or absence of an empty wall sign should also be evaluated. This is performed by visualizing the lateral intercondylar notch wall and the normal insertion site of the anterior cruciate liga-ment. This may be enhanced by placing the knee into a figure-four position with the knee flexed 90° and varus force applied. The visualization of the anterior cruciate ligament origin can sometimes be enhanced by placing the scope into the anteromedial portal. In addition, the presence or absence of cyclops lesions should be verified by visualizing the most anterior portion of the anterior cruciate ligament footprint. Occasionally a portion of the anterior cruciate ligament stump may heal in an an-terior oriented position and may not be initially seen on inspection of the intercondylar notch. Anterior inspec-tion of the intercondylar notch may also demonstrate evidence of anvil osteophytes, which may limit terminal extension of the knee.

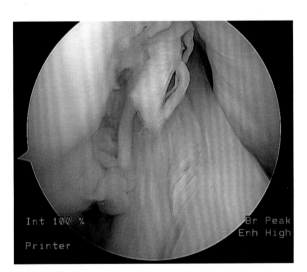

FIGURE 54.9. Intercondylar notch.

POSTERIOR CRUCIATE LIGAMENT

The posterior cruciate ligament should also be carefully inspected. The origin on the distal medial intercondylar notch can typically be well visualized, although there may be a synovial lining covering this (Fig. 54.12). The an-terolateral and posteromedial bundles of the anterior cruci-ate ligament fibers can usually be identified. Often there is no direct evidence of trauma to the posterior cruciate liga-ment, or there has been a posterior cruciate ligament injury.

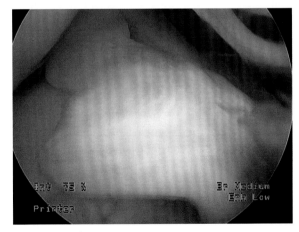

FIGURE 54.10. Ligamentum mucosum.

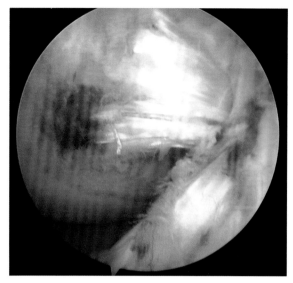

FIGURE 54.12. Posterior cruciate ligament.

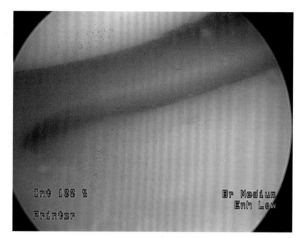

FIGURE 54.13. Meniscus.

This may be related to the overlying synovium. Secondary signs of posterior cruciate ligament insufficiency that can be identified at the time of arthroscopy include pseudolaxity of the anterior cruciate ligament. The posterior cruciate ligament should be carefully inspected and palpated during the course of the arthroscopic evaluation. An anterior and posterior drawer force can also be used to assess the presence or absence of a posterior cruciate ligament laxity.

LATERAL COMPARTMENT

Anatomic structures of interest in the lateral compartment include the articular cartilage, the distal lateral femoral condyle, the lateral tibial plateau, the lateral meniscus, and the popliteal hiatus. Again, the compartment should be opened up by a varus stress. This is typically performed by placing the knee into a figure-four position with the knee flexed to approximately 90° and gently flexed. It is often easiest to enter into the lateral compartment by placing the scope over the anterior insertion of the lateral meniscus and then gently sweeping the scope toward the lateral side visualizing laterally. The meniscus should be carefully palpated and inspected (Fig. 54.13). The normal popliteal hiatus should be visualized with the popliteus tendon passing obliquely through the hiatus (Fig. 54.14). A probe placed through a medial portal can be used to palpate the meniscus. The meniscus should be carefully palpated on its superior and inferior surfaces for the presence or absence of meniscal tears. It should be noted that the posterior horn of the lateral meniscus is much more mobile than the medial meniscus. Careful inspection of the area immediately adjacent to the popliteal hiatus should be performed because tears can extend from the popliteal hiatus.

The lateral compartment can be assessed for the amount of a lateral site opening. During this period of varus stress the amount of lateral site opening is somewhat more variable than the medial site and can be as much as 4 to 5 mm in some patients.

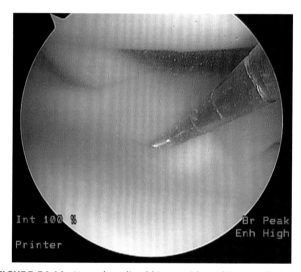

FIGURE 54.14. Normal popliteal hiatus with popliteus tendon passing obliquely through hiatus.

Palpation of the meniscus should be very carefully performed, in particular the undersurface of the posterior portion of the lateral meniscus. The convex nature of the lateral plateau lends itself to loose bodies hiding behind the posterolateral tibial plateau. Careful inspection and palpation of this area can occasionally reveal loose bodies trapped in this area. It is important for the articular cartilage surfaces to be carefully inspected and palpated. The articular cartilage of the lateral femoral condyle should be carefully inspected throughout a full range of motion. It should be noted that the sulcus terminalis, which is an indentation at the distal femur, is a normal anatomical finding marking the end of the lateral femoral tibial articulation and should not be confused with an osteochondral impaction fracture.

POSTEROMEDIAL COMPARTMENT

The posteromedial compartment consists of the recess behind the posteromedial femoral condyle. Anatomic structures that can be visualized in this area include the posterior capsule, posterior aspect of the medial femoral condyle, the posterior capsule, and the posterior horn and medial meniscus as well as the posterior cruciate ligament. Typically, entrance into the posteromedial compartment of the knee is performed by a Gillquist maneuver (7, 8), where the arthroscope is placed between the posterior cruciate ligament and the medial intercondylar notch wall. This is often easiest to perform with the knee in approximately 90° of flexion with the scope coming from either the anterior lateral portal or the Gillquist portal, which is a trans patella tendon central portal (7, 8). The scope can be gently placed into this opening directly. Alternatively, it may be easier to place the scope into the anterior medial portal with the knee flexed to 90° and visualize a switching stick placed through the anterolateral portal by using the Gillquist maneuver underneath the posterior cruciate ligament into the posteromedial compartment. The scope and scope sheath can then be removed, the sheath passed over the switching stick, and the scope passed into the posteromedial compartment. Owing to the anatomy of some knees, it may be quite difficult to access this posteromedial compartment. This is particularly true in patients with significant tibial eminence osteophytes.

In the posteromedial compartment the arthroscope can be gently rotated to visualize the various elements of the posterior capsule, the posterior horn of the medial meniscus and the posterior femoral condyle. Occasionally a synovial fold or small opening contiguous with a posterior Baker's cyst can be identified in the posterior capsule (Fig. 54.15). A posteromedial portal can be atraumatically created, as described in the previous chapter, and instrumentation can be placed into the posteromedial compartment. A switching stick can also be placed into the posteromedial compartment from the posteromedial portal, and then the scope can be placed over the switching stick and used to visualize the posteromedial compartment from a different approach. This will typically allow improved visualization of

the posterior cruciate ligament and, in particular, its tibial insertion which lies below the tibial plateau. Alternatively evaluation of the posterior cruciate ligament tibial insertion and the posteromedial compartment can be enhanced by using a 70° scope instead of a 30° scope in this area. In the posteromedial compartment loose bodies in addition to synovitis or meniscal fragments can also be identified.

POSTEROLATERAL COMPARTMENT

Anatomical features in the posterolateral compartment that can be identified are the posterolateral capsule, posterior horn of the lateral meniscus, the posterolateral capsule, and the posterior aspect of the lateral femoral condyle (Fig. 54.16). Placement of the arthroscope into the posterolateral compartment can be accomplished either from the anterior medial portal or occasionally from the anterior lateral portal. The scope is placed underneath the posterolateral bundle of the anterior cruciate ligament and the lateral intercondylar notch wall (9). A 70° scope can provide increased visualization of this compartment compared with the 30° scope. Typically, the posterolateral root insertion can be identified as well as the posterior aspect of the lateral meniscus. Loose bodies, synovitis, or meniscal fragments can be identified in this area. Instrumentation of this posterolateral compartment can be performed using a posterolateral portal and the scope can be placed in the posterolateral portal to visualize the posterior horn of the lateral meniscus and posterior capsule. The septum dividing the posteromedial and posterolateral compartments can be arthroscopically divided, which allows the posterior capsule to float posterior along and increasing the separation from between the posterior cruciate ligament and posterior neurovascular structures. This technique has been used by some authors to perform posterior cruciate ligament reconstruction from a posterior approach (10). In evaluation of the posterior cruciate ligament and the posterior horn of the lateral meniscus, it can be noted that

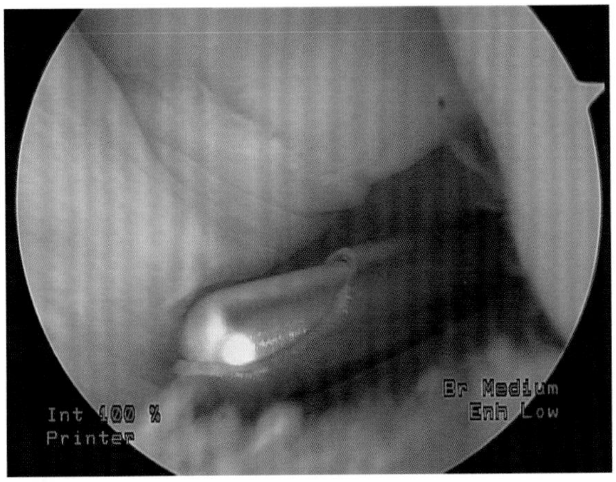

FIGURE 54.15. Synovial fold or small opening contiguous with a posterior Baker's cyst in the posterior capsule.

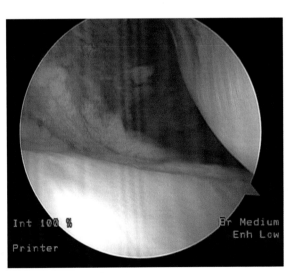

FIGURE 54.16. Posterolateral compartment.

V. A. The Knee General

the meniscal femoral ligaments can be sometimes identified including ligament of Wrisberg or Humphrey.

COMPLICATIONS, CONTROVERSIES, AND SPECIAL CONSIDERATIONS

Complications associated with diagnostic arthroscopy or evaluation of an arthroscopic anatomy include iatrogenic damage to the articular cartilage. Great care should be taken while maneuvering the arthroscope or instrumentation around the knee joint to avoid excessive pressure on articular cartilage. Vigorous or forceful movements, particularly while working in the medial lateral compartments or in the patellofemoral articulation, should be carefully avoided. The clinical significance of small areas of articular cartilage scuffing or partial thickness defects remains unknown; however it is quite clear that these do not heal. From a PubMed search there is no literature describing significant effects from arthroscopic scuffing.

Careful placement of arthroscopic portals is also critical to avoid iatrogenic damage. The author recommends the use of a spinal needle to enter into the joint prior to the creation of any arthroscopic portal. For instance, the spinal needle should be carefully observed to see whether it is above or below the anterior horn of the meniscus. Careful portal creation should also avoid placement of the instruments cutting through the anterior horn of the medial lateral menisci. Other complications associated with diagnostic arthroscopy include medial collateral ligament sprain during the course of diagnostic arthroscopy of the knee joint. The medial collateral ligament can be disrupted, resulting in a sudden pop and opening of the medial compartment. Typically, this is of relatively low clinical significance postoperatively, and these lesions typically will heal without subsequent need for significant intervention. It is recommended that postoperative bracing be applied if this is a concern postoperatively.

Other pathology related to diagnostic arthroscopy includes missed pathology such as missed loose body. This can be avoided by careful inspection of all the compartments of the knee joint, including posteromedial and posterolateral. It can also be enhanced at times by avoidance of use of outflow directly attached to the scope. In cases where a loose body is clinically suspected, inflow of arthroscopic fluid can be placed on a separate cannula or the inflow on the scope can be temporarily turned off while the new joint is being inspected. Arthrofibrosis is rare but can be a devastating complication following knee arthroscopy.

Controversies associated with diagnostic knee arthroscopy typically involve the area of antibiotic prophylaxis and venous thromboembolism prophylaxis. There is no definitive standard of care for antibiotic prophylaxis during knee arthroscopy (11). The prophylactic use of antibiotics has not been demonstrated to prove to decrease the risk of perioperative infection (12). There is also no current standard of care for the prevention of

thromboembolic disease following knee arthroscopy (13). Clinically significant thromboembolic events following knee arthroscopy in most studies are quite minimal, on the order of 0.25% (14). However, a number of prospective studies using duplex ultrasound or venogram have demonstrated the incidence of deep vein thrombosis from 8% to 18% (15). Tourniquet application is also somewhat controversial in the context of diagnostic knee arthroscopy. There does appear to be some increased incidence of complication in patients who have tourniquet application for more than 60 minutes (16). This author prefers not to use a tourniquet in view of the potential risk of deep vein thrombosis and also some limited evidence demonstrating some delay in return of quadriceps activation following the use of the tourniquet (17).

Other complications associated with diagnostic knee arthroscopy include infection. Infection rates following knee arthroscopy remain quite low. These are of the order of approximately 15% (12).

PEARLS AND PITFALLS

Pearls

1. Use a spinal needle to aim arthroscopic portals and instrumentation.
2. Move the arthroscope to an alternative portal to improve visualization.
3. Recognize that the capsular opening and skin incision change relative position with the knee flexion and extension.
4. A central patella tendon portal can increase access to the posterior compartment.
5. Posteromedial and posterolateral compartments of the knee with minimal morbidity.
6. Loose bodies are often found in the posteromedial or posterolateral compartments of the knee as well as underneath the posterior horn of the lateral meniscus.
7. The 70° scope may increase visualization of the posteromedial and posterolateral compartments.
8. Rehabilitation following diagnostic arthroscopy typically consists of range of motion, strengthening, and gait training. Attention should be paid to patella and patella tendon mobility because anterior fat pad scarring can create adhesions or loss of range of motion anteriorly.

CONCLUSIONS AND FUTURE DIRECTION

The anatomy of the knee can be more clearly and completely visualized using arthroscopic surgical techniques compared with open surgical approaches while reducing the morbidity associated with these evaluations. Increasingly sophisticated tools may allow visualization of the knee joint in three dimensions as well as evaluation of the articular cartilage at a structural level using optical coherence tomography (18). This may allow the evaluation of biomechanical parameters as well as gross visualization of articular cartilage arthroscopically. Further description of the arthroscopic anatomy of the knee joint will undoubtedly continue.

REFERENCES

1. Hardaker WT, Whipple TL, Bassett FH. Diagnosis and treatment of the plica syndrome of the knee. *J Bone Joint Surg Am.* 1980;62(2):221–225.

2. Ewing JW. Plica: pathologic or not? *J Am Acad Orthop Surg.* 1993;1:117–121.

3. Outerbridge RE. The etiology of chondromalacia patellae. *J Bone Joint Surg Br.* 1961;43:752–757.

4. Brittberg MN, Peterson L. Introduction of an articular cartilage classification. *ICRS Newsletter.* 1998;1:5–8. Available at ICRS Cartilage Evaluation Package 2000. http://www.cartilage.org/Evaluation_Package/ICRS_Evaluation.pdf. Accessed August 6, 2002.

5. Insall J, Falvo KA, Wise DW. Chondromalacia Patellae. A prospective study. *J Bone Joint Surg Am.* 1976;58(1):1–8.

6. Amis AA, Dawkins GP. Functional anatomy of the ACL. *J Bone Joint Surg Br.* 1991; 73:260–267.

7. Gillquist J, Hagberg G. New modification of the technique of arthroscopy of the knee joint. *Acta Chir Scand.* 1976;142(2):123–130.

8. Gillquist J, Hagberg G, Oretorp N. Arthroscopic examination of the posteromedial compartment of the knee joint. *Orthopedics.* 1979;3(1):13–18.

9. Morin WD, Steadman JR. Arthroscopic assessment of the posterior compartments of the knee via the intercondylar notch: the arthroscopist's field of view. *Arthroscopy.* 1993;9(3):284–290.

10. Ahn JH, Ha CW. Posterior trans-septal portal for arthroscopic surgery of the knee joint. *Arthroscopy.* 2000;16(7):774–779.

11. Kurzweil PR. Antibiotic prophylaxis for arthroscopic surgery. *Arthroscopy.* 2006;22(4):452–454.

12. Bert JM, Giannini D, Nace L. Antibiotic prophylaxis for arthroscopy of the knee: is it necessary? *Arthroscopy.* 2007;23(1):4–6.

13. Ramos J, Perrotta C, Badariotti G, et al. Interventions for preventing venous thromboembolism in adults undergoing knee arthroscopy. *Cochrane Database Syst Rev.* 2008;8(4):CD005259.

14. Maletis GB, Reynolds S, Inacio MCS. Incidence of thromboembolism after knee arthroscopy. Paper no. 340. Presented at: the American Academy of Orthopaedic Surgeons 76th Annual Meeting; February 25–28, 2009; Las Vegas, NV.

15. Ilahi OA, Reddy J, Ahmad I. Deep venous thrombosis after knee arthroscopy: a meta-analysis. *Arthroscopy.* 2005;21(6):727–730.

16. Sherman OH, Fox JM, Snyder SJ, et al. Arthroscopy—"no-problem surgery." An analysis of complications in two thousand six hundred and forty cases. *J Bone Joint Surg Am.* 1986;68(2):256–265.

17. Kirkley A, Rampersaud R, Griffin S, et al. Tourniquet versus no tourniquet use in routine knee arthroscopy: a prospective, double-blind, randomized clinical trial. *Arthroscopy.* 2000;16(2):121–126.

18. Zheng K, Martin SD, Rashidifard CH, et al. In vivo micronscale arthroscopic imaging of human knee osteoarthritis with optical coherence tomography: comparison with magnetic resonance imaging and arthroscopy. *Am J Orthop (Belle Mead NJ).* 2010;39(3):122–125.

Meniscus

Meniscus Resection

Emilio Lopez-Vidriero • Donald H. Johnson

CLINICAL EVALUATION

Pertinent History

The meniscus is commonly injured in sports, but can also occur as a sequela of age-related degeneration. In these cases, there may be no trauma, but more typically, patients report a twisting hyperflexion injury followed by pain. This acute episode may involve locking of the knee, with the development of moderate swelling over the first 24 hours. With recurrent episodes of pain and swelling, mechanical symptoms such as catching, popping, or locking are reported. The pain tends to localize along the joint line, especially with deep flexion and twisting motions.

It is important to establish symptoms of instability, because the menisci are a secondary restraint to anteroposterior translation, and certain tears can worsen in cases of an Anterior Cruciate Ligament (ACL) deficient knee.

Physical Examination

The patient is examined for signs of an effusion, loss of quadriceps bulk, and decreased range of motion (ROM). Tenderness to palpation along either the medial or the lateral joint line is among the most significant sign of a meniscal tear (Fig. 55.1A), reported statistically at 74% with a positive predictive value of 50%. The collateral and cruciate ligaments must be assessed to rule out additional injury. With an ACL-deficient knee, the sensitivity of joint line tenderness has been shown to decrease to around 50%.

Special tests for assessing the meniscus, such as the McMurray, Steinmann, and Apley tests, can aid in the diagnosis, but the McMurray test is preferred because it is easy, fast, and reliable. Also, complementary knee tests may be done in the same position. The McMurray test is performed with the patient supine, the hip flexed to 90°, and the knee in forced maximal flexion. One hand grasps the heel, the knee is steadied, and the joint line palpated with the other hand. As the knee is slowly taken into extension, external rotation stress will test the medial meniscus, whereas internal rotation stress tests the lateral meniscus (Fig. 55.1B). As a mnemonic rule, the heel of the foot points toward the injured meniscus. The result of the test is considered positive when the patient feels pain in the appropriate joint line accompanied by a thud or click. When the clunk is present, the test has a sensitivity of 98% but, due to the fact that not always is possible to evoke the clunk, its specificity is only 15%.

In conclusion, the hallmarks of a meniscal tear are presence of an effusion, joint line tenderness, and positive McMurray test. When history and physical examination are used together, the overall sensitivity to diagnose a meniscal tear, confirmed with arthroscopy, is around 95% with a specificity of 88%.

Diagnostic Imaging

Evaluation of a meniscal tear should include routine AP and lateral X-rays of the knee. If degenerative changes are expected, standing views including a 45° flexion PA view should be performed to assess the degree of joint space narrowing. Assessing osteoarthritis is important to counsel the patient about expectations of success, because the degree of arthrosis before surgery predicts poorer postoperative results in the short and long term.

Although not clinically indicated in all patients, MRI is valuable in evaluating the full range of meniscal pathology. This includes the primary diagnosis of a meniscal tear, detection of a recurrent tear after resection or repair, and demonstration of associated injuries. MRI shows the relative locations of the tears and determines the presence of a meniscal tear with an accuracy of over 90%. It provides an accurate noninvasive technique for evaluating meniscal tears, especially when combined with pertinent history, and physical examination. This is particularly important when treating young adults, where tears can be completely asymptomatic.

Decision Making: Indications and Contraindications

Meniscectomy is indicated when the type of tear will not heal spontaneously, or in those cases where a repair is not possible. Although the technology is improving and the indications for repair are increasing, arthroscopic partial meniscectomy is still indicated in 80% of the tears (Table 55.1).

FIGURE 55.1. A: Palpating for joint line tenderness. The most sensitive sign for meniscal tear. **B:** The Mc-Murray test. As a mnemonic rule, the heel of the foot points toward the injured meniscus. The result of the test is considered positive when the patient feels pain in the appropriate joint line accompanied by a thud or click.

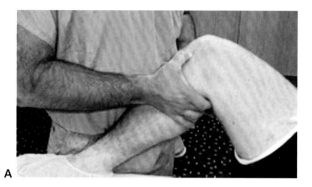

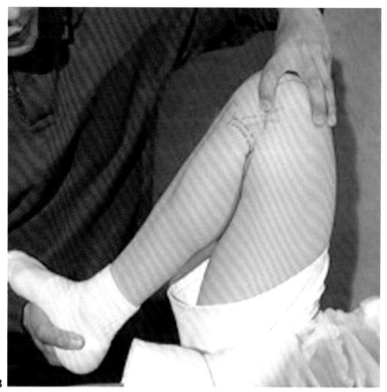

Factors to consider when deciding whether to resect or to repair a meniscal tear are location of the tear, morphology, size, chronicity, and inherent patient factors.

In terms of location, tears in the white–white zone are resected because, according to Arnoczky, they have a low degree of vascularity and their chances of healing are very low. If the tear is in the white–red zone, the other abovementioned factors will inform the decision.

When morphology is taken into account, horizontal cleavage tears, radial lateral tears, and degenerative bucket handle tears of the meniscus are not usually considered repairable. Tears larger than 20 mm in size are normally resected.

Generally, tears are considered chronic after 8 to 12 weeks. Usually the meniscus becomes shredded, or degenerative with time, and is no longer suitable for repair.

In terms of the patients' age, there may be less vascularity and cellularity in the older meniscus and thus less healing potential. The older patient often has a degenerative tear that is not repairable. There is no age limit to a meniscus repair, but most surgeons would favor resection over repair in patients over 40 to 50 years of age.

Patients with an acute ACL injury often have a small posterior flap tear of the lateral meniscus. Although there is some controversy, most people feel that this should simply be resected.

In the chronic unstable ACL-deficient knee, a meniscus tear should be resected, unless the ACL is reconstructed. Due to the abnormal kinematics of the ACL-deficient knee, the failure rate of meniscal repair in the unstable knee is much higher than the stable or reconstructed knee.

Table 55.1

Indications for meniscectomy. This table summarizes clinical situations where meniscectomy is preferred over repair

Meniscal Tear Factors	
Location	White–white
Morphology	Horizontal clavage Radial lateral Degenerative bucket handle
Size	>20 mm
Chronicity	>8–12 wk
Patient factors	
Age	>40 y old
ACL acute-deficient knee	Small posterior flap tear in lateral meniscus
ACL chronic-deficient knee	All types of tears
Rehabilitation	Noncompliant patient

Where patients are noncompliant with rehabilitation programs, resection is the better option.

Classification

Meniscus tears may be classified by the location of a tear relative to its blood supply and its vascular appearance. The peripheral and central surfaces can be clinically graded as white (relatively avascular) or red (vascular) at the time of arthroscopy. This classification is based on anatomic studies that have depicted a peripheral vascular zone. [*Include a line drawing*]

A red–red tear is defined as a peripheral capsular detachment, and it has the best prognosis for healing. Unfortunately, a significant portion of tears occur in the white–white zone, the central, avascular portion of the meniscus, and theoretically are unable to heal. The red–white (Fig. 55.2) are meniscal rim tears through the peripheral vascular zone of the meniscus. While the central portion of this tear exists in the avascular zone, theoretically, these lesions should have sufficient vascularity to heal by fibrovascular proliferation.

Conventional wisdom dictates that meniscal repairs be limited to the peripheral vascular area of the meniscus (i.e., the red–red and red–white tears). Both experimental and clinical evidence suggests that white–white tears are incapable of healing, even in the presence of surgical suturing, and has provided the rational for partial meniscectomy. In an effort to extend the zone of repair more peripherally, techniques such as the creation of vascular access channels by trephination, synovial abrasion, and the use of a fibrin clot have been developed.

Meniscal tears can also be classified by their *stability* (Table 55.2). A tear is considered unstable when it is more than half the length of the meniscus and subluxes under the femoral condyle when probed with a hook (Fig. 55.3). This concept is especially important in deciding treatment options: leave alone, trephinate, resect, or repair.

Table 55.2

Criteria of stability defined arthroscopically using the probe

Cannot be displaced into the intercondylar notch
The inner edge of the meniscus cannot touch the central part of the femoral condyle
Length of the tear less than 10 mm

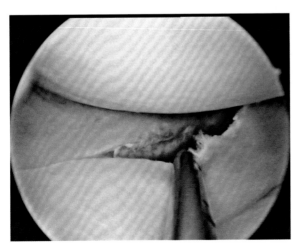

FIGURE 55.2. Longitudinal vertical tear in the red–white zone.

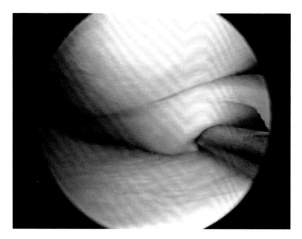

FIGURE 55.3. Unstable longitudinal vertical tear. Note how it subluxes under the femoral condyle when probed.

Stable tears, which occur particularly in the posterior aspect of the meniscus and which do not subluxate into the joint, may be left alone (Fig. 55.4A–C).

Tears can be described according to their *morphology* and based on their *configuration*. Under these criteria, tears can be vertical or horizontal, depending on whether the line of the lesion goes from superior to inferior (vertical) (Figs. 55.3 and 55.4), or from inside to outside (horizontal), and commonly called "open book" or "fish mouth" (Fig. 55.5). Moreover, tears can be described as longitudinal (Figs. 55.3 and 55.4) if the pattern is from anterior to posterior, or transverse, and are also called radial or "parrot beak" (Fig. 55.6). Combinations of these four basic patterns make up the others types of tears: the oblique, being vertical and radial or the so-called bucket handle, which is a vertical-longitudinal tear that is unstable, and subluxes completely under the condyle (Figs. 55.3 and 55.7A–C). Lastly, the complex tear is a combination of all, usually in the degenerative setting, and located in the posterior horn of the medial meniscus (Fig. 55.8).

Longitudinal-vertical tears usually occur in younger patients, in association with an ACL tear, and more frequently in the medial meniscus because it is less mobile. Oblique tears tend to appear between the medial and the posterior third of the meniscus. They may cause mechanical symptoms of entrapment and pain, due to the tension on the meniscus–capsule junction.

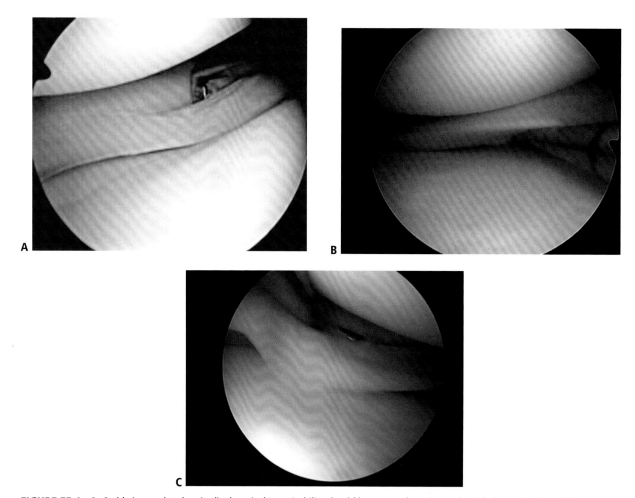

FIGURE 55.4. A: Stable incomplete longitudinal vertical tear. Stability should be assessed continuously with the probe. **B:** Stable incomplete longitudinal vertical tear. Probing under the meniscus is a key to assess stability. **C:** Stable complete longitudinal vertical tear. Probing over the meniscus may show a complete tear. Some longitudinal-vertical tears although complete may also be stable.

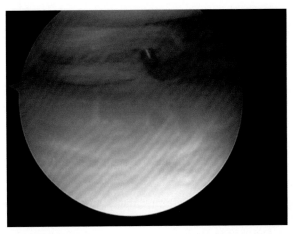

FIGURE 55.5. Horizontal degenerative tear. Note how it opens with the use of the probe. Some of these tears may reach the meniscocapsular junction.

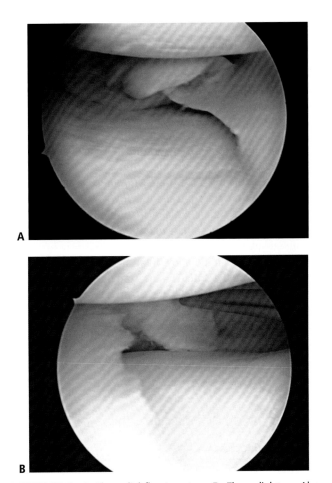

FIGURE 55.6. A: The radial flap-type tear. **B:** The radial tear. Also called "parrot beak."

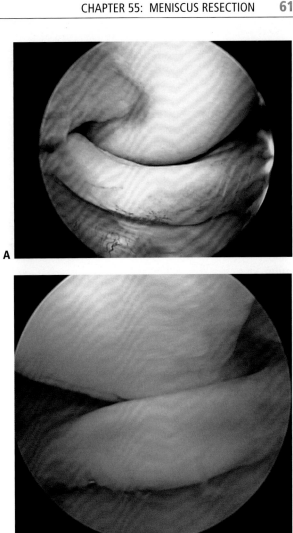

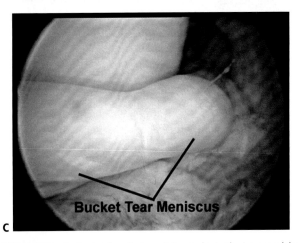

FIGURE 55.7. A: Bucket handle tear dislocated into the intercondylar notch. This meniscus is torn in the red–white zone. Note the vascular supply to the dislocated fragment. Some of these tears are amenable to repair. **B:** Bucket handle tear that dislocates into the intercondylar notch when probed. Note the chondral lesion on the condyle. **C:** Irreducible bucket handle tear.

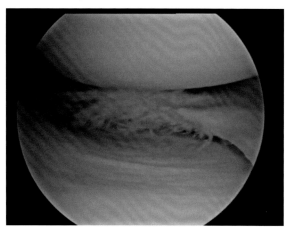

FIGURE 55.8. Complex tear. These tears are usually located in the posterior horn of the medial meniscus and are associated with degeneration.

Horizontally shaped tears usually begin as intrasubstance degeneration in the middle of the meniscus and migrate toward the free surface. Often, they extend to the capsular junction and can cause the formation of a cyst. As the cyst grows, the patient may experience pain and tenderness. Cysts appear more frequently in the lateral meniscus, and are filled with a gel-like substance, chemically similar to synovial fluid. These cysts have been reported to be 1% to 10% of the meniscal pathology.

Complex tears appear mainly in older patients and are usually associated with cartilage degeneration. They are considered to be part of the process of arthrosis and degenerative arthropathy. Due to their complex pattern, the fragments can be unstable and cause mechanical symptoms. The associated histologic pathology is myxoid degeneration, hyaline acellular degeneration, and dystrophic calcification.

Timing is also important in decision making. Tears can be either acute, with a greater chance of healing, or chronic, associated with complex patterns and degeneration and requiring resection. In general, a tear is considered chronic 8 to 12 weeks after the lesion occurred.

The *cause or mechanism* of the tear should be determined. If the tear is traumatic, as commonly found in young, active patients and is diagnosed acutely, there is a greater chance of success. Conversely, degenerative complex tears usually occur in older patients, and are associated with arthrosis. Whether they are a cause or a consequence of the osteoarthritic process is still unknown.

Finally, tears can be classified by whether they are medial or lateral. Metcalf observed that 69% of the tears affected the medial meniscus, whereas the lateral was affected 24% of the time. In his review, both menisci were torn at the same time in 7% of the patients. Moreover, 80% of the tears were vertical or oblique and affected the posterior medial part of the meniscus.

In summary, the most common meniscal tears are

- Chronic, degenerative, horizontal, or complex in medial meniscus (Fig. 55.5). They usually occur insidiously in older patients and need resecting.
- Acute, traumatic, longitudinal, and vertical in medial meniscus (Fig. 55.2). Seen more often in the younger patient, they can potentially be repaired.

TREATMENT OPTIONS

Conservative

The patient should be informed that some meniscal tears become asymptomatic after several months of protection of the joint. During this period, conservative treatment consists of ice, nonsteroidal anti-inflammatory drug (NSAID), modified activities, and protected weight bearing. The best activity is an exercise bike with the seat in a high position. The patient should also be counseled to avoid full squats. If the patient is willing to modify activities and has no pain or swelling, then conservative management of the tear may be successful.

ARTHROSCOPIC TECHNIQUE

If the patient continues to have pain, swelling, locking, or catching symptoms and wants surgical treatment, then operative intervention is indicated.

There are several surgical principles that should be followed to achieve good outcomes. First, and following the Hippocratic principle of "primum non nocere" (First do no harm), do not make the situation worse. If there is a stable, vertical tear in a young patient, it should be left alone and not resected. Second, portal placement should be accurate enough to allow good visualization of the entire meniscus. In addition, portals should allow instruments to be introduced without scuffing the articular surface. Third, when resection is performed, the main objective is to achieve a stable peripheral rim by removing any unstable fragments that could cause mechanical symptoms or pain (Fig. 55.9). During meniscectomy, it is important to contour the edges in order to have a smooth border and avoid progression to a second tear. The probe should be used in order to assess stability of

Surgical principles for meniscectomy
Surgical principles
Primum non nocere (firstly do not harm)
Good access for viewing and instruments
Achieve stable rim: remove any unstable fragments of meniscus
Smooth border: to contour the edges
Use the probe constantly
Protect meniscocapsular junction
Stimulate healing: rasp, trephination, marrow, plasma rich in growth factors

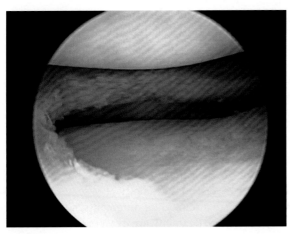

FIGURE 55.9. Post-meniscectomy appearance. Note the stable rim and the smooth shape of the remnant of the meniscus.

the rim. Twenty-five percent of bucket handle tears have a secondary tear of the rim that might be missed. If a complete meniscectomy is performed, care should be taken to prevent excessive bleeding from the meniscocapsular junction. Last, after meniscectomy, or when the tear is left alone, stimulation of healing helps to improve the results. This can be done by rasping the synovium, trephinating the meniscus to allow vascularization, and perforating the notch to cause bleeding. The penetration of the subchondral bone in the notch allows bone marrow mesenchymal cells into the field. Finally, adding autologous plasma rich in growth factors, and cytokines may optimize the healing environment.

Preparation and Portal Placement

Patient positioning must allow circumferential access to the affected knee. The leg should be prepped and draped to allow posteromedial and posterolateral incisions, should they be required in the case of a repair (Fig. 55.10). This can be done with the patient supine, such that the break in the table is at the level of the tourniquet, and the knee can be flexed to 90°. Alternatively, a leg holder can be used

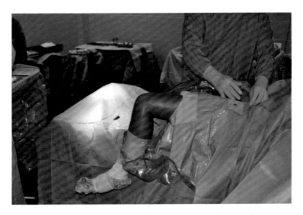

FIGURE 55.10. Setup for meniscectomy. Note that it allows circumferential access to the affected knee. The knee can be positioned in figure of four on the table to access the lateral meniscus and in valgus on the surgeons waist to access the medial meniscus.

that allows the surgeon to abduct the leg from the operating table, allowing the knee to flex for access.

The anterolateral portal is used to place the scope for visualization. The portal is vertical at the edge of the patellar tendon and at the inferior border of the patella. This high lateral portal allows the scope to be above the fat pad, avoiding putting the tip of the scope into the fat pad, "fat padoscopy." It is also central enough to allow visualization of the posterior notch. A superolateral portal is made in the pouch to allow drainage and lavage and improve visualization.

Diagnostic arthroscopy is performed using a 30° arthroscope. This includes an evaluation of the suprapatellar pouch, both menisci, articular cartilage, and cruciate ligaments. After diagnosis, and based on the type of the tear, the medial portal is established. With the help of the finger, the medial soft spot is located. A spinal needle is placed to confirm the position of the new portal. The tip of the needle should be able to reach the area of the meniscal tear. The scope is rotated to view the needle. It is essential to avoid cutting the meniscus or damaging the articular surface of the medial condyle. The medial portal is made with an 11 blade in an oblique direction to allow increasing the size of the portal, if needed. Making the incision obliquely also reduces the risk of cutting the articular surface with the blade. After the portals are established, the menisci are probed on the inferior and superior surfaces to identify any tears. In assessing meniscal stability, it is important to remember that the lateral meniscus is normally more mobile, up to 10 mm. The definition of an unstable meniscal tear is one that is half the length of the meniscus, and subluxes under the condyle when probed with a hook (Table 55.1).

Although a tourniquet may be used to improve visualization during the procedure, some surgeons prefer to leave it deflated for the diagnostic arthroscopy, in order to assess the vascularity of the meniscal tear after rasping. Resection of the medial meniscus is usually done close to extension and with valgus stress (Fig. 55.11A). In ACL-deficient patients, note that the lateral compartment will sublux anteriorly in internal rotation. The medial spine will obscure the visualization of the posterior horn of the medial meniscus. In order to get to the posterior horn of the medial meniscus, the assistant should perform external rotation of the tibia by holding the ankle or the foot (Fig. 55.11B).

In the case of a very tight knee, an 18G needle may be used to "pie crust" the medial ligament over the tibia. When valgus stress is placed on the MCL, sufficient opening will allow access to the posterior horn.

On the lateral side, the best visualization is obtained with the knee flexed, and the leg placed in the figure-of-four position. This position is also key in protecting the peroneal nerve, which lies posterior to the biceps femoris tendon, and farthest from the joint capsule with the knee in flexion.

Resection Techniques

The technique is determined by the type of tear. The success of the resection is significantly affected by instrument

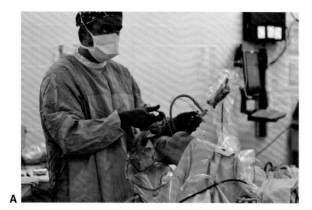

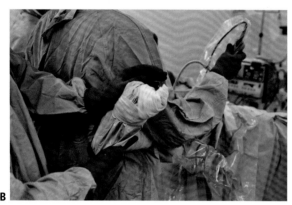

FIGURE 55.11. A: Positioning of the surgeon for medial meniscectomy on a left knee. The leg is placed in valgus and 10° of flexion. Note that the scope is held on the very end allowing the surgeon to use the elbow to hold the leg in case needed. **B:** Meniscectomy in the ACL-deficient knee. The access to the medial compartment is difficult due to the anteriorly and internal rotation pivoted knee. In order to improve visualization, the assistant may reduce the subluxated knee by externally rotating the affected knee.

access to the surgery site. The most common limiting factors are poor portal placement, a tight compartment, or instrument geometry. In general, the principles of partial meniscectomy are to remove as little tissue as possible to maintain stability of the remaining meniscal rim.

Approach to the Medial Meniscus

Begin at the extreme posterior attachment. To view the resection directly, the scope is passed into the medial compartment. The tip of the scope is kept positioned toward the tibia, and the telescope rotated to look up under the condyle. This throws light into the posterior area and prevents scuffing of the femoral condyle with the scope tip. Then, a meniscal up-curved punch designed to fit under the curve of condyle is used on tears of the posterior horn of the medial meniscus. When inserting the punch, it should be left closed until it is in place next to the meniscal tear and posterior to the curve of the condyle. It is then advanced posteriorly. This way the insertion is easier, and iatrogenic lesions to the cartilage are avoided. Next, advance the upper jaw of the instrument just above the

superior surface of the area intended for resection. Once positioned with the selected segment between the jaws, they are closed, resecting the tear vertically. This step should be repeated circumferentially until the leaflet is resected completely. The side-angled basket is also used as the resection proceeds anteriorly. In order to prevent the pushing away effect of the basket, certain maneuvers can be performed by the assistant. One maneuver is to apply digital pressure on the posterior capsule, stabilizing the superior leaflet so it can be seen and resected.

Moving to the anterior aspect, a straight large basket is used to resect the length of a segment of about 1 cm. Then, the remaining fragments adjacent to the medial collateral ligament are resected with an angled basket. When the mid-portion of the medial meniscus is approached, it may be resected by changing the scope to the medial portal and inserting the basket through the lateral portal. Between resections with hand instruments, a small diameter intra-articular shaver can be used to smooth any rough scalloping and develop a well-contoured rim between resected areas. The shaver with suction also removes semi-attached fragments from the rim border to improve visualization and determine if further resection is needed. Angled small and large baskets can also be used to resect the posterior one-third. It is advisable to carefully monitor the process to ensure adequate resection.

Ideally, resection of the posterior medial meniscus leaves an approximate 2 to 3 mm rim, which is gradually beveled through the middle to the anterior one-third.

Where resection of the anterior horn is required, back-biting cutters are available. Alternatively, place the arthroscope in the medial portal and the instruments in the lateral portal. Rotary basket cutters can also be used for resection of the anterior horn. Isolated anterior horn tears are relatively rare, occurring most often in combination with bucket handle tears.

Approach to the Lateral Meniscus

The arthroscope is inserted through the anterolateral portal. The basket cutters are used through the medial portal to resect the mid-portion of the lateral meniscus. The posterior horn cannot be approached this way. Thus, the lateral portal is used for instruments and the medial portal for the scope. Resection of the anterior one-third of the meniscus of right knee is performed by using the left rotary basket, inserted through the medial portal. The intra-articular shaver is used frequently, interspersed with the left or right rotary baskets.

Resecting a Displaced Bucket Handle Tear

In tears of the medial meniscus, the anteriorly displaced fragment (Fig. 55.7A–C) obscures visualization of the medial compartment and the posterior region of the tear. Assessment of the rim may be done before the tear is reduced to ascertain if a repair is possible.

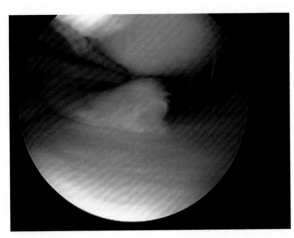

FIGURE 55.12. Bucket handle tear once resected its posterior attachment. The flap is still attached to the anterior horn avoiding it to move freely in the joint.

The first step is to improve visualization by reducing the fragment with the probe or the blunt trocar from the arthroscope. Valgus stress must be applied to perform the reduction.

Next, use the arthroscopic scissors to cut the posterior horn attachment. Cutting this first prevents the fragment from displacing into the posterior compartment after cutting the anterior horn. The scope may have to be placed into the intercondylar notch and the depth of the cut assessed from there (Fig. 55.12).

The anterior attachment is cut as close to the axilla of the tear as possible, leaving a minuscule attachment to prevent the fragment from moving away.

Finally, the end of the fragment is grasped and removed from the joint. The rim should be contoured with the 4-mm shaver. Be sure to hook the remaining rim, as there is a secondary tear in 25% of cases.

If there is a tear in the rim, resect any unstable portion.

If it is impossible to reduce the chronic displaced bucket handle on the medial side, the anterior attachment may be cut first. A grasper is used to place tension on the end of the bucket handle fragment, and cutting scissors are inserted through the same portal to cut under the posterior horn attachment. This cut is "blind" and careful monitoring of the depth of the cut is important to prevent posterior neurovascular injury.

The technique is similar for lateral displaced bucket handle tears.

Resection of a Radial Lateral Meniscus Tear

A radial tear (Fig. 55.6A, B) of the lateral meniscus is approached with instruments from the medial portal. The straight basket is used to resect the posterior edge, and the 90° basket is used to resect the anterior edge. The small shaver is used to further contour the meniscus. This has to be resected back to a normal appearing rim. The body of the meniscus will often have a degenerative mucoid appearance that must be resected.

Resection of the Lateral Meniscal Tears Associated with a Cyst

This tear is approached in much the same fashion as described for the radial tear. The entrance to the cyst is usually below the meniscus and can be entered with a small shaver. External digital palpation of the cyst will cause some ganglion-like fluid to enter the joint through the entrance made by the shaver. The suction on the shaver is used to evacuate the cyst. No external excision of the cyst is necessary if the meniscectomy is adequate.

Resection of the Discoid Lateral Meniscus

Often the central tear of the discoid meniscus will be difficult to visualize. The center of the meniscus is probed with a hook, and the delamination or tear is then palpated. The basket forceps are brought through the medial portal and the central portion is resected back to a normal appearing rim of lateral meniscus. It is important to probe the rim to be certain that it is attached and not unstable. Rarely, a Wrisberg type of lateral meniscus will be encountered that does not have any peripheral attachments, and a suture repair of the rim must be performed.

Bakers Cyst and Degenerative Medial Meniscal Tears

In most instances, once the degenerative medial meniscus is resected, recurrent effusions are controlled, and the symptoms of pain and swelling due to the Baker's cyst will diminish. Occasionally, with a very large symptomatic cyst, and a degenerative medial meniscal tear associated with degeneration of the medial compartment, the Baker's cyst must be addressed. A posteromedial portal is made with the scope in the lateral portal and then advanced, under the Posterior Cruciate Ligament (PCL), into the posteromedial compartment. The overlapping flaps of the Baker's cyst are identified, and with a shaver through the posteromedial portal, the inferior flap is resected to leave an opening into the cyst. The cyst will then drain into the joint and remain decompressed. Once joint effusion is controlled, the Baker's cyst will gradually shrink.

In cases of a chronic Baker's cyst, the shaver may have to be introduced into the cyst through a separate percutaneous puncture, and the cyst walls resected. The scope is introduced into the cyst through the opening made in the posterior capsule to monitor the progress of the cyst wall excision.

SPECIAL CONSIDERATIONS: ACL RECONSTRUCTION AND MENISCECTOMY

Finding a meniscal tear during ACL surgery is not an uncommon situation, with studies showing rates of 30% to 57%. A predominance of lateral meniscal tears has been demonstrated with acute ACL rupture, whereas the incidence of medial meniscal tears increases significantly with chronic ACL deficiency. This suggests that lateral meniscal tears occur at the time of injury to the ACL or very soon after injury, whereas medial meniscal tears are acquired after the knee has been ACL deficient.

Treatment decisions are especially important in these cases. Deciding to leave certain types of tears can shorten the duration of the procedure and yet, still produce good outcomes. Stability is the key and an arthroscopic definition of stability is a tear that does not sublux under the condyles, or one less than 10 mm long. The bleeding environment, along with the stable knee, facilitates healing after surgery. Taking that into account, some surgeons consider that the radial tear of the lateral meniscus can also be saved during ACL reconstruction. Shelbourne advocates leaving the short stable vertical tear located posterior to the popliteus tendon and the posterior horn avulsion. He has shown in his long-term follow-up that they are asymptomatic. In his series of stable peripheral vertical tears of the medial meniscus treated with trephination and abrasion, he has a 94% success rate.

Based on a systematic review of the literature, Pujol et al. have proposed to leave the stable tears on the lateral side. On the other hand, they found that the literature shows that medial meniscus tears left untreated have failed in about 50% of the cases. Failure is defined as pain, locking, or any other clinical meniscal symptoms, and proof of nonhealing in any image test, such as arthro-MRI, normal MRI, or arthroscopy. Therefore, they advise either repair or resection. In cases of ACL reconstruction with a tear in the lateral meniscus that could not be left, repair is preferable to resection, due to the lateral meniscus's important role in stability. A repaired lateral meniscus has a potential role in reducing anterior translation, thereby protecting the graft from undesirable stresses that could lead to failure.

In terms of timing, ACL surgery with concomitant meniscal tear, should be performed before the 3rd month postinjury, according to the findings of Papastergiou et al. They found that the prevalence of a meniscal tear needing treatment increases significantly after this period. In their study, the prevalence of a meniscal tear in the first 3 months after the traumatic injury was around 45%, increasing up to 69% after the 6th month. Considering that the prevalence of medial meniscal tears increases with time, they concluded ACL reconstruction in the early period would reduce the risk of secondary meniscal tears.

POSTOPERATIVE REHABILITATION

The goals of rehabilitation after meniscectomy are to diminish the swelling, regain full ROM, and obtain thigh strength similar to the nonoperative knee.

Some studies support physical therapy after partial meniscectomy versus no treatment. The studies that measured the isokinetic knee extensor strength have shown that the speed of strength recovery is significantly faster with physiotherapy (3 weeks) compared with no treatment (7 to 12 weeks).

Although controlled physiotherapy is advisable after surgery, especially in noncompliant patients, a systematic literature review has shown that a supervised physiotherapy program, plus written and verbal advice after arthroscopic partial meniscectomy, is no more effective than written and verbal advice alone. In this same study, the authors conclude that for those patients who have undergone an uncomplicated arthroscopic partial meniscectomy, physical therapy is not necessary, as it will have little or no effect on their return to activities of daily living.

Rehabilitation after meniscectomy can be as aggressive as is tolerated by the patient, but as such, pain management during surgery and in the early postoperative period is crucial. The use of intra-articular, and portal injection with long-lasting anesthetics (bupivacain or ropivacain), combined with oral analgesics and anti-inflammatories facilitates early ROM exercises. The use of local anesthetics is also beneficial to minimize the use of opioids. If no other procedures have been performed, the patient is allowed partial weight-bearing immediately after the surgery. In cases of concomitant chondral treatment or ACL surgery, individualized protocols should be followed.

The first days are focused on decreasing swelling. This can be performed with the assistance of a physiotherapist, using draining massage, ROM exercises, electrotherapy, and cryotherapy. The use of self-controlled continuous passive motion (CPM) devices can also be helpful to control swelling. Following uncomplicated meniscectomies, some surgeons do not refer patients to physiotherapists. Rather, the patient is instructed to use cryotherapy intermittently in the early postoperative period, with elevation of the leg and ambulation as tolerated. Oral anti-inflammatories are used for 5 days after surgery, and other analgesics, such as acetaminophen, are allowed as needed.

In addition to swelling control, ROM exercises are encouraged. Once full ROM is achieved, strengthening exercises are introduced to rebuild muscle mass in the thigh, equal to the other thigh. Our protocol for meniscectomy is to examine the patient 1 week after surgery to check the portals for infection, assess the ROM, and evaluate for deep venous phlebitis or septic arthritis. If there are no complications and the ROM is good, the patient is advised to ride a stationary bike, resume strengthening of quadriceps and hamstrings in the gym, and return to normal activities. Usually, the use of the bicycle is better tolerated in the first phase, and muscle-specific exercises are recommended after several weeks. Once full strength compared with the other knee is obtained, sports-specific activities are authorized.

In the case of problems such as stiffness or weakness, the patient is sent to controlled physiotherapy, and individualized rehabilitation protocols are begun.

COMPLICATIONS

The overall complication rate of knee arthroscopy is relatively low. It has been estimated in retrospective series of 118,590 and 395,566 arthroscopies to be 0.8% and 0.5%, respectively.

In a prospective study reviewing 10,262 procedures, Small found an overall complication rate of 1.68%. The most common complications in this study were hemarthrosis (60.1%), infection (12.1%), thromboembolic disease (6.9%), anesthetic complications (6.4%), instrument failure (2.9%), complex regional pain syndrome 1 (CRPS 1) (2.3%), ligament injury (1.2%), and fracture or neurologic injury (0.6% each).

Operative complications are usually iatrogenic and may be avoided with a careful surgical technique. During surgery, several structures may be damaged, such as the medial collateral ligament, neurovascular structures, meniscal, and cartilage tissues.

Medial collateral injury during arthroscopic maneuvers may occur. Leg holders or posts are commonly used to aid exposure, particularly of the posterior horn of the medial meniscus. In order to achieve better exposure, valgus force is applied. If the force is not applied judiciously, a medial collateral ligament injury may result. This is especially true of a tight medial compartment in middle-aged or elderly patients having less-flexible soft tissue.

Small reported a 0.003% of medial collateral injury in his series, where 90% were attributed to the use of the leg holder. Usual treatment is functional bracing with initial restriction of extension

Neurologic damage can occur during arthroscopic meniscectomy. Rodeo et al. reported four possible mechanisms for it. These are (1) direct trauma, (2) pressure secondary to compartment syndrome occurring as a result of extravasation of fluid, (3) damage related to the use of a tourniquet, and (4) dysfunction due to the ill-understood condition of CRPS 1.

Nerve injury to the sensitive branches innervating the knee can cause numbness and/or neuropathic pain. This can happen in the anterior part of the knee when preparing the portals. On the medial side, the infragenicular branches of the saphenous nerve (IGBSN) are most vulnerable to injury.

Although "safe zones" have been advocated, the wide variability in the course of the nerve precludes the absolute avoidance of damage. Mochida et al. recommended that arthroscopic portals should be positioned close to both the patella and the patellar tendon if injury to the IGBSN is to be avoided.

Another complication that can occur during portal preparation is iatrogenic section of the anterior horn of menisci. This can be avoided by palpating the soft point for the anterolateral portal and creating the anteromedial portal under direct arthroscopic visualization. It is advisable to cut upward with the knife away from the meniscus rather than downward.

Iatrogenic lesions to the cartilage can also occur when inserting instruments. It is important not to use a sharp trocar to introduce the arthroscope into the knee. A portal of adequate size should be made so that a blunt obturator can be used. To avoid cartilage damage during an arthroscopic procedure, always direct instruments to the intercondylar notch gently. After that, control the instrument's position with the scope and then direct it where needed.

Postoperative complications may also occur, such as joint effusion, residual pain, infection, and thromboembolism.

Joint effusion after surgery can be due to either hydrarthrosis or hemarthrosis. Hydrarthrosis is usually a consequence of synovitis. This could be due to previous knee osteoarthritis or to aggressive use of the joint during rehabilitation or the daily activities.

On the other hand, hemarthrosis is usually a consequence of extended meniscal excisions reaching the vascular zone or even the capsule. This complication can cause intense pain and loss of ROM in the knee. If the joint is under high tension, evacuation might be needed. Preoperatively, infiltrating with local anesthetic and adrenalin may be of help. Rarely, a second arthroscopy is needed to cauterize the bleeding vessel. To avoid this complication, some surgeons do not use the tourniquet or they deflate it before finishing the arthroscopy. This way bleeding points can be controlled and cauterized with the aid of electrical devices. In addition, preserving as much of the meniscal tissue as possible, mainly the rim, and avoiding sectioning the capsule will prevent bleeding.

Joint effusion, in general, is managed with evacuation, rest, elevation, and ice. If it persists, the judicious use of a cortisone injection is indicated.

Infection rates of arthroscopic meniscectomy are similar to other basic arthroscopic procedures. Kirchhoff reported an incidence of infection in elective arthroscopy of 0.42%. In knee arthroscopy, Sherman et al. reported an incidence of 0.1%, DeLee of 0.08%, D'Angelo et al. of 0.23%, and Armstrong et al. of 0.42%. This serious complication may be avoided with the use of antibiotic prophylaxis; however, Bert has shown that routine antibiotic administration does not reduce the rate of post-op septic arthritis.

The appearance of a septic arthritis postmeniscectomy must be treated aggressively. The most common infecting organism is *Staphylococcus aureus*. In the treatment protocol, arthroscopic debridement and intravenous antibiotics should be included. CPM is recommended, as soon as the patient tolerates it.

The overall incidence of thromboembolic disease in knee arthroscopy is approximately 0.1%. Thromboembolism is even more infrequent after meniscectomy, due to the short duration of the procedure and the immediate mobility after surgery. There is no indication for routine thromboprophylaxis in arthroscopic surgery, but the operating and tourniquet times should be kept to a minimum, and postoperative mobilization should be as rapid as possible. Chemoprophylaxis should be considered only in patients with high risk, particularly those with previous thromboembolism.

PEARLS

1. Use drainage from the superolateral portal to improve visualization
2. Use vertical/oblique incisions in case portal augmentation will be needed
3. Use external rotation and valgus to view the posthorn of the medial meniscus
4. Use figure of four to view the lateral compartment
5. Use the "pie crusting" technique on the MCL to open the medial compartment in a tight knee
6. Use the probe constantly

CONCLUSIONS AND FUTURE DIRECTIONS

The arthroscopic technique offers advantages and better outcomes over the open procedure, as does partial over total meniscectomy. In general, the literature has shown consistently good to excellent results in 80% to 95% of patients who have undergone arthroscopic partial meniscectomy, in the short term. In the long term, results are more controversial.

Although meniscectomy is still the most frequent procedure nowadays, there is an increasing interest in preserving techniques because of a better understanding of the role of the menisci. Moreover, the new biologic enhancing techniques and tissue engineering may be the near future of the treatment of meniscal pathology.

ACKNOWLEDGEMENTS

Fundacion Caja Madrid

SUGGESTED READINGS

Levy IM, Torzilli PA, Warren RF. The effect of medial meniscectomy on anterior-posterior motion of the knee. *J Bone Joint Surg Am.* 1982;64(6):883–888.

King D. The healing of semilunar cartilages. 1936. *Clin Orthop Relat Res.* 1990;252:4–7.

Arnoczky SP, Warren RF. Microvasculature of the human meniscus. *Am J Sports Med.* 1982;10(2):90–95.

Fitzgibbons RE, Shelbourne KD. "Aggressive" nontreatment of lateral meniscal tears seen during anterior cruciate ligament reconstruction. *Am J Sports Med.* 1995;23(2):156–159.

Shelbourne KD, Benner RW. Correlation of joint line tenderness and meniscus pathology in patients with subacute and chronic anterior cruciate ligament injuries. *J Knee Surg.* 2009;22(3):187–190. *Am J Sports Med.* 1995;23(2): 166–169.

Fabricant PD, Rosenberger PH, Jokl P, et al. Predictors of short-term recovery differ from those of long-term outcome after arthroscopic partial meniscectomy. *Arthroscopy.* 2008;24(7):769–778.

Englund M, Lohmander LS. Risk factors for symptomatic knee osteoarthritis fifteen to twenty-two years after meniscectomy. *Arthritis Rheum.* 2004;50(9):2811–2819.

Papastergiou SG, Koukoulias NE, Mikalef P, et al. Meniscal tears in the ACL-deficient knee: correlation between meniscal tears and the timing of ACL reconstruction. *Knee Surg Sports Traumatol Arthrosc.* 2007;15(12):1438–1444.

Shelbourne KD, Rask BP. The sequelae of salvaged nondegenerative peripheral vertical medial meniscus tears with anterior cruciate ligament reconstruction. *Arthroscopy.* 2001;17(3):270–274.

Pujol N, Beaufils P. Healing results of meniscal tears left in situ during anterior cruciate ligament reconstruction: a review of clinical studies. *Knee Surg Sports Traumatol Arthrosc.* 2009;17(4):396–401.

Goodwin P, Morrisey M. Physical therapy after arthroscopic partial meniscectomy: is it effective? *Exerc Sport Sci Rev.* 2003;2:85–90.

Roos H, Laurén M, Adalberth T, et al. Knee osteoarthritis after meniscectomy: prevalence of radiographic changes after twenty-one years, compared with matched controls. *Arthritis Rheum.* 1998;41(4):687–693.

Burks RT, Metcalf MH, Metcalf RW. Fifteen-year follow-up of arthroscopic partial meniscectomy. *Arthroscopy.* 1997;13(6):673–679.

Higuchi H, Kimura M, Shirakura K, et al. Factors affecting long-term results after arthroscopic partial meniscectomy. *Clin Orthop Relat Res.* 2000(377):161–168.

Kirkley A, Griffin S, Whelan D. The development and validation of a quality of life-measurement tool for patients with meniscal pathology: the Western Ontario Meniscal Evaluation Tool (WOMET). *Clin J Sport Med.* 2007;17(5):349–356.

Englund M. The role of the meniscus in osteoarthritis genesis. *Med Clin North Am.* 2009;93(1):37–43.

Fabricant PD, Jokl P. Surgical outcomes after arthroscopic partial meniscectomy. *J Am Acad Orthop Surg.* 2007;15(11): 647–653.

Fauno P, Nielsen AB. Arthroscopic partial meniscectomy: a long-term follow-up. *Arthroscopy.* 1992;8(3):345–349.

Small NC. Complications in arthroscopy: the knee and other joints, committee on complications of the Arthroscopy Association of North America. *Arthroscopy.* 1986;2:253–258.

Sherman OH, Fox JM, Snyder SJ, et al. Arthroscopy—"no-problem surgery". An analysis of complications in two thousand six hundred and forty cases. *J Bone Joint Surg Am.* 1986;68(2):256–265.

All-Inside Arthroscopic Meniscal Repair

Matthew J. Goldstein • Nicholas A. Sgaglione

Meniscal preservation is essential for maintaining articular cartilage homeostasis, joint congruence, stability, and proprioception (1). In younger and more active patients, meniscal repair remains the preferred method of treatment for unstable meniscal tears and may play an important role in optimizing knee function (2, 3) and delaying the progression of degenerative disease. Owing to the important physiologic role that meniscal tissue plays in the knee, meniscal repair is advocated in young athletically active patients (4). The indications for repair may be heightened in those patients who present with meniscal tears and associated concomitant pathology such as anterior cruciate ligament tears or those requiring articular cartilage resurfacing or axial realignment osteotomies (5). Furthermore, as our knowledge and understanding of meniscal pathophysiology, healing, biomechanics, and minimally invasive repair improve, indications for repair are likely to expand. All-inside arthroscopic methods using novel suture-based devices represent a potentially effective and minimally invasive approach to meniscal repair. Adjuvant biologic therapies, such as platelet-rich plasma also appears promising and may increase the potential of repairing "irreparable meniscal tears" and improve the clinical success of surgically repaired "biologically-at-risk" tears.

CLINICAL EVALUATION

Knee kinematics predicts that internal rotation of the femur on the tibia forces the medial meniscus posteriorly and toward the center of the joint. If a meniscal attachment is abnormally loaded (peripheral or otherwise), as the posterior portion of the meniscus is forced toward the center of the joint, it may be caught between the femur and tibia, and resultant meniscal tearing can occur with further extension of the joint.

Patients with meniscal injuries typically present with clinical symptoms of focal joint line pain, swelling, and discomfort at the extremes of motion as well as specific mechanical symptoms such as catching, locking, and loss of extension. Physical examination should include evaluation and assessment of anatomic and mechanical axial alignment as well as signs of effusion, antalgia, loss of motion, focal joint line point tenderness, joint locking/clicking, and pain with squatting in terminal flexion and with axial compression. Manual examination for meniscal pathology has been reported to have a sensitivity and specificity of 55% to 85% and 29% to 67%, respectively (6). Provocative maneuvers for meniscal pathology include McMurray's test, the Apley grind or compression test, the Thessaly test, the Steinmann test, and Childress (squat) test (6–8). McMurray's test is performed by placing a varus or valgus stress to a flexed knee while extending, and is a reliable examination maneuver for diagnosing meniscal tears. The sensitivity of McMurray's test has been reported at 16% to 37%, with specificity at 77% to 98%, and a positive predictive value of 83% (6, 7). Similarly, the Apley grind or compression test, performed by flexing the knee, rotating, and compressing, has been reported to have a sensitivity of 13% to 16%, a specificity of 80% to 90%, and overall accuracy of 28%. The Thessaly test, in which the patient stands flatfooted on the floor and rotates at the knee in 20° of flexion internally and externally, has been reported to have a sensitivity, specificity, and overall accuracy of 89%, 97%, and 94%, respectively for medial meniscus tears and 92%, 96%, 96%, respectively for lateral meniscus tears (8). The Steinmann test is performed as a flexed knee is internally and externally rotated at the foot, whereas the Childress (squat) test elicits symptoms with the patient fully squatting with feet in internal and external rotation. The Bounce home test is performed with the patient supine by holding the great toe or forefoot and then attempts to identify a sharp endpoint as a fully flexed knee is taken to full extension or even hyperextension. A positive test occurs when full extension is unable to be obtained.

Clinical assessment for meniscal tears should always include plain roentgengrams, which should be evaluated to assess for crystal arthropathy, osteoarthritis, osteonecrosis, osteochondral defects, and calcification. Radiographs should include extension weight bearing anteroposterior, lateral, notch, and patella skyline views. Weight-bearing 45° flexion posteroanterior comparison views should also obtained to assess a narrowed joint space in cases where articular cartilage wear is suspected. Routine magnetic resonance imaging is often not necessary for diagnosis of meniscal injury but may prove valuable in a more comprehensive evaluation of the knee.

TREATMENT

The meniscus is mainly composed of type I collagen fibers (although types II, III, V, and VI have been identified) oriented in circumferential, radial, and perforating (random) directions. Classic tear patterns have been described and classified as vertical longitudinal, horizontal cleavage, radial, oblique, flap or parrot beak tears, and bucket handle tears (Fig. 56.1). The ultrastructural anatomic distribution of these fibers provides rigidity and tensile resistance and accounts for the characteristic tear patterns observed with failure. For example, ultrastructural failure at the junction of the circumferential bands characteristically results in a vertical tear, whereas failure along the radial tie fibers results in a radial tear (Fig. 56.2).

In a case series of 378 knees in 364 young athletes (285 males, 79 females, mean age 22.3, range 16 to 32) described by Terzidis et al. (9), meniscal tears were reported more often in the medial meniscus (69.3%) than in the lateral meniscus (30.7%). Although the majority of tears involved only the inner half of the meniscus (70.2% in the medial meniscus, 91.4% in the lateral meniscus), 23.3% of overall tears extended into the peripheral half of the meniscus. In addition, 74.8% tears involved the posterior horn (22.7% in the middle body and 2.5% in the anterior horn). Bucket handle tears occurred most often (23.1%), followed by longitudinal (18.2%), horizontal (17.4%), oblique (16.4%), radial (14.4%), and flap tears (10.5%).

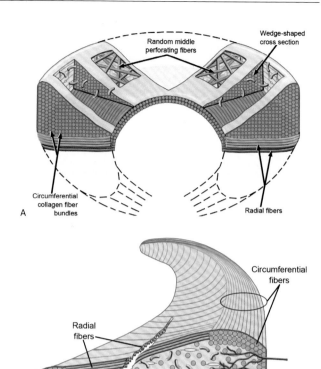

FIGURE 56.2. Meniscus ultrastructure

DECISION MAKING—REPAIR VERSUS RESECT

Decision making regarding meniscal repair is dependent upon tear characteristics (i.e., tear pattern, geometry, location, vascularity, size, stability, tissue viability, or quality), associated pathology, previous surgeries, and patient expectations and goals (10). Vertical longitudinal tears (77.5% of medial meniscal tears and 59.4% of lateral meniscal tears (9)) with minimal deformation in the vascularized peripheral meniscus are generally considered anatomically optimal for repair owing to their vascular potential for healing. Deformed or frayed oblique flaps, radial, horizontal cleavage, or degenerative complex tears within the avascular white–white zone have traditionally been treated with resection (10). Patient age, activity level, and postoperative rehabilitation compliance must also be taken into account before a decision is made regarding repair versus resection (Table 56.1).

Small, peripheral tears less than 7 mm in length and incomplete tears noted in the posterior horn of the lateral meniscus in a relatively asymptomatic patient (such as a patient undergoing concurrent anterior cruciate ligament reconstruction) can be left alone and be expected to heal. Shelbourne and Heinrich (11). concluded that posterior horn lateral meniscus tears, stable incomplete radial flap tears, or peripheral or posterior third tears within 1 cm of the popliteus tendon can be treated successfully and left in situ.

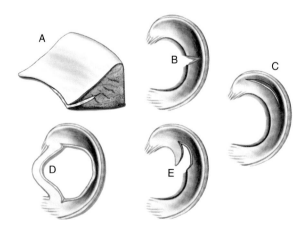

FIGURE 56.1. Tear types, **(A)** horizontal, **(B)** vertical radial, **(C)** vertical longitudinal, **(D)** bucket handle, **(E)** flap.

Table 56.1

Indications for meniscal resection, rasping, and repair (10)

	Resect	Rasp	Repair
Chronicity	Degenerative, nonclinically correlative tears in older patients	NA	Acute, symptomatic tears
Pattern	Oblique flaps, radial, degenerative complex, horizontal	Incomplete longitudinal	Longitudinal/vertical bucket handles
Site	Inner (white–white)	Red–red posterior horn, lateral meniscus	Peripheral (red–red), middle (red–white), inner (white–white)
Size	NA	<7–10 mm	>7–10 mm
Excursion	NA	Stable, incomplete tears, <3–5 mm displaced into notch	Unstable, >5 mm displaced into notch
Tissue viability	Deformed, frayed, nonviable	Viable	Minimal deformation, holds repair device, viable
Prognosticators	ACL intact, no malalignment or chondral lesions; associated infectious, rheumatoid, or collagen vascular diseases	ACL intact, well-aligned, no chondral lesions	Associated ACLR or chondral procedure, axially malaligned
Patient Compliance/ Preference	Recovery or rehabilitation is an issue	NA	Patient preferred

Abbreviations: ACL, anterior cruciate ligament; ACLR, anterior cruciate ligament repair; NA, not applicable.
Adapted from Sgaglione NA, Steadman JR, Shaffer B, et al. Current concepts in meniscus surgery: resection to replacement. *Arthroscopy.* 2003;19(suppl 1):161–188.

In contrast, surgical intervention is indicated in patients with unstable tissue, substantial peripheral longitudinal tears, mechanical symptoms, or when nonoperative measures (modification of activities, inflammation reduction, and physical therapy) fail.

Meniscal excision may alter load transmission, contact stresses, and tibiofemoral patholaxity (particularly in knees with associated anterior cruciate ligament [ACL] deficiency). Posterior root tears of the medial meniscus have been shown to increase peak contact pressure by 25% in the medial compartment and 13% in the lateral compartment than with an intact meniscus (12). Repair of the tear site returned peak contact pressures to baseline and showed significant improvement in medial compartment contact pressures, tibial external rotation, and lateral tibial translation. In addition, meniscectomy in athletes has been shown to lead to knee instability, radiographic changes, and reduction in functional activities as early as 4.5 years postsurgery (13). Clinical outcomes following partial meniscectomy reveal that radiographic progression of medial compartment osteoarthritis after medial meniscectomy was greater than lateral compartment osteoarthritis after lateral meniscectomy (14). Furthermore, when less than 50% of the meniscal rim remains, radiographic progression may be seen.

Fabricant et al. (15) reported on a level 1 prognostic prospective study of 126 arthroscopic partial meniscectomies evaluating first year postoperative recovery revealed that female gender and extent of chondral pathology affected knee pain, knee function, and overall physical knee status (effusion, flexion, extension, gait, and general progress) significantly. Age, body mass index, depth of meniscal excision (amount of meniscus removed from any zone), involvement of one or both menisci, and extent of meniscal tear (total number of zones involved) showed no association. Extent of the meniscal tear affected overall physical knee status but not knee pain or function. Meniscal excision and involvement of one or both menisci had no impact on recovery. McDermott and Amis (16) pointed out that negative factors affecting long-term prognosis include the amount of tissue resected, the location of resection (posterior horn worse than anterior horn or bucket-handle tears), the disruption of retained circumferential fibers, lateral meniscectomy (worse than medial), a preexisting chondral lesion, varus alignment of the affected knee, ACL deficiency or ligamentous pathoplaxity, and increased postmeniscectomy activity levels. Further support is provided by a retrospective comparative study of medial versus lateral arthroscopic partial meniscectomies suggesting that a more optimal prognosis can be predicted with patients less than age 35, vertical tears, absence of cartilage damage, and an intact meniscal rim following meniscectomy (17). In addition to the consideration of the natural history of meniscal resection, patient counseling of the procedural risks, benefits, expected recovery and rehabilitation as well as the outcomes of selected treatment options are essential. Recovery time and re-tear risks should also be addressed and may play a role in decision making when an expeditious and more predictable return to work or sport is preferred.

Timing

Controversy remains regarding what the ideal interventional period for isolated meniscal tears is. Tenuta and Arciero (18) evaluated 51 patients with 54 meniscal repairs with second-look arthroscopy at an average of 11 months after repair. Time to surgery did not effect healing; however, meniscal repairs that did not heal when carried out with ACL reconstruction had a longer time to repair (60 weeks) than those that healed (19 weeks). Henning et al. (19) reported a significant difference in repair outcomes within 8 weeks of injury to those performed later, although the repairs performed later may have been more complex. Cannon and Vittori (5) evaluated 90 meniscal repairs, 68 in conjunction with ACL reconstructions. Isolated meniscal tears repaired within 8 weeks were more clinically successful (57%) than those carried out later than 8 weeks (47%). Similarly, those repaired in conjunction with ACL reconstruction had a 96% healing rate within 8 weeks of injury versus 91% for repairs carried out later than 8 weeks postinjury.

Scott et al. (20) reported on 260 meniscal repairs at an average of 47.3 weeks from initial injury (median 19 weeks). They found no difference in healing rates in patients with a span of more than 3 weeks from injury to surgery to those operated on within 3 weeks of injury. They concluded that chronicity of symptoms did not alter prognosis of healing. Noyes and Barber-Westin (4) evaluated 30 meniscal repairs in patients 40 years of age or older, 20 chronic, and 10 acute (within 10 weeks of injury), for tears extending into the central one-third of the meniscus or with a rim width of 4 mm or more. Chronicity of the injury also yielded no significant effect on repair. Noyes and Barber-Westin (21) later evaluated 71 meniscal tears that extended into the avascular region in patients 19 years of age and younger. Average time from injury was 40 weeks (range 1 to 256 weeks). Forty repairs were performed acutely (1 to 12 weeks) and 31 for a chronic

condition. No difference was found between success (or failure) of repair and length of time from injury to repair.

TECHNIQUES

Meniscus repair techniques include open, arthroscopically assisted, and all-arthroscopic methods. Currently, arthroscopic-assisted meniscal repair techniques are considered preferable owing to shorter operative times and reduced patient morbidity.

The outside-in technique initially described by Rodeo and (22), is best indicated in meniscal tears involving the mid- and anterior one-third portions of the meniscus and for provisional fixation and stabilization of unstable tear fragments (use of traction and reducing stitch). An 18G spinal needle is passed percutaneously from outside to inside the joint through the meniscal tear. The technique allows for placement of variable suture patterns for repair while maintaining a safe vector, well anterior to the posterior neurovascular bundle.

The inside-out technique popularized by Henning and others (5, 20, 23), is considered by some to be the "gold standard" meniscal repair method and combines arthroscopic suture passage with open tensioning and cinching of knots down to the corresponding capsule. Inside-out suture techniques require the use of a several centimeter accessory posteromedial or posterolateral incision to capture the exiting repair needles and sutures under direct visualization. It allows the placement of vertical mattress sutures in the middle one-third and posterior horns while protecting the posterior neurovascular structures using a popliteal tissue retractor placed within the accessory incision.

All-arthroscopic methods include the use of all-inside fixators, which are largely based on a reverse-barbed fishhook design that reapproximates and reduces tear fragments (24). Fixators are placed perpendicular to the tear and serve to effectively lag tear fragments. Multiple fixator devices exist that differ in shape, size, composition, insertion, and delivery technique. Biomechanical strength concerns and complications associated with fixators including inferior pullout, delayed resorption, breakage, retained polymer fragments, foreign body reactions, surrounding soft-tissue inflammation, and chondral injury have led these devices to fall out of favor.

More recently, all-arthroscopic, all-inside suture-based device techniques have been introduced and have increased in popularity. These methods offer a less invasive, suture-integrated design with the strength of a traditional vertical mattress pattern (25). Most devices incorporate suture and anchors within a single integrated needle delivery system. All-arthroscopic suture repair devices provide a number of advantages over previous fixator designs, as braided suture is compressible, less rigid, and may result in a safer profile as far as adjacent articular cartilage surfaces are concerned. Furthermore, the two-point fixation construct allows adjustable, tensionable compression across the tear site yielding a more optimal biomechanical strength profile. Furthermore, all-inside suture techniques obviate the need for posteromedial or posterolateral dissection, thereby resulting in a truly arthroscopic, minimally invasive methodology. This translates to a less invasive and less painful procedure that is theoretically easier and safer as far as surgical morbidity is concerned. Disadvantages include the learning curves associated with the use of these newer generation devices, lack of longer-term clinical outcome data, extracapsular implant placement and/or prominence, soft-tissue inflammation, and the significant cost of these devices.

SUTURE-BASED DEVICES

ULTRA FasT-Fix and FasT-Fix 360

Smith and Nephew Endoscopy (Andover, MA) released the FasT-Fix Meniscal Repair System in 2001 as an updated version of the T-Fix meniscal repair system introduced in 1994. The ULTRA FasT-Fix Meniscal Repair System, introduced in 2008, incorporates two 5-mm bioinert anchors (poly-ether-ether-ketone [PEEK] or bioabsorbable anchors [PLLA]) with attached high strength nonabsorbable no. 0 Ultrabraid suture integrated with a preloaded and pretied, self-sliding knot delivered via a 16.5G insertion needle (27° curved or 15° reverse-curved). The system includes a split-sheath insertion cannula, adjustable depth penetrator, separate curved knot pusher/suture cutter, and metallic portal insertion skid. Vertical mattress suture configurations and the versatility for variable insertion points are two advantages of the ULTRA FasT-Fix (Fig. 56.3A and B) (24). The newer, enhanced FasT-Fix 360 has been

introduced incorporating a stiffer delivery device with circular (360°) implant deployment trigger, ergonomic depth gauge ratchet, and lower-profile implants with 2-0 Ultrabraid suture (Fig. 56.4A and B).

Meniscal Cinch

In 2008, Arthrex Inc. (Naples, FL) introduced the Meniscal Cinch. The dual-trocar, pistol-grip device has two PEEK anchors connected to one another with 2-0 FiberWire on a horseshoe-shaped, slotted open, ergonomic delivery cannula. A sliding knot is preloaded on the second deployment cannula for final tensioning. The system provides an adjustable external depth stop with 2-mm ruler for intraoperative tear measurement and for greater protected deployment of the implant. A free suture tail remains following deployment of the second anchor, which allows further tensioning and countersinking of the sliding knot with a knot pusher (Fig. 56.5).

MaxFire and MaxFire MarXmen

Biomet Sports Medicine (Warsaw, IN) introduced the Max-Fire Meniscal Repair Device in 2008. The system provides two preloaded no. 5 polyester "suture" pledget anchors on ergonomic disposable needle insertion and deployment slide trigger devices. The "suture" anchors are connected to one another using proprietary knotless ZipLoop

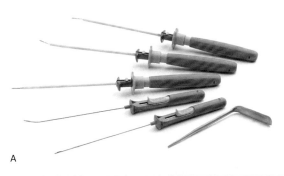

A

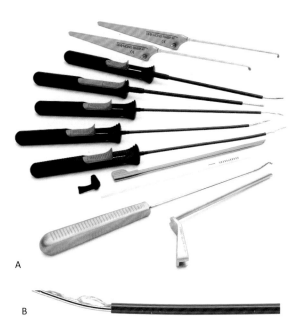

FIGURE 56.3. A: ULTRA FasT-Fix meniscal repair system. **B:** ULTRA FasT-Fix meniscal repair needle delivery device and implant. (Courtesy of Smith and Nephew Endoscopy.)

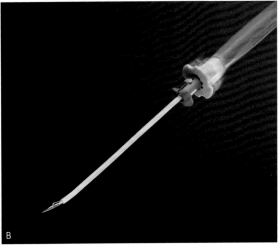

FIGURE 56.4. A: FasT-Fix 360 meniscal repair system. **B:** FasT-Fix 360 meniscal repair needle delivery device and implant. (Courtesy of Smith and Nephew Endoscopy.)

technology that is a single polyethylene suture woven through itself twice in opposite directions and allows for predictable suture loop cinching. In effect, the system is two loops, connected with a sliding suture crimp. Sutures can be positioned 5- to 10-mm apart in either horizontal or vertical mattress configurations. Once the two anchors are deployed, a free strand of suture remains, which allows tensioning of sliding knot (Fig. 56.6). The MaxFire MarX-men has been recently introduced that now incorporates a pistol grip device for single-handed MaxFire deployment. The pistol grip is designed with a single trigger, thumb wheel for deployment and retraction of a needle protection cannula, and a needle depth indicator (Fig. 56.7A and B).

CrossFix

Cayenne Medical (Scottsdale, AZ) introduced the Cross-Fix Meniscal Repair System in 2009 as a suture-only device consisting of an integrated 2-prong, 15G needle (24 mm in length) delivery system. A 3-mm, 10° oblique suture construct with No. 0 nonabsorbable high strength polyethylene sutures are deployed with single piercing of

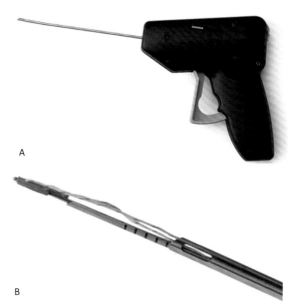

FIGURE 56.7. A: MaxFire MarXmen mechanical delivery device. **B:** MaxFire MarXmen needle delivery tip and soft tissue anchors. (Courtesy of Biomet Sports Medicine.)

the meniscus through the use of an integrated crossing needle. A pretied sliding knot then cinches the repair. A knot pusher/suture cutter is available to further tension the repair if necessary. The delivery needles are available in straight or 12° up-curved options (Fig. 56.8A and B).

Omnispan

The DePuy Mitek, Inc. (Raynham, MA) OMNISPAN Meniscal Repair system consists of a disposable, multiuse surgeon loaded dual trigger, pistol-grip applicator and delivery needles preloaded with 2 PEEK anchors connected with proprietary 2-0 ORTHOCORD suture (55% PDS). The knotless repair is tensioned through the use of a probe and a free suture tail. Once tensioned, the remaining suture is cut with the arthroscopic cutter. The calibrated delivery needles are available in straight, 12°, and 27°; vertical, horizontal, and oblique repairs are possible (Fig. 56.9A and B).

Sequent

Conmed Linvatec (Largo, FL) recently introduced the Sequent Meniscal Repair Device, which allows for a "running" knotless meniscal repair using a combination of PEEK-Optima anchors and no. 0 Hi-Fi Suture. The device is multiply loaded, allowing for multiple individually tensioned configurations. First, a depth stop sheath is cut to size and placed over the needle prior to insertion of the needle into the joint. The needle pierces the meniscus and using the Freewheel, trigger, and 720° device rotation, the implants are deployed and the stitch is tensioned. A suture cutter is used to remove the excess suture. Straight or curved needles preloaded with either four or seven implants are available (Fig. 56.10A and B).

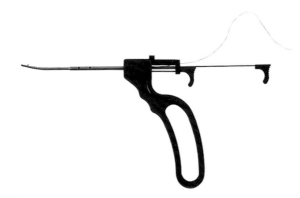

FIGURE 56.5. Meniscal cinch. (Courtesy of Arthrex Inc.).

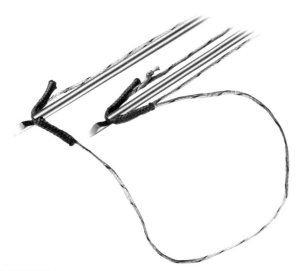

FIGURE 56.6. MaxFire meniscal repair device and soft tissue anchors. (Courtesy of Biomet Sports Medicine.)

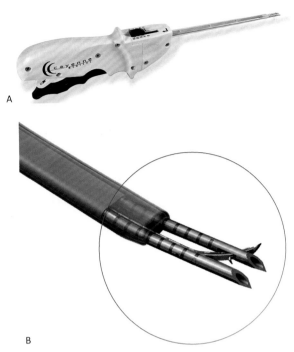

FIGURE 56.8. A: Crossfix meniscal repair mechanical delivery device. **B:** Crossfix meniscal repair integrated needle delivery tip. (Courtesy of Cayenne Medical.)

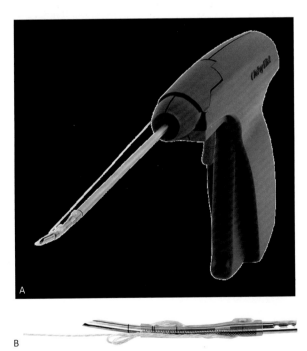

FIGURE 56.9. A: OMNISPAN meniscal repair mechanical delivery device. **B:** OMNISPAN meniscal repair needle delivery tip and soft tissue anchors. (Courtesy of DePuy Mitek, Inc.)

Biomechanics

Numerous ex vivo mechanical studies have concluded that vertical mattress suture constructs result in the strongest fixation (26–28). Biomechanical testing of many of the currently available all-arthroscopic meniscal repair

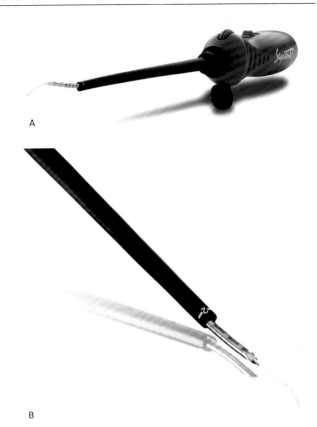

FIGURE 56.10. A: Sequent meniscal repair mechanical delivery device. **B:** Sequent meniscal repair needle delivery tip and soft tissue anchors. (Courtesy of Conmed Linvatec.)

systems reveal that displacement and stiffness closely approximate vertical mattress sutures (26, 29), whereas previous fixator design strength profiles were associated with less optimal pullout, ultimate load to failure, and stiffness.

In a porcine model, Barber et al. (26) investigated the load to failure in strength of vertical and horizontal 2-0 Mersilene (Ethicon, Sommerville, NJ) sutures, vertical and horizontally oriented FasT-Fix, Arthrex meniscal darts, Arthrotek meniscal screw (Biomet, Warsaw, IN), and RapidLoc devices. Vertical 2-0 Mersilene suture remained strongest, but FasT-fix results approached mattress suture. Borden et al. (25) in a cadaveric knee model, studied load to failure, displacement, and stiffness of the horizontal FasT-Fix, Vertical 0 Ti-Cron (Ethicon, Somerville, NJ) sutures, and 13-mm Meniscus Arrows (ConMed Linvatec, Largo, FL). Horizontal FasT-Fix and vertical mattress sutures significantly exceeded the Meniscus Arrow in all three parameters. Horizontal FasT-Fix and vertical mattress sutures provided comparable levels of the parameters measured. In a bovine model, Zantop et al. (27) studied initial fixation strength, stiffness, and failure mode of the FasT-Fix, RapidLoc, Meniscus Arrow, and horizontal and vertical 2-0 Ethibond sutures. The vertical and horizontal FasT-Fix sutures were the strongest devices in pullout strength and showed no difference from vertical Ethibond sutures. The mattress sutures and FasT-Fix specimen failed at the suture, whereas the RapidLoc failed at the backstop' and the arrow failed by pullout of the barbs.

Zantop et al. (28) later studied cyclic loading of the FasT-Fix, RapidLoc, and horizontal and vertical 2-0 Ethibond sutures to attempt to mirror in vivo loading under 1,000 cycles of load. No difference was found in displacement of any of the repair techniques. Furthermore, no difference in vertical suture, horizontal FasT-Fix, and vertical FasT-Fix was noted in ultimate failure load after 1,000 cycles; however, horizontal suture and RapidLoc showed significantly lower failure loads. Both FasT-Fix devices were significantly stiffer than the sutures and RapidLoc.

In a comparison study, Chang et al. (30) evaluated the Meniscal Viper, vertical FasT-Fix, and vertical no. 0 Ethibond suture for cyclic loading and load-to-failure differences. The study revealed less mean displacement and greater mean stiffness of the vertical suture with cyclic loading, but found no difference between the FasT-Fix and vertical suture (both significantly greater than Meniscal Viper) with load-to-failure testing. However, the FasT-Fix and Meniscal Viper both displayed greater mean stiffness than vertical mattress suture in load-to-failure testing, with the Meniscal Viper achieving statistical significance.

AUTHORS' PREFERRED TREATMENT

Patients are usually treated at an outpatient ambulatory surgery center with local anesthesia, intravenous sedation, and general anesthesia with a laryngeal mask airway. A femoral nerve block with general endotracheal or epidural anesthesia is recommended when concomitant procedures are planned. A lateral post or leg holder is used to apply valgus stress for medial meniscal pathology. Meniscal pathology is addressed and treated first if ACL or articular cartilage procedures are to be performed concurrently.

The meniscal tear is identified; size, stability, and excursion (how displaceable), ease of reduction; and tissue viability are assessed. The length and geometry of the tear site should be assessed to provisionally select the needed number of sutures and the length of the devices that may be needed with regard to patient size, meniscal size, variance, distance of the tear from the periphery and capsule, and technique to be used. A contralateral portal approach is commonly used to increase the margin of safety (i.e., posterior horn medial meniscus tears are approached from a contralateral inferolateral portal with the suture repair device) when directing the suture repair vectors.

Following initial assessment and if an ACL reconstruction will not be required, a fibrin clot technique is initiated. Immediate sterile autologous blood is requested and obtained from the anesthesiologist and centrifuged to produce a platelet-rich fibrin matrix (PRFM) clot (31). Preparation of the tear site is completed by debridement of the meniscal tear site, its edges, and the peripheral meniscal–capsular junction using a motorized shaver blade or low-profile meniscal rasp. An 18G spinal needle or meniscal trephine can be used to create vascular access channels for healing augmentation and to induce a vascular response

(Fig. 5.6.11A and B). After preparation is complete, the tear is then reduced. Provisional reduction of unstable displaced bucket-handle tears may be obtained via an 18G spinal needle inserted in an inside-out or outside-in direction or with the use of an outside-in 0-PDS traction stitch. Vertical mattress sutures are placed 3 to 5 mm apart for optimal fixation and when sufficient tissue is available, double vertical configurations theoretically allow for greater resistance to the tensile and compressive femoral and tibial sides of the repair (Fig. 56.12). An outside-in hybridized approach is used for anterior- and middle-third tears in thinner patients. Post-operative protocols emphasize immediate motion, protected weight bearing, and individualized approached to modification of activities (see section Rehabilitation).

Outcomes

Results of all-inside meniscal repair supplemented with hybridized arthroscopic suture techniques have been reported to be successful in selected patients. Krych et al. (32) in a level 4 case series study, reported a 62% overall clinical success rate for arthroscopic isolated meniscal repair upon retrospective review in patients 18 years and younger. An 80%

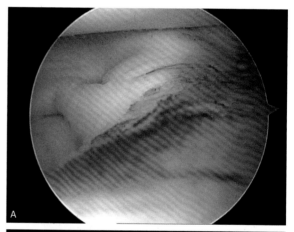
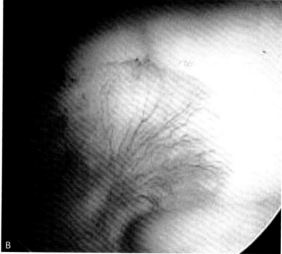

FIGURE 56.11. A, B: Hypervascular meniscal healing response seen 6 weeks after repair upon second look arthroscopy.

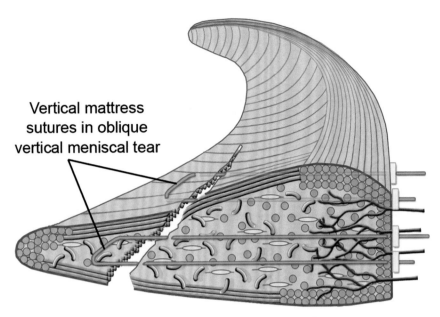

Vertical mattress
sutures in oblique
vertical meniscal tear

FIGURE 56.12. Vertical longitudinal tear repair with double vertical mattress pattern.

clinical success rate is reported for simple meniscal tears, 68% for displaced bucket-handle tears, and 13% for complex tears. A rim width of 3 to 6 mm from the meniscosynovial junction and increasing tear complexity are reported as potential risk factors for obtaining a successful repair.

Pujol et al. (33) in a level 4 case series, reported overall healing rate of 73.1% as determined with postoperative CT arthrography. In addition, Feng et al. (34) in a level 4 case-series study, reported an 89.6% overall meniscal healing rate for large bucket-handle meniscus tears upon second-look arthroscopy at an average of 26-month follow-up using an arthroscopic hybrid suture technique with inside-out vertical mattress and 45° suture hook (Suture Hook Corkscrew; Conmed Linvatec, Largo, FL) with associated ACL reconstruction.

In a prospective level 4 case-series study of the FasT-Fix repair system at 18-month average follow-up of 61 longitudinal tears in the red–red or red–white zones (36% isolated, 64% with concurrent ACL reconstruction), successful repairs were reported in 88% (as measured by improved Lysholm knee scores) (35). No chondral injury was noted in two relooks. Similarly, in a prospective level 4 case-series study evaluating the success of the FasT-Fix repair system in 41 repairs associated with an accelerated rehabilitation program, Barber et al. (36) reported clinically effective meniscal repair in 83% at a mean of 30.7-month follow-up as measured by Lysholm, Tegner, Cincinnati, and the International Knee Documentation Committee form (IKDC) activity scores. Preliminary case-series data evaluating all-inside meniscal repair using the FasT-Fix meniscal repair system, Sgaglione et al. (unpublished data) reported an 88% clinical success rate of 81 meniscal repairs in 73 patients (52 males, 21 females, 71.2% with concomitant ACL reconstruction) at

an average 72-month follow-up as measured by the Modified Lysholm, Cincinnati, Tegner, and visual analog scale (VAS) scores. Complications included one painful implant requiring removal.

In a prospective level 4 case-series study evaluating meniscal repair with the RapidLoc during concurrent ACL reconstruction of 38 meniscal tears, Billante et al. (37) reported an 86.8% success rate as measured by the IKDC and the Knee Disorders Subjective visual analog scale (KDS-VAS) at a mean follow-up of 30.4 months (range, 21 to 56 months). In a level 4 case-series retrospective review of 54 meniscal repairs (all associated with ACL reconstruction) in 46 patients for a mean follow-up of 34.8 months, using the Rapid-Loc device, Quinby et al. (38) reported a 90.7% success rate measured by IKDC and VAS at a mean follow-up of 34.8 months (range, 24 to 50 months).

Kalliakmanis et al. (39), in a level 3 comparative study, reported success rates of 92.4% for FasT-Fix, 87% for T-Fix (Acufex Microsurgical, Mansfield, MA), and 86.5% for RapidLoc in patients with Cooper radial zone 1 or 2 meniscal tears and concurrent ACL reconstruction at a mean follow-up of 24.5 months (range, 20 to 26 months). IKDC and Lysholm scores improved significantly postrepair with no difference elicited between device used. Furthermore, tear chronicity, length, site, and patient age were not found to affect healing rate.

COMPLICATIONS, CONTROVERSIES, AND CONSIDERATIONS

In a multicenter survey of 395,566 arthroscopies including 375,069 knee arthroscopies, Small et al. (40) reported the overall complication rate for arthroscopy at 0.56%

with a complication rate specific to meniscal repair at 2.4%. Common complications included saphenous nerve injury. Other studies have reported rates of complications specific to meniscal surgery in a similar range from 1.7% for meniscectomy to 1.29% for meniscal repair (41). Austin et al. (41) however, reported an 18% overall complication rate of meniscal tears (19% for medial repairs and 13% for lateral repairs). Many of the complications of all-inside repair regard the use of fixators and include reports of broken implants, retained foreign bodies, inflammatory reactions, fixator migration or prominence, and chondral injury (Fig. 13A and B) (41). All-inside repair techniques

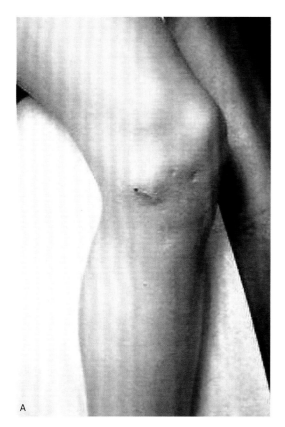

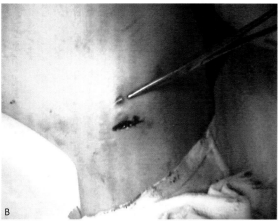

FIGURE 56.13. A: Painful medial knee implant 15 months postoperatively prior to removal. **B:** Painful medial knee implant site postremoval.

using suture-based designs limit risk to chondral surfaces; however, painful implants have been reported. Similarly, risks to neurovascular structures are limited with all-inside techniques, but vascular structures have been reported to be as close as 3 mm to the needle tip when repairing the posterior horn of the lateral meniscus (42). Peroneal nerve injury from lateral side repairs can also occur but is less common (41). Cost-effectiveness must be taken into consideration when using many of these newer generation suture devices. Furthermore, improper deployment of these devices can lead to time-consuming retrieval in an effort to dispose of the wasted implants and added cost per case for "dropped implants (43)."

REHABILITATION

Several authors have reported success with accelerated rehabilitation programs emphasizing immediate range of motion, weight bearing, and return to pivoting sports. Others suggest a more conservative approach as accelerated programs yielded lower healing rates (18). The author's preferred postoperative regimen for isolated meniscal repairs remains similar to the protocol used for ACL reconstruction and emphasizes an individualized approach depending on the type of tear and repair construct. This patient-specific approach takes into consideration patient comfort as well as the repair characteristics. Patients are placed postoperatively into a brace or knee immobilizer in the operating room, locked in extension for comfort and facilitated ambulation and transfers. The brace is discontinued when the patient demonstrates adequate leg control, proprioception, and is comfortable without it or at about 4 weeks. Weight bearing in extension is initially limited to crutches to prevent undue compressive and shear forces about the repair. Weight bearing is advanced as tolerated with full weight bearing encouraged at 4 weeks when effusion and antalgia have subsided and quadriceps firing is adequate. Immediate range of motion is encouraged 0° to 90° on postoperative day 1 (if an associated ACL reconstruction is performed as patients are placed in a continuous passive motion machine at home set 0° to 90°). Progression of motion, particularly terminal flexion (to limit flexion/roll back compression) is dependent on repair characteristics including site, size, and geometry, and also strength of the repair. Tears considered "at risk" may be protected for a greater period, and rehabilitation is progressed with regard to comfortable range of motion, flexibility, strengthening, and conditioning. Return to sports activities is considered at 4 to 6 months based on the successful attainment of functional goals and absence of symptomatic point tenderness over the repair site.

FUTURE DIRECTIONS

Biologic augmentation of tissue repair and regeneration remains the future of current repair techniques to broaden the indications of meniscal repair and potentially increase and enhance healing rates and clinical success. Early research is underway regarding the use of growth factor and morphogen-coated sutures (platelet-derived growth factor [PDGF] and growth factor differentiation factor-5 [GDF-5]), PRFM gels/membranes including PDGF, bioadhesive polyphenolic proteins, and bioscaffolds using collagen-GAG as adjuvants to meniscal healing. Results of GDF-5 coated sutures in repaired tendons have shown improved biomechanical strength at earlier time points than uncoated sutures (44). PRFM as an autologous source of bioactive growth factors with a concentrated fibrin matrix has shown promise and may have utility in the avascular white–white zone of the meniscus (31). The addition of healing adjuvants and biologic promoters of the healing process may allow for a stronger and more predictable repair results in the less vascularized zones of the meniscus and in turn, may further broaden anatomic considerations for meniscal repair and improve surgical outcomes (Fig. 56.14A–C).

CONCLUSIONS

All-inside all-arthroscopic meniscal repair is a safe and effective minimally invasive method. As meniscal repair technology continues to improve, surgeons can expect more versatile, easier, and quicker arthroscopic suture insertion and delivery repair systems. Improvements in load-to-failure strength, stiffness, and more predictable tissue anchors are certainly on the horizon. Hybridization of arthroscopic techniques, whether outside-in or inside-out, remains a useful supplement to all-inside all-arthroscopic suture techniques. Biologic augmentation of the meniscal repairs is currently evolving and may represent an opportunity to broaden the indications for repair and provide more predictable and timely healing process and resultant clinical outcomes.

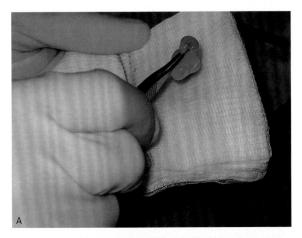

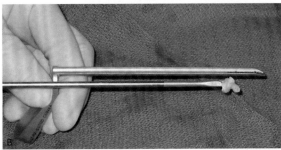

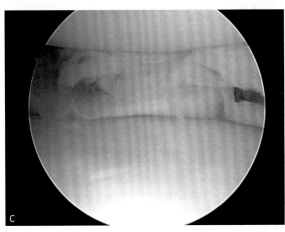

FIGURE 56.14. A: Autogenous PRFM prepared after centrifugation. **B:** Autogenous PRFM, arthroscopic introducer, and delivery device. **C:** Arthroscopic image of PRFM incorporated into all-inside meniscus repair.

REFERENCES

1. Levy IM, Torzilli PA, Warren RF. The effect of medial meniscectomy on anterior–posterior motion of the knee. *J Bone Joint Surg Am.* 1982;64(6):883–888.
2. Faunø P, Nielsen AB. Arthroscopic partial meniscectomy: a long-term follow-up. *Arthroscopy.* 1992;8(3):345–349.
3. Sturnieks DL, Besier TF, Mills PM, et al. Knee joint biomechanics following arthroscopic partial meniscectomy. *Orthop Res.* 2008;26(8):1075–1080.
4. Noyes FR, Barber-Westin SD. Arthroscopic repair of meniscus tears extending into the avascular zone with or without anterior cruciate ligament reconstruction in patients 40 years of age and older. *Arthroscopy.* 2000;16(8):822–829.
5. Cannon WD Jr, Vittori JM. The incidence of healing in arthroscopic meniscal repairs in anterior cruciate ligament-reconstructed knees versus stable knees. *Am J Sports Med.* 1992;20(2):176–181.
6. Malanga GA, Andrus S, Nadler SF, et al. Physical examination of the knee: a review of the original test description and scientific validity of common orthopedic tests. *Arch Phys Med Rehabil.* 2003;84(4):592–603.
7. Evans PJ, Bell GD, Frank C. Prospective evaluation of the McMurray test. *Am J Sports Med.* 1993;21(4):604–608.
8. Karachalios T, Hantes M, Zibis AH, et al. Diagnostic accuracy of a new clinical test (the Thessaly test) for early detection of meniscal tears. *J Bone Joint Surg Am.* 2005;87(5):955–962.
9. Terzidis IP, Christodoulou A, Ploumis A, et al. Meniscal tear characteristics in young athletes with a stable knee: arthroscopic evaluation. *Am J Sports Med.* 2006;34(7):1170–1175.
10. Sgaglione NA, Steadman JR, Shaffer B, et al. Current concepts in meniscus surgery: resection to replacement. *Arthroscopy.* 2003;19(suppl 1):161–188.

11. Shelbourne KD, Heinrich J. The long-term evaluation of lateral meniscus tears left in situ at the time of anterior cruciate ligament reconstruction. *Arthroscopy*. 2004;20(4):346–351.

12. Allaire R, Muriuki M, Gilbertson L, et al. Biomechanical consequences of a tear of the posterior root of the medial meniscus. Similar to total meniscectomy. *J Bone Joint Surg Am*. 2008;90(9):1922–1931.

13. Jørgensen U, Sonne-Holm S, Lauridsen F, et al. Long-term follow-up of meniscectomy in athletes. A prospective longitudinal study. *J Bone Joint Surg Br*. 1987;69(1):80–83.

14. Fabricant PD, Jokl P. Surgical outcomes after arthroscopic partial meniscectomy. *J Am Acad Orthop Surg*. 2007;15(11):647–653.

15. Fabricant PD, Rosenberger PH, Jokl P, et al. Predictors of short-term recovery differ from those of long-term outcome after arthroscopic partial meniscectomy. *Arthroscopy*. 2008;24(7):769–778.

16. McDermott ID, Amis AA. The consequences of meniscectomy. *J Bone Joint Surg Br*. 2006;88(12):1549–1556.

17. Chatain F, Adeleine P, Chambat P, et al; Société Française d'Arthroscopie. A comparative study of medial versus lateral arthroscopic partial meniscectomy on stable knees: 10-year minimum follow-up. *Arthroscopy*. 2003;19(8):842–849.

18. Tenuta JJ, Arciero RA. Arthroscopic evaluation of meniscal repairs. Factors that effect healing. *Am J Sports Med*. 1994;22(6):797–802.

19. Henning CE, Lynch MA, Yearout KM, et al. Arthroscopic meniscal repair using an exogenous fibrin clot. *Clin Orthop Relat Res*. 1990;(252):64–72.

20. Scott GA, Jolly BL, Henning CE. Combined posterior incision and arthroscopic intra-articular repair of the meniscus. An examination of factors affecting healing. *J Bone Joint Surg Am*. 1986;68(6):847–861.

21. Noyes FR, Barber-Westin SD. Arthroscopic repair of meniscal tears extending into the avascular zone in patients younger than twenty years of age. *Am J Sports Med*. 2002;30(4):589–600.

22. Rodeo SA. Arthroscopic meniscal repair with use of the outside-in technique. *Instr Course Lect*. 2000;49:195–206.

23. Henning CE, Lynch MA, Yearout KM, et al. Arthroscopic meniscal repair using an exogenous fibrin clot. *Clin Orthop Relat Res*. 1990;(252):64–72.

24. Sgaglione NA. New generation meniscus fixator devices. *Sports Med Arthrosc Rev*. 2004;12(1):44–59.

25. Borden P, Nyland J, Caborn DN, et al. Biomechanical comparison of the FasT-Fix meniscal repair suture system with vertical mattress sutures and meniscus arrows. *Am J Sports Med*. 2003;31(3):374–378.

26. Barber FA, Herbert MA, Richards DP. Load to failure testing of new meniscal repair devices. *Arthroscopy*. 2004;20(1):45–50.

27. Zantop T, Eggers AK, Weimann A, et al. Initial fixation strength of flexible all-inside meniscus suture anchors in comparison to conventional suture technique and rigid anchors: biomechanical evaluation of new meniscus refixation systems. *Am J Sports Med*. 2004;32(4):863–869.

28. Zantop T, Eggers AK, Musahl V, et al. Cyclic testing of flexible all-inside meniscus suture anchors: biomechanical analysis. *Am J Sports Med*. 2005;33(3):388–394.

29. Borden P, Nyland J, Caborn DN, et al. Biomechanical comparison of the FasT-Fix meniscal repair suture system with vertical mattress sutures and meniscus arrows. *Am J Sports Med*. 2003;31(3):374–378.

30. Chang HC, Nyland J, Caborn DN, et al. Biomechanical evaluation of meniscal repair systems: a comparison of the Meniscal Viper Repair System, the vertical mattress FasT-Fix Device, and vertical mattress ethibond sutures. *Am J Sports Med*. 2005;33(12):1846–1852.

31. Angel MJ, Sgaglione NA, Grande DA. Clinical applications of bioactive factors in sports medicine: current concepts and future trends. *Sports Med Arthrosc*. 2006;14(3):138–145.

32. Krych AJ, McIntosh AL, Voll AE, et al. Arthroscopic repair of isolated meniscal tears in patients 18 years and younger. *Am J Sports Med*. 2008;36(7):1283–1289.

33. Pujol N, Panarella L, Selmi TA, et al. Meniscal healing after meniscal repair: a CT arthrography assessment. *Am J Sports Med*. 2008;36(8):1489–1495.

34. Feng H, Hong L, Geng XS, et al. Second-look arthroscopic evaluation of bucket-handle meniscus tear repairs with anterior cruciate ligament reconstruction: 67 consecutive cases. *Arthroscopy*. 2008;24(12):1358–1366.

35. Kotsovolos ES, Hantes ME, Mastrokalos DS, et al. Results of all-inside meniscal repair with the FasT-Fix meniscal repair system. *Arthroscopy*. 2006;22(1):3–9.

36. Barber FA, Schroeder FA, Oro FB, et al. FasT-Fix meniscal repair: mid-term results. *Arthroscopy*. 2008;24(12):1342–1348.

37. Billante MJ, Diduch DR, Lunardini DJ, et al. Meniscal repair using an all-inside, rapidly absorbing, tensionable device. *Arthroscopy*. 2008;24(7):779–785.

38. Quinby JS, Golish SR, Hart JA, et al. All-inside meniscal repair using a new flexible, tensionable device. *Am J Sports Med*. 2006;34(8):1281–1286.

39. Kalliakmanis A, Zourntos S, Bousgas D, et al. Comparison of arthroscopic meniscal repair results using 3 different meniscal repair devices in anterior cruciate ligament reconstruction patients. *Arthroscopy*. 2008;24(7):810–816.

40. Small N. Complications in Arthroscopy: The knee and other joints; committee on complications of the arthroscopy association of North America. *Arthroscopy*. 1986; 2: 253–258.

41. Austin KS, Sherman OH. Complications of arthroscopic meniscal repair. *Am J Sports Med*. 1993;21(6):864–868.

42. Cohen SB, Boyd L, Miller MD. Vascular risk associated with meniscal repair using Rapidloc versus FasT-Fix: comparison of two all-inside meniscal devices. *J Knee Surg*. 2007;20(3):235–240.

43. Miller MD, Kline AJ, Jepsen KG. "All-inside" meniscal repair devices: an experimental study in the goat model. *Am J Sports Med*. 2004;32(4):858–862.

44. Dines JS, Weber L, Prajapati R, et al. The effect of growth differentiation factor-5-coated sutures to enhance tendon healing in a rat model. *J Shoulder Elbow Surg*. 2007;16(5 suppl):S215–S221.

Inside-Out and Outside-In Meniscus Repair

Peter R. Kurzweil

As our knowledge of the role the meniscus plays in knee function increases, preserving it becomes increasingly important. Even a small partial meniscectomy can significantly alter joint biomechanics. Removing less than a third of the meniscus will increase contact pressure greater than 350%. Arthroscopic inside-out repair techniques gained popularity in the early 1980s. Outside-in procedures were subsequently developed to decrease the risk of neurovascular injury. All-inside methods are increasingly performed due to ease of technique, reduced operative times, and even lower risk of injury to the neurovascular structures. The goal of this chapter is to provide a comprehensive overview of suture repair of the meniscus with the outside-in and inside-out techniques.

The medial and lateral menisci are not mirror images of each other. The medial meniscus has extensive peripheral attachments to the capsule and medial collateral ligament (MCL). The lateral meniscus has fewer capsular attachments, none at the popliteal hiatus, and no contact with the lateral collateral ligament (LCL). The lateral meniscus is more mobile and can translate up to 1 cm with knee range of motion.

The meniscus is 90% type I collagen, with the majority of the fibers aligned circumferentially (Fig. 57.1). This orientation permits absorption of the hoop stresses generated when the joint is loaded. Radially oriented fibers act to bundle together the circumferential fibers, adding strength to the overall construct. The vertical mattress stitch configuration, which mimics the path of the radially oriented fibers, has a greater repair strength than other suture orientations.

It is important to understand the vascularity of the meniscus when considering the healing potential of a tear. It is generally thought that increased vascularity correlates with better healing potential. Branches of the medial and lateral genicular arteries perforate the menisci at the capsular attachments. In the lateral meniscus, the popliteal hiatus lacks any peripheral blood supply and is essentially avascular in this region. For clinical purposes, the repairable zone of the meniscus is generally within 5 mm of the peripheral rim. This is the so-called red–red or red–white zone.

CLINICAL EVALUATION

A thorough evaluation including the patient's history, physical exam, and imaging studies can lead to an accurate diagnosis of a meniscus tear in most cases. Meniscal tears in younger patients are typically caused by a traumatic event that involves twisting or hyperflexion. Older patients may have degenerative changes in the menisci, resulting in tears with less dramatic events or even no history of injury. Symptoms typically include knee pain, swelling, locking, catching, and giving out. In the acute phase patients often limp and cannot squat.

Although several tests focus specifically on meniscal injuries, no single physical exam finding can reliably predict the presence of a tear. A recent meta-analysis found a sensitivity and specificity of 60% to 70% for the McMurray's and Apley's tests and joint line tenderness. Nevertheless, taken all together, these specific meniscal tests can give the examiner a fairly reliable method to determine whether a tear is present.

The first finding to observe is knee extension. A locked knee (with a fixed flexion contracture) is typically caused by mechanical block and is commonly seen with a bucket-handle meniscus tear. Specific focal joint line tenderness can be another clue, particularly when an effusion is present. Joint line tenderness is best assessed with the patient relaxed (sitting or supine) and the knee gently flexed close to 90°. There are three provocative maneuvers that we routinely use, although doing them depends on the patients level of guarding. The McMurray test may be too painful with an acute knee injury. In chronic situations, it can reproduce the patient's symptoms. However, if knee pain and guarding precludes performing a McMurray test, then we do an Apley's test. The patient sits with the legs dangling over the side of the exam table, and the knee is twisted internally and externally by rotating

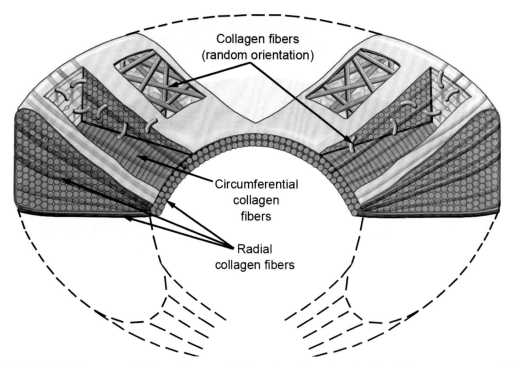

FIGURE 57.1. Three types of collagen fibers: radial, circumferential, and random. Vertical mattress sutures mimic the radial fibers and better capture the circumferential fibers that comprise the majority of the meniscus. collagen.

the foot and ankle. A positive test refers pain to the joint line. Finally, in more chronic cases, the Thessaly test is extremely helpful. This test requires a single leg stance with the leg slightly bent. The patient is then asked to twist back and forth through the knee. This frequently reproduces the knee symptoms. We typically ask the patient to perform this maneuver on the good leg first, to make sure they can do it and that it is painless.

Diagnostic Imaging

Imaging begins with the standard 4-view series of the knee, which includes weight-bearing anteroposterior (AP) and tunnel (45° posterior–anterior view), lateral, and sunrise views. Unless there is chondrocalcinosis, the menisci are not visualized. Nevertheless, plain radiographs provide valuable information regarding knee alignment, preservation of joint space, and other possible sources of knee pain.

MRI has become the gold standard for meniscal imaging, although it should be remembered when interpreting the study that the number of patients with asymptomatic tears increases with age. The MRI can also provide information regarding tear size, location, and configuration. A recent retrospective review showed that the preoperative MRI scan could accurately predict more than 90% of the time when a tear is reparable. We typically prefer not to use intra-articular contrast when imaging the menisci for tears on routine studies. The one situation that we request its use is when there is a need for assessing whether a prior meniscal repair may have retorn.

TREATMENT

Once a patient has been diagnosed with a symptomatic tear of the meniscus, several parameters should be considered when assessing the reparability of the tear. Many of these factors are best judged arthroscopically, including vascularity, size, instability, tear orientation, and tissue quality. Knee stability is another factor to consider when contemplating meniscal repair. Studies have repeatedly shown that a concomitant anterior cruciate ligament (ACL) reconstruction enhances the success rate of meniscus repair while healing rates are less than 30% in an ACL-deficient knee.

Nonoperative

Not all meniscus tears require surgery. As discussed, several studies have shown that the incidence of asymptomatic meniscal tears increases with age. If one such patient sustains a knee injury and an MRI is obtained, the scan will show a meniscus tear. However, there was no way to discern whether or not the tear was preexisting from the scan. It is important to correlate the patient's symptoms, mechanism of injury, and exam with the MRI. Patient education is also important in this scenario, as patients have come to suppose that the diagnosis from the MRI reading is "right" and subsequently expect an arthroscopic surgery. We have successfully treated numerous patients in this situation, where we concluded that the symptoms were not arising from the meniscus tear seen on MRI.

Once in surgery, not all meniscus tears are repaired or resected. Partial or small (<5 mm) tears that are judged to be stable are typically left alone, especially when located near the peripheral rim. Also, stable tears posterior to the popliteus tendon generally do not need to be resected or repaired when seen at the time of ACL reconstruction.

The protocol for nonsurgically treated meniscus tears includes a short period of restricted weight bearing and immobilization. Following resolution of the effusion and pain from the acute injury, a rehabilitation protocol is implemented that includes strengthening and range of motion. We restrict squatting and twisting activities until symptoms have resolved.

Operative

Before considering a repair, the patient should understand the postoperative restrictions that will be necessary for a successful outcome. We counsel patients and their families that despite adhering to the rehabilitation protocol, there is a 20% chance of failure that would require a second procedure. The possibility of needing additional small incisions and neurovascular risks is also discussed. Furthermore, despite the best intentions of repairing the meniscus, not all tears are reparable, and the ultimate decision regarding treatment is made in surgery. If these factors are not acceptable to the patient, they may request a meniscectomy, with a more reliable short-term outcome and quicker recovery.

TECHNIQUE

With the goal of avoiding scuffing of the articular cartilage, complete relaxation with general anesthesia facilitates instrumentation of the tear site. It would not be possible to apply a significant valgus force to the knee to open the medial compartment with local anesthesia. There would also be concern about discomfort when making accessory incisions for the repair if patients were awake. Prolonged positioning in the Figure 57.4 position, which opens up the lateral side would also be uncomfortable. Local anesthetics containing epinephrine are injected around the portals and accessory incision sites, but we are reluctant to use large doses of intra-articular local anesthetics, which would be required for surgery under local anesthesia.

A nonsterile tourniquet is applied to the proximal thigh, but rarely inflated. Avoiding tourniquet use allows better assessment of the vascularity of the tear. Gravity inflow is used, as the higher pressure from the fluid pumps may hinder bleeding at the tear site and could also lead to excessive joint swelling postoperatively.

Meniscal Preparation

Preparation of the tear, like a fracture, includes freshening the edges, reducing it anatomically, and (sometimes) insertion of provisional fixation prior to final fixation.

A rasp is used to scrape the edges of the tear down to a fresh surface. We use a small motorized shaver with minimal suction to help remove the "nonunion" tissue between the meniscal fragments. In cases of questionable vascularity, the tear site is trephinated with multiple perforations from outside-in using an 18G needle.

With unstable tears, a probe is used to reduce and hold the two fragments in anatomic alignment. The probe applies counterpressure on the inner fragment as an 18G needle is introduced from outside-in, and across the tear, to provide initial fixation.

We try to insert the meniscal fixation devices or sutures so that they apply compression perpendicular to the orientation of the tear. This typically requires instrumentation of the tear through the contralateral portal while viewing through the ipsilateral portal. The main exception to this rule is with posterior horn tears repaired with fixators. These are generally inserted through the ipsilateral portal, although this requires particular care to avoid injury to the posterior neurovascular structures.

Sutures repairs are delivered with the aid of needles or cannulas, which allow the surgeon to create vertical mattress repairs. The number of sutures used depends on the length and stability of the tear. We tend to place sutures every 6 to 8 mm. If when the knee is ranged, gapping at the repair site is observed, then additional sutures may be required.

AUTHOR'S PREFERRED METHOD OF REPAIR

We typically fix the meniscus tears with several methods, depending upon location. This "hybrid" repair utilizes both sutures and fixators. All-arthroscopic fixators are used in the most posterior aspect of the tear, as accessing this are with outside-in or inside-out suture techniques is quite difficult. For anterior third tears, outside-in sutures are used. For tears in the middle third, we will use either outside-in or inside-out sutures.

Inside-Out Repair

Inside-out repairs are best suited for middle or posterior tears. Medially, the saphenous nerve is at risk. There are several techniques we use to avoid injury to the nerve. The first is transillumination. With the lights in the operating room set low, the skin on the medial side of the knee can be transilluminated with the arthroscope, allowing visualization of a dark linear streak, which is the saphenous vein. The nerve lies just posterior to the vein. Second, by flexing the knee to 90°, the nerve moves posteriorly, away from the area of the intended incision. This 3- to 4-cm incision is made just posterior to the MCL and parallel to the posteromedial border of the tibia. The interval between the joint capsule and the medial head of the medial head of the gastrocnemius is developed mostly with blunt dissection. A retractor or spoon is inserted to protect the posterior neurovascular structures, even as the knee is brought into extension. The retractor also helps capture the needles as they are passed.

A major reason that surgeons are reluctant to undertake outside-in repair of the lateral meniscus is the risk of injury to the common peroneal nerve. The accessory incision is designed to avoid this and is typically done with the knee in 90° of flexion. The incision is made just posterior to the LCL, essentially in the "soft spot" where one would place a posterolateral portal. The iliotibial band and biceps femoris tendon are identified. The retractor is inserted anterior to the biceps, protecting the peroneal nerve that lies posterior to the biceps. Once the lateral head of the gastrocnemius is peeled of the capsule, one can begin passing the sutures.

Zone-specific cannulas are usually available in most ORs and surgery centers. The appropriate cannula is placed through the contralateral portal and can aid with reducing the tear while the sutures are passed. One should be careful when placing the cannulas intra-articularly as the tips are fairly sharp to allow purchase on the meniscus without slipping, but this can lead to iatrogenic injury to the articular cartilage of the femoral condyle as it is passed into the joint and onto the meniscus.

We typically used 2-0 nonabsorbable sutures for the repair. These can be delivered with double armed flexible needles or reusable nitinol needles, which are loaded with the suture of choice. Inside-out suture repair typically requires an assistant to hold the retractor in place and retrieve the needles as they exit the posterolateral incision. Needle sticks can occur at this stage, so extra care is required as the sutures emerge from the joint. Once the first suture is retrieved, the cannula is moved slightly to create the desired repair configuration and then the second arm of the suture is passed. Each suture is tagged and the process is repeated with as many sutures are required to

create a stable repair. Efforts are made to avoid capturing the popliteus tendon with the sutures, if possible.

Outside-In Repair

This is my preferred method for repairing tears located in the anterior two-thirds of the meniscus. Although no formal posterior incision is made, it does require one or two additional portal-sized incisions along the joint line. We typically percutaneously pass the needle into the joint until the best location is achieved. This needle is often left in place to provide initial provisional fixation to hold the reduction (Fig. 57.2). At this point, the portal-like incision is made, and a clamp is used to bluntly dissect down to the capsule.

There are several simple ways to perform and outside-in repair. There are kits commercially available from for this. If no kit is available, one can simply use the needle from an 18G angiocatheter. A long suture—either braided or nonbraided—is passed through the barrel of the needle, leaving 10 cm of the stitch extending beyond the tip of the needle. Through the accessory portal, the needle is passed across the meniscus tear from outside-in. A probe can be used for counterpressure and to maintain the reduction of the tear as the needle is passed. A grasper is sometimes needed to hold the created loop of suture inside the joint as the needle is withdrawn. A second pass with a similarly loaded needle is directed so it comes out just above the meniscus. This needle should be directed so that it passes through the loop of the first suture. Alternatively, a grasper can simply go through loop then grasp the protruding second suture and deliver it out the portal. The second needle is gently pulled out, unloading the suture. Pulling the loop of the first suture will bring the second suture

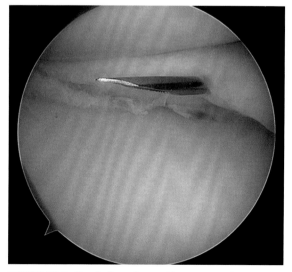 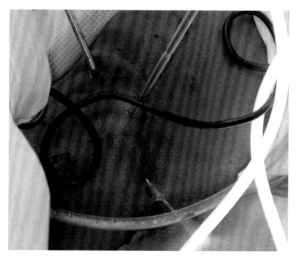

FIGURE 57.2. Needle brought outside-in to provide provisional fixation and hold reduction to facilitate meniscal repair. The photo on the right shows the probe holding the reduction through the medial portal as the needle is introduced. The arthroscope is in the anterolateral portal.

through its track, creating a vertical mattress configuration (Fig. 57.3). The sutures are then retrieved through the accessory portal and then tied (Fig. 57.4). Through each accessory portal two or three outside-in sutures can be delivered.

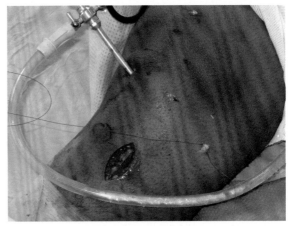

FIGURE 57.4. Right knee with hamstring harvest incision. The two suture ends are exiting the accessory portal. They will be retrieved and then tied down over the capsule. The arthroscope is in the anterolateral portal.

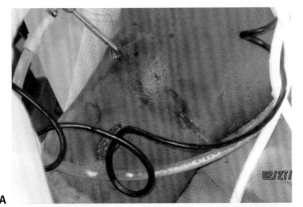

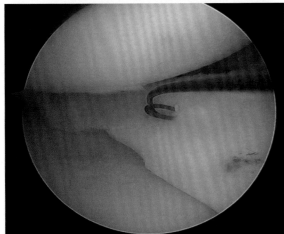

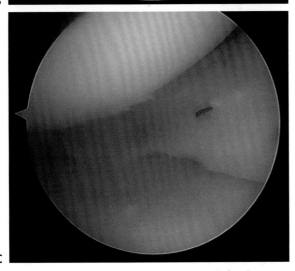

FIGURE 57.3. Outside-in meniscus repair. **A:** Strand of prolene exiting medial portal with the other end in needle. **B:** Intra-articular view of Figure A shows strand of prolene exiting medial portal after passing between second suture loop. **C:** Suture loop is pulled, bringing strand of suture through meniscus and creating oblique suture configuration.

COMPLICATIONS, CONTROVERSIES, AND SPECIAL CONSIDERATIONS

Early complications in meniscal repairs arise mainly from adverse events associated with knee arthroscopy in general. To prevent infection, we routinely give preoperative, prophylactic antibiotics (typically 1 g of cefazolin intravenously prior to the case).

As we try to enhance vascularity of the repair site, we are promoting bleeding into the knee. This does increase the risk of a hemarthrosis postoperatively. There is a fine line between appropriate and excessive bleeding. Nevertheless, we still prefer to avoid the use of postoperative drains. Patients are cautioned about this ahead of time and if the hemarthrosis is significant, the knee may be aspirated in the post-op period.

A higher rate of arthrofibrosis can be seen when meniscal repairs. Classically, this has been attributed to inside-out sutures that also capture and pinch the capsule. This has led some authors to recommend early aggressive rehabilitation protocols. Once again, a balancing act is needed since too aggressive motion may lead to gapping at the repair site.

Although this is considered a low-risk procedure for developing a deep vein thrombosis (DVT), it still can occur, especially if patients are to remain nonweight bearing for several weeks. We typically ask about family history for DVTs and pulmonary emboli. If negative, then patients are placed on one 81 mg aspirin daily or every other day for 6 weeks. If the family history is positive, or the patients themselves have had a prior blood clot, then more formal anticoagulation measures would be initiated.

Failure of the meniscus repair in the short-term is probably the most common complication. If it occurs in the first few weeks after surgery, it may be due to a loss in fixation at the repair site. This can occur for various reasons including loss of fixation, overly aggressive physical therapy, or blatant noncompliance with the protocol. In cases where a repair has failed and the patient is having mechanical symptoms, a reoperation is indicated. There are several studies in the literature demonstrating successful outcomes following initial failures of meniscus repairs, although sometimes a partial or subtotal meniscectomy as necessary.

If peroneal nerve damage is encountered, then an open exploration of the nerve is recommended. If the case involved sutures, one needs to determine whether the nerve was compressed when tying the knots for the repair. Saphenous nerve injury is more controversial. As this nerve is purely sensory, some authors recommend observation with the anticipation that the nerve may slowly regenerate. Nevertheless, it may still be worthwhile to immediately explore it just to rule out damage secondary to a suture tied directly over the nerve.

PEARLS AND PITFALLS

If vascularity of the tear site is equivocal, the motorized shaver that is used to remove the scar tissue at the repair site can be used a bit more aggressively on the peripheral fragment. In this way, the tear site is brought a bit closer to the rim, bringing vascularity to the repair.

It is not uncommon for the medial compartment to be tight, especially with locked bucket-handle medial meniscus tears. This can make reduction and instrumentation of the tear more difficult. In these situations, we routinely recess the MCL to open up the medial compartment a few extra millimeters. This is done by applying a valgus pressure to the knee joint while introducing a 14G angiocatheter needle from outside-in with multiple passes. This is continued until the joint pops open a few millimeters (Fig. 57.5). The danger is that the entire MCL is popped, but in either case, the patient is braced postoperatively. The extra room will allow better visualization, improving the reduction and insertion of fixation devices or sutures.

Sometimes the best location for making an accessory incision is gauged by setting up for an inside-out repair and actually passing the first needle out the skin percutaneously. Seeing where the needle penetrates the skin helps the surgeon judge the optimal location for the more formal accessory incision.

After the sutures have been placed, we recommend tying them before proceeding with the next part of the procedure, such as the ACL reconstruction. Sutures should be tied while arthroscopically visualizing the meniscus tear. This will help avoid overtensioning or undertensioning the knots of each suture. Cyclic loading studies demonstrate that all fixators and knots slip a little. Therefore, we prefer to err on making the tension of the repair slightly too tight rather than slightly too loose.

After completing the repair, one final step remains, which is ensuring stability of the repair site. We remove

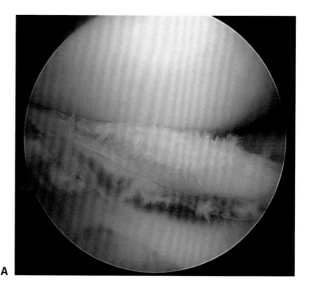
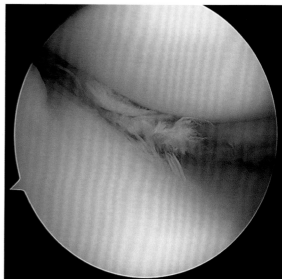
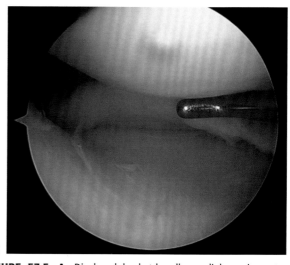

FIGURE 57.5. A: Displaced bucket-handle medial meniscus tear. **B:** Meniscus malreduced and still rotated due to tight compartment. **C:** Anatomic reduction after recessing MCL and opening tight medial compartment.

the arthroscope and range the knee several times. The scope is then reinserted and the repair site visualized and probed. If any areas of gapping or instability are seen, then more fixation may be required. We generally recommend completing the meniscus repairs fully before proceeding onto the ACL reconstruction, if one is to be performed. If the repair is not stable enough to withstand instrumentation in the OR, it will not survive the early post-op period.

POSTOPERATIVE REHABILITATION PROTOCOL

Patients use crutches during the first 2 weeks after surgery to maintain toe-touch weight bearing. A knee immobilizer or hinged brace is worn locked in extension is used for 4 weeks. Patient discontinue crutches beginning week 3 and walk in the brace with the knee held in full extension. Supine or nonweight bearing range of motion is allowed from 0° to 90° immediately. By 1 month unrestricted walking out without a brace is permitted and use of the stationary bike is encouraged. We keep away from aggressive protocols as it may lead to gapping at the repair site. Squatting beyond 90° is restricted until after 4 months. Patients can typically return to cutting and pivoting sports by 6 months. If an ACL reconstruction is done at the same time, the protocol for the meniscal repair takes precedence.

CONCLUSIONS AND FUTURE DIRECTIONS

Although the short-term results of meniscectomy are good, loss of meniscus tissue can lead to degenerative changes in the long term. When treating a symptomatic meniscus tear, every effort should be made to preserve as much of the meniscus as possible. Although suture repairs have been labeled the "gold standard," the recent trend has been to address tears with all-inside meniscus fixators. Suture repairs typically require small accessory incisions. There has been a reluctance to make accessory incisions in the knee, although it seems to be an accepted part of arthroscopic procedures in the shoulder. It is our opinion that the same attitude should pertain to knees, as suture repairs are more cost-effective and biomechanically superior to fixators.

With improved biomechanical strength of repairs, the failure of meniscal repairs appears to be biologic. One reason that there is a higher success rate of meniscus repair when done with a concomitant ACL reconstruction may be the growth factors released into the joint from exposed bone marrow of the bone tunnels. This has led others to try to simulate this milieu by performing a microfracture in the intercondylar notch during isolated meniscus repairs. Other methods to biologically enhance healing of meniscal repairs will be sought. There is increased use of adjuncts such as Platelet Rich Plasma (PRP), although my personal preference has been to use blood clot. Blood clot has been shown to be effective with meniscus tears and is much more cost-effective.

Finally, replacement of the lost meniscal tissue with a scaffold is on the horizon is already being done by our European colleagues. Currently, there are two scaffolds available, although not currently Food and Drug Administration (FDA) approved for use in the United States. The Menaflex (need name of company and city) is made of specially treated bovine collagen, whereas the Actifit (need name of company and city) is made of a biosynthetic polyurethane. The defect in the meniscus is filled with a custom-shaped implant, which is sutured to the remaining normal meniscal tissue using arthroscopic meniscus repair techniques. It differs from a meniscal allograft as normal meniscal tissue does not have to be removed, no bone tunnels are required, and the risks and hassles of using allograft tissue are avoided.

Repair of the meniscus can be a satisfying procedure with a high chance of a successful outcome when performed for the right indications and with strict adherence to the postoperative rehabilitation protocols.

SUGGESTED READINGS

Arnoczky SP, Warren RF. Microvasculature of the human meniscus. *Am J Sports Med.* 1982;10:90–95.

Barber FA, Herbert MA, Schroeder FA, et al. Biomechanical testing of new meniscal repair techniques containing ultra high–molecular weight polyethylene suture. *Arthroscopy.* 2009;25(9):959–967.

Barber FA, McGarry JE. Meniscal repair techniques. *Sports Med Arthrosc.* 2007;15(4):199–207.

Boden SD, Davis DO, Dina TS, et al. A prospective and blinded investigation of magnetic resonance imaging of the knee: abnormal findings in asymptomatic subjects. *Clin Orthop Relat Res.* 1992;282:177–185.

Chang HC, Nyland J, Caborn DN, et al. Biomechanical evaluation of meniscal repair systems: a comparison of the Meniscal Viper Repair System, the vertical mattress FasT-Fix Device, and vertical mattress ethibond sutures. *Am J Sports Med.* 2005;33(12):1846–1852.

DeHaven KE. Decision-making features in the treatment of meniscal lesions. *Clin Orthop Relat Res.* 1990;252:49–54.

Hegedus EJ, Cook C, Hasselblad V, et al. Physical examination tests for assessing a torn meniscus in the knee: a systematic review with meta-analysis. *J Orthop Sports Phys Ther.* 2007;37(9):541–550.

Laupattarakasem W, Sumanont S, Kesprayura S, et al. Arthroscopic outside-in meniscal repair through a needle hole. *Arthroscopy.* 2004;20(6):654–657.

McDevitt CA, Webber RJ. The ultrastructure and biochemistry of the meniscal cartilage. *Clin Orthop Relat Res.* 1990;252:8–18.

Nguyen TB, Kurzweil PR. Avoiding and managing complications in meniscus repair. In: Meislin RJ, Halbrecht J, eds. *Complications in Knee and Shoulder Surgery, Management and Treatment Options for the Sports Medicine Orthopedist.* London: Springer; 2009.

Stärke C, Kopf S, Petersen W, et al. Meniscal repair. *Arthroscopy.* 2009;25(9):1033–1044.

Thoreux P, Rety F, Nourissat G, et al. Bucket-handle meniscal lesion: magnetic resonance imaging criteria for reparability. *Arthroscopy.* 2006;22(9):954–961.

Meniscus Transplantation

Samuel P. Robinson • Kevin F. Bonner

The function of the meniscus in load sharing, shock absorption, joint stability, joint nutrition, and overall protection of the articular cartilage is well known (Fig. 58.1) (1–3). As a result of our increased understanding of meniscus function, the treatment of meniscal injuries has evolved from complete resection to meniscal preservation when possible. Although meniscus preservation through repair or limited resection is always preferable, specific meniscal pathology often dictates treatment. Relatively large resections to include subtotal or total meniscectomy are not uncommon, even in young patients.

Articular contact stresses increase as a function of the amount of meniscus resected. Complete medial meniscectomy decreases contact area by 50% to 70% and doubles the joint contact stress of the medial compartment (4). Segmental meniscectomy may have a similar effect on contact area and contact stress when compared with complete meniscectomy (5). Complete lateral meniscectomy decreases contact area 40% to 50% and increases joint contact stress 200% to 300% in part due to the relative convexity of the lateral tibial condyle (4). For this reason, lateral meniscectomy is considered to have a poorer prognosis than medial meniscectomy with regard to the development of osteoarthritis and pain. Since the medial meniscus is also the primary secondary stabilizer to anterior tibial translation in an anterior cruciate ligament (ACL)-deficient knee, a large posterior horn resection in this setting often increases tibial translation and instability symptoms.

Although many postmeniscectomy patients do very well and remain relatively asymptomatic for long periods, some patients develop pain earlier in the meniscal-deficient compartment as the result of increased articular contact stresses. It also must be remembered, however, that a degenerative meniscal tear may be the earliest symptomatic clinical event that signals a complicated degenerative pathway has been initiated, which is affected by more factors than just the status of the meniscus. Nonetheless, meniscal allograft transplantation has been developed to provide symptomatic relief to select patients and potentially slow the progression of degenerative changes. Since

the first meniscus transplantation in 1984 by Milachowski was reported, the technique and its indications continue to be modified and improved. Contemporary meniscus allograft transplantation after meniscectomy has been shown to decrease peak stresses and improve contact mechanics, but does not restore perfect knee mechanics (6, 7). Despite these potential benefits, this remains a difficult patient population to treat. Physicians must carefully evaluate potential meniscus transplant patients and help them maintain realistic outcome expectations.

CLINICAL EVALUATION

History

Potential transplant patients are typically less than 50 years of age with an absent or nonfunctional meniscus who are symptomatic from their meniscal insufficiency. A detailed history regarding a patient's specific symptoms, prior injuries, and subsequent surgery should be obtained. Recent arthroscopy pictures can be very helpful in determining the degree of meniscal resection and condition of the articular cartilage. Symptomatic postmeniscectomy patients typically present with joint line tenderness, swelling, and activity-related pain. Symptoms may sometimes be subtle and can be associated with barometric pressure changes.

Patients with combined ACL instability and a deficient medial meniscus may complain soley of instability or combined instability and medial-sided pain. They may have a history of an ACL injury treated nonoperatively or may have recurrent instability following ACL reconstruction in the setting of a deficient medial meniscus.

Physical Examination

Physical examination should focus on location of the pain, alignment, gait, ligament stability, range of motion, muscle strength, and ruling out alternative pathology as the primary source of pain. Joint line tenderness is critical in determining the location and cause of the symptoms while ruling out other causes of pain. The pain or tenderness from meniscal deficiency is often dull and diffuse along the involved compartment. Sharp pain on McMurray test

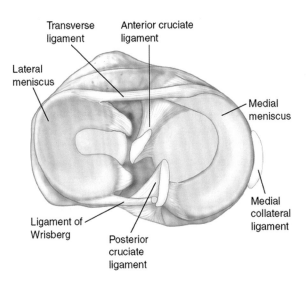

FIGURE 58.1. Illustration of proximal tibial soft tissue attachments.

may indicate recurrent meniscal injury or chondral lesion. Be sure to assess the knee for alternate causes of symptoms such as pes tendonitis. Evaluating a patient's overall alignment and gait is important in determining if a corrective osteotomy needs to performed initially or potentially in combination with other procedures. Ligamentous stability should be assessed to determine the integrity and function of both the native ligaments and the prior reconstructions. Before considering a patient for meniscal transplant, the patient should have full symmetric range of motion and adequate muscle strength.

Imaging

Imaging starts with plain radiographs that include weight-bearing anteroposterior full extension views of both knees, weight-bearing posteroanterior views in 45° of flexion (Rosenberg view), Merchant view, and a nonweight-bearing flexion lateral view (Fig. 58.2). These films are helpful to assess the degree of degenerative changes and subtle joint space narrowing. If malalignment is suspected clinically, long-leg alignment films are indicated to provide an objective evaluation. MRI is often helpful to assess the integrety of the menisci, articular cartilage, and subchondral bone (Fig. 58.2). Bone scan may reveal increased activity in the involved compartment, but the sensitivity of bone scan in this setting unknown.

If the last arthroscopy occurred over 6 months to 1 year before evaluation, diagnostic arthroscopy is useful to evaluate the meniscus and articular cartilage before ordering meniscal allograft tissue (Fig. 58.2). Arthroscopy in this setting will accurately define extent of prior meniscectomy and the degree of arthrosis in cases where previous arthroscopic images are unavailable or unclear. When evaluating the knee for a possible meniscal transplant, the integrity of the articular cartilage is critical. Patients with less than Outerbridge grade 3 articular cartilage changes are optimal candidates for a meniscus transplant although small areas of grade 3 can sometimes

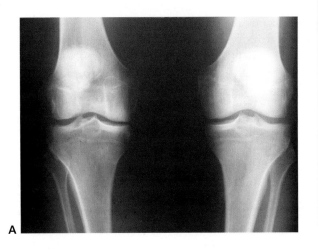

A

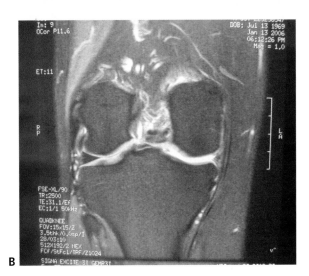

B

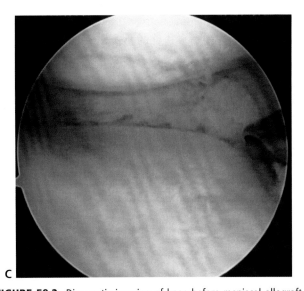

C

FIGURE 58.2. Diagnostic imaging of knee before meniscal allograft transplant. **A:** Weight-bearing anteroposterior full extension views of both knees showing early medial compartment joint space narrowing following meniscal resection. **B:** MRI of knee showing medial meniscal deficiency. **C:** Arthroscopy image of meniscus-deficient medial compartment.

V. B. The Knee **Meniscus**

be accepted. In the setting of a focal grade 4 lesion, this focal area may be addressed with a concurrent cartilage resurfacing procedure.

Differential Diagnosis

The differential diagnosis that should be considered includes recurrent meniscal tear, chondral or osteochondral lesion, advanced bipolar degenerative chondrosis, synovitis, pain emanating from the patellofemoral compartment, extra-articular knee sources (pes tendonitis/bursitis, neuroma), and hip or spine pathology. Any of these conditions may be the primary cause of symptoms rather than the proposed meniscal deficiency. However, in our experience, a small meniscal re-tear in the setting of a prior substantial meniscectomy rarely causes the patients primary symptoms. Although it may be difficult, a good examination combined with careful assessment of the studies can typically delineate who would be likely to benefit from a meniscus transplant. Injections can be helpful to differentiate intra-articular from extra-articular sources of pain. Certainly one of the most challenging aspects of meniscus transplant surgery is determining when moderate chondrosis has advanced to the point where a meniscal transplant is unlikely to yield a good clinical outcome. Although a chondral or osteochondral lesion may be the primary cause of pain in a meniscal-deficient compartment, meniscal deficiency may need to be addressed concurrently (i.e., chondroprotection of meniscus transplant).

TREATMENT

Nonoperative Treatment

Patients typically undergo a trial of conservative management. This may include activity modification to include nonimpact activities and exercises, appropriate pharmacologic therapy (Non-steroidal anti-inflammatory medications [NSAID], etc.), injection therapy, and unloader braces. These treatment options may also be helpful for diagnostic purposes while trying to work through the differential diagnosis. A possible exception to initial nonsurgical management may be in the setting of medial meniscal deficiency combined with chronic ACL deficiency or a failed prior ACL reconstruction. A concomitant reconstruction of the ACL with meniscal allograft replacement may improve joint stability, ACL graft survival, and eventual clinical outcome (8).

Surgical Indications

Meniscal allograft transplantation is an option in the carefully selected patient with symptomatic meniscal deficiency. The procedure is typically indicated in patients less than 50 years of age with an absent or nonfunctional meniscus with symptoms of moderate-to-severe pain due to meniscal insufficiency before the development of advanced chondrosis. Younger individuals (often in their teens and twenties) presenting with joint space narrowing

following meniscectomy associated with more mild pain may be considered a relative indication. Contraindications to surgery include age above 50 years (relative, not absolute), skeletal immaturity, immunodeficiency, inflammatory arthritis, prior deep knee infection, osteophytes indicating bony architectural changes, marked obesity, generalized Outerbridge grade 3 to 4 articular changes (focal chondral defects may be addressed concurrently), knee instability (unless concurrently corrected), or marked malalignment (unless concurrently corrected). A point of interest is that some authors have had success with combined medial meniscus transplant, cartilage repair, and osteotomy in select patients with unicompartment arthritis under the age of 50 (9).

Patient selection is a critical factor in achieving a successful clinical result. Meniscal transplantation improves the contact forces across the joint, which may potentially limit or slow the progression of osteoarthritic changes. Certainly a patient that has already developed severe degenerative changes will not benefit from the chondroprotective effects of a meniscal transplant. Long-term data is not currently available to justify the procedure as a prophylatic treatment in young *asymptomatic* patients with significant meniscal deficiency. Until further data is available to help elucidate which asymptomatic meniscectomy patients would benefit in the long term from a transplant, there is currently a subset of patients who will present within a "window of opportunity" between the onset of symptoms and the development of prohibitive degenerative arthritic changes.

An evolving indication involves patients with combined medial meniscal insufficiency and chronic ACL instability or prior ACL reconstruction failure. Patients with increased anterior translation due to loss of the posterior horn of the medial meniscus and increased laxity of the other secondary restraints may potentially have improved outcomes from the ACL reconstruction when combined with a medial meniscus transplant (8). Our experience has also shown that we are able to more reliably restore stability to a chronically ACL/medial meniscus-deficient knee in either a primary or a revision setting with the combined procedure.

Preoperative Planning

Although size matching of meniscal allografts to recipient knees is thought to be critical, the tolerance of size mismatch is unknown. Authors generally recommend that meniscal transplant allografts be within 5% of the patients' native meniscal size. Various sizing methods have been proposed, but measurements based on plain radiographs utilizing magnification markers and MRI are most commonly used clinically. On anteroposterior radiographs, the meniscal width is calculated based on the width of the compartment from the peak of the medial or lateral eminence to the boarder of the tibial plateau. The lateral radiograph is used to determine the meniscal length based on the length of the tibial plateau. After correction for magnification, the values are multiplied by 0.8 for the medial meniscus and 0.7 for the lateral meniscus. This technique, described by Pollard (10), has been shown to successfully match the meniscus in at least 95% of cases (11).

Meniscal allografts are procured under strict aseptic conditions within 12 hours of cold ischemic time in accordance with standards established by the American Association of Tissue Banks for donor suitability and testing. Meniscal allografts have been available as fresh, freeze dried, cryopreserved, or fresh frozen although cryopreserved and fresh frozen are the most common. Fresh allografts are logistically difficult because they must be used within 7 to 14 days of harvest, but still maintain cell viability. Freeze-dried allograft preparation not only alters the biomechanical properties of the tissue, but this processing (lyophilization) has been implicated in meniscal graft shrinkage. Thus, these grafts are no longer used clinically. The cryopreservation preparation process does not affect the structural and tensile properties of the meniscus, but cell viability in the meniscus is only 10% to 40% (11). Although shown to work well and safely, cryopreserved grafts have not proved to be superior to fresh frozen in clinical trials. Fresh-frozen allografts, which do not maintain cell viability, are easier to manage clinically and are the most commonly utilized grafts at this time. Unlike osteochondral allografts, maintenance of cell viability is not believed to have clinical significance related to outcomes. Meniscal allografts become repopulated with recipient cells within 4 weeks of transplantation (12, 13).

AUTHORS' PREFERRED TECHNIQUE

Lateral Meniscus Graft Preparation

A previously size-matched lateral meniscus with the attached tibial plateau is thawed in a saline/antibiotic solution. The excess capsular tissue is removed from donor meniscal tissue. The bone bridge-in-slot technique, which maintains a bridge of bone between anterior and posterior inseretion sites, is always used. The most common bone preparation techniques include keyhole, dovetail, and slot configurations (Fig. 58.3). Commercially available meniscus workstations can facilitate bone bridge preparation into various shapes, which will match tibial recipient sites (Arthrex, Naples, FL; Stryker, Kalamazoo, MI). Care is used during bone preparation not to injure the meniscus insertion sites. The superior surface of the meniscus and the popliteal hiatus are marked with a surgical marker. Utilizing 10-in flexible meniscus repair needles (Ethibond, Somerville, NJ), a vertical mattress suture are placed through the posterior horn of the meniscus, which

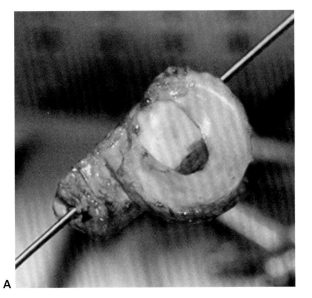

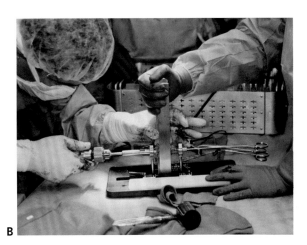

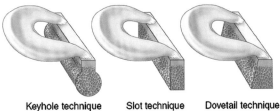

C   Keyhole technique   Slot technique   Dovetail technique

FIGURE 58.3. Lateral meniscal allograft preparation. **A:** Lateral meniscal allograft before preparation. **B:** Allograft preparation station—keyhole (Arthrex, Naples, FL). **C:** Illustration of meniscal allograft bone block preparation techniques (keyhole, slot, and dovetail). **D:** Intraoperative preparation of meniscal bone block (dovetail). **E:** Lateral meniscal allograft just before transplantation (keyhole).

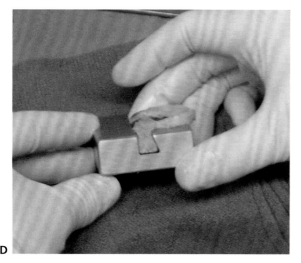

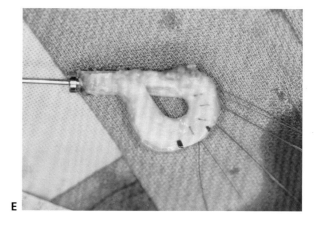

FIGURE 58.3. (continued)

will serve as a passage suture to aid in the reduction of the meniscus. The needles are left intact on the sutures.

Lateral Approach and Tibial Preparation

The patient is placed supine on the operating table with the knee at the table break. After induction of anesthesia, an examination under anesthesia is performed. A nonsterile touniquet is placed around the patient's thigh and a post is placed along the lateral aspect of the affected thigh. For a lateral meniscal transplant, the lower extremity is placed in figure-four position during various steps of the procedure to aid in distraction of the lateral compartment. The procedure begins with an arthroscopy to address any concommitant pathology and to confirm the patient is still a good candidate for the procedure. Once the medial compartment is examined, the lateral post is typically removed so that it does not get in the way throughout the remainder of the procedure.

A combined arthroscopic, lateral parapatellar arthrotomy, and posterolateral approach is used for the procedure. It is helpful to make the lateral portal just adjacent to the patellar tendon so that it will be close to being in line to the anterior and posterior horn insertion sites. An arthroscopic debridement and excoriation to the far peripheral meniscal rim or joint capsule is performed with a combination of upbiters, shavers, and meniscal rasps. Typically, a small 1 to 2 mm rim of meniscal tissue is maintained, if present. A scalpel blade may be placed through the anterolateral portal to assist in excising the anterior horn of the lateral meniscus. Initially, the attachment sites of the anterior and posterior horns are preserved as they will serve as a guide for placement of the recipient trough. An arthroscopic burr is used through the anterolateral portal to create a small trough in line with the anterior and posterior horn attachments to function as a guide for the recipient site (Fig. 58.4). If the anterolateral portal is not in an optimal position, the scope is placed in the anteromedial portal and a new lateral portal is established with the aid of a spinal needle.

The proximal tibia is exposed with a small lateral parapatellar arthrotomy extended in line with the trough (Fig. 58.5). Commercially available instrumentation (Arthrex, Naples, FL; Stryker, Kalamazoo, MI) is used to create the tibial recipient site in line with the anterior and posterior horn attachments as previously identified with the trough. Care is taken to advance the trough to, but not penetrating, the posterior tibial cortex. Intraoperative fluoroscopy can be helpful, if needed. The recipient site is prepared so that it is large enough to easily accept the graft. A posterolateral exposure is performed to receive inside-out sutures as performed with a meniscus repair. With the knee in 90° of flexion, the skin incision is made just posterior to the lateral collateral ligament; two-thirds of the incision is made distal to the joint line. The interval

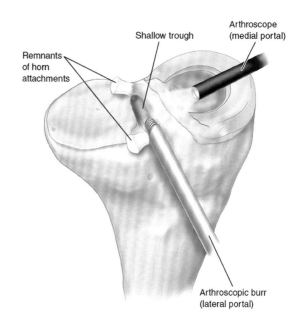

FIGURE 58.4. Illustration of arthroscopic burr being used to create bone trough along lateral meniscus insertion sites.

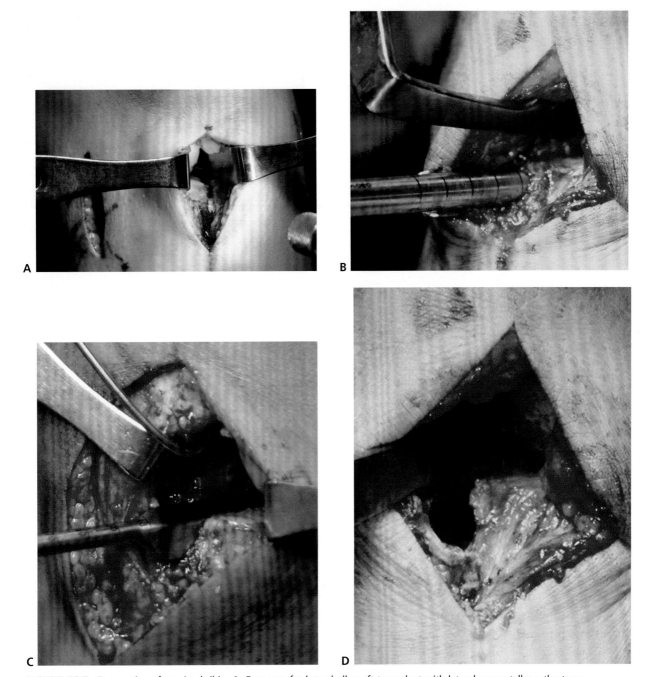

FIGURE 58.5. Preparation of proximal tibia. **A:** Exposure for lateral allograft transplant with lateral parapatellar arthrotomy and posterolateral approach. **B and C:** Preparation of tibial trough with commercially available instrumentation (B-keyhole, C-dovetail). **D:** Completed keyhole tibial preparation (not tibial as stated).

between the iliotibial band and the biceps femoris is developed. The posterolateral joint capsule is exposed with a deep dissection between the lateral collateral ligament and the lateral gastrocnemius tendon. It is often easier to develop the interval between the gastrocnemius and the joint capsule by starting distally.

Delivery and Fixation of the Lateral Meniscus

The inside-out passage suture, which was previously placed in the posterior horn of the graft, is first passed through

the miniarthrotomy and posterolateral capsule to assist in delivery of the graft (Fig. 58.6). Optimal placement of these sutures through the capsule is based on their relative position in the meniscus. The popliteus tendon and the popliteal hiatus in the graft are used as guides for proper placement. With the knee in figure-four position to keep a varus stress on the knee, the shape-matched donor graft is simultaneously inserted into the tibial recipient site while the posterior inside-out sutures are pulled to advance the graft and reestablish the normal insertion sites. Similar

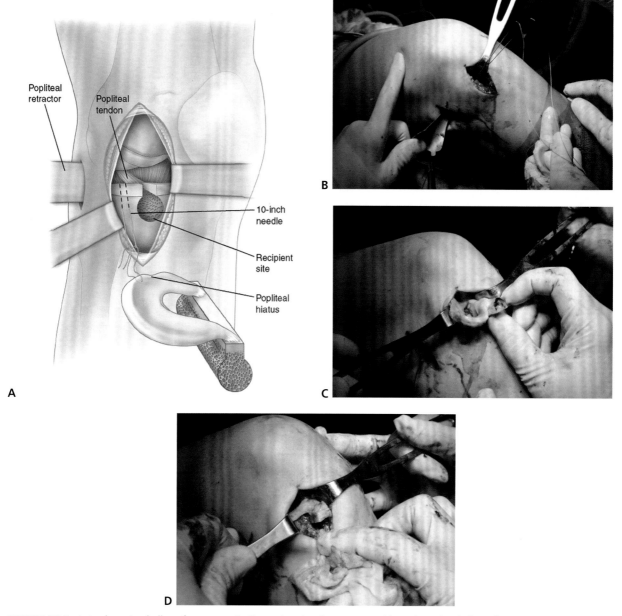

FIGURE 58.6. Lateral meniscal allograft passage. **A:** Illustration showing passage of lateral meniscal allograft. **B:** Inside-out sutures passed through the posterolateral capsule are placed to facilitate graft passage. **C and D:** Intraoperative photograph showing insertion of a dovetail lateral meniscal allograft.

to a bucket-handle meniscal tear, a probe or blunt trocar may assist in reducing the posterior horn under the lateral femoral condyle. Matching the anterior cortices of the graft and the recipient while bringing the knee through a full range of motion assists in final anterior–posterior positioning. Proper final positioning should be confirmed by visualizing the posterior horn with the arthroscope. With a suture cannula placed through the medial portal and the scope is placed into the lateral arthrotomy incision, additional inside-out meniscal sutures are placed (Fig. 58.7). Sutures are delivered and tied through the posterolateral meniscal repair incision with the knee in flexion. The slot technique may use an interference screw or transosseous

suture fixation to secure the bone portion of the graft in the donor slot, but this fixation is typically unecessary with the dovetail and keyhole techniques.

Medial Meniscus Graft Preparation

A previously size-matched medial meniscus allograft with the attached tibial plateau is thawed in a saline/antibiotic solution. The soft tissues are removed as described previously for the lateral meniscus. Although some authors utilize a bone-bridge technique for the medial side, due to the location of the ACL tibial insertion site and the distance between the insertion sites, we typically utilize a bone plug-tunnel technique for the medial meniscus. The

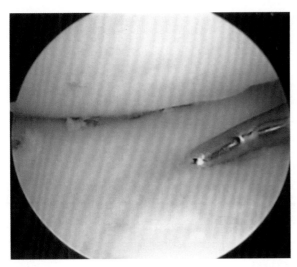

FIGURE 58.7. Arthroscopic view of reduced and repaired lateral meniscal allograft transplant.

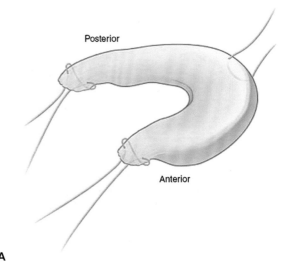

A

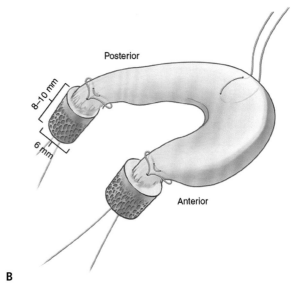

B

FIGURE 58.8. Illustration of medial meniscal allograft preparation options. **A:** Without bone plugs. **B:** With bone plugs.

anterior and posterior horns of a medial meniscal allograft may be fashioned with or without bone plugs, which is currently a point of controversy (Fig. 58.8). For preparation without bone plugs, detach the anterior and posterior horns from the bone block and whipstitch each horn with heavy nonabsorbable suture. Our preferred technique utilizes a preparation with bone plugs, which are prepared by placing a beath guidepin through the insertion sites on the bone block. A 6- to 7-mm bone plug is prepared for the posterior horn by using commercially available collared pins and coring reamers (Arthrex, Naples, FL) (Fig. 58.9). The beath pin, which was drilled into the insertion site, is removed and the collared pin is placed into the hole. The coring reamers, which are placed over their respectively sized collared pins, are used to harvest the bone plugs (Fig. 58.9B). For sizing purposes, a 7-mm collared pin/coring reamer will produce a 6-mm bone plug. The anterior horn is fashioned in a similar fashion, but can be slightly larger. The bone plugs are trimmed and tapered until the length of each measures 6 to 8 mm. A heavy nonabsorbable suture is placed up the hole in the bone plug, whipstitched through the meniscal root tissue, and placed back down the bone plug hole. Each bone plug is prepared in a similar fashion. Similar to the lateral meniscus, a vertical inside-out passing stitch utilizing 10-in needles with nonabsorbable suture is placed in the posterior horn of the medial meniscus. This not only aids in passage and reduction of the meniscus, but also for fixation to the joint capsule. The posterior horn is marked on the superior meniscal surface for in vivo visualization (Fig. 58.9D).

Medial Meniscus Approach and Tibial Preparation

The positioning, evaluation under anesthesia, and arthroscopy of a medial meniscus transplant is identical to that previously described for the lateral meniscus. The case is performed through arthroscopic, medial parapatellar, and posteromedial meniscal repair approaches. The medial parapatellar portal is made in line with the anterior and posterior insertion sites. Alternatively, an accessory portal can be made by going under the posterior cruciate ligament (PCL) insertion site in order to access the posterior horn insertion site. Arthroscopically, the meniscal remnant, if present, is debrided back to a 1- to 2-mm meniscal rim. The surrounding capsule and meniscal bed is abraded with the shaver and meniscal rasps. In order to visualize and access the posterior horn insertion site, a small notchplasty is performed under the femoral insertion of the PCL (Fig. 58.10). This can be performed with a combination of currettes and bone shavers without damaging the PCL. The medial tibial spine is also resected until there is adequate space for placement of the posterior tunnel guide and subsequent delivery of the bone plug.

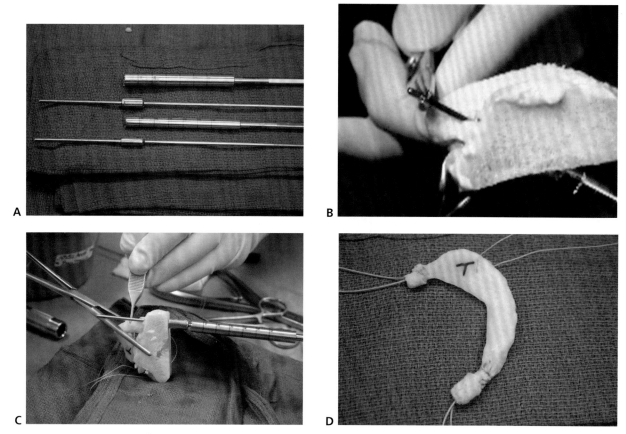

FIGURE 58.9. A: Commercially available collared pins and coring reamers (Arthrex, Naples, FL). **B:** Reaming over collared pin placed in posterior horn insertion site. **C:** Reaming over collared pin placed in anterior horn insertion site. **D:** Medial meniscal allograft with bone plugs prepared for transplant.

Under arthroscopic visualization, a variable angle ACL tibial drill guide is used to place a guidepin in the center of the native posterior horn insertion site footprint (Fig. 58.11). A 7- to 8-mm tibial tunnel is drilled using a cannulated reamer while the guidepin is cupped using a

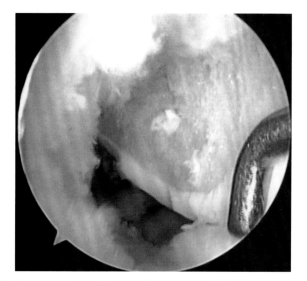

FIGURE 58.10. Notchplasty under native PCL facilitates exposure to insertion site of posterior horn of medial meniscus.

curved currette to avoid inadvertant advancement. After completion, the intraarticular aperture of the tunnel is debrided and chamfered. A medial parapatellar incision is made to allow access to the anteromedial proximal tibia (Fig. 58.12). It is important, however, to complete the posterior tibial tunnel before making the arthrotomy. A shuttle suture is placed up the posterior tibial tunnel exiting out the arthrotomy. We typically use a commercially made looped PDS suture; alternatively, a wire loop can be used. A posteromedial exposure for an inside-out medial meniscal repair is performed. During this exposure, the infrapatellar branch of the saphenous nerve must be protected.

Delivery and Fixation of the Medial Meniscus

The knee is flexed 20° and a valgus stress applied with adequate posterior exposure and retractor placement. The delivery suture needles are placed through the medial arthrotomy and out through the posteromedial capsule. The posterior bone plug sutures are delivered through the arthrotomy, out the posterior horn tunnel through the previously placed suture shuttle. The posterior bone plug suture and midportion allograft suture are advanced into the knee with the previously placed suture shuttles. Through the medial parapatellar arthrotomy, the meniscal allograft

V. B. The Knee Meniscus

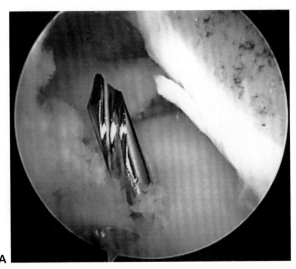

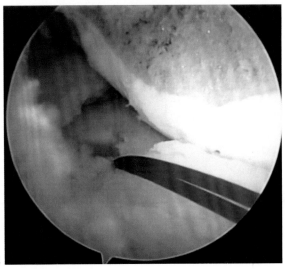

FIGURE 58.11. Preparation of posterior tibial insertion site for medial meniscal transplant. **A:** Arthroscopic placement of guidepin in center of native posterior horn medial meniscus insertion site. **B:** Passage suture in posterior bone tunnel exiting anterior through medial arthrotomy.

is delivered into the knee by simultaneously pulling traction on the posterior bone plug sutures through the tibial tunnel and the posterior horn suture through the posteromedial incision (Fig. 58.13). With the scope through the anterolateral portal, a hemostat is placed through the arthrotomy to grasp the bone plug and assist in delivering the plug posteriorly under the PCL. A hemostat or probe can assist in delivering the posterior horn under the medial femoral condyle. It is often difficult to fully seat the posterior bone plug until the posterior horn is reduced. A valgus stress is required to reduce the posterior horn while simultaneously pulling on the posteromedial suture. Before continuing, the posterior bone plug should be fully seated into the posterior tunnel. Using an inside-out meniscal repair technique, the posterior half to two-thirds of the allograft is sutured to the periphery. Through the parapatellar arthrotomy, the anterior horn insertion site is determined and a beath guidepin is placed in its center. A 9-mm tunnel is drilled vertically to a depth sufficient

to accept the anterior allograft bone plug (approximately 10 mm). A 2.5-mm hole is drilled perpendicular to the tunnel from the anterior tibial cortex. A large free needle loaded with the sutures from the anterior bone plug can be used to shuttle the sutures through the anterior tunnel exiting the anterior cortex. Alternatively, a Hewston suture passer can be passed through the 2.5-mm hole to shuttle the bone plug sutures. The anterior bone plug suture is advanced and used to deliver the anterior bone plug in the tunnel such that it is fully seated (Fig. 58.14). The bone plug can also be impacted under direct visualization through the arthrotomy. The anterior bone plug sutures are tied to the posterior bone plug sutures over the bone bridge in the anterior cortex. Another option for fixation is a ligament button or Endobutton (Smith & Nephew, Warsaw, IN) on the anterior tibial cortex. The meniscal allograft repair for the anterior horn is completed using additional inside-out sutures through an open repair technique through the miniarthrotomy (Fig. 58.15).

PEARLS AND PITFALLS

A practical dilemma in meniscus transplant surgery is properly identifying patients who will benefit and be happy with their outcome following surgery. It is sometimes difficult to be sure that meniscal deficiency is the main cause of the patient's symptoms or that a meniscal transplant will significantly improve a patient's outcome when performed with a concomitant procedure such as a cartilage resurfacing or ACL reconstruction. Patients often do not present within the window between onset of symptoms and development of advanced degenerative changes.

Preoperative planning is crucial to optimize operating room efficiency and organize the steps of the procedure. When combined with other procedures, tunnel or troughs

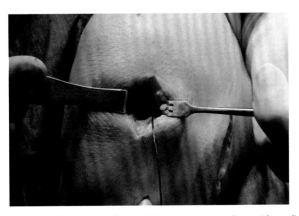

FIGURE 58.12. Exposure for medial meniscus transplant with medial parapatellar arthrotomy.

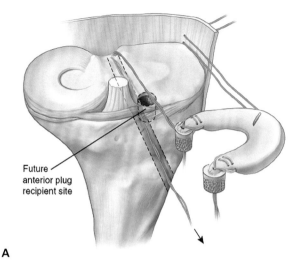

A

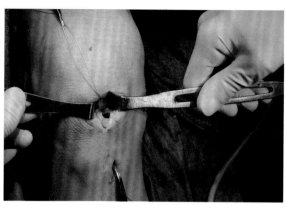

FIGURE 58.14. Intraoperative photograph of the anterior horn bone plug just before insertion into the recipient site.

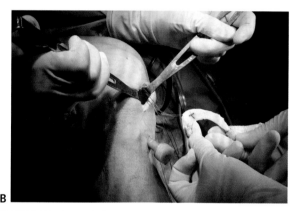

B

FIGURE 58.13. Medial meniscal allograft passage. **A:** Illustration of medial meniscal allograft passage. **B:** Preparing to deliver posterior bone plug and meniscus through the medial arthrotomy. Note the passage suture going through the cannula and up the posterior tunnel exiting the anterior arthrotomy.

may need to be adjusted to avoid tunnel convergence. Proper preparation of the host compartment and the meniscal allograft is essential. If possible, it is important to leave a 1- to 2-mm vascularized peripheral rim of host meniscus. A limited release of the MCL in a tight medial compartment may not only help with visualization, but can often be critical in facilitating meniscus delivery and instrumentation access. However, it is important to make sure this is done either proximal or distal (preferred) to the joint line, so as to not interfere with the capsule where the inside-out sutures need to be secured. When preparing the graft for a medial transplant, it is important to undersize bone plugs by at least 1 mm relative to the tunnels. Making the posterior plug as small as possible while maintaining the bone integrity of the plug facilitates passage of the plug. For a lateral meniscal transplant, we recommend commercially available graft preparation instrumentation for a bone block technique.

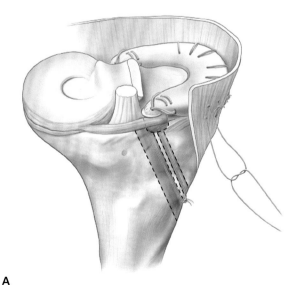

A

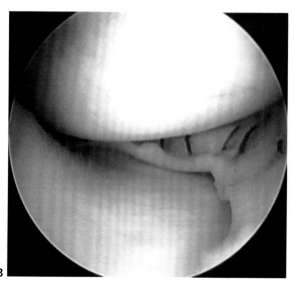

B

FIGURE 58.15. Completion of medial meniscal allograft transplant. **A:** Illustration showing final medial meniscal allograft transplant construct. **B:** Arthroscopic photograph of the completed medial meniscal transplant.

For a medial transplant, inadvertent bone plug detachment or fracture can be corrected by reattachment with suture or conversion to a plugless technique. Although we favor the utilization of bone plugs, it is currently controversial if bone plug fixation significantly improves the outcome of meniscal transplantation.

REHABILITATION

Guidelines after meniscus transplantation often need to be altered based on concommitant procedures. In an isolated meniscal transplant, weight bearing as tolerated is generally permitted with a hinged knee brace locked in full extension and crutch assistance. The hinged knee brace is used for a total of 6 weeks. Crutches are discontinued when the patient has full extension without quadriceps lag and is able to ambulate without a flexed-knee gait. A continuous passive motion machine may be helpful for 3 to 6 weeks. Non-weight-bearing range of motion is limited from 0° to 90° for the first 6 weeks after which flexion is increased as tolerated. Closed chain exercises, cycling, and swimming start 6 weeks after surgery. Patients may start straight line running between 4 and 6 months. Deep squatting is not allowed for 6 to 9 months. Pivoting sports, if patients return at all, are not permitted until 6 to 12 months after surgery, depending on concommitant procedures and overall knee pathology.

COMPLICATIONS

Before proceeding with surgical intervention, it is important to discuss potential complications and realistic outcome expectations with patients considering this procedure. Meniscal allograft transplantation carries a risk of persistent or progressive symptoms, surgical site infection, viral or bacterial disease transmission, neurovascular injury, meniscus tear or extrusion, nonhealing or incomplete healing of the allograft, and arthrofibrosis. Typically, recurrent or progressive symptoms are related to further degeneration of the articular cartilage.

CONTROVERSIES AND SPECIAL CONSIDERATIONS

Fixation of the meniscal allograft to the tibia is a source of debate among orthopedic surgeons familiar with this procedure. Although the procedure is technically less demanding without bone plugs, some authors currently feel that bone plug fixation may improve outcomes through enhanced fixation (14). There is debate regarding the differences in stability, healing, and fixation strength between bone plug fixation and soft tissue fixation. Further study is needed to fully evaluate the long-term in vivo healing, stability, and clinical results of various fixation methods. Certainly some authors routinely do not utilize bone plugs with good reported success. In cases where our posterior bone plug has become compromised, we have converted to soft tissue fixation of the meniscal root and have not noted differences in clinical success in these cases.

Another area of controversy involves indications and timing of surgery. Currently, we do not generally recommend this procedure in an asymptomatic patient. However, it is important to educate young patients on the early, sometimes subtle, symptoms of meniscal deficiency and early chondrosis. Progression of joint space narrowing with very early onset of symptoms in a very young patient with a large meniscal resection warrants consideration of a meniscal transplant.

Patients with combined medial meniscal insufficiency and chronic ACL instability or failure of a prior ACL reconstruction are an area of special consideration. Patients with increased anterior translation due to loss of the posterior horn of the medial meniscus and increased laxity of the secondary restraints may potentially have improved outcomes from the ACL reconstruction when combined with a medial meniscus transplant (8). Our experience has also shown that we have had more reliable results with the combined procedure, but this has yet to be shown in a randomized trial.

Although meniscal transplant is generally contraindicated in compartments with advanced chondrosis, some authors have reported some success in this group when combined with other procedures (9). The extent of chondrosis and ability to potentially restore this area, assessment, and potential correction of alignment, as well as the age and activity levels of patients, are factors when determining if this is a reasonable treatment option. As patients get older, we must not forget that unicompartmental arthroplasty may offer a more reliable alternative.

Research into these areas of controversy will continue to improve our understanding, clarify our indications, and modify our techniques related to meniscal transplantation. Further study is needed to determine if meniscal transplantation, when performed for the proper indications, will change the natural history of progressive degenerative arthritis in the meniscal-deficient compartment and to what degree clinical outcomes are improved.

CONCLUSIONS AND FUTURE DIRECTIONS

With appropriate indications, current success rates for allograft meniscus transplantation range between 75% and 85% (15–17). The ideal candidate is a younger patient with a well-aligned, stable knee who has activity-related pain from meniscal deficiency, but has not yet progressed to significant degenerative changes. Since poor results are typically associated with more advanced articular cartilage degeneration, and many patients do not present until this time, it is important to carefully assess the articular cartilage before considering meniscal allograft transplantation (18, 19). Patient selection is critical and patient expectations should be reasonable.

When meniscus transplants are combined with articular cartilage resurfacing, ligament reconstruction, and/or realignment procedures, favorable outcomes can be obtained. One study reported that 86% of patients with a combined ACL reconstruction and meniscus transplant had normal or near-normal International Knee Documentation Committee (IKDC) scores with an average maximum KT arthrometer side-to-side difference of 1.5 mm (20). Cole et al. found that meniscal allograft transplantation alone or with concurrent articular cartilage reconstructive procedure had improvements in knee pain and function at 2-year follow-up. They found that 90% of patients were classified as normal or nearly normal using the IKDC knee examination score (16).

Despite the technical difficulty associated with meniscal allograft transplantation, appropriately indicated patients have shown moderate-to-high levels of satisfaction. There is no question; however, this is often a difficult patient poplulation to manage, and outcome expectations need to be reasonable. Patients need to realize that you are not giving them back a normal knee. Additional study into the indications, techniques, and outcomes of meniscal allograft transplantation is required to refine the controversial aspects of the surgery and improve clinical outcomes.

The future use of biologic scaffolds that may be implanted arthroscopically into the meniscal defect at the time of meniscectomy is currently under investigation. Early clinical use of a bioresorbable collagen matrix implant has been used for both acute and chronic meniscal deficiency. Although there may be some promise to improving outcomes in more chronic cases, further study needs to be done to determine if biomechanically competent meniscal-like tissue can predictably form, function, and improve outcomes to justify its use. Other matrix type implants are currently under investigation in animal models as well. Certainly the theory of implanting an off-the-shelf biologic scaffold-type implant is atttractive if proven to be effective. Only future study will determine if these or similar technologies will play a clinical role in our treatment of patients with meniscal deficiency.

REFERENCES

1. Fairbanks TJ. Knee joint changes after menisectomy. *J Bone Joint Surg.* 1948;30B:664–670.
2. Levy IM, Torzilli PA, Warren RF. The effect of medial meniscectomy on anterior posterior motion of the knee. *J Bone Joint Surg.* 1982;64A:883–887.
3. Walker PS, Erkman MJ. The role of the meniscus in force transmission across the knee. *Clin Orthop.* 1975;109:184–192.
4. Baratz ME, Fu FH, Mengato R. Meniscal tears: the effect of meniscectomy and of repair on intra-articular contact areas and stress in the human knee: a preliminary report. *Am J Sports Med.* 1986;14:270–275.
5. Lee SJ, Aadalen KJ, Malaviya P, et al. Tibiofemoral contact mechanics after serial medial meniscectomies in the human cadaveric knee. *Am J Sports Med.* 2006;34:1334–1344.
6. Markolf KL, Mensch JS, Amstutz HC. Stiffness and laxity of the knee—the contributions of supporting structures. *J Bone Joint Surg.* 1976;58A:583–594.
7. Allen PR, Denham RA, Swan AV. Late degenerative changes after meniscectomy: factors affecting the knee after the operation. *J Bone Joint Surg.* 1984;66B:666–671.
8. Sekiya JK, Giffin RJ, Irrgang JJ, et al. Clinical outcomes after combined meniscal allograft transplantation and anterior cruciate ligament reconstruction. *Am J Sports Med.* 2003;31(6):896–906.
9. Gomoll AH, Kang RW, Chen AL, et al. Triad of cartilage restoration for unicompartmental arthritis treatment in young patients: meniscus allograft transplantation, cartilage repair and osteotomy. *J Knee Surg.* 2009;22(2):137–141.
10. Pollard ME, Kang Q, Berg EE. Radiographic sizing for meniscal transplantation. *Arthroscopy.* 1995;11:684–687.
11. Verkonk R, Kohn D. Harvest and conservation of meniscal allografts. *Scand J Med Sci Sports.* 1999;87:715–724.
12. Jackson DW, Windler GE, Simon TM. Cell survival after transplantation of fresh meniscal allografts: DNA probe analysis in a goat model. *Am J Sports Med.* 1993;21:540–549.
13. Verdonk PM, Demurie A, Almqist KF, et al. Transplantation of viable meniscal allograft. Survivorship analysis and clinical outcome of one hundred cases. *J Bone Joint Surg Am.* 2005;87:715–724.
14. Rodeo SA. Meniscal allografts-where do we stand? *Am J Sports Med.* 2001;29:246–261.
15. Cole BJ, Carter TR, Rodeo SA. Allograft meniscal transplantation: background, techniques, and results. *J Bone Joint Surg.* 2002;84A:1236–1250.
16. Cole BJ, Dennis MG, Lee S, et al. Prospective evaluation of allograft meniscus transplantation: minimum 2-year follow-up. *Am J Sports Med.* 2006;13:1–9.
17. Kang RW, Lattermann C, Cole BJ. Allograft meniscus transplantation: background, indication, techniques, and outcomes. *J Knee Surg.* 2006;19:220–230.
18. Shelton WR, Dukes AD. Meniscus replacement with bone anchors: a surgical technique. *Arthroscopy.* 1994;10:324–327.
19. Garrett JC. Meniscal transplantation: review of forty-three cases with two-to-seven year follow up. *Sports Med Arthrosc Rev.* 1993;1:164–167.
20. Sekiya JK, Ellingson CI. Meniscal allograft transplantation. *J Am Acad Orthop Surg.* 2006;14:164–174.

PART C
Patellofemoral

Clinical Approach to the Patellofemoral Joint

John P. Fulkerson

CLINICAL EVALUATION

Diagnosis of the patellofemoral joint has been challenging for orthopedic surgeons and other musculoskeletal clinicians. Because diagnosis around the anterior knee can be complicated, the prudent clinician will allow the time necessary to acquire a full history of the problem and also time for a thorough clinical evaluation. Designing proper treatment is only possible with a thorough understanding of each patient's problem.

History

Of paramount importance with regard to diagnosis in patients with anterior knee, pain is establishing the nature of the problem. Has the patient experienced instability? Has the patient had predominantly pain or instability and pain? Confusing this issue, at times, is the fact that instability or imbalance of forces around the anterior knee can also lead to pain. It is the clinician's responsibility to discern the differences here and determine what is going on.

Listening to the patient has proven very important. William Post (1) published an article regarding the importance of pain diagrams, he established through asking patients to fill in a picture of the knee, specifically identifying location of pain, that patients will generally point the clinician in the right direction. By the same token, if pain is not the primary consideration, then patient may not be able to complete the pain diagram and therefore the clinician must help the patient to better address the nature of his/her problem, usually instability. So, a careful series of questions for the patient regarding the nature of his/her problem will be most helpful. In particular, the clinician should ask the location of pain, timing of pain (is it activity related?), and initial onset (was there an injury?). Any pattern of referral above or below the knee is important. One should recall also that a problem in the hip can cause pain radiating down to anterior thigh and sometimes to the region immediately above or around the patella. I have found that approaching diagnosis of the anterior knee with a few provocative questions often leads to important insights. For instance, trying to define the

nature of the pain (sharp, dull, tingley, localized, diffuse, etc.) will provide some clues.

If the patient has instability, one must determine causes of instability events and whether the problem is really instability of the patella or giving away of the knee related to weak quadriceps, a meniscus tear, ligament deficiency, or some other dysfunction of the knee.

In the patient who has had previous surgery, one should be aware of the possibility of *medial patella* instability after lateral release or realignment of the anterior knee. Patients with medial patella instability will often give a history of *very sudden* collapse of the knee. The nature of these episodes is slippage of the patella from too far medial back laterally into the trochea, very suddenly. This can be misleading, as such patients experience their patella going laterally when in fact it is indeed going laterally but from too *far medial*. Failing to recognize this may cause the clinician to believe that the patient still has lateral patella instability and potentially lead to additional surgery aimed at moving the patella further medially. The only way to make this differentiation is to understand the problem and the nature of the episodes. A proper history aimed at differentiating these problems is of paramount importance. So regarding history, most important is listening to the patient. It is surprising how many times the patient will lead the clinician to accurate diagnosis simply by having a chance to express details of the problem, prompted by targeted questions. I had an overweight patient in my office yesterday who had twisted his knee 2 years ago. He had had extensive (and expensive) physical therapy and was miserable with pain. No one had put a finger on his tender semimembranosus tendon. After injecting it, his pain vanished for the first time in 2 years.

Physical Examination

Optimal physical examination with regard to the anterior knee should involve examination of the patient supine, prone, standing, and moving.

First, notice patient's affect and body habitus. Particularly in adolescents and young adults, excessive attachment to the parent or domination by a parent may pertain as well.

With the patient supine, evaluate flexion and extension in the knee to see if there is any visible sign of lateral patella tracking. The J sign in particular will become evident at this time. In patients with patellofemoral, pain or ongoing pain is not uncommon for the apparent mechanical function of the patellofemoral joint to seem normal. On the contrary, many patients with an instability problem will manifest some evidence of lateral patella tracking or patella tilt. Of course, there are patients who complain of pain who have evidence of malalignment (a net imbalance of the patellofemoral joint, usually caused by multiple structural factors, leading to suboptimal or inappropriate load distribution in the patellofemoral articulation) and patients without any evidence of malalignment who have recurrent instability episodes. All of this will pertain to the nature of the specific deficiency or imbalance.

Next, the examiner should palpate the entire anterior knee methodically and precisely oriented to anatomic detail. Particularly in patients with a complaint of anterior knee pain, the examiner should search for tender spots and should again ask the patient to identify any specific source of pain. Together, the examiner and the patient may be able to "zero in" on a source of pain. It is surprising how often a patient will point directly to a source of pain in the peripatellar retinaculum that has been missed, sometimes for years. So, peripatellar examination is extremely important, particularly as small nerve injury, presumably related to aberrant retinacular stress, is common in the retinaculum of patellofemoral pain patients (2, 3). Palpate everything including the vastus lateralis tendon, lateral retinaculum, the patella tendon, the retro patella tendon region, the medial retinaculum particularly vastus medialis obliques (VMO) tendon insertion, and the quadriceps tendon itself. Any of these areas can be a source of anterior knee pain. If the patient has had previous surgery, be sure to palpate every portal and incision to identify if there might be a neuroma or tender scar causing pain. If a primary source of pain can be identified, this area should be prepped and injected with a local anesthetic to see if the pain disappears upon specific injection. If this is successful, adding corticosteroid to the injected site maybe warranted, and ultimately, resection of the painful tissue may be curative (4).

Once the retinacular examination is finished, the clinician should use palpation also to help with intra-articular diagnosis. Particularly, the medial infrapatella space should be palpated upon flexion and extension of the knee, looking for evidence of a pathologic plica (Fig. 59.1). Typically, patients who have a symptomatic plica will identify the *nature* of pain with this area palpated partially if there is a click associated with palpation.

Some examiners like to palpate the lateral facet of the patella by displacing the patella laterally and palpating. I have found this particular method to be confusing as the retinaculum is also stretched quite tensely with this technique. It is important to *differentiate* the nature of any pain noted on palpation.

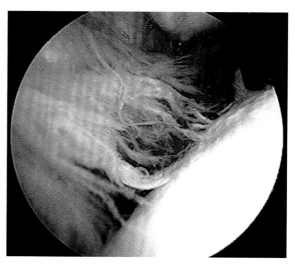

FIGURE 59.1. Irritated medial infrapatellar plica.

Following this, patient should be displaced supine with the knee extended, pushing the patella medially, and then the knee is flexed suddenly. Contrarily, the patella should be displaced laterally and the knee flex abruptly. Using this particular method, the examiner would identify if there is a problem with *relocation* pain or instability such as is experienced in patient with medial patella subluxation (5). Such patients have a patella that "wanders" to far in one direction or the other and relocates suddenly. This is particularly striking in the patient with medial patella instability. In such patients, the patella sits slightly medial then immediately relocates very abruptly upon flexion of the knee, sometimes on stairs and unexpectedly causing the patient to fall to the ground as the patella relocates from too far medial back into the central trochlea with sharp intense pain and giving away. I have found this method to be helpful in differentiating medial from lateral patella instability.

To examine for integrity of the medial patellofemoral ligament (MPFL), the patella is pushed laterally while palpating medially, and then the knee is slowly flexed to see if the MPFL is pulling the patella into the central trochlea. Normally, this occurs promptly and completely by 30° of knee flexion. If the patella stays lateral, the MPFL is deficient. One must be careful not to dislocate the patella (Fig. 59.2).

Following this, the patella should be compressed against the trochlea while the knee is flexed and extended looking for crepitus or pain. Using this method, the examiner can determine to what extent the pain may be elicited from articular compression, and the location of the painful articular lesion may be determined as well. In a distal pole patella articular lesion, the pain will be elicited in early flexion, whereas in a crush, proximal pole patella lesion, crepitus, and pain will more typically be found upon compression of the patella with the knee flexed 70° to 110°. This differentiation becomes very important in surgical planning. One must determine how best to unload a specific, painful lesion on the patella.

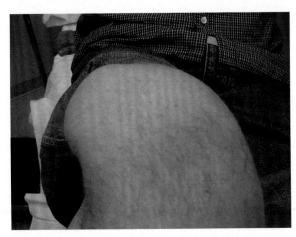

FIGURE 59.2. Habitually dislocating patella secondary to severe trochlea dysplasia.

Some sense of laxity around the anterior knee should also be acquired looking at "quadrant laxity." Essentially one is testing overall ligament laxity, and this, together with an appraisal of general joint laxity of the elbow thumb and fingers will help in determining quality of the patient's connective tissue.

Patient's hamstring flexibility should be examined and then place the patient prone to evaluate rotation of the hips and quadriceps tightness. With the knee extended in the prone position, one can also palpate the peripatellar retinacular tissue as the extensor mechanism relaxes well in this position.

The patient is then asked to walk while the examiner evaluates gait to see if there is evidence of antalgia pertaining to the hip or knee. A single leg knee bend is important both to establish quadriceps support but most importantly to evaluate core stability at the hip level as well as pronation at the foot and ankle. It is surprising how many patients will show evidence of inadequate support of the lower extremity with excessive internal rotation at the hip. Be sure to establish the level of lower extremity support in any patient with patellofemoral instability or pain such that physical therapy may be guided appropriately to improve over all lower extremity function and balanced tracking of the patella during activity.

I like to have the patient do a "step down" test in which the patient stands on a small step and steps down on one side and then the other, looking specifically for evidence of pain, the patient who experiences intense pain upon early step down may well have a distal patella articular lesion as a source of pain. This distal pole articular lesion will often be missed if this test is not done. In the patient with reproduction of pain upon doing this test, unloading the distal pole of the patella may be necessary by anterior or anteromedial tibial tubercle transfer at some point if other measures fail including a full program of core stability. Further evaluating core stability, the patient should jump down from a step while the examiner watches to see if there is excessive

internal rotation at the hip level producing functional valgus at the knee and pronation at the foot and ankle level. Core stability training may be what is needed in such patients.

Imaging

In most patients with anterior knee pain or instability, I recommend four radiographic views, taken with precision, in the office. In addition to standard AP views, I like to take a 30° knee flexion weight-bearing PA radiograph of the knee. Third is the precise lateral, posterior condyles overlapped. Finally is the axial view. My preference is the 30° knee flexion Merchant axial view.

The lateral (6) and Merchant axial (7) are most important in the patient with anterior knee pain and instability. Without fluoroscopy, it is difficult to obtain a true lateral radiograph but our technicians developed a technique of palpating the posterior condyles while the patient stands next to the X-ray cassette. This technique has been surprisingly accurate in determining when the knee is truly lateral such as the posterior condyle will overlap on the radiograph. Although every picture will not be perfect, we have found that for screening purposes in the office, this has worked out quite well. Evaluating the lateral requires some experience. One must learn to identify the medial and lateral trochlear condyles in the central trochlea as seen on lateral radiograph. One must also learn to identify the appearance of a patella that is tilted, subluxated, and or subluxated versus normal on the lateral view.

Good office radiographs are all that is needed in the majority of patients. Ninety degrees knee flexion axial views are of very limited value in my experience. In order to obtain a good axial view, one will need either bolsters cut to the appropriate angle or a Merchant frame that will place the knee in a desired amount of flexion.

One can readily see evidence of subluxation and/or tilt on a standard radiograph. Ronald Grelsamer (8) has made the point that a simple visual impression is most helpful as well as understanding how to interpret the lateral radiograph. For most orthopedic surgeons, it will be apparent when the patella is grossly tilted or laterally displaced in the trochlea.

The precise lateral (9) is really a better index of patella displacement, particularly tilt, as the lateral edge of the patella and the center ridge of the patella will overlap, producing a single line when the patella is clinically tilted. This is a good objective parameter. Also, on the lateral radiograph, one can appreciate the depth and structures of the trochlea.

Displacing the patella laterally, one might also consider the axial linear displacement view advocated by Urch et al. (10) In this case, a Merchant axial view is taken with the patella displaced laterally, documenting displaceability of the patella as an index of propensity for dislocation.

Tomographic Imaging

MRI can be helpful in a detailed analysis of patella alignment; however, these studies are often *not* necessary in my experience. Good office radiographs, put together with accurate clinical, physical examination are all that is necessary in most patellofemoral patients. In more difficulty cases, and in cases when one wants to rule out other intra-articular pathology, MRI may be helpful. Essentially, I recommend obtaining MRI only very selectively. It has been useful for determining the medial–lateral distance between the tibial tubercle and the central trochlear groove (commonly known as the TT–TG index). Too often MRI is used instead of proper physical examination and when radiographs have not been done properly or evaluated thoroughly. Tomographic images with progressive knee flexion has been possible in some centers, even weight-bearing, but this is expensive and generally not available.

CT of the patellofemoral joint has been studied well, patellofemoral CT, with midpatella transverse images at 0°, 15°, 30°, and 45° flexion (reproducing normal standing alignment in the scanner gantry) will give a detailed impression of the patella tracking. CT is also optimal for identifying patellofemoral osseous injury (Fig. 59.3), as well as trochlear morphology (11). One must remember, however, that such studies are not taken weight-bearing and therefore, in this way, computerized studies are typically less accurate than a good standing lateral radiograph at 30° knee flexion with the patient weight-bearing radionuclide imaging as described by Dye (12), is helpful in localizing articular lesions with subchondral bone response. As in the case of MRI and CT, radionuclide imaging should be reserved for difficult or complex cases in which diagnosis is difficult. Radionuclide imaging or even SPECT scan (tomography of a bone scan) may be invaluable in a patient with blunt trauma to identify or follow the progress of an impact injury. Subchondral bone response may be followed over time by repeat study in an effort to avoid intervention surgically.

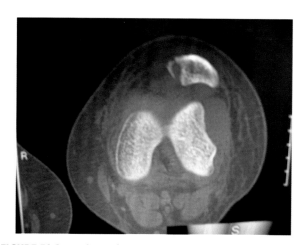

FIGURE 59.3. Avulsion of medial patella at time of dislocation.

PUTTING IT ALL TOGETHER

Approaching the patellofemoral joint, one must keep an open mind and be prepared to correlate the history, physical examination, and images available. The patterns must produce a coordinated and a clear picture of the problem. The examiner should be open to unusual findings, as anterior knee pain and instability problems vary significantly. It is best if the clinician has an impression of what is going on based on clinical examination and history alone looking for support through images, rather than relying on images alone to give an answer. In the final analysis, a good physical examination is the key to understanding patients with anterior knee pain and instability.

TREATMENT

In designing a proper treatment plan, one must first determine if the problem is primarily one of patellofemoral pain or of patellofemoral instability. If the problem is pain, it behooves the examiner to identify whether the pain source is articular, synovial, referred, or peripatellar. Similarly, if the problem is one of instability, one must identify the nature of this instability, whether it can be corrected by enhanced lower extremity core stability or whether the problem is related to substantial structural or alignment deficiency such that surgical intervention will be required.

Retinacular Pain

Simply, if the clinician can identify a source of pain around the patella whether it be patella tendon, medial retinaculum, lateral retinaculum, vastus lateralis tendon, vastus medialis tendon, or quadriceps tendon, the treatment should be very specific. Once identified, it is often helpful to inject the retinacular pain source with lidocaine or marcaine to see if the pain can be eradicated. Then the treatment will follow logically. Sometimes stretching and local treatment with physical therapy modalities will work, sometimes corticosteroid injection is necessary, and sometimes resection of the painful tissue will be required (4).

Infrapatella Pain

When physical diagnosis has established that the patient has a painful infrapatellar plica (see Fig. 59.1) or fat pad syndrome, corticosteroid injection initially may be helpful, but often the painful plical tissue must be resected arthroscopically.

Articular Patellofemoral Pain

Most important is to establish location through physical diagnosis and then design treatment appropriately. Local chondroplasty may give good symptomatic relief when there are loose fragments of cartilage (13). If the particular lesion is lateral and associated with patella tilt, lateral release is appropriate if nonoperative measures fail. One must be careful on the other hand not to do a lateral release adding load to a medial articular lesion as this may well be counterproductive, particularly if the patient does not have underlying tilt causing the problem in the first place. Proximal, crush type lesions of the patella are difficult to treat. In some cases, articular resurfacing using autogenous osteochondral core transplantation or other resurfacing will be necessary (14). Anteriorizing procedures should be avoided in patients with proximal lesions, as anteriorizing the tibial tubercle actually adds load to the proximal patella earlier in the flexion cycle.

In more severe cases with more advanced lateral facet articular breakdown (excessive lateral pressure syndrome—Fig. 59.4) or intractable pain related to a distal and/or articular lesion, anteromedial tibial tubercle transfer is the treatment of choice (15–17). If the articular lesion is distal and the patient has no evidence of any malaligned lateral tracking, straight anteriorization may be needed using either a Maquet procedure or a sagittal plane tibial tubercle slide (straight anteriorization of the tibial tubercle).

In some more extensive patella articular lesions, selective osteochondral transplant may be the best solution (14). This is true particularly when the articular lesion is proximal and/or medial (such that anteromedial tibial tubercle transfer is not appropriate) and in trochlea lesions over 1.5 cm in diameter. Synthetic (Fig. 59.5) and allogeneic osteochondral resurfacing can provide effective pain relief in treating medial and proximal articular lesions, but consistent long-term results with this treatment are not yet available. Smaller trochlear lesions are best treated by arthroscopic microfracture arthroplasty (Fig. 59.6). Larger areas of trochlear breakdown may require replacement arthroplasty.

Patellofemoral replacement should be reserved for patients in whom joint preservation is not possible by

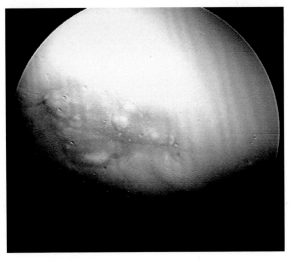

FIGURE 59.5. Patella resurfaced with synthetic OBI (Smith and Nephew, Andover, MA).

transferring load off of articular lesions or using osteochondral transplantation because the lesion is too extensive patellofemoral replacement is most appropriate in patients with diffuse patella articular loss particularly when the trochlea is also involved (Fig. 59.7). In such patients, allograft osteochondral resurfacing may also be considered.

In extreme cases, patellectomy can be appropriate, and hemipatellectomy (lateral facetectomy) has proven effective in some patients. In general, such procedures are indicated in younger patients in whom patellofemoral replacement is not possible or desirable. It is most important to maintain extensor mechanism integrity when a patella is removed, and one must be particularly careful if a patient has had extensive lateral release previously as this may weaken the extensor mechanism such that allograft tendon reinforcement is necessary after patellectomy.

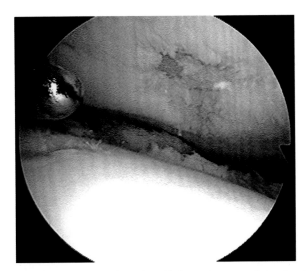

FIGURE 59.4. Excessive lateral patellofemoral pressure from chronic lateral malalignment often results in eventual lateral facet breakdown.

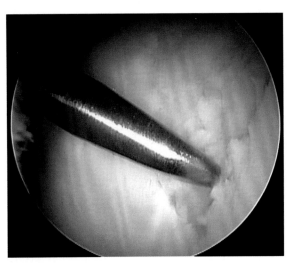

FIGURE 59.6. Microfracture arthroplasty is often all that is needed for smaller trochlea articular lesion.

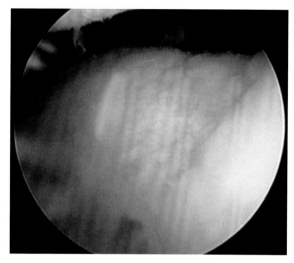

FIGURE 59.7. When trochlear lesion is large and uncontained, replacement arthroplasty may be necessary, particularly when the patella is extensively degenerated.

Larger osteochondral allografts play a limited role in the seriously deficient patellofemoral joint and can provide pain relief and improved function. Little is known however about long-term results and consequences.

Patellofemoral Instability

Many patients with patella instability can be treated nonoperatively with CORE stability training, emphasizing external hip rotator support and new design patellofemoral braces (Fig. 59.8). Such patellofemoral braces are lighter with design features that make them more effective than the previous generation. Patellofemoral taping can also be helpful but requires relatively frequent retaping and can be hard on the skin. Nonoperative treatment of patella instability should focus on restoring lower extremity alignment and strength as well as external support of the patella.

After acute dislocation, aspiration of hemarthrosis followed by patella brace support and rehabilitation of the quadriceps, and lower extremity balance is most appropriate to control patella instability. This may require immobilization in some patients for 4 to 6 weeks. Osteochondral fragments should generally be replaced with open surgery when possible.

MPFL will heal elongated after a patella dislocation such that recurrent instability is more likely. In patients without significant underlying malalignment, imbrication or advancement of the healed MPFL 3 to 6 months after the dislocation, often combined with lateral release to relieve excessive lateral tightness and/or tilt will restore adequate support in many people. Arthroscopic MPFL imbrication (18) can be effective in patients without lateral tracking in whom the trochlea is reasonably well formed (Fig. 59.9). It is imperative, however, that MPFL heal before being advanced or imbricated. Success rates regarding stability alone following medial imbrication by any means are generally less

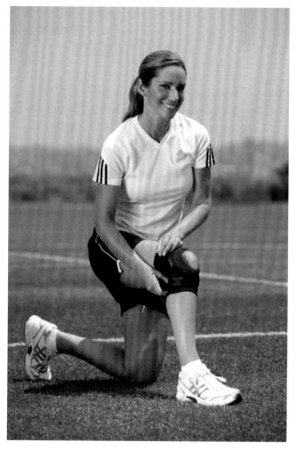

FIGURE 59.8. Trupull lite brace patellofemoral brace (Picture courtesy of DJ Ortho, Vista, CA). Newer patellofemoral braces are much more effective and comfortable.

satisfactory than with tendon graft MPFL reconstruction. Nonetheless, advancing the healed medial capsule/retinaculum uses existing healed anatomic structures, thereby reconstituting the entire medial complex (not just the MPFL). Most important is to balance patellofemoral tracking as

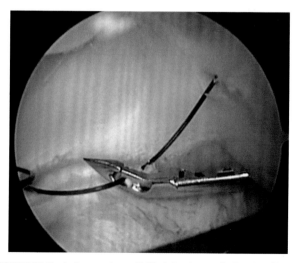

FIGURE 59.9. Arthroscopic medial imbrications will often be effective in patients without trochlea dysplasia or patella malalignment.

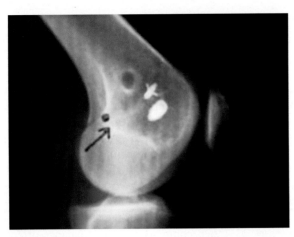

FIGURE 59.10. Poorly placed MPFL graft resulted in severe patella breakdown and chronic pain in this patient. Arrow designates proper location for posterior aspect of MPFL graft fixation on the femur.

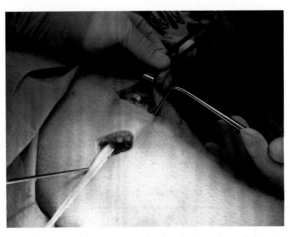

FIGURE 59.12. MPFL tendon graft placed through medial retinaculum, under VMO, and suture securely to underside of VMO tendon as well as through the quadriceps tendon.

needed, releasing deforming forces and correcting incongruities such as abnormal Q angle or elevated TT–TG by tibial tubercle transfer before doing medial imbrications. In addition, imbrication or advancement of the medial capsule is safer for surgeons who are not intricately involved in the study and mechanics of the MPFL. Tragic destruction of the patellofemoral joint will occur as a result of an improperly placed MPFL tendon graft (Fig. 59.10). Revision of a failed medial imbrications is much more forgiving than revision of an improperly placed MPFL tendon graft.

Acute repair of the MPFL is questionable (19) and, in general, it is usually best to let the ligament heal and advance or imbricate it later, as the MPFL is a very thin ligament, difficult to suture when acutely disrupted. The MPFL has been shown to heal consistently, 91% of the time, albeit elongated (Fig. 59.11) (20).

MPFL tendon graft reconstruction is appropriate in more severe cases when medial structure has been more severely disruptive and when there is more serious dysplasia of the extensor mechanism. I have developed a method of suturing the MPFL tendon graft deep to the native,

disrupted MPFL, passing it directly through the Vastus Medialis Obliquus tendon insertion at the proximal half of the patella. The tendon graft is then sutured with no. 2 ethibond into the VMO tendon where it comes through, and then anchored above it by passing it through and suturing to the adjacent quadriceps tendon (Fig. 59.12). This avoids drilling the patella and the risk if fracture associated with this. I have also used the technique described by Schepsis and Farr of using suture anchor fixation into a trough on the patellar side. In either case, the graft must be secured (I use the Arthrex biotenodesis screw) at the precise anatomic femoral origin of MPFL with the patella centered at 30° knee flexion. This point should be carefully located by following the adductor tendon to the adductor tubercle, identifying the medial epicondyle precisely and placing the femoral end of the graft precisely between these two anatomic landmarks. Radiographic criteria defined by Schoettle and associates are also useful and advised for those less familiar with the anatomy of this region (21). In complex cases with more severe trochlear dysplasia and/or distal medial patella articular injury, articular resurfacing (14, 22) and/or anteromedialization of the tibial tubercle may also be advisable at the time of MPFL reconstruction.

When there is more severe lateral tracking then the presence of a high Q-angle and elevated TT–TG relationship (distance between the tibial tubercle and the trochlear groove in the medial–lateral plane), medial transfer of the tibial tubercle is often the best and most straightforward alternative to stabilize the extensor mechanism. I prefer a simple Elmslie-Trillat medial rotation of the tibial tubercle. Medial rotation of the entire proximal tibia, as described initially by Cameron and recently reviewed by Paulos, is also effective in such patients but is a much larger operation, which poses some risk to the peroneal nerve. I have not found this procedure to be necessary. Tibial tubercle transfer is effective and less likely to create a serious complication when used for the right indications

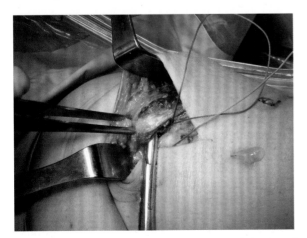

FIGURE 59.11. Open advancement of a healed medial retinaculum and VMO in a patient without trochlea dysplasia.

to centralize the extensor mechanism and compensate for trochlea deficiency, keeping the patella tracking centrally and off the dysplastic, deficient lateral trochlea. The best objective measurements for determining the need for tibial tubercle transfer is the TT–TG index (>20 mm from tibial tubercle to central trochlear groove is abnormal).

Distal femur derotation has also been proposed to correct excessive internal rotation of the femur, but I have not found this necessary and prefer compensatory surgery oriented to restore balanced central tracking of the patella in the trochlea with the least risky approach possible. Moving the tibial tubercle has proven highly effective for balancing patella tracking in the central trochlea when alignment requires correction.

When there is significant distal medial patella articular disruption (Fig. 59.13, very common after dislocation), anteromedial tibial tubercle transfer (15–17) is desirable to raise the distal pole off damaged articular cartilage while centralizing the extensor mechanism to optimize balanced tracking.

In instability patients, lateral release does not play any useful role except as needed to supplement other stabilization procedures and to relieve patellar tilt. Lateral release does not move the patella medially and can actually make some instability patients worse.

Beware of medial patella instability in patients who have excessive lateral release or excessive medial tubercle transfer. These patients have sudden giving away, usually much more severe than the initial instability problem that has already been treated. In such patients, repair or reconstruction of the disrupted lateral retinaculum and possibly transfer the tibial tubercle back laterally to a balanced location will be necessary. Sometimes a tendon graft is necessary to supplement the lateral reconstruction.

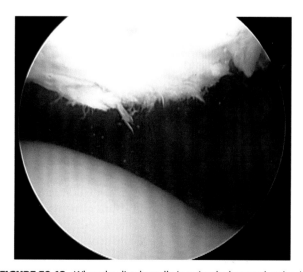

FIGURE 59.13. When the distal patella is seriously damaged, unloading it by anteromedialization reduces risk of postoperative pain.

Trochleoplasty

Trochleoplasty procedures stabilize patella tracking by capturing the patella into a deepened proximal trochlear groove. The procedure will usually stabilize the patella, but unacceptable incidences of pain and even arthrofibrosis are reported. Available procedures focus on the proximal trochlea and fail to create a uniform depth to the trochlea further into flexion. Although trochlear deficiency is common in patients with patella instability as a result of chronic lateral tracking developmentally (this author believes that most trochlea dysplasia is secondary), deepening the trochlea requires severe, irreversible subchondral bone and articular damage and has rarely been necessary as other compensatory and balance-oriented surgery appears to work well.

AUTHOR'S PREFERRED TREATMENT

As a matter of approach, I like to minimize treatment whenever possible, relying on physical therapy and bracing, but it is very important to recognize when surgery is necessary, as many people suffer greatly with patellofemoral problems. Surgical treatment is always very specific for the problem identified using objective evaluation and very careful clinical examination, as it is easy to be fooled or to miss something very important.

I use lateral release only for documented tilt. In patella instability patients, I use minimal procedures whenever possible to stabilize the patella (arthroscopic or miniopen MPFL retensioning/imbrication) but always looking critically to see if the alignment (elevated Q angle or TT–TG) and/or trochlea dysplasia are such that something more is necessary. I like medial tibial tubercle transfer (Elmslie-Trillat style) through a 3-in incision as a means of compensation for malalignment (high Q angle, J tracking, elevated TT–TG index) and trochlear dysplasia. In addition, when patella alta is present, the tubercle may be advanced slightly to correct this and get the patella into the trochlea sooner upon knee flexion. Well-done tibial tubercle transfer with secure fixation allows immediate motion and centralization/balancing of contact forces in the PF joint. Sometimes, then, I will retension the medial capsulo-retinacular complex arthroscopically or miniopen, but this is not always necessary once the tracking is corrected accurately by tibial tubercle transfer. In more severe instability cases, I will add a tendon graft reconstruction of the MPFL, particularly when there is a more profound trochlea dysplasia for which to compensate. If a minimally invasive proximal procedure fails to provide long-term stabilization, I will redo the procedure adding MPFL tendon graft and/or tibial tubercle transfer as needed. If someone has recurrent instability after a stabilizing procedure, I look critically for medial instability also, and correct that by adding lateral support for the patella. Optimal surgery requires careful balancing of patella tracking, correcting underlying malalignment as needed. I prefer to avoid femoral and tibial derotation as I believe I can achieve good and excellent results consistently with less risky, compensatory, balance-oriented procedures.

PEARLS

1. Examine the peripatellar retinaculum in every patient and look for hidden findings, which may end up being the keys to successful treatment.

2. Use standard 45° knee flexion axial views, always the same, and insist on precise standing lateral radiographs.

3. Insist on a comprehensive rehabilitation program including core stability training in all patients with anterior knee pain or instability.

4. Let the MPFL heal after a patella dislocation so that it can be advanced or imbricated later if necessary.

5. Always be sure that you know the source of pain.

6. If pain is articular, unload the painful area by tibial tubercle transfer when appropriate.

7. If pain is retinacular, inject, release or resect the painful lesion when appropriate.

8. Move the patellofemoral joint early after surgery.

9. If you do MPFL surgery, anatomic precision in placement of the graft is imperative.

10. If you do tibial tubercle transfer, add obliquity in order to achieve anteriorization (for anteromedialization) of the distal patella to unload a distal patella articular lesion. Move the tubercle only as far as necessary. Correct patella alta at this time as needed. Always use secure fixation such that immediate motion will be possible.

11. Use tomographic imaging in tough cases in order to measure the TT–TG index and to assess cartilage lesions more precisely.

Disclosure: The author receives royalties on sales of the Trupull brace produced by DJ Ortho, Vista, CA.

REFERENCES

1. Post WR. Anterior knee pain: diagnosis and treatment. *J Am Acad Orthop Surg.* 2005;13(8):534–543.

2. Fulkerson JP, Tennant R, Jaivin JS, et al. Histologic evidence of retinacular nerve injury associated with patellofemoral malalignment. *Clin Orthop Relat Res.* 1985;(197):196–205.

3. Biedert RM, Stauffer E, Friederich NF. Occurrence of free nerve endings in the soft tissue of the knee joint. A histologic investigation. *Am J Sports Med.* 1992;20(4):430–433.

4. Kasim N, Fulkerson JP. Resection of clinically localized segments of painful retinaculum in the treatment of selected patients with anterior knee pain. *Am J Sports Med.* 2000;28(6):811–814.

5. Fulkerson JP. A clinical test for medial patella tracking. *Tech Orthop.* 1997;12(3):144.

6. Malghem J, Maldague B. Profile of the knee. Differential radiologic anatomy of the articular surfaces. *J Radiol.* 1986;67(10):725–735.

7. Merchant AC, Mercer RL, Jacobsen RH, et al. Roentgenographic analysis of patellofemoral congruence. *J Bone Joint Surg.* 1974;56(7):1391–1396.

8. Grelsamer R. A roentgenographic analysis of patellar tilt. *J Bone Joint Surg.* 1993;75B:822–824.

9. Grelsamer R. The lateral trochlea sign. *Clin Orthop.* 1992;281:159–162.

10. Urch S, Tritle B, Shelbourne D, et al. Axial linear patellar displacement. *Am J Sports Med.* 2009;37:970–973.

11. Dejour H, Walch G, Neyret P, et al. Dysplasia of the femoral trochlea. *Rev Chir Orthop Reparatrice Appa Mot.* 1990;76(1):45–54.

12. Dye S. Radionuclide imaging of the PF joint in young adults with anterior knee pain. *Orthop Clin North Am.* 1986;17:249–262.

13. Federico DJ, Reider B. Results of isolated patellar debridement for patellofemoral pain in patients with normal patellar alignment. *Am J Sports Med.* 1997;25(5):663–669.

14. Farr J. Patellofemoral articular cartilage treatment. Radiographic Landmarks for Femoral Tunnel Placement in Medial Patellofemoral Ligament Reconstruction. In: *AAOS Monograph Series 29.* AAOS; 2005:85–99:chap 9.

15. Farr J, Schepsis A, Cole B, et al. Anteromedialization, review and technique. *J Knee Surg.* 2007;20:120–128.

16. Fulkerson JP. Alternatives to patellofemoral arthroplasty [Review]. *Clin Orthop Relat Res.* 2005;(436):76–80.

17. Saleh KJ. Arendt EA, Eldridge J, et al. Symposium. Operative treatment of patellofemoral arthritis. *J Bone Joint Surg Am.* 2005;87(3):659–671.

18. Halbrecht JL. Arthroscopic patella realignment: an all-inside technique. *Arthroscopy.* 2001;17(9):940–945.

19. Silianpaa P, Maenpaa H, Mattila V, et al. Arthroscopic surgery for primary patellar dislocation. *Am J Sports Med.* 2008;36(12):2301–2309.

20. Tom A, Fulkerson JP. Restoration of native MPFL support after patella dislocation. *Sports Med Arthrosc Rev.* 2007;15(2):68–71.

21. Schöttle PB, Schmeling A, Rosenstiel N, et al. *Am J Sports Med.* 2007;35(5):801–804. Epub 2007 Jan 31.

22. Minas T. Autologous chondrocyte implantation for focal chondral defects of the knee. *Clin Orthop Relat Res.* 2001;(391 suppl):S349–S361.

Surgical Approaches to Patellar Malalignment

Donald C. Fithian • Robert A. Teitge • Samuel Ward • Robert Afra

BACKGROUND

The patellofemoral joint (PFJ) is a unique articulation with a complex architecture. Its motion differs from that of most other joints, in that, it is mostly comprised of sliding rather than rolling. This places unique challenges on the articular cartilage. The most common disorders of the PFJ are thought to occur as a result of alterations in the mechanics of this joint, leading to cartilage overload or gross instability.

It is worth pointing out that the objective of "offloading the patella" is very difficult to achieve by surgical means. The patella exists to improve the leverage of the knee extensor system, and it is necessary that the PFJ support compressive loads in order for the knee to function properly. Although it is true that anteriorization of the tibial tuberosity (TT), as described by Maquet (1), can reduce PFJ force while maintaining quadriceps-generated extension torque, the practical limitations of this procedure are well known. Surgical realignment in most cases, then, is directed at redistributing forces so that all joint surfaces and soft tissues in the knee wear out at a similar acceptable rate.

DEFINITIONS OF ALIGNMENT AND MALALIGNMENT

There are two common uses for the term "alignment" as it relates to the patellofemoral articulation: (1) position of the patella in the femoral groove, and (2) position of the patella *and* groove between the body and the foot. It is a common oversimplification to consider alignment as referring only to the position of the patella on the femoral trochlea. Although alignment of the patella on the trochlea (e.g., medial/lateral shift, alta/infera, and tilt) is important, this assessment should not distract us from the equally important consideration of how the position of the knee in space affects the location and magnitude of forces within the PFJ. Thorough workup requires evaluation of knee extensor alignment from *both* perspectives.

The concept of malalignment is based on several assumptions:

1. Mechanical systems have a theoretical optimal alignment, in which forces are well balanced, and no part of the mechanism wears out before any other part.
2. Forces that are applied off-center can be magnified many times by the moments they generate.
3. Any variation from optimal skeletal alignment may increase the force vectors acting on the PFJ, causing either ligament failure with subsequent subluxation or dislocation or cartilage failures as in chondromalacia or arthrosis.

Malalignment distributes abnormal stresses to both the ligaments and the joint surfaces in the misaligned limb. Ligament overload and subsequent failure may occur with a single traumatic episode or with chronic repetitive episodes of minor trauma. Skeletal malalignment may cause chondromalacia patella and subsequently arthrosis by generating forces on the PFJ that exceed the load-carrying capacity of the cartilage. Even if forces are not excessive, reduction in contact surface area caused by a small patella, patella alta, or patellar subluxation can increase the force per unit area (stress) beyond the load capacity of the articular cartilage, leading to cartilage failure (arthrosis). Similarly, excessive or abnormal gliding of the joint can increase shear stresses beyond the capacity of the articular cartilage, leading to cartilage failure. Anterior knee pain in the setting of a malaligned lower extremity may be the result of abnormal compression, tension or shear in the capsule, ligaments, synovium, or subchondral bone.

EFFECT OF ROTATIONAL MALALIGNMENT ON PFJ POSITION IN SPACE

Maximum gait efficiency with minimal stress is affected by normal limb alignment. Any deviation from normal limb alignment in any plane can lead to pain, much like when twisting a knee. These include femoral anteversion or retroversion, excess internal or external tibial torsion (ETT), genu valgum or varum, hyperpronation and Achilles contracture. Twisting of the knee away from the limb mechanical axis (inward or outward) will change the direction and magnitude of the patellofemoral compression force, and will also add a side-directed vector to the patella. This vector is resisted by the soft tissues (both medial and lateral patellofemoral ligaments as well as accessory capsular ligaments). It is also resisted by the femoral trochlea, to a degree determined by its depth, length, and shape. The distribution of these constraining forces between retinaculum and trochlea is determined primarily by the shape of the trochlea: the greater its depth and length, and the steeper its medial and lateral walls (i.e., sulcus angle), the lower the resulting force in the soft tissues.

The foot progression angle (FPA) is generally defined as the angle between the long axis of the foot and the direction of body progression. It varies from 10° to 20° (2). It has been shown that despite congenital or acquired (after fracture) torsional deformities in the lower limb bones, the FPA remains unchanged (3–5). It is hypothesized that the hip musculature plays a role in accommodating these deformities during gait. For example, in the presence of an internal femoral or external tibial rotational deformity with a normal FPA (Fig. 60.1A, B), the knee joint axis rotates inward and a side force vector is produced, acting on the patella so that both the strain on the medial patellofemoral ligament (MPFL) and compression on the lateral patellofemoral facet are increased. It is not well understood how the body accommodates rotational deformities during gait. Importantly, the compensatory options are limited and none of them is optimal from a mechanical point of view. For example, in the setting of pure femoral anteversion (Fig. 60.1C, D), if the body seeks to restore

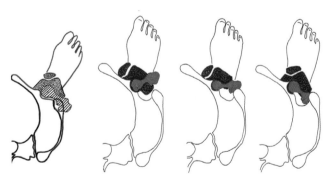

FIGURE 60.1. A, B: The drawings show a limb with excess ETT. Assuming a normal FPA, the knee points inward. As a result, there is a compensatory hip internal rotation, placing the hip abductors at a mechanical disadvantage, causing functional weakness and possibly leading to easy fatigue. **C:** In the setting of pure femoral anteversion, if the body seeks to restore normal femoroacetabular alignment, the knee (and trochlea) will point medially across the midline. **D:** If the body seeks the normal sagittal alignment of the knee joint and foot, the greater trochanter will be posteriorly positioned, which places the hip abductors at a mechanical disadvantage.

normal femoroacetabular alignment, the knee (and trochlea) will point medially across the midline. In this case, we see either an in-toeing gait and/or a compensatory foot pronation in order to achieve a normal FPA. If the body seeks the normal sagittal alignment of the knee joint and foot, the greater trochanter will be posteriorly positioned, which places the hip abductors at a mechanical disadvantage. In this case, we may see medial collapse (adduction and internal rotation) of the hip during weight-bearing.

ASSOCIATION BETWEEN SKELETAL MALALIGNMENT AND PFJ PATHOLOGY

In the frontal plane, malalignment has been shown to influence the progression of PFJ arthritis (6, 7). Varus alignment increases the likelihood of medial patellofemoral arthrosis progression, whereas valgus alignment increases the likelihood of lateral patellofemoral arthrosis progression. Fujikawa et al. (8) in a cadaveric study found a marked alteration of patellar and femoral contact areas with the introduction of increased varus alignment produced by a varus osteotomy.

Lerat et al. (9) noted a statistically significant correlation between increased femoral internal torsion (i.e., femoral anteversion) and both patellar chondrosis and instability. Janssen (10) also found that patients with a history of patellar dislocation had increased odds of internal femoral torsion compared with control subjects. They speculated that internal femoral torsion was responsible for the development of dysplasia of the trochlea and of the patella. Takai et al. (11) measured femoral and tibial torsion in patients with patellofemoral, medial, and lateral unicompartmental osteoarthrosis. They noted that patellofemoral osteoarthrosis was associated with increased femoral torsion (23° vs. 9° in controls), and concluded that excessive femoral torsion contributed to patellofemoral wear in these patients.

Turner (12) studied the association of tibial torsion and knee joint pathology. He observed that patients with patellofemoral instability had greater than normal ETT (25° vs. 19° in controls). Eckhoff et al. (13) found that the tibia in the extended knee was 6° more externally rotated than normal controls in a group of patients with anterior knee pain. Whether this represented an abnormal skeletal torsion or an abnormal rotation of the tibia on the femur due to knee joint soft tissue laxity or abnormal muscle pull is unknown.

EFFECTS OF ROTATIONAL MALALIGNMENT ON PFJ CONTACT AND MPFL STRAIN

Fixed rotation of either femur or tibia has been shown to have a significant influence on PFJ contact areas and pressures. Hefzy et al. (14) used a cadaveric model to study the effects of tibial rotation on PFJ contact areas. The authors found that internal tibial rotation increased medial PFJ contact areas, whereas external tibial rotation increased lateral PFJ contact areas at all flexion angles. More recently, Lee et al. (15–17) investigated the effects of rotational deformities of the lower extremity on PFJ contact pressures in a cadaver model. They simulated various types of rotational deformities of the femur and tibia by internally and externally rotating cadaver knees around the axis representing the distal third of the femur and the shaft of the tibia. They found that 30° of either internal or external femoral rotation created a significantly greater peak contact pressure respectively on the lateral or medial facet of the patella.

Lee's findings have been confirmed in an independent study in whole cadaver limbs (including the femoral head and foot) stabilized by simulated quadriceps contraction. When the distal femur was internally rotated 30°, there was increased contact pressure on the lateral aspect of the PFJ and decreased contact pressure on the medial aspect of the joint. When the distal femur was rotated 30° externally, the opposite effect was observed (18).

Kijowski (Teitge et al., unpublished work) also studied the effects of femoral rotational osteotomy on strain in the MPFL. They found that 30° of experimentally induced internal femoral rotation (rotating the distal femur inward, simulating anteversion) of the femur resulted in significant increases in the strain of the MPFL. It is interesting to note that the effect of bony alignment on MPFL strain was much greater at 30° than at 60° or 90° of flexion. These observations corroborated Lee's findings that medial patellofemoral retinacular strains were significantly affected only at low angles of knee flexion (16). The results of this study and Lee's studies show that variations in femoral torsion cause alterations in the patterns of force transmission across the PFJ, including strain in the MPFL. Weight-bearing activity in individuals with an internally rotated femur could cause pain either by overload of the cartilage laterally or by abnormal strain in the MPFL. The MPFL could fail either acutely or by chronic overload in such knees.

Trochlear dysplasia alters the contact relationship between patella and trochlea. Since the contact area and thus the contact pressures are altered, trochlear dysplasia and patella shape should be evaluated when assessing malalignment. Trochlear dysplasia is an abnormality of the shape and depth of the trochlear groove (TG) mainly at its cephalad part, which has been associated with patellar instability, anterior knee pain, and early patellofemoral arthrosis (19, 20). Brattström (21) and others (22, 23) have studied trochlear geometry in recurrent dislocation of the patella and concluded that a shallow femoral groove (i.e., trochlear dysplasia) was the most common finding (Fig. 60.2). These and other authors, mostly in Europe,

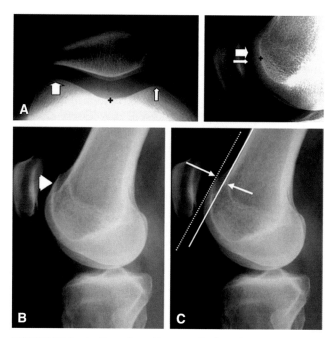

FIGURE 60.2. A: Normal trochlea. On the lateral view, the profile shows a sclerotic curved white line that corresponds to the floor of the trochlea (+). The curves representing the trochlear ridges *(arrows)* do not cross the curve of the trochlear floor. Note that accurate interpretation of the lateral view requires that the posterior condyles be aligned **(B)** and **(C)**. **B:** The crossing sign is a simple and characteristic image, a qualitative criterion of trochlear dysplasia. The arrowhead indicates the point where the curve of the trochlear floor crosses the anterior contour of the lateral femoral condyle. By definition, the trochlea is flat at this level. This sign is of fundamental importance in the diagnosis. **C:** The prominence (bump) is a quantitative characteristic that is particularly significant in trochlear dysplasia. The prominence represents the distance between the most anterior point of the trochlear floor *(dashed line)* and a line drawn along the distal 10 cm of the anterior femoral cortex *(solid line)*. (From Fithian DC, Neyret P, Servien E. Patellar instability: the lyon experience. *Tech Knee Surg.* 2007;6(2):112–123, with permission.)

worked to develop strict and reliable protocols for radiographic evaluation in order to provide guidelines for the treatment of patients with patellar instability (24, 25). In the 1980s, Dejour et al. (23) defined several specific morphologic features commonly seen on radiographs of patients with patellar instability that were rarely seen in a population of control subjects (26–29). The fundamental anatomic feature distinguishing the two populations was the presence of trochlear dysplasia—a flattening or occasionally a convexity of the upper part of the TG—in a high percentage of recurrent patellar dislocators and in only 2% of control subjects.

These studies provide strong circumstantial evidence to suggest that abnormal skeletal alignment of the lower extremity is an important factor in the pathogenesis of various disorders of the PFJ.

CLINICAL EVALUATION

Pertinent History

The knee extensor mechanism is a complicated and delicate system, the treatment of which is only further complicated by surgery if the surgeon has not clearly defined the pathologic basis of the presenting complaint. The chief complaint should guide the workup and the discussion of treatment options; this will help the physician to focus on the patient's needs and expectations. For example, the patient who seeks help for relief of daily pain has a very different problem than one complaining of occasional sharp pain and giving-way. Although pain itself can result in knee instability (a symptom), it is important to differentiate painful knee giving-way from episodic pain due to patellofemoral laxity. Pain and catching in early flexion points to an articular lesion at the inferior patella or proximal trochlea; pain throughout the range indicates a more diffuse, perhaps extra-articular process. As the clinician develops an understanding of the symptoms and complaints, he or she can begin to develop one or more hypotheses, which can be tested in the physical examination and with subsequent imaging studies. The isolated complaint of pain, with no objective findings to suggest a specific source (pathology) representing an indication for surgery, should be treated nonoperatively.

Physical Examination

Owing to the complex and delicate interactions between the knee extensor system and the lower limb function, clinical evaluation of patellofemoral complaints can be challenging. After other disorders have been ruled out, specific testing for disorders of the PFJ can be performed. The patient should be first evaluated standing, walking, and stepping up and down from a small step, squatting, sitting, supine, running, and jumping (Fig. 60.3). Any hindfoot valgus, forefoot pronation, and/or heel cord tightness should be noted as they can affect tibial rotation and patellofemoral alignment (30).

Femoral and tibial rotation can be estimated by examining the patient prone with the hips extended, the knees flexed 90°, and the feet and ankles in a neutral, comfortable position with the soles of the feet parallel to the floor after the method of Staheli et al. (31) This position allows

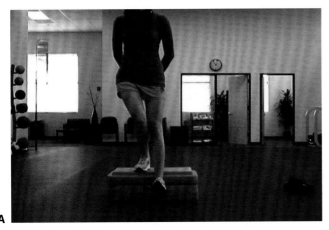

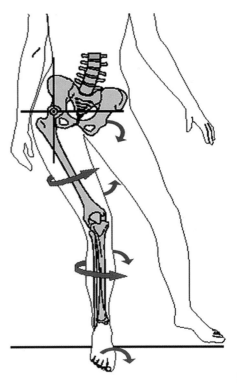

FIGURE 60.3. The step-down test is a simple test that can be done in the clinic to evaluate core and hip control. **A:** The patient on the left demonstrates pelvic weakness with hip adduction and medial collapse of the knee. **B:** Schematic showing the potential contributions of the various lower-extremity segments to abnormal alignment: *(1)* contralateral pelvic drop, *(2)* femoral internal rotation, *(3)* knee valgus, *(4)* tibia internal rotation, and *(5)* foot pronation. (From Powers CM. The influence of altered lower-extremity kinematics on patellofemoral joint dysfunction: a theoretical perspective. *J Orthop Sports Phys Ther.* 2003;33(11):639–646, with permission.)

A

B

estimation of femoral internal and external rotation limits as well as the foot-thigh angle (FTA) and/or transmaleolar axis (TMA). Kozic et al. (32) showed that on physical examination, femoral anteversion should be suspected if prone hip internal rotation exceeds external rotation by at least 45°. With respect to estimating FTA and TMA, Staheli et al. (31) reported a wide range of normal values, with mean values of 10° for FTA and 20° for TMA. Souza and Powers (33) also confirmed the reliability of the Staheli method for estimating femoral anteversion, though axial imaging was more precise. Our preferred approach is to use the prone physical examination to screen for torsion of the tibia and femur, and to obtain CT scan to assess rotational alignment if hip IR exceeds ER by at least 20° or if the prone foot-thigh axis or TMA is greater than 20°.

The lines of action of the quadriceps and the patellar tendon are not collinear. The angular difference between the two is the quadriceps angle, or "Q-angle." Because of this angle, the force generated by the quadriceps serves both to extend the knee and to drive the patella laterally, compressing the femoral trochlea in order to convert tension in the quadriceps into extension torque at the knee. The relative magnitude of the laterally directed force is related to the Q-angle. External rotation of the tibia, internal rotation of the femur, and increasing knee valgus all cause an increase in the Q-angle and thus an increase in the laterally directed force within the PFJ (Fig. 60.4) (30). However, use of the Q-angle alone grossly underestimates the complexity of patellofemoral alignment and often leads to errors of diagnosis and treatment. Furthermore, the Q-angle is highly variable and unreliable as a measurement (34, 35). These considerations have led

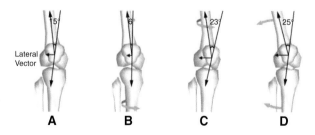

FIGURE 60.4. A: The Q angle is measured as the angle formed by the intersection of the line drawn from the anterior superior iliac spine to the midpoint of the patella and a proximal extension of the line drawn from the TT to the midpoint of the patella. Normal alignment of the tibia and femur results in an offset in the resultant quadriceps force vector (proximal) and the patellar tendon force vector (distal), creating a lateral vector acting on the patella. **B:** tibia internal rotation decreases the Q angle and the magnitude of the lateral vector acting on the patella. **C:** femoral internal rotation increases the Q angle and the lateral force acting on the patella. **D:** knee valgus increases the Q angle and the lateral force acting on the patella. (From Powers CM. The influence of altered lower-extremity kinematics on PFJ dysfunction: a theoretical perspective. *J Orthop Sports Phys Ther.* 2003;33(11): 639–646, with permission.)

the International Patellofemoral Study Group (IPSG) to recommend abandonment of clinical measurement of Q angle, preferring imaging studies to estimate the lateralizing vector at the PFJ (see TT-TG offset below under "Imaging").

Careful palpation of both medial and lateral retinaculum is helpful to localize tenderness. Studies have shown that 90% of patients with patellofemoral pain syndrome (PFPS) had pain in some portion of the lateral retinaculum (36). Palpation of the specific site of pain can help guide further investigation of what mechanical overload, if any, has occurred. The patella should be displaced to the side undergoing examination so that while fibers are being palpated, they are also brought away from underlying structures in order to avoid confusion about the site of tenderness.

The term "patellar tracking" refers to the change in position of the patella relative to the femur during active knee flexion and extension. Although it is obviously important, no clinically useful tracking measurement systems exist. The J sign is a useful but nonspecific sign of patellofemoral pathology. It represents a patella that does not seat immediately as the knee is flexed, as well as the rotational torque between the extensor hood (tendons, retinaculum, and patella) and the femur. But many factors can contribute to abnormal tracking, such as trochlear dysplasia, patella alta, and medial retinacular laxity. Thus, the clinical usefulness of abnormal tracking in the assessment of alignment remains unclear because its relationship to the loading characteristics of the joint is not a simple one.

Normal tracking of the patella within the TG has been described by translation and tilt, both of which change with knee flexion angle (37). As the normal knee begins to flex, the patella becomes engaged in the trochlea, causing it to translate medially approximately 4 mm by 20° of knee flexion. With progressive flexion it then follows the TG approximately 7 mm laterally by 90° of knee flexion. Although it is translating laterally, it also tilts medially in a progressive linear fashion about 7° at 90 of flexion. Deep in flexion, it is more medially tilted with the odd (far medial) facet articulating with the medial trochlea. The patella flexes with the knee at a rate of about 0.7° per degree of knee flexion (37).

Abnormal patellar tracking may be caused by muscle weakness, soft tissues deficiencies, abnormal joint geometry, or limb malalignment. Early in flexion the medial retinaculum (specifically the MPFL) provides much of the restraint to lateral displacement of the patella. Its contribution to patellar restraint decreases with flexion from 50% at 0° of flexion to 30% at 20° knee flexion, as the patella begins to engage the femoral trochlea. The lowest force required to displace the patella laterally occurs at 30° of flexion. With further flexion, the patella engages the TG and trochlear geometry becomes the primary constraint to mediolateral patellar motion. In cadaver studies where the trochea has been modified (flattened) to simulate a dysplastic trochlea, the constraint of the patella is reduced by 70% (38).

Patellar mobility is best assessed both at 0° and at 30° of flexion. The checkrein often is easier to recognize at 0° because in this position the trochlea does not constrain the patella, so it is easier to feel an "endpoint" as you displace the patella laterally. At 30° of flexion, the patella is seated in the TG, and it is easier to quantify the amount of mobility in each direction. Normal translation should be symmetric in each direction and not exceed 7 to 10 mm with a 5-lb (2.26 kg) load. Alternatively, the patella can be divided into four quadrants, and the displacement can be recorded in quadrants. Particularly in heavy patients, stress X-rays may be more useful for assessing patellar mobility (see imaging below) (39). If patients are apprehensive as the patella is moved, an exam or stress X-rays under anesthesia can be very helpful to confirm pathologic laxity prior to proceeding with surgical stabilization. Stabilization is never indicated unless excess laxity has been documented either in the clinic or under anesthesia.

Imaging

Imaging begins with plain radiographic views of the knee including anteroposterior (AP), true lateral and axial views. Of these standard X-ray views, the true lateral view yields by far the most useful information when evaluating for instability. Axial images are helpful to evaluate the patellofemoral chondral interval (joint space).

Sagittal Plane Alignment

A true lateral means that the posterior and distal femoral condyles are superimposed as in Figures 60.2 and 60.5. No more than 2 mm of offset between the condyles should be accepted between the condyles, because any more obliquity in the X-ray projection will make it impossible to read the films correctly. The lateral is performed in approximately 30° of flexion in order to ensure that passive tension in the quadriceps pulls the patellar tendon to its full length, because several radiographic measures of patella alta assume that the tendon is at its full length. In the sagittal plane, two important osseous factors to be evaluated include length and depth of the trochlea, and patellar height. Trochlear length relative to patellar height is of particular importance, as this relationship governs the timing of patellar engagement within the groove in early flexion. The higher the patella, and the shorter the groove, the later the patella will engage in the trochlea. This puts the retinacular tissues under higher loads and places the patella at risk for subluxation and dislocation (Fig. 60.5A, B).

Figure 60.2 illustrates the difference between normal and dysplastic trochlea. Normal knees have prominent sloping medial and lateral trochlear walls enclosing a deep V-shaped groove. The proximal end of the floor of this V-shaped groove is continuous with the anterior femoral

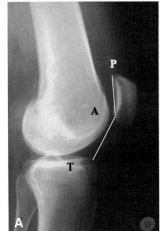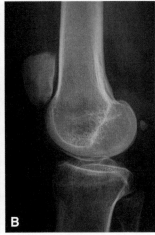

FIGURE 60.5. A: The height of the patella is surprisingly difficult to measure reliably. One of the more reliable methods is the index of Caton and Deschamps. This is the ratio between the distance of the lower edge of the patellar joint surface to the upper corner of the tibial plateau (AT) and the length of the patellar articular surface (AP). **B:** In cases of severely dysplastic trochlea or severe patella alta, the Bernageau view may be useful. The Bernageau view is a true lateral view taken in full knee extension with the quadriceps contracted. (From Fithian DC, Neyret P, Servien E. Patellar instability: the lyon experience. *Tech Knee Surg.* 2007;6(2):112–123, with permission.)

cortex at the trochlear inlet. On the strict lateral view, the floor of the groove is visible in profile as a distinct sclerotic line curving distally and posteriorly, starting from the anterior cortex and ending at the anterior end of Blumensaat's line. In its entire course, this line should never pass anterior to a line extending down the anterior femoral cortex. In contrast, patients with recurrent patellar instability often have a flat or shallow groove. This may result either from deficient walls or a groove that is not "dug out" sufficiently. An abnormally prominent floor of the groove passes anterior to the anterior femoral cortex, and eventually it rises anterior to one or both side walls. Mechanically, this deformity results simultaneously in a reduction of mediolateral constraint and an increase in PFJ contact loads. These mechanical effects are why many European surgeons consider trochlear dysplasia to be the fundamental abnormality in patellar instability as well as an important factor in isolated patellofemoral arthrosis.

On the lateral X-ray, the crossing sign represents the point at which the floor of the trochlea is in line with the most anterior rims of the medial and lateral trochlear walls. A small distance between the floor and the anterior rims reflects flatness of the groove and, by definition, absence of trochlear constraint against medial or lateral patellar displacement. Trochlear prominence is present when the most cephalad aspect of the groove is anterior to the anterior femoral cortex. The prominence represents the bump that the patella must climb over in order to enter the groove. Remember that "prominence" refers to the bottom and not the sides of the TG. Prominent medial and lateral walls are desirable because they constrain medio-lateral patellar displacement and guide its movement in flexion and extension. But if the bottom of the groove is prominent, it negates the height of the walls and presents an obstruction to passage of the patella as the knee flexes.

To summarize, on the true lateral X-ray, two features are needed to identify trochlear dysplasia:

1. The depth of the TG, or gorge, with respect to the height of the medial and lateral trochlear walls (the "crossing" sign), which represents the flattening of the groove as it is viewed from the side (Fig. 60.2B).
2. The prominence (also called the trochlear "boss," "bump," or "eminence") of the floor of the groove with respect to the anterior cortex of the distal femur (Fig. 60.2C).

These two findings on the lateral X-ray, the crossing sign and/or a prominence greater than 4 mm, indicate the presence of trochlear dysplasia.

The shape of the TT is best seen on the lateral radiograph. A hypoplastic tuberosity may be identified. The prominence of the TT alters the angle of patellar flexion and the lever arm of the extensor mechanism in producing torque at the knee (1). These alterations may be expected to affect compressive forces and contact areas in the distal patella.

After evaluating trochlear development, the next task in assessing sagittal plane alignment is to measure patellar height (alta or infera). In patella alta, the patella engages the trochlea later than normal as the knee flexes. This causes greater strain in the retinacular soft tissues (ligaments and muscles) and higher stress in the zone of articular contact because the contact area is smaller than normal (40). What is of interest, then, is the height of the distal patellar articular surface relative to the upper trochlea. However, it is difficult to standardize knee flexion angles for routine lateral knee X-rays, and just a small change in knee flexion can have a significant effect the position of the patella relative to the trochlear inlet. The result is that, for practical reasons, measuring patellar height relative to the tibia, instead of the femur, is much more reliable when using plain X-rays. Also, magnification on regular X-rays makes direct measurement of dimensions impossible without routine of scaling markers, so that ratios rather than crude patellar height is typically reported. Traditionally, using X-rays, patellar height has been measured using the Insall–Salvati, Blackburne–Peel, or Caton–Deschamps ratio because they are most reproducible on standard X-ray views. The Caton–Deschamps ratio evaluates distance from the inferior patellar articular margin to the tibial plateau to the length of the patellar articular surface (Fig 60.5A). Given the desirability of precise surgical planning and the unmet need for easy and reproducible direct measurement of patello-trochlear positioning in the sagittal plane (Fig. 60.5B), it seems likely that patellar height measurements taken from MR images will eventually supplant traditional ratios (see "Future Directions").

Frontal Plane Alignment

This is best determined using long (full-length) standing AP radiographs including hip, knee, and ankle joint (41, 42). To determine the mechanical axis, a line is drawn from the center of the femoral head to the center of the ankle joint (Fig. 60.6). Typically, normal alignment is defined as the mechanical axis passing just medial to the center of the knee (43). Valgus alignment refers to the mechanical axis passing lateral to the center of the knee, whereas varus refers to the mechanical axis passing medial to the center of the knee.

Two commonly measured angles are the mechanical tibiofemoral angle (center of femoral head to center of knee to center of talus) and the anatomical tibiofemoral angle (line down center of femoral shaft and line down center of tibial shaft). The mechanical tibiofemoral angle is the angle between the mechanical axis of the femur and the tibia. An angle of $1.2° \pm 2°$ is considered normal (i.e., the limb mechanical axis falls just medial to the center of the knee joint) (43–46). The anatomical tibiofemoral angle is the angle between the femoral shaft and the tibial shaft and is usually $5.5° \pm 2°$. Several studies have found no difference in these angles between males and females (46–49).

Rotational (Axial) Plane Alignment

As stated previously under physical examination, imaging for rotational alignment is performed only when physical examination suggests excessive femoral or tibial torsion. In

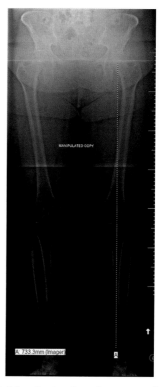

FIGURE 60.6. Full-length standing alignment radiograph with mechanical axis added showing neutral alignment. (Show only the left limb and enhance the line for contrast.)

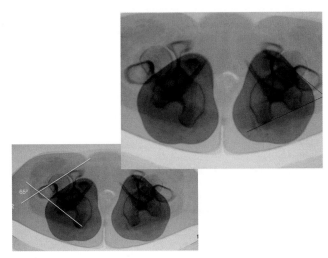

FIGURE 60.7. Two clinical examples of measuring femoral torsion (anteversion). A CT slice through the femoral head, a CT slice through the inferior greater trochanter, and a CT slice through the knee joint are superimposed. One line is drawn from the center of the femoral head through the greater trochanter and a second is tangent to the posterior femoral condyles at the knee joint.

assessing rotational alignment of the limb, axial computed tomography is needed (either CT or MRI). Measurements that can be of interest include torsion of the femur, torsion of the tibia, version or the relationship of the distal femur and proximal tibia, and the relationship between the femoral TG and the TT, known as the TT-TG distance or offset.

Femoral torsion is defined as the angle formed between the axis of the femoral neck and the distal femur; this is measured in degrees. To assess femoral torsion with CT scan, a line is drawn from the center point of the femoral head to the center point of the base of the femoral neck. This second point is more easily selected by locating the center of the femoral shaft at the level of the base of the neck where the shaft becomes round. Based on the classic tabletop method, the condylar axis is defined as the line between the two most posterior aspects of the femoral condyles. Alternatively a line connecting the epicondyles can be used. Then the angle formed by the intersection of these two lines is measured (Fig. 60.7).

For assessment of tibial torsion, a line is drawn across the center of the tibial plateau (47). As this line is not easy to locate, some authors use the tangent formed by the posterior cortical margin of the tibial plateau (Fig. 60.8). The femoral epicondylar axis might also be selected because it is easier to locate, and it is valid because what is of interest to the surgeon is the relationship of the knee joint axis to the ankle joint axis. Because different authors have used different reference lines at the upper tibia for establishing their ranges, it is important to realize that the line chosen will affect the measurement, and therefore, the appropriate source should be referenced in deciding how much correction is needed. Next, a line connecting the center point of the medial malleolus with the center point of the lateral malleolus is drawn. The angle formed by the intersection of these two lines is measured to determine tibial torsion (Fig. 60.8).

Strecker et al. (50, 51) reported the largest series of torsion measurements in normal individuals using CT scan. The authors measured torsion in 505 femurs and 504 tibias. They found normal measures of femoral anteversion to be $24.1° \pm 17.4°$ and normal measures of ETT to be $34.85° \pm 17.4°$. No correlation to sex could be established. Yoshioka and Cooke (48) made direct skeletal measurements of femur and tibia and found femoral anteversion of 7° using the epicondylar axis; with a standard deviation of 8°. There was no significant difference between males and females for femoral torsion. However, lateral tibial torsion averaged 24° with a significant difference

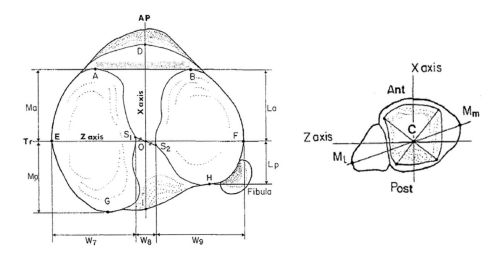

FIGURE 60 8. Tibial torsion may be measured using several different proximal tibial reference lines. Yoshioka used the angle between the line spanning the widest distance on the tibial plateau (EF) and the line connecting the malleoli ($M_m – M_l$). Yoshioka reported mean ETT for Males = 21°, and for Females = 27°. (From Yoshioka Y, Siu DW, Scudamore RA, et al. Tibial anatomy and functional axes. *J Orthop Res.* 1989;7(1):132–137, with permission.)

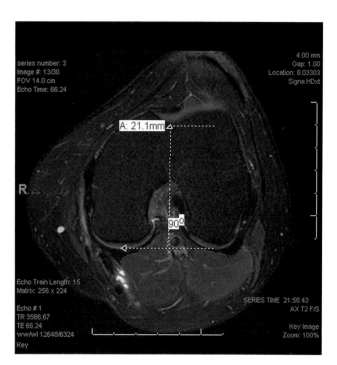

FIGURE 60.9. The MR images show a method of TT-TG measurement. The TT-TG offset is defined as the lateral distance of the TT with
respect to the center of the TG, measured parallel to a line connecting
the posterior condyles. One way to measure the offset is as follows:
1. Connect posterior condyles of femur. 2. Draw perpendicular reaching
apex of femoral groove. 3. Scroll to apex of TT and leave cursor there.
4. Scroll back to trochlear slice. 5. Draw a line to the first perpendicular
and measure. This line is parallel to the posterior femoral condylar line.

between males (21° ± 5°) and females (27° ± 11°). These
gender differences have not been corroborated by other
studies (52, 53) and their significance is uncertain. Again,
whatever reference line is used at the upper tibia in determining tibial torsion, the normal range should be taken
from the specific paper in which that line was used.

TT-TG Distance or Offset

Axial tomographic imaging (CT or MRI) is used to determine tibial tubercle offset (TT-TG distance). TT-TG
distance is a measure of the lateralizing vector that would
be applied to the patella by the tibia through the patellar
tendon during quadriceps contraction. The measurement
method is summarized in Figure 60.9. MRI is more helpful
than CT scan in identifying patterns of wear or overload
of the patellofemoral articulation. This can be useful in
planning surgical intervention.

TREATMENT

Whatever the bony architecture of the limb may be,
it serves only as a backdrop during functional activities. Given the degree of motion available and the

wide range of uses for the lower limb, neuromuscular
control, strength, and conditioning play an important
role in protecting the limb from injury during weight-
bearing activity. It is important then that any surgeon
contemplating correction of lower limb malalignment
needs to be fully familiar with the assessment and correction of common disorders of trunk and lower limb
control in patients presenting with patellofemoral
complaints.

Nonoperative Approaches

Many patients with patellofemoral disorders have defiin
proximal limb neuromuscular control that can contribute
to dynamic knee valgus, hip adduction, and hip internal
rotation (30, 54–56), all of which accentuate any underlying bony malalignment of the lower limb. It is important
to recognize that with mechanical overload, the most prudent treatment should be an overall reduction of loading
by activity restriction or modification, weight loss, and
flexibility and strength training. In general, rehashould focus on range of motion, pain control, quadriceps strengthening and conditioning, and proximal limb control (core
strengthening).

Operative Indications, Timing, and Technique

For the surgeon considering surgical intervention for
patellofemoral malalignment, two things should be understood from the outset. First, humans are not capable
of making a knee "normal." It is not within a surgeon's
power to make all aspects of a knee function optimally
in all respects. Even if the usual complications are
avoided and the patient heals as planned, there will be
a cost to the patient of having had surgery. Second, few
surgical procedures have yet been devised that prevent
the development of arthrosis; and to our knowledge,
no operation of the knee has ever been shown to prevent arthrosis. It is self-evident that successful procedures reduce symptoms and may improve function in
the short term, but it is not realistic to do any surgical procedure in the knee for the purpose of preventing
arthrosis.

Treatments are best based on an accurate diagnosis
and analysis of the predisposing factors presented in the
sections above. In the analysis of the pathogenesis, it is
important to establish a cause and effect. If a primary
abnormality is identified, the treatment should be directed
to correcting this abnormality if possible. Any soft tissue
or intra-articular procedure that does not properly identify
the underlying cause is destined to fail. In the vast majority of cases, a combination of predisposing factors exists.
James et al. (57) in 1978 described a "miserable malalignment syndrome," a combination of femoral anteversion,
squinting patellae, genu varum, patella alta, increased
Q-angle, external tibial rotation, tibia varum, and "compensatory" foot pronation. A single common surgical procedure such as lateral release or TT transfer is not likely

to cure anterior knee pain in this setting. It is essential to try to detect all of the bony and soft tissue factors present. When multiple malalignment factors are present, the relative contribution of each one is difficult to quantify. In a case with only one variable believed to be responsible for the pathogenesis, that variable should be corrected if possible. For cases with multiple abnormalities, our approach is either to correct the deformity that is most abnormal or to correct the factor that we believe contributes most to the symptoms.

Multiplane osteotomy can be useful when bone geometry is abnormal, but it is a difficult and demanding procedure. It might seem too aggressive in some cases to perform a femoral or tibial osteotomy to treat anterior knee pain; however, it has to be understood that the patellofemoral pain is often the expression of a complex problem of skeletal geometry. Following a well done femoral rotational osteotomy, patients may see not only improvement in their pain, but also improvement in their gait pattern, disappearance of foot pronation and bunions, disappearance of muscle tightness in the thigh and calf, and even improvement in the posture and lumbar pain (Fig. 60.10).

AUTHORS' PREFERRED TREATMENT

If history and experience have taught us anything, it is that a prudent approach to patellofemoral pain and arthrosis begins and ends with a specific rehabilitation program aimed at maximizing limb control, balance, and coordination. It seems wise to institute this program prior to surgery, even if workup reveals obvious anatomical predispositions. Surgery is indicated when rehabilitation fails to resolve symptoms and an anatomical defect explains that failure of response. For example, significant femoral anteversion can reduce the lever arm of the hip abductors when the foot follows a normal FPA (Fig. 60.1B), compromising strength and/or endurance, and contributing to faulty limb control. If therapeutic exercise fails to restore limb control, then rotational osteotomy in this case is indicated in order to improve the mechanical advantage of the gluteus muscles.

Osteotomy is performed at the level of the deformity whenever possible (Table 60.1) in order to produce the most effective derotation with minimal side effects. In the femur, the absence of landmarks between the lesser

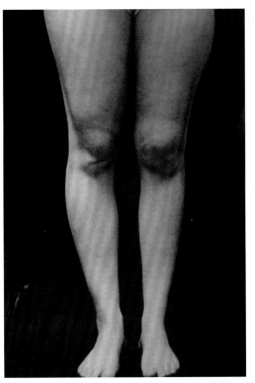
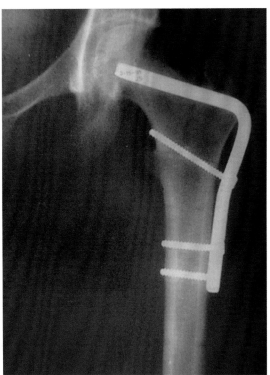

FIGURE 60.10. A: Picture shows a patient with excess femoral anteversion. On the patient's left side, a proximal intertrochanteric femoral derotational osteotomy has been performed. The right lower extremity has had no surgery. Observe the difference between right and left in the alignment of the extremity. On the right side, the patella points inward, the calf muscles are more prominent, giving a "pseudovarus" appearance, and the foot is more pronated. **B:** Postoperative X-ray of the femur derotational osteotomy. (From Teitge RA, Torga-Spak R. Failure of patellofemoral surgery: analysis of clinical cases. In: Sanchis-Alfonso V, ed. *Anterior Knee Pain and Patellar Instability*. London, UK: Springer; 2006:337–352.)

Surgical options for correction of skeletal malalignment associated with patellofemoral pathology

Deformity	Procedure
Frontal plane	
Genu valgum	Femoral osteotomy (supracondylar)
Genu varum	Tibial osteotomy
Sagittal plane	
Prominent trochlea	Trochleoplasty
Shallow trochlea	Lateral condyle osteotomy
Patella alta	Distal tuberosity transfer
Aplastic tuberosity	Maquet osteotomy (without medicalization)
Horizontal plane	
Increased femoral anteversion (>25°)	Proximal femoral external rotation osteotomy (intertrochanteric)
Tibial external torsion (>40°)	Proximal tibial internal rotation osteotomy (infratuberosity)
Increased TT-TG (≥20 mm)	Tuberosity medialization
Decreased TT-TG (<10 mm)	Tuberosity lateralization
Combined deformities	
Valgus + femoral anteversion	Distal femoral varus external rotation osteotomy
Varus + vemoral anteversion	Distal femoral valgus external rotation osteotomy
Tibial torsion + increased TT-TG	Proximal tibial osteomtomy (supratuberosity)
Femoral anteversion + tibial torsion (miserable malalignment)	Proximal femoal external rotation osteotomy + proximal tibial internal rotation osteotomy

trochanter proximally and the condyles distally allows us to choose a level at which the surgeon is comfortable and can make an accurate correction. The senior one of us (RAT) prefers proximal femoral osteotomy for pure rotational correction in order to avoid a sudden change in direction of the quadriceps if the osteotomy is done at the supracondylar level (Fig. 60.10B). In cases of multiplanar deformity, the osteotomy is performed at the distal femur (Table 60.1).

With excessive external torsion of the tibia and the foot moving in the line of a normal FPA, the patella is pulled laterally in the TG. This increases the displacement or subluxation force and the lateral patellofemoral articular compression force. If the TT-TG distance is normal, the derotation osteotomy should be performed below the TT so as not to medialize the tuberosity as an unwanted side effect (Fig. 60.11A–C).

Distal TT transfer is a relatively simple technique that is done commonly in Europe to correct patella alta, but in the United States, few surgeons feel comfortable performing it. There are several concerns specific to distalization osteotomy: (1) inadequate fixation with loss of correction due to shearing forces on the fragment; (2) gap formation at the distal interface, leading to a stress riser and slow healing, which can produce late tibial fracture at the distal end of the osteotomized fragment (Fig. 60.12A); (3) loss of knee flexion due to increased passive quadriceps tension;

and (4) increased PFJ pressures due to increased quadriceps tension. Fixation of the fragment to overcome shear forces is achieved with two 4.5 cortical screws placed in lag screw technique and offset in the anterior cortical hole so that dynamic compression drives the fragment distally, compressing the fragment against the intact anterior tibial cortex (Fig. 60.12B).

COMPLICATIONS

Strict adherence to the principles of osteosynthesis leads to prompt healing in most cases. Wound complications are avoidable with good surgical technique and gentle handling of the soft tissues. Multiplanar osteotomies and trochleoplasties are complex geometrical problems and should be done only by experienced surgeons at this time. It seems likely that this is an area in which navigational software will help to improve the accuracy of the correction (see "Future Directions").

REHABILITATION

It is important that osteotomies be well fixed in order to support immediate motion whenever possible. This avoids stiffness and loss of motor control. Limited weight-bearing in a brace is appropriate for most osteotomies in the first

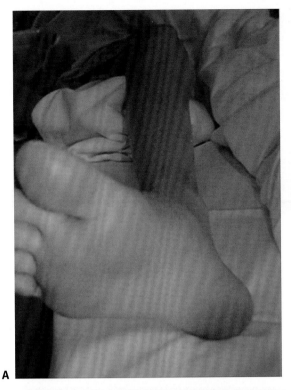

A

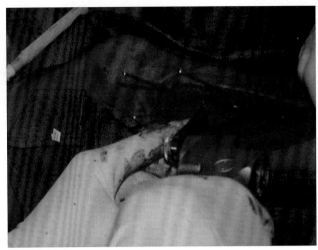

B

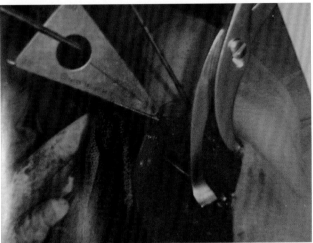

C

FIGURE 60.11. A: A patient with excess ETT. **B:** The deformity is corrected by an internal rotation osteotomy below the level of the TT. A blade of a blade plate has been inserted into the proximal fragment in a direction to prevent changes in varus or valgus, flexion, or extension. It is inserted 30° in a posterior medial direction relative to the flat surface on the lateral tibial diaphysis. Two K-wires that were placed parallel before the osteotomy now are changed to an angle of 30° with the distal wire in the distal or shaft fragment having been rotated internally 30°. A clamp is holding the side plate to the lateral tibial cortex while the tension device will be applied. (From Teitge RA, Torga-Spak R. Failure of patellofemoral surgery: analysis of clinical cases. In: Sanchis-Alfonso V, ed. *Anterior Knee Pain and Patellar Instability.* London, UK: Springer; 2006:337–352.)

6 weeks postoperatively, but controlled exercises are instituted as soon as pain allows and are progressed as soon as possible. The goal is to restore functional limb control with optimal load distribution, so that the surgeon and therapist are working toward the same ultimate return to full function.

Active knee extension is prevented by immobilization in an extension brace for 6 weeks. Passive heel slides, medial–lateral patellar mobilization exercises and gentle quad set exercises prevent loss of knee motion and quadriceps control during this period of protected healing. Loss of knee flexion should be expected, but it is only a functional limitation in patients who have overtight quadriceps. Prone knee flexion (with the hip extended) will detect tight quadriceps, which should be corrected both preoperatively and postoperatively with exercise. Finally,

it has been asserted that increased passive quadriceps tension caused by distalization could elevate PF loads, but this has not been shown to be true. In any case, as was mentioned earlier, surgery is done to *redistribute* load. Distalization redistributes loads more proximally on the patella, often bypassing diseased distal patellar cartilage. It can be argued that any incremental increase in net PF loading would contribute to knee extension. Any need to counter the potentially small increased loading would then be addressed by therapeutic exercise and weight management.

CONCLUSIONS AND FUTURE DIRECTIONS

Malalignment is best defined more broadly than has traditionally been the case in the United States. High Q angle or TT-TG offset represents only one dimension of

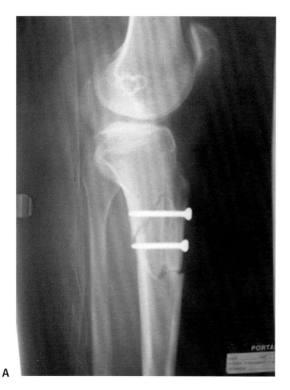

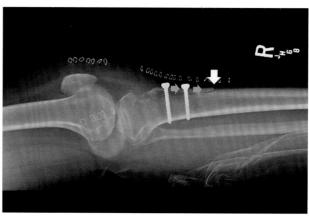

FIGURE 60.12. **A:** After distalization, slow-healing anterior cortex can leave a stress riser, leading to potential fracture. **B:** To help prevent this, distal compression is achieved with offset drilling of the far (posterior) cortex to apply dynamic compression at the junction of the osteotomized fragment and the intact cortex. Alternatively, the screws can be directed in a slightly distal direction or a plate can be used for rigid fixation.

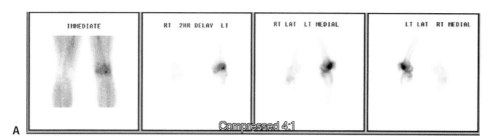

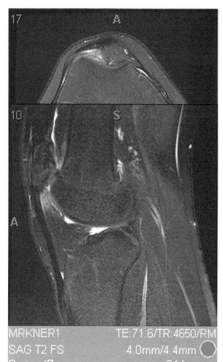

FIGURE 60.13. **A:** Bone scan and (**B**) MR imaging are useful to identify abnormalities of bone turnover or presence of edema within the soft tissues that can be evidence of abnormal loading.

malalignment and is overly simplistic. Focus on lateralized quadriceps force alone can lead to a dogmatic approach with medialization of the TT as an incorrect mainstay of treatment. An important study recently has shown that patella alta is associated with high contact stress near full knee extension, associated with lateral shift and increased tilt of the patella (40). The patella and femur relate to one another in three dimensions, therefore, alignment could conceivably be measured in 6° of freedom (rotation and displacement with respect to any of three axes). Any abnormal rotation or displacement represents potential malalignment.

Malalignment is believed to cause symptoms by uneven distribution of forces that may result in overload of a particular region of the patellofemoral articulation. Evidence of significant overload can usually be documented on imaging studies that demonstrate physiologic stress. These include SPECT, MRI, and bone scan. Bone scan is an excellent study to localize a presumed area of overload showing increased metabolic activity (Fig. 60.13A). MRI can also show evidence of abnormal loading of the soft tissues such as the fat pad (Fig. 60.13B). If surgical correction is being considered, objective evidence should be sought using these modalities. Besides confirming the hypothesis that local articular overload is in fact the cause of the pain, this approach can help the surgeon to develop a rationale for off-loading the stressed area.

Multiplanar corrections and deformities of trochlear geometry remain extremely challenging problems even for experienced surgeons. At this time, they are best left to surgeons with a great deal of experience. However, navigational techniques have already contributed to correction of multiplanar abnormalities in knee surgery and are becoming easier and cheaper to incorporate into the routine setting. Newer approaches to trochleoplasty are likely to make this difficult problem more accessible to the community surgeon.

At this time, patella alta represents one of the more frequently identified forms of malalignment that is ignored in treating patellofemoral disorders. Distalization of the TT is a relatively simple procedure that can yield major improvements in PFJ force distribution, but there are technical principles that will yield optimal outcomes (see above).

REFERENCES

1. Maquet P. Advancement of the tibial tuberosity. *Clin Orthop Relat Res.* 1976;(115):225–230.
2. Losel S, Burgess-Milliron MJ, Micheli LJ, et al. A simplified technique for determining foot progression angle in children 4 to 16 years of age. *J Pediatr Orthop.* 1996;16(5):570–574.
3. Jaarsma RL, Ongkiehong BF, Grüneberg C, et al. Compensation for rotational malalignment after intramedullary nailing for femoral shaft fractures. An analysis by plantar pressure measurements during gait. *Injury.* 2004;35(12):1270–1278.
4. Seber S, Hazer B, Köse N, et al. Rotational profile of the lower extremity and foot progression angle: computerized tomographic examination of 50 male adults. *Arch Orthop Trauma Surg.* 2000;120(5–6):255–258.
5. Tornetta P III, Ritz G, Kantor A. Femoral torsion after interlocked nailing of unstable femoral fractures. *J Trauma.* 1995;38(2):213–219.
6. Cahue S, Dunlop D, Hayes K, et al. Varus-valgus alignment in the progression of patellofemoral osteoarthritis. *Arthritis Rheum.* 2004;50(7):2184–2190.
7. Elahi S, Cahue S, Felson DT, et al. The association between varus-valgus alignment and patellofemoral osteoarthritis. *Arthritis Rheum.* 2000;43(8):1874–1880.
8. Fujikawa K, Seedhom BB, Wright V. Biomechanics of the patello-femoral joint. Part II: a study of the effect of simulated femoro-tibial varus deformity on the congruity of the patello-femoral compartment and movement of the patella. *Eng Med.* 1983;12(1):13–21.
9. Lerat JL, Moyen B, Galland O, et al. Morphological types of the lower limbs in femoro-patellar disequilibrium. Analysis in 3 planes. *Acta Orthop Belg.* 1989;55(3):347–355.
10. Janssen G. Chondropathy of the patella as pre-arthrosis of the knee. Its causes and treatment, based on results after "abrasio patellae" (author's transl). *Z Orthop Ihre Grenzgeb.* 1974;112(5):1036–1044.
11. Takai S, Sakakida K, Yamashita F, et al. Rotational alignment of the lower limb in osteoarthritis of the knee. *Int Orthop.* 1985;9(3):209–215.
12. Turner MS. The association between tibial torsion and knee joint pathology. *Clin Orthop Relat Res.* 1994;(302):47–51.
13. Eckhoff DG, Brown AW, Kilcoyne RF, et al. Knee version associated with anterior knee pain. *Clin Orthop Relat Res.* 1997;(339):152–155.
14. Hefzy MS, Jackson WT, Saddemi SR, et al. Effects of tibial rotations on patellar tracking and patello-femoral contact areas. *J Biomed Eng.* 1992;14(4):329–343.
15. Lee TQ, Morris G, Csintalan RP. The influence of tibial and femoral rotation on patellofemoral contact area and pressure. *J Orthop Sports Phys Ther.* 2003;33(11):686–693.
16. Lee TQ, Yang BY, Sandusky MD, et al. The effects of tibial rotation on the patellofemoral joint: assessment of the changes in in situ strain in the peripatellar retinaculum and the patellofemoral contact pressures and areas. *J Rehabil Res Dev.* 2001;38(5):463–469.
17. Lee TQ, Anzel SH, Bennett KA, et al. The influence of fixed rotational deformities of the femur on the patellofemoral contact pressures in human cadaver knees. *Clin Orthop Relat Res.* 1994;11(302):69–74.
18. Kijowski R, Plagens D, Shaeh SJ, et al. The effects of rotational deformities of the femur on contact pressure and contact area in the patellofemoral joint and on strain in the medial patellofemoral ligament. Presented at the Annual Meeting of the International Patellofemoral Study Group, Napa Valley, CA, USA; 1999.
19. Fithian D, Neyret P, Servien E. Patellar instability: the lyon experience. *Tech Knee Surg.* 2007;6(2):112–123.
20. Lin YF, Jan MH, Lin DH, et al. Different effects of femoral and tibial rotation on the different measurements of patella tilting: An axial computed tomography study. *J Orthop Surg.* 2008;3:5.

21. Brattstrom H. Shape of the intercondylar groove normally and in recurrent dislocation of patella: a clinical and X-ray anatomical investigation. *Acta Orthop Scand Suppl.* 1964;68:134–148.

22. Malghem J, Maldague B. Depth insufficiency of the proximal trochlear groove on lateral radiographs of the knee: relation to patellar dislocation. *Radiology.* 1989;170(2):507–510.

23. Dejour H, Walch G, Nove-Josserand L, et al. Factors of patellar instability: an anatomic radiographic study. *Knee Surg Sports Traumatol Arthrosc.* 1994;2(1):19–26.

24. Maldague B, Malghem J. Radiology of patellar instability: contribution of the lateral radiography and the 30-degree axial view with external rotation. *Acta Orthop Belg.* 1989;55(3):311–329.

25. Raguet M. Mesure radiologique de la hauteur trochléene. *J Traumatol Sport.* 1986;3:210–213.

26. Walch G, ed. Morphologic factors in patellar instability: clinical, radiologic, and tomographic data. In: *Journees du Genou.* 6th ed. Lyon, France; 1987:25–35.

27. Walch G, Dejour H. Radiology in femoro-patellar pathology. *Acta Orthop Belg.* 1989;55(3):371–380.

28. Walch G, Dejour H, eds. Radiology in pathology of the patellofemoral joint. In: *Journees du Genou.* 6th ed. Lyon, France; 1987:25–35.

29. Dejour H, Walch G, Neyret P, et al. Dysplasia of the femoral trochlea. *Rev Chir Orthop Reparatrice Appar Mot.* 1990;76(1):45–54.

30. Powers CM. The influence of altered lower-extremity kinematics on patellofemoral joint dysfunction: a theoretical perspective. *J Orthop Sports Phys Ther.* 2003;33(11):639–646.

31. Staheli LT, Corbett M, Wyss C, et al. Lower-extremity rotational problems in children. Normal values to guide management. *J Bone Joint Surg Am.* 1985;67(1):39–47.

32. Kozic S, Gulan G, Matovinovic D, et al. Femoral anteversion related to side differences in hip rotation. Passive rotation in 1,140 children aged 8–9 years. *Acta Orthop Scand.* 1997;68(6):533–536.

33. Souza RB, Powers CM. Concurrent criterion-related validity and reliability of a clinical test to measure femoral anteversion. *J Orthop Sports Phys Ther.* 2009;39(8):586–592.

34. Greene CC, Edwards TB, Wade MR, et al. Reliability of the quadriceps angle measurement. *Am J Knee Surg.* 2001;14(2):97–103.

35. Tomsich DA, Nitz AJ, Threlkeld AJ, et al. Patellofemoral alignment: reliability. *J Orthop Sports Phys Ther.* 1996;23(3):200–208.

36. Fulkerson JP. The etiology of patellofemoral pain in young, active patients: a prospective study. *Clin Orthop.* 1983;(179):129–133.

37. Amis AA, Senavongse W, Bull AM. Patellofemoral kinematics during knee flexion-extension: an in vitro study. *J Orthop Res.* 2006;24(12):2201–2211.

38. Senavongse W, Amis AA. The effects of articular, retinacular, or muscular deficiencies on patellofemoral joint stability. *J Bone Joint Surg Br.* 2005;87(4):577–582.

39. Teitge RA, Faerber WW, Des Madryl P, et al. Stress radiographs of the patellofemoral joint. *J Bone Joint Surg Am.* 1996;78(2):193–203.

40. Ward SR, Terk MR, Powers CM. Patella alta: association with patellofemoral alignment and changes in contact area during weight-bearing. *J Bone Joint Surg Am.* 2007;89(8):1749–1755.

41. Felson DT, Cooke TD, Niu J, et al; OAI Investigators Group. Can anatomic alignment measured from a knee radiograph substitute for mechanical alignment from full limb films? *Osteoarthritis Cartilage.* 2009;17(11):1448–1452.

42. Sled EA, Sheehy LM, Felson DT, et al. Reliability of lower limb alignment measures using an established landmark-based method with a customized computer software program. *Rheumatol Int.* 2011;31(1):71–77.

43. Moreland JR, Bassett LW, Hanker GJ. Radiographic analysis of the axial alignment of the lower extremity. *J Bone Joint Surg Am.* 1987;69(5):745–749.

44. Cooke TD, Li J, Scudamore RA. Radiographic assessment of bony contributions to knee deformity. *Orthop Clin North Am.* 1994;25(3):387–393.

45. Chao EY, Neluheni EV, Hsu RW, et al. Biomechanics of malalignment. *Orthop Clin North Am.* 1994;25(3):379–386.

46. Hsu RW, Himeno S, Coventry MB, et al. Normal axial alignment of the lower extremity and load-bearing distribution at the knee. *Clin Orthop Relat Res.* 1990;(255):215–227.

47. Yoshioka Y, Siu DW, Scudamore RA, et al. Tibial anatomy and functional axes. *J Orthop Res.* 1989;7(1):132–137.

48. Yoshioka Y, Cooke TD. Femoral anteversion: assessment based on function axes. *J Orthop Res.* 1987;5(1):86–91.

49. Yoshioka Y, Siu D, Cooke TD. The anatomy and functional axes of the femur. *J Bone Joint Surg Am.* 1987;69(6):873–880.

50. Strecker W, Keppler P, Gebhard F, et al. Length and torsion of the lower limb. *J Bone Joint Surg Br.* 1997;79(6):1019–1023.

51. Strecker W, Franzreb M, Pfeiffer T, et al. Computerized tomography measurement of torsion angle of the lower extremities. *Unfallchirurg.* 1994;97(11):609–613.

52. Reikeras O, Hoiseth A. Torsion of the leg determined by computed tomography. *Acta Orthop Scand.* 1989;60(3):330–333.

53. Sayli U, Bölükbasi S, Atik OS, et al. Determination of tibial torsion by computed tomography. *J Foot Ankle Surg.* 1994;33(2):144–147.

54. Souza RB, Powers CM. Differences in hip kinematics, muscle strength, and muscle activation between subjects with and without patellofemoral pain. *J Orthop Sports Phys Ther.* 2009;39(1):12–19.

55. Souza RB, Powers CM. Predictors of hip internal rotation during running: an evaluation of hip strength and femoral structure in women with and without patellofemoral pain. *Am J Sports Med.* 2009;37(3):579–587.

56. Kulig K, Harper-Hanigan K, Souza RB, et al. Measurement of femoral torsion by ultrasound and magnetic resonance imaging: concurrent validity. *Phys Ther.* 2010;90(11):1641–1648.

57. James SL, Bates BT, Osternig LR. Injuries to runners. *Am J Sports Med.* 1978;6(2):40–50.

Surgical Management of Patellar Instability

Alex Dukas • Michael Pensak • Cory Edgar • Thomas DeBerardino

CLINICAL EVALUATION

Pertinent History

Predisposing anatomical factors and/or traumatic events are both common findings among patients who cite a history of multiple patella dislocations (1). A comprehensive history should focus on the onset and duration of symptoms, the mechanism of injury, provocative maneuvers/activities, and any prior patellofemoral joint symptoms. Patients with trochlear dysplasia or significant limb malalignment typically present at a very young age and have minimal history of trauma. In this patient, it is common to have failed past procedures and requires a meticulous workup to ensure successful outcome, as a single procedure is usually not enough. Patients who have recurrent dislocations frequently report diffuse pain around the knee that is aggravated by going up and down stairs or getting up from a seated position, as well as feelings of insecurity about their knee with episodes of giving way, crepitation, and/or swelling. If treatment was unsuccessful, it is necessary to determine whether it was in part due to a diagnostic error, inappropriateness of the treatment modality, issues with patient compliance or perhaps a new event that exacerbated the patient's symptoms. It is important to delineate the difference between symptomatic instability and pain due to cartilage lesions, overload, or osteoarthritis.

Physical Exam

A focused physical exam should begin with adequate inspection of both lower extremities, preferably with the patient wearing shorts. The presence of an effusion and whether or not the patella is ballotable should be noted. Repetitive flexion/extension of the knee with the patient relaxed and the physician's palm centered over the patella will help gauge if the patella tracks normally in the center of the trochlea. The presence of the "J sign" should be sought in which the patella subluxates from its centered position in the trochlea at 30° of flexion to a lateral position at full extension.

If the patient presents with acute subluxation, ballottement and effusion should be evaluated. Aspiration of

joint fluid might reveal serosanguinous fluid. The presence of fat droplets may indicate the presence of osteochondral fragment(s) within the joint (2).

The Q-angle, defined as the angle formed between intersecting lines from the anterior superior iliac crest to the midpatella and from the midpatella to the midtibial tuberosity with the patient supine, should be measured. This angle provides an estimate of tibial and femoral torsion about the knee joint. Normal Q-angles are 14° and 17° for males and females, respectively. Angles greater than these can predispose patients to patellar instability. When making this measurement, it is critical to ensure that the patella is centered over the trochlear groove as slight subluxation owing to a deficient medial patellofemoral ligament (MPFL) or medial structures can falsely decrease the Q-angle.

The extent to which the patella glides medially and laterally can offer valuable information about the soft-tissue structures around the patella. The main static soft-tissue stabilizer of the patella is the MPFL, accommodating approximately 53% of patellar tension (3). Lesser contributions come from the medial patellar retinaculum. The integrity of the MPFL can be evaluated by assessing the extent of lateral patellar glide. This maneuver is performed with the patient supine, relaxed and the leg in extension. The examiner then shifts the patella laterally from the midline. Excursion of three quadrants or more indicates a hypermobile patella and possible damage to the MPFL and medial-sided structures (2). Failure of the patella to move more than quadrant in the medial direction suggests a tight lateral retinaculum.

Patellar tilt refers to the examiner's ability to raise the lateral edge of the patella past the horizontal in the axial plane with the patient supine, relaxed and the knee flexed approximately 20°. Patients with tight lateral structures may have chronic overload of the lateral patellar facet and have tenderness to palpation along the lateral border of the patella upon physical exam (4).

The patellar apprehension test is an attempt to elicit the same sensations experienced by a patient who previously suffered a patella dislocation. With the patient supine, relaxed and the knee flexed 20° to 30°, the examiner carefully glides the patella laterally looking for any quadriceps contraction, indicating a positive test for the apprehension sign.

If crepitus is felt with patellar compression during full ROM, patellar arthrosis or chondral lesions should be suspected. Compression of the patella during full range of motion of the knee may reproduce the associated pain. Approximate location of cartilage lesions can be made on the basis that the distal chondral surface of the patella articulates with the femoral trochlea early in flexion and more distally as the knee is flexed. Posterior drawer stability should also be examined, as the presence of a PCL deficiency is associated with degenerative patellar arthritis (5). Valgus stability should also be assessed, as MCL injury is associated with MPFL tears (4).

IMAGING

Radiographs

A set of standard knee radiographs should be obtained consisting of weight-bearing posteroanterior (PA) views of both knees in extension and 45° of flexion, lateral views, and Merchant views. Aside from patella-specific measurements, all radiographs should be scrutinized for located joints (patellofemoral and tibiofemoral) and the presence of subtle fractures.

True lateral radiographs with the knee in 30° of flexion are of utmost importance in evaluation as assessment of trochlear dysplasia, tilt, and patellar height can be made from this view. Patellar height is valuable as an abnormally high patella, patella alta, has been implicated in 25% of patellar dislocations (6). Patella height can be measured by many methods namely, the Blackburne–Peel, Insall–Salvati, or Caton–Deschamps ratios (7) (Figs. 61.1 to 61.3). The Insall–Salvati index is calculated by dividing the length of the patellar tendon by the diagonal length of the patella (B/A), normal being in the range of 0.8 to 1.2. The Blackburne–Peel index is calculated by measuring the perpendicular distance from the lower end of the articular surface of the patella to a line projected forward along the tibial plateau (the tibial plateau line) and then dividing that distance by the length of the articular surface of the patella (B/A), normal range being 0.54 to 1.06. The Caton–Deschamps index is calculated by measuring the distance between the lower end of the (spacing) articular surface of the patella and the designated superior anterior angle of the tibia and then dividing that distance by the length of the articular surface of the patella (B/A), normal range being 0.6 to 1.2. Escala et al. (8) reported a 78% sensitivity and 68% specificity when using the Insall–Salvati

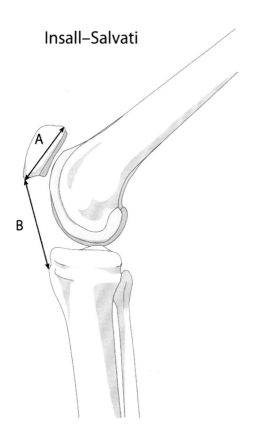

FIGURE 61.1. The Insall–Salvati index is calculated by dividing the length of the patellar tendon by the diagonal length of the patella. Normal values are within the range of 0.8 to 1.2.

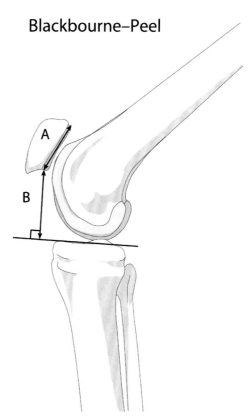

FIGURE 61.2. The Blackburne–Peel index is calculated by measuring the perpendicular distance from the lower end of the articular surface of the patella to a line projected along the tibial plateau and then dividing that distance by the length of the articular surface of the patella. Normal values are within the range of 0.54 to 1.06.

Canton–Deschamps

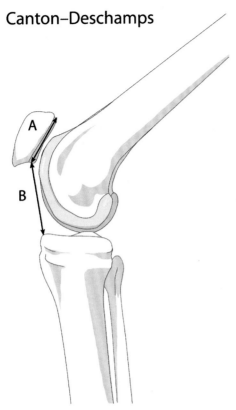

FIGURE 61.3. The Caton–Deschamps index is calculated by measuring the distance between the lower end of the articular surface of the patella and the designated superior anterior angle of the tibia and then dividing that distance by the length of the articular surface of the patella. Normal values are within the range of 0.6 to 1.2.

ratio. However, it has been shown that the Blackburne–Peel is the most reproducible ratio and has been preferred in more recent literature (9–11).

Evidence of trochlear dysplasia has been implicated in up to 96% of patients with a true history of patellar dislocation (12). The degree of trochlear dysplasia can be gauged from the lateral radiograph by the presence of a supratrochlear spur, double contour (hypoplastic medial condyle), or crossing sign (floor of the trochlear groove crosses the anterior outline of the lateral femoral condyle). Evidence of patellar tilt can be seen if there is overlap of the medial condylar ridge and lateral patellar facet, but this is more definitively evaluated on axial views (13, 14).

The Merchant view is the preferred axial view rather than the skyline view because as the knee is hyperflexed in the latter, the patella fully engages within the trochlear groove and subtle variations of patellar tilt or subluxation get lost (15). Merchant views allow for the assessment of patellar tilt, subluxation, and trochlear dysplasia. Traction spurs and thinning of the lateral facet–lateral trochlear interval can be evaluated using this view. The most objective measurement of instability in this view is patellar tilt, the angle formed by lines tangential to the longest transverse dimension of the patella and to the most posterior aspect of both femoral condyles (8, 16, 17). Escala et al. (8) observed that evidence

of patellar tilt above 11° provides a sensitivity of 92.7% and specificity of 63.3% for recurrent patellar instability.

Computed Tomography

CT scans are valuable for measuring the tibial tubercle-trochlear groove distance (TT-TG). The TT-TG distance is a measure of lateral offset of the tibial tubercle relative to the trochlear groove. Jones et al. (18) described a value of 2 to 9 mm as normal, 10 to 19 mm as abnormal and more than 20 mm as highly abnormal and indicative of surgical correction.

Magnetic Resonance Imaging

MRI is most helpful in the setting of an acute dislocation as soft tissue structural damage, and the presence of osteochondral fragments can be detected, the latter of which often warrants surgical intervention. The presence of bone bruising on the medial patellar facet and lateral femoral condyle can also be appreciated on MRI. Lastly, separation of marrow fat and blood can be visualized on MRI and serve as another indicator of a subtle or overt fracture.

NONOPERATIVE MANAGEMENT

Recurrent Subluxation

Chronic patellar instability can often be successfully treated by nonoperative means. The principal goals in rehabilitation are to decrease symptoms, increase quadriceps strength and endurance, and return the individual to maximal function. Accordingly, the mainstay of rehabilitation in these patients has been quadriceps strengthening, with special focus on the vastus medialis obliquus, which has been implicated to play a role in dynamic stabilization of the knee (19). Closed-chain exercises have been advocated by Stensdotter et al. (20) to promote a more synchronous firing of the quad musculature and decrease patella contact stresses as compared with open-chain exercises. Patellar taping or bracing can be utilized as an adjunct during rehabilitation to limit patellar motion. Failure of conservative management warrants a discussion of the available surgical options to alleviate symptoms.

TREATMENT OF ACUTE PATELLA DISLOCATION

Acute Primary Dislocation

Surgical treatment of acute patella dislocations has been the subject of much debate within the orthopedic community. Although it has been shown that the MPFL is almost universally torn upon dislocation, nonoperative treatment has been the mainstay of management (21). It has been shown that 15% to 25% of patients who dislocate will inevitably dislocate again (1, 22). Although there are proponents of early reconstruction of the MPFL in young or professional athletes or high functioning individuals, a randomized control trial by Nikku et al. (23, 24) published results at 2 and 7 years and found no significant difference in functional outcome scores or the rate of subluxations/dislocations. In light of such evidence, the senior author does not routinely address acute patellar dislocations with surgical intervention. However, surgery is acutely indicated in the presence of a mechanical block to full knee range of motion, loose osteochondral fragments, fractures requiring fixation, persistent patellar subluxation or bony detachment of the medial retinaculum/MPFL from the patella. In these instances, a diagnostic arthroscopy in conjunction with a mini-open/open approach to the knee is usually required to address the offending pathology.

Standard medial and lateral knee arthroscopy portals are established, and the knee is systematically evaluated. Careful attention should be paid to the medial patellar facets and lateral femoral condyle for the presence of any chondral/osteochondral damage as these sites are frequently affected during the dislocation event. Loose cartilage and osteochondral fragments should be removed and the latter preserved and more carefully scrutinized for possible fixation with a host of devices, the senior author prefers absorbable headless compression screws to secure repairable osteochondral lesions. Large, irreparable, cartilage voids are usually addressed at a later date and are beyond the scope of this chapter. After thorough inspection of the knee's articulating surfaces, the region of the MPFL should be evaluated. However, being an extra-articular structure, arthroscopy is more of an adjunct for fully evaluating the extent of MPFL damage.

Medial Imbrication

The traditional two-incision imbrication procedure described by Insall has fallen out of favor with the development of smaller, mini-open procedures that tend to reduce contact stresses and postoperative stiffness (25). A less extensive imbrication of the medial retinaculum can be accomplished arthroscopically using percutaneously passed sutures (26). However, it is the opinion of the senior author that a mini-open approach is the best way to visualize and palpate the region of the MPFL and medial retinaculum to determine whether a repair is feasible. Key points to consider when evaluating the MPFL are whether its bony insertion sites are preserved, whether the ligamentous tissue is of adequate quality, strength, and orientation to repair/imbricate, whether any intrasubstance scar tissue has formed. Of utmost importance is ensuring that an imbrication will not overly constrain the MPFL, thereby overloading the medial patellar facet. These points are critically important in deciding whether to repair the medial-sided structures or reconstruct them with a tendon graft, the latter option to be discussed in a separate chapter. The senior author currently favors a mini-open imbrication of the MPFL in isolation as the proximal realignment procedure of choice when the narrow indications are met for an acute surgical exploration of the knee following a patellar

dislocation. Vastus medialis obliquus (VMO) advancement is not performed as it is a nonanatomic technique.

Imbrication of the MPFL begins with a small longitudinal midline incision over the patella. The VMO is isolated and elevated with 3 to 5 mm of tendon from its interdigitations with the MPFL. Next, the deep surface of the MPFL is palpated. In the true acute setting (within 48 hours of injury), no scar tissue will be present if there is a midsubstance attenuation or tear, the latter of which is palpable by sweeping a finger along the posterior surface of the MPFL. Grasping the MPFL in its midsubstance or juxta-patellar insertion region and pulling laterally is an indirect means of checking the integrity of the ligament's femoral attachment. If the ligament becomes taut with this maneuver, then proximal anchorage can be confirmed. If tibial or femoral avulsions are present and the quality of the MPFL is good, then the bony insertions are anatomically restored with suture anchors and the MPFL is repaired. If the tissue quality is poor, an MPFL reconstruction is warranted.

For symptomatic patients undergoing a delayed surgical procedure following their first patella dislocation, a taut, elongated, but properly oriented MPFL is often present (4). Figure-of-eight stitches using nonabsorbable suture are placed in the midsubstance of the MPFL, tension is held and the knee is ranged to ensure that the knee is not overly constrained, the patella tracks normally and there is appropriate tension in the region of the repair. The stitches are usually tied with the knee at 90° of flexion. The number of imbrication stitches placed and the knee flexion angle can be titrated to achieve the desired goal of restoring the balance of forces that enable the patella to be safely and consistently delivered into the femoral trochlea during the initial 10 to 30 of knee flexion.

LATERAL RETINACULAR RELEASE

Isolated lateral releases for addressing patellar instability have fallen out of favor owing to the high rates of complications and lack of clinical improvement cited in numerous studies (27–29). At the present time, the senior author only performs a limited lateral release to address residual patellar tilt following repair and/or reconstruction of the medial-sided structures. Standard arthroscopic portals are utilized. With the arthroscope in the standard inferolateral portal, the preferred radiofrequency device is introduced into the inferomedial portal. Starting proximally on the joint capsule juxtaposed to the superior margin of the patella, sequential passes are made with the radiofrequency device from proximal to distal until the deep layers of the capsule begin to divide. Cautery is used liberally on the cut surfaces so as to maintain hemostasis and visualization. As the tissue begins to spread upon release, progressively deeper passes from proximal to distal are made until visual evidence confirms complete release of the lateral capsule. The vector of the release is essentially horizontal with the knee in the extended position beginning at the desired start position about 5 to 10 mm below the lateral edge of the patellar cartilage and extending down to the lateral portal through which the arthroscope is located. Visualization is optimized if the internal synovitic pericapsular tissue is debrided back to the smooth, tight lateral capsular tissue. In order to ensure the release is complete distally, the arthroscope may be moved to the inferomedial portal, and any residual bands of tissue between the nearly completed release and the lateral portal can be easily released with the radiofrequency device introduced into the inferolateral portal.

Indirect feedback of a completed release is noted via the external view of the knee, whereby a complete lack of tethering or banding is noted across the lateral aspect of the knee joint. Additional indirect evidence of a completed release occurs when no shadows are noted via direct visual observation of the outside of the knee from residual lateral capsular tissue bands as the arthroscope light source is aimed laterally.

DISTALIZATION FOR PATELLA ALTA

Patella alta has been traditionally underappreciated as a contributor to chronic patellar instability. It has been shown to be present in approximately 25% of patients with chronic instability and only 3% of patients without such symptoms (6). Even with traditional nonoperative treatment or isolated MPFL reconstruction patients with patella alta are at risk for recurrent instability (30). Reasons for this connection are still being studied and are likely due to several contributing factors. With patella alta, there is decreased contact between the patella and the trochlea. With less contact, the lateral trochlea does not contribute its normal resistance to the lateral component of pull from the quadriceps complex. This in combination with dysplasia of the trochlea further puts the patients at risk for subluxation. Patella tendon length specifically at lengths of 50 mm or greater have been shown to correlate with increased subluxation risk (8).

A longitudinal incision of about 6 cm in length is made just lateral to the tibial tubercle down through the skin and subcutaneous tissue. The proximal point of insertion of the patella tendon is identified. Two drill holes (4.5-mm drill) are made through the anterior tubercular cortex about 1.5 cm apart down the midline of the tubercle starting about 1 cm from the proximal border of the tubercle (Fig. 61.4 A, B).

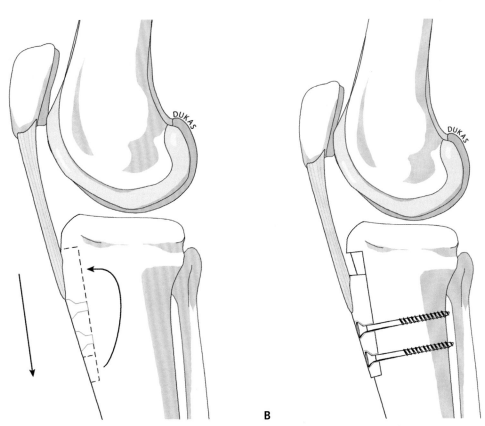

A   **B**

FIGURE 61.4. A: When distalizing the tibial tubercle, predrill two 4.5 mm holes approximately 1.5 cm apart 1 cm distal to distal insertion of the patella tendon. **B:** After making a vertical 1-cm depth cut just proximal to the patella tendon insertion, a sagittal saw is utilized to fashion a flat horizontal tubercle osteotomy of length 6 cm. Depending on the predetermined amount of needed distalization, the same length is cut horizontally from the leading end of the free tubercle and relocated proximal to the freed tubercle to act as a bony backstop preventing proximal migration of the tubercle. The tubercle is temporarily secured and the knee taken through range of motion. Finally, a 3.2-mm drill bit is placed in the 4.5-mm predrilled holes and drilled bicortically and appropriately-sized lag screws are placed.

A proximal vertical cut is made into the tibia from lateral to medial at the point of initial tendon insertion to a depth of about 1 cm. This provides a bony backstop preventing proximal sliding of the tubercle during early healing. Allowing for a 1-cm thick tibial tubercle, a small sagittal saw is utilized to fashion a flat horizontal tubercle osteotomy of length 6 cm. A terminal cut is made across the tubercle orthogonal to the longitudinal cut to free the tubercle from the tibia. The terminal 1 cm (more or less as determined by the surgeon) of the tubercle is removed with the saw. This allows for an in situ distalization up to the same amount of resected tubercle bone (1 cm). The removed piece of distal tubercle can be placed at the proximal aspect of the osteotomy between the initial proximal vertical cut and the tibial tubercle to serve as a mechanical block to prevent proximal tubercle migration. No fixation is required as it is kept in place by the overlying tension and compression of the patella tendon. Prior to final tubercle fixation, two 3.2-mm drills are placed via the predrilled tubercle holes to temporarily secure the tubercle in the desired new distalized position. The knee is taken through a full range of motion to ensure adequate tracking of the patella and confirm that full flexion is obtainable. Once the corrected position is determined, the 3.2-mm drills are drilled bicortically and appropriate length lag screws are placed to secure the tubercle in the new position.

AFTERCARE

Postoperative rehabilitation is similar for all procedures mentioned above. After ensuring that a full range of motion is obtainable intraoperatively, the rehabilitation plan is to begin physical therapy immediately after surgery. After wound closure a hinged knee brace is applied over the final ace wrap and locked in extension. Patients are allowed to fully weight bear initially with the brace locked in extension. At 4 weeks, closed-chain quadriceps strengthening is initiated and patients are allowed to resume walking when adequate quad strength has been achieved. Patients are not allowed to return to full activity or sports until 4 to 6 months postoperatively.

REFERENCES

1. Colvin AC, West RV. Patellar instability. *J Bone Joint Surg Am.* 2008;90:2751–2762.
2. Boden BP, Pearsall AW, Garrett WE Jr, et al. Patellofemoral instability: evaluation and management. *J Am Acad Orthop Surg.* 1997;5:47.
3. Conlan T, Garth WP Jr, Lemons JE. Evaluation of the medial soft-tissue restraints of the extensor mechanism of the knee. *J Bone Joint Surg Am.* 1993;75:682.
4. Redziniak DE, Diduch DR, Mihalko WM, et al. Patellar instability. *J Bone Joint Surg Am.* 2009;91:2264.
5. Torg JS, Barton TM, Pavlov H, et al. Natural history of the posterior cruciate ligament-deficient knee. *Clin Orthop Relat Res.* 1989;208.
6. Dejour H, Walch G, Nove-Josserand L, et al. Factors of patellar instability: an anatomic radiographic study. *Knee Surg Sports Traumatol Arthrosc.* 1994;2:19–26.
7. Blackburne JS, Peel TE. A new method of measuring patellar height. *J Bone Joint Surg Br.* 1977;59:241.
8. Escala JS, Mellado JM, Olona M, et al. Objective patellar instability: MR-based quantitative assessment of potentially associated anatomical features. *Knee Surg Sports Traumatol Arthrosc.* 2006;14:264–272.
9. Berg EE, Mason SL, Lucas MJ. Patellar height ratios. A comparison of four measurement methods. *Am J Sports Med.* 1996;24:218.
10. Simmons E Jr, Cameron JC. Patella alta and recurrent dislocation of the patella. *Clin Orthop Relat Res.* 1992;265.
11. Seil R, Müller B, Georg T, et al. Reliability and interobserver variability in radiological patellar height ratios. *Knee Surg Sports Traumatol Arthrosc.* 2000;8:231–236.
12. Dejour D, Le Coultre B. Osteotomies in patello-femoral instabilities. *Sports Med Arthrosc.* 2007;15:39.
13. Laurin CA, Dussault R, Levesque HP. The tangential x-ray investigation of the patellofemoral joint: x-ray technique, diagnostic criteria and their interpretation. *Clin Orthop Relat Res.* 1979;144:16.
14. Merchant AC, Mercer RL, Jacobsen RH, et al. Roentgenographic analysis of patellofemoral congruence. *J Bone Joint Surg Am.* 1974;56:1391.
15. Fulkerson JP, Buuck DA. Disorders of the patellofemoral joint. Philadelphia: Lippincott Williams & Wilkins, 2004.
16. Grelsamer RP, Bazos AN, Proctor CS. Radiographic analysis of patellar tilt. *J Bone Joint Surg Br.* 1993;75:822.
17. Bollier M, Fulkerson JP. The role of trochlear dysplasia in patellofemoral instability. *J Am Acad Orthop Surg.* 2011;19:8.
18. Jones RB, Bartlett EC, Vainright JR, et al. CT determination of tibial tubercle lateralization in patients presenting with anterior knee pain. *Skeletal Radiol.* 1995;24:505–509.
19. Larsen E, Lauridsen F. Conservative treatment of patellar dislocations: influence of evident factors on the tendency to redislocation and the therapeutic result. *Clin Orthop Relat Res.* 1982;171:131.
20. Stensdotter AK, Hodges PW, Mellor R, et al. Quadriceps activation in closed and in open kinetic chain exercise. *Med Sci Sports Exerc.* 2003;35:2043.
21. Mäenpää H, Lehto MU. Patellar dislocation. The long-term results of nonoperative management in 100 patients. *Am J Sports Med.* 1997;25:213.
22. Fithian DC, Paxton EW, Stone ML, et al. Epidemiology and natural history of acute patellar dislocation. *Am J Sports Med.* 2004;32:1114.
23. Nikku R, Nietosvaara Y, Aalto K, et al. Operative treatment of primary patellar dislocation does not improve medium-term outcome: a 7-year follow-up report and risk analysis of 127 randomized patients. *Acta Orthop.* 2005;76:699–704.
24. Nikku R, Nietosvaara Y, Kallio PE, et al. Operative versus closed treatment of primary dislocation of the patella. Similar 2-year results in 125 randomized patients. *Acta Orthop Scand.* 1997;68:419–423.
25. Insall J, Falvo KA, Wise DW. Chondromalacia patellae. A prospective study. *J Bone Joint Surg Am.* 1976;58:1.
26. Halbrecht JL. Arthroscopic patella realignment: an all-inside technique. *Arthroscopy.* 2001;17:940–945.

27. Kolowich PA, Paulos LE, Rosenberg TD, et al. Lateral release of the patella: indications and contraindications. *Am J Sports Med.* 1990;18:359.

28. Lattermann C, Toth J, Bach BR Jr. The role of lateral retinacular release in the treatment of patellar instability. *Sports Med Arthrosc.* 2007;15:57.

29. Fulkerson JP. Diagnosis and treatment of patients with patellofemoral pain. *Am J Sports Med.* 2002;30:447.

30. Thaunat M, Erasmus PJ. Recurrent patellar dislocation after medial patellofemoral ligament reconstruction. *Knee Surg Sports Traumatol Arthrosc.* 2008;16:40–43.

Indications and Technique for MPFL Reconstruction

Derek F. Papp • Bashir A. Zikria • Andrew J. Cosgarea

The medial patellofemoral ligament (MPFL) has garnered attention in the literature as the primary static ligamentous checkrein, preventing lateral patellar subluxation and/or dislocation. It is estimated that the MPFL resists 53% to 60% of the force required to cause lateral subluxation of the patella (1, 2), and it usually ruptures with patellar dislocation (3). This latter finding is important because the MPFL heals in an elongated fashion approximately 90% of the time after rupturing (4), compromising its normal function. Reconstruction of the MPFL reestablishes the primary soft-tissue restraint to lateral subluxation of the patella.

CLINICAL EVALUATION

Evaluation of the patient with patellar instability begins with obtaining a complete history. The physician should determine what types of activities cause painful subluxation or dislocation and the number of episodes. Indirect mechanisms account for most patellar dislocations; for instance, a right-handed softball player might feel a "pop" in her right knee as her body rotates to the left while trying to hit a pitch. Less commonly, a direct blow to the medial aspect of the patella causes the injury.

Physical examination begins with assessment of the tibiofemoral alignment with the patient standing. Excessive valgus alignment may predispose the patient to patellar instability. With the patient supine, the surgeon performs a thorough ligamentous examination. Patients with an elevated "Q" angle have an increased lateral force vector and greater risk for patellar instability, and those with a prominent "J" sign have bony malalignment. The physician tests for patellar apprehension by manually placing a laterally directed force on the medial edge of the patella. The patellar glide test is used to assess patellar laxity by quantifying patellar translation in quadrants. The examiner measures lateral retinacular tightness by using the patellar tilt test. Other pertinent parts of the examination include assessment for tibial torsion, femoral anteversion and vastus medialis weakness. It is also important to identify the area of maximum tenderness

of the MPFL because this point usually correlates with the location of the ligament rupture. A standard series of radiographs of the knee includes anteroposterior, lateral (in 30° of flexion), tunnel, and sunrise (in 45° of flexion) views. The lateral view best shows patella alta and trochlear dysplasia, the tunnel view commonly reveals loose bodies in the notch or osteochondritis dissecans lesions, and patellar tilt, and the degree of subluxation is best appreciated on the sunrise view. CT imaging of the knee defines the amount of subluxation and tilt more accurately than does conventional radiography. A characteristic bone bruise pattern involving the medial patellar facet and the lateral femoral condyle is often seen in patients who sustain a patellar dislocation. This pattern is easily detected with MRI, which can also ascertain the extent of articular cartilage damage. The surgeon can use CT or MRI to measure the distance between the tibial tuberosity and the trochlear groove, which is a manifestation of bony malalignment.

INDICATIONS AND TREATMENT

The main indication for MPFL reconstruction is recurrent instability in patients with medial soft-tissue deficiency. The literature has shown that nonoperative treatment of acute patellar dislocations provides good-to-excellent outcomes (5). Initial episodes of patellar dislocation should usually be treated nonoperatively; a closed reduction may be necessary if the patella remains dislocated on presentation. The patient can progress quickly (within 1 to 2 weeks) away from the use of crutches and a knee immobilizer through a rehabilitation program that focuses on pain management, soft-tissue swelling control, core and quadriceps strengthening, and proprioception. The patient can return to normal activities when strength and agility allow for functional progression.

Some clinical situations necessitate acute surgical intervention. For instance, patients with a large loose body, concurrent intra-articular abnormality (e.g., meniscal tear), or persistent subluxation after a course of therapy benefit from early surgical treatment. Patellar dislocations often cause osteochondral loose bodies and should be suspected in patients who experience mechanical symptoms. The loose bodies are often visualized on MRI or even conventional radiographs ordered at the time of initial presentation. Asymptomatic, diminutive loose bodies are treated with observation; larger fragments that could cause mechanical symptoms require removal.

When acute surgical intervention is warranted, the surgeon should consider concomitant MPFL repair. Acute repair affords an opportunity to repair the static restraint, which is torn in most cases. Direct repair does present several challenges that the surgeon should appreciate. For example, it is not always possible to identify the exact location of the MPFL tear and its repair. Although MPFL avulsions from the origin or insertion sites can be treated with suture anchor fixation, correcting midsubstance tears can be more difficult. Imbricating the tissues in the proper location and determining the correct tension is crucial. Overtensioning the tissue leads to pathologic increases in joint reactive forces or ligament failure as a result of overload (6).

In cases of recurrent instability, patients with bony malalignment as the primary abnormality may be better served with isolated or concomitant osteotomy of the tibial tuberosity. The surgeon must account for patient factors that contribute to recurrent patellar dislocation and understand that MPFL reconstruction alone does not provide adequate treatment in all cases. From a practical standpoint, the surgeon must examine whether the primary pathophysiology is bony malalignment or soft tissue insufficiency. Failure to address a bony abnormality during a soft-tissue procedure could lead to failure. An excessive Q angle increases lateral forces, predisposing the patella to dislocation. The surgeon should consider medializing the tibial tubercle if the angle exceeds 20°. Using the preoperative CT or MRI sequences, the surgeon can measure the distance between the tibial tuberosity and the trochlear groove; measurements greater than 15 mm indicate excessive tuberosity lateralization and should make the surgeon consider the addition of a distal realignment procedure (7). The presence of high-grade chondral defects may also predispose the patient to pain and progressive arthrosis. Depending on the location of the lesion, the patient may benefit from an osteotomy to decrease loading forces. Although MRI often shows damage to the articular cartilage, intraoperative arthroscopic examination is the best way to truly determine the extent of the lesion, at which point the surgeon can decide whether or not to proceed with before osteotomy. Patients without excessive bony malalignment who have recurrent symptomatic subluxation or dislocation are the best candidates for MPFL reconstruction (Fig. 62.1).

TECHNIQUE

Numerous techniques have been described for MPFL reconstruction, and the literature does not indicate that any one method is clearly superior to the others (8–13). The techniques differ, depending on the source of the graft and the method of fixation. There are various graft options, including semitendinosus (11), gracilis (14), fascia lata (9), adductor longus (15), adductor magnus (8, 16), quadriceps (13, 15), allograft (17), and even artificial mesh (10). Methods of patellar fixation described include tunnels (15, 16, 18), suture anchors (9), and more recently, a docking technique (19). For femoral side fixation, authors have described using sutures to attach the graft to soft tissues (13), staples (10), a bone tunnel with endobutton fixation (18), soft-tissue slings (8), and interference screws (14).

AUTHORS' PREFERRED TREATMENT

In the preoperative holding area, the patient is identified, the affected knee is marked, and prophylactic antibiotic is infused. The patient is positioned supine with a tourniquet on the thigh. For the diagnostic arthroscopy portion of the procedure, a vertical post is used, which can later be removed. General or regional anesthesia is administered according to institution or surgeon preference.

Examination of the patient under anesthesia provides the surgeon an opportunity to better characterize the degree of pathologic translation using the patellar glide test (Fig. 62.2). With the patient's knee in full extension, the surgeon applies a lateral force; this procedure occasionally results in frank dislocation. The degree of tightness in the lateral retinaculum should then be measured using the patellar tilt test (Fig. 62.3), and a lateral release is performed if the lateral retinaculum is deemed to be excessively tight.

Standard superolateral, inferomedial, and inferolateral portals are used for the arthroscopic examination. Loose bodies often hide in the suprapatellar pouch, the medial and lateral gutters, and the posteromedial and posterolateral compartments. Any damage to the articular cartilage should be noted, especially any high-grade lesions that may benefit from unloading. If identified, chondral lesions should be addressed with debridement, microfracture, or repair, depending on surgeon preference. The decision whether to proceed solely with MPFL reconstruction or distal bony realignment, or with a combination thereof, is based on imaging findings, physical examination, and arthroscopic observations.

Next, the tibial tuberosity, adductor tubercle, medial femoral epicondyle, and medial border of the patella are marked (Fig. 62.4). The leg is exsanguinated with a compression wrap, and the tourniquet is inflated. We prefer a hamstring autograft for reconstruction of the MPFL because of the proximity of the graft within the prepped

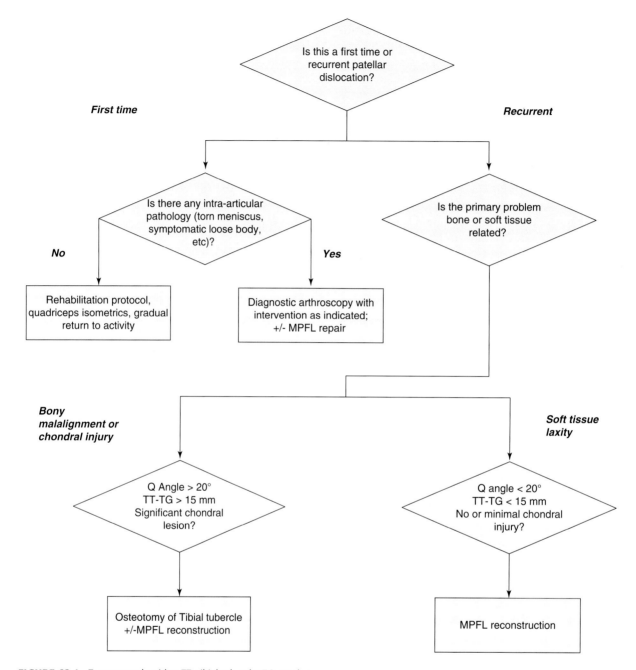

FIGURE 62.1. Treatment algorithm TT, tibial tubercle; TG, troclear groove.

surgical field and because the strength of a hamstring autograft exceeds that of the native MPFL (1, 20). A 3- to 4-cm incision is made obliquely over the pes anserinus insertion, carefully exposing the sartorial fascia. The hamstring tendons are exposed by incising the superior attachment of the fascia. Using standard tendon harvesting technique, the semitendinosus tendon is isolated from the gracilis. We usually use a single-stranded semitendinosus graft. Alternatively, a single or a double-stranded gracilis tendon can be used. We then repair the sartorial fascia to its insertion site before closing the wound. Heavy scissors or another instrument should be used to

remove any remaining muscle or other soft tissues from the harvested graft (Fig. 62.5A), and the tendon is then measured with a tunnel sizer (Fig. 62.5B). Grafts that are less than 5 mm in diameter can be doubled over to provide sufficient strength. A number-2 FiberLoop suture (Arthrex, Inc., Naples, FL) is then woven into the end of the graft and subsequently used to pull the graft through the femoral tunnel.

A 3- to 4-cm longitudinal incision is made over the MPFL, midway between the patella and the medial femoral epicondyle. The native MPFL is identified where it lies adjacent to the inferior border of the vastus medialis

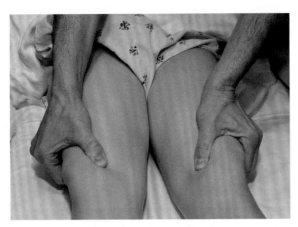

FIGURE 62.2. Before beginning the diagnostic arthroscopy, the surgeon should examine the affected and unaffected limbs under anesthesia. Patellar translation is commonly tested using the patellar glide test, which is measured in quadrants.

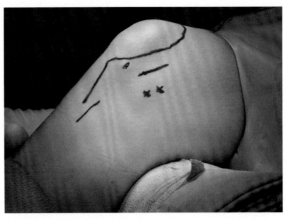

FIGURE 62.4. Before making the incision, the surgeon should identify and mark the appropriate surface landmarks, including the tibial tuberosity, adductor tubercle, medial femoral epicondyle, and medial border of the patella. The graft harvest incision is made over the pes insertion site.

obliquus. The superior and inferior margins of the MPFL are exposed (Fig. 62.6).

Preparation of the patellar tunnel begins with identification of the insertion site of the MPFL. The correct starting point for the patellar tunnel is in the superior half of the patella, which the surgeon clears using a rongeur. At the midpoint of the MPFL insertion site, a 2.0-mm eyelet Kirschner wire (K-wire) is drilled from medial to

lateral. The surgeon must not violate the articular surface or the patella's anterior cortex, which could predispose to fracture with a subsequent injury. A small arthrotomy is made through the capsule along the medial border of the patella, allowing introduction of a finger to help guide

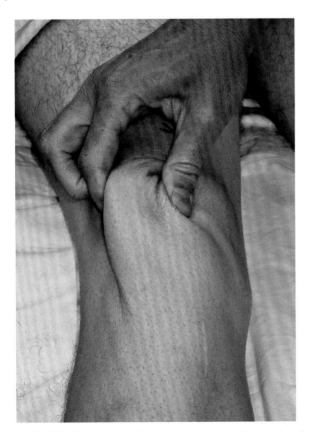

FIGURE 62.3. Tightness of the lateral retinaculum is tested under anesthesia by assessing the amount of lateral tilt of the patella and comparing it with that of the other side.

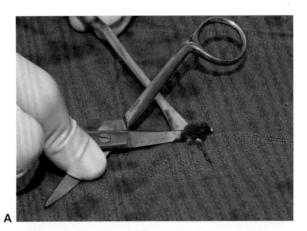

A

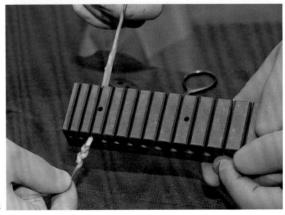

B

FIGURE 62.5. Excess soft tissue and muscle is debrided from the semitendinosus autograft using scissors or a knife. Surgeons should plan on using 9 to 10 cm of graft **(A)**. The diameter of the graft is measured so that the tunnel can be drilled to the appropriate size **(B)**.

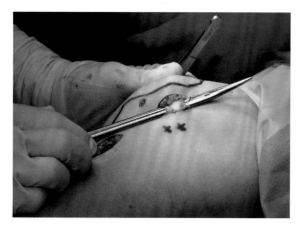

FIGURE 62.6. An incision is made midway between the medial border of the patella and the medial femoral epicondyle. The superior and inferior borders of the MPFL are identified.

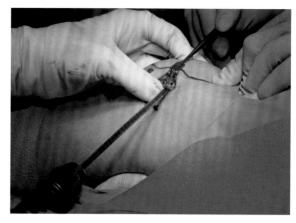

FIGURE 62.8. A cannulated drill bit 0.5 mm larger than the graft size is used to overdrill the K-wire, creating a blind patellar tunnel approximately 15 mm deep.

placement of the K-wire and confirm that the articular cartilage is not violated (Fig. 62.7). We use fluoroscopy to confirm K-wire position. The K-wire is then overdrilled to a depth of approximately 15 mm with the correct cannulated drill bit as measured earlier (Fig. 62.8). A second eyelet K-wire is then placed in the blind tunnel and drilled to diverge from the first through the base of the blind patellar tunnel. The suture ends are then passed through the eyes of the 2-mm K-wires, and the graft is pulled into the blind tunnel (Fig. 62.9A,B). Fixation of the patellar end of the graft is obtained by tying the suture through the superolateral arthroscopic portal directly over the patella (Fig. 62.9C).

Next, the femoral tunnel is prepared. A K-wire is placed just anterior to the medial femoral epicondyle and just distal to the adductor tubercle (Fig. 62.10). We

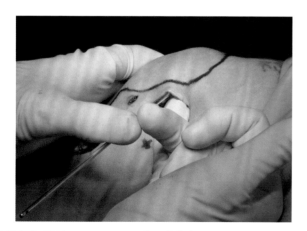

FIGURE 62.7. A K-wire is used to drill the patellar tunnel; careful attention should be paid to finding the correct starting point in the superior half of the patella. While drilling, care must be taken to avoid violating the articular surface or the anterior cortex. A small arthrotomy allows for placement of a finger on the articular surface to help guide placement of the K-wire and prevent violation of the articular cartilage.

use fluoroscopy to confirm correct position. The graft is passed through a soft-tissue tunnel deep to the medial retinaculum and superficial to the capsule. To test for isometry, the free end of the graft is then wrapped about the K-wire, and the knee is then ranged (Fig. 62.11). The graft should not be placed too far proximally because doing so will increase tension in the graft and concomitantly increase joint reactive forces in the patellofemoral joint. If isometry is not optimal, the position of the K-wire should be altered. The K-wire is then overdrilled with a cannulated drill bit that measures 0.5 mm larger than the graft diameter, to a depth of 25 mm (Fig. 62.12). The remaining graft is then cut so that a length of 15 to 20 mm will fit within the femoral tunnel. The K-wire is directed slightly anteriorly and proximally so that it exits the lateral femur in a safe area away from the common peroneal nerve. After threading the eye with the suture ends, the graft is brought into the tunnel by pulling on the K-wire (Fig. 62.13).

With one hand, the surgeon grasps the ankle to take the knee through its range of motion and with the other hand, places tension on the graft sutures exiting the lateral thigh. In this fashion, the surgeon can determine the correct graft tension and confirm the patella is not overconstrained. The importance of not overtensioning the graft cannot be overstated. A graft that is fixed too tight will lead to increased patellofemoral articular cartilage pressure and predispose the patient to future arthrosis. The surgeon then repeats the patellar glide test, providing another opportunity to check the graft tension. With the leg in full extension, the patella is pushed laterally and compared with the amount of translation on the unaffected side. Lateral patellar translations should be a little larger than on the contralateral side to prevent an overly tight graft. Fixation of the femoral side is obtained with a 7-mm bioabsorbable cannulated femoral interference screw and may be augmented by suturing the graft to

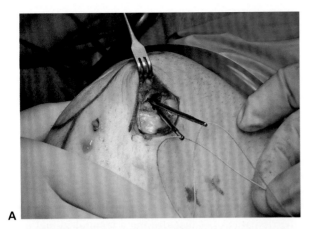

A

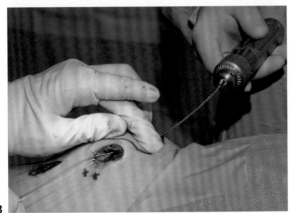

B

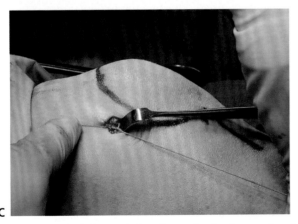

C

FIGURE 62.9. The docking technique for patellar fixation uses two diverging K-wires passed through the blind end of the patellar tunnel (**A**). The surgeon then docks the graft into the blind tunnel by pulling the K-wires with their sutures through the superolateral arthroscopy portal (**B**). The sutures are then tied with the knot placed directly on the surface of the bone (**C**).

adjacent soft tissue (Fig. 62.14). The wound is closed in layers (Fig. 62.15). We routinely use cryotherapy to help with pain control and ameliorate swelling, and we then apply a compressive dressing, followed by a hinged range-of-motion brace locked in extension.

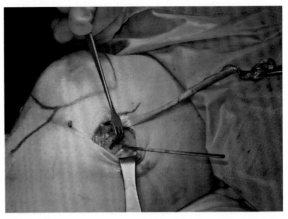

FIGURE 62.10. The appropriate starting point for the femoral tunnel is identified by passing a K-wire just anterior to the medial femoral epicondyle.

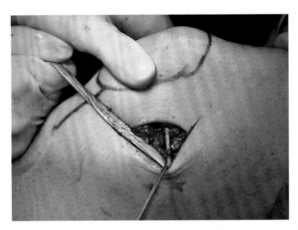

FIGURE 62.11. By wrapping the graft around the K-wire and carefully ranging the knee, the surgeon can test for the appropriate graft tension and isometry.

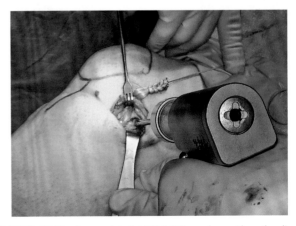

FIGURE 62.12. A cannulated drill bit 0.5 mm larger than the diameter of the graft is used to overdrill the K-wire and create the femoral tunnel.

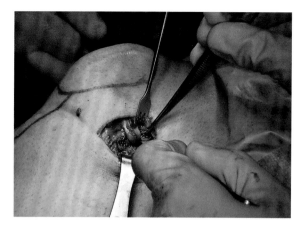

FIGURE 62.13. The graft is pulled into the tunnel.

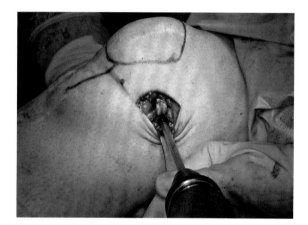

FIGURE 62.14. Femoral tunnel fixation is achieved with an interference screw.

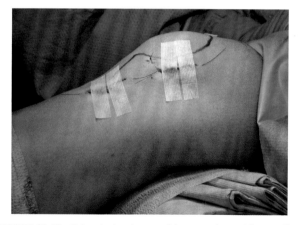

FIGURE 62.15. Subcuticular closure of the wounds provides excellent cosmesis.

COMPLICATIONS, CONTROVERSIES, AND SPECIAL CONSIDERATIONS

Postoperative stiffness remains the most common complication of MPFL reconstruction. To avoid this complication, the surgeon must ensure that the patient receives adequate pain medication and begins range-of-motion exercises soon after surgery. Physical therapy should focus on immediate quadriceps activation, range of motion, and progressive weightbearing. The surgeon must also recognize that technical errors, such as tunnel malpositioning or overtensioning of the graft, can also lead to loss of motion and premature patellofemoral arthrosis. Malpositioning the graft proximally or using a graft that is too short (thereby increasing graft tension) causes increasing pressure on patellofemoral cartilage; in combination, these situations can increase patellofemoral articular pressure by more than 50% (6). Other complications include patella fracture (18), graft failure, recurrent instability, and painful hardware (14).

Of special consideration is femoral fixation in the pediatric patient because drilling a femoral tunnel places the open distal physis at risk for growth arrest. Surgeons can use standard patellar fixation, but alternative femoral fixation is necessary. The femoral end of the graft can be wrapped around the distal end of the adductor magnus or the proximal end of the superficial medial collateral ligament. Correct graft tension should be obtained by the methods mentioned previously.

PEARLS AND PITFALLS

1. Fluoroscopy is beneficial in locating the correct femoral **and patellar tunnel positions**.
2. The patellar articular surface or anterior cortex should not be violated. Violating the anterior cortex could predispose the patella to fracture.
3. A capsular window adjacent to the patellar tunnel allows digital access to the articular surface. By sliding a finger underneath the patella, the surgeon can have better control when placing the K-wire.
4. When preparing the graft, the final distal suture passage is made orthogonal to the previous suture. This procedure "bullets" the graft, making it easier to pass into the tunnel.
5. The adductor tubercle and the medial femoral epicondyle, which is located 1 cm distal to the adductor tubercle, need to be differentiated. Proximal placement of the graft will increase pressure in the patellofemoral joint.
6. Great care should always be taken to avoid overtensioning the graft. Grafts that are too tight increase pressure across the patellofemoral articular cartilage and could lead to arthrosis. If anything, the graft should be left slightly looser than the native MPFL.

REHABILITATION

Immediately after surgery, a physical therapist teaches the patient the correct technique for quadriceps sets, straight-leg raises, and toe-touch weightbearing. Outpatient rehabilitation begins after 1 week. The therapist unlocks the brace and the patient then begins to work on range of motion as tolerated. Most patients are full weightbearing by 1 week, have 120° of flexion at 4 weeks, and have full range of motion at 8 weeks. They can usually discontinue the brace after approximately 6 weeks. Jogging can resume at approximately 12 weeks, followed by initiation of sport-specific drills. After 4 to 5 months, most athletes are able to return to their regular sports.

CONCLUSIONS AND FUTURE DIRECTIONS

Most studies of MPFL reconstruction report good to excellent results. One study using semitendinosus autograft with patellar fixation performed through a tunnel and endobutton fixation of the femoral side showed an increase in mean Kujala score from 30.5 preoperatively to 95.2 postoperatively [18]. Patellar apprehension was relieved in all patients, and over three-fourths of their patients returned to preinjury sports levels [18]. In another study in which an adductor tendon autograft, a bone-quad tendon autograft, and a bone-patellar tendon allograft were used, the authors reported an increase in Kujala scores from 53.3 preoperatively to 90.7 postoperatively. They estimated their good-to-excellent results to be between 85.3% and 91.1%, depending on which outcome instrument was used [16].

We are unaware of any long-term studies or randomized control studies of MPFL reconstruction. Most studies have been limited by small samples, lack of adequate controls, retrospective designs, and nonuniform measures of clinical outcome [3, 14]. Colvin and West [5] found that although level I evidence exists showing the efficacy of nonoperative treatment measures for acute patellar dislocation, most studies describing surgical treatment for chronic patellar instability provide only level IV evidence. Although the approach described in this chapter has produced successful and reproducible results in our hands, we cannot necessarily advocate it as the single best technique for MPFL reconstruction. Randomized controlled studies, long-term follow-up, and ongoing biomechanical analysis are needed to optimize treatment in the future.

REFERENCES

1. Conlan T, Garth WP Jr, Lemons JE. Evaluation of the medial soft-tissue restraints of the extensor mechanism of the knee. *J Bone Joint Surg Am.* 1993;75:682–693.
2. Desio SM, Burks RT, Bachus KN. Soft tissue restraints to lateral patellar translation in the human knee. *Am J Sports Med.* 1998;26:59–65.
3. Smith TO, Walker J, Russell N. Outcomes of medial patellofemoral ligament reconstruction for patellar instability: a systematic review. *Knee Surg Sports Traumatol Arthrosc.* 2007;15:1301–1314.
4. Fulkerson JP. Mini-medial patellofemoral ligament advancement. *Tech Knee Surg.* 2008;7:2–4.
5. Colvin AC, West RV. Patellar instability. *J Bone Joint Surg Am.* 2008;90:2751–2762.
6. Elias JJ, Cosgarea AJ. Technical errors during medial patellofemoral ligament reconstruction could overload medial patellofemoral cartilage. A computational analysis. *Am J Sports Med.* 2006;34:1478–1485.
7. Schoettle PB, Zanetti M, Seifert B, et al. The tibial tuberosity-trochlear groove distance; a comparative study between CT and MRI scanning. *Knee.* 2006;13:26–31.
8. Deie M, Ochi M, Sumen Y, et al. A long-term follow-up study after medial patellofemoral ligament reconstruction using the transferred semitendinosus tendon for patellar dislocation. *Knee Surg Sports Traumatol Arthrosc.* 2005;13:522–528.
9. Drez D Jr, Edwards TB, Williams CS. Results of medial patellofemoral ligament reconstruction in the treatment of patellar dislocation. *Arthroscopy.* 2001;17:298–306.
10. Nomura E, Horiuchi Y, Kihara M. A mid-term follow-up of medial patellofemoral ligament reconstruction using an artificial ligament for recurrent patellar dislocation. *Knee.* 2000;7:211–215.
11. Nomura E, Inoue M. Hybrid medial patellofemoral ligament reconstruction using the semitendinous tendon for recurrent patellar dislocation: minimum 3 years' follow-up. *Arthroscopy.* 2006;22:787–793.
12. Burks RT, Luker MG. Medial patellofemoral ligament reconstruction. *Tech Orthop.* 1997;12:185–191.
13. Steensen RN, Dopirak RM, Maurus PB. A simple technique for reconstruction of the medial patellofemoral ligament using a quadriceps tendon graft. *Arthroscopy.* 2005;21:365–370.
14. Cosgarea AJ. Medial patellofemoral ligament reconstruction and repair for patellar instability. In: Cole BJ, Sekiya JK, eds. *Surgical Techniques of the Shoulder, Elbow, and Knee in Sports Medicine.* Philadelphia, PA: Saunders (Elsevier); 2008:733–747.
15. Teitge RA, Torga-Spak R. Medial patellofemoral ligament reconstruction. *Orthopedics.* 2004;27:1037–1040.
16. Steiner TM, Torga-Spak R, Teitge RA. Medial patellofemoral ligament reconstruction in patients with lateral patellar instability and trochlear dysplasia. *Am J Sports Med.* 2006;34:1254–1261.
17. Anbari A, Cole BJ. Medial patellofemoral ligament reconstruction: a novel approach. *J Knee Surg.* 2008;21:241–245.
18. Mikashima Y, Kimura M, Kobayashi Y, et al. Clinical results of isolated reconstruction of the medial patellofemoral ligament for recurrent dislocation and subluxation of the patella. *Acta Orthop Belg.* 2006;72:65–71.
19. Ahmad CS, Brown GD, Stein BS. The docking technique for medial patellofemoral ligament reconstruction: surgical technique and clinical outcome. *AMJ Sports Med,* 37, 2009, 2021–7.
20. Amis AA, Dowson D, Wright V. Elbow joint force predictions for some strenuous isometric actions. *J Biomech.* 1980;13:765–775.

Articular Cartilage

Clinical Approach to Articular Cartilage Pathology

Andrea L. Bowers • Thomas L. Wickiewicz

Articular cartilage pathology in the knee is commonly encountered and may vary significantly in etiology and symptomatology and therefore management. Many cartilage irregularities are incidental findings and may be best treated with observation. Others are a source of significant pain and mechanical symptoms that warrant surgical intervention. Decision making in the management of articular cartilage lesions depends on a multitude of factors including lesion-specific etiology, location, chronicity, and size, concomitant pathologies, as well as patient-specific age, activity level, physical demands, and rehabilitation potential. A thorough understanding of articular cartilage composition, function, and injury patterns as well as a comprehensive clinical evaluation is necessary for successful management of such lesions.

STRUCTURE, FUNCTION, AND METABOLISM OF ARTICULAR CARTILAGE

Articular cartilage is a complex, highly organized biologic lining of the ends of articulating surfaces. In the knee, it surfaces with varying thickness the underside of the patella, trochlea, femoral condyles, and tibial plateau. Its main functions are to provide a smooth, durable surface for near-frictionless gliding and to withstand and distribute forces transferred across the joint.

Histologically, articular cartilage is composed of distinct layers (Fig. 63.1). The superficial 10% to 20%, called the tangential zone, consists of flattened chondrocytes and collagen fibers lined parallel to the joint surface. In the intermediate 40% to 60%, or transitional zone, cells are round and sporadically dispersed among obliquely oriented collagen fibers. The deepest 30%, comprising the basal zone, features more densely packed chondrocytes aligned in vertical columns. Proteoglycan concentration is greatest in this zone. Collagen fibrils extend from the basal zone across a tidemark, which separates this deep layer from the underlying calcified cartilage, and ultimately subchondral and cancellous bone.

The cartilage function is a reflection of its intricate morphology and biologic activity. This avascular, alymphatic tissue is a composite of chondrocytes suspended within a collagen and proteoglycan-rich extracellular matrix. Chondrocytes, which comprise 1% to 10% of articular cartilage volume, are derived from undifferentiated mesenchymal marrow stem cells. Chondrocytes maintain matrix homeostasis through synthesis and degradation of matrix material in response to local tissue composition, growth factor and cytokine effect, mechanical load, aging, and injury. Another 60% of cartilage dry weight is composed of collagen, 90% of which is highly cross-linked type II fibrils, and the remainder types IX and XI. This collagenous portion contributes to the form and tensile properties of articular cartilage. The ability to withstand compression, however, is attributed to proteoglycans, which comprise

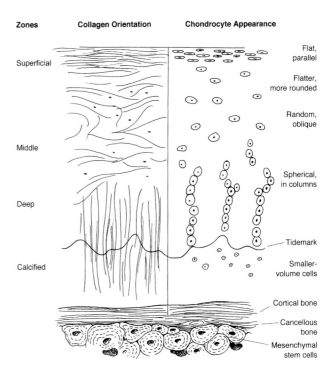

FIGURE 63.1. Basic structural anatomy of articular cartilage. (Reprinted from Browne JE, Branch TP. Surgical alternatives for treatment of articular cartilage lesions. *J Am Acad Orthop Surg.* 2000;8:180–189, with permission.)

the remaining 35% of the tissue's dry weight. Proteoglycan structure includes a core protein, aggrecan, which is produced by chondrocytes and is unique to hyaline cartilage. A single aggrecan unit can have up to 60 keratin sulfate and 100 chondroitin sulfate glycosaminoglycan chains attached; these sulfated disaccharides lend a large negative charge to the aggrecan molecule. Aggrecan strands are polar, and their N-terminal globular domains attach, or aggregate, through link proteins to a hyaluronic acid chain. The negatively charged proteoglycans interspersed within the collagen matrix increases tissue osmolality, thereby attracting water molecules. Water comprises 75% to 80% of the wet weight of articular cartilage. The interplay of proteoglycans and water in maintaining an osmolal balance allows the tissue to withstand high pressures seen with compression. Swelling of the tissue is in turn prevented by the highly organized type II collagen matrix. The matrix is further stabilized by smaller proteoglycan units including decorin, biglycan, and fibromodulin; greater concentrations of these smaller, stabilizing proteoglycans have been observed in response to increased physiologic stress (1).

Cell surface-binding proteins termed integrins link chondrocytes to the extracellular matrix and allow the cells to be stimulated by mechanical forces imparted to the matrix. Cellular metabolism, including matrix secretion and degredation, is thereby regulated in great part by local forces. As articular cartilage is devoid of vascular and lymphatic channels, oxygen and nutrients needed to maintain homeostasis are obtained instead by diffusion from synovial fluid. Due to low local oxygen tension, anaerobic metabolism of glucose through glycolysis serves as the major source of fuel for chondrocytes. Metabolites accumulate in the interstitial fluid, which is expressed from the permeable collagen–proteoglycan matrix in response to a compressive load. When the compression is withdrawn, the matrix is reconstituted with nutrient-rich fluid. Further, metabolic activity in the chondrocyte stagnates in the face of static pressure but is upregulated in response to changes in hydrostatic pressure seen with dynamic loading. Mechanical stimulation is therefore paramount to maintaining chondrocyte health.

CARTILAGE INJURY AND HEALING RESPONSE

The lack of direct blood supply also impedes the articular cartilage's ability to mount a healing response in the face of injury. Spontaneous repair is seldom seen without violation of the tidemark, which allows egress of reparative cells originating from subchondral bone. Partial-thickness cartilage injury, observable only on the microscopic level, is frequently the result of a blunt trauma imparting a compressive load that exceeds the tissue's tolerance. Local cells undergo apoptosis. A transient metabolic and enzymatic response leads to collagen degradation and proteoglycan loss. A zone of necrosis develops that does not remodel

over time (2). Partial-thickness injury may also result from repetitive microtrauma. Chronic increased stress affects thinning of the cartilage and, in response, a thickening of the calcified cartilage layer. Since the cartilage layer is aneural, pain signals are not appreciated until enough microdamage has accumulated to expose underlying subchondral bone.

A full-thickness cartilage injuries can be limited to the cartilage itself (transchondral fracture) or extend to the underlying subchondral bone (osteochondral fracture). Chondral fractures, like partial thickness injuries, result in chondrocyte necrosis and apoptosis. Surviving cells attempt to repair the tissue by proliferating into clusters and upregulating collagen and matrix production at the periphery of zone of injury. This response is short lived, however, and fails to bridge the chondral fracture (3). Propagation of the injury over time damages a greater surface area and leads to progressive and symptomatic joint deterioration.

CLASSIFICATION OF ARTICULAR CARTILAGE LESIONS

The most commonly used classification system for articular cartilage lesions was described by Outerbridge (4) in 1961 for grading of patellar lesions. Four grades of progressive size and depth of injury by gross appearance are described. Many employ a "modified" Outerbridge classification (Fig. 63.2), which describes partial-thickness fissuring as grade 2 and full-thickness fissuring as grade 3, regardless of size of area involved. Grade 4 injuries result in exposure of subchondral bone.

A newer classification system has been set forth by the International Cartilage Repair Society (ICRS), founded in 1997 to facilitate collaborative research endeavors (5). The ICRS recommends specific systems for articular cartilage injury mapping, articular cartilage injury classification, osteochondritis dissecans (OCD) classification, and a cartilage repair assessment system. The articular cartilage injury classification involves five grades, and the OCD classification four grades (Table 63.1).

Regardless of the classification system employed, depth, size, shape, location, and quality and morphology of the shouldering tissue are all important factors to note when describing cartilage lesions and determining a management plan.

INCIDENCE

A great challenge in the evaluation of articular cartilage lesions is determining which lesions are incidental findings versus true symptom generators. A retrospective review of more than 30,000 knee arthroscopies identified a 63% incidence of articular cartilage lesions, most commonly involving the patella and the medial femoral condyle. Forty-one percent were Outerbridge grade 3 and 19.2% Outerbridge grade 4 chondral injuries (6). With

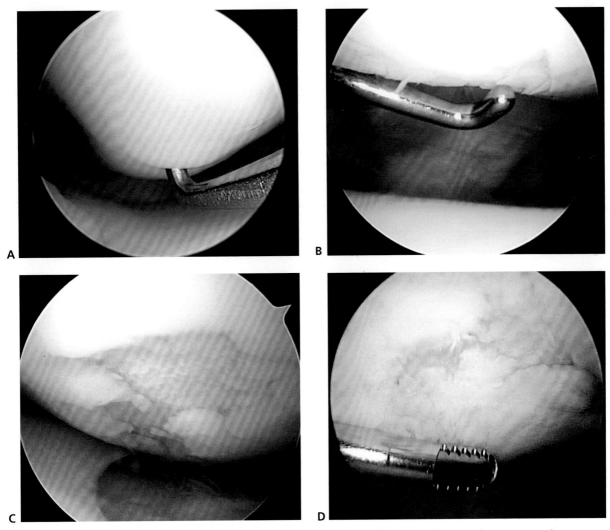

FIGURE 63.2. Arthroscopic photographs of articular cartilage lesions using modified Outerbridge classification. **A:** Grade 1 softening. **B:** Grade 2 partial-thickness fissuring. **C:** Grade 3 full-thickness fissuring and fibrillation. **D:** Grade 4 articular changes with exposed bone centrally surrounded by diffuse grade 3 articular cartilage.

vast improvements in MRI in the past two decades, articular cartilage can now be scrutinized with great detail. The goal is to be able to detect, through history, physical examination, and MRI evaluation, clinically relevant cartilage injuries requiring treatment.

HISTORY

History varies with etiology of the articular cartilage lesion. Chronicity of symptoms must be considered. Traumatic lesions typically give a history of a distinct mechanism, such as a direct blow, twist, or dislocation event. Palpable or audible "snaps" may be described. Immediate pain is the most common chief complaint. A retrospective review of 76 patients found that 67% reported an acute trauma, 95% complained of pain, 76% swelling, and 18% locking (7). Swelling and mechanical symptoms, including locking, clicking, catching, or giving way can result from cartilaginous loose bodies and may be difficult to differentiate

from meniscal or ligamentous injury. Articular cartilage injuries may also coexist with other intra-articular pathology, to further complicate the clinical picture.

In the setting of a discrete lesion, the patient may describe certain positions or activities that preferentially load the region of interest and aggravate the pain. For example, squatting or hyperflexion will engage a posterior condylar lesion, whereas forceful extension can irritate a patellar or trochlear disease.

Cartilage injuries resulting from degenerative or inflammatory arthrosis may have more subtle or vague presentations. Pain, aching, and intermittent swelling may be the patient's only complaints. Detailed history regarding other joint involvement and systemic symptoms (i.e., fatigue, weight loss, generalized arthralgias, and rash) should be elicited. Cartilage destruction may also stem from avascular necrosis, and risk factors, including steroid use, alcohol, HIV and anti-retroviral use, dysbarism, Gaucher disease, among others, should be explored.

Table 63.1

Classification schemes for cartilage lesions

Grade	Outerbridge	Modified Outerbridge	ICRS—Cartilage Lesions	ICRS—OCD Lesions
0	Normal	Normal	Normal	
1	Softening and swelling of surface	Softening and swelling of surface	Nearly normal; superficial lesions, soft indentation, and/or superficial fissures and cracks	Stable, continuity: softened area covered by intact cartilage
2	Fissuring, diameter <½″	Partial-thickness fissuring	Abnormal; lesions extending down to <50% of cartilage depth	Partial discontinuity, stable on probing
3	Fissuring, diameter >½″	Full-thickness fissuring	Severely abnormal; defects extending >50% of cartilage depth, down to calcified layer, down to but not through subchondral bone, includes blisters	Complete discontinuity, "dead in situ," not dislocated
4	Erosion down to bone	Erosion down to bone	Severely abnormal	Dislocated fragment, loose within the bed or empty defect; >10 mm in depth is B-subgroup

Adapted, in part, from Williams RJ. *Cartilage Repair Strategies.* Totowa, NJ: Humana Press; 2007:41.

The knee symptomatology must be evaluated in the context of the individual patient. Many factors need to be taken into account, including the patient's age, anthropomorphic measures, vocation, comorbidities, medications, prior surgeries, social habits, worker's compensation, or pending litigation. If the patient has previously undergone surgery for this joint, an attempt is made to obtain prior operative notes and pertinent images. Activity level, and in particular, change in activity, is critically important. Patients commonly modify the type or intensity of activities in which they participate to accommodate or mitigate their lesion-related knee discomfort. Use of a validated activity rating scale, such as the Marx activity score, can be helpful to measure baseline activity and function and track progress through the treatment process. Similarly, this assessment helps to gauge patient expectations and guide treatment decisions.

PHYSICAL EXAMINATION

Routine physical examination of the knee should always be performed. Height, weight, and body mass index (BMI) should be measured and calculated, as BMI greater than 30 has been associated with poorer outcomes in management of cartilage injuries (8). Gait should be inspected for alterations due to pain, mechanical blockage, or limb malalignment that may ultimately need to be addressed in conjunction with management of the cartilage lesion. Muscle atrophy may be appreciated in instances of chronic, degenerative, or inflammatory disease and measurement of bilateral thigh and calf circumference should be noted. Palpation or ballottement of a fluid wave is performed to assess for effusion and estimate the volume. In the setting of a traumatic effusion, for example, with patella dislocation, aspiration of hemarthrosis or lipohemarthrosis can be suggestive of osteochondral fracture.

Knee motion should be assessed for range, symmetry, and points at which the lesion is aggravated (extension or hyperflexion, as discussed above). Any loss of passive extension, hyperextension, or flexion should be quantified with a goniometer and compared with the contralateral knee. The anterior, medial, and lateral compartments are individually assessed for crepitation with range of motion and whether there is associated pain. It is necessary to assess the region of pathology as well as the status of a possible harvesting site if cartilage transfer is being considered.

Palpation of the patellar facets, distal condyles, and joint line is performed to identify discrete sites of pain. Loading of sites of suspected chondral injury can elicit pain. Wilson's sign, first described for OCD in the classic lateral aspect of the medial femoral condyle, is pain with internal rotation and extension relieved with external rotation of the knee.

Ligamentous integrity should be assessed to understand concomitant injury patterns and help guide management. We routinely evaluate the Lachman exam, anterior drawer, posterior drawer, posterior sag, pivot shift, reverse pivot shift, prone dial (external rotation) test at 30° and 70°, and joint opening with varus or valgus stress at 0° and 30°, as well as more detailed provocative maneuvers as warranted by examination findings.

Functional testing may also be included. We commonly test gait, single-leg squat, controlled step-down off an 8" step, and single leg hop in comparison with performance by the contralateral knee. More subtle deficits, particularly muscle weakness and proprioceptive imbalance, may be discerned.

IMAGING

Standard plain radiographs fail to visualize cartilage defects, but can identify OCD lesions, avascular necrosis (AVN), progressive osteoarthritis, or contributing malalignment. Weight-bearing PA images with the knee in 45° of flexion provide a view of the notch that may identify classic OCD lesions in the lateral aspect of the medial femoral condyle. The patellar/trochlear articulation and may be scrutinized with Merchant or Laurin views for tilt, which may indicate facet overload, or classic injury patterns to the medial facet of the patella and lateral trochlea, as seen in dislocation. Hip-to-ankle full-length films should be obtained when malalignment is suspected based on physical examination or standard knee views.

MRI historically has been most useful for assessment of cartilage at the patellofemoral articulation. Extensive advances in MRI technology in the past two decades have led to the development of cartilage-specific sequences, which allow detailed scrutiny of the tibiofemoral articular surfaces as well. Signal properties depend on collagen, proteoglycans, and water; orientation of collagen in the different laminae (superficial vs. deep) provides for characteristic gray-scale stratification within healthy cartilage.

Low signal at the bone with increasing signal toward articular surface is characteristic of healthy cartilage.

T1rho sequences evaluate for proteoglycan content; values increase as proteoglycan concentration decreases. Quantitative T2 mapping, in general, is useful for evaluation of collagen orientation and can be useful in assessing lesion fill after microfracture or other cartilage-stimulating technique. Proteoglycan content, and thereby compressive strength, can be assessed through newer dGEMRIC technology in which delayed T1rho-weighted images are obtained after intravenous injection of negatively charged gadolinium; dGEMRIC is particularly useful in assessing results of cartilage restoration techniques such as autologous cartilage transplant. Fat-suppressed images are evaluated for bony edema often seen adjacent to traumatic cartilage lesions or chronic lesions where cartilage deficiency alters stress patterns to the underlying bone.

Fast- or turbo-spin echo sequencing best visualizes the articular layer itself. The cartilage volume should be scrutinized for thickness and surface area. Hyperintensity at the bone–cartilage interface, where water should be most restricted, is suggestive of impending delamination. Chronic cartilage lesions may exhibit depression or undulation of the subchondral plate at the cartilage/bone interface.

In situ OCD lesions are evaluated for the presence of fluid beneath the lesion, suggestive of loosening and instability. The donor bed is also evaluated for sclerosis or collapse of the subchondral plate as signs of chronicity. The maturity of the physes is taken into account when considering the potential for the OCD to heal. Better outcomes have been identified when there is a favorable presentation (<2 cm, no dissection on imaging, no effusion) and the physes remain open (9). Old, healed OCD lesions commonly exhibit depression of subchondral bone with localized thickening of the cartilage.

Loose cartilaginous bodies can be identified by MRI and need to be evaluated for morphology (Fig. 63.3). The location of the tidemark—on the loose fragment or at the

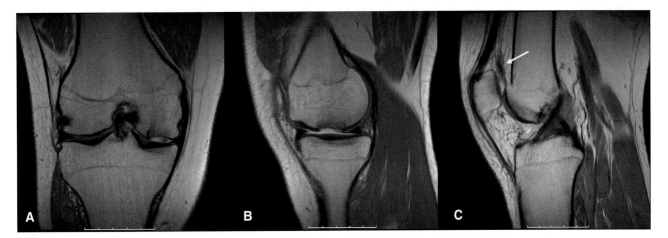

FIGURE 63.3. Coronal **(A)** and sagittal **(B, C)** MRI images demonstrate and osteochondral lesion over the medial femoral condyle resulting in depression of the subchondral bone and areas devoid of cartilage, with a fragment of devitalized bone and attached cartilage *(white arrow)* in the suprapatellar pouch.

donor site—is critical in assessing potential for repair. Sclerosis of the subchondral bone, both on the side of the fragment and on the donor bed, indicates chronicity with remodeling and suggests poor healing potential.

DECISION MAKING

Ultimately, the thorough assessment of articular cartilage lesions determines management strategies. The practitioner needs to weigh patient-specific pathology and symptomatology with anticipated natural history of the disease process, which is often difficult to predict. The goal in management, surgical or nonsurgical, is mitigation of pain and restoration of function.

The first major decision-making point is whether this can be achieved conservatively. Indications, techniques, and outcomes of surgical management are discussed in detail in subsequent chapters. In general, in the absence of discrete trauma, frank mechanical symptoms, or a locked knee, a patient presenting for the first time with an articular lesion is commonly initially managed with noninvasive techniques.

Treatment begins with patient education regarding the relevant anatomy and function, the nature of the pathology, the anticipated natural history, goals of treatment, and the gamut of available interventions. Emphasis is placed on a multimodal approach to management of symptoms and improving knee function. Nonoperative interventions include activity modification, physical therapy, cryotherapy, bracing, nonsteroidal anti-inflammatory medications, intra-articular steroid injections, or viscosupplementation. Frequent reassessment may be warranted to gauge response to or optimize such therapeutic measures. Surgery is then considered for persistent pain or the development of mechanical symptoms despite compliance with the treatment plan for up to 3 to 6 months.

When contemplating surgical options, the goal is to bring about relief of symptoms while minimizing morbidity and maximizing cost-effectiveness and long-term efficacy. Successful management of cartilage injury requires defect fill and restoration of congruity with tissue that will prove durable and stand the test of time. Table 63.2 provides a brief overview of how the first-line treatment options available in the United States meet these parameters.

Briefly, when selecting surgical intervention, we first consider the size of the lesion and the demands of the patient. Focal lesions less than 2 cm (2) are primarily treated with debridement and/or microfracture in the low-demand patient, with consideration for synthetic plugs or mosaicplasty (osteochondral autograft) in the high-demand patient (a laborer or one who desires to resume athletic activities). For lesions greater than 2 cm (2), debridement is reserved only for certain low-demand patients, and synthetic plugs, mosaicplasty, or even osteochondral allograft may be employed for low- or high-demand patients. Allogenic or autogenous osteochondral grafting is our treatment of choice in the revision setting. For lesions greater than 5 cm (2), we prefer allograft due to the limitation in the amount of donor tissue available and possible morbidity with autograft harvesting.

CONCLUSIONS

Articular cartilage pathology is common in the knee. The practitioner is challenged to determine if the cartilage irregularity is indeed a generator of pain or disability. Clinical approach to the patient with articular cartilage pathology involves eliciting a detailed history, comprehensive lower extremity physical examination, and judicious use of plain radiographs or MRI. Patient-specific data is synthesized in the context of known structure and function of cartilage and the absence of intrinsic healing capabilities. Treatment goals of pain relief and restoration of function can often be achieved with nonoperative means. Surgical management is indicated for traumatic injuries, mechanical symptoms,

Table 63.2			
First-line treatment options for surgical management of cartilage lesions			
Treatment	Repair Tissue	Fill	Durability
Lavage	None	None	Poor
Chondroplasty/debridement	None	None	Poor
Microfracture	Fibrocartilage	Variable	2+ years
Synthetic Osteoarticular Plugs	Normal bone, Isointense cartilage	Variable	Unknown
Mosaicplasty/OATS	Hyaline cartilage	Near total	5+ years; unknown beyond

or the lesion refractory to conservative management and is discussed in detail in subsequent chapters.

REFERENCES

1. Visser NA, de Koning MH, Lammi MJ, et al. Increase of decorin content in articular cartilage following running. *Connect Tissue Res*. 1998;37:295–302.
2. Mankin HJ. The response of articular cartilage to mechanical injury. *J Bone Joint Surg Am*. 1982;64:460–466.
3. Lotz M. Cytokines in cartilage injury and repair. *Clin Orthop Relat Res*. 2001;391(suppl):S108–S115.
4. Outerbridge RE. The etiology of chondromalacia patellae. *J Bone Joint Surg Br*. 1961;43-B:752–757.
5. Brittberg M, Winalski CS. Evaluation of cartilage injuries and repair. *J Bone Joint Surg Am*. 2003;85(suppl 2):58–69.
6. Curl WW, Krome J, Gordon ES, et al. Cartilage injuries: a review of 31,516 knee arthroscopies. *Arthroscopy*. 1997;13:456–460.
7. Johnson-Nurse C, Dandy DJ. Fracture separation of articular cartilage in the adult knee. *J Bone Joint Surg Br*. 1985;67:42–43.
8. Mithoefer K, Williams RJ III, Warren RF, et al. The microfracture technique for the treatment of articular cartilage lesions of the knee. A prospective cohort study. *J Bone Joint Surg Am*. 2005;87(9):1911–1920.
9. Hefti F, Beguiristain J, Krauspe R, et al. Osteochondritis dissecans: a multicenter study of the European Pediatric Orthopedic Society. *J Pediatr Orthop B*. 1999;8(4):231–245.

Osteochondritis Dissecans of the Knee and Articular Cartilage Fractures

Alberto Gobbi • Massimo Berruto • Giuseppe Filardo • Elizaveta Kon • Georgios Karnatzikos

Osteochondritis dissecans (OCD) is a disorder of one or more ossification centers, characterized by sequential degeneration or aseptic necrosis and recalcification. An OCD lesion involves both bone and cartilage but appears to affect the subchondral bone primarily and the articular cartilage secondarily.

The condition was first described by Ambrosio Pare' and was named by Franz König (1) in 1888 describing it as a knee subchondral inflammatory process, resulting in a loose fragment of cartilage from the femoral condyle. Incidence of OCD has been stated to be between 0.02% and 0.03% on radiographs and 1.2% on arthroscopy (2). Linden (3) stated the incidence of OCD in Sweden, between 15 and 21 cases per 100,000. It most commonly occurs in patients aged 10 to 15 years, with a male-to-female ratio of 2:1 and occurs bilaterally (4) in 15% to 30%.

ETIOLOGY

The pathogenesis of OCD is still controversial: various theories have been proposed throughout the years but no theory is markedly superior over the other.

Theories can be divided into three major groups: genetic, vascular, and traumatic.

Genetic theory shows variation or subgroup of epiphyseal dysplasia and thus may display a similar inheritance pattern.

OCD has been found with a variety of inherited conditions, including dwarfism, tibia vara, Legg-Calvé-Perthes disease, Stickler syndrome (5–9) and that there is a familial predisposition to the occurrence of OCD in other joints.

Other authors (10–12) have suggested a vascular etiology with the occurrence of a vascular event such as embolism, thrombosis, or venous stasis, which can cause a secondary osteonecrosis; however, others (13) have demonstrated that the presence of an abundant vascularization does not end at the femoral epiphysis, which refuted the vascular etiology.

The traumatic etiology (14–16) is by far the oldest and the most well established and is based on clinical history of previous trauma, predominantly affecting men,

and the probability of reproducing similar lesions in other parts of the body.

According to the theory of repeated microtrauma, as described by Fairbank (17) and validated by Smillie (18) in the 1960s, the OCD is caused by contact of a hypertrophied tibial spine on the medial femoral condyle. This theory, despite being the most credited, does not allow an explanation of the localization of the disease in different locations of the knee. Nowadays, repetitive microtrauma correlated with a possible vascular insufficiency and other inherited factors are still under investigation.

OCD CLASSIFICATION

There are several types of classifications of OCD that is based on the following:

1. Age of onset of the disease
2. Radiographic localization
3. Patho-anatomy
4. Arthroscopic evaluation

Age of Onset

Smillie (18) distinguished two forms of OCD, juvenile and adult, and suggested unique etiologies.

The juvenile form OCD was supposed to be related to a disturbance of the epiphyseal development, whereas in the adult a more direct traumatic causation was supposed. Other authors (19) suggested a distinction based on the osseous age of the patient at the time of symptom onset: juvenile OCD, which affects patients with open growth of cartilage in a general age group of between 10 and 16 years, and OCD in adults, when the cartilage physis is closed.

Radiographic Localization

The location of OCD can be defined topographically on standard radiographic projections of the knee (19). In the anteroposterior view, it is typically located centrally on the medial condyle, whereas on the lateral view, it is most commonly in the anterior or middle segments (Fig. 64.1).

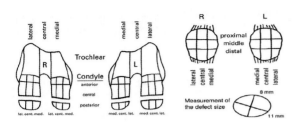

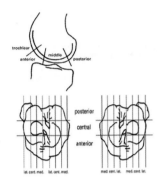

FIGURE 64.1. ICRS mapping system.

Anatomo-pathologic Classification

Proposed by Conway and subsequently amended by Guhl (20), this classification, which was useful in the past to address the type of treatment, taking into account the anatomical characteristics of the lesion and subdivided into five stages:

- Stage I: Lesion evident at radiography, the CT or the MRI, with the presence of a sclerotic line, cartilage intact, and, only in some cases, slightly softened but only in some points.
- Stages II and III: Cartilage not intact, with the presence of fissures and fragments in situ or partially detached.
- Stage IV: Complete detachment but normal joint.
- Stage V: The fragment is displaced and there are findings of degenerative cartilage damage.

Classification by Arthroscopy

Recently, the board of the International Cartilage Repair Society (ICRS) (21) defined a classification of OCD arthroscopy in four stages:

- Stage I: Stable lesion with a continuous but softened area covered by intact articular cartilage.
- Stage II: Lesion with partial articular cartilage discontinuity but stable when probed.
- Stage III: Lesion with an unstable but not dislocated fragment "dead in situ."
- Stage IV: Empty defect with a dislocated fragment (loose body).

CLINICAL EVALUATION

Juveniles and adolescents will complain of vague, non-specific, poorly localized anterior knee pain with variable intermittent amount of swelling, locking of the knee, grinding, or catching; pain is aggravated by activity and relieved by rest (22). While others may be asymptomatic, a high level of suspicion should be exhibited with these type of symptoms. Symptoms are usually preceded by trauma in 40% to 60% of the cases (15, 23). Others may present with Wilsons (24) sign, which is performed by flexing the knee to 90° then slowly internally rotating the leg and extending it. Patients will complain of pain at 30° of flexion, and the pain is relieved by external rotation. Pain is exhibited because the tibial spine impinges on the medial femoral condyle. This test, albeit unreliable, has been shown to have an accuracy of only 70% (2, 25).

Radiographic Evaluation

The radiographic examination of a patient suspected to have OCD should always begins with plain radiographs. Standard request should be an anteroposterior, lateral, notch, and Merchant view of the knee. Notch view is specifically recommended because it demonstrates the most common areas for the occurrence of OCD, and it increases the percentage of detection. Classic findings of OCD on plain film are a well-circumscribed area of subchondral bone, separated by a crescent shaped sclerotic radiolucent outline of the OCD fragment (14, 25). In pediatric patients and adolescents, contralateral views should be requested to avoid confusion with the growth plates. Plain radiographs, however, cannot visualize for us the stability and status of the overlying cartilage; hence, additional diagnostic procedures may be necessary for us to treat these lesions.

CT Scan

The use of the CT scan has fallen out of favor with the advent of the MRI because the MRI gives a more detailed picture of the disease entity. CT scanning is helpful in determining lesion size and loose bodies but is rarely used nowadays as part of the treatment strategy.

Scintigraphy

Technetium bone scans have been previously used to localize the lesion of a specific joint and follow the progression of healing in juvenile patients. This imaging modality provides no information on the status of the cartilage and has been replaced by MRI. Some authors have proposed serial bone scanning of juvenile patients (but have not been widely adopted due to the time required for the study, invasive venous access, and the risk of introducing a radioactive isotope).

Magnetic Resonance Imaging

MRI has proven superior in providing valuable information as compared with other diagnostic modalities.

It generally gives us the dimensions of the lesion, as well as the status of the cartilage and subchondral bone. The most appropriate MRI protocol for evaluating OCD lesions is fast spin echo, proton density, and T2-weighted image (25). MRI-arthrography with gadolinium has been shown to have 100% accuracy, determining the status of articular cartilage using gradient echo techniques (26).

TREATMENT

The advent of arthroscopy has outright revolutionized the treatment of OCD. Using standard arthroscopic portals and techniques, surgeons are now visualizing lesions previously missed on standard diagnostic procedures. Open techniques have not fallen out of favor and are still utilized for lesions requiring greater exposure and visualization. Treatment options largely depend on age of the patient, lesion size, and stability. Unstable lesions must be treated surgically.

Nonoperative Treatment

Nonoperative treatment is still used in a select group of patients with OCD. The goal of nonsurgical treatment is to promote healing of lesions in situ and prevent lesion displacement. Skeletally, immature patients usually have a better prognosis. Lesions on weight-bearing surfaces and those that are greater than 1 cm in size have shown to have an unsuccessful outcome (15, 20, 27, 28). The mainstay of nonsurgical treatment has been cessation of athletic activity and lifestyle modification. This is done for a period of 3 to 6 months with an initial 6 to 8 weeks of nonweight bearing and daily range-of-motion exercises. If at the 6th month there are no signs of radiographic healing, then operative treatment should be considered (29, 30). A healing rate of 50% to 94% has been noted with nonoperative treatment (4, 19, 29).

Operative Treatment

Excision of Fragments

Previously considered the most common treatment for these lesions have fallen out of favor due to the dismal long-term results in juvenile and adult patients (31–34). The addition of a debridement and curettage of the lesion bed has shown to improve the results in juvenile patients (31, 35).

Arthroscopic Drilling

Considered as one of the first surgical treatments for OCD, either arthroscopic or open, is still one of the most common treatment methods for OCD. The rationale behind this procedure is that the OCD is treated as a fracture nonunion, and by penetrating the subchondral bone, it will instigate an inflammatory healing cascade, creating channels for subsequent revascularization (27). It is started on juveniles with a failed trial of conservative management. Drilling can be done in an antegrade or retrograde fashion;

the former is more technically challenging in trying to center the drill and gaining the right depth over the lesion, and the latter is easier to perform but violates the continuity of the articular cartilage. Anderson et al. (36). noted a 90% healing potential in the skeletally immature group, whereas the skeletally mature group had a 50% healing potential. This technique is generally reserved for ICRS stage I lesions.

Open Reduction of the Fragment

Reduction and stabilization of the OCD fragment can be done with a multitude of devices such as K-wires, variable pitch screws, cannulated screws, bioabsorbable pins, tacks nails, and screws. This should be reserved for lesions less than 2 cm. Anderson and Pagnani (33) reported that long-term results for large lesions is poor-developing, early onset arthritis.

Thorough evaluation of the underlying subchondral bone should be performed and assessment of stability done if in situ fixation is amenable to the lesion. Lesions with little anchoring to the base usually have abundant scar tissue, which needs to be debrided prior to reduction and fixation of the fragment. Drilling or microfracture can be employed to stimulate the healing potential prior to reduction. In cases of fragment, mismatch during reduction bone grafting can be employed. This can be taken from the proximal tibia or the intercondylar notch of the femur.

A multitude of fixation materials can be used each with its own advantages and disadvantages. Till date, there is a lot of controversy as to which is the implant of choice. Pins and K-wires can achieve multiple points of fixation with less risk of an iatrogenic fracture to the fragment; disadvantage is that they provide no compression and usually loosen, which eventually require removal. The advent of biomaterials has revolutionized the way in fixing the fragments. The concept of having to put an implant that could provide compression and be absorbed by the body was novel, but it was not without problems. Postoperative complications ranged from inflammatory reactions with effusion to loose bodies secondary to implant not being absorbed by the body at all (37, 38).

Osteochondral Grafting

Transplanting of either autografts or allografts to the OCD defect has the advantage of restoring hyaline cartilage providing a biomechanically stronger and more resilient tissue. Osteochondral autograft transfer (OAT) is used for lesions smaller than 2 cm. It is a single-step procedure, which can be done arthroscopically or as a mini-open procedure. This entails harvest of cylindrical plugs from the nonweight bearing aspect of the notch of the medial trochlear ridge. Where either single or multiple plugs are harvested and transferred back to the defect. OAT can be a technically demanding procedure and any mismatch in

V. D. The Knee Articular Cartilage

articular surface can cause an increase in contact pressures and shear. Wu et al. (39). showed that plugs that are 1 mm prominent caused an increase in contact pressures and shear, whereas a 0.25-mm recess decreased pressure by 50%. This is also limited by the amount of graft a donor site can give, creating a situation such as "robbing from Peter to pay Paul."

Fresh osteochondral allograft designed to treat larger lesions (>2 cm in diameter) this could be done in either a pressfit plug technique or a shell graft technique. Advantages are the flexibility of sizing the grafts, ability to use a single plug for a defect and the lack of donor site morbidity. The disadvantages include reduced viability of the graft due to storing and processing, immunogenicity, transmission of diseases, and the availability of the grafts (not available in many countries worldwide).

First- and Second-Generation Autologous Chondrocyte Implantation

In lesions larger than 2 to 3 cm², the transplantation of autologous chondrocytes can now be considered the technique of choice. Peterson et al. (40) reported successful clinical results at 2 to 10 years follow-up in more than 90% of patients with OCD treated with ACI. They showed that autologous chondrocyte implantation (ACI) produced an integrated repair tissue with successful clinical results.

In the experience of Peterson, a pioneer of the technique of ACI, the OCD was and along with isolated lesions of the medial femoral condyle these injuries have obtained the best results with this method.

In the first phase of his experience, Peterson performed the simple transplantation of chondrocytes in suspension. Successively, he has perfected his technique for treating OCD lesions deeper than 10 mm involving significant subchondral bone loss with his "sandwich technique" in which cancellous bone is used to fill the defect and closed with a periosteal flap, the grafted chondrocytes are then suspended in between the first periosteal flap and are then closed with a second periosteal flap.

The recent introduction of bioengineered tissues with chondrocytes seeded on the scaffold represents another possibility to fill the lesion. However, when the lesion is deep, it is necessary to reconstitute a bone on the floor and then paste the scaffold on it to reconstitute cartilage.

SECOND-GENERATION ACI: OUR EXPERIENCE

Since being introduced in 1987, the cell-based approach has gained increasing acceptance, and recent studies highlight the long-term durable nature of this form of treatment due to the production of hyaline-like cartilage that is mechanically and functionally stable and integrates into the adjacent articular surface. However, these good results have to be weighed against the number of problems that

can be observed with the standard ACI methods. First-generation ACI has been associated with several limitations related to the complexity and morbidity of the surgical procedure. This technique requires a large joint exposure with a high risk of joint stiffness and arthrofibrosis. Moreover, there is a frequent occurrence of periosteal hypertrophy that often requires revision surgery. To these problems related to the surgical procedure, we must add the technical problems of the culture and transplantation procedure, such as maintenance of chondrocyte phenotype, nonhomogeneous cell distribution in the three-dimensional (3D) spaces of the defect, and cell loss using liquid suspension.

Taking into consideration all these factors, a new generation procedure for cartilage transplantation was developed. The so-called matrix-assisted or second-generation ACI technique uses a new tissue-engineering technology to create a cartilage-like tissue in a 3D culture system with the attempt to address all the concerns related to the cell culture and the surgical technique. Essentially, the concept is based on the use of biodegradable polymers as temporary scaffolds for the in vitro growth of living cells and their subsequent transplantation onto the defect site. On the basis of published results, the matrix-assisted chondrocyte implantation guarantees results comparable with, or even better than, the traditional ACI technique and simplify the procedure with marked advantages from a biologic and surgical point of view.

Our experience with the treatment of OCD through the implant of a bioengineered tissue regards a scaffold entirely based on the benzylic ester of hyaluronic acid (HYAFF 11, Fidia Advanced Biopolymers Laboratories, Padova, Italy). It consists of a network of 20-µm-thick fibers with interstices of variable sizes, which has been demonstrated to be an optimal physical support to allow cell–cell contacts, cluster formation, and extracellular matrix deposition (Fig. 64.2).

The cells harvested from the patient are expanded and then seeded onto the scaffold to create the tissue-engineered product Hyalograft C. Seeded on the scaffold

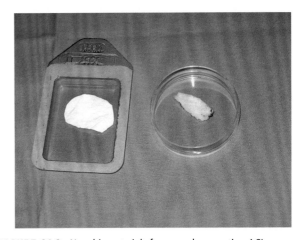

FIGURE 64.2. New biomaterials for second-generation ACI.

the cells are able to redifferentiate and to retain a chondrocytic phenotype even after a long period of in vitro expansion in monolayer culture. The efficacy of the cell-scaffold construct was also proven by in vivo implantation in an animal model. This 3D scaffold for autologous chondrocyte culture can improve the biologic performance of autologous cells and overcome some of the difficulties of the ACI surgical technique. Hyalograft C constructs can be implanted by press fitting directly into the lesion, thus avoiding suturing to surrounding cartilage and obviating the need for a periosteal flap, thereby also avoiding the possibility of periosteal hypertrophy (Figs. 64.3 and 64.4). Moreover, the features of this device have permitted the development of an arthroscopic surgical technique, reducing patient morbidity, surgical and recovery time, and complications related to open surgery (Fig. 64.5).

Since 2001, we used this tissue-engineering approach for the treatment of OCD, and we implanted the bioengineered cartilage tissue in more than 50 patients. We believe that surgical goals should always try to reestablish the joint surface in the most anatomical way possible. In fact, as underlined by Linden (3) in a long-term retrospective outcome study (average follow-up 33 years) of patients with OCD of the femoral condyle, the natural history of

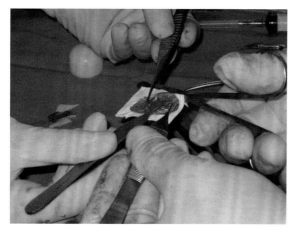

FIGURE 64.3 Preparation of the scaffold.

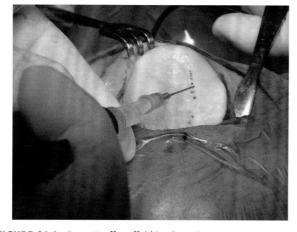

FIGURE 64.4. Open Hyaff scaffold implantation.

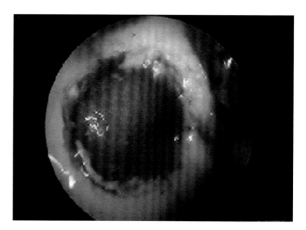

FIGURE 64.5. Arthroscopic implantation.

this osteochondral joint pathology is an earlier degeneration process. Patients with adult OCD showed radiographically to develop osteoarthritis about 10 years earlier in life than primary osteoarthritis. The use of the autologous bioengineered tissue Hyalograft C in OCD lesions presents the problem of promoting only the cartilage but not the bone regeneration. For this reason, in case of deep lesions, we utilized a two-step technique. When necessary, second-generation autologous transplantation was preceded by an autologous bone grafting, in order to restore the entire osteochondral structure, and, therefore, a more anatomical articular surface. The first arthroscopic surgical step consists of the implant of a bone graft harvested from the ipsilateral tibia to fill the bone loss. In the same surgical procedure, healthy cartilage is harvested from the intercondylar notch for the autologous chondrocyte culture expansion. The second surgical procedure is performed 4 to 6 months later after the integration of the autologous bone graft is achieved and consists of the second-generation arthroscopic autologous chondrocyte transplantation according to the technique described by Marcacci et al. (41).

We have reviewed the patients with at a minimum follow-up of 3 years. A total of 38 OCD of the knee was treated and evaluated at a mean follow-up of 4 years. The mean age was 21.2 years (range 15 to 46), 84% of patients were active and practiced sports at least at amateur level, and 42% underwent previous surgery. The most common location of the lesion was the medial femoral condyle (76%), and the mean size was 2.9 cm^2 (range 1.5 to 4 cm^2). The mean number of Hyalograft C patches used was 2.8 (range 1 to 4), and in 62% of the cases, the additional bone graft step was required to restore the articular surface. The results were evaluated with the International Knee Documentation Committee (ICRS–IKDC 2000) and the Tegner scores. No complications related to the Hyalograft C implant and no serious adverse events were observed during the treatment and follow-up period.

ICRS and Tegner scores showed an overall satisfactory clinical outcome. At mean 4 years' follow-up, the average ICRS–IKDC 2000 was increased from 41.4 to 74.9 in cases of OCD of the femoral condyle (increase 80.4%). In cases of OCD of the patella, a lower but still significant improvement was observed: the mean score increased from 47 to 68. The Tegner score passed from 1.5 preoperatively to 5 at the latest follow-up with a significant improvement, even if still lower than the previous sport activity level of 6.

Second-look arthroscopy was performed in five cases, and results were graded according to ICRS scale two were normal and three almost normal.

MRI examination showed a good appearance in the anatomical location of the transplant, with a concentration of glycosaminoglycans (GAGs) similar to that of a normal cartilage (Figs. 64.6 and 64.7). In few cases were observed persistent irregularities of the subchondral bone, which were not filled at the time of (Fig. 64.7).

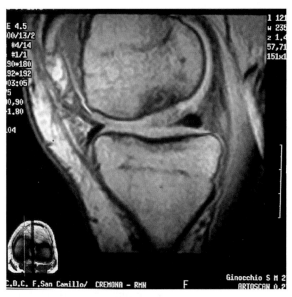

FIGURE 64.6. Preoperative MRI.

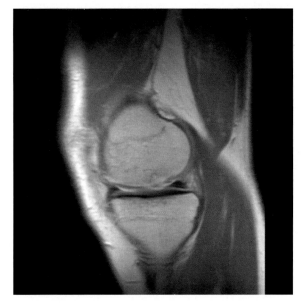

FIGURE 64.7. Second-genderation ACI: 3 years post-op. MRI.

New Osteochondral Cell-free Scaffold: Preliminary Experience

Various biodegradable polymers for the second-generation ACI technique, such as hyaluronan, collagen, fibrin glue, alginate, agarose, and various synthetic polymers have been proposed during recent years for the treatment of articular cartilage lesions. However, the results obtained for the treatment of cartilage lesions are still controversial, and the treatment of osteo-cartilaginous lesions is even more problematic because tissue damage is also extended to the subchondral bone, involving two different tissue types characterized by different intrinsic healing capacities. In the case of OCD, a more complex surgical procedure is often required: in deep damages, the full thickness of the defect needs to be replaced in order to restore the joint surface. For the repair of the entire osteochondral unit, several authors have highlighted the need for biphasic scaffolds to reproduce the different biologic and functional requirements for guiding the growth of the two tissues (42). Moreover, both from a surgical and commercial standpoint, an ideal graft for osteochondral defect repair would be an off-the-shelf product able to induce in situ cartilage and bone regeneration after direct transplantation onto the defect site. The possibility to create a cell-free implant to be sufficiently "intelligent" to bring into the joint the appropriate cues to induce orderly and durable tissue regeneration is still under investigation in numerous animal studies. Following this rationale, we studied a new bicomposite, multilayer, biomimetic scaffold, which can mimic the osteocartilaginous structure in all of its components. This scaffold comprising type I collagen and nanostructured hydroxyapatite, has been designed for the treatment of cartilaginous and osteocartilaginous defects. The osteochondral nanostructured biomimetic scaffold developed (Fin-Ceramica Faenza S.p.A., Faenza, Italy) has a porous 3D composite trilayered structure, mimicking the whole osteochondral anatomy. The cartilaginous layer, consisting of type I collagen, has a smooth surface. The intermediate layer (tide-mark-like) consists of a combination of type I collagen (60%) and HA (40%), whereas the lower layer consists of a mineralized blend of type I collagen (30%) and HA (70%), reproducing the subchondral bone layer. The structure of the scaffold is conceived with the aim to confine the bone formation into the deepest portion of construct without involving any superficial layer, where the process of cartilaginous-like connective tissue formation should begin. We tested this novel biomaterial in vitro and animal studies (horse and sheep model) and obtained good results with cartilage and bone tissue formation. The implant of the gradient biomimetic scaffold led to a reconstruction of both hyaline-like cartilage and structured bone tissue anchored to the interface of adjacent healthy tissues, even with no other bioactive agents added. We observed same macroscopic, histologic, and radiographic results when implanting scaffold loaded with autologous chondrocytes or scaffold alone. The scaffold demonstrated the ability to induce an in situ regeneration, likely through a process mediated by mesenchymal precursor cells resident in the subchondral bone, recruited within the material and differentiated in osteogenic and chondrogenic lineages.

Thus, we applied this innovative scaffold as a cell-free approach for osteochondral reconstruction into clinical practice. We performed a clinical pilot study, whereby the newly developed biomimetic scaffold was used for the treatment of chondral and osteochondral lesions of the knee joint, in order to evaluate the safety and feasibility of the surgical procedure and to test the intrinsic stability of the device without any other fixation techniques. For the early postoperative evaluation of graft attachment, invasive methods are not appropriate, whereas MRI represents a well-accepted powerful tool for postoperative monitoring of osteochondral lesions and repair tissues. Therefore, we use MRI to determine the early postoperative adherence rate at 4 to 5 weeks and 25 to 26 weeks in all the patients (43). MRI evaluation at short-term follow-up demonstrated a good stability of the scaffold without any other fixation device. In a further MRI evaluation at 12 months, the complete filling of cartilage defect was noted in 86.2% of the patients, and the congruency of the articular surface was seen in the same percentage. Moreover, clinical evaluation at 2-year follow-up confirmed the good initial findings, and we observed encouraging clinical results with a satisfactory outcome even in big osteochondral defects (44). The implant of biomaterials for in situ cartilage and bone regeneration represent an innovative promising approach for the restoration of the articular surface, especially in case of osteochondral defects.

Table 64.1

Location and size of knee cartilage lesions treated with MSC implantation

Patient / Side	Location & Size of lesions (mm x mm)	Size (cm²)	CFU MSC/mL	Concomitant procedures
1 / Right	MFC 50 x 20	10	4700	ACLR
2 / Right	Patella 40 x 20	8	2600	Patellar realignment (Fulkerson)
3 / Left	Trochlea 25 x 20	5	4600	Opening wedge osteotomy
4 / Right	Trochlea 20 x 12	2.4	4550	none
5 / Right	Patella 45 x 15	6.75	4600	Opening wedge osteotomy
6 / Left	MTP 20 x 10	3	4650	none
7 / Left	MFC 20 x 30 MTP 13 x 10	7.3	3650	Opening wedge osteotomy
8 / Right	Patella 40 x 20	8	5700	ACLR
9 / Right	Trochlea 30 x 25 Patella 25 x 25 MFC 25 x 20	18.75	5700	Patellar realignment (Fulkerson)
10 / Left	Patella 12 x 8 Patella 20 x 15	3.95	2640	Lateral release
11 / Left	Trochlea 40 x 30 MCF 18 x 23	16.15	3100	none
12 / Left	MTP 20 x 30 MFC 40 x 30 Trochlea 20 x 20	22	2435	Opening wedge osteotomy
13 / Left	MTP 20 x 10 MFC 40 x 30 Trochlea 15 x 10	15.5	2808	Opening wedge osteotomy
14 / Left	Patella 40 x 25	10	4900	ACLR (Allograft)
15 / Right	LFC 11 x 11	1.5	2000	ACLR

Note: MSC = mesenchymal stem cells; CFU = colony-forming unit (CFU/mL) of MSC per patient; MFC = medial femoral condyle; MTP = medial tibial plateau; LFC = lateral femoral condyle; ACLR = anterior cruciate ligament reconstruction.

The potential advantages of the treatment of OCD through this surgical approach are very attractive. The properties of the graft are specifically tailored to introduce the structural, biologic, and biomechanical cues into the affected joints, leading to a reproducible and durable repair, and imply further advantages, such as the need of a one-step surgery, reduced costs, and a simplified procedure.

FUTURE TRENDS: THE ROLE OF MESENCHYMAL STEM CELLS

Recent directions in cartilage repair are moving towards the possibility of performing one-step surgery; several groups are analyzing the possibility of using mesenchymal stem cells (MSC) with chondrogenic potential and growth factors (GF), thus avoiding the first surgery for cartilage biopsy and subsequent chondrocyte cell cultivation (45-47). MSC have a self-renewal capacity and multi-lineage differentiation potential and they can be characterized by their cultivation behavior and their differentiation potential into adipogenic, osteogenic and chondrogenic cells; therefore, once MSC are cultured in the appropriate microenvironment, they can differentiate to chondrocytes and form cartilage (48–50). In this regard, the use of bone marrow aspirate concentrated cells (BMAC), which contain pluripotent MSCs and growth factors, can represent a possible alternative for regenerating cartilage tissue.

We prospectively followed up for 2 years a group of 15 non-professional athletes with 15 knees operated on for grade IV large cartilage lesions, measuring up to a total lesion area of 22 cm2 per patient (average size 9.2 cm^2) (Table 65.1); all have been implanted using BMAC covered with a collagen I/III matrix (ChondroGide®- Geistlich Wolhusen, CH) in a one-step procedure (51). Bone marrow was harvested from ipsilateral iliac crest using a dedicated aspiration kit and centrifuged using a commercially available system (BMAC Harvest Smart PreP2 System, Harvest Technologies, Plymouth, MA). In order to concentrate the baseline value of the bone marrow cells 4 to 6 times, we followed the method recommended by the manufacturer. Using a Batroxobin enzyme (Plateltex®act-Plateltex SRO Bratislava, SK), the bone marrow concentrate was activated in order to produce a sticky clot, which was implanted into the prepared cartilage defect. The patients followed the same specific rehabilitation program for a minimum of 6 months. All patients showed significant improvement in evaluation scores. Mean pre-op values were: Visual Analogue Scale for pain (VAS) 5, IKDC subjective 41.7, Knee injury and Osteoarthritis Outcome Score (KOOS) Pain=66.6/ Symptoms=68.3/ ADL=70/ Sorts=41.8/ QOL=37.2), Lysholm 65 and Tegner 2.07. At final follow up mean scores were: VAS 0.8, IKDC subjective 75.5, KOOS P=89.8/ S=83.6/ ADL=89.6/ SP=58.9/ QOL=68, Lysholm 87.9 and Tegner 4.1. No adverse reactions or post-op complication were noted. MRI showed good coverage of the lesions. Four patients gave their consent for second-look arthroscopy but only 3 for a concomitant biopsy. Good histological findings were reported for all the specimens analyzed which presented many hyaline-like features (51).

The good clinical outcome showed that the use of BMAC in full-thickness large articular cartilage lesions repair can be a promising option for the treatment of knee cartilage defects; however, an increased sample size and longer term prospective randomized studies are needed to confirm these preliminary results.

CONCLUSION

OCD is still a challenge for the orthopedic both diagnostically and therapeutically. No one single technique has been deemed appropriate for this very tricky condition. Recent techniques with new biomaterials have shown good medium-term results but still needs to be followed up for more than 10 years.

REFERENCES

1. König F. Ueber freie Körper in den Gelenken. *Deutsche Zeitschr Chir.* 1888;27:90–109.
2. Schenck RC Jr, Goodnight JM. Osteochondritis dissecans. *J Bone Joint Surg Am.* 1996;78:439–478.
3. Lindén B. The incidence of osteochondritis dissecans in the condyles of the femur. *Acta Orthop Scand.* 1976 Dec;47(6):664–667.
4. Hefti F, Beguiristain J, Krauspe R, et al. Osteochondritis dissecans: a multicenter study of the European Pediatric Orthopedic Society. *J Pediatric Orthop B.* 1999;8:231–245.
5. Ribbing S. The hereditary multiple epiphyseal disturbance and its consequences for the aetiogenesis of local malacias- particularly the osteochondritis dissecans. *Acta Orthop Scand.* 1955;24:286–299.
6. Gardiner TB. Osteochondritis dissecans in three members of one family. *J Bone Joint Surg Br.* 1955;37:139–141.
7. Mubarak SJ, Carroll NC. Familial osteochondritis of the knee. *Clin Orthop.* 1979;140:131–136.
8. Stougart J. Familial occurrence of osteochondritis dissecans. *J Bone Joint Surg Br.* 1964;46:542–543.
9. Stougart J. The hereditary factor in osteochondritis dissecans. *J Bone Joint Surg Br.* 1961;43:256–258.
10. Campbell CJ, Ranawat CS. Osteochondritis dissecans: the question of etiology. *J Trauma.* 1966;6:201–221.
11. Chiroff RT, Cooke CP. Osteochondritis dissecans: a histologic and microradioographic analysis of surgical excised lesions. *J Trauma.* 1975;15:689–696.
12. Green WT, Banks HH. Osteochondritis dissecans in children. *J Bone Joint Surg Am.* 1953;35:26–47.
13. Rogers WM, Gladstone H. Vascular foramina and arterial supply of the distal end of the femur. *J Bone Joint Surg Am.* 1950;32:867–874.
14. Fisher AG. A study of loose bodies composed of cartilage and bone occurring in joints. With special reference to their aethiology and pathology. *Br J Surg.* 1921;8:493–523.
15. Garret JC. Osteochondritis dissecans. *Clin Sports Med.* 1991;10:569–593.
16. Wolbach SB, Allison N. Osteochondritis dissecans. *Arch Surg.* 1928;16:67–82.

17. Fairbank HA. Osteochondritis dissecans. *Br J Surg.* 1933;21:67–82.

18. Smillie IS. Treatment of osteochondritis dissecans. *J Bone Joint Surg Br.* 1957;29:248–260.

19. Cahill BR. Osteochondritis dissecans of the knee: treatment of juvenile and adult forms. *J Am Acad Orthop Surg.* 1995;3:237–247.

20. Guhl JF. Arthroscopic treatment of osteochondritis dissecans. *Clin Orthop Relat Res.* 1982;167:65–74.

21. I.C.R.S. Meeting. 2000; Gothenburg, Sweden.

22. Caffey J, Madell SH, Royer C, et al. Ossification of the distal femoral epiphysis. *J Bone Joint Surg Am.* 1958;40:647–654.

23. Garrett JC, Kress KJ, Mudano M. Osteochondritis dissecans of the lateral femoral condyle in the adult. *Arthroscopy.* 1992;8:474–481.

24. Wilson JN. A diagnostic sign in osteochondritis dissecans of the knee. *J Bone Joint Surg Am.* 1967;49-A:477–480.

25. Schwarz C, Bilazina ME, Sisto DJ. The results of operative treatment of osteochondritis dissecans of the patella. *Am J Sports Med.* 1988;16:522–529.

26. Aglietti P, Buzzi R, Bassi PB, et al. Arthroscopic drilling in juvenile osteochondritis dissecans of the medial femoral condyle. *Arthroscopy.* 1994;10:286–291.

27. Cain EL, Clancy WG. Treatment algorithm for osteochondral injuries of the knee. *Clin Sports Med.* 2001;20:321–342.

28. Kocher MS, Micheli LJ, Yaniv M, et al. Functional and radiographic outcomes of juvenile osteochondritis dissecans of the knee treated with transarticular drilling. *Am J Sports Med.* 2001;29:562–566.

29. Wall E, Von Stein D. Juvenile osteochondritis dissecans. *Orthop Clin North Am.* 2003;34:341–353.

30. Robertson W, Kelly BT. Green DW. Osteochondritis dissecans of the knee in children. *Curr Opin Pediatr.* 2003;15:38–44.

31. Frederico DJ, Lynch J, Jokl P. Osteochondritis dissecans of the knee: a historical review of etiology and treatment. *Arthroscopy.* 1990;6:190–197.

32. Wright RW, Mclean M, Matava MJ, et al. Osteochondritis dissecans of the knee: long term results of excision of the fragment. *Clin Orthop Relat Res.* 2004;424:239–243.

33. Anderson AF, Pagnani M. Osteochondritis dissecans of the femoral condyles: long term results of excision of the fragment. *Am J Sports Med.* 1997;25:830–834.

34. Twyman RS, Desai K, Aichroth PM. Osteochondritis dissecans of the knee: a long term study. *J Bone Joint Surg Br.* 1991;73:461–464.

35. Aglietti P, Ciardullo A, Giron F, et al. Results of arthroscopic excision of the fragments in the treatment of osteochondritis dissecans of the knee. *Arthroscopy.* 2001;17:741–746.

36. Anderson AF, Richards D, Pagani MJ, et al. Antegrade drilling for osteochondritis dissecans of the knee. *Arthroscopy.* 1997;13:319–324.

37. Bradford G, Svendsen R. Synovitis of the knee after intra articular fixation with biofix: report of two cases. *Acta Orthop Scand.* 1992;63:680–681.

38. Freidrichs MG, Greis PE, Burks RT. Pitfalls associated with fixation of osteochondritis dissecans fragments using bioabsorbable screws. *Arthroscopy.* 2001;17:542–545.

39. Wu JZ, Herzog W, Hasler EM. Inadequate placement of osteochondral plugs may induce abnormal stress strain distributions in articular cartilage—finite element stimulations. *Med Eng Phys.* 2002;24:85–97.

40. Peterson L, Minas T, Brittberg M, et al. Treatment of osteochondritis dissecans of the knee with autologous chondrocyte transplantation: results at two to ten years. *J Bone Joint Surg Am.* 2003;85:17–24.

41. Marcacci M, Zaffagnini S, Kon E, et al. Arthroscopic autologous chondrocyte transplantation: technical note. *Knee Surg Sports Traumatol Arthrosc.* 2002;10(3):154–159.

42. Mano JF, Silva GA, Azevedo HS, et al. Natural origin biodegradable systems in tissue engineering and regenerative medicine: present status and some moving trends. *J R Soc Interface* 2007, 4:999–1030.

43. Kon E, Delcogliano M, Filardo G, et al. A novel nanocomposite multi-layered biomaterial for treatment of osteochondral lesions: technique note and an early stability pilot clinical trial. *Injury.* 2010 Jul;41(7):693–701.

44. Kon E, Delcogliano M, Filardo G, et al. Novel nano-composite multilayered biomaterial for osteochondral regeneration: a pilot clinical trial. *Am J Sports Med.* 2011 Jun;39(6):1180–90.

45. Mackay AM, Beck SC, Murphy JM, et al. Chondrogenic differentiation of cultured human mesenchymal stem cells from marrow. *Tissue Eng.* 1998 Winter;4(4):415–428.

46. Fortier LA, Mohammed HO, Lust G, Nixon, AJ. Insulin-like growth factor-I enhances cell-based repair of articular cartilage. *J Bone Joint Surg Br.* 2002 ;84(2):276–288.

47. Nixon AJ, Wilke MM, Nydam DV. Enhanced early chondrogenesis in articular defects following arthroscopic mesenchymal stem cell implantation in an equine model. *J Orthop Res.* 2007. Jul; 25(7): 913–225.

48. Nakamura Y, Sudo K, Kanno M, et al. Mesenchymal progenitors able to differentiate into osteogenic, chondrogenic, and/or adipogenic cells in vitro are present in most primary fibroplast like cell populations. *Stem Cells.* 2007 Jul; 25(7): 1610–1617.

49. Wakitani S, Yokoyama M, Miwa H, et al. Influence of fetal calf serum on differentiation of mesenchymal stem cells to chondrocytes during expansion. *J Biosci Bioeng.* 2008 Jul; 106(1): 46–50.

50. Grigolo B, Lisignoli G, Desando G, et al. Osteoarthritis treated with mesenchymal stem cells on hyaluronan-based scaffold in rabbit. *Tissue Eng Part C Methods.* 2009 Dec;15(4):647–658.

51. Gobbi A, Karnatzikos G, Scotti C, et al. One-step cartilage repair with bone marrow aspirate concentrated cells and collagen matrix in full- thickness knee cartilage lesions: results at 2-year follow-up. *Cartilage.* 2011;2(3):286–299.

Chondral Injuries in the Knee

Onur Hapa • F. Alan Barber

INTRODUCTION AND OVERVIEW

Articular cartilage damage is common with sports-related injuries and often observed at arthroscopic surgery. Articular cartilage damage was found in 63% of more than 31,000 arthroscopies. The medial femoral condyle and the patellar surface were the most frequently injured sites (1). Although these articular cartilage lesions seem to be localized and limited in scope, what they represent for the future of the knee may not be innocuous.

The treatment of articular cartilage injury in the athlete presents several challenges. Not only does the average athlete wish to return to full activity as quickly as possible but the expectation that this will happen through the normal course of medical treatment also sometimes raises unrealistic expectations. In addition, more individuals are currently continuing their athletic activities longer, with the result that older patients are now included in the population sustaining athletic articular cartilage damage.

The knee articular cartilage has a complex structure and plays a vital role in normal athletic activity. It transmits loads uniformly across the joint and provides a smooth, low-friction, gliding surface. The lack of a vascular response and the relative absence of an undifferentiated cell population to respond to injury make damage to the articular cartilage a problem and limit its healing capacity. Localized full-thickness defects and contusions can cause significant symptoms and are especially problematic because of the potential for these lesions to progress. This is compounded by the natural environment of athletic participation during which the knee is repeatedly loaded, and the potential for violent contact with the ground or other participants exists.

Articular cartilage is a smooth, viscoelastic, hypocellular structure providing a low coefficient of friction. It has the ability to withstand significant recurring compressive loads. Articular cartilage has a large extracellular matrix composed principally of type II collagen (60% of the dry weight of cartilage) (2). The collagen fibers provide form and tensile strength, and water gives it substance by comprising 75% to 80% of the extracellular matrix. The cellular component (chondrocytes) synthesizes and degrades proteoglycans and is the metabolically active portion of this structure.

The articular cartilage injury can occur from shear forces associated with an anterior cruciate ligament (ACL) tear or blunt force trauma to the joint surface. This may result in the injury or death of articular chondrocytes. Although this can play a role in the development of articular cartilage degeneration after injury, such an injury may not be readily apparent at first. Areas of chondral injury and subchondral bone edema (bruising) are often seen on MRI with ACL tears.

The extent and implications of this injury may not be initially appreciated and may be one explanation for the late appearance of degenerative change after ACL reconstruction. If the articular cartilage is damaged, a defect may develop. Increased contact pressure is then placed on the edges of the articular cartilage defect and any exposed subchondral bone. This leads to overloading and degeneration of the defect with an expansion of the lesion. As this progresses, the exposed bone contacts the opposing articular cartilage, leading to bipolar injury and ultimately a bone-on-bone lesion.

The goal of the treatment of articular cartilage injury is to remove any tissue that is creating a problem and if needed replace it with durable tissue that not only fills the defect but also integrates well with the adjacent articular cartilage and does not deteriorate over time. One challenge of treating articular cartilage injury is its lack of a blood supply or an endogenous source of new cells, resulting in very limited spontaneous healing. The reparative process may result in fibrous tissue, degenerating hyaline tissue, fibrocartilage, or bone (3). The type of tissue created will determine the long-term clinical success. Factors affecting the repair quality include the patient's age, lesion size, lesion depth, associated ligament instability, meniscus loss, angular malalignment, and the acuteness of the injury when treatment occurs.

CLINICAL EVALUATION

History

Chondral damage can be caused by various mechanisms of injury including a pivoting twisting fall, a direct impact on the knee, ACL tear, or a patellar dislocation. A traumatic hemarthrosis can be associated with chondral injury. Sometimes, no specific traumatic event is recalled and the patient only reports pain with weight bearing.

Pain is usually localized to one knee compartment. A persistent dull aching pain is often reported that worsens after activity and may be most noticeable when the patient attempts to fall asleep. Loaded activities such as running, stair climbing, rising from a chair, and squatting may aggravate these symptoms. Sitting for prolonged times such as in an automobile, a theater, or on an airplane may aggravate pain from a patellar lesion. In addition to pain, the patient may complain of swelling, crepitus, giving way, catching, and locking of the knee. This tends to be activity induced, but varies widely from patient to patient.

Physical Examination

Joint line tenderness, an effusion, and quadriceps atrophy are sometimes present, depending on the patient's activity prior to the evaluation. It is important to evaluate limb alignment looking for varus or valgus change, hyperextension, or flexion contractures. For patellar or trochlear lesions, subpatellar crepitus, patellar grind, and pull-through sensitivity are often observed. Patellar tracking, the Q angle, and lateral retinaculum tightness should be evaluated. Associated lesions should be considered and meniscal signs and joint instability should be evaluated as well.

Imaging

A standard radiographic office evaluation should include the standing anterior–posterior view of both legs in full extension to look for angular changes and to compare joint space height. If this is not revealing, a 45° flexion posterior–anterior weight-bearing view to identify subtle joint space narrowing that the extension view does not demonstrate should be obtained. A nonweight-bearing lateral view obtained in 45° flexion in which the posterior femoral condyles overlap, an axial view of both patellae to help evaluate the patellar alignment, and an anterior–posterior knee flexion view to outline the femoral intercondylar notch should also be routinely obtained.

MRI can help outline the articular cartilage surface and demonstrate localized full-thickness lesions in a patient with otherwise normal standard radiographs. A layer of fluid or edema surrounding an articular cartilage lesion suggests that it may be detached. The two most widely used imaging techniques are the T1-weighted fat-suppressed three-dimensional (3D) spoiled gradient echo technique and the T2-weighted fast spin-echo technique. Software advances and newer MRI techniques with intravenous or intra-articular enhancement continue to improve the evaluation of articular cartilage.

Three-dimensional pulse sequence techniques are being used for preoperative assessments of articular cartilage defects to determine defect size and cartilage volume. The use of quantitative MRI to detect changes in the ultrastructure and biochemistry of articular cartilage is a developing technique for the evaluation of cartilage repair as well. These techniques assess either the proteoglycan content (sodium imaging, delayed gadolinium enhanced imaging, T1ρ mapping) or the collagen orientation (T2 mapping) within the cartilage repair tissue. In addition, higher field strengths (3.0-T magnets) with higher in-plane resolution are being used. Preoperative and postoperative cartilage assessment should be done with magnets having a 1.5-T strength or greater.

Classification

A consistent method of evaluating articular cartilage lesions is important to facilitate communication, arrive at a prognosis, and devise an appropriate treatment plan. This evaluation should consider the size and depth of the lesion as well as its location, any subchondral bone damage, and associated knee pathology such as an ACL or meniscal tear.

The Outerbridge classification system is commonly used for articular cartilage lesions (4). In this system, articular cartilage damage of grade 1 shows surface softening or blistering, grade 2 shows fibrillation or superficial fissures less than 1 cm in diameter, grade 3 shows deep fissuring extending into the subchondral bone without exposed bone, measuring more than 1 cm in diameter, and grade 4 shows exposed subchondral bone (Fig. 65.1). The modified International Cartilage Repair Society (ICRS) chondral injury classification system (5) was more recently developed (Fig. 65.2). This system is based on the depth and amount of the cartilage injury. ICRS grade 1 injuries are superficial with a soft indentation or superficial fissures and cracks. ICRS grade 2 lesions involve less than half of the cartilage depth, whereas ICRS grade 3 lesions involve half or more of the cartilage depth, but not into the subchondral bone. ICRS grade 4 lesions extend to include the subchondral bone.

Decision-Making Algorithms

Articular cartilage treatment algorithms depend on the size and the depth of a lesion. The possibility for reattachment of a mobile fragment associated with the lesion exists only if the subchondral bone is viable. Some type IV lesions have associated bone loss. If the depth of loss is greater than 8 mm, marrow-stimulating techniques and autologous chondrocyte implantation (ACI) are not suitable choices and bone grafting to fill the defect should be performed either as part of an autograft or allograft procedure or as an independent initial step prior to ACI. Figure 65.3 outlines the treatment options based on these factors.

Osteochondritis Dissecans

Osteochondritis dissecans (OCD) is the term used for the separation of the articular cartilage with underlying

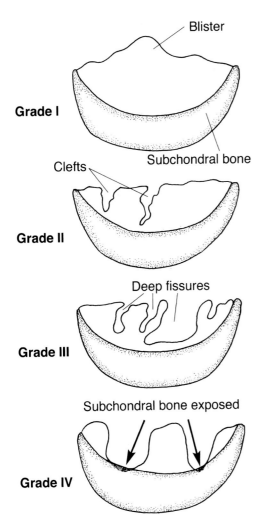

FIGURE 65.1. The Outerbridge classification for articular cartilage lesions. (From Browne JE, Branch TP. Surgical alternative for treatment of articular cartilage lesions. *J. Am Acad Orthop Surg.* 2000;8:180–189.)

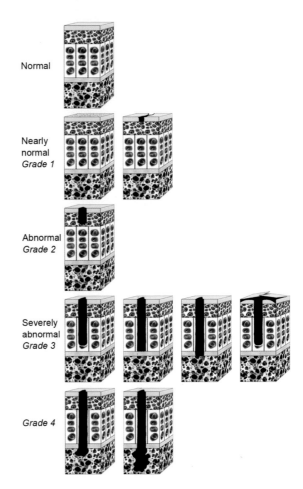

FIGURE 65.2. The ICRS chondral injury classification system. (Adapted from Brittberg M, Winalski CS. Evaluation of cartilage injuries and repair. *J Bone Joint Surg Am.* 2003;85(suppl 2):58–69.)

subchondral bony segment. It is divided into the juvenile (open physis) and the adult (closed physis) forms. Its etiology is unclear. It is more frequently seen in adolescent males with an increase in its prevalence and a decrease in the mean age of OCD patients noted in recent years. OCD is **most commonly located** in the posterolateral aspect of the medial femoral condyle. It usually manifests itself with vague, nonspecific symptoms. For diagnosis, comparative plain radiographs including the notch view are required. However, differentiating this condition from anatomical variations of normal ossification is difficult. An MRI helps distinguish between these two conditions and helps estimate the lesion size, status of the cartilage, and "stability of the OCD lesion" for deciding the treatment option. Treatment options consist of nonoperative (immobilization, isometric muscle strengthening, range-of-motion exercises, and nonweight bearing for 8 to 12 weeks) and operative treatment. The stability of the lesion is the most important consideration in selecting the appropriate treatment option. Size, weight-bearing surface, and the affected condyle

are also important determinants of the prognosis. Operative treatment options include drilling of the OCD fragment in situ or operative fragment reduction followed by fixation using either Kirschner wires, compression screws, bone pegs, bioabsorbable screws, or fibrin glue. In the presence of a devitalized free fragment or a multifragmented piece that is not amenable to fixation, the techniques used for repair of focal chondral defects, such as microfracture, osteochondral autograft, autologous chondrocyte transfer, and fresh osteochondral grafting, can be used.

TREATMENT

Nonoperative

Arthroscopically, it is not uncommon to find Outerbridge type I or II chondral damage that does not require intervention. Smaller type III lesions that are asymptomatic can be observed and treated nonoperatively especially in athletes participating in low-impact activities. Small painful type III lesions may become asymptomatic once the acute synovitis resolves. Long-term studies suggest that isolated

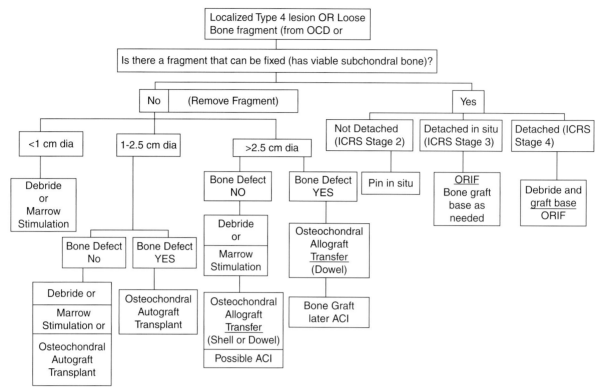

FIGURE 65.3. Articular Cartilage Treatment Algorithm.

chondral lesions less than 1 cm in diameter have an excellent or good prognosis without treatment and may be left alone (6). Intervention should be postponed as long as these areas do not cause symptoms.

Nonoperative care includes nonsteroidal anti-inflammatory drugs, physical therapy, activity modification, and possibly bracing. Bracing options include patellar-stabilizing braces for patellofemoral instability and load shifting shoe orthotics or knee braces for valgus or varus changes observed radiographically not responding to activity modification. Intra-articular injection of hyaluronic acid or steroid can be helpful.

Evaluating the particular position the athlete plays may provide opportunities for continued participation while "resting" the joint. Changes in an exercise program or technique may also prove helpful. Nonoperative treatment for an athlete is often based on the player's position and the sport's seasonal cycle. Operating on a player in the middle of his season can be a difficult choice and it is often better to wait until the season is over before surgery is performed. Although less than ideal, the future impact of such a choice on the knee's prognosis and the potential consequences of the various treatment options should be thoroughly discussed with the athlete and the athlete's family.

Operative Indications

The surgical indications for articular cartilage injury include significant, symptomatic type III and type IV

lesions that have failed an appropriate nonoperative trial, the presence of loose bodies, and symptomatic OCD lesion not responding to nonoperative treatment. The goal of this surgery is to relieve symptoms including pain, swelling, catching, locking, and giving way, stabilize areas of irregular articular cartilage hopefully preventing further deterioration, to stabilize mobile or loose osteochondritis dessicans lesions, and to remove any unstable or loose fragments of articular cartilage and bone.

Unstable OCD fragment with viable subchondral bone or fresh traumatic fragments with viable bone can be primarily repaired (fixed to the bone bed). Articular cartilage lesions with loose osteochondral fragments (especially those >2 cm diameter) require immediate intervention to assess the potential to reattach a viable fragment. The chances of successful nonoperative treatment for these cases are low and the risks of progressive damage are high if allowed to go untreated.

TECHNIQUES

Debridement

Debridement of Outerbridge type III and IV lesions is an appropriate primary treatment for smaller lesions, especially in older, low-demand patients, and for those lesions associated with few symptoms (Fig. 65.4). The best results seem to be in younger patients with symptoms less than 1 year in duration, a specific history of trauma, no prior

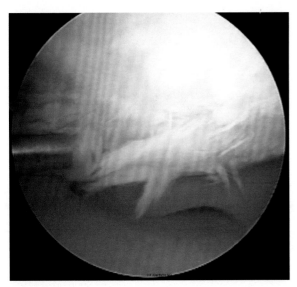

FIGURE 65.4. Debridement of Outerbridge type III and IV lesions is appropriate for smaller lesions, low-demand patients, and incidentally observed lesions with few symptoms.

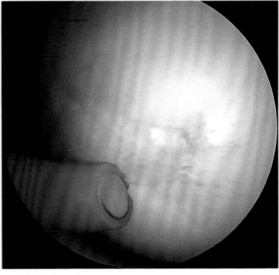

FIGURE 65.5. A monopolar thermal probe is used to treat Outerbridge type III damage on the medial femoral condyle.

surgery, little to no malalignment, and a low BMI (7). The debridement should only remove unstable chondral fragments causing mechanical symptoms and that are likely to become detached with additional activity or trauma. Mechanical debridement does not stimulate articular cartilage repair, and there is a risk that the adjacent hyaline cartilage can be damaged (8). With additional trauma, these additional areas can progress to osteoarthritis.

Mechanical debridement using a motorized shaver may use blades varying from an aggressive open-faced blade to one with small fenestrations (whisker blade) that is less likely to dig into normal articular cartilage. Damaged articular cartilage should be carefully probed to assess the extent of the softening and fragmentation before shaving. Only fragmented areas (Outerbridge type III) should be debrided. Any unstable edges of type IV lesions should also be debrided. On occasion, the shaver blade may not be able to completely debride a flap of articular cartilage and a basket punch is needed.

Once the extent and location of the lesion is appreciated, the shaver is inserted and brought into contact with the damaged articular cartilage. Little pressure on the shaver blade and a moderate amount of suction is required to perform this procedure. A back-and-forth sweeping motion is used to remove the prominent fragments. It is helpful to turn the cutting face of the shaver on its side so that the open face is at a 90° angle to the articular cartilage surface. The suction will lift the fragments into the rotating shaver blade that amputates them. Additional portals may be needed (especially for the patella) to address all the damaged areas without digging into the tissue excessively. Once a stable base is achieved, the debridement is terminated.

The use of thermal treatment for type III damage has been advocated in the past but has fallen into disfavor (Fig. 65.5).

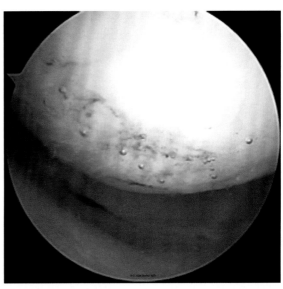

FIGURE 65.6. Thermal treatment of type III chondral lesions seals the cartilage, provides a smoother surface, and may prevent the extension of the lesion.

Advocates of the thermal technique suggested that thermal treatment seals the cartilage, provides a smoother surface as seen with scanning electron microscopes, and may prevent the extension of the lesion (Fig. 65.6). If thermal treatment is selected, it should be applied to the area after the mechanical debridement is concluded. Concerns about heat damage to the adjacent macroscopically undamaged articular cartilage and subchondral bone have been raised. Treatment of the articular cartilage with heat causes immediate chondrocyte death. In addition, the type of heat application may be significant. Bipolar devices penetrate 78% to 92% deeper than monopolar systems and reach the subchondral bone when a paintbrush pattern is utilized (9). Although concerns about the long-term safety and effectiveness of this technique have lead to a significant reduction in its use, there are some data which suggest it is more effective than shaver debridement (10).

Rehabilitation

Progressive weight bearing is allowed starting immediately after surgery using crutches as needed. An aggressive exercise program is allowed, and depending on the extent of the articular cartilage damage, high-impact activities may begin as early as 3 to 4 weeks after surgery if the swelling has resolved and strength and pain permit. However, if full-thickness articular cartilage loss or extensive type III damage exists in the weight-bearing areas, high-impact activities such as running should be avoided.

Marrow Stimulation (Drilling, Microfracture, Abrasion)

Subchondral marrow-stimulation techniques have been utilized for many years. Initially this consisted of penetrating the subchondral bone with multiple drill holes (Pridie) (11) and later the technique of abrasion arthroplasty. Recently the use of variously angled picks was found to be easier than the more cumbersome drilling technique (microfracture). These techniques facilitate access to the vascular system and result in the development of a fibrocartilage scar that deteriorates over time. The initial reports of drilling were by Pridie[11] who observed that treated areas became covered by a fibrous scar and resulted in clinical improvement. Later Johnson (12) advocated an arthroscopic variation of the technique called abrasion arthroplasty. This technique was principally indicated for extensive osteoarthritic knee surfaces. It required the abrasion of the entire surface removing 1 to 2 mm of bone in the involved area followed by a period of nonweight bearing of up to 8 weeks. Most of the subjects were older with degenerative arthritic changes and some reports of this technique showed poor clinical outcomes. This technique has few advocates today and was controversial even at its greatest popularity.

Penetrating the subchondral bone by either a drill or a pick is a common option for smaller localized areas (Fig. 65.7) (13). This technique provides a healing vascular response, leading to a fibrocartilage scar in the defect. Any chondral flaps are removed and the calcified cartilage layer is lightly debrided without damaging the underlying subchondral bone. Although there is no direct scientific proof about the exact origin of the healing tissue, the process by which this scar forms is thought by some to be through an influx of undifferentiated, mesenchymal cells from the subchondral marrow. It is recognized that this tissue response can be both unpredictable and variable. In addition, it is unclear whether this repair tissue responds well to compression and shear loads or whether it can withstand these stresses over time. The reported clinical results indicate an 80% "improved" status at an average of 7 years after treatment (13). However, no control group has been studied.

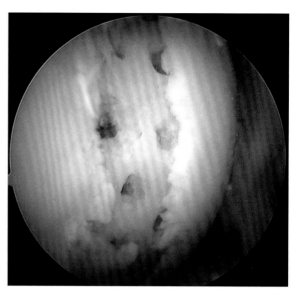

FIGURE 65.7. For smaller, more localized areas penetrating the subchondral bone by either a drill or a pick is a common option.

Various angled picks are used for this technique (13) to perforate the subchondral bone. These picks are said to be superior to subchondral penetration by drilling because of less heat generation, which is suggested to be less destructive to the bone, by providing better access to the curved portions of the femoral condyle, a consistent depth of penetration, and the creation of holes that are perpendicular to the subchondral plate. Although the use of an angled pick certainly permits an easier access to the more posterior lesions, whether the depth and angle of penetration make any difference and whether, considering the cool aqueous arthroscopic environment, any significant heat difference exists between that created by the use of a pick and a small smooth drill is not established.

Technique

The marrow-stimulation techniques require bed preparation by using a curette or a full-radius shaver blade to remove any remaining fragments of articular cartilage. Loose fragments should also be removed at the lesion's margin and vertical walls of well-attached healthy cartilage should be created. The subchondral plate should not be penetrated, but the calcified cartilage layer above it removed with the curette. Multiple penetrating holes are placed 3 to 4 mm apart throughout the bed of the lesion (Fig. 65.8).

The indications for marrow-stimulation techniques include grade 4 degenerative areas or focal traumatic full-thickness lesions. Contraindications for this technique are areas with significant subchondral bone loss, malaligned knees, and noncompliant patients.

Positive prognostic factors for the marrow-stimulation techniques are an age below 30, a nonweight bearing, condylar location, lesions less than 2 cm², a BMI (14) of less than 25 kg per m², a duration of symptoms of less than 12 months, no prior surgical interventions, and the degree

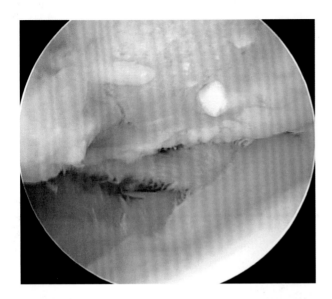

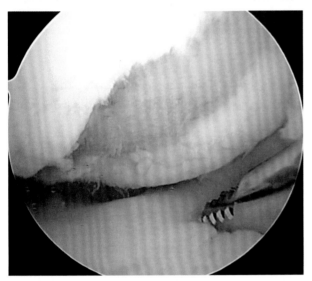

of subsequent defect filling at MRI (15). Results of microfracture may deteriorate in high-demand athletes.

Rehabilitation

The initially described postoperative treatment for the microfracture technique included continuous passive motion (CPM) for up to 8 hours a day and nonweight bearing for 8 weeks. A stationary bicycle program began 1 to 2 weeks after surgery. Full weight bearing was allowed starting 8 weeks after surgery followed by a progressive strengthening program. The rehabilitation program for the patellofemoral lesions was more aggressive. Controversy exists about the necessity of using CPM or limiting weight bearing. Some reports suggest that microfracture outcomes are equivalent after allowing weight bearing as tolerated and without the use of a CPM.

Osteochondral Autograft Transfer

Osteochondral autografting transfers a cylindrical plug of osteochondral material that includes normal articular cartilage with viable chondrocytes and the underlying attached viable subchondral bone from a nonarticulating portion of the joint into a full-thickness articular cartilage defect. Several different equipment systems are available to accomplish this transfer and various brand names include COR (DePuy Mitek, Raynham, MA), OATS (Arthrex, Naples, FL), and Mosaicplasty (Smith & Nephew Endoscopy, Andover, MA).

Focal full thickness, traumatic defects of the femoral condyle are the principal indication for this technique (Fig. 65.9). The lesion should be unipolar, between 1 and 2.5 cm in diameter, and in a stable normally aligned joint. Generalized osteoarthritic change or lesions in multiple sites are contraindications.

The advantages of the osteochondral autograft transplantation are that it provides noninflammatory healing

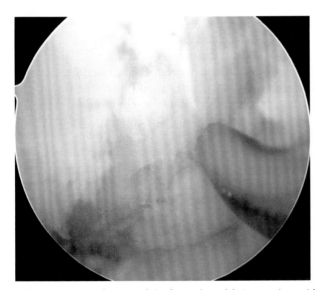

FIGURE 65.8. Microfracture of the femoral condyle in a patient with an acute ACL injury and chondral injury. **(A)** Initial lesion **(B)** debridement of the margins and calcified cartilage layer **(C)** microfracture of the base using angled awls.

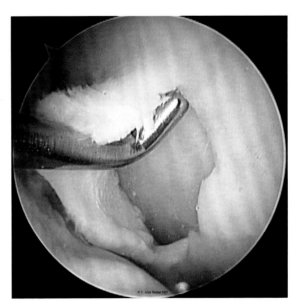

FIGURE 65.9. Focal symptomatic, full-thickness, traumatic defects of the femoral condyle are the principal indication for chondral osseous transplantation.

with a potentially arthroscopic technique using 3D autologous materials that are readily available and can address lesions that also have bone loss. The single-step procedure carries a much lower cost than allografting or cartilage cloning techniques and can be done in an outpatient setting. The disadvantages include the limited number of autograft plugs that can be obtained from a single knee making the treatment of lesions greater than 2.5 cm in diameter difficult, the technically challenging nature of the arthroscopic technique, the requirement to remove normal articular material for the repair, and the difficulty in restoring a surface congruent with the convex condylar surface.

The results of chondral osseous autograft transplantation were compared with abrasion arthroplasty, microfracture, and subchondral drilling of lesions between 1 and 9 cm^2. Subchondral bone penetration resulted in a deterioration of results over time. Marrow-stimulating procedures demonstrated improvements ranging from 48% to 62%, whereas the improvement achieved by chondral osseous autograft transplantation remained at 86% to 90% for 5 years (16).

A recent study reported significant clinical improvement with patellar resurfacing, but they reported that the plug cartilage did not incorporate fully and that "fissures at the interface" with the host cartilage remained whereas the bony part of the plug incorporated readily with the adjacent bone (17). Another study reported slower recovery for autologous chondrocyte implantation (ACI) patients compared with an autologous osteochondral transplantation group. Histologically the ACI group healed with fibrocartilage while the autologous osteochondral transplantation group retained hyaline articular cartilage tissue but with a persistent gap between the host and the implanted graft tissue (18).

Autologous osteochondral transplants are reported to clinically improve at 7-year follow-up; however, there was a trend toward decreased sports activity between the 2nd and the 7th year. Smaller defect sizes and fewer grafts offered better clinical outcomes (19). Another study comparing autologous osteochondral transplantation with microfracture indicated that in highly competitive, athletic patients better clinical, histologic, and radiographic healing was observed after autologous osteochondral transplantation than microfracture (20).

Technique

The technique requires the careful evaluation and preparation of the lesion to determine the number of grafts needed. The defect base should be debrided of articular cartilage flaps and the margins of the lesion shaped with a curette to create vertical walls of healthy articular cartilage (Fig. 65.10). Various plug sizes are available, but the 6-mm -diameter size offers the advantages of conforming better to the contour of the femoral condyle than larger grafts and leaving a smaller donor lesion less likely to cause problems of its own. Considering that a lesion of 10 mm

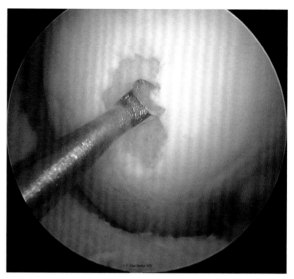

FIGURE 65.10. The defect base should be debrided of articular cartilage flaps and the margins of the lesion shaped with a curette to create vertical walls of healthy cartilage.

diameter is an indication for grafting, harvesting a 10-mm graft defeats the purpose of using this grafting technique.

Once the size and number of the grafts to be used is determined, using the DePuy Mitek system, the recipient sites in the defect are drilled with the appropriately sized COR drill bit under direct arthroscopic visualization, keeping the drill perpendicular to the articular surface. The projecting tooth at the drill tip keeps the drill from "walking" and allows for precise recipient site placement by creating a starter hole. The fluted drill's concave sides remove bone during drilling and reduce both friction and heat.

The drill is advanced to the appropriate depth using the graduated laser markings varying from 5 to 20 mm found on the side of the drill. The selected line is compared with the level of the adjacent articular cartilage. In cases of subchondral bone loss, the depth should be under drilled to restore the contour and height of the articular surface. This is accomplished by aligning the laser mark with the desired articular cartilage height. All recipient holes can be drilled at the same time or sequentially after autograft insertion (Fig. 65.11). Once the desired depth is achieved, the drill is removed and the debris removed with a motorized shaver. Care should be taken to maintain a bone bridge between recipient sites of 2 to 3 mm and to avoid recipient site convergence.

Harvesting of osteochondral plugs from the donor site can be an arthroscopic or open procedure. The donor sites commonly used are the superior lateral intercondylar notch (Fig. 65.12), the lateral femoral trochlea, or the medial femoral trochlea above the linea terminalis. Contact pressures are lower in the intercondylar notch and medial trochlea, but available harvest material is limited. Higher contact pressures are found in the lateral trochlea, but these decrease more posteriorly.

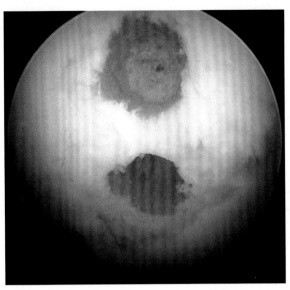

FIGURE 65.11. The drilled recipient sites should be placed immediately adjacent to the vertical articular wall of normal cartilage.

Once the number of plugs to be obtained is determined and the recipient sites prepared, the harvester is inserted into the disposable cutter. The retropatellar fat pad should be completely debrided to improve visualization and avoid soft tissue entrapment. The COR Harvester Delivery Guide comes with the cutting tool preassembled as a single unit. The perpendicularity rod should be inserted into this Harvester/Cutter assembly prior to its insertion into the joint. The perpendicularity rod will function as an obturator and minimize both soft tissue capture and fluid loss as the assembly is inserted into the knee. The Harvester Delivery Guide/Cutter/perpendicularity rod assembly is positioned on the donor site in preparation for the graft harvest. The perpendicularity rod is used to confirm the perpendicular position of the cutter and then removed. The arthroscope can be rotated to view this alignment from several angles and confirm this alignment.

Using a mallet and continuing to hold the harvester perpendicular to the articular cartilage in all planes, the Harvester Delivery Guide/Cutter is tapped to the desired depth based on the laser markings on the side of the harvester. A unique feature of the COR system is the tooth on the cutting face of the harvester. This tooth underscores the cancellous bone at the distal end of the harvester tube and creates a precise and consistent depth cut. The T-handle of the harvester is rotated clockwise at least two full rotations, underscoring the distal end of the bone plug and creating a precise harvest depth. The plug is then removed by gently twisting the T-handle while withdrawing the plug. Care should be taken to avoid toggling the donor hole.

It is important to consider the potential deleterious effects of what is called a "zone of influence," which in turn can lead to defect increase, collapse of the surrounding bone, and the articular cartilage at the periphery, due to the unsupported walls of a defect. These grafts should not be large and it is better to obtain two smaller grafts than one large graft.

Once the graft is harvested, the Harvester Delivery Guide/Cutter is placed on a firm surface. The Harvester Delivery Guide/Cutter is inserted into the graft loader and pushed down until it makes contact with the bottom of the loader. The harvested graft will be pushed from the cancellous bone side of the graft plug upward into the Harvester/Delivery Guide and out of the cutter section (Fig. 65.13).

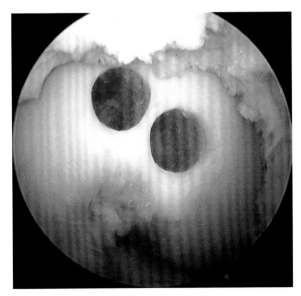

FIGURE 65.12. The superior lateral intercondylar notch is a common donor site.

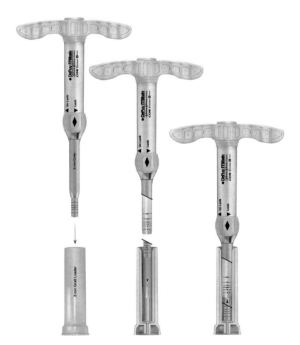

FIGURE 65.13. Loading of the harvested graft onto the harvester/delivery device is accomplished without the application of force onto the articular cartilage surface.

A load noise usually accompanies this transfer. Notably, this transfer places no pressure on the articular cartilage surface. This is significant because the effects of impact load during surgical harvesting and transfer of osteochondral plugs must be considered and kept to a minimum. Blunt trauma consistently results in articular chondrocyte death. When the harvester is disconnected from the cutter the graft plug remains inside the harvester until it can be implanted. This transfer system eliminates any load to the articular surface of the graft and eliminates the danger of chondrocyte damage in this step.

Once the harvester tube is removed from the delivery assembly, the graft plug can be observed in the clear plastic insertion tube. The harvested plug is then inserted into the defect, keeping a vertical insertion orientation and being aware of any variation in the articular cartilage contour (Fig. 65.14).

The plastic plunger is placed in the harvester delivery system and the loaded harvester–clear plastic delivery guide system is inserted into the knee. It may be necessary to enlarge this portal slightly to permit passage of the delivery guide system. The clear end of the delivery system is held perpendicular to the recipient site outlet, and aligning the articular cartilage of the autograft with the adjacent articular cartilage, implanted with gentle tapping until it is flush with the articular cartilage. A minimal amount of pressure is required with this system for this transfer minimizing chondrocyte damage.

If more than one graft is needed to repair an articular cartilage defect, the Harvester/Delivery Guide and Cutter are reassembled and the process repeated until the defect is completely filled. A 2- to 3-mm bone bridge should be maintained between the drilled holes to allow for a secure graft press fit. The osteochondral autograft plug should

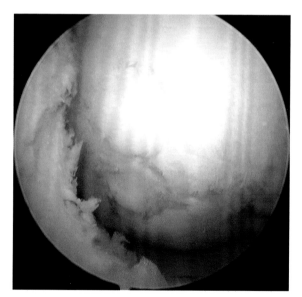

FIGURE 65.14. The osteochondral autograft plugs should be flush with the adjacent surface. A tamp can be used to adjust the height to match the adjacent articular cartilage level.

not stand proud and if it is after insertion, a tamp should be used to adjust the height to match the adjacent articular cartilage surface.

Rehabilitation

The postoperative protocol for autograft transplantation includes immediate early motion and nonweight bearing for 3 weeks. These grafts are held in place by the press fit design. They heal into position rapidly and progressive weight bearing is allowed starting at 3 and continuing through 6 weeks after surgery. Full weight bearing is permitted after 6 weeks. At that point a progressive rehabilitation program can be initiated.

Osteochondral Allograft Transfer

The implantation of composite fresh cadaveric allografts can also address full-thickness articular cartilage defects. These allografts come in various shapes and sizes and have both intact articular cartilage and subchondral bone. Optimizing the survival of the transplanted chondrocytes is a challenge. The grafts cannot be frozen, but maintaining them at 4°C for up to 4 days will preserve 100% viability of the cartilage cells along with the cellular elements of the subchondral bone. Implantation within the first week after harvest is recommended, but this creates a potential antigenic exposure and viral transmission risk (21).

As with osteochondral autograft transplantation, allografts are indicated for focal traumatic defects (only larger) of the femoral condyle and large osteochondral lesions such as those seen with osteochondritis dessicans, osteonecrosis, large fractures, and for salvage procedures where other techniques have failed. Full-thickness lesions on the patella and tibia may also be treated. Although usage in the patellofemoral region yields favorable results, the results seem not as good as for the other knee compartments.

Allograft reconstructions are recommended for lesions greater than 3 cm in diameter and with substantial bone loss of 1 cm in depth or more (21). Contraindications include an unstable joint, generalized osteoarthritic changes, and lesions in multiple sites. Relative contraindications include meniscal insufficiency, axial malalignment, inflammatory diseases, and crystal induced arthritis. Osteochondral allografts provide good long-term results, are suitable for larger defects, cause no donor site morbidity, and are appropriate for any size or shape of defect (22). In addition, articular cartilage contours can be more accurately matched. The allograft technique is typically an open rather than arthroscopic procedure. Although it is a single-step procedure, obtaining a well-matched donor femoral condyle requires careful preoperative planning and depends on donor availability.

The disadvantages of allograft transplantation include the potential immune response or disease transmission, limited graft availability, a slower rehabilitation than with autografts, significantly increased costs, and increased pain resulting in an inpatient procedure. Prolonged storage of the fresh allograft decreases chondrocyte viability, but may be required to verify graft safety. A recent clinical study of cases with prolonged graft storage (average 24 days) demonstrated results consistent with previous studies using fresh implanted graft studies with an 84% satisfaction rate at a mean of 3 years follow-up (23). The short-term failure of fresh allograft material depends on chondrocyte viability, which can be addressed by harvesting and storage methods, whereas long-term graft survival depends on the mechanical stability of the implant, precise site matching, and the graft fit with the host bed (22).

Technique

The process for insertion of an allograft starts by determining the correct size requirements. An MRI of the knee should be obtained and is often sent to the tissue bank to aid in sizing an appropriate donor graft. Once a suitable fresh graft is obtained, surgery is scheduled. An arthroscopic procedure has usually been performed previously and any associated lesions already corrected.

Two types of allografts are commonly available: dowel grafts (Fig. 65.15) and shell grafts. Using a dowel plug is similar to that of an osteochondral autograft and is best for well-defined lesions up to 3.5 cm in diameter on the femoral condyle. A circular coring device creates a recipient site encompassing the lesion and the prepared donor plug is press fit into this hole. A shell graft works better for lesions with an irregular shape or contour such as those on the patella, trochlear, or tibia.

Shell grafts are technically more challenging and require fixation. The defect is identified and an outline drawn around it using straight lines. A regular geometric shape is preferred because it is easier to reproduce when cutting the graft by hand. As with other grafting techniques, vertical walls of normal articular cartilage adjacent to the lesion are created using a knife or curette. Once the recipient site is prepared, a template is created using some readily available paper from the back table. This could be from a suture package or sterile cardboard. This template is cut to match the defect and then the template is placed on the allograft. The allograft is marked with a pen and then the cuts are made. The shell graft should retain 5 mm of subchondral bone, and it is better for the graft to be slightly larger than needed at first. The graft is carefully trimmed to the exact size using several trial fittings until the best match is achieved. The articular cartilage of the graft should fit flush or slightly recessed with the adjacent normal articular cartilage. Biodegradable absorbable pins can be used to fix the shell graft in place.

Rehabilitation

The postoperative protocol for allograft transplantation starts with extensive preoperative counseling about what to expect. Immediately after surgery, the patient should emphasize quadriceps activation and achieving full extension. A supervised physical therapy program should be included as well as the use of a constant passive motion machine and nonweight bearing for from 6 to 12 weeks with dowel grafts or nonweight bearing from 8 to 16 weeks for shell grafts. These ranges depend on graft size and location. Full activity may begin at 6 months for femoral condyle grafts and 12 months for tibial plateau grafts. In either case, activity progression is determined by radiographic evidence of healing.

Chondrocyte Implantation

ACI is designed to address traumatic focal lesions on the weight-bearing surface primarily of the femoral condyle and attempts to replace a full-thickness articular cartilage defect with hyaline-like tissue. It is indicated for localized, symptomatic full-thickness articular cartilage lesions of at least 2 cm in diameter in younger patients with good alignment, stability, and otherwise nonarthritic joints. Lesions with bone loss greater than 8 mm are not suitable for cell implantation until bone grafting of the defect is performed and completely heals. Multiple lesions are a contraindication. Any malalignment or ligament instability should be corrected at the time of ACI. ACI is not indicated for the treatment of osteoarthritis including bipolar bone-on-bone lesions and opposing grade 3 chondral damage.

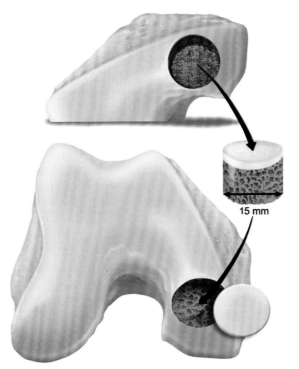

FIGURE 65.15. Allograft dowel graft for implantation into a femoral defect.

15 mm

Good to excellent results with ACI were reported in 92% of isolated femoral condyle lesions, 65% of patellar lesions, and 89% with OCD lesions at 2 to 9 years follow-up (24). One concern about these outcome studies is that the reported success may be due in part to the natural history of chondral injuries or that the debridement performed as part of the procedure rather than the chondrocyte transplantation resulted in the improvement (25). The clinical reports are mixed when ACI is compared with osteochondral autograft transplantation although ACI patients have a slower recovery.[18]

ACI can provide clinical improvement even after previous failed cartilage treatments such as marrow stimulation or debridement (26). A recent prospective study failed to find differences in histologic or clinical scores 5 years postoperatively when ACI-treated patients were compared with microfracture patients (27). A different multicenter, prospective study reported better structural and histologic healing (more chondrocyte-like cells, less fibrous, higher proteoglycan content tissue) with ACI compared with microfracture, but the clinical outcomes were not different for the two groups (28). A second-generation ACI technique demonstrated better clinical improvement and return to sports at 5 years follow-up compared with microfracture patients (27).

Periosteal patch hypertrophy is the most common finding at reoperation and the most common early postoperative complication and can cause mechanical symptoms. Debridement of the hypertrophied tissue is also detrimental to the results at later follow-up (30).

Technique

The ACI technique requires the arthroscopic harvesting of 200 to 300 mg of viable autologous articular cartilage as a separate initial procedure. A gouge or ring curette is used to take a 5 by 10 mm full-thickness segment of articular cartilage. The subchondral bone is not violated to reduce the fibrovascular response. Harvest sites include the superior lateral or medial femoral condyle or the superior lateral intercondylar notch. The harvested articular cartilage is placed in a special sterile container provided by the company filled with a culture medium and sent to the company laboratory where the harvested cells are cultured and induced to increase in number and volume. This process requires at least 3 weeks. When finished, a suspension of autologous chondrocytes containing 12 million cells per 0.4 mL of culture medium is prepared.

Once cloned, the cells are implanted later during a separate procedure using a medial or lateral parapatellar arthrotomy (Fig. 65.16). As with other cartilage repair procedures, clean vertical walls of normal articular cartilage are prepared adjacent to the lesion. Care should be taken not to penetrate the subchondral bone and to prevent bleeding into the defect. It is important that a vertical articular cartilage wall completely surround the lesion to provide a rim to which the periosteum can be sewn. If that is not possible, small suture anchors may be used to

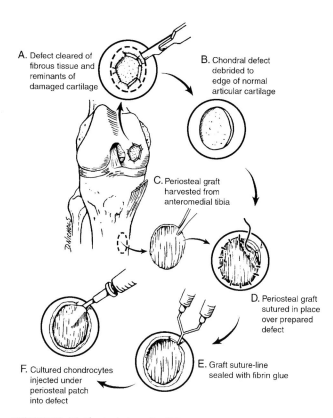

A. Defect cleared of fibrous tissue and reminants of damaged cartilage

B. Chondral defect debrided to edge of normal articular cartilage

C. Periosteal graft harvested from anteromedial tibia

D. Periosteal graft sutured in place over prepared defect

E. Graft suture-line sealed with fibrin glue

F. Cultured chondrocytes injected under periosteal patch into defect

FIGURE 65.16. The technique for ACI.

suture that portion of the patch to the periphery. Bleeding must be completely controlled before proceeding to the next step. The defect is precisely measured and a template prepared using some sterile disposable paper from the back table.

A medial tibial border incision is made and the periosteum exposed. The proximal medial tibia distal to both the pes anserine and the medial collateral ligament insertion is the best periosteal graft harvest site. The periosteum is thicker on the posterior tibial cortex. Remove the overlying fat and fascia from the periosteum before it is harvested leaving the periosteum white and glistening. The periosteum harvested should be oversized by 2 mm in each dimension than the template that was created because the periosteum tends to shrink after harvesting. The periosteal patch should be kept moist and a mark placed on the outer surface to distinguish it from the inner cambium layer that should be sutured to face the bone surface. The tourniquet is then released and hemostasis obtained.

The periosteal patch is sutured to the adjacent articular cartilage with no. 6-0 absorbable sutures on a P-1 cutting needle over the cartilage defect with the cambium layer down and trimmed to fit. The periosteal graft should be taut without wrinkles. A circumferential watertight closure should be performed except at the top of the lesion where the cells will be inserted. The suture knots should be tied on the periosteal side rather than the articular cartilage side and cut with short tails. Injecting saline under the patch can test the watertight status. Once a watertight seal is confirmed, the saline is removed by aspiration through the remaining defect at the top of the patch and the edges sealed with fibrin glue.

The autologous chondrocyte suspension should be carefully removed for the nonsterile vial after the cells are resuspended in the fluid by aspirating and injecting several times. The catheter attached to the syringe containing the cells is inserted through the defect at the top of the patch and the cells slowly injected into the lesion. The opening is then closed with additional sutures and sealed with fibrin glue. The wounds are closed and the knee immobilized for 8 hours to allow the cells to adhere to lesion base (Fig. 65.17).

Rehabilitation

The rehabilitation program slowly returns the patient to full activity. A CPM machine is used 6 to 8 hours a day for up to 6 weeks and nonweight bearing or light touch weight bearing is required for 6 weeks. Patellofemoral mobilization is used to avoid adhesions with the goal of achieving full motion and full weight bearing by 6 weeks. Strengthening exercises are started and progressed between 6 and 12 weeks. Active knee extension should be avoided for the first 12 weeks. A return to full activity is allowed at 8 months.

FUTURE DIRECTIONS

Synthetics

Synthetic materials are a potentially easy and cost-effective alternative to the biologic repair of focal chondral defects. They would present minimal concerns about disease transmission, a single-stage implantation, which could be performed arthroscopically or by a mini-open technique. Such synthetic material properties would include chondroconductivity, osteoconductivity, fixation strength to withstand weight-bearing forces with low friction, a durable surface, and good biocompatibility. From a biomechanical perspective, most synthetics have adequate strength, but the challenge is overcoming the lack of a tissue interface conducive to host tissue ingrowth and replacement. Other issues include wear debris and micromotion, which may lead to the implant loosening. A polyvinyl alcohol-hydrogel is in clinical use in Europe. This implant is available in different diameters and is implantable using an osteochondral press-fit technique. Other synthetics made from biocompatible polyurethane and polyhydrogel are being studied.

Minced cartilage is being investigated as a potential repair technique. Autologous cartilage cells are harvested, minced, and then loaded onto a biodegradable scaffold for insertion into a cartilage defect. The cartilage autograft implantation system (CAIS, DePuy Mitek, Raynham, MA) homogenously distributes the harvested cartilage fragments onto a 3D polyglycolide/polycaprolactone scaffold reinforced by polydioxanone (PDS) mesh, which is secured to the defect with resorbable PDS staples.

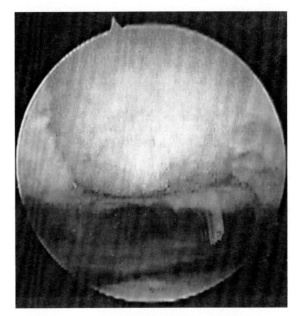
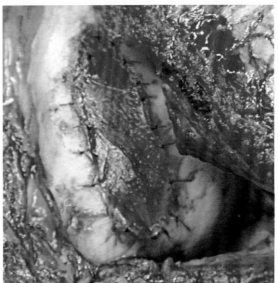
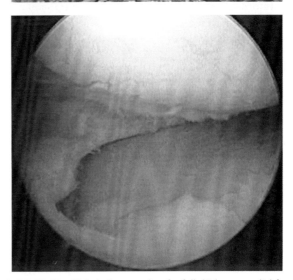

FIGURE 65.17. Clinical photographs of a full-thickness medial femoral condyle defect **(A)** after ACI **(B)** and at arthroscopic reevaluation 18 months postoperatively **(C)**.

A minimum of 200 mg of articular cartilage is required for two 13 × 5 mm grafts. Fibrin sealant is used to stabilize the graft on the scaffold and then the oversized implant is trimmed and secured with staples. The DeNovo ET graft (Zimmer Inc., Warsaw, and ISTO Technologies Inc., St Louis, MO) is another cartilage graft consisting of 1-mm juvenile allograft cartilage cubes that are minced without any enzymatic digestion or biologic manipulation (Fig. 65.18). No marrow stimulation is performed. Fibrin glue adhesive is applied to secure the cartilage pieces and to form secondary fibrin adhesive layer at the defect.

Second-Generation ACI

Original method of ACI relied on a sutured periosteal cover (PACI) to keep the chondrocytes in the desired location. A second-generation autologous chondrocyte technique is collagen-membrane covered ACI (or CACI to distinguish it from the periosteal covered version). In this technique, the implanted chondrocytes are covered with a specialized bilayer collagen membrane instead of a periosteal patch. This appears to reduce graft hypertrophy, results in better results than the periosteal covered version, and decrease the need for reoperation. Matrix-induced autologous chondrocyte implantation (MACI) technique uses a porcine collagen membrane as a substrate for chondrocyte implantation. As with the conventional ACI technique the first surgical step requires articular cartilage harvesting from a nonweight-bearing zone. These chondrocytes are cultured for approximately 4 weeks, which then seeded onto a porcine type I/III matrix membrane that acts as a cell carrier. At a second operation, the defect area is debrided and cleaned. The matrix with the cellular face toward the subchondral bone is implanted and secured to the defect with fibrin glue. Comparable results have been reported in a comparison of PACI and MACI techniques although better results are reported in patients younger than 35 years of age (31).

The Hyalograft C (Fidia Advanced Biopolymers Laboratories, Padova, Italy) is another second-generation ACI technique. It uses a hyaluronan-based scaffold based on the benzyl ester of hyaluronic acid and consists of fibers which allow the chondrocytes to retain their phenotypes. Similar to other cell based repair procedures 150 to 200 mg cartilage tissue is harvested and processed for 6 weeks. At a second procedure, the lesion is debrided and a circular area with regular margins for graft implantation created. The graft is inserted using a press-fit technique. Fibrin glue can be used to augment the fixation of larger lesions (Fig. 65.19). No differences were shown at 5 years follow-up between the conventional PACI and the hyaluronic acid scaffold technique although the conventional open group reported more complications such as graft hypertrophy, delamination, and secondary operations (32). The hyaluronic acid scaffold technique also showed more durable good clinical results and better sports activity resumption compared with microfracture (29).

The Bioseed C technique loads cultured autologous chondrocytes onto a scaffold of polyglactin/poly-*p*-diaxanon fleece using the fibrin glue. The graft can be implanted arthroscopically or by mini-arthrotomy. The graft corners are fixed with sutures transosseously. Complications including graft hypertrophy, delamination, and insufficient tissue regeneration were similar to that of conventional ACI (33).

Fibrin is a normal scaffold for wound healing. BioCart II is a fibrin–hyaluronan matrix (ProChon BioTech Ltd, Ness Ziona, Israel) produced by copolymerization of homologous human fibrinogen and recombinant hyaluronan and is subsequently freeze-dried to produce a sponge-like 3D structure. Similar to the conventional PACI technique, 150 mg of cartilage tissue is harvested and cultured. Afterward it is implanted onto a fibrin–hyaluronan matrix 3 to 4 days preoperatively. Human serum and fibroblastic growth factors are used for supplementation. Three to four weeks after chondrocyte harvest, implantation of the graft

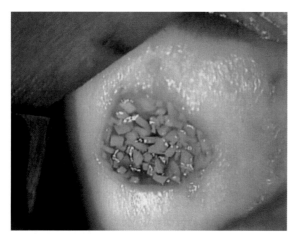

FIGURE 65.18. Intraoperative picture of the minced articular cartilage in a defect. (McCormick F, Yanke A, Provencher MT, et al. Minced articular cartilage. Basic science, surgical technique, and clinical application. *Sports Med Arthrosc Rev.* 2008;16:219, Figure 4.)

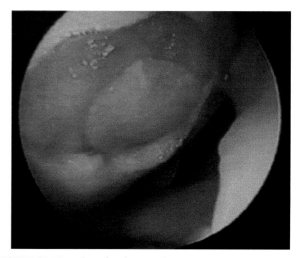

FIGURE 65.19. Hyalograft C (a second-generation ACI technique) uses a hyaluronan-based scaffold impregnated with chondrocytes. Similar to other cell based repair techniques 150 to 200 mg cartilage tissue is harvested and processed for 6 weeks. (Kerker JT, Leo AJ, Sgaglione NA. Cartilage repair: synthetics and scaffolds. *Sports Med Arthrosc Rev.* 2008;16:213, Figure 2).

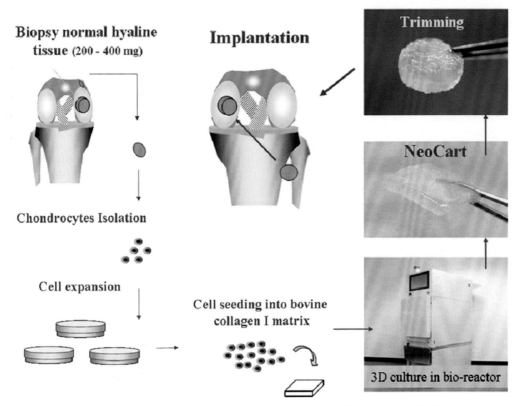

FIGURE 65.20. With the NeoCart process, harvested autologous chondrocytes are processed for a minimum of 7 days to enhance the material properties of the cultured chondrocytes. In a second operation, the cartilage tissue is implanted and secured with bioadhesive using a mini-arthrotomy. (Hettrich CM, Crawford D, Rodeo SA. Cartilage repair: third-generation cell based technologies. *Sports Med Arthrosc Rev.* 2008;16:232, Figure 1).

is performed by mini-arthrotomy, and implant is fixed to the defect by press-fitting and the application of fibrin glue.

Other techniques have been introduced that use different structures for implanting and holding cultured autologous chondrocytes. The Cartipatch (TBF Banque de tissues, France) is an implant composed of agarose and alginate on hydrogel for autologous chondrocyte suspension. The Novocart 3D (TETEC Tissue Engineering Technologies AG, Reutlingen, Germany) places autologous chondrocytes on a collagen-based biphasic scaffold with a dense protective layer preventing synovial cell invasion and improving the biomechanical properties of the implant. Autologous chondrocytes cultured on fibrin glue (Tissue-col, Baxter International Inc.) has also used clinically as well as autologous chondrocytes cultured with atelocollagen solution (3% type-I collagen; Koken, Tokyo, Japan) for 3 weeks to create an opaque, jelly-like gel for implantation.

Recently Developed Products

VeriCart (Histogenics Corporation, Waltham, MA) is a honeycomb, acellular collagen scaffold that is rehydrated with the patient's dilute bone marrow aspirate and implanted into a cartilage defect. Once implanted, it is said to attract chondrocytes and stem cells into the scaffold to form neocartilage. *Neocart* (Histogenics Corporation, Waltham, MA) takes a different approach. In an initial procedure, autologous chondrocytes are harvested. These

harvested autologous chondrocytes are processed for a minimum of 7 days to increase the material properties of the cultured chondrocytes. In a second operation, the cartilage tissue is implanted and secured with the bioadhesive using a mini-arthrotomy (Fig. 65.20). The difference between these two approaches is that it is hoped that the cultured chondrocytes will produce more matrix molecules, leading to a more mature or hyaline-like tissue.

CONCLUSION

Full-thickness chondral injuries in the knee present a unique challenge principally because of the limited capacity of articular cartilage to heal. The operative treatment options include marrow-stimulation, autografting, allografting, and **cell-based repair methods**. Various techniques have been developed to facilitate these treatments, but level-one prospective studies with appropriate control groups and sufficient power are lacking. The ultimate goal is to repair the damaged area with either normal articular cartilage or tissue which will have most of the mechanical properties of articular cartilage and prove durable over time. As new cartilage repair techniques are introduced, care should be taken to critically evaluate their outcomes. Synthetic biocompatible scaffolds and cell-based repair methods hold considerable promise and excite the imagination, yet until there is rigorous and reproducible clinical data supporting their utilization, caution should be exercised.

REFERENCES

1. Curl WW, Krome J, Gordon ES, et al. Cartilage injuries: a review of 31,516 knee arthroscopies. *Arthroscopy.* 1997;13:456–460.
2. Buckwalter JA, Mankin HJ. Articular cartilage: tissue design and chondrocyte-matrix interactions. *Instr Course Lect.* 1998;47:477–486.
3. Nehrer S, Spector M, Minas T. Histologic analysis of tissue after failed cartilage repair procedures. *Clin Orthop Relat Res.* 1999;365:149–162.
4. Outerbridge RE. The etiology of chondromalacia patellae. *J Bone Joint Surg Br.* 1961;43-B:752–757.
5. Brittberg M, Winalski CS. Evaluation of cartilage injuries and repair. *J Bone Joint Surg Am.* 2003;85-A(suppl 2):58–69.
6. Messner K, Maletius W. The long-term prognosis for severe damage to weight-bearing cartilage in the knee: a 14-year clinical and radiographic follow-up in 28 young athletes. *Acta Orthop Scand.* 1996;67:165–168.
7. Harwin SF. Arthroscopic debridement for osteoarthritis of the knee: predictors of patient satisfaction. *Arthroscopy.* 1999;15:142–146.
8. Kim HK, Moran ME, Salter RB. The potential for regeneration of articular cartilage in defects created by chondral shaving and subchondral abrasion. An experimental investigation in rabbits. *J Bone Joint Surg Am.* 1991;73:1301–1315.
9. Lu Y, Edwards RB III, Cole BJ, et al. Thermal chondroplasty with radiofrequency energy. An in vitro comparison of bipolar and monopolar radiofrequency devices. *Am J Sports Med.* 2001;29:42–49.
10. Spahn G, Kahl E, Muckley T, et al. Arthroscopic knee chondroplasty using a bipolar radiofrequency-based device compared to mechanical shaver: results of a prospective, randomized, controlled study. *Knee Surg Sports Traumatol Arthrosc.* 2008;16:565–573.
11. Pridie KH. A method of resurfacing osteoarthritic knee joints. *J Bone Joint Surg Br.* 1959;41:618–619.
12. Johnson LL. Arthroscopic abrasion arthroplasty historical and pathologic perspective: present status. *Arthroscopy.* 1986;2:54–69.
13. Steadman JR, Briggs KK, Rodrigo JJ, et al. Outcomes of microfracture for traumatic chondral defects of the knee: average 11-year follow-up. *Arthroscopy.* 2003;19:477–484.
14. Asik M, Ciftci F, Sen C, et al. The microfracture technique for the treatment of full-thickness articular cartilage lesions of the knee: midterm results. *Arthroscopy.* 2008;24:1214–1220.
15. Mithoefer K, Williams RJ III, Warren RF, et al. High-impact athletics after knee articular cartilage repair: a prospective evaluation of the microfracture technique. *Am J Sports Med.* 2006;34:1413–1418.
16. Hangody L, Kish G, Karpati Z, et al. Mosaicplasty for the treatment of articular cartilage defects: application in clinical practice. *Orthopedics.* 1998;21:751–756.
17. Nho SJ, Foo LF, Green DM, et al. Magnetic resonance imaging and clinical evaluation of patellar resurfacing with press-fit osteochondral autograft plugs. *Am J Sports Med.* 2008;36:1101–1109.
18. Horas U, Pelinkovic D, Herr G, et al. Autologous chondrocyte implantation and osteochondral cylinder transplantation in cartilage repair of the knee joint. A prospective, comparative trial. *J Bone Joint Surg Am.* 2003;85-A:185–192.
19. Marcacci M, Kon E, Delcogliano M, et al. Arthroscopic autologous osteochondral grafting for cartilage defects of the knee: prospective study results at a minimum 7-year follow-up. *Am J Sports Med.* 2007;35:2014–2021.
20. Gudas R, Stankevicius E, Monastyreckiene E, et al. Osteochondral autologous transplantation versus microfracture for the treatment of articular cartilage defects in the knee joint in athletes. *Knee Surg Sports Traumatol Arthrosc.* 2006;14:834–442.
21. Shasha N, Aubin PP, Cheah HK, et al. Long-term clinical experience with fresh osteochondral allografts for articular knee defects in high demand patients. *Cell Tissue Bank.* 2002;3:175–182.
22. Gross AE, Kim W, Las Heras F, et al. Fresh osteochondral allografts for posttraumatic knee defects: long-term followup. *Clin Orthop Relat Res.* 2008;465:1863–1870.
23. McCulloch PC, Kang RW, Sobhy MH, et al. Prospective evaluation of prolonged fresh osteochondral allograft transplantation of the femoral condyle: minimum 2-year follow-up. *Am J Sports Med.* 2007;35:411–420.
24. Peterson L, Minas T, Brittberg M, et al. Two- to 9-year outcome after autologous chondrocyte transplantation of the knee. *Clin Orthop Relat Res.* 2000:212–234.
25. Newman AP. Articular cartilage repair. *Am J Sports Med.* 1998;26:309–324.
26. Zaslav K, Cole B, Brewster R, et al. A prospective study of autologous chondrocyte implantation in patients with failed prior treatment for articular cartilage defect of the knee: results of the Study of the Treatment of Articular Repair (STAR) clinical trial. *Am J Sports Med.* 2009;37:42–55.
27. Knutsen G, Drogset JO, Engebretsen L, et al. A randomized trial comparing autologous chondrocyte implantation with microfracture. Findings at five years. *J Bone Joint Surg Am.* 2007;89:2105–2012.
28. Saris DB, Vanlauwe J, Victor J, et al. Characterized chondrocyte implantation results in better structural repair when treating symptomatic cartilage defects of the knee in a randomized controlled trial versus microfracture. *Am J Sports Med.* 2008;36:235–246.
29. Kon E, Gobbi A, Filardo G, et al. Arthroscopic second-generation autologous chondrocyte implantation compared with microfracture for chondral lesions of the knee: prospective nonrandomized study at 5 years. *Am J Sports Med.* 2009;37:33–41.
30. Henderson I, Gui J, Lavigne P. Autologous chondrocyte implantation: natural history of postimplantation periosteal hypertrophy and effects of repair-site debridement on outcome. *Arthroscopy.* 2006;22:1318–1324.e1.
31. Bartlett W, Skinner JA, Gooding CR, et al. Autologous chondrocyte implantation versus matrix-induced autologous chondrocyte implantation for osteochondral defects of the knee: a prospective, randomised study. *J Bone Joint Surg Br.* 2005;87:640–645.
32. Ferruzzi A, Buda R, Faldini C, et al. Autologous chondrocyte implantation in the knee joint: open compared with arthroscopic technique. Comparison at a minimum follow-up of five years. *J Bone Joint Surg Am.* 2008;90(suppl 4):90–101.
33. Niemeyer P, Pestka JM, Kreuz PC, et al. Characteristic complications after autologous chondrocyte implantation for cartilage defects of the knee joint. *Am J Sports Med.* 2008;36:2091–2099.

Revision Procedures and Complex Articular Cartilage Surgery

Brian J. Cole • Robert C. Grumet • Nicole A. Friel

The management of traumatic and degenerative articular cartilage injuries is a known challenge given the lack of a pluripotent cell line and poor vascularity, resulting in limited capacity for healing. The surgical management of these cartilage lesions may be further complicated by injuries, which include large and/or deep, multiple lesions, or patients with associated pathology, which may have contributed to failure of previous surgeries. These comorbid conditions may include ligamentous instability, malalignment, and meniscal deficiencies. The appropriate management of a patient with a revision or complex articular cartilage lesion requires a stepwise approach on a case-by-case basis with careful attention to patient and lesion-specific variables and the patient's expectations for postoperative outcome.

CLINICAL EVALUATION

History

Chondral lesions are often difficult to diagnose due to their variable presentation. Most often, acute injuries to the cartilage are caused by direct trauma with articular cartilage impact or involve a twisting or shearing movement associated with axial loading. This mechanism of injury often causes an injury to the surrounding soft tissues and capsuloligamentous structures. For example, condylar lesions may result from an acute or chronic anterior cruciate ligament (ACL) deficiency. Similarly, trochlear or patellar cartilage lesions may result from patellar instability.

A thorough history should include a discussion of the patient's pain, swelling, and instability or mechanical symptoms. Pain is the most often the patient's primary complaint. Pain is usually described at the associated compartment; ipsilateral medial or lateral joint line for condylar injury and anterior for trochlear or patellar lesions. Chondral lesions may be aggravated by certain positions or activities, such as weight-bearing activities for femoral condyle lesions and climbing stairs or squatting for patellofemoral lesions. An effusion usually accompanies the pain in the same location and is noted during activity. Possible concomitant injury to other soft tissue structures

of the knee joint requires careful questioning regarding knee stability or meniscal symptoms. Meniscal pain can often be difficult to discern from pain due to an articular cartilage lesion. In this case, a history of previous meniscectomy can help guide the surgeon toward the possibility of meniscal deficiency as a cause for continued pain and disability.

Prior attempts at treatment should be reviewed with the patient. Previous knee surgeries should be discussed, including the type of surgery, when the surgery took place, the type of rehabilitation followed and whether postoperative symptomatic relief occurred initially with subsequent recurrence of symptoms or not at all following the prior intervention. Nonsurgical management, such as oral medications, injections, bracing, physical therapy, and lifestyle modification, should also be discussed as an important part of the patient's prior treatment.

Physical Exam

Observation of body habitus and the patient's gait is an important aspect of the physical examination. An antalgic gait as well as evidence of malalignment with a valgus or varus thrust should be noted. Inspection of the lower extremity should include visualization of incisions from previous surgeries, as well as assessment of quadriceps circumference. An effusion can often be appreciated as fullness in the suprapatellar pouch at the anterolateral joint line with knee flexion.

Palpation of the knee joint elicits pain in the involved compartment. Patients with chondral injuries of the condyles often have joint line tenderness at the ipsilateral side of the knee. Meniscal injury also presents as pain at the joint line, but this pain is often more posterior than pain due to chondral injury. Patellofemoral lesions are usually associated with anterior pain and crepitation. Patellar tilt and glide should be assessed to evaluate for tightness of the lateral retinaculum and potential patellar instability.

Range of motion should be evaluated in both knees. Normally patients have full extension to a few degrees of hyperextension. Any evidence of a flexion contracture in the affected extremity should be noted as it is associated with a poor environment for postoperative rehabilitation.

Identification of associated pathology is critical to the successful outcome of revision and complex articular cartilage restoration. Persistent instability, malalignment, or meniscal deficiency is often a cause of premature failure of articular cartilage repairs and poor outcomes. Stability of the ACL, posterior cruciate ligament (PCL), medial collateral ligament (MCL) as well as lateral collateral ligament (LCL) and posterolateral complex (PLC) should be a routine part of any knee examination. Notably, a rotational component can be accentuated in the setting of meniscal deficiency.

Imaging

Standard radiographs for cartilage injury include bilateral knees, AP weight bearing, nonweight bearing 45° flexion lateral, and an axial (Merchant) view of the patellofemoral joint. Additional views include 45° flexion posteroanterior(PA) to identify subtle joint space narrowing that may be missed in an extension view and long-leg alignment view to assess the mechanical axis. In the case of patellar instability, a CT scan may be helpful to further assess the patellofemoral joint and associated tibial tubercle-trochlear groove (TT-TG) distance (1, 2). An MRI is useful to characterize the size, depth, and location of the cartilage lesion, the quality of subchondral bone or the presence of bony fractures, and associated pathology to ligaments, menisci, and other soft tissues.

Documentation of Previous Procedures

Patient's that have undergone previous knee procedures should be asked about the details of the chondral lesion and procedure. Documentation, including the operative report, intraoperative photographs, and pre- and postoperative clinic notes, are all important in determining the most appropriate treatment options for the patient.

TREATMENT

Goals

Expectations should always be reviewed with the patient, especially with complex or revision procedures that may not completely resolve the patient's pain and/or totally restore functional level. Overall, the treatment goals for cartilage restoration are reduction of symptoms, improvement in joint congruency, elimination of instability, and protection of the cartilage repair.

Treatment Options and Decision Making

Several options are available for treatment of cartilage lesions, depending upon the location, size, depth, geometry, and containment of the lesion. In addition, each patient should be considered on a case-by-case basis as age, activity level, response to prior therapies, and comorbidities such as malalignment, instability, and meniscal deficiency weigh heavily in the decision-making process.

Nonoperative Treatment

Despite the complexity of the cartilage injury, all nonoperative options should be fully explored before surgery. Indications for nonoperative treatment include asymptomatic lesions and small, incidental lesions. Several modalities are used to treat these lesions. Oral glucosamine and chondroitin supplementation may reduce knee pain. Acetaminophen, nonsteroidal anti-inflammatory drugs(NSAID) (including selective cyclooxygenase-2 inhibitors), and intra-articular steroid or viscosupplementation injections are also used to reduce symptoms. Physical therapy is another modality to rehabilitate a patient according to their functional activity goals and it must include a comprehensive proximal core-strengthening program in addition to traditional distal strengthening.

Operative Treatment

The surgical management of articular cartilage lesions can be grouped into three categories. Palliative procedures include arthroscopic debridement and lavage to provide symptomatic relief to the patient with little potential for cartilage regeneration. Reparative procedures include marrow-stimulation techniques, which create a pluripotent fibrin clot, ultimately resulting in fibrocartilage replacement. Finally, restorative procedures attempt to restore the natural hyaline surface of articular cartilage through the use of cultured chondrocytes or osteochondral grafts. These procedures may be considered as part of an algorithm for the management of focal cartilage defects from least invasive to more invasive. The goal of surgery is to restore the patient's function and ameliorate the patient's symptoms with the least invasive method possible. In the setting of revision or complex articular cartilage surgery, many patients have had a simple microfracture or debridement and the surgeon may need to consider more aggressive management to achieve their goals.

Lesion and patient-specific factors are important determinants of the type of procedure indicated. Lesion-specific variables include size, depth, geometry, and bone quality. Patient specific variables include the patient's physiologic age, activity level, and previous surgeries.

Perhaps the most important consideration in the setting of revision and complex articular cartilage restoration is a firm understanding of the reason for failure. There is often a comorbid condition such as malalignment, instability, or meniscal deficiency, which has either failed to protect a previous attempt at cartilage restoration or led to premature degradation of the replacement tissue. In addition, the patient's expectations after the prior surgery must be discussed as a potential cause for dissatisfaction or failure. The timing of return to sport, interval symptom relief after return, change in the character or nature of the symptoms, and the patient's future activity level and goals should be discussed as well. A thorough preoperative examination should include a standing-limb-alignment radiograph and oftentimes a diagnostic arthroscopy to evaluate the integrity of the cartilage lesion and potential concomitant pathology such as meniscal or ligamentous deficiency in an effort to appropriately plan or stage the necessary corrective procedures.

INDICATION

The indication for revision or complex articular cartilage restoration is a symptomatic focal cartilage defect, which has failed to improve with conservative measures or previous palliative or reparative surgical techniques. Additional indications include comorbid conditions such as malalignment and ligament or meniscal deficiency, which have contributed to a premature failure of the surgical procedure and can be appropriately addressed concomitantly or in a staged fashion. Osteotomies should be considered in any patient with varus or valgus alignment whose mechanical axis passes through the affected compartment

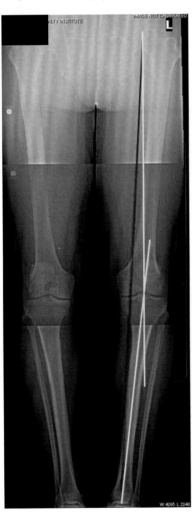

FIGURE 66.1. Standing full-length alignment radiograph in a patient with varus deformity. The mechanical axis is approximated by a line drawn from the center of the femoral head to the center of the talus *(red)*. The mechanical axis passes medial to the medial tibial spine correlating with varus deformity. The angle of correction to restore neutral alignment is the angle between the hip center to neutral knee and the ankle center to neutral knee *(yellow)*.

on a standing-AP-alignment radiograph (Fig. 66.1). The osteotomy should be planned to correct the mechanical axis to neutral in the case of cartilage preservation (Fig. 66.1). However, slight correction beyond neutral alignment should be planned in the setting of pain and arthrosis. Alternatively, in the setting of anterior or posterior cruciate ligament deficiency a sagittal plane osteotomy may be considered to improve joint kinematics and decrease tibial translation. Finally, a tibial tubercle osteotomy should be considered in any patient with patellofemoral lesions. The degree of anteriorization versus medialization can be titrated based on the patient's history of instability, maltracking (TT-TG distance), or arthrosis.

TIMING

In the setting of complex and revision cartilage surgery, patients may require osteotomies, meniscal transplants, and/or ligament reconstruction in an effort to preserve joint function and protect the cartilage-restorative procedure. The ideal timing of these procedures, whether undertaken simultaneously or in a staged fashion, is an important part of the preoperative planning and affects patient expectations regarding time to recovery and possible need for multiple surgeries.

Cartilage or Meniscus Deficiency and Malalignment

A focal cartilage defect or meniscal deficiency in the medial or lateral tibiofemoral compartment, with varus or valgus alignment, respectively, may be managed either simultaneously or staged. In general, young, active patients can be treated simultaneously with a high-tibial osteotomy or distal femoral osteotomy (DFO) and concomitant cartilage procedure (Fig. 66.2). Older, less active patients may benefit from an osteotomy first, followed by a period of observation. These patients may have satisfactory symptomatic relief from the osteotomy such that an additional cartilage procedure may not be warranted. Patients with previously failed patellofemoral lesions are often treated with a distal realignment procedure of the tibial tubercle to decrease the contact pressure of the patellofemoral joint (Fig. 66.3) along with the cartilage procedure.

Cartilage or Meniscus Deficiency and Ligament Deficiency

Patients with cartilage lesions or meniscal deficiency and instability due to ACL deficiency are managed with an ACL reconstruction and cartilage restoration or meniscal transplantation in an effort to restore joint kinematics and decrease shear across the joint surface. Cartilage lesions in the setting of a previously failed ACL reconstruction are common. Patients requiring a revision ACL

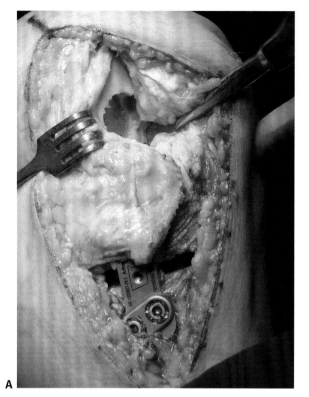

A

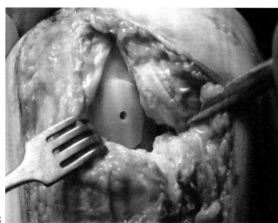

B

FIGURE 66.2. Cartilage restoration with realignment. This patient is a 36-year-old male with a history of multiple surgeries for a medial femoral condyle (MFC) defect. The initial evaluation revealed a 20-by-20-mm defect and varus deformity. Definitively underwent osteochondral allograft (OA) of MFC and HTO. **A:** High tibial osteotomy done with hardware in place. The socket for the osteochondral allograft on the femoral condyle has been prepared. **B:** The osteochondral allograft has been placed.

reconstruction with extensive bony tunnel expansion should be managed with a staged bone-grafting procedure followed by ACL reconstruction when the grafted tunnels have matured. We typically use bone-patellar tendon-bone or Achilles tendon allografts for revision treatment to reduce patient morbidity and provide versatility in graft-fixation techniques when combined procedures are performed.

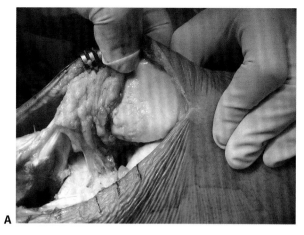

A

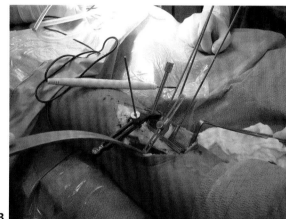

B

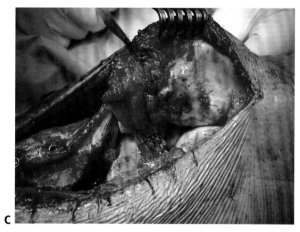

C

FIGURE 66.3. Cartilage restoration with realignment. This patient is a 22-year-old male with a history of a dislocated patella 1 year prior. At that time had a loose body removal and debridement of the chondral lesion. The patient had persistent symptoms (pain, swelling, and instability). **A:** Chondral lesion on inferior pole of patella. **B:** He underwent a tibial tubercle osteotomy (AMZ) using the T3 Tibial Tubercle Osteotomy System (Arthrex, Inc.). **C:** A concomitant patellar ACI was performed.

Ligament Deficiency Plus Malalignment Plus Cartilage Lesion

Perhaps the most difficult patient to manage is a young patient with a focal cartilage lesion, affected compartment malalignment and concomitant meniscal deficiency. These patients often require multiple procedures in an effort to restore join function. The ideal sequence of procedure is considered on a case-by-case basis with careful attention to the patient's expectations, goals, and symptoms (instability versus pain). Patients whose primary symptom is pain may be managed primarily by a corrective osteotomy with an attempt to reduce load in the affected compartment. Alternatively, patients with the primary symptom of instability may be managed with a primary ligament reconstruction. Future procedures in these patients are then guided by the patient's symptoms and ability to return to their desired activity level. Those patients with both pain and instability are typically managed in a staged fashion, with ACL reconstruction first followed by alignment and cartilage resurfacing procedures at 4 to 6 months postoperative.

Additional Situations

Patients with a known ACL deficiency and malalignment may be managed with an ACL reconstruction alone, osteotomy alone or an ACL plus osteotomy. The decision is again guided by the patient's symptoms, goals, and expectations. If a high-tibial osteotomy is to be performed in isolation, the surgeon may consider a biplanar osteotomy whereby the varus alignment is addressed with an opening wedge medially; however, the ACL deficiency may be aided by also decreasing the tibial slope with the osteotomy cut. Alternatively, patients who are PCL deficient with a concomitant malalignment may have the tibial slope increased with an anterior-based opening-wedge osteotomy to aid in posterior tibial translation.

Finally, perhaps the most common scenario is the patient with a known focal cartilage defect and a history of previous meniscectomy who now has persistent joint line pain. As previously discussed, it can often be difficult to discern whether the source of pain is the cartilage lesion or the loss of meniscal tissue. These patients are then managed with a concomitant meniscal transplantation and cartilage restorative procedure. These patients have generally been treated with a previous primary cartilage procedure such as marrow stimulation or debridement and are often revised with an osteochondral allograft in addition to the meniscal transplantation as a salvage procedure (Fig 66.4).

TECHNIQUES

Cartilage lesions that have been previously treated with marrow stimulation techniques, osteochondral grafting or autologous chondrocyte implantation are generally amenable to an autologous chondrocyte implantation or osteochondral allograft as a revision procedure. Lesions on the patella or trochlea may require a distal realignment procedure using the T3 Tibial Tuberosity System (Arthrex, Inc., Naples, FL) of the tibial tubercle in addition to the cartilage procedure. These procedures have been discussed in previous sections and will not be extensively covered in this chapter.

Osteotomies

High tibial osteotomy (HTO) is performed through a medially based incision beginning 1 cm below the joint line and extending approximately 5 cm distally positioned between the tibial eminence and the medial tibial border. A longitudinal incision is made adjacent to the pes anserinus and continues obliquely posteriorly along the top edge of the gracilis tendon to the level of the MCL, which is elevated rather than incised. The junction between the fat pad and the patellar tendon insertion is exposed and protected with a right-angle retractor. Under fluoroscopic guidance, a guide pin is placed obliquely across the tibia beginning slightly distal to the origin of the tibial tubercle, crossing the midtibia at the origin of the tibial tubercle and ending 1 cm below the joint line at the level of the proximal fibula. A second guide pin is placed posteriorly parallel to the first and also with the tibial slope unless a correction is desired in the sagittal plane. The cut is made with an oscillating saw, taking care not to violate the posterior or lateral cortex. The osteotomy, including the posterior cortex, can be completed with the use of osteotomes. Gradual opening of the osteotomy site is performed using the wedge osteotomes, and a plate (Arthrex HTO Plate, Arthrex, Inc.) is placed to the desired level of correction. A bone graft is typically used to fill the osteotomy void in the form of iliac crest, cortical ring allograft, or demineralized bone matrix supplements.

DFO is used to correct varus malalignment (Fig. 66.5). Similar to a HTO, a DFO is used in combination with a cartilage procedure in an effort to neutralize the mechanical axis and protect the joint-preserving procedure. A DFO is approached through a lateral incision from just distal to the lateral epicondyle extending approximately 10 cm proximally. Under fluoroscopic guidance, a guide pin is placed obliquely across the distal femur to the level of the MCL origin. The osteotomy is performed using a combination of an oscillating saw and flexible osteotomes. Care must be taken to protect the neurovascular structures posteriorly when performing the osteotomy. An appropriately sized femoral locking plate (Arthrex DFO Plate, Arthrex, Inc.) and wedge are placed to achieve the preoperatively templated correction (Fig. 66.5).

A distal patellar realignment procedure (anteromedialization [AMZ]) may be performed with previously failed cartilage defects about the patellofemoral joint. AMZ should be considered in patients with a lateral tilt and resultant lateral patellar overload or distal and lateral chondral injuries of the patella. Care should be taken when performing a distal realignment procedure in patients with proximal pole, medial, or pan patellar lesions as well as patients with bipolar lesions. Patients with a normal Q angle and therefore a normal TT-TG distance may benefit

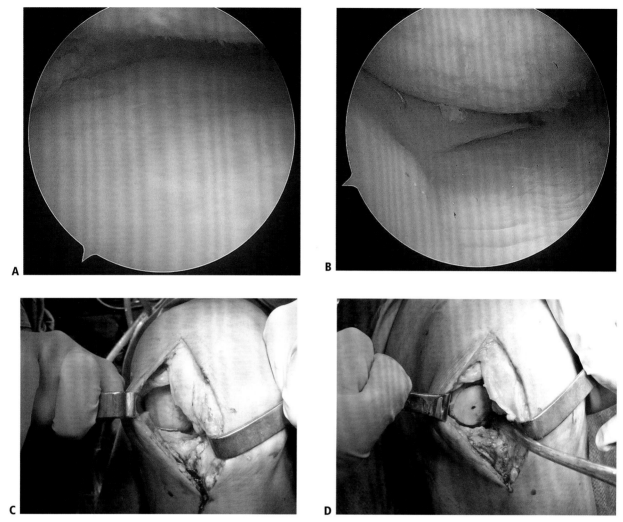

FIGURE 66.4. A: Arthroscopic images of 36-year-old active female with a history of medial meniscectomy and debridement of chondral injury. Patient had persistent symptoms due to meniscal deficiency and focal cartilage defect. **B:** Arthroscopic image after meniscal transplantation. The area of cartilage injury on the femoral condyle is again appreciated. **C:** An open approach shows the extent of the focal cartilage injury. **D:** An osteochondral allograft was performed in conjunction with the meniscal transplantation.

from a more vertically directed osteotomy with little medialization in an effort to decrease patellofemoral contact pressure. This is facilitated with a T3 Tibial Tubercle Osteotomy System (Arthrex, Inc.), which will objectively determine the angle of inclination of the osteotomy cut.

Hemiplateau Transplant

Select patients with a history of traumatic cartilage and bony loss to the lateral tibial plateau due to a tibial plateau fracture may benefit from an osteochondral allograft transplant of the hemiplateau with associated meniscal transplantation. This procedure is performed through a lateral parapatellar arthrotomy. A guide used for resecting the tibial plateau in unicompartmental knee arthroplasty is used to resect the hemiplateau. This guide allows appropriate coronal and sagittal resection to the level of the ipsilateral tibial spine (Fig 66.6). Care must be taken to

preserve the natural tibial slope. The allograft tibial plateau is then contoured to restore the normal joint space, taking care to evaluate the flexion and extension spaces similar to a unicompartmental arthroplasty (Fig. 66.6). The graft is held in position using headless Bio-compression screws (Arthrex Inc.) around the periphery. A standard meniscal repair is performed to the remaining synovium.

AUTHORS' PREFERRED TREATMENT

Our preferred treatment for previously failed or complex articular cartilage lesions is a stepwise approach to the patient's treatment and extensive preoperative planning as mentioned previously. Isolated femoral condyle cartilage lesions with no additional copathology (malalignment, instability, and meniscal deficiency) are generally treated with an osteochondral allograft after a previously

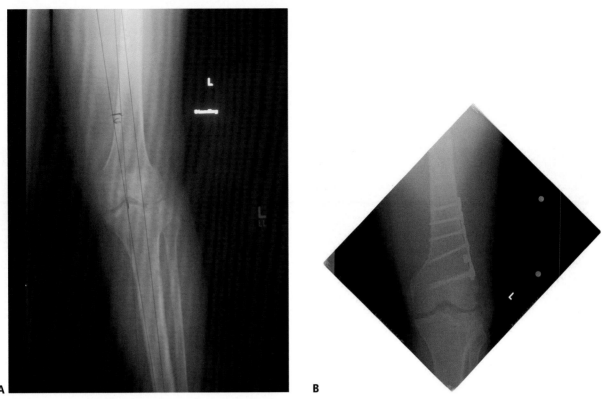

FIGURE 66.5. **A:** Preoperative radiographs of patient with history of lateral tibial plateau fracture with resultant valgus deformity. **B:** A distal femoral osteotomy has been performed to restore neutral alignment.

failed marrow-stimulation technique, debridement or ACI (Fig 66.7). Those lesions that are present on the patella or trochlea are often treated with ACI with an objectively calculated AMZ of the tibial tubercle after a failed primary treatment. In addition, concomitant pathology such as instability, meniscal deficiency, or malalignment are planned for and addressed in a staged fashion or in combination with the cartilage procedure.

COMPLICATIONS, CONTROVERSIES, AND SPECIAL CONSIDERATIONS

Complications from complex cartilage surgery are similar to those experienced with primary treatment of cartilage lesions including infection, bleeding, and deep venous thrombosis. Perhaps most common among complex cartilage reconstruction is the possibility of postoperative stiffness. This is seen more often when concomitant surgery is performed and can be addressed with early range-of-motion exercises, oral steroids in the early postoperative period (3) or possibly arthroscopy and lysis with gentle manipulation under anesthesia if no improvement is seen. Patients undergoing an osteotomy must be appropriately counseled on the risk of infraoperative fracture, intra-articular screw placement, nonunion, hardware failure, hematoma, and compartment syndrome. With the popularity of opening-wedge ostetomies, there

is theoretically less risk of developing a neuropraxia from the realignment procedure as compared with previous closing-wedge ostetomies. (4) Patients revised with ACI must be warned about the possibility of graft hypertrophy requiring up to 40% reoperation rate when a periosteal patch is used. (5) Graft hypertrophy is believed to be less of an issue with the use of newer synthetic patches. (6) Finally, patients having an osteochondral allograft must be cautioned about the possibility of graft dislodgement. This complication is less commonly seen when fixation is used to hold the grafts. In addition, risk of graft resorption or collapse has been described. However, this risk has been minimized through the use of fresh osteochondral grafts in comparison with frozen. (7)

Controversies surrounding complex cartilage restoration include the ideal procedure for a given cartilage lesion. In keeping with the principles previously outlined regarding treatment, the simplest, most predictable, and least invasive surgery to alleviate the patients symptoms and restore function should be performed first. In the setting of complex cartilage restoration, the more difficult cases or patient's with refractory symptoms often need larger, more invasive surgeries. Unfortunately, this setting makes it difficult to predict the clinical outcome and patient satisfaction with a given salvage procedure. In addition, the patient's age is often a point of contention regarding cartilage restoration. We submit that it is not the patient's chronologic age that matters, but rather their physiologic age, and therefore their desired activity level, which must be considered when predicting the ability of a cartilage procedure to restore function and alleviate symptoms.

Special considerations include those previously discussed. Perhaps the most significant consideration is appropriate timing of procedures, especially when multiple procedures may be needed. In general, comorbid conditions may be treated at the same time or a staged approach can be undertaken. Oftentimes, a single procedure can alleviate much of the symptomatology and obviates the need for additional stages. For example, a patient with significant varus malalignment in addition to a focal cartilage defect in the medial femoral condyle (MFC) and meniscal deficiency may benefit from a corrective HTO to offload

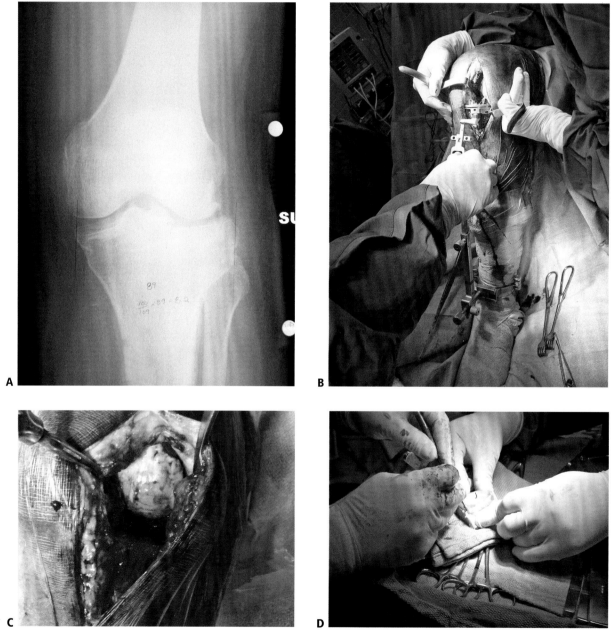

FIGURE 66.6. This patient is a 32-year-old male with a history of a lateral tibial plateau fracture. Despite removal of hardware, the patient described significant weight-bearing pain and recurrent swelling on the lateral side of his knee. **A:** Preoperative radiographs showing loss of joint space at the lateral joint line, healed depressed tibial plateau fracture. **B:** Unicompartmental knee jig is placed to resect the lateral tibial plateau taking care to maintain the natural tibial slope. **C:** View of the lateral compartment following resection of the tibial plateau. **D:** Osteochondral graft and meniscus prepared on the back table, contoured to fit the level of tibial plateau resection. **E:** The graft in place, held in position with circumferential bio-compression screws, a standard meniscal repair is performed. **F:** Postop radiographs after a concomitant distal femoral osteotomy, with restoration of the lateral joint space.

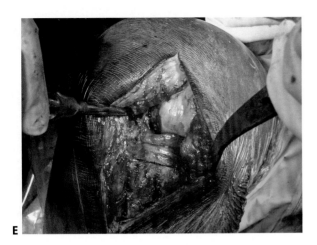

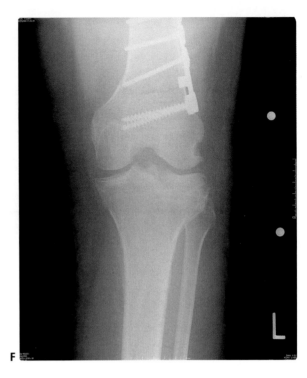

FIGURE 66.6. (continued)

the affected compartment, alleviating symptoms and restoring function sufficiently.

PEARLS AND PITFALLS

When approaching a patient with a previously failed cartilage-restorative procedure, avoid linear thinking. Each individual patient must be considered on a case-by-case basis, with particular attention to the patient-and lesion-specific factors previously outlined. Always consider the potential cause for cartilage failure and asses for comorbid pathology such as malalignment, instability, and meniscal deficiency.

Preoperative planning should include an evaluation of not only the cartilage lesion but also the integrity of the underlying bone. Focal cartilage lesions with underlying

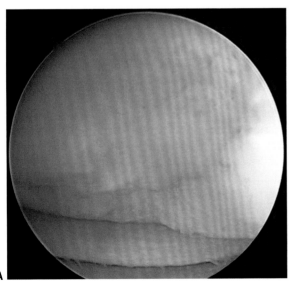

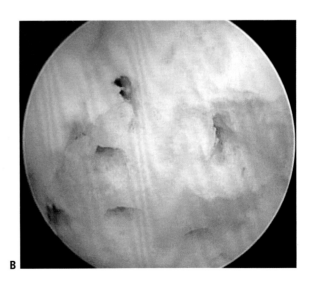

FIGURE 66.7. Failed ACI with revision to osteochondral allograft. This patient is a 38-year-old male with a history of ACI of the lateral femoral condyle for a grade 4 lesion measuring 16 by 38 mm. The patient's symptoms improved but then returned at 18 months postoperative **(A)**. The patient was taken back to the operating room where debridement and marrow stimulation was performed **(B)**. This procedure provided the patient some symptomatic relief but recurrent symptoms lead to an osteochondral allograft with excellent symptomatic relief **(C, D)**.

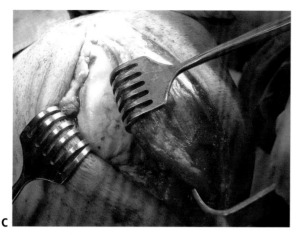

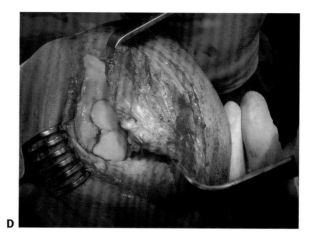

FIGURE 66.7. (continued)

bone loss require a bone-filling procedure. Large bone deficiencies may be managed by bone grafting primarily or in a single stage under the collagen membrane in the setting of ACI. Alternatively, osteochondral grafts may be fashioned to compensate for underlying bony deficiency.

Patients requiring a meniscal transplant with concomitant ACL reconstruction are another important consideration. When performing a meniscal transplant and using bony tunnels to pass and secure the meniscal allograft, care must be taken not to communicate the ACL tibial tunnel with the bone tunnels of the meniscal allograft. Alternatively, a bridge in slot technique as described by the senior author with interference screw fixation or with transosseous sutures may be utilized instead of bone tunnels to secure the meniscal allograft. (8–10) The posterior bone and meniscal insertion should be passed and secured prior to the ACL graft in order to aid in visualization.

HTO with concomitant ACL reconstruction may be a technically challenging procedure due to the complex interaction of tunnels, graft passage, and graft tunnel mismatch. A stepwise approach to this pathology includes arthroscopic intra-articular preparation first. This is followed by tibial tunnel preparation. The tibial tunnel must be shorter than a typical ACL tunnel to avoid communication with the proposed osteotomy site or in the very least, performed proximal to a more distal starting point for the HTO on the medial tibia. Alternatively, retro-drill (Arthrex, Inc.) technology may allow an all-inside ACL reconstruction minimizing concern for tibial tunnel interference with the osteotomy site. Next, the femoral tunnel is prepared, taking care to deepen the femoral socket to avoid significant graft-tunnel mismatch due to the shortened tibial tunnel. The HTO is performed next with plate fixation and bone grafting as previously described. The ACL graft is passed, recessing the femoral plug to compensate for the graft-tunnel mismatch. The femoral plug and tibial plug are then securely fixed with the desired method.

Additional pearls for HTO of the knee include adequate exposure of the patellar tendon at the tibial tubercle to ensure the appropriate resection level. Fluoroscopic guidance is essential to ensure the appropriate placement of the osteotomy, hardware, and desired level of correction. A more horizontal osteotomy should be considered in patients requiring a large correction to improve fixation stability.

REHABILITATION

The specific rehabilitation protocol used varies according to the procedure(s) performed. In general, patients are placed in a hinged knee brace postoperatively. All patients with intra-articular cartilage work are placed in a continuous passive motion machine postoperatively for 4 to 6 weeks. Patients with femoral condyle lesions and osteotomies are protected from full-weight bearing for 4 to 6 weeks and utilize a specialized postoperative hinged unloading brace (TROM Adjustor, DJ Orthopedics, LLC, Vista, CA). Patients with patellofemoral lesions are placed weight bearing as tolerated with the knee brace locked in extension unless a tibial tubercle osteotomy is performed whereby patients undergo a period of protected weight bearing to prevent a tibial stress fracture. The goals of early rehabilitation are range of motion, patellar mobilization, quadriceps sets, isometrics, and proximal core strengthening. Six to 12 weeks postoperatively, patients begin to focus on a functional strengthening program. Beginning about 3 months postoperatively, patients are advanced to muscular endurance with progressive running activities, advanced closed-chain strengthening, and plyometrics.

CONCLUSIONS

The variable algorithm and concomitant procedures often performed in revision cartilage restoration result in less predictable patient outcomes when compared with primary procedures. Zaslav et al. (5) in a prospective multicenter cohort study, evaluated the outcome of 154 patients undergoing ACI after a previous cartilage-repair procedure. The authors reported a 76% success rate with no difference observed among patients with a prior history of marrow stimulation as compared with those with debridement. There was a statistically significant improvement of outcome measures at an average of 48 months postoperatively compared with preoperative. A statistically significant improvement in the duration of the symptom-free interval postoperative was an average of 31 months longer when compared with the primary procedure. Finally, a rather high reoperation rate was noted at 49%, 40% of which was related to the ACI procedure including graft hypertrophy due to periosteal patch use.

Osteochondral allografting after previously failed primary cartilage restoration (debridement, fixation, and marrow stimulation) has also been described in the literature. McCulloch et al. (11) evaluated the outcome of 25 patients who underwent fresh osteochondral grafting of the femoral condyle. Ninety-six percent of patients had a history of previous surgery (debridement, fixation, ACI, or marrow stimulation). Fifty-six percent of patients had a concomitant procedure (osteotomy, meniscal transplant, or ligament reconstruction). There were no significant outcome differences between patients with isolated osteochondral grafting as compared with those with multiple procedures. Patients overall reported an 84% satisfaction with their knee and subjectively rated their knee function to be 79% of the unaffected knee. Recently, LaPrade et al. (7) prospectively evaluated 23 patients with osteochondral allografts at an average of 3 years, follow-up. Similarly, 20 of the 23 patients had a history of prior surgery. Significant improvements in Cincinnati and International Knee Documentation Committee (IKDC) outcome measures were observed.

Rue et al. (12) evaluated patients with a meniscal transplant in combination with an articular cartilage restorative procedure. Thirty patients were prospectively followed after a meniscal transplant plus cartilage restoration (52% ACI, 48% OCA) at a minimum of 2 years, follow-up. Overall, 76% of patients reported being completely or mostly satisfied with their outcome and 48% scored as normal or near-normal functional outcome by IKDC. Finally, patients with articular cartilage lesions, malalignment, and meniscal deficiency are not as commonly seen. However, Gomoll et al. (13) evaluated seven patients at an average of 2 years with evidence of early unicompartmental arthritis due to the loss of articular cartilage, meniscus, and malalignment. The authors reported that six of the seven patients were able to return to their previous level of activity unrestricted. A statistically significant improvement in outcome measures was observed with the exception of KOOS pain ($p = 0.053$), KOOS symptom ($p = 0.225$), and SF12 ($p = 0.462$).

Complex and revision articular cartilage restoration remains a challenge in the young active patient in an effort to preserve joint function, alleviate symptoms, and return patients to their desired level of activity. A stepwise approach to these patients with careful consideration of the reasons for failure (concomitant pathology), patient-and lesion-specific factors, and most importantly patient expectations, help guide our patients through the treatment of these difficult situations. Previous literature serves as a guide to discuss the desired patient outcomes. However, extreme caution should be taken when counseling as there are many confounding variables (additional procedures) that may positively or negatively affect these outcomes.

REFERENCES

1. Ando T, Hirose H, Inoue M, et al. A new method using computed tomography scan to measure the rectus femoris-patellar tendon Q-angle comparison with conventional method. *Clin Orthop Relat Res*. 1993;289:213–219.
2. Inoue M, Shino K, Hirose H, et al. Subluxation of the patella. Computed tomography analysis of patellofemoral congruence. *J Bone Joint Surg Am*. 1998;70(9):1331–1337.
3. Rue JP, Ferry AT, Lewis PB, et al. Oral corticosteroid use for loss of flexion after primary anterior cruciate ligament reconstruction. *Arthroscopy*. 2008;24(5):554–559.e1.
4. Miller BS, Downie B, McDonough EB, et al. Complications after medial opening wedge high tibial osteotomy. *Arthroscopy*. 2009;25(6):639–646.
5. Zaslav K, Cole B, Brewster R, et al. A prospective study of autologous chondrocyte implantation in patients with failed prior treatment for articular cartilage defect of the knee: results of the Study of the Treatment of Articular Repair (STAR) clinical trial. *Am J Sports Med*. 2009;37(1):42–55.
6. Gomoll AH, Probst C, Farr J, et al. Use of a type I/III bilayer collagen membrane decreases reoperation rates for symptomatic hypertrophy after autologous chondrocyte implantation. *Am J Sports Med*. 2009;37(1):S20–S23.
7. LaPrade RF, Botker J, Herzog M, et al. Refrigerated osteoarticular allografts to treat articular cartilage defects of the femoral condyles. A prospective outcomes study. *J Bone Joint Surg Am*. 2009;91(4):805–811.
8. Cole BJ, Fox JA, Lee SJ, et al. Bone bridge in slot technique for meniscal transplantation. *Op Tech Sports Med*. 2003;11(2):144–155.
9. Farr J, Cole BJ. Meniscus transplantation: bone bridge in slot technique. *Op Tech Sports Med*. 2002;10(3):150–156.
10. Alford W, Cole B. Failed ACL reconstruction and meniscus deficiency. Background, indications, and techniques for revision ACL reconstruction with allograft meniscus transplantation. *Sports Med Arthrosc Rev*. 2005;13(2):93–102.
11. McCulloch PC, Kang RW, Sobhy MH, et al. Prospective evaluation of prolonged fresh osteochondral allograft transplantation of the femoral condyle: minimum 2-year follow-up. *Am J Sports Med*. 2007;35(3):411–420.
12. Rue JP, Yanke AB, Busam ML, et al. Prospective evaluation of concurrent meniscus transplantation and articular cartilage repair: minimum 2-year follow-up. *Am J Sports Med*. 2008;36(9):1770–1778.
13. Gomoll AH, Kang RW, Chen AL, et al. Triad of cartilage restoration for unicompartmental arthritis treatment in young patients: meniscus allograft transplantation, cartilage repair and osteotomy. *J Knee Surg*. 2009;22(2):137–141.

Arthroscopic Treatment of Degenerative Arthritis of the Knee

Jack M. Bert

Significant controversy exists regarding the arthroscopic treatment of osteoarthritis (OA) of the knee. The indications for arthroscopic treatment of OA of the knee alone and in conjunction with other arthroscopic procedures will be reviewed.

HISTORICAL PERSPECTIVE

Arthroscopic debridement for OA of the knee was initially reported by Burman et al. (1) in 1934. The authors reviewed the first 30 cases where knee arthroscopy was used to diagnose a "possible meniscal injury, arthritis in the knee, or suspected tumor (1–3)". In the group of arthritic cases, they had "the pleasant surprise of seeing a marked improvement in the joint following arthroscopy." The authors stated that "arthroscopy involves only minimal risk, and in some cases has actually had a beneficial therapeutic effect, probably due to the thorough flushing and distention of the joint, which it necessitated." (1) In 1941, Magnuson introduced the term "joint debridement" to describe an operation of the knee in which "all the accessible synovial membrane, osteophytes, diseased cartilage, and normal soft tissues were removed in an effort to relieve the symptoms of OA." This was performed as an open procedure in which he stated that "complete recovery of symptoms" occurred in 60 of 62 patients (4).

During and after World War II, arthroscopy waned, and the open Magnuson procedure consisting of total synovectomy, osteophyte resection, cruciate ligament excision (if torn), as well as patellectomy was performed in most cases with reported symptomatic improvement in 66% of patients. This procedure became widely accepted as the treatment of choice for OA of the knee as published by Haggart (5) in 1947 and Isserlin (6) in 1950. These open debridement procedures, therefore, became the treatment of choice for arthritis of the knee until the resurgence of arthroscopy in the early 1970s.

CARTILAGE REPAIR

In 1743, William Hunter (7) stated, "From Hippocrates to the present age, it is universally allowed that ulcerated cartilage is a troublesome thing and that once destroyed it is not repaired." In 1849, Leidy (8) confirmed this principle stating that "a rupture of cartilage fragments is never united and that articular cartilage lacks regenerative power and fracture gaps extending into the joint become filled with tough fibrous tissue (9)."

Redfern (10), in 1851, described the histology of induced wounds of the articular cartilage of dog joints and stated that the wound "healed perfectly by the ingrowth of fibrous tissue," which he believed arose from the intercellular substance of the chondrocytes of the articular cartilage. However, as Mankin concluded in 1952, superficial lacerations of cartilage "neither heal nor progress to more serious disorders if they are small lesions." On the basis of multiple animal studies, these superficial lacerations, therefore, are generally limited in progression and do not lead to clinical OA (11). He furthermore noted that deep lacerations may be clearly visible years after injury (12–14). When the subchondral bone is thus disrupted, interosseous blood vessels expose bone matrix growth factors, causing fibrin clot formation. Inflammation introduces new cells into the cartilage defect and these cells proliferate and begin matrix repair (15). The matrix of articular cartilage has extraordinary biochemical characteristics. It is a hyperhydrated tissue, with estimates of water content ranging as high as 80%. It contains type I collagen consisting of two α and one α_2 chains. The collagen of cartilage contains three α_1 (type II) chains. Furthermore, the α_1 (type II) chains of type II collagen have a different structure from those of type I. It is this type I collagen that is formed when fibrous tissue regenerates in attempts at forming normal hyaline articular cartilage (11–14, 16–22). Furthermore, mature repair tissue has a relatively low proteoglycan concentration, and the proteoglycans do not resemble the large elaborate molecules found in the articular cartilage. These reparative cells, therefore, do not produce tissue with the unique composition, structure, and biochemical properties of normal articular cartilage (15, 18, 23). After cartilage injury or during the progression of OA, some chondrocytes do proliferate but do not migrate through the matrix to enter the site of tissue injury. The repair tissue matrix, which is usually formed by undifferentiated cells containing primarily type I collagen, thus cannot restore normal articular cartilage properties. These reparative cells fail to organize the molecules they produce to create a strong cohesive structure like that of articular cartilage and they produce other types of molecules that may interfere with the assembly of the cartilage matrix. This abnormal matrix with its different composition and structure, therefore, adversely alters the material properties of the tissue (24–26). These alterations compromise the ability of cartilage to survive and function in the highly stressed mechanical environment found in load-bearing joints and may lead to further cartilage degeneration and OA. Disruption of collagen cross-linking causes cartilage to lose its intrinsic tensile stiffness, strength, and shear stiffness, and this loss of proteoglycans and increased water content compromise its compressive and permeability properties (27–29).

Multiple treatments have been attempted to stimulate repair or reformation of the articular surface of the knee joint. Arthroscopically, these treatments include marrow stimulation procedures, debridement and shaving of fibrillated cartilage, and joint lavage. Other arthroscopic biologic articular cartilage treatment including osteochondral autografting or allografting will be described by other authors.

MARROW-STIMULATION PROCEDURES

The concept of drilling through eburnated bone to stimulate reparative cartilage formation was originally described by Pridie in 1959 (Fig. 67.1). Seventy-four percent of 62 patients believed their operation was a success and stated they would "have the operation again under similar circumstances (30)." To reconfirm the findings of Pridie, Akeson surgically removed the articular cartilage of the femoral heads of dogs and drilled the subchondral bone. He noted that after 1-year at the time of retrieval, "excessive loading destroyed the initial repair tissue or prevented formation of repair tissue." The results also indicated that 1 year after surgery, the concentration of proteoglycans in the reparative cartilage was less than half of that found in normal cartilage (31). Mitchell and Shepard found that multiple small drill holes made in the subchondral bone of rabbit-knee-joints-stimulated repair from large areas of the articular surface. They found that repair tissue grew from the drill holes and spread over the exposed bone. However, large areas of repair tissue that had the appearance of hyaline cartilage began to fibrillate and deteriorate within 1 year. These experiments were the first that showed that abrasion or perforation of subchondral bone

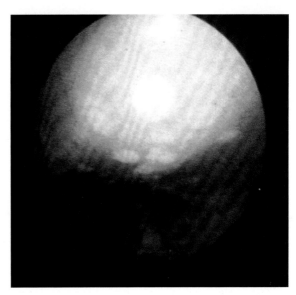

FIGURE 67.1. Picture of patient S/P Pridie procedure illustrating fibrocartilage formation in medial femoral condylar drill holes.

could stimulate repair of large areas of joint surface with fibrocartilaginous tissue, but the retrieved repair tissue lacked the proteoglycan concentration found in previously published studies of normal hyaline cartilage (32, 33).

Abrasion arthroplasty of grade 4 eburnated chondral lesions using motorized instrumentation was introduced by Johnson in 1981. This procedure is essentially an extension of the Pridie procedure except that in abrasion arthroplasty a superficial layer of subchondral bone, approximately 1 to 3 mm thick, is removed to expose interosseous vessels (Fig. 67.2). Theoretically, the resulting hemorrhagic exudate forms a fibrin clot and allows for formation of fibrous repair tissue over the eburnated bone (Fig. 67.3). In some patients, this fibrocartilaginous tissue

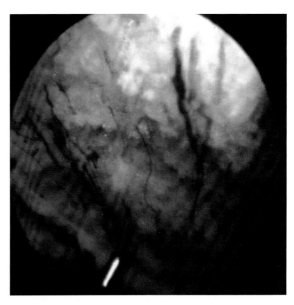

FIGURE 67.2. Abrasion arthroplasty illustrating bleeding bone.

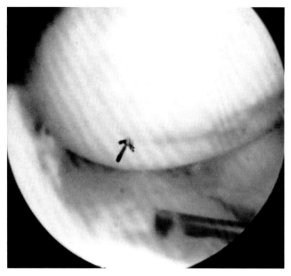

FIGURE 67.3. Arthroscopic view of patient 4 years after abrasion arthroplasty illustrating resurfacing with fibrocartilage.

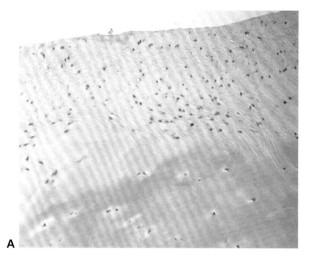

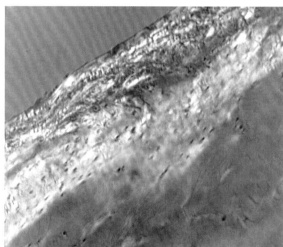

FIGURE 67.4. Electron microscopic view of regenerated fibrocartilage **(A)** with polarized light view **(B)** of same section illustrating the disorganized surface fibrocartilage compared with the hyaline cartilage cells beneath. (Courtesy of Dr. Steven Arnoczky, Laboratory for Comparative Orthopedic Research, Michigan State University, East Lansing, MI.)

lasted up to 4 years but in Johnson's (34) series, only one of eight biopsy specimens showed any type II collagen typical of hyaline cartilage at the time of arthroscopic review and biopsy, and the rest had types I and III collagen. In a series of patients at our institution who had abrasion arthroplasty, at 5-year follow-up exams, 15 had been converted to total knee replacement (TKA) and biopsies were obtained at the time of TKA. All patients had fibrocartilage and type I collagen on their biopsy specimens (Fig. 67.4A,B). In our series of 126 patients who had treatment of unicompartmental gonarthrosis with either abrasion arthroplasty or arthroscopic debridement alone, at 5-year follow-up examinations, 51% had good to excellent results with abrasion arthroplasty. Sixty-six percent had good to excellent results with arthroscopic debridement alone. However, all of these patients had complete obliteration of the medial joint space preoperatively. The results in our series were unrelated to age, presence of previous surgery, weight, extent of unicompartmental disease, presence or absence of joint space widening after surgery, and extent of residual varus or valgus deformity (35). Coventry and Bowman (36) noted that formation of hyaline-like cartilage occurred in the unloaded medial compartment of several patients after valgus upper tibial osteotomy (Fig. 67.5). This finding was confirmed arthroscopically by Fujisawa et al. (37) 12 to 18 months after upper tibial osteotomies, which implies that regeneration of reparative cartilage can occur secondary to unloading of bone alone without additional surgery.

MICROFRACTURE

Blevens et al. (38) recommended a "microfracture" technique in which they used an arthroscopic awl to create multiple perforations into the subchondral bone arthroscopically. They reported 266 patients between

1985 and 1990, with 3.7-year follow-up using a similar grading system to the Outerbridge classification (39, 40). The indications for the microfracture technique includes a full-thickness, well-circumscribed cartilage defect on a weight-bearing surface of the knee with exposed subchondral bone (i.e., grade 4 lesions). After chondral surface debridement, the bone is perforated to a depth of 3 to 4 mm using an awl and the holes placed approximately 4 to 5 mm apart (Fig. 67.6). Blood should be seen emanating from the microfracture holes after perforation is complete. A postoperative rehabilitation program was used to provide motion without applying high-load stress to the treated chondral defect. Repeat arthroscopies were performed in 80 patients. In the "majority" of chondral defects, subchondral bone was covered with cartilage of "varying quality" and the term "hyaline-like" was introduced to describe the fibrocartilage surface. There was absolutely no evidence that hyaline cartilage was present

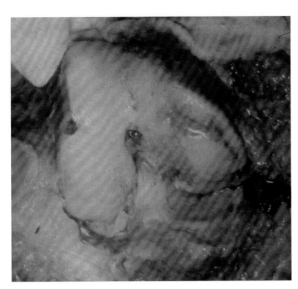

FIGURE 67.5. Picture of patient S/P valgus producing upper tibial osteotomy illustrating formation of fibrocartilage on medial femoral condyle. (Courtesy of Dr. Mark Coventry, Dept. of Orthopedics, Mayo Clinic, Rochester, MN.)

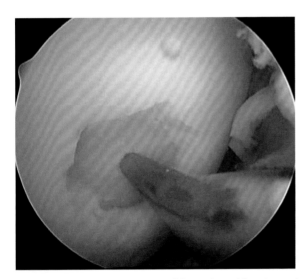

FIGURE 67.6. Intraoperative photo of femoral condyle using awl to begin microfracture technique.

at the second-look arthroscopy, and the authors confirmed that the only type of tissue that has been seen to regenerate over these surfaces was fibrocartilaginous repair tissue. The authors furthermore stated that the "biochemical composition and durability of the presumed fibrocartilage repair tissue is unanswered." Clearly, there is no evidence that hyaline cartilage is regenerated by marrow stimulation.

ARTHROSCOPIC DEBRIDEMENT

Arthroscopic debridement as a treatment option for OA was initially reported by Sprague in 1981. He arthroscopically debrided 330 knees diagnosed as having

"degenerative arthritis… in two or more compartments of the knee." Meniscectomy, chondroplasty of all surfaces, loose body and "debris" removal was performed. Seventy-four percent of the patients stated that the "knee was improved and more functional" than before surgery at 1-year follow-up. The extent of arthritis, however, was not correlated clinically or roentgenographically with success rates (41). Several authors in the early to mid-1980s reported that the results of arthroscopic debridement were not correlated with age, extent of arthritis either roentgenographically or arthroscopically with up to 11-year follow-ups (42, 43). Gross (44) and Ogilvie-Harris (45) concluded in the early 1990s that OA severity was the best predictor of success after arthroscopic debridement and that normally aligned knees with mild arthritis had the best results with 8-year follow-ups. It is certainly not clear, however, that shaving damaged articular cartilage relieves pain. O'Donoghue (46) reported that chondroplasty in rabbit knees did not stimulate cartilage repair nor did it result in joint deterioration. Bentley (47, 48) reported that chondroplasty during arthrotomy produced unpredictable results, and only 25% of patients treated with patellar chondroplasty had satisfactory results beyond 1 year. Timoney retrospectively reviewed 109 patients in 1990 who had arthroscopic debridement for degenerative arthritis of the knee with 4.2-year follow-up. Only 45% reported good results and 21% of patients experienced worsened symptoms and subsequently had TKA (49). Moseley in 1996 was one of the first authors to suggest that arthroscopic debridement for OA of the knee was no better than placebo. He randomized 10 patients with OA of the knee into a placebo group, an arthroscopic lavage group, and an arthroscopic debridement group. All 10 patients at 6 months reported improvement in their pain scores and satisfaction with their surgery, with the exception of one placebo patient, after their 6-month follow-up (50). He repeated this study in 2002 and with a larger patient group at a VA hospital. Seventy percent of these patients had moderate to severe OA. He found no significant differences between the three groups who had arthroscopy with debridement, arthroscopy with lavage, and placebo knee surgery. Of interest was that those patients who had positive MRIs with meniscal tears were excluded from his study. He concluded that there was no clear role for arthroscopy in knees with OA (51). Steadman et al. (52) recently reported a 71% success rate at 2 years for arthroscopic debridement of OA using the WOMAC and Lysholm scoring system. Wai et al. (53) and Hawker et al. (54) reported that up to 9.2% of patients had a TKA after 1 year and 18.4% had a TKA after 3 years subsequent to arthroscopic debridement indicating the transient nature of improvement in some patients subsequent to arthroscopic debridement for OA. Multiple authors claim that arthroscopic debridement and shaving help to relieve the symptoms of OA of the knee, but it is not clear why these patients improve and equally unclear as to why they stay improved for as long as 5 years post-operatively (33, 34, 45, 47, 48, 55–60).

ALIGNMENT AND ARTHROSCOPIC DEBRIDEMENT

Correlation of preoperative angular deformity with the results of arthroscopically debrided knees was originally reported by Salisbury et al. in 1985. In patients with residual varus deformity, 32% noted improvement in pain at 1 year. Normal knee alignment was considered 1° to 7° of femorotibial valgus alignment preoperatively (61). Harwin et al. (47) and Baumgartner et al. (62) concluded that abnormal varus or valgus angulation was a statistically significant factor in predicting a failed result after arthroscopic debridement. Similar findings were reported by Ogilvie-Harris and Fitsialos (45). Those patients who have varus or significant valgus knee deformities with medial or lateral compartment disease, respectively, will have worse results than those with postoperative neutral or mild valgus alignment.

ARTHROSCOPY, RADIOGRAPHY, AND DEGENERATIVE JOINT DISEASE

The correlation between degenerative joint disease viewed on X-ray films and at arthroscopy was reported by Lysholm in 1987. Chondral damage was graded arthroscopically according to Outerbridge (39) and radiographic examination was evaluated according to the Ahlback classification (63). In one group of patients, there were Outerbridge grade 2 changes involving both the tibia and the femur with space narrowing consistent with Ahlback grade 1 changes on X-ray. In a second group with Outerbridge grade 3 and 4 changes, complete joint space obliteration occurred consistent with Ahlback grade 2 changes. Involvement of the lateral compartment as assessed on arthroscopy was significantly more common in patients with medial compartment Outerbridge grade 2 and 3 changes as well as Ahlback grade 2 and 3 changes on X-ray (64).

ARTHROSCOPY AND LAVAGE

In 1978, Bird and Ring reported on a series of 14 patients who had arthroscopic lavage of the knee. Thirteen (93%) patients improved by 1 week, but by 4 weeks only, seven (50%) had noted mild to moderate improvement (65). Jackson reported on more than 207 patients with "femoral tibial arthritic disease in either the medial or lateral compartment" who had lavage versus arthroscopic debridement with 2-year follow-ups in 1988. The authors found that debridement of chondral and meniscal tissue produced "68% improvement." Lavage alone resulted in 45% symptomatic improvement (66). Livesley in 1991 compared 37 knees with OA treated by arthroscopic lavage and

physiotherapy with a control group of 24 knees treated by physiotherapy alone. Those treated by joint lavage improved to a greater degree than the control group and the improvement lasted longer. The physiotherapy group initially experienced an improvement, but by the end of the study, they had returned to their pretreatment state (55). Ike in 1992 compared a group of patients treated with standard medical treatment (nonsteroidal anti-inflammatory drugs, steroid injections, physical therapy, and analgesics) with those receiving tidal lavage in the office using local anesthesia. One thousand cubic centimeters of saline was injected into the joint in multiple stages and aspirated, and the patient was sent home. At the conclusion of this prospective 12-week study, 62% of the tidal irrigation group patients and 36% of the medically managed patients were improved functionally and symptomatically (67). In 1993, Chang reported on two groups of patients, one that received arthroscopic surgery and debridement and another needle joint lavage. At 1-year, 44% of patients who underwent arthroscopic surgery reported improvement, and 58% of patients who underwent joint lavage noted improvement. Patients with tears of the medial or lateral meniscus had a higher probability of improvement after arthroscopic surgery as opposed to closed-needle lavage. Only 2 of the 27 measures of outcome showed statistically significant differences between the arthroscopy and lavage groups. The authors concluded that the removal of soft-tissue abnormalities through arthroscopic surgery did not generally improve pain and knee dysfunction associated with non-end-stage OA any more than did simple joint lavage unless a meniscal tear was present (68). Multiple explanations for symptomatic relief secondary to arthroscopic lavage have been postulated such as removal of cartilage debris, crystals, and inflammatory factors. Temporary improvement in signs of inflammation may support the hypothesis that lavage removes inflammatory agents, although it is not known what these inflammatory agents specifically and objectively are (69–72).

CONCLUSIONS

Arthroscopic debridement of the degenerative knee has been described as a worthwhile procedure in young patients and in older patients who desire symptomatic improvement and do not wish to risk the morbidity of a TKA. Success rates for arthroscopic debridement vary between 50% and 67% depending on many factors, including patient age, degree of arthritis, activity level, and extent of follow-up. Arthroscopic lavage success rates vary between 45% and 51% and do not appear to have the same longevity of success as arthroscopic debridement. Furthermore, it is apparent from at least two studies comparing arthroscopic debridement alone to abrasion arthroplasty in conjunction with arthroscopic debridement that abrasion arthroplasty and the Pridie procedure do not appear to offer any greater benefit in the treatment of degenerative arthritis of the knee than debridement alone (35, 59). There does not appear to be any advantage in performing arthroscopy in conjunction with upper tibial osteotomy compared with upper tibial osteotomy alone. The results are similar. Furthermore, the results of upper tibial osteotomy in conjunction with abrasion arthroplasty were identical to those in a similar series of patients who had upper tibial osteotomy alone (73). Arthroscopic procedures therefore in conjunction with upper tibial osteotomy seem to be of limited value. Furthermore, the prognostic value of the arthroscope in determining whether to proceed with upper tibial osteotomy is minimally helpful as noted by both Fujisawa et al. (37) and Keene et al (74). They concluded there was no correlation in terms of prognosis and arthroscopic evaluation prior to tibial osteotomy compared with the clinical results subsequent to osteotomy.

Since the Moseley (51) study published in 2002, the center for Medicare and Medicaid services has disallowed the arthroscopic code for debridement in a patient on Medicare. This is due to Moseley's conclusion that success rates for arthroscopic debridement are no greater than other "sham" operations for OA in elderly patients. This opinion was reaffirmed by Kirkley et al. (75) in 2008 when they published a similar study. In this patient group at 2 years, they compared 86 patients who had arthroscopic lavage for grade 2 to 4 changes with a larger group that had PT, NSAID's steroid injections and viscosupplementation. They excluded patients with meniscal lesions or mechanical symptoms and concluded using WOMAC and SF-36 scoring systems that there was no role for arthroscopic debridement in OA of the knee. Recently, Bin reported on 68 patients, with a mean age of 63 years, with grade 4 medial compartment OA. In this group, 90% improved after surgery using VAS and Lysholm scoring systems yet 5% required TKA at 4 years post-op and 25% required further surgery at a mean 6.3 years (76).

The three clinical variables associated with improvement after arthroscopic debridement are preoperative medial joint line tenderness and a positive Steinman test indicative of a torn medial meniscus and with the unstable meniscal tissue at the time of arthroscopy (77). The reported predictors of improved outcomes from arthroscopic debridement are preoperative mechanical symptoms resulting from loose bodies, displaced articular chondral lesions, and meniscal tears (78). In contrast, the reported predictors for poor outcomes after arthroscopic debridement for OA of the knee are marked malalignment, restricted range of motion, prior surgery, and severe OA in most published articles (79). The American Academy of Orthopedic Surgeons (AAOS) (80) guideline titled "treatment of OA of the knee" adopted by the AAOS board of directors published on December 6, 2008 agreed that in joints with mechanical symptoms including locking, catching, or giving way, arthroscopic removal of loose bodies, chondral flaps, and/or unstable meniscal tissue with debridement in the arthritic joint improves symptoms and is clearly indicated.

In conclusion, the arthroscope is useful in the treatment of degenerative arthritis of the arthritic knee when a patient has preoperative symptoms indicating a mechanical abnormality. It has an extremely low morbidity. However, based on the series reviewed in the literature, arthroscopic debridement has minimal value in association with upper tibial osteotomy or marrow-stimulation procedures.

REFERENCES

1. Burman MS, Finkelstein H, Mayer L. Arthroscopy of the knee joint. *J Bone Joint Surg.* 1934;16:255–261.
2. Burman MS. Arthroscopy for the direct visualization of joints. An experimental cadaver study. *J Bone Joint Surg.* 1931;13:669–673.
3. Finkelstein H, Mayer L. The arthroscope, a new method of examining joints. *J Bone Joint Surg.* 1931;13:583–589.
4. Maguson PB. Joint debridement: surgical treatment of degenerative arthritis. *Surg Gynecol Obstet.* 1941;73:1–7.
5. Haggart GE. Surgical treatment of degenerative arthritis of the knee joint. *J Bone Joint Surg Br.* 1947;22:717–723.
6. Isserlin LB. Joint debridement for osteoarthritis of the knee. *J Bone Joint Surg Br.* 1950;32:302–309.
7. Hunter W. On the structure and diseases of articulating cartilage. *Philos Trans R Soc Lond B Biol Sci.* 1743;9:267–273.
8. Leidy J. On the intimate structure and history of articular cartilage. *Am J Med Sci.* 1849;17:277–282.
9. Jackson RW. The role of arthroscopy in the management of the arthritic knee. *Clin Orthop.* 1974;101:28–36.
10. Redfern P. On the healing of wounds and articular cartilage. *Monthly J Med Sci.* 1851;13:201–207.
11. Mankin HJ. Localization of tritiated thymidine in articular cartilage of rabbits: II. Repair in immature cartilage. *J Bone Joint Surg Am.* 1962;33:638–649.
12. Mankin HJ. Reaction of articular cartilage to injury and osteoarthritis: Part I. *N Engl J Med.* 1974;291:1285–1297.
13. Mankin HJ. Reaction of articular cartilage to injury and osteoarthritis: part II. *N Engl J Med.* 1974;291:1335–1344.
14. Mankin HJ. Response of articular cartilage to mechanical injury. *J Bone Joint Surg Am.* 1982;64:460–472.
15. Buckwalter JA, Rosenberg LC, Hunziker EB. Articular cartilage: composition, structure, response to injury and methods of facilitating repair. In: Ewing JW, ed. *Articular Cartilage and Knee Joint Function: Basic Science in Arthroscopy.* New York, NY: Raven Press; 1990:19.
16. Buckwalter JA. Articular cartilage. *Instruct Course Lect.* 1983;32:349–357.
17. Buckwalter JA. Cartilage. In: Dulvecco R, ed. *Encyclopedia of Human Biology.* Vol 2. San Diego, CA: Academic Press; 1991:201.
18. Buckwalter JA, Cruess R. Healing of musculoskeletal tissues. In: Rockwood CA, Green DP, Bucholz RW, eds. *Fractures in Adults.* 3rd ed. Philadelphia, PA: JB Lippincott; 1991:181.
19. Buckwalter JA, Woo SL. Articular cartilage: composition and structure. In: Woo SL, Buckwalter JA, eds. *Injury and Repair of the Musculoskeletal Soft Tissues.* Park Ridge, IL: American Academy of Orthopaedic Surgeons; 1988:405.
20. Buckwalter JA, Woo SL. Articular cartilage: injury and repair. In: Woo LS, Buckwalter JA, eds. *Injury and Repair of the*

Musculoskeletal Soft Tissues. Park Ridge, IL: American Academy of Orthopaedic Surgeons; 1988:465.

21. Muir H, Bullough P, Marodas A. The distribution of collagen in human articular cartilage with some of its physiologic implications. *J Bone Joint Surg Br*. 1970;52:554–562.

22. Poole CA, Flint MH, Bearumont BW. Morphological and functional interrelationships of articular cartilage matrices. *J Anat*. 1984;138:113–119.

23. Mow VC, Rosenwasser MP. Articular cartilage: biomechanics. In: Woo SL, Buckwalter JA, eds. *Injury and Repair of the Musculoskeletal Soft Tissues*, Park Ridge, IL: American Academy of Orthopaedic Surgeons; 1988:427.

24. Donohue JM, Buss D, Oeyema TR, et al. The effects of indirect blunt trauma on adult canine articular cartilage. *J Bone Joint Surg Am*. 1983;65:948–956.

25. Radin EL, Martin RB, Burr DB, et al. Effects of mechanical loading on the tissue of the rabbit knee. *J Orthop Res*. 1984;2:221–227.

26. Repo RU, Finlay JV. Survival of articular cartilage after controlled impact. *J Bone Joint Surg Am*. 1977;59:1068–1074.

27. Armstrong CG, Mow VC. Variations in the intrinsic mechanical properties of human articular cartilage with age: degeneration of water content. *J Bone Joint Surg Am*. 1982;64:88–96.

28. Mansour JM, Mow VC. The permeability of articular cartilage under compressive strain and high pressures. *J Bone Joint Surg Am*. 1976;58:509–517.

29. Woo SL-Y, Mow VC, Lai WM. Biomechanical properties for articular cartilage. In: Skalik R, Chein S, eds. *Handbook of Bioengineering*. New York, NY: McGraw-Hill; 1987:41.

30. Pridie AH. The method of resurfacing osteoarthritic knee joints. *J Bone Joint Surg Br*. 1959;41:618–623.

31. Akeson WH. Experiment cup arthroplasty of the canine hip. *J Bone Joint Surg Am*. 1969;51:149–156.

32. Mitchell N, Shepard N. Resurfacing of adult rabbit articular cartilage by multiple perforations of the subchondral bone. *J Bone Joint Surg Am*. 1976;58:230–239.

33. Mitchell N, Shepard N. Effects of patellar shaving in the rabbit. *J Orthop Res*. 1987;5:388–396.

34. Johnson LO. Arthroscopic abrasion arthroplasty. Historical and pathological perspective: present status. *Arthroscopy*. 1986;2:54–63.

35. Bert JM, Maschka K. The arthroscopic treatment of unicompartmental gonarthrosis: a five-year follow-up study of abrasion arthroplasty plus arthroscopic debridement and arthroscopic debridement alone. *Arthroscopy*. 1989;5:25–34.

36. Coventry MB, Bowman PW. Long-term results of upper tibial osteotomy for degenerative arthritis of the knee. *Acta Orthop Belg*. 1982;48:139–156.

37. Fujisawa Y, Masuhara K, Shiomi S. The effect of high tibial osteotomy in osteoarthritis of the knee: an arthroscopic study in 54 knee joints. *Orthop Clin North Am*. 1979;10:585–591.

38. Blevens FT, Steadman R, Rodrigo J. Treatment of articular cartilage defects in athletes: an analysis of functional outcome and lesion appearance. *J Orthop*. 1998;21(7):761–767.

39. Outerbridge RE. The etilology of chondromalacia of patellae. *J Bone Joint Surg Br*. 1961;43:752–760.

40. Rodrigo J, Stedman JR, Silliman JE, et al. Improvement of full thickness chondral defect healing in the human knee after debridement and microfracture using continuous passive motion. *Am J Knee Surg*. 1994;4:109–116.

41. Sprague NF III. Arthroscopic debridement for degenerative knee joint disease. *Clin Orthop*. 1981;160:118–125.

42. Jackson RW, Silver R, Marans R. The arthroscopic treatment of degenerative joint disease. *J Arthrosc*. 1986;2:11–19.

43. Shahriaree H, O'Connor RF, Nottage W. Seven years follow-up arthroscopic debridement of degenerative knee. *Filed View*. 1982;1:1–7.

44. Gross DE. The arthroscopic treatment of degenerative joint disease in the knee. *J Orthop*. 1991;14:1317–1326.

45. Ogilvie-Harris DJ, Fitsialos DP. Arthroscopic management of the degenerative knee. *Arthroscopy*. 1991;7:151–159.

46. O'Donoghue DH. Treatment of chondral damage to the patella. *Am J Sports Med*. 1981;9:12–21.

47. Bentley G. The surgical treatment of chondromalacia of the patellae. *J Bone Joint Surg Br*. 1978;60:74.

48. Bentley G. The surgical treatment of chondromalacia of the patellae. *J Bone Joint Surg Am*. 1980;52:221–229.

49. Timoney JM, Kneisl JS, Barrack RL, et al. Arthroscopy in the osteoarthritic knee. *Orthop Rev*. 1990;19(4):371–379.

50. Moseley B. Arthroscopic treatment of osteoarthritis of the knee: a prospective randomized placebo controlled trial. *Am J Sports Med*. 1996;24(1):28–36.

51. Moseley B, O'Malley K, Petersen N, et al. A controlled trial of arthroscopic surgery for osteoarthritis of the knee. *N Engl J Med*. 2002;347:81–88.

52. Steadman R, Ramappa A, Maxwell B, et al. An arthroscopic treatment regimen for osteoarthritis of the knee. *Arthroscopy*. 2007;23(9):948–955.

53. Wai E, Kreder J, Williams J. Arthroscopic debridement of the knee for osteoarthritis in patients fifty years of age or older: utilization and outcomes in the Province of Ontario. *J Bone Joint Surg Am*. 2002;84:17–22.

54. Hawker G, Guan J, Judge A, et al. Knee arthroscopy in England and Ontario: patterns of use, changes over time and relationship to total knee replacement. *J Bone Joint Surg Am*. 2008;90:2337–2345.

55. Livesley PJ, Doherty M, Needoff M, et al. Arthroscopic lavage of osteoarthritic knees. *J Bone Joint Surg Br*. 1991;73:922–926.

56. Harwin SF, Stein A, Stern R, et al. Arthroscopic debridement of the osteoarthritic knee: a step toward patient selection. *Arthroscopy*. 1991;1:7–15.

57. Harwin S. Arthroscopic debridement for osteoarthritis of the knee: predictors of patient satisfaction. *Arthroscopy*. 1999;15:142–146.

58. McGinley B, Cushner F, Scott W. Debridement arthroscopy. 10 year follow-up. *Clin Orthop Relat Res*. 1999;367:190–194.

59. Rand JA. Role of arthroscopy in osteoarthritis of the knee. *Arthroscopy*. 1991;7:358–363.

60. Yang S, Nisonson B. Arthroscopic surgery of the knee in the geriatric patient. *Clin Orthop Relat Res*. 1995;316:50–58.

61. Salisbury RB, Nottage WM, Gardner D. The effect of alignment on results in arthroscopic debridement of the degenerative knee. *Clin Orthop*. 1985;198:268–275.

62. Baumgartner M, Cannon W, Vittori J, et al. Arthroscopic debridement of the arthritic knee. *Clin Orthop Relat Res*. 1990;253:197–202.

63. Ahlback S. Osteoarthrosis of the knee. A radiographic investigation (thesis). Stockholm, Swedan: Karolinska Institute; 1968:11–15.

64. Lysholm J, Hamberg P, Gilquist J. The correlation between osteoarthritis as seen on radiographs and arthroscopy. *Arthroscopy*. 1987;3:161–169.

65. Bird HA, Ring EF. Therapeutic value of arthroscopy. *Ann Rheum Dis*. 1978;37:78–83.

66. Jackson RW, Marans HJ, Silver RS. The arthroscopic treatment of degenerative arthritis of the knee. *J Bone Joint Am*. 1988;33:42–51.

67. Ike RW, Arnold WJ, Rothschild EW, et al. Tidal Irrigation versus conservative medical management in patients with osteoarthritis of the knee: a prospective randomized study. *J Rheumatol*. 1992;19(5):772–781.

68. Chang RW. A randomized controlled trial of arthroscopic surgery vs. closed-needle joint lavage for patients with osteoarthritis of the knee. *Arthritis Rheum*. 1993;36:289–295.

69. Byers PH. Complement as a mediator of inflammation in acute gouty arthritis. *J Ala Clin Med*. 1973;81:761–768.

70. Dieppe PT, Muskinson BC, Willoughby DA. The inflammatory component of osteoarthritis. In: Nuki ED, ed. *An Etiopathogenesis of Osteoarthritis*. London, UK: Pitman Medical; 1980:117.

71. Goldenberg DL, Egan MS, Cohen AS. Inflammatory synovitis in degenerative joint disease. *J Rheumatol*. 1982;9:205–214.

72. Halverson PB, McCarty DJ. Identification of hydroxyapatite crystals in synovial fluid. *Arthritis Rheum*. 1979;22:389–395.

73. Fanelli GC, Rogers VP. High tibial valgus osteotomy combined with arthroscopic abrasion arthroplasty. *Contemp Orthop*. 1989;19:547–556.

74. Keene J, Dyravy J. High tibial osteotomy in the treatment of osteoarthritis of the knee: the role of preoperative arthroscopy. *J Bone Joint Surg Am*. 1983;65:36–44.

75. Kirkley A, Birmingham T, Litchfield R. A randomized trial of arthroscopic surgery for osteoarthritis of the knee. *N Engl J Med*. 2008;359:1097–1107.

76. Bin S, Lee S, Kim C, et al. Results of arthroscopic medial meniscectomy in patients with grade IV osteoarthritis of the medial compartment. *Arthroscopy*. 2008;24(3):264–268.

77. Dervin G, Stiell I, Rody K, et al. Effect of arthroscopic debridement for osteoarthritis of the knee on health related quality of life. *J Bone Joint Surg*. 2008;85A(1):10–17.

78. Fond J, Rodin R, Ahmad S, et al. Arthroscopic debridement for the treatment of osteoarthritis of the knee: 2 and 5 year results. *Arthroscopy*. 2002;18(8):829–834.

79. Hunt S, Jazrawi L, Sherman O. Arthroscopic management of osteoarthritis of the knee. *J Am Acad Orthop Surg*. 2002;10:356–363.

80. Richmond J, Hunter D, Irrgang J, et al. AAOS Clinical Practice Guideline Summary: Treatment of Osteoarthritis of the Knee (Nonarthroplasty). *J Am Acad Orthop Surg*. 2009; 17:591–600.

V. D. The Knee Articular Cartilage

Complex Approaches to the Diffuse Arthritic Knee: Including Corrective Osteotomy and Prosthetic Resurfacing

Christian Sybrowsky • Annunziato Amendola

The treatment of active patients who develop progressive or untimely osteoarthritis of the knee remains a taxing clinical challenge for physicians. As many patients continue to participate in high-demand and rigorous physical activities well into later age, the opportunity for repetitive or traumatic chondral injury similarly increases. Consequently, an increasing number of patients present with activity-limiting knee pathology, coupled with a strong desire to remain as active as possible. The current treatments for osteoarthritis range from simple activity modification and pharmacologic therapy to more invasive surgical procedures such as total knee arthroplasty (TKA). Although TKA has been a successful procedure for the treatment of osteoarthritis in elderly patients, many physiologically young patients are hesitant to pursue this as a treatment due to activity restrictions and cautionary recommendations associated with this procedure.

CLINICAL EVALUATION

The evaluation and treatment of arthritis should include a comprehensive evaluation including multiple clinical and patient-specific factors. Medical history, age, body mass index (BMI), current functional level, and patient expectations and goals must be considered when counseling patients. Prior injury, a history of surgery and radiographic appearance will also guide treatment, as the location, size, and chronicity of cartilage defects, as well as the degree of underlying degenerative joint disease, may exclude some treatments. If an osseous procedure such as high tibial osteotomy (HTO) is planned, diffuse disease is a contraindication, and bone quality must also be considered, as it may be challenging to obtain robust fixation in patients with osteoporosis and other diseases that affect bone density and quality. Consideration must also be given to other risk factors for failure, including smoking, corticosteroid dependency, chronic illness, immunosuppressants, etc.

NONOPERATIVE TREATMENT

Conservative treatment of osteoarthritis of the knee encompasses a broad spectrum of modalities and pharmaceuticals. Before considering surgical intervention, many patients are offered conservative therapies as a means to delay invasive procedures. Often, multiple modalities are used in concert to maximize benefit. These treatments can provide symptomatic relief as well as alter the knee environment to attempt to limit the progression of the disease. Conservative possibilities include nonsteroidal anti-inflammatory drugs (NSAIDs), cyclooxygenase-2 (COX-2) inhibitors, steroid injections, viscosupplementation, bracing and other orthoses, physical therapy and other exercise, and weight loss.

Weight Loss

Two randomized trials have demonstrated that even a modest reduction in weight (5% to 10% decrease in total body weight) can improve both pain and physical function in patients with osteoarthritis of the knee (1, 2). Although these studies did not specifically evaluate physiologically "young," active patients, they support the notion that dietary weight loss is an important adjunct in the treatment of this disorder. More recently, the American Academy of Orthopaedic Surgeons (AAOS) has published a clinical practice guideline for the treatment of osteoarthritis of the knee, strongly recommending (grade A) that patients with a BMI >25 should be encouraged to lose a minimum of 5% of body weight (3).

Physical Therapy and Exercise

A number of randomized trials have supported regular, low-impact aerobic exercise as an effective modality for decreasing both pain and disability from knee OA (4, 5). Targeted physical therapy and home-based exercises for muscle strengthening and flexibility have also been supported by several studies (6–8). The beneficial effects of exercise therapy, however, may diminish over time (9, 10). The AAOS clinical practice guidelines strongly support (grade A) a low-impact fitness program, with lesser recommendations for targeted therapies (3).

Acetaminophen and NSAIDs

Acetaminophen is commonly prescribed for the analgesic treatment of arthritis due to its relative safety and efficacy. Hepatic toxicity secondary to acetaminophen overdose has been associated with dosages exceeding 4,000 mg per day. NSAIDs are also widely prescribed for degenerative joint disease. NSAIDs inhibit the enzyme cyclooxygenase, which subsequently results in decreased prostaglandin synthesis. Prostaglandins mediate the inflammatory response, which accounts for the anti-inflammatory effect of this class of drugs. However, some prostaglandins also increase protective gastric mucosal secretions and decrease gastric acid release, accounting for the nontrivial risk of gastrointestinal (GI) toxicity and bleeding associated with NSAIDs. Some studies suggest that GI toxicity is present in more than 25% of patients and treatment of GI side effects accounts for more than 30% of the total cost of arthritis care (11). Selective COX-2 inhibitors have been developed to decrease the GI toxicity and bleeding associated with conventional NSAIDs (12). COX-2 inhibitors are associated with fewer GI side effects and decreased gastroduodenal ulcers (13, 14). Topical NSAIDs have also been used in some patients to avoid systemic toxicity, but these may be effective only for a few weeks when compared with oral NSAIDs and may include side effects of rashes, burning, and itching (15). Some NSAIDs appear to stimulate collagen synthesis, which may aid in soft-tissue healing (16). However, NSAIDs and COX-2 inhibitors have also been shown to decrease bone ingrowth and may delay fracture healing (17). The AAOS clinical practice guidelines support (grade B) the use of these medications in the symptomatic treatment of osteoarthritis (3).

Braces and Orthoses

Knee braces and foot orthoses are commonly employed treatments for patients with early osteoarthritis who wish to maintain an active lifestyle and defer surgical treatment (18). Candidates for bracing include patients with early degenerative disease, particularly medial compartment osteoarthritis, focal posttraumatic arthritis, and meniscal deficiency resulting in unicompartmental disease. Brace design can range from simple neoprene sleeves to custom-fit hinged unloader braces, with the ultimate goal being a reduction in mechanical load in the affected compartment with a subsequent decrease in pain perception and increase in function. Unloader braces differ from traditional functional braces by the addition of an internal valgus angle (for medial compartment disease) or varus angle (for lateral compartment disease), which can, in theory, shift the weight-bearing axis toward the less affected

compartment (19). Unloader bracing has been shown to be beneficial in patients with passively correctible coronal plane deformity of less than 10°, without excessive ligamentous laxity. Several studies report improvement of pain symptoms in more than 75% of patients (20, 21). with measurable reduction in both coronal moments and compartmental loads (22). Reduced muscle contractions about the knee, mediated by the stabilization of the brace, may also contribute to decreased pain in some patients (23).

Lateral wedge orthoses (both heel wedges and lateral-wedge insoles) have also been shown to be beneficial in patients with symptomatic medial compartment disease (19). Pain relief and functional improvement in these patients are likely achieved by a reduction in external varus moment and medial compartment load (24). However, a recent systematic review suggests that the benefit gained from these orthoses is modest at best (25), and the AAOS clinical practice guidelines caution against their use (3).

Steroid Injections

Intra-articular corticosteroid injections are commonly used for anti-inflammatory relief in knee osteoarthritis. Although water-soluble formulations are available, depot formulations, which are less soluble and retain crystals in the injected area, are most commonly used in the treatment of osteoarthritis. Methylprednisolone and triamcinolone are the most commonly used depot preparations (26). Side effects are generally mild and can include postinjection flare, facial flushing, and skin or fat atrophy. A recent randomized, double-blind, controlled trial compared triamcinolone with saline injections in the knee repeated every 3 months for up to 2 years. Findings demonstrated improved clinical scores and range of motion in the corticosteroid group, with no progression of joint space narrowing (27). Intra-articular corticosteroid injections are supported (grade B) by the recent AAOS clinical practice guidelines for the treatment of osteoarthritis (3).

Viscosupplementation

Intra-articular viscosupplementation refers to the injection of hyaluronic acid (HA) into the affected joint. With both viscous and elastic properties, HA is produced by the synovial membrane and is a major component of joint synovial fluid. HA has anti-inflammatory, anabolic, analgesic, and chondroprotective effects (28). In a recent meta-analysis of randomized controlled trials comparing HA injections with placebo, there were significant improvements in pain and functional outcomes with HA, although the effects were inversely proportional to age and the degree of joint degeneration (29). Several preparations of HA are available, including products from both avian and bacterial origins (28). The material properties of HA can be influenced by molecular weight, and cross-linking of the molecules can increase average molecular weight. Hylan G-F 20 is the only form of injectable HA in the United States that has cross-linked hyaluronan. In one study, hylan G-F 20 was shown to delay total knee replacement by 2 years or more (30). Side effects can include hypersensitivity and cutaneous anaphylaxis, and erythema (pseudo-sepsis) (31). The AAOS clinical practice guidelines could not make a recommendation for or against their use, due to inconclusive evidence (3).

ARTHROSCOPY

The role of arthroscopy in the treatment of osteoarthritis of the knee remains controversial (18). Fifty percent or more of patients who undergo arthroscopy for osteoarthritis will report symptomatic relief (32). However, other studies have shown that only 44% of patients maintain decreased pain scores at 2-year follow-up (33), and up to 18% of patients undergo TKA within 3 years (34). Despite these findings, arthroscopic debridement remains a commonly performed procedure for osteoarthritis, and generalizability of the literature is limited by the heterogeneity of patient populations in these studies (18).

Several more recent randomized trials, however, have challenged the role of arthroscopic debridement in the treatment of osteoarthritis. In a randomized, controlled trial comparing arthroscopic lavage, debridement, or placebo surgery, Moseley et al. (32) evaluated 180 male veterans for a mean of 2 years following arthroscopy for treatment of osteoarthritis. Throughout the 2-year follow-up period, there were no statistically significant changes in pain scores among the three groups, leading the authors to conclude that the beneficial results of arthroscopy were no better than placebo in this homogenous patient population. In a subsequent study of a civilian population with moderate-to-severe osteoarthritis, Kirkley et al. (35) randomized 188 patients to either surgical debridement with medical/physical therapy or medical/physical therapy in isolation. At 2-year follow-up, there were no differences in Western Ontario and McMaster Universities Osteoarthritis Index (WOMAC) or Short Form-36 (SF-36) scores between the two groups. The authors concluded that arthroscopic debridement was no better than optimized medical/physical therapy.

These randomized studies, however, largely excluded patients with large meniscal tears or mechanical symptoms, suggesting that some subpopulations of patients, particularly those with mechanical symptoms from degenerative meniscal pathology, would benefit from arthroscopy. For example, in a study of 68 patients with Outerbridge grade IV osteoarthritis and a medial meniscal tear, up to 82% of patients reported a reduction of pain at 52 months after debridement, with 75% of patients requiring no further surgery up to 75 months after arthroscopy (36). Other authors have shown that up to 81% of patients with advanced arthritis might benefit from aggressive arthroscopic lysis of adhesions to increase joint volume and thereby decrease joint reactive forces (37). Despite these findings, however, other studies have demonstrated difficulty predicting

which patients might benefit from arthroscopic debridement (33, 38). Dervin et al. (33) evaluated 126 patients with primary osteoarthritis who had failed initial medical management. Unstable chondral flaps and meniscal tears were addressed at the time of arthroscopy. Only 44% of patients maintained decreased WOMAC scores at 2 years. However, the presence of medial joint line tenderness preoperatively coupled with the debridement of a corresponding meniscal tear at the time of surgery seemed to portend better outcomes. Despite this, the authors concluded that physicians were unable to reliably predict which patients would benefit from surgery, based on preoperative clinical findings.

The role of arthroscopy in physiologically young patients with osteoarthritis is also unclear. The AAOS clinical practice guideline for treatment of osteoarthritis of the knee recommends against routine arthroscopy with debridement/lavage in patients with primary osteoarthritis (3). However, a corollary to this stipulation specifies that this recommendation does not apply to patients with a primary diagnosis of meniscal tear, loose body, or other mechanical symptoms in the setting of concomitant osteoarthritis. In the absence of specific studies targeting these subgroups, clinical judgment and proper patient selection are critical for surgical decision making. Younger patients with mechanical symptoms and less severe disease are the most likely to benefit from a trial of arthroscopy. It is important, however, to have a candid discussion regarding expectations, cautioning patients that any postoperative gains may be of limited benefit.

OSTEOTOMY

For more than 50 years, HTO and distal femoral osteotomy (DFO) have been used for correction of lower extremity malalignment and alleviation of unilateral compartment gonarthrosis (39, 40). Lower extremity alignment has been shown to be a significant factor in the progression of osteoarthritis of the knee (41). Coventry (42) initially defined indications for HTO and suggested that the optimal candidate was relatively active, with a stable knee, good range of motion, localized (unicompartmental) osteoarthritis, and age less than 65 years. Due to concomitant surgical procedures, contemporary indications for HTO have expanded to encompass coronal and sagittal malalignment, unicompartmental overload with prearthritic change, anteroposterior and varus/valgus instability, lateral or hyperextension thrust from posterolateral instability, and ligamentous deficiency (43–47). Osteotomies are also commonly used for limb realignment in concert with meniscal transplantation or articular resurfacing procedures (48–51). The medial compartment is the most common site of deformity in both primary knee osteoarthritis and secondary arthritis resulting from osteochondral lesions, postmeniscectomy change, or chronic anterior cruciate ligament (ACL) deficiency. The lateral compartment can also be involved, often in concert with a valgus deformity, particularly in the context of lateral meniscal deficiency, as the lateral compartment is highly reliant on meniscal integrity to avoid overload and secondary osteoarthritis. Varus deformity is usually secondary to proximal tibia vara, and is best addressed with HTO. Valgus deformity of the knee is usually secondary to deformity of the distal femur, and therefore DFO is often more appropriate.

As opposed to arthroplasty procedures, which often require avoidance of certain activities, patients who have undergone osteotomy are generally allowed to continue at their desired activity level. Osteotomy is therefore appropriate for patients with isolated (unicompartmental) arthritis and coronal/sagittal malalignment who desire to continue participation in high-impact activities. Osteotomy can also be useful as an adjunctive treatment for focal cartilaginous lesions. Since an osteotomy procedure will often shift the weight-bearing axis from an overloaded compartment to another area of the knee, patient selection is paramount to achieve a satisfactory result. Patients with global osteoarthritis or inflammatory disease may not benefit from a shift of the weight-bearing axis. Additionally, shifting of the mechanical axis into a compartment that has previously undergone meniscectomy would also be a relative contraindication to osteotomy.

Osteotomies may be performed by either an opening wedge or a closing wedge technique. Closing wedge techniques involve the removal of a wedge of bone, and therefore require a high degree of precision to obtain the desired correction. Opening wedge osteotomies require only a single cut, and are therefore technically easier to perform. Furthermore, opening wedge osteotomies of the proximal tibia require only a single tibial cut and avoid a secondary osteotomy of the proximal fibula with its concomitant risk of peroneal nerve and posterolateral corner injury (52–54). Additionally, opening wedge techniques allow for correction in both the coronal and sagittal planes, as hinging through the intact proximal tibiofibular joint decreases the posterior tibial slope (55). Alteration of the posterior tibial slope can also be achieved by distracting the osteotomy more posteriorly or anteriorly, which changes the resting position of the tibia with respect to the femur. In general, the more posterior the slope, the more anterior the resting position will be, although cruciate-intact knees may be less susceptible to these alterations (56, 57). Giffin et al. (57) noted increased tibial translation with increasing posterior tibial slope, but did not demonstrate altered cruciate kinematics. They concluded that inadvertent alterations of tibial slope during HTO would not alter knee stability or cruciate forces in situ. These findings have been supported by a recent cadaveric study suggesting that large variations of tibial slope can influence the resting position of the tibiofemoral articulation, but do not appear to adversely influence the strain environment of the ACL (56). This sagittal orientation of the osteotomy is of particular importance in patients with symptomatic hyperextension-varus thrust (45).

Preoperative Templating

Radiographic evaluation begins with standard knee radiographs, including weightbearing A/P, lateral, posteroanterior tunnel views in 30° of flexion, and merchant patellar views. The surgeon should assess the extent of knee arthrosis, fractures, retained hardware, etc. Lateral radiographs are important to evaluate tibial slope. Standing long-leg alignment films (pelvis-to-ankle) are necessary for estimation of the mechanical axis, with the axis commonly passing through the compartment exhibiting signs and symptoms of overload (Fig. 68.1A–C). The HTO correction can also be calculated from these radiographs (58). The mechanical and weight-bearing axes are estimated, and the correction to be made is then calculated by shifting this axis just lateral to the lateral tibial spine, at a point representing approximately 62% of the joint surface as referenced from the medial joint line.

Surgical Technique

For medial opening wedge HTO, a medial incision is made halfway between the anterior tibial spine and the posteromedial border of the tibia. Dissection is carried through skin and subcutaneous tissue to bone. Subperiosteal elevation is performed, elevating the medial collateral ligament and pes anserinus if necessary. A guide wire is inserted into the proximal tibia from medial to lateral, under fluoroscopic guidance. The wire is oriented obliquely from the superior aspect of the tibial tubercle to a point approximately 1 cm below the far lateral joint line. This position allows for the osteotomy to avoid the patellar ligament insertion, yet remain remote enough to minimize the risk of intra-articular extension. An oscillating saw is used to create shallow cortical cuts, and the osteotomy is subsequently deepened with flexible and rigid osteotomes under fluoroscopic guidance. It is important to leave a lateral hinge. A soft bump is placed under the leg in order to hyperextend the knee and assist with closing the osteotomy anteriorly, if necessary. The osteotomy is then opened to the predetermined amount and fixation achieved with an opening wedge plate. Positioning the plate more anteriorly or posteriorly can modify the tibial slope to match preoperative templating. Corticocancellous allograft wedges (harvested from femoral head allograft) or synthetic allograft wedges are employed to fill the osteotomy site. The wounds are then closed in layers.

Lateral closing wedge HTO employs an anterolateral incision just anterior to the fibular head. Dissection is carried to the fibular head, with subperiosteal dissection of a sleeve containing the lateral collateral ligament and biceps femoris attachment. The fibula is cut at the level of the fibular neck and the head and neck are excised. Exposure of the proximal tibia is achieved by subperiosteal elevation. The proximal osteotomy is made parallel to the joint line, at a point approximately 2 cm distal to the joint. The oblique distal osteotomy is then made to allow for a

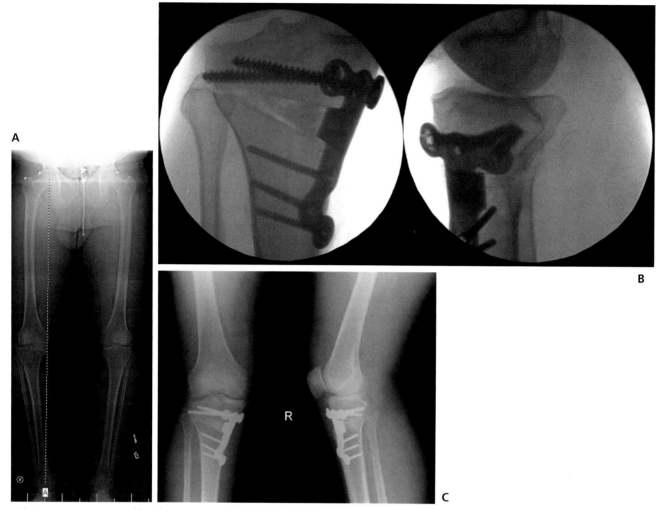

FIGURE 68.1. A 43-year-old male with right-sided medial joint line pain. **A:** Preoperative radiographs demonstrating approximately 14° varus malalignment and medial joint degenerative disease. **B:** Intraoperative fluoroscopic views demonstrating correction of the varus deformity with medial opening-wedge osteotomy, backfilled with tricortical allograft. **C:** Postoperative radiographs at 12 weeks showing consolidation of the osteotomy site.

closing wedge. A plate or staple can be used to cross the osteotomy site and provide fixation.

Distal femoral opening wedge osteotomy is achieved via a lateral approach to the distal femur. A longitudinal incision is made over the iliotibial band, beginning distal to the lateral epicondyle and extending proximally. Dissection is carried down through the iliotibial band to the vastus lateralis, which is retracted anteriorly to expose the distal femoral metaphysis. A guide wire is placed obliquely through the metaphysis at approximately 20° to the joint surface and confirmed fluoroscopically. The oblique osteotomy is then performed by cutting the lateral cortex with the oscillating saw and completing the osteotomy with serial osteotomes. Again, it is important to leave a medial hinge. The osteotomy is then opened to the correct amount and fixation achieved with a lateral plate and tricorticocancellous graft.

Medial femoral closing wedge osteotomy is performed via a medial longitudinal incision carried down to the

vastus medialis, which is retracted anteriorly to expose the distal medial femur. Subperiosteal dissection exposes the femur. Guide pins are inserted proximally and distally according to preoperative templating. Cuts are made parallel in the coronal plane to avoid alterations in the flexion/extension alignment of the distal femur. The wedge of bone is excised and the osteotomy is closed. Fixation is usually achieved with a blade plate or other fixed-angle device.

Postoperative Rehabilitation

For both tibial and femoral osteotomies, it is important to allow bone healing to occur prior to initiating weight-bearing. A hinged knee brace is employed to allow progressive recumbent knee range-of-motion to 90° within the first week. Radiographs are taken at 6 weeks, with progression to 50% weight-bearing if there is evidence of bony consolidation of the osteotomy. Partial progressive weight-bearing is continued until full weight-bearing is achieved at approximately 12 weeks. Physical therapy and quadriceps strengthening exercises are prescribed concurrently. Interval radiographs confirm healing of the osteotomy.

Results

Osteotomy for physiologically young patients with early osteoarthritis remains controversial. Survivorship of the osteotomy is generally not as predictable as unicompartmental or TKA in this patient population. Additionally, conversion or revision of a prior osteotomy to a TKA can present several technical challenges including malalignment, instability, component fixation, and extensor mechanism maltracking (59–61). Despite these issues, however, osteotomy can be a successful procedure in many patient populations, and several authors have reported excellent results with osteotomy. Survivorship of HTO, as measured by conversion to TKA, has been reported to be as high as 98% at 10 years (62) and 70% at 20 years (63). Survivorship of DFO has been reported to be as high as 82% at 10 years, but drops to 45% at 15 years (64). Osteotomy should not be viewed as the ultimate solution to joint degeneration, but rather as a means to delay arthroplasty in physiologically young patients, sometimes for more than 20 years (18).

Complications associated with osteotomy include nonunion, hardware failure, fracture, infection, prominent/symptomatic hardware, peroneal nerve palsy, compartment syndrome, vascular injury, thromboembolic disease, and others. Intraoperative fracture of the proximal tibia has been reported to be as high as 18% in HTO (65). Staying distal to the guide pin placed as described in our operative technique can minimize this complication. Instances of intra-articular fracture require anatomic reduction and rigid fixation.

Summary

The correction of mechanical malalignment in young, active patients may allow for increased function and decreased pain in patients with unicompartmental gonarthrosis. Furthermore, corrective osteotomy is a critical adjunct in the treatment of focal osteochondral lesions, meniscal transplantation, etc., where there is overload of the affected compartment. Both HTO and DFO have been shown to be effective methods of correcting coronal and/or sagittal malalignment, with a consequent decrease in the progression of osteoarthritis. Proper patient selection, meticulous preoperative planning, and precise surgical technique are essential to successful outcomes.

UNICONDYLAR AND PATELLOFEMORAL ARTHROPLASTY

Introduction

Unicompartmental knee arthroplasty (UKA) has been in use for several decades; however, contemporary developments in materials and the publication of several long-term outcome studies have led to an expansion of indications and an increase in popularity of this procedure for unicompartmental degenerative disease. UKA can involve prosthetic replacement of unicondylar disease (medial or lateral compartments) or patellofemoral disease, and there are several advantages to UKA in the treatment of arthritis in the physiologically young patient. In general, UKA preserves tibiofemoral bone stock, which allows for a much simpler revision procedure. Additionally, UKA allows for a more natural and physiologic range of motion when compared with TKA (66). Furthermore, UKA is associated with reduced blood loss, shorter inpatient stays, and decreased costs compared with TKA (67).

Proper patient selection is the most important factor for the success of UKA. Traditional indications for UKA include osteoarthritis or posttraumatic arthritis with unicompartmental pain, relatively sedentary occupation, lack of obesity, minimal coronal malalignment (<10° of varus/valgus deformity), preoperative range of motion of at least 90° without a flexion contracture, and intact cruciate ligaments (67, 68). Additional indications for UKA include physiologically young patients who are unwilling to undergo realignment osteotomy for unicompartmental overload, yet still desire a reliable procedure. Patients with isolated and radiographically proven patellofemoral degenerative disease may benefit from patellofemoral resurfacing. Contraindications to UKA include inflammatory arthritis, nonlocalizable knee pain, flexion contracture, ligamentous instability, and participation in high-impact sports. In contrast, some contemporary authors have suggested that ACL-deficiency is not a strict contraindication to *medial* compartment UKA (68). This is not the case, however, with lateral compartment UKA, as this compartment has more inherent motion, and relies on an intact ACL to avoid untoward translation.

Surgical Technique

The surgical approach relies heavily on the instrumentation of the chosen implant system. Both traditional and minimally invasive approaches have been described, and the choice, again, is dependent on the preferred implant manufacturer recommendations and surgeon preference.

For medial compartment unicondylar arthroplasty, an incision is made just medial to the midline. A medial parapatellar arthrotomy is performed, and the compartment is exposed. Medial retractors protect the fibers of deep medial collateral ligament, and a Hohmann or similar retractor is used in the intercondylar notch to protect the notch contents and retract the patella laterally. An extramedullary jig is then used to make a tibial cut, with no more than 4 to 5 mm of bone removed. This cut must be orthogonal to the tibial shaft and extend laterally to the ACL insertion. The femoral sizing and cutting jigs are then applied to the femur, referencing the tibial cut. Trial components are placed once all the appropriate bone has been removed and peg holes have been drilled. The knee should be examined for appropriate alignment, tracking, and stability in both flexion and extension, with component alterations made as necessary. Bony surfaces are then prepared for cement, and the components are cemented in place. Care must be taken to remove extraneous cement from the periphery of the implants. The incision is then closed in layers (Fig. 68.2A, B). These principles are similar for lateral compartment unicondylar arthroplasty, although a slightly longer incision and lateral parapatellar arthrotomy are employed to gain access to the lateral compartment.

For patellofemoral arthroplasty, many surgeons begin with arthroscopy to address concomitant pathology and to perform a lateral release, if indicated. The skin incision

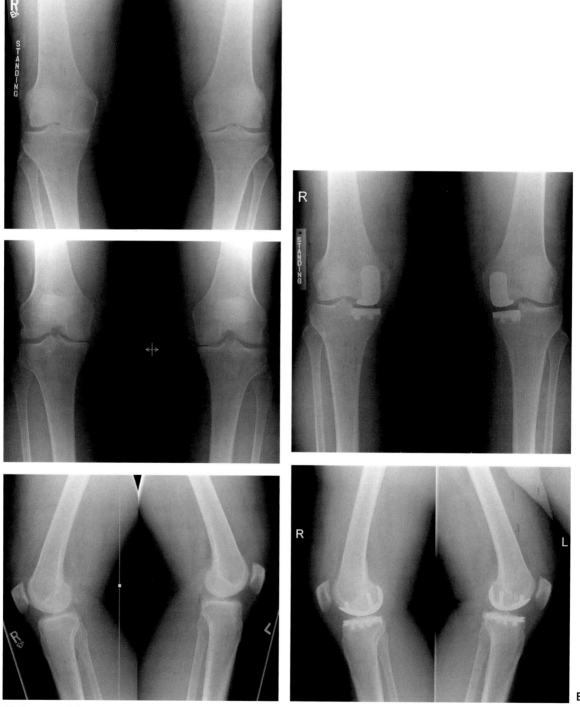

FIGURE 68.2. A: Weightbearing anteroposterior, posteroanterior views in 30° of flexion, and lateral radiographs of a 56-year-old male with bilateral medial knee pain. **B:** Postoperative radiographs following bilateral unicompartmental arthroplasty of the medial knee.

can be either a longitudinal incision made in the midline over the patella, or a medial incision that incorporates the medial arthroscopy portal. Dissection is carried to the medial retinaculum, and a medial parapatellar arthrotomy is performed. Exposure of the trochlea can be achieved by placing a retractor over the lateral femoral condyle, which reflects the patella laterally. Exposure of the articular surface of the patella is achieved by everting the patella into the surgical incision. The anteroposterior trochlear axis (Whiteside's line) and transepicondylar axis (perpendicular to Whiteside's line) are identified. The trochlear alignment and cutting/milling jigs specific to the chosen implant system are then applied. The appropriate bone cuts are made, and trial components, if applicable, are placed. The patella is then everted and resurfacing ensues, specific to the chosen implant. With trial components in place, the knee range of motion and patellar tracking is examined, with component adjustments as necessary. The components are then cemented in place. The skin is then closed in layers (Fig. 68.3A–F).

Postoperative Rehabilitation

Similar to TKA, full weight-bearing is permitted postoperatively, with rehabilitation emphasizing range of motion. Physical therapy for gait training and quadriceps strengthening is initiated, with advancement of activity as tolerated by the patient.

Results

Survivorship of unicondylar UKA as measured by conversion to TKA has been reported in recent studies to be as high as 90% to 94% at 15 years (69, 70). In patients younger than 60 years, clinical outcome scores for pain and function were good or excellent in 90% of patients at up to 6 years (71). In a separate study of unicondylar UKA in a physically active patient population, the overall survival was 92% at 11 years (72). Isolated patellofemoral arthroplasty has shown more modest results, with some studies reporting successful results in 80% of patients at 5 years (73), with survivorship as high as 84% at 10 years

V. D. The Knee Articular Cartilage

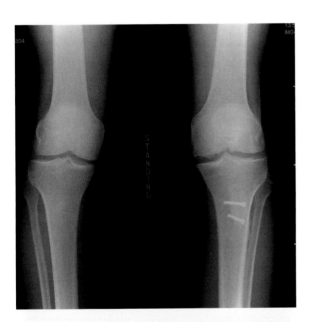

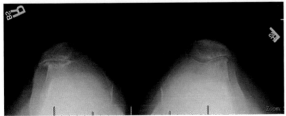

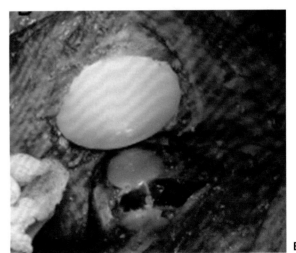

FIGURE 68.3. **A:** Preoperative radiographs demonstrating isolated bilateral patellofemoral degenerative disease. The patient has previously undergone a unilateral tibial tubercle transfer. **B:** Intraoperative view demonstrating an onlay-type patellofemoral arthroplasty. **C:** Postoperative radiographs. **D:** Preoperative radiographs from a separate patient with recalcitrant left-sided patellofemoral pain and degenerative disease. This patient has also previously undergone a unilateral tubercle transfer. **E:** Intraoperative view demonstrating an inlay-type patellofemoral resurfacing. **F:** Postoperative radiographs.

(Continued)

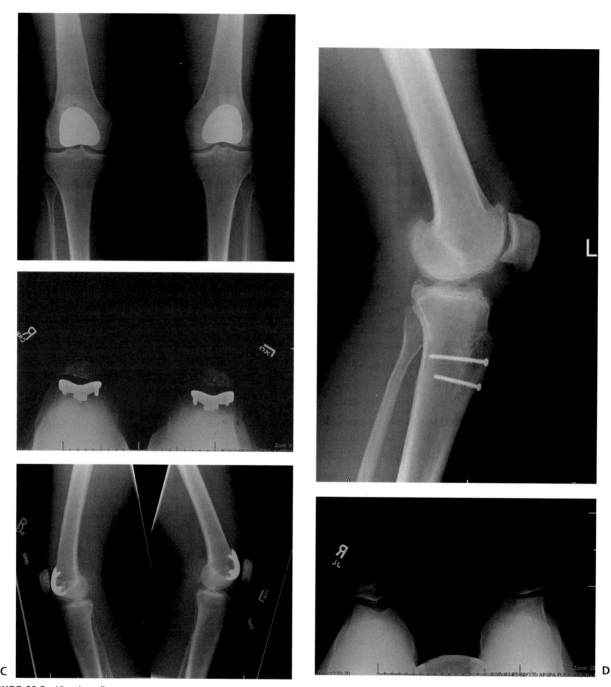

FIGURE 68.3. (Continued)

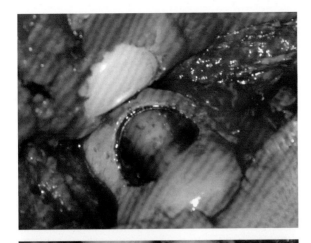

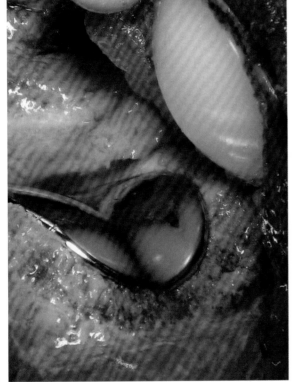

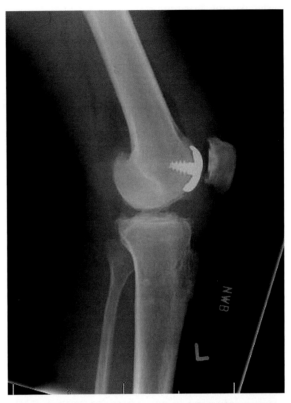

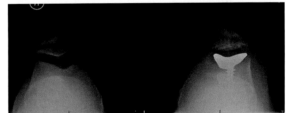

E

F

FIGURE 68.3. (Continued)

and 69% at 20 years (74). Randomized clinical trials are currently underway to compare isolated patellofemoral arthroplasty with TKA.

Complications of UKA include component wear and loosening, progression of osteoarthritis, malalignment, infection, mechanical clicking, etc (68). Complications of UKA often require revision to TKA.

Summary

UKA is a useful surgical procedure for patients with isolated unicompartmental disease in which conservative measures have failed. Although there may be some activity limitations with these procedures, unicondylar arthroplasty has demonstrated excellent short- and long-term outcomes and survivorship. Patient selection and proper

surgical technique are of utmost importance to avoid complications and early failures.

TOTAL KNEE ARTHROPLASTY

TKA has been used for many years to provide pain relief and functional improvement to patients with varying degrees of posttraumatic or degenerative osteoarthritis. Significant advances in implant design and improved material properties of the components have led to excellent long-term survivorship and clinical function. However, despite these encouraging results in elderly patients, TKA is usually reserved as a final option, especially for physiologically younger, active patients (18). For many years, age less than 60 years was seen as a contraindication to total knee replacement. However, as many patients continue to participate in high-demand and rigorous physical activities well into later age, the indications for TKA are being expanded to include this younger population.

Although there is compelling evidence that relatively inactive patients with TKA will exhibit less wear than that of an active patient, it is important to balance concerns of component wear with maintaining a healthy and fulfilling lifestyle in patients who have undergone TKA. As such, the appropriate level of activity following TKA remains a topic of great controversy. In a retrospective review of 160 TKA patients, Bradbury et al. (75) found that less than half of patients regularly participated in sports prior to surgery, and only 65% of this group returned to sports participation following TKA. Most of these activities were low-impact sports such as bowling, with only 20% of this group returning to impact sports such as tennis. Healy et al. (76) polled 58 members of The Knee Society to determine recommendations for appropriate activities following TKA. Kuster (77) expanded upon and provided scientific guidelines for these recommendations, stressing a conservative approach to activities that involve high joint loads in flexion. A summary of these recommendations is provided in Table 68.1. Some studies suggest that up to 16% of TKA patients will participate in "nonrecommended" activities contrary to their physician's recommendations (78). Other studies have suggested that there is no difference in failure rates between "high-activity" versus "low-activity" patients with TKA (79). The correct balance between activity level and concerns for implant wear must be patient-specific. Patients must understand that certain activities have a theoretical risk of accelerated wear, which is of particular importance to the young or physiologically younger patient who has undergone TKA.

A discussion of surgical considerations in TKA is beyond the scope of this chapter. In the care of the active patient with degenerative disease of the knee, however, TKA must be part of the clinical armamentarium. When other options have failed, TKA may provide a reliable method for improving quality of life in this patient population.

CONCLUSIONS AND FUTURE DIRECTIONS

The treatment of diffuse arthritis in active patients is a challenging problem for clinicians who want to help the patient achieve pain control while maintaining a high level of activity. Nonoperative modalities have clinical applicability throughout the treatment algorithm of this disorder and are used concurrently with many of the surgical procedures discussed. Furthermore, as our understanding of the basic mechanisms of osteoarthritis improves, new avenues of medical therapy may open to not only prevent, but also treat the biochemical processes that accelerate joint degeneration.

Arthroscopy, in isolation, has a limited role in the treatment of diffuse arthritis but can be a useful adjunct with other procedures. It has a role in the treatment of concomitant intraarticular pathology encountered during osteotomy and UKA. It is also employed in certain situations following TKA. Osteotomy is paramount to restoring mechanical alignment and alleviating joint overload. Similar to arthroscopy, osteotomy can also be a useful adjunctive procedure in the treatment of focal cartilaginous lesions. Contemporary indications for osteotomy have broadened to include ligamentous deficiencies, and several techniques for concomitant osteotomy/ligamentous reconstruction procedures have been described.

Table 68.1

Recommendations for activity following TKA

Recommended	Allowed with Experience	Not Recommended	No Conclusion
Low-impact aerobics	Road bicycling	Racquetball	Fencing
Stationary bicycling	Canoeing	Squash	Inline skating
Bowling	Hiking	Rock climbing	Downhill skiing
Golf	Rowing	Soccer	Weightlifting
Dancing	Cross-country skiing	Singles tennis	
Horseback riding	Stationary skiing	Volleyball	
Croquet	Speed walking	Football	
Walking	Tennis	Gymnastics	
Swimming	Weight machines	Lacrosse	
Shooting	Ice skating	Hockey	
Shuffleboard		Basketball	
Horseshoes		Jogging	
		Handball	

Indications for unicondylar and patellofemoral arthroplasty have also expanded to include concomitant cruciate reconstruction in cruciate-deficient knees with unicompartmental disease. Patellofemoral arthroplasty can be combined with tubercle osteotomy procedures to maximize patellar alignment. Combination procedures involving unicondylar and patellofemoral arthroplasties have also been described. TKA is also a useful adjunct in the treatment of diffuse arthritis. Although many physiologically younger patients are reluctant to pursue TKA due to cautionary recommendations related to this procedure, TKA can be a reliable procedure for alleviating pain and improving quality of life in patients who have exhausted other options.

REFERENCES

1. Christensen R, Astrup A, Bliddal H. Weight loss: the treatment of choice for knee osteoarthritis? A randomized trial. *Osteoarthritis Cartilage.* 2005;13(1):20–27.

2. Messier SP, Loeser RF, Miller GD, et al. Exercise and dietary weight loss in overweight and obese older adults with knee osteoarthritis: the Arthritis, Diet, and Activity Promotion Trial. *Arthritis Rheum.* 2004;50(5):1501–1510.

3. Richmond J, Hunter D, Irrgang J, et al. Treatment of osteoarthritis of the knee (nonarthroplasty). *J Am Acad Orthop Surg.* 2009;17:591–600.

4. Zhang W, Moskowitz RW, Nuki G, et al. OARSI recommendations for the management of hip and knee osteoarthritis, part II: OARSI evidence-based, expert consensus guidelines. *Osteoarthritis Cartilage.* 2008;16(2):137–162.

5. Zhang W, Nuki G, Moakoqir RW, et al. OARSI recommendations for the management of hip and knee osteoarthritis: part III: Changes in evidence following systematic cumulative update of research published through January 2009. *Osteoarthritis Cartilage.* 2010;18(4):476–499.

6. Bennell K, Hinman R. Exercise as a treatment for osteoarthritis. *Curr Opin Rheumatol.* 2005;17(5):634–640.

7. Kon E, Filardo G, Drobnic M, et al. Non-surgical management of early knee osteoarthritis. *Knee Surg Sports Traumatol Arthrosc.* 2012;20(3):436–449.

8. McCarthy CJ, Mills PM, Pullen R, et al. Supplementation of a home-based exercise programme with a class-based programme for people with osteoarthritis of the knees: a randomised controlled trial and health economic analysis. *Health Technol Assess.* 2004;8(46):iii–iv, 1–61.

9. Pisters MF, Veenhof C, Schellevis FG, et al. Long-term effectiveness of exercise therapy in patients with osteoarthritis of the hip or knee: a randomized controlled trial comparing two different physical therapy interventions. *Osteoarthritis Cartilage.* 2010;18(8):1019–1026.

10. van Baar ME, Dekker J, Barnaart LF, et al. Effectiveness of exercise in patients with osteoarthritis of hip or knee: nine months' follow up. *Ann Rheum Dis.* 2001;60(12):1123–1130.

11. Bloom BS. Direct medical costs of disease and gastrointestinal side effects during treatment for arthritis. *Am J Med.* 1988;84(2A):20–24.

12. Lane JM. Anti-inflammatory medications: selective COX-2 inhibitors. *J Am Acad Orthop Surg.* 2002;10(2):75–78.

13. Rostom A, Muir K, Dube C, et al. Prevention of NSAID-related upper gastrointestinal toxicity: a meta-analysis of traditional NSAIDs with gastroprotection and COX-2 inhibitors. *Drug Healthc Patient Saf.* 2009;1:47–71.

14. Silverstein FE, Faich G, Goldstein JL, et al. Gastrointestinal toxicity with celecoxib vs nonsteroidal anti-inflammatory drugs for osteoarthritis and rheumatoid arthritis: the CLASS study: a randomized controlled trial. Celecoxib Long-term Arthritis Safety Study. *JAMA.* 2000;284(10):1247–1255.

15. Mason L, Moore RA, Edwards JE, et al. Topical NSAIDs for chronic musculoskeletal pain: systematic review and meta-analysis. *BMC Musculoskeletal Disord.* 2004;5:28.

16. Dahners LE, Mullis BH. Effects of nonsteroidal anti-inflammatory drugs on bone formation and soft-tissue healing. *J Am Acad Orthop Surg.* 2004;12(3):139–143.

17. Goodman SB, Jiranek W, Petrow E, et al. The effects of medications on bone. *J Am Acad Orthop Surg.* 2007;15(8):450–460.

18. Feeley BT, Gallo RA, Sherman S, et al. Management of osteoarthritis of the knee in the active patient. *J Am Acad Orthop Surg.* 2010;18(7):406–416.

19. Krohn K. Footwear alterations and bracing as treatments for knee osteoarthritis. *Curr Opin Rheumatol.* 2005;17(5):653–656.

20. Dennis DA, Komistek RD, Nadaud MC, et al. Evaluation of off-loading braces for treatment of unicompartmental knee arthrosis. *J Arthroplasty.* 2006;21(4)(suppl 1):2–8.

21. Giori NJ. Load-shifting brace treatment for osteoarthritis of the knee: a minimum 2 1/2-year follow-up study. *J Rehabil Res Dev.* 2004;41(2):187–194.

22. Pollo FE, Otis JC, Backus SI, et al. Reduction of medial compartment loads with valgus bracing of the osteoarthritic knee. *Am J Sports Med.* 2002;30(3):414–421.

23. Ramsey DK, Briem K, Axe MJ, et al. A mechanical theory for the effectiveness of bracing for medial compartment osteoarthritis of the knee. *J Bone Joint Surg.* 2007;89(11):2398–2407.

24. Crenshaw SJ, Pollo FE, Calton EF. Effects of lateral-wedged insoles on kinetics at the knee. *Clin Orthop Relat Res.* 2000;(375):185–192.

25. Brouwer RW, Jakma TS, Verhagen AP, et al. Braces and orthoses for treating osteoarthritis of the knee. *Cochrane Database Syst Rev.* 2005;(1):CD004020.

26. Cole BJ, Schumacher HR. Injectable corticosteroids in modern practice. *J Am Acad Orthop Surg.* 2005;13(1):37–46.

27. Raynauld JP, Buckland-Wright C, Ward R, et al. Safety and efficacy of long-term intraarticular steroid injections in osteoarthritis of the knee: a randomized, double-blind, placebo-controlled trial. *Arthritis Rheum.* 2003;48(2):370–377.

28. Watterson JR, Esdaile JM. Viscosupplementation: therapeutic mechanisms and clinical potential in osteoarthritis of the knee. *J Am Acad Orthop Surg.* 2000;8(5):277–284.

29. Wang CT, Lin J, Chang CJ, et al. Therapeutic effects of hyaluronic acid on osteoarthritis of the knee. A meta-analysis of randomized controlled trials. *J Bone Joint Surg Am.* 2004;86-A(3):538–545.

30. Waddell DD, Bricker DC. Total knee replacement delayed with Hylan G-F 20 use in patients with grade IV osteoarthritis. *J Manag Care Pharm.* 2007;13(2):113–121.

31. Goomer RS, Leslie K, Maris T, et al. Native hyaluronan produces less hypersensitivity than cross-linked hyaluronan. *Clin Orthop Relat Res.* 2005;(434):239–245.

32. Moseley JB, O'Malley K, Petersen NJ, et al. A controlled trial of arthroscopic surgery for osteoarthritis of the knee. *N Engl J Med.* 2002;347(2):81–88.

33. Dervin GF, Stiell IG, Rody K, et al. Effect of arthroscopic débridement for osteoarthritis of the knee on health-related quality of life. *J Bone Joint Surg Am.* 2003;85-A(1):10–19.

34. Wai EK, Kreder HJ, Williams JI, et al. Arthroscopic débridement of the knee for osteoarthritis in patients fifty years of age or older: utilization and outcomes in the Province of Ontario. *J Bone Joint Surg Am.* 2002;84-A(1):17–22.

35. Kirkley A, Birmingham TB, Litchfield RB, et al. A randomized trial of arthroscopic surgery for osteoarthritis of the knee. *N Engl J Med.* 2008;359(11):1097–1107.

36. Bin SI, Lee SH, Kim CW, et al. Results of arthroscopic medial meniscectomy in patients with grade IV osteoarthritis of the medial compartment. *Arthroscopy.* 2008;24(3):264–268.

37. Steadman JR, Ramappa AJ, Maxwell RB, et al. An arthroscopic treatment regimen for osteoarthritis of the knee. *Arthroscopy.* 2007;23(9):948–955.

38. Aaron RK, Skolnick AH, Reinert SE, et al. Arthroscopic débridement for osteoarthritis of the knee. *J Bone Joint Surg Am.* 2006;88(5):936–943.

39. Jackson JP, Waugh W. Tibial osteotomy for osteoarthritis of the knee. *Proc R Soc Med.* 1960;53(10):888.

40. Jackson JP, Waugh W. Tibial osteotomy for osteoarthritis of the knee. *J Bone Joint Surg Br.* 1961;43-B:746–751.

41. Sharma L, Song J, Felson DT, et al. The role of knee alignment in disease progression and functional decline in knee osteoarthritis. *JAMA.* 2011;286(2):188–195.

42. Coventry MB. Upper tibial osteotomy for osteoarthritis. *J Bone Joint Surg Am.* 1985;67(7):1136–1140.

43. Dejour H, Bonnin M. Tibial translation after anterior cruciate ligament rupture. Two radiological tests compared. *J Bone Joint Surg Br.* 1994;76(5):745–749.

44. Dejour H, Neyret P, Boileau P, et al. Anterior cruciate reconstruction combined with valgus tibial osteotomy. *Clin Orthop Relat Res.* 1994;(299):220–228.

45. Naudie DD, Amendola A, Fowler PJ. Opening wedge high tibial osteotomy for symptomatic hyperextension-varus thrust. *Am J Sports Med.* 2004;32(1):60–70.

46. Noyes FR, Barber-Westin SD, Hewett TE. High tibial osteotomy and ligament reconstruction for varus angulated anterior cruciate ligament-deficient knees. *Am J Sports Med.* 2000;28(3):282–296.

47. Phisitkul P, Wolf BR, Amendola A. Role of high tibial and distal femoral osteotomies in the treatment of lateral-posterolateral and medial instabilities of the knee. *Sports Med Arthrosc.* 2006;14(2):96–104.

48. Amendola A. Knee osteotomy and meniscal transplantation: indications, technical considerations, and results. *Sports Med Arthrosc.* 2007;15(1):32–38.

49. Gross AE, Shasha N, Aubin P. Long-term followup of the use of fresh osteochondral allografts for posttraumatic knee defects. *Clin Orthop Relat Res.* 2005;(435):79–87.

50. Jamali AA, Emmerson BC, Chung C, et al. Fresh osteochondral allografts: results in the patellofemoral joint. *Clin Orthop Relat Res.* 2005;(437):176–185.

51. McCulloch PC, Kang RW, Sobhy MH, et al. Prospective evaluation of prolonged fresh osteochondral allograft transplantation of the femoral condyle: minimum 2-year follow-up. *Am J Sports Med.* 2007;35(3):411–420.

52. Chun YM, Kim SJ, Kim HS. Evaluation of the mechanical properties of posterolateral structures and supporting posterolateral instability of the knee. *J Orthop Res.* 2008;26(10):1371–1376.

53. Laprade RF, Engebretsen L, Johensan S, et al. The effect of a proximal tibial medial opening wedge osteotomy on posterolateral knee instability: a biomechanical study. *Am J Sports Med.* 2008;36(5):956–960.

54. Tunggal JA, Higgins GA, Waddell JP, et al. Complications of closing wedge high tibial osteotomy. *Int Orthop.* 2010;34(2):255–261.

55. Amendola A, Rorabeck CH, Bourne RB, et al. Total knee arthroplasty following high tibial osteotomy for osteoarthritis. *J Arthroplasty.* 1989;4(suppl):S11–S17.

56. Fening SD, Kovacic J, Kambic H, et al. The effects of modified posterior tibial slope on anterior cruciate ligament strain and knee kinematics: a human cadaveric study. *J Knee Surg.* 2008;21(3):205–211.

57. Giffin JR, Vogrin TM, Zantop T, et al. Effects of increasing tibial slope on the biomechanics of the knee. *Am J Sports Med.* 2004;32(2):376–382.

58. Dugdale TW, Noyes FR, Styer D. Preoperative planning for high tibial osteotomy. The effect of lateral tibiofemoral separation and tibiofemoral length. *Clin Orthop Relat Res.* 1992;(274):248–264.

59. Katz MM, Hungerford DS, Krackow KA, et al. Results of total knee arthroplasty after failed proximal tibial osteotomy for osteoarthritis. *J Bone Joint Surg Am.* 1987;69(2):225–233.

60. Nelson CL, Saleh KJ, Kassim RA, et al. Total knee arthroplasty after varus osteotomy of the distal part of the femur. *J Bone Joint Surg Am.* 2003;85-A(6):1062–1065.

61. Parvizi J, Hanssen AD, Spangehl MJ, et al. Total knee arthroplasty following proximal tibial osteotomy: risk factors for failure. *J Bone Joint Surg Am.* 2004;86-A(3):474–479.

62. Akizuki S, Shibakawa A, Takizawa T, et al. The long-term outcome of high tibial osteotomy: a ten- to 20-year follow-up. *J Bone Joint Surg Br.* 2008;90(5):592–596.

63. Tang WC, Henderson IJ. High tibial osteotomy: long term survival analysis and patients' perspective. *Knee.* 2005;12(6):410–413.

64. Backstein D, Morag G, Hanna S, et al. Long-term follow-up of distal femoral varus osteotomy of the knee. *J Arthroplasty.* 2007;22(4)(suppl 1):2–6.

65. Spahn G. Complications in high tibial (medial opening wedge) osteotomy. *Arch Orthop Trauma Surg.* 2004;124(10):649–653.

66. Laurencin CT, Zelicof SB, Scott RD, et al. Unicompartmental versus total knee arthroplasty in the same patient. A comparative study. *Clin Orthop Relat Res.* 1991;(273):151–156.

67. Bert JM. Unicompartmental knee replacement. *Orthop Clin North Am.* 2005;36(4):513–522.

68. Borus T, Thornhill T. Unicompartmental knee arthroplasty. *J Am Acad Orthop Surg.* 2008;16(1):9–18.

69. Newman J, Pydisetty RV, Ackroyd C. Unicompartmental or total knee replacement: the 15-year results of a prospective randomised controlled trial. *J Bone Joint Surg Br.* 2009;91(1):52–57.

70. Price AJ, Waite JC, Svard U. Long-term clinical results of the medial Oxford unicompartmental knee arthroplasty. *Clin Orthop Relat Res.* 2005;(435):171–180.

71. Schai PA, Suh JT, Thronhill TS, et al. Unicompartmental knee arthroplasty in middle-aged patients: a 2- to 6-year follow-up evaluation. *J Arthroplasty.* 1998;13(4):365–372.

72. Pennington DW, Swienckowski JJ, Lutes WB, et al. Unicompartmental knee arthroplasty in patients sixty years of age or younger. *J Bone Joint Surg Am.* 2003;85-A(10):1968–1973.

73. Ackroyd CE, Newman JH, Evans R, et al. The Avon patellofemoral arthroplasty: five-year survivorship and functional results. *J Bone Joint Surg Br.* 2007;89(3):310–315.

74. van Jonbergen HP, Werkman DM, Barnaart LF, et al. Long-term outcomes of patellofemoral arthroplasty. *J Arthroplasty.* 2010;25(7):1066–1071.

75. Bradbury N, Borton D, Spoo G, et al. Participation in sports after total knee replacement. *Am J Sports Med.* 1998;26(4):530–535.

76. Healy WL, Iorio R, Lemos MJ. Athletic activity after joint replacement. *Am J Sports Med.* 2001;29(3):377–388.

77. Kuster MS. Exercise recommendations after total joint replacement: a review of the current literature and proposal of scientifically based guidelines. *Sports Med.* 2002; 32(7):433–445.

78. Dahm DL, Barnes SA, Harrington JR, et al. Patient-reported activity level after total knee arthroplasty. *J Arthroplasty.* 2008;23(3):401–407.

79. Mont MA, Marker DR, Syler TM, et al. Knee arthroplasties have similar results in high- and low-activity patients. *Clin Orthop Relat Res.* 2007;460:165–173.

Knee Ligament

Evolving Concepts in Tunnel Placement for ACL Reconstruction

Chlodwig Kirchhoff • Peter U. Brucker • Andreas B. Imhoff

Rupture of the anterior cruciate ligament (ACL) is one of the most frequent injuries of the knee joint in nowadays field of orthopedic surgery (1, 2). The ACL consists of at least two functional bundles (3–5) with its unique stabilizing effect represented by the anteromedial (AM) bundle for predominantly anterior stability and the posterolateral (PL) bundle for predominantly rotational stability. A complete rupture of the ACL usually results in a decreased stability in both the anterior–posterior (a-p) and the rotational axis, which can be tested during the clinical examination performing the two main examination maneuvers, the Lachman test (6–8) and the pivot-shift test (9, 10),

The standard operation technique for ACL reconstruction continues to evolve over the last decades. Advances in the treatment of ACL injuries include extensive investigations of injury, technical improvements providing more anatomic reconstructions, considerations of the relative success rate of the variety of graft options, and effects of different rehabilitation and training methods.

Single-bundle ACL reconstruction techniques were routinely performed over the last decades and progressively modified in an anatomical manner performing more centrally placed tunnels within the widely spread anatomical footprint of both bundles at the femur as well as the tibia to maintain adequate anterior and rotational stability. Recent attempts have focused on recapitulating the AM and PL bundles using a variety of double-bundle techniques to improve the results of surgical reconstruction of the ACL. These double-bundle techniques were introduced to respect the complex anatomy of the native ACL more closely.

Independently of single- or double-bundle ACL reconstruction techniques, the most critical factor for successful ACL reconstruction is the correct placement of the femoral and tibial tunnel(s). Indeed, incorrect placement of the tunnels may result in loss of extension and/or flexion causing improper graft tension resulting in premature graft failure by elongation or rerupture. Due to relevant alterations in knee kinematics, long-term consequences of incorrect tunnel placement may induce early increased cartilage degeneration and osteoarthritis. The essential

factor for a successful ACL reconstruction is graft fixation within the tunnels (11). Various anatomic aperture and extra-anatomic fixation techniques have been described. Combinations of anatomic and extra-anatomic fixation techniques were introduced as hybrid techniques. All fixation techniques include advantages and disadvantages.

Typical potential disadvantages such as graft-tunnel motion (12), windshield wiper effect (13), and/or suture stretch-out (14) might result from indirect extra-anatomical and extra-articular fixation techniques (11).

Since various rupture patterns of the ACL have been recognized (15), these different rupture types might need differentiated reconstruction techniques especially when autologous hamstring tendon graft techniques were considered. This seems of importance since the hamstring muscles are known for protecting the ACL graft by their synergistic function (16). Thus, the logic consequence is an implementation of a concept of differentiated tunnel placement with hamstring autografts.

CLINICAL EVALUATION

Physical Examination

The clinical evaluation of the joint is important in the diagnostic phase of pathology and in the assessment of surgical technique. The appraisal of ACL reconstruction is usually based on objective clinical examinations; many tests are dedicated to objectively determining an ACL lesion, each with its own specificity and sensitivity. In this context, the Lachman test and the pivot-shift test are the most important clinical tests for detection of an ACL rupture. For performing the *Lachman test*, one hand fixes the distal femur of the patient laying in a supine position, whereas the knee is flexed at approximately 20°. The other hand pulls the proximal tibia in an anterior direction. If the tibia reacts like a drawer anteriorly with no abrupt stopping, a rupture of the ACL is presumable (6). In some cases, 4 to 6 weeks following an ACL injury, the Lachman test may be more or less negative, caused by scar tissue among the stumps of the ACL (17).

The *pivot-shift test* is another manual test to identify ACL ruptures or relevant underlying laxity of the knee joint. The test's name comes from the pivot (axis), shift (dislocation) and was first described by the group of Macintosh (10) in 1972. To perform this test, the patient lies in a relaxed supine position. The examiner takes the heel with one hand by slightly rotating the shank internally, whereas the other hand is used to conduct a valgus stress to the tibial head. In case of an ACL rupture, the tibial head slides anteriorly in a subluxation position. At 30° to 40° knee flexion, the tibial head jumps back into the physiologic position. Normally, this appears with a snapping sensation or a visible bounce emitted by the iliotibial band sliding over the lateral femoral epicondyle to its posterior location. If the examiner feels this effect, the test is positive with a high specificity of a ruptured ACL (18). The test can be falsified, if a medial-capsule-ligament instability or a ruptured iliotibial band is present (9, 10).

The *drawer test* is also used to examine the ACL's integrity. The patient is placed in a supine position on the table with a 90° flexed knee and 45° flexed hip joint. The examiner places the hands around the proximal tibia with the thumbs crossing the anterior joint line. The patient's foot is anchored in a neutral position by the examiner's thigh. The examiner tells the patient to relax the hamstrings. Once the patient is relaxed, the examiner attempts to pull the tibia anteriorly. Instability is determined by examining both sides and comparing the amount of present excursion. Overall, however, this test is not as sensitive as the aforementioned tests.

Imaging

Preoperative Examination

The magnetic resonance imaging (MRI) examination of the injured knee has been established as the gold standard imaging examination to identify musculoskeletal pathologies in acute or chronic knee damage. The cruciate ligaments are located intracapsularly and extrasynovially. Acute ACL tears are mostly associated with hemarthros (19). For the routine MRI of the knee, the positioning of the knee is in 10° to 15° external rotation, performing 3-mm-slice-thick images. On MRI, the collateral damage of the knee in terms of meniscal lesions, additional ligamentous injuries, and bone bruise can be detected as well and may lead to different therapy. In this context, the detection of a bone bruise can be helpful and is most commonly cumulated, deeper, and more intense in the lateral compartment after ACL rupture and persists at least for 4 months (20, 21). The appearance of a deep sulcus in the lateral femur condyle on MRI in patients with torn ACLs is deeper (>1.5 mm) compared with the sulcus of ACL sufficient knees (1.2 mm). The deep sulcus sign of the lateral condyle is used as an indirect sign of a torn ACL (22) in cases where the MRI do not allow for a detailed view of the ACL.

Postoperative Examination

Misplaced tunnels cause unfavorable results, therefore, precise postoperative analysis of tunnel placement is essential. Conventional radiographs in two planes represent the standard method for assessing the position of both the femoral and the tibial tunnels in a-p and lateral projections. If a bone–tendon–bone graft is used, the bone blocks within the tunnels and metal implants such as interference screws or crosspins are visible. However, in the case of exclusive soft-tissue tendon grafts, such as the hamstrings, tunnel, and graft positions are more difficult and often impossible to assess.

MRI in contrast allows for a precise assessment of tendon grafts and their position to anatomical landmarks. Determination of the femoral and tibial tunnels is hardly susceptible to mistakes. The relationship of the tendon grafts to the surrounding bone and the posterior cruciate ligament (PCL) can be evaluated three dimensionally. Impingement of the graft against the roof (notch impingement), the lateral femoral condyle (lateral impingement), or the PCL can be diagnosed directly on the sagittal, oblique coronal, or horizontal scans, respectively. This means that those patients may be reoperated early (e.g., by a notchplasty) before graft failure occurs. In addition, the position of bioabsorbable fixation devices can be detected, which is limited using conventional radiographs.

TIMING AND TECHNIQUE

The treatment of ACL ruptures depends on different patients' factors such as age, profession, sporting activity, comorbidities, and compliance. The single-bundle ACL reconstruction techniques were performed in the beginning and also modified performing more centrally placed tunnels within the widely spread anatomical footprint of both bundles at the femur as well as the tibia.

Recent attempts to improve the results of surgical reconstruction of the ACL have focused on recapitulating the AM and PL bundles using a variety of double-bundle techniques. These double-bundles techniques were introduced to be able to respect the complex anatomy of the native ACL more closely. The advantages of the double-bundle technique include an improved stability of the knee joint, especially for internal rotation of the tibia, less bone loss due to smaller tunnels, but also aperture fixation to prevent tunnel enlargement. However, this rather novel technique incorporates some disadvantages such as higher surgical and technical demands on the surgeon, higher implant costs due to the insertion of four bioresorbable interference screws and the possibility of more complicated revision surgery.

Moreover, recent interest has been focused on symptomatic partial ACL tears in order to perform a selected and individualized augmentation of the AM or PL bundle.

Independently of performing a single-, double-bundle ACL reconstruction, or AM-/PL-augmentation reconstruction techniques, the femoral tunnel(s) are drilled via the anteromedial portal(s), which results in a more reliable positioning of the femoral tunnel(s).

SINGLE-BUNDLE TECHNIQUE

Surgical setup and portal placement as well as diagnostic arthroscopy and ACL footprint preparation in ACL single-bundle reconstruction are equivalent to the ACL double-bundle reconstruction technique. However, the accessory secondary AM portal is not required for single-bundle ACL reconstruction. Graft harvesting and preparation is also similar to the double-bundle ACL technique, although harvest of only the semitendinosus tendon by leaving the gracilis tendon intact and subsequent triple- or quadruple-strand semitendinosus tendon graft preparation is sufficient. In cases of a semitendinosus tendon length of >32 cm, a double-bundle ACL reconstruction is feasible with only harvesting of the semitendinosus tendon.

Femoral and Tibial Tunnel Placement of the Single-Bundle Technique

During single-bundle ACL reconstruction, the tunnel aperture is positioned in the anatomical center of the ACL footprint, which is different to the anatomical placement of the femoral and tibial AM and the PL tunnels in double-bundle ACL reconstruction.

In more detail, the AM portal at a knee angle of 130° flexion is used for the placement of a 5-mm offset drill guide (Arthrex, Naples, FL) in the femoral site at the posterior aspect of the notch at the 2 o'clock (left knee) or at the 10 o'clock position (right knee) followed by an overdrilling and notching performed in a similar way for the AM tunnel in the double-bundle ACL technique.

For the tibial tunnel, the tip of the tibial drill guide is placed within the tibial ACL stump anteriorly to the posterior cruciate ligament in between the anatomical center of the tibial insertion of the AM and the PL bundle. Before overdrilling of the tibial tunnel, an arthroscopic impingement test is performed for evaluation of correct placement of the tibial tunnel aperture.

DOUBLE-BUNDLE TECHNIQUE

Depending on the size of the femoral and the tibial insertion area, a single- or a double-bundle ACL reconstruction technique is performed. In the double-bundle technique, the standard instruments are used for autologous hamstring tendons (semitendinosus and gracilis) as ACL grafts. An initial diagnostic arthroscopy may be necessary to differentiate between complete and partial rupture of the ACL, which—in the latter case—may only need an

ACL augmentation technique (AM or PL augmentation by leaving the intact bundle in situ).

In 2006, our group has published the arthroscopic aperture fixation technique in anatomic ACL double-bundle reconstruction (23). Since then, we have modified this double-bundle ACL reconstruction technique only with respect to the femoral tunnel drilling using an AM portal technique for the AM tunnel instead of a transtibial technique for the aforementioned AM tunnel.

Femoral Tunnel Placement for the Anteromedial and Posterolateral Bundle

At first, the femoral tunnel for the AM bundle is drilled via the AM portal, whereas in most cases, a 4-mm offset drill guide (Arthrex) is used. To provide a more detailed description, the drill guide is positioned at 1:30 o'clock at the posterior aspect of the notch (left knee) or at 10:30 o'clock position (right knee) with respect to the coronal plane. Then, the guide wire is positioned in 130° flexion and consecutively it is overdrilled by an acorn drill of the corresponding graft size to a depth of at least 25 mm. To avoid a later tunnel blowout, an at least 1-mm bony bridge between the posterior wall of the AM tunnel and the posterior cortex of the notch should be preserved. With a notching device (Arthrex), an osseous notch at the anterior-superior edge of the tunnels for aperture fixation by bioabsorbable interference screws is carried out.

However, the accessory AM portal is used to drill the femoral tunnel for the PL bundle. Therefore, a modified 5-mm offset drill guide (see Fig. 69.1) is placed in the anterior-inferior aspect of the already established femoral tunnel aperture for the AM bundle representing a 2:30 o'clock in the left or a 9:30 o'clock position in the right knee for the PL bundle (see Fig. 69.2). To preserve the

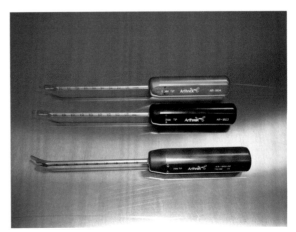

FIGURE 69.1. Modified angled 5-mm offset drill guide (red handle, in front) for drilling of the femoral PL tunnel compared to a conventional 5-mm (red handle) and 6-mm (green handle) offset drill guide (in the background) for drilling of the femoral AM tunnel (Arthrex, Naples, FL).

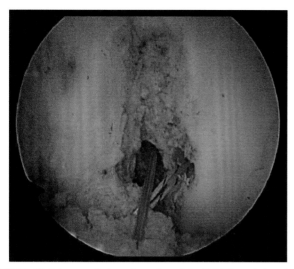

FIGURE 69.2. Intra-articular orientation of the AM (FiberWire) and PL bundles (TigerWire) on arthroscopic visualization with use of a standard AM portal in 90° of flexion.

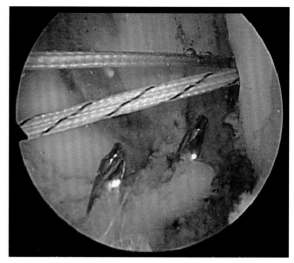

FIGURE 69.3. Arthroscopic view of the tibial tunnels for the AM and PL bundles.

peroneal nerve and the chondral surface of the lateral femoral condyle from iatrogenic damage, the PL tunnel placement is performed in 90° of flexion. Then, the guide wire is overdrilled with an acorn drill of the corresponding graft size as well to a depth of 25 mm allowing for a bony bridge of approximately 1 mm between both femoral tunnels.

Since for each femoral tunnel placement the AM portal is utilized separately, the divergence of both femoral tunnels permits additional stability of the bone bridge. Notching reduce drive failure and screw breakage by decreasing peak screw insertion torque. A FiberWire and a TigerWire no. 2 (Arthrex) are pulled through the femoral tunnels of the AM and the PL bundle via standard AM and accessory AM portal, respectively.

Tibial Tunnel Placement for the Anteromedial and Posterolateral Bundle

For the tibial site, first the tunnel for the PL bundle followed by the tunnel for the AM bundle is drilled. The oblique transversal AM incision of the hamstrings donor site is routinely used for the positioning of both tibial tunnels. The tibial tunnel's diameter for the AM bundle usually varies between 6 and 7 mm and for the PL bundle between 4 and 5 mm. For the drilling of the tunnel for the PL bundle, the tip of the drill guide is placed 3 mm anteriorly with respect to the anterior border of the posterior cruciate ligament when the tunnel diameter is between 4 to 5 mm at the PL aspect of the tibial footprint of the ACL, whereas the drilling start point for the PL bundle tunnel is positioned inferiorly to the tibial insertion of the superficial medial collateral ligament. In contrast, the AM bundle tunnel is placed more anteriorly and centrally (see Fig. 69.3). While the first drill guide wire for the PL bundle is kept in situ, the tibial drill guide's tip is placed within the AM aspect of the tibial ACL footprint with respect to

an adequate distance to the PL tibial tunnel. Consecutively, an arthroscopic impingement test is performed in extension to prevent the knee from a notch impingement.

In case of a correct positioning of both guide wires, these guide wires are overdrilled one after the other in compliance with the grafts' size. To describe the tunnel configuration in more detail, the tibial tunnel for the PL bundle has a more oblique direction (45° to the sagittal plane), whereas the tibial tunnel for the AM bundle has a more sagittal orientation (20° to the sagittal plane). Both tibial tunnels discharge in approximation of the oval anatomical footprint of the native ACL. However, for maintenance of a sufficient bony bridge, a distal bony bridge of at least 2 to 2.5 cm should be preserved.

An arthroscopic grasper is used to pull the FiberWire and the TigerWire no. 2 sutures through their corresponding tibial tunnels in a retrograde way.

COMPLICATIONS, CONTROVERSIES, AND SPECIAL CONSIDERATIONS

Besides graft rerupture and extension deficit due to wrong tunnel placement, the common postoperative phenomenon in ACL reconstruction is tunnel widening. Recent investigations promote the theory of a combination of mechanical and biologic factors. It is idle to allocate the one or other fixation method as the only reason for tunnel widening, since this abnormality is described for all fixation methods. This tunnel widening usually occurs between the sixth and the eighth week after the operation (24–26). Mechanical causes might play a major part in the dilatation of the tunnels. In this context besides the drilling technique, the bungee effect and the windshield wiper effect may be an explanation. The windshield wiper effect, firstly described by L'Insalata et al. (13), accuses the remote extra-anatomic fixation of the graft in the femoral tunnel.

Current findings favor the point of graft fixation as the main reason of tunnel widening. Using this remote fixation method like cortical buttons, the graft in the femoral tunnel allows for micromotions in the longitudinal direction. Because the fixation construct is more elastic than interference screws, the longitudinal motion has been described as the bungee effect and is at least partially responsible for femoral tunnel widening (12, 27, 28). After these findings, the idea of a fixation technique congruent to the joint line became more popular and promising to avoid tunnel widening. In fact, the investigation of Simonian et al. (29) showed a significant reduction of tunnel expansion by usage of an aperture fixation. Using the aperture fixation method with interference screws, it has to be mentioned that the tunnel needs an adequate diameter. If the diameter is too small, the compression of bony walls due to a too strong screw fixation may appear in tunnel widening (30). In contrast, too large tunnel diameters may cause insufficient fixation strength and synovial fluid leakage. Besides mechanical factors, even biologic reasons may increase tunnel widening or graft failure. Several studies showed that the composition of the synovial fluid varies after ACL rupture and ACL reconstruction (31–33). The amount of proinflammatory enzymes and transmitters (TNF-α, IL-6, and IL-1) increase weeks after ACL reconstruction (33). Related to their influence on osteoclastic cells, a reduction of bone substance was found (34). Zysk et al. (33) found increased concentrations of IL-6 and TNF-α 7 days after ACL rupture and also 38 days postoperatively after bony tunnel widening was described radiologically.

To summarize, mechanical and biologic factors may play a major part in tunnel widening. The danger of graft insufficiency and persisting instability may be the result. The fixation of the graft at the articular surface level of the surrounding bony tunnel aperture seems to be advantageous compared with remote fixation using plates, buttons, or pins.

Injury to the posterior vessel and nerve bundle represents a very rare complication due to an inadequate flexion angle during drilling: If this injury is suspected because of the position of the guide wire, the tourniquet should be released and the pulses of the dorsalis pedis and tibialis posterior arteries should be evaluated by visualization using Doppler sonography. This may be followed by angiography and vascular exploration if needed.

If notch impingement occur postoperatively which inhibits extension due to a mechanically based graft or tibial ACL stump hypertrophy, trimming of the graft and/or the ACL stump may be necessary. In addition, if the tibial tunnel was placed in a far anterior position, it may be possible to shift the AM bundle slightly toward posterior by removing and reinserting the tibial screw anteriorly so that the bundle lies posteriorly to the screw. An incorrectly placed tunnel medially or laterally can also be adjusted

to some extent in this way. Another option to be considered in cases of superior or lateral notch impingement is notchplasty with elevation of the notch roof or lateral wall of the notch.

REHABILITATION

Surgical reconstruction of the ACL and the early-rehabilitation phase have undergone a rapid evolution over the past 25 years. However, there is a controversy of standardized, objective criteria to accurately assess an athlete's ability to progress through the end stages of rehabilitation and safe return to sportive activity (35). Reviewing the last years' rehabilitation protocols, they can be divided e.g. into an acute or a subacute phase or into return to activity (36). These protocols usually focus on acute and subacute management with relatively stringent guidelines regarding progression of weight bearing, increase of range of motion (ROM), and introduction of specific types of exercises in early rehabilitation. The guidelines and supervised therapy can significantly improve the early postsurgical outcome (37). Late-stage rehabilitation and return to sportive activity in terms of training after ACL reconstruction without guideline followed training may lead to deficits in lower extremity neuromuscular control, strength, and ground reaction attenuation. These deficits may increase the risk of reinjury or limit the achievement of optimal performance levels (38–40). The "release for full activity" is a potentially sensitive landmark for the athlete who has a strong desire to immediately return to high-level sports participation.

Over the last years, we developed and modified our own postoperative rehabilitation scheme starting with postoperative continuous cooling of the elevated limb as well as compression and physiotherapeutic exercise program from the first postoperative day including reduction of swelling. From the first day after the operation, there are no restrictions for flexion and extension but full weight bearing is restricted. In detail, 20-kg weight bearing adapted to individual pain levels and effusion for at least 2 weeks postoperatively is recommended. After week 7 postoperatively, sensomotoric exercises are started, and approximately after the 8th week, we recommend treadmill, cycle, or crawling training. Three months after surgery, impacting activities such as jogging can be started. The individual sport specific training can usually begin after 6 months. But body contact or pivoting sports such as soccer, skiing, and martial arts should be started not until 8 to 9 months postoperatively.

REFERENCES

1. Gianotti SM, Marshall SW, Hume PA, et al. Incidence of anterior cruciate ligament injury and other knee ligament injuries: a national population-based study. *J Sci Med Sport.* 2009;12(6):622–627.

2. Parkkari J, Pasanen K, Mattila VM, et al. The risk for a cruciate ligament injury of the knee in adolescents and young adults: a population-based cohort study of 46 500 people with a 9 year follow-up. *Br J Sports Med.* 2008;42(6):422–426.

3. Petersen W, Zantop T. Anatomy of the anterior cruciate ligament with regard to its two bundles. *Clin Orthop Relat Res.* 2007;454:35–47.

4. Zantop T, Herbort M, Raschke MJ, et al. The role of the anteromedial and posterolateral bundles of the anterior cruciate ligament in anterior tibial translation and internal rotation. *Am J Sports Med.* 2007;35(2):223–227.

5. Zantop T, Wellmann M, Fu FH, et al. Tunnel positioning of anteromedial and posterolateral bundles in anatomic anterior cruciate ligament reconstruction: anatomic and radiographic findings. *Am J Sports Med.* 2008;36(1):65–72.

6. Benjaminse A, Gokeler A, van der Schans CP. Clinical diagnosis of an anterior cruciate ligament rupture: a meta-analysis. *J Orthop Sports Phys Ther.* 2006;36(5):267–288.

7. Ferretti M, Ekdahl M, Shen W, et al. Osseous landmarks of the femoral attachment of the anterior cruciate ligament: an anatomic study. *Arthroscopy.* 2007;23(11):1218–1225.

8. Prins M. The Lachman test is the most sensitive and the pivot shift the most specific test for the diagnosis of ACL rupture. *Aust J Physiother.* 2006;52(1):66.

9. Anderson AF, Rennirt GW, Standeffer WC Jr. Clinical analysis of the pivot shift tests: description of the pivot drawer test. *Am J Knee Surg.* 2000;13(1):19–23.

10. Galway HR, MacIntosh DL. The lateral pivot shift: a symptom and sign of anterior cruciate ligament insufficiency. *Clin Orthop Relat Res.* 1980;(147):45–50.

11. Harner CD, Giffin JR, Dunteman RC, et al. Evaluation and treatment of recurrent instability after anterior cruciate ligament reconstruction. *Instr Course Lect.* 2001;50:463–474.

12. Höher J, Livesay GA, Ma CB, et al. Hamstring graft motion in the femoral bone tunnel when using titanium button/polyester tape fixation. *Knee Surg Sports Traumatol Arthrosc.* 1999;7(4):215–219.

13. L 'Insalata JC, Klatt B, Fu FH, et al. Tunnel expansion following anterior cruciate ligament reconstruction: a comparison of hamstring and patellar tendon autografts. *Knee Surg Sports Traumatol Arthrosc.* 1997;5(4):234–238.

14. Scheffler SU, Südkamp NP, Göckenjan A, et al. Biomechanical comparison of hamstring and patellar tendon graft anterior cruciate ligament reconstruction techniques: the impact of fixation level and fixation method under cyclic loading. *Arthroscopy.* 2002;18(3):304–315.

15. Zantop T, Brucker PU, Vidal A, et al. Intraarticular rupture pattern of the ACL. *Clin Orthop Relat Res.* 2007;454:48–53.

16. Solomonow M, Baratta R, Zhou BH, et al. The synergistic action of the anterior cruciate ligament and thigh muscles in maintaining joint stability. *Am J Sports Med.* 1987;15(3):207–213.

17. Strobel MJ, Schulz MS, Petersen WJ, et al. Combined anterior cruciate ligament, posterior cruciate ligament, and posterolateral corner reconstruction with autogenous hamstring grafts in chronic instabilities. *Arthroscopy.* 2006;22(2):182–192.

18. Scholten RJ, Opstelten W, van der Plas CG, et al. Accuracy of physical diagnostic tests for assessing ruptures of the anterior cruciate ligament: a meta-analysis. *J Fam Pract.* 2003;52(9):689-94.

19. Johnson DL, Warner JJ. Diagnosis for anterior cruciate ligament surgery. *Clin Sports Med.* 1993;12(4):671–684.

20. Bretlau T, Tuxøe J, Larsen L, et al. Bone bruise in the acutely injured knee. *Knee Surg Sports Traumatol Arthrosc.* 2002;10(2):96–101.

21. Viskontas DG, Giuffre BM, Duggal N, et al. Bone bruises associated with ACL rupture: correlation with injury mechanism. *Am J Sports Med.* 2008;36(5):927–933.

22. Cobby MJ, Schweitzer ME, Resnick D. The deep lateral femoral notch: an indirect sign of a torn anterior cruciate ligament. *Radiology.* 1992;184(3):855–858.

23. Brucker PU, Lorenz S, Imhoff AB. Aperture fixation in arthroscopic anterior cruciate ligament double-bundle reconstruction. *Arthroscopy.* 2006;22(11):1250.e1–6.

24. Clatworthy MG, Annear P, Bulow JU, et al. Tunnel widening in anterior cruciate ligament reconstruction: a prospective evaluation of hamstring and patella tendon grafts. *Knee Surg Sports Traumatol Arthrosc.* 1999;7(3):138–145.

25. Fink C, Zapp M, Benedetto KP, et al. Tibial tunnel enlargement following anterior cruciate ligament reconstruction with patellar tendon autograft. *Arthroscopy.* 2001;17(2):138–143.

26. Peyrache MD, Djian P, Christel P, et al. Tibial tunnel enlargement after anterior cruciate ligament reconstruction by autogenous bone-patellar tendon-bone graft. *Knee Surg Sports Traumatol Arthrosc.* 1996;4(1):2–8.

27. Segawa H, Omori G, Tomita S, et al. Bone tunnel enlargement after anterior cruciate ligament reconstruction using hamstring tendons. *Knee Surg Sports Traumatol Arthrosc.* 2001;9(4):206–210.

28. Webster KE, Feller JA, Hameister KA. Bone tunnel enlargement following anterior cruciate ligament reconstruction: a randomised comparison of hamstring and patellar tendon grafts with 2-year follow-up. *Knee Surg Sports Traumatol Arthrosc.* 2001;9(2):86–91.

29. Simonian PT, Monson JT, Larson RV. Biodegradable interference screw augmentation reduces tunnel expansion after ACL reconstruction. *Am J Knee Surg.* 2001;14(2):104–108.

30. Buelow JU, Siebold R, Ellermann A. A prospective evaluation of tunnel enlargement in anterior cruciate ligament reconstruction with hamstrings: extracortical versus anatomical fixation. *Knee Surg Sports Traumatol Arthrosc.* 2002;10(2):80–85.

31. Cameron ML, Fu FH, Paessler HH, et al. Synovial fluid cytokine concentrations as possible prognostic indicators in the ACL-deficient knee. *Knee Surg Sports Traumatol Arthrosc.* 1994;2(1):38–44.

32. Cameron M, Buchgraber A, Passler H, et al. The natural history of the anterior cruciate ligament-deficient knee. Changes in synovial fluid cytokine and keratan sulfate concentrations. *Am J Sports Med.* 1997;25(6):751–754.

33. Zysk SP, Fraunberger P, Veihelmann A, et al. Tunnel enlargement and changes in synovial fluid cytokine profile following anterior cruciate ligament reconstruction with patellar tendon and hamstring tendon autografts. *Knee Surg Sports Traumatol Arthrosc.* 2004;12(2):98–103.

34. Jacobs JJ, Roebuck KA, Archibeck M, et al. Osteolysis: basic science. *Clin Orthop Relat Res.* 2001;(393):71–77.

35. Myer GD, Paterno MV, Ford KR, et al. Neuromuscular training techniques to target deficits before return to sport after anterior cruciate ligament reconstruction. *J Strength Cond Res.* 2008;22(3):987–1014.

36. Wilk KE, Reinold MM, Hooks TR. Recent advances in the rehabilitation of isolated and combined anterior cruciate ligament injuries. *Orthop Clin North Am.* 2003;34(1):107–137.

37. Howe JG, Johnson RJ, Kaplan MJ, et al. Anterior cruciate ligament reconstruction using quadriceps patellar tendon graft. Part I. Long-term follow up. *Am J Sports Med.* 1991;19(5):447–457.
38. Ageberg E, Zätterström R, Moritz U, et al. Influence of supervised and nonsupervised training on postural control after an acute anterior cruciate ligament rupture: a three-year longitudinal prospective study. *J Orthop Sports Phys Ther.* 2001;31(11):632–644.
39. DeVita P, Hortobagyi T, Barrier J. Gait biomechanics are not normal after anterior cruciate ligament reconstruction and accelerated rehabilitation. *Med Sci Sports Exerc.* 1998;30(10):1481–1488.
40. Hewett TE, Paterno MV, Myer GD. Strategies for enhancing proprioception and neuromuscular control of the knee. *Clin Orthop Relat Res.* 2002;402(402):76–94.

Two-Tunnel Single-Bundle ACL Reconstruction

Mark E. Steiner • Aaron Gardiner

ACL reconstruction techniques have undergone an evolution over the past few decades both in terms of graft choice and in surgical techniques. The historical "gold standard" technique was considered by many to be a patellar tendon autograft placed with a transtibial drilling technique. The transtibial technique replaced the older technique of outside-in femoral drilling and certainly increased the ease of femoral tunnel placement. However, this ease came at the expense of significant constraint in femoral tunnel placement. Over the past several years, there have been two major technical developments in ACL reconstruction. The first is the use of medial portal drilling for the femoral tunnel that gives the surgeon increased flexibility in tunnel placement compared with a transtibial technique. The second is the improved understanding of the native ACL anatomy, which has led to both a refinement of the single-bundle technique and the development of the double-bundle technique, which may more closely reproduce the native ACL anatomy.

Good results can be achieved using various grafts including patellar tendon autografts, hamstring autografts, quadriceps tendon autografts, and various allografts. More

critical than graft selection appears to be surgical technique including tunnel placement, graft tensioning, and fixation technique. An accelerated rehabilitation with no restrictions on range of motion and weight bearing as tolerated are standards for all reconstruction techniques.

Despite the overall success of getting most patients back to athletic activity, several areas of concern remain with current ACL reconstruction techniques. First is that an estimated 10% to 30% have residual symptomatic instability (1, 2). This is the patient who has a Lachman test with a solid end point, but a mildly positive pivot shift test and functional instability during athletic activity. Second, there is a relatively high reinjury rate among young athletic patients for whom a reoperation rate of over 25% has been reported (3). Third, despite a successful ACL reconstruction and a stable knee that allows a return to pivoting activities, many patients develop degenerative changes in the long term (4). Fourth, modern analysis has shown that kinematic abnormalities remain in clinically stable knees (5–7). Certainly, despite intensive study and many years of refinement, the current techniques of ACL reconstruction leave room for significant improvement.

Recent research has raised significant concerns with conventional transtibial drilling in regard to knee stability. Howell (8) in 2001 demonstrated that conventional transtibial drilling often produced vertical grafts that resulted in loss of motion and residual anterior laxity. Similarly, a cadaver study by Woo (9) in 2002 showed that a single-bundle reconstruction placed with a conventional transtibial drilling technique was unable to restore normal laxity.

Subsequent biomechanical studies have demonstrated that the residual laxity of transtibial techniques may be avoided with a double-bundle graft. The biomechanical rationale for this procedure is that while a conventional transtibial single-bundle graft may restore anterior laxity and produce a knee with an end point during Lachman examination, there may still be residual laxity with a positive pivot shift and instability due to rotatory loads (10–12).

One limitation of some of the comparisons of double-bundle reconstructions to single-bundle reconstructions is that these studies used a conventional transtibial drilling with single-bundle grafts that did not optimize tunnel placement in the center of the anatomic footprints. Recent work by the senior author (M.E.S.) in a cadaver model has shown that a single-bundle graft placed with independent drilling in the center of the anatomic footprints can improve stability compared with a transtibial graft and can provide stability equivalent to a double-bundle graft (13, 14).

The premise of a single-bundle anatomic reconstruction is that the limitations of transtibial drilling are the basis for single-bundle grafts not restoring functional stability. Anatomic placement of a single-bundle graft is a means of increasing stability rather than increasing the number of grafts crossing the knee joint. In order to place single-bundle grafts centered in the anatomic footprints, independent drilling of the tibial and femoral tunnels is required (15). This chapter will review the technique for single-bundle ACL reconstruction, including patient selection, operative techniques, and rehabilitation.

CLINICAL EVALUATION

Most patients with an ACL injury will give a history of acute trauma. Patients often report hearing a "pop" at the time of injury. Often this will be a noncontact injury during a deceleration and rotation maneuver. Patients generally are unable to continue their activity, develop a hemarthrosis within 24 hours, and seek medical attention. Patients with a chronic ACL tear will often give a history of recurrent episodes of instability, especially with cutting or pivoting activities.

On examination, an effusion will usually be present. This may not be the case during an initial on-field examination or in chronic cases. A Lachman test will reveal increased anterior translation with no firm end point. This examination should be performed on both knees for comparison. The pivot shift test will reveal a greater shift in the ACL injured knee compared with the contralateral normal knee, but muscle spasm may impair the examination.

A complete knee examination should be performed as many associated injuries may also be present. Evaluation of the collateral ligaments, posterolateral corner, posterior cruciate ligament (PCL), and menisci is important. Particularly in chronic or revision cases, an evaluation of limb alignment should be performed, as undiagnosed malalignment is a potential cause of failure of reconstruction.

Patients with a suspected ACL injury should initially be evaluated with a series of plain radiographs. Although these will generally be normal, they are useful in ruling out fracture in the setting of an acute injury with hemarthrosis. A Segond fracture, a small bony avulsion of the lateral tibial plateau, can sometimes be seen and is strongly associated with ACL injury. Generally, anteroposterior (AP), lateral, and sunrise views are sufficient in the case of an acutely injured knee. In cases of chronic ACL tears or in revision cases, the surgeon should be alert

to the possibility of malalignment and full-length standing films of both lower extremities should be evaluated if malalignment is suspected.

CT scan does not have a major role in cases of acute ACL injury, but it may be helpful in revision cases to accurately identify tunnel positions and possible tunnel widening.

MRI is the most useful imaging modality for diagnosis of ACL injury. The torn ACL is usually identified by the interruption of the fibers and the abnormal horizontal alignment of the ligament. Associated injuries, including meniscal tears, chondral injuries, and ligamentous injuries, can also be identified. In over 80% of patients, a bone bruise will be identified, usually in the lateral compartment. If these bone bruises are absent, the clinician may suspect the injury is chronic or the possibility of another injury.

TREATMENT, OPERATIVE INDICATIONS, AND TIMING

Treatment for ACL tears should be individualized to the patient. In general, ACL reconstruction allows a return to sports and other activities that require cutting and pivoting. For some patients, especially older patients that do not participate in these activities, a nonoperative approach may be the preferred treatment. Certainly, a trial of nonoperative treatment, consisting of physical therapy and a gradual return to activity, is appropriate for the older, low-demand patient. If this patient has instability during their normal activities after completing a rehabilitation program, at that point they would be a candidate for ACL reconstruction. The decision to undergo ACL reconstruction should be individualized after a thoughtful discussion between the surgeon and the patient regarding the risks, benefits, and expected outcomes of the procedure.

Operative treatment should be offered to all patients who desire to return to cutting or pivoting athletic activities. An ACL tear is a season-ending injury and allowing an athlete to return to competition with an unstable knee exposes the patient to a significant risk of meniscal and chondral injury that could likely be avoided by ACL reconstruction.

Timing of ACL reconstruction has received attention in the sports medicine literature with some conflicting reports as to when it is safe to perform ACL reconstruction after an injury. It is important to assess the "personality" of the knee injury and to recognize the large variation among patients. Prior to performing ACL reconstruction, the knee effusion and swelling should have largely resolved, and the range of motion, particularly extension, should be regained. A strong quadriceps contraction is critical to the return of full extension and some patients have severe quadriceps inhibition with this injury. There is a rare patient who will have an impinging torn ACL that requires debridement in a separate arthroscopic procedure to facilitate the return of full extension. A continuous passive motion (CPM) machine can also be helpful in rare cases where loss of flexion and parapatellar fibrosis limits flexion. If patients are progressing slowly with their recovery prior to surgery, reconstruction may be delayed for a period of weeks to allow the soft tissues around the knee to recover.

AUTHORS' PREFERRED TREATMENT

Our preferred technique is an anatomic single-bundle reconstruction with independent drilling of the tibial and femoral tunnels. Based on the clinical situation, either autograft (either hamstring or patellar tendon) or an allograft (usually tibialis anterior tendon) may be used. The decision on graft is based on patient preference, but a patellar tendon graft is preferred for very unstable knees or in a young athlete with a strong quadriceps who plays the most demanding sports. Allografts are used when an early return to daily activities is important and the demands on the knee are less. Hamstring grafts are used for competitive and recreational athletes who prefer autograft and may not rehabilitate well with the disability of a patellar tendon autograft harvest. The same anatomic single-bundle technique can be used regardless of graft choice.

A standard operating table is used with the foot of the bed left extended. A leg holder is not used as it often prevents adequate flexion of the knee when drilling through the anteromedial portal. Instead, we use three posts to support the operative leg in either 90° or full flexion (Fig. 70.1A,B). A vertical post is placed on the lateral side of the thigh to allow access to the medial compartment as well as to prevent hip abduction when the knee is flexed. Two posts are placed across the bed to serve as footrests to maintain the two flexion angles most often needed during the procedure (90° and >125°). This setup allows the knee to be held in either position without any assistance, which frees the hands of both the surgeon and the assistant. Regardless of the setup, if an anteromedial portal drilling technique will be used, it is essential that the knee can be flexed adequately.

Arthroscopically, most of the torn ACL fibers are removed with a motorized shaver leaving some fibers for precise identification of the footprints. Pay close attention to the borders of the notch and its relationship to the planned ACL graft. Depending on the particular anatomy encountered, a small amount of bone may need to be removed from the lateral side of the notch and from the superior aspect of the notch. The amount of bone removed varies greatly from patient to patient. This step is important to prevent graft impingement. The native ACL is hourglass shaped, which helps to avoid impingement; however, the grafts used in reconstruction are cylindrical. The best way to assess for possible impingement is to observe the relationship of the notch to the anatomic center of the tibial footprint with the knee in extension. It is important to remember that the potential impingement

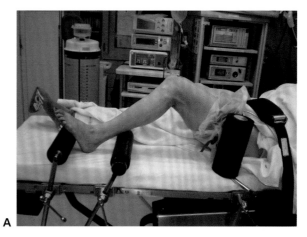

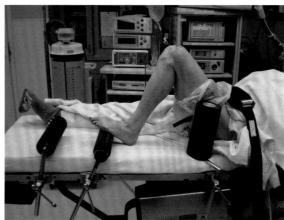

FIGURE 70.1. The operative setup is shown. The foot of the table is left up and three posts are used. Two posts allow the foot to rest with the knee in either 90° **(A)** or 125° of flexion **(B)**. A third post is positioned vertically next to the lateral thigh to prevent hip abduction when the knee is flexed.

will be exaggerated by any anterior tibial translation that is present due to ACL deficiency, and that this will resolve with proper graft tensioning.

The key to an anatomic single-bundle technique is accurately identifying the center of the ACL footprints. A reproducible point based on anatomic studies is to center the tibial tunnel 15 mm anterior to the PCL notch (15, 16) (Fig. 70.2). The tunnel should be biased approximately one-half tunnel width anteriorly and medially because the graft will tend to fall posteriorly and laterally in the tunnel. A second method for determining intra-articular placement of the tibial tunnel is to identify the medial tibial eminence (17). The entire native tibial ACL insertion is anterior to the posterior border of the medial tibial eminence. In practice the tibial tunnel will enter the joint within the anterior half of the medial tibial eminence. The center of the tibial footprint varies between patients, but an approximation of 15 mm anterior to the PCL is a good approximation (Fig. 70.3).

Externally, the starting point for the tibial tunnel may be placed relatively close to the tibial tubercle. Because the femoral tunnel position is not dependent on the tibial

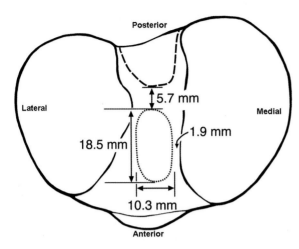

FIGURE 70.2. The oval-shaped tibial insertion of the ACL is illustrated. The posterior fibers of the ACL are 5.7 mm anterior to the PCL notch. The center of the footprint is 15 mm anterior to the PCL notch. The final, definitive version of this figure has been published in *The American Journal of Sports Medicine,* Vol 35 / Issue 10, Oct. 2007 by SAGE Publications Ltd./SAGE Publications, Inc., All rights reserved. © 2007

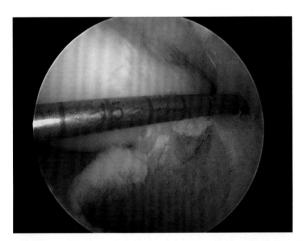

FIGURE 70.3. The completed tibial tunnel is viewed arthroscopically from a lateral portal. The arthroscopic probe is placed in the PCL notch, showing the tunnel placement approximately 15 mm anterior to the PCL notch.

tunnel position, there is no need to place the tunnel on the medial side of the tibia. This avoids damage to the medial collateral ligament (MCL) and allows for longer tunnel lengths. The tunnel should be drilled at an angle that creates tunnels with a length of at least 30 to 40 mm.

After the tibial footprint has been identified, a guide pin is placed using a commercially available aiming guide. Prior to reaming, the placement of the pin is carefully evaluated relative to the native footprint. If the center of the tunnel needs to be moved a few millimeters, the guide pin is left in place and a reamer several sizes smaller than the final tunnel size is used. After this preliminary step, the guide pin can be repositioned eccentrically in the preliminary tunnel to move the center of the final tunnel to

the proper position prior to reaming up to the final size. A rasp is used to contour the posterolateral corner of the tunnel to avoid sharp bone edges contacting the graft. Soft tissue is cleared from the tunnel opening on the anterior aspect of the tibia, as soft tissue here may impair graft passage.

In order to safely and properly drill the femoral tunnel, an adequate medial arthroscopy portal must be created. In order to reach the anatomic footprint, this portal should be just superior to the medial meniscus and close enough to the midline to avoid the articular surface of the medial femoral condyle (Fig. 70.4). If a portal has already been created earlier during the procedure that is not ideally positioned, an accessory medial portal should be created at this point.

A small amount of native ACL fibers on the femoral attachment serve as a guide for tunnel placement. In chronic or revision cases, these fibers will most likely not be present. A small ridge is present on the lateral wall of the notch, which lies just anterior to the ACL fibers. However, this is not always a consistently easy landmark to identify.

Another preparatory step is to remove any portion of the fat pad that impairs visualization. Slightly more fat pad needs to be removed with medial portal drilling compared with transtibial drilling, as the higher flexion required of the knee brings more of the fat pad into the notch during drilling.

In order to identify the location of the femoral footprint, the knee is positioned in 90° of flexion. This is a reproducible way to achieve a known orientation of the femoral footprint that has been described by anatomic studies (15–18) (Fig. 70.5). Next, the posterior border of the notch is identified from its highest point at the apex of the notch to its lowest point on the lateral wall of the notch at the articular cartilage margin. The midpoint between these two points is the central point of the ACL femoral insertion (Fig. 70.6A–C).

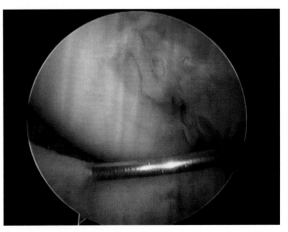

FIGURE 70.4. A spinal needle is placed in the planned position of the medial portal showing the safe position just above the medial meniscus and entering the notch without damaging the medial femoral condyle.

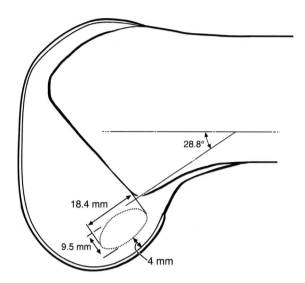

FIGURE 70.5. The oval-shaped femoral insertion of the ACL is illustrated as viewed in the sagittal plane. The footprint is approximately 18.4 mm long and 9.5 mm wide and is oriented along an axis approximately 28.8° off the shaft of the femur. The final, definitive version of this figure has been published in *The American Journal of Sports Medicine,* Vol 35 / Issue 10, Oct. 2007 by SAGE Publications Ltd./SAGE Publications, Inc., All rights reserved. © 2007

A 7-mm offset guide is introduced through the antero-medial portal to start the guide pin. This pin is drilled a few millimeters into the insertion site with the knee at 90° of flexion (Fig. 70.7). At this point, the tip of the guide pin should not easily slip away from the starting point. The knee is then flexed to over 125° and the guide pin is advanced through the lateral cortex of the femur and through the skin of the lateral thigh (Fig. 70.8). It is essential that the knee be adequately flexed to over 125° during this step to ensure that the tunnel is of adequate length and to maintain adequate distance between the guide pin and the peroneal nerve as the pin exits the lateral femur (19). It is sometimes helpful for the surgeon to step back for a moment during this part of the procedure to visualize the angle of the guide pin prior to drilling. A tunnel with a minimum length of 30 mm should be created. In some cases, especially with smaller legs, this is not possible. It is acceptable to drill a few millimeters shorter than this, as a 23-mm interference screw is typically used on the femoral side. Occasionally the drill will penetrate the far cortex of the femur. This does not change the strength of the reconstruction, but the surgeon must be aware of this prior to passing the graft as the graft may be pulled into the soft tissue of the lateral thigh.

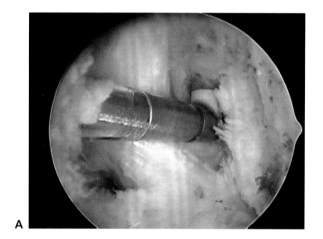

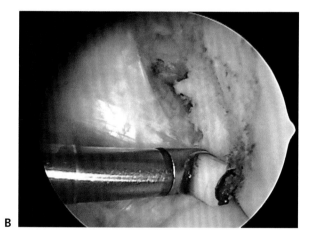

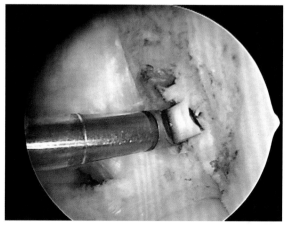

FIGURE 70.6. The femoral footprint is outlined in the three arthroscopic photos shown. The probe is positioned at the superior border of the footprint **(A)** the inferior border **(B),** and the center of the femoral footprint **(C)**. All photos are of a left knee viewed from a lateral portal with the knee in approximately 90° of flexion.

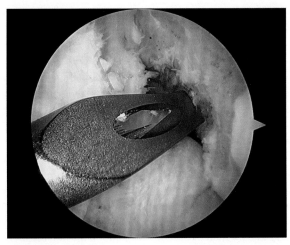

FIGURE 70.7. The guide pin for the femoral tunnel is placed at a point midway between the apex of the notch and the articular margin at the lowest point on the lateral wall. The guide pin is brought into the knee at 90° of flexion and is drilled a few millimeters into the femur at which point the knee is flexed to 125° as shown in the next figure.

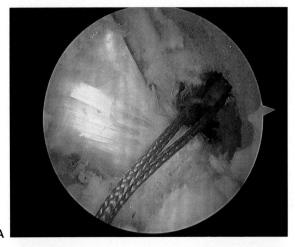

A

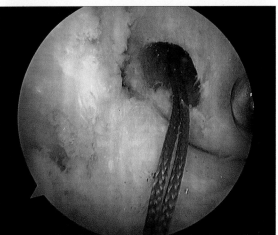

B

FIGURE 70.9. These arthroscopic photographs show the completed femoral tunnel after a passing suture has been passed through the femoral tunnel and subsequently retrieved through the tibial tunnel. The femoral tunnel is seen from both the lateral **(A)** and the medial-viewing portals **(B)**. At this point, the knee is prepared for graft passage.

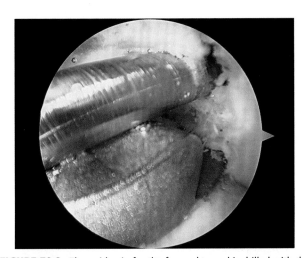

FIGURE 70.8. The guide pin for the femoral tunnel is drilled with the knee flexed to 125°. At this amount of flexion the aiming guide rotates underneath the femoral condyle, and the normal perspective of the notch is lost.

A passing suture (usually a braided no. 5 suture) is then passed using a beath pin through the medial portal, into the femoral tunnel, and out the lateral thigh. The loop end of the passing suture is retrieved through the tibial tunnel using an arthroscopic grasper. This suture is used to pull the graft through both the tibial and the femoral tunnels (Fig. 70.9A,B). The graft is watched arthroscopically as it passes across the joint and into the femoral tunnel. It is helpful to mark the graft prior to passage at a known length to ensure that the graft has fully seated in the femoral tunnel.

Prior to fixation, the graft is inspected with the knee flexed and extended to detect any impingement. It is far easier to remove any impinging bone at this stage rather than after fixation. However, there is rarely any significant

impingement after graft passage with precise tunnel placement and adequate notch preparation.

Bioabsorbable interference screw fixation is used for both the femoral and the tibial sides of the graft. The femoral side is fixed first. A 23-mm long screw that is the same diameter as the tunnel is used. A flexible nitinol guidewire is passed into the femoral tunnel through the medial portal. The knee is flexed to the same position as during drilling, which will avoid a divergent screw pathway. Care should be taken during screw introduction through the medial portal to avoid damage to the medial femoral condyle. Also, care should be taken to avoid twisting the graft around the screw when this technique is used with soft tissue grafts. The guidewire should be removed prior to fully seating the screw to avoid incarcerating the guidewire.

After fixation of the femoral side, a guidewire is passed up the tibial tunnel from the anterior tibia into the joint. The arthroscope is removed from the joint and the knee is brought into full extension. Because an anatomically centered grafts will often lengthen in extension similar to the native ACL, it is important to not overconstrain the knee by overtensioning the graft in flexion. An anatomic graft placement is very effective at restoring physiologic laxity and this obviates any need to overtension the graft. The graft is tensioned to approximately 15 lb (6.8 kg) while the screw is placed. A 30-mm long screw with a diameter of 1 mm larger than the tunnel size is used. If soft tissue grafts are used, it is important for the construct strength to ensure that all strands of the graft are tensioned equally (20). The joint and all incisions are then irrigated thoroughly and closed using standard techniques.

COMPLICATIONS, CONTROVERSIES, AND SPECIAL CONSIDERATIONS

The various graft choices available for use in ACL reconstruction have led to some debate over the past few years. The anatomic single-bundle technique can be used irrespective of the graft chosen. At this time, conclusive data is lacking demonstrating a clear advantage of one graft type over another.

We use interference screw fixation on both the femoral and the tibial sides of the reconstruction. A wide variety of ACL graft fixation devices are commercially available at this time and many can be used for the anatomic single-bundle technique. Unfortunately, many cross pin-type fixation devices require a transtibial technique for their instrumentation and the surgeon should be aware of this limitation. Many device manufacturers have recently introduced new instrumentation that can be used with independent tunnel drilling.

A second concern relates to femoral fixation with a cortical suspensory system. The femoral tunnel may be shorter with an independent drilling technique compared with a transtibial technique, particularly if maximum flexion is not sought during reaming. With suspensory fixation and a short tunnel, there is the potential to have a relatively short length of graft in the femoral tunnel. If this is excessively short, this could theoretically impair graft to bone healing. If the surgeon uses suspensory fixation, he or she should be aware of this possibility and be prepared to employ alternative fixation methods if needed.

With regard to complications specific to the tibial tunnel, an anatomic single-bundle technique is technically very similar and perhaps slightly safer and easier than a transtibial technique. There is more flexibility in the starting point and no need to compromise the tunnel position in order to accommodate a femoral drill. The starting point can be closer to the tibial tubercle and the drill angle kept steeper, which prevents injury to the medial collateral ligament and allows for a longer tunnel with perhaps stronger bone for fixation. Also, the tunnel can be placed through the anatomic footprint with less risk of impingement as the graft will lie lower in the notch.

The femoral tunnel is more challenging technically with the key being high knee flexion during drilling.

Lower flexion angles will lead to a shorter tunnel and will lead to the guide pin exiting the lateral side of the femur closer to the peroneal nerve (19). Visualization can be challenging as well during femoral drilling and resection of fat pad is necessary. When the knee is flexed over 125°, the usual landmarks become distorted and it appears that the guide pin has been placed anteriorly in the notch. In order to reference normal landmarks, the guide pin is started a few millimeters into the bone with the knee at 90° and then the knee is flexed to over 125° for passage through the femur.

The entry of the drill through the medial portal also introduces some potential complications. The meniscus is at risk for iatrogenic damage, as a properly positioned portal allows instruments to pass just superior to the meniscus. Also, the articular surface of the medial femoral condyle is at risk during the introduction of the reamer. Care should be taken to place the anteromedial portal appropriately and to bring the drill carefully into the notch to avoid any articular damage.

Revision cases are particularly suited to using the anatomic single-bundle technique. The method provides freedom to place the new tunnels separate from the prior tunnels. Specifically, in cases where the femoral tunnel was placed with a transtibial technique during the index procedure, independent femoral drilling will allow a tunnel that is divergent from the original tunnel and fixation can be performed as in a primary reconstruction. In cases of severe tunnel widening this is not possible and these revisions are performed as a two-stage procedure with bone grafting to restore bone stock prior to revision reconstruction.

REHABILITATION

ACL reconstruction is performed as an outpatient procedure. Patients are allowed to be weight bearing as tolerated with crutches from the time of surgery. A knee immobilizer or hinged knee brace is not routinely used. An emphasis is placed on range of motion and quadriceps-driven full extension. Patients progress through a standard ACL rehabilitation program. Simple jogging begins at approximately 3 months and return to competition is generally allowed at 6 months.

PEARLS AND PITFALLS

1. The ability to achieve adequate knee flexion during femoral drilling is critical to the safety and success of this procedure. Flexion should be checked prior to draping. Breaking the foot of the bed and using leg holders may limit knee flexion.
2. Proper placement of the medial portal is essential. Care should be taken not to damage the medial meniscus or medial femoral condyle during portal creation or during instrument passage. If a medial portal has been created

earlier during the procedure for another purpose, such as meniscal repair, then an accessory medial portal may be necessary.

3. Visualize the anatomic footprints using known landmarks. The center of the femoral footprint is located halfway between the apex and the base of the notch on the lateral wall of the notch 7 mm anterior to the posterior border of the condyle. The center of the tibial footprint is located approximately 15 mm anterior to the PCL notch.

4. Check for bony impingement and adjust bone preparation and graft placement accordingly. Reconstruction of an hourglass-shaped ACL with a cylindrical graft requires some adjustments to prevent impingement.

CONCLUSIONS AND FUTURE DIRECTIONS

The recent wave of research defining the anatomy of the native ACL has allowed for an improvement in the technique of single-bundle ACL reconstruction. A single-bundle reconstruction centering a single-bundle graft within the anatomic footprints of the native ACL allows for improved mechanics compared with a transtibial reconstruction. Anatomically placed grafts can restore physiologic knee laxity in response to translational and rotatory forces. Future research and long-term follow-up studies will be necessary to determine if an anatomically placed single-bundle reconstruction can improve outcomes compared with a conventional single-bundle reconstruction. Also, similar comparative studies between anatomic single-bundle reconstruction and double bundle reconstructions will help determine whether clinical outcomes will be affected by the addition of a second bundle.

REFERENCES

1. Biau DJ, Tournoux C, Katsahian S, et al. ACL reconstruction: a meta-analysis of functional scores. *Clin Orthop Relat Res.* 2007;458:180–187.

2. Freedman KB, D'Amato MJ, Nedeff DD, et al. Arthroscopic anterior cruciate ligament reconstruction: a metaanalysis comparing patellar tendon and hamstring tendon autografts. *Am J Sports Med.* 2003;31:2–11.

3. van Dijck RA, Saris DB, Willems JW, et al. Additional surgery after anterior cruciate ligament reconstruction: can we improve technical aspects of the initial procedure? *Arthroscopy.* 2008;24:88–95.

4. Øiestad BE, Engebretsen L, Storheim K, et al. Knee osteoarthritis after anterior cruciate ligament injury: a systemic review. *Am J Sports Med.* 2009;37:1434–1443.

5. Georgoulis AD, Papadonikolakis A, Papageorgio CD, et al. Three-dimensional tibiofemoral kinematics of the anterior cruciate ligament-deficient and reconstructed knee during walking. *Am J Sports Med.* 2003;31:75–79.

6. Ristanis S, Stergiou N, Patras K, et al. Excessive tibial rotation during high-demand activities is not restored by anterior cruciate ligament reconstruction. *Arthroscopy.* 2005;21:1323–1329.

7. Tashman S, Collon D, Anderson K, et al. Abnormal rotational knee motion during running after anterior cruciate ligament reconstruction. *Am J Sports Med.* 2004;32:975–983.

8. Howell SM, Gittins ME, Gottlieb JE, et al. The relationship between the angle of the tibial tunnel in the coronal plane and loss of flexion and anterior laxity after anterior cruciate ligament reconstruction. *Am J Sports Med.* 2001;29:567–574.

9. Woo SL, Kanamori A, Zeminski J, et al. The effectiveness of reconstruction of the anterior cruciate ligament with hamstrings and patellar tendon. A cadaveric study comparing anterior tibial and rotational loads. *J Bone Joint Surg Am.* 2002;84A:907–914.

10. Mae T, Shino K, Miyama T, et al. Single-versus two-femoral socket anterior cruciate ligament reconstruction technique: biomechanical analysis using a robotic simulator. *Arthroscopy.* 2001;17:708–716.

11. Yagi M, Wong EK, Kanamori A, et al. Biomechanical analysis of an anatomic anterior cruciate ligament reconstruction. *Am J Sports Med.* 2002;20:660–666.

12. Yamamoto Y, Wei-Hsiu H, Woo SL, et al. Knee stability and graft function after anterior cruciate ligament reconstruction: a comparison of a lateral and an anatomical femoral tunnel placement. *Am J Sports Med.* 2004;32:1825–1832.

13. Steiner ME, Battaglia TC, Heming JF, et al. Independent drilling outperforms conventional transtibial drilling in anterior cruciate ligament reconstruction. *Am J Sports Med.* 2000;37:1912–1919.

14. Ho JY, Gardiner A, Shah V, et al. Equal kinematics between central anatomic single bundle and double bundle anterior cruciate ligament reconstructions. *Arthroscopy.* 2000;25:464–472.

15. Heming JF, Rand J, Steiner ME. Anatomical limitations of transtibial drilling in anterior cruciate ligament reconstruction. *Am J Sports Med.* 2007;35:1708–1715.

16. Colombet P, Robinson J, Christel P, et al. Morphology of anterior cruciate ligament attachments for anatomic reconstruction: a cadaveric dissection and radiographic study. *Arthroscopy.* 2006;22:984–992.

17. Girgis FG, Marshall JL, Monajem A. The cruciate ligaments of the knee joint. Anatomical, functional and experimental analysis. *Clin Orthop Relat Res.* 1975;106:216–231.

18. Amis AA, Jakob RP. Anterior cruciate ligament graft positioning, tensioning and twisting. *Knee Surg Sports Traumatol Arthrosc.* 1998;6(suppl 1):s2–s12.

19. Nakamura M, Deie M, Shibuya H, et al. Potential risks of femoral tunnel drilling through the far anteromedial portal: a cadaveric study. *Arthroscopy.* 2009;25:481–487.

20. Hamner DL, Brown H, Steiner ME, et al. Hamstring tendon grafts for reconstruction of the anterior cruciate ligament: biomechanical evaluation of the use of multiple strands and tensioning techniques. *J Bone Joint Surg Am.* 1999;81:549–557.

Double-Bundle ACL Reconstruction

James R. Romanowski • Verena M. Schreiber • Freddie H. Fu

Anterior cruciate ligament (ACL) injuries continue to be one of the most common problems that orthopedic surgeons encounter. With an annual incidence of about 1 in 3,000 knees, approximately 100,000 ACL reconstructions are performed each year (1, 2). Management of these ligament ruptures varies, but ranges from nonoperative modalities to various methods of surgical reconstruction. Significant resources have been committed toward studying every aspect of the ACL including the anatomy, biomechanics, intra- and extraarticular reconstruction methods, as well as synthetic ligament substitutes and optimization of allograft and autograft sources. With such a multifaceted commitment toward research, it is not surprising that the management of these injuries has evolved as the understanding of the ACL has improved.

A primary tenant of orthopedic surgery is anatomy. Without a clear understanding of the affected structure and the associated function, accurate restoration of function with surgical reconstruction will fail. Originally described in 1938, the ACL consists of two bundles: the anteromedial (AM) and the posterolateral (PL) (3) (Fig. 71.1). An occasionally recognized anatomic variant includes a third,

or intermediate (IM) bundle. The nomenclature is based on the tibial insertion of each bundle. These individual areas of insertion provide important functional contributions to both anterior–posterior (AM bundle) and rotational stability (PL bundle) (4).

The primary goal of surgical intervention is to restore function. Every patient has a unique ACL footprint, therefore, it is of paramount importance to respect anatomic landmarks for proper identification of the origins and insertions of each ACL bundle. It is this uniqueness that precludes generalization to a particular "o'clock" or set millimeter reference for tunnel placement. Furthermore, there is a significant risk of tunnel mismatch, that is, PL tibial tunnel to AM femoral tunnel. Most surgical reconstructions for ruptured or dysfunctional ACLs have been single-bundle reconstructions. Single-bundle techniques have enjoyed relatively successful outcome in terms of stability and return to sport, but long-term results have revealed several shortcomings and only approach normal International Knee Documentation Committee (IKDC) scores in 61% to 67% of patients (5).

As the understanding of the ACL evolves, optimizing each functional component will allow for continued improve patient outcomes.

CLINICAL EVALUATION

As with any patient complaint, it is necessary to perform a thorough history and physical evaluation.

Pertinent History

The patient with a torn ACL typically presents with one of two scenarios. A noncontact injury sustained during pivoting or cutting activities, or from traumatic contact. Establishing the mechanism of injury remains important as it may suggest other pathologies, particularly with varus or valgus loads with subsequent injury to the MCL, LCL, PL corner, and menisci. Failure to recognize additional structural injuries will result in higher failure rates regardless of the reconstructive method (6). Oftentimes, a "pop" is described and an effusion present. Some patients

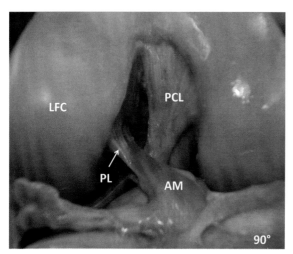

FIGURE 71.1. Right knee showing the ACL with the AM and PL bundles. LFC, lateral femoral condyle; PCL, posterior cruciate ligament.

will attempt to return to activities before seeking treatment and may complain of persistent instability. For those that deny instability but have an isolated ACL tear, this may be a significant factor in the decision-making process and avoid surgery.

Age is also an important consideration. Within the preadolescent and teenager population, it is critical to evaluate growth plates, and those with advanced age have increased risk of degenerative joint disease that may preclude surgical intervention.

Lifestyle should also be evaluated as a sedentary individual may not have the same functional demands as an elite athlete. Prior surgical procedures or infections of the affected extremity must be considered as there are associated surgical risks.

Physical Examination

Most patients are evaluated in the office setting, however, evaluation at the time of injury can provide valuable information as there is little/no swelling present. The patient is asked to wear shorts to allow for direct visualization of both lower extremities and comparison throughout the examination. The affected knee is first inspected noting any joint effusion, bruising, or atrophy. The overall alignment is also observed as significant angular deformities may need to be addressed. The range of motion is measured and followed as this needs to be optimized prior to any surgical intervention. Palpation of all bony prominences as well as the joint line and parapatellar region helps identify associated meniscal, ligamentous, and patellofemoral injuries. Tests specific for the ACL ruptures are performed including the Lachman, anterior drawer, and pivot shift maneuvers. Although more sensitive, the pivot shift may be difficult as patients tend to guard especially in the acute setting. Supplementing the examination, the McMurray, varus and valgus stress at 0° and 30°, Dial, reverse pivot shift, and posterior drawer testing are performed for completion.

Objective methods are also employed as part of the evaluation and include the KT-2000 arthrometer. Dysfunction or disruption of the ACL is suggested with side-to side differences greater than 3 mm.

Imaging

Radiographs remain a key component during the workup of ACL-injured patient and help to identify tibial spine avulsions or rule out associated fractures, evaluate limb malalignment, and assess with open growth plates. Standard radiographs include the weightbearing full extension and 45° posteroanterior X-rays, nonweightbearing lateral, and merchant views. For patients where the physical examination suggests lower extremity malalignment, a bilateral long cassette view is obtained for further assessment. The need for an MRI is arguable, but patients often present having already had the study and within our practice an MRI is obtained for further identification associated injuries.

CT scans are not necessary for primary ACL reconstruction, but have a preoperative role in revision cases.

Decision Making

Persistent instability that causes functional limitations with either activities of daily living or with sports remain critical aspects when deciding whether or not to pursue surgical intervention.

TREATMENT

Nonoperative

Sedentary or low demand patients who can modify their activities may pursue conservative management.

Operative Indications

Surgery is typically reserved for individuals with persistent instability or symptoms associated with the ACL tear or dysfunction. Candidates include patients with functionally demanding employment, high-level athletes, and individuals who are limited in their activities of daily living secondary to the ligamentous compromise. Age is a consideration that is related to the presence of open growth plates in children and adolescents, and the potential for degenerative arthritis in older individuals. Double-bundle reconstructions should be avoided with open growth plates because the technique involves a larger area of the tibia, theoretically increasing the risk of growth arrest. Double-bundle constructs should also be avoided in multiligamentous injuries, advanced knee arthritis, active sepsis, and in noncompliant patients that cannot follow postoperative rehabilitation protocols.

Timing

Considerable debate remains over the appropriate timing of surgical reconstruction after injury to the ACL (8). Although there is no consensus, it is generally agreed upon that the patient should regain range of motion (0° to 120°) and reestablish quadriceps control preoperatively to avoid postoperative arthrofibrosis (9). Acute reconstruction (<3 weeks) has been associated with significantly increased rates of arthrofibrosis, with some series reporting up to 37% of patients experiencing loss of motion versus only 5% in individuals with delayed intervention (10, 11). Delay in surgical intervention has been found to increase the risk of cartilage damage 1% per month of surgical delay (8). Furthermore, there is a higher risk of secondary meniscal tears and degenerative arthritis in individuals that delay surgery greater than 12 months from the time of injury (12). Our current practice is to perform subacute reconstruction (>3 weeks) after successful preoperative rehabilitation.

TECHNIQUE

Anesthesia

Prior to surgery, the surgeon identifies, initials, and marks the operative site with a "yes." A discussion is held between the surgeon, anesthesiologist, and the patient to develop an appropriate anesthesia regimen. Typically, peripheral nerve blocks involving the femoral and sciatic nerves are performed by an experienced anesthesiologist utilizing ultrasound guidance. In combination with "light" sedation, these temporary nerve blocks provide adequate intraoperative pain control and helps minimize postoperative narcotic use.

Setup and Examination under Anesthesia

The patient is brought back to the operating suite and placed supine on the OR table. After adequate anesthesia and analgesia, an examination under anesthesia is performed. Specific tests include the Lachman, pivot shift, anterior drawer, posterior drawer, varus/valgus stress, Dial testing, and range of motion. The foot of the table is maximally flexed, allowing for. The nonoperative limb is comfortably place in a well-padded leg holder with the hip and knee flexed to 80° to 90° and positioned in abduction. A tourniquet is placed proximally on the operative thigh and secured with a bolster. All neurovascular and bony prominences are cushioned and protected. Securing the leg in slight hip flexion (10° to 20°) allows for increased knee flexion for later femoral tunnel creation. The operative knee should have a range of motion from 0° to at least 120° (Fig. 71.2).

Surface Landmarks and Incisions

Critical to the success and limited invasiveness of arthroscopic ACL reconstruction are appropriately placed

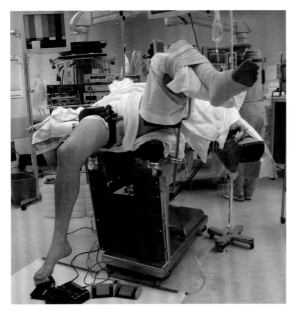

FIGURE 71.2. Patient setup using a leg holder.

skin incisions. With properly placed portals, a notchplasty is not required and all tunnels may be created with careful portal placement. The anatomic landmarks are identified and marked, including the inferior pole of the patella, medial, and lateral borders of the patellar tendon, medial joint line, tibial tubercle, and anterior and posteromedial borders of the tibia. Additional incisions may be required for meniscal repair depending on the chosen technique. The leg is elevated and an esmarch is used to exsanguinate the leg for tourniquet insufflation.

With the knee in 90° of flexion, the anterolateral portal (LP) is established just lateral to the origin of the patellar tendon on the inferior pole of the patella. A no. 11 blade scalpel is used to make the vertical incision. The arthroscopic trocar is then used to enter the joint and sweep under the medially lying fatpad. This portal is used primarily for visualization of the tibial ACL footprint.

Again with the knee in 90° of flexion, the central medial portal (CMP) is established. A no. 18G spinal needle is used to determine the trajectory of the instrumentation and visualization pathway from the CMP. The needle typically follows the course of the normal ACL. The skin incision should be tangential to the medial border of the patellar tendon and just superior to the anterior horn of the medial meniscus. This position allows for optimal visualization of the notch and femoral footprint. It also allows for adequate working space for the third arthroscopic portal—the Accessory medial portal (AMP). A no. 11 blade scalpel is used to make a vertical incision in the skin, carefully cutting away from the underlying medial meniscus. Prior to placement of the AMP portal, it is often necessary to debride the fatpad and improve arthroscopic visualization to optimize the portal placement (Fig. 71.3). The accessory medial portal is perhaps the most critical of all the portals as the trajectory must capture the AM and PL ACL origins of the femur while avoiding damage to the cartilage surface of the medial femoral condyle. If the portal is placed too medial, then the femoral AM tunnel entrance angle may be too acute and risk posterior wall blowout of the lateral femoral condyle.

The skin incision for the tibial tunnels may now be established. Centered between the anterior and the posteromedial borders of the tibia, and no. 10 blade scalpel is used to make a vertical incision starting proximally at the level of the tibial tubercle and extending distally approximately 4 cm. Sharp dissection is carried through the underlying periosteum, sweeping it gently both medially and laterally with a periosteal elevator. Careful attention is paid toward leaving a cuff of tissue for later repair and eventual coverage of the AM and PL tibia tunnels.

Diagnostic Arthroscopy

With the arthroscope in the LP, a diagnostic arthroscopy is performed inspecting the patellofemoral joint, medial, and lateral compartments. Meniscal and cartilage pathology is addressed as needed at this time prior to reconstruction

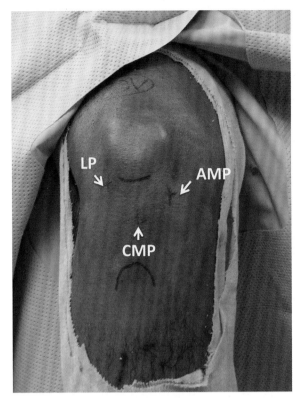

FIGURE 71.3. Portal establishment with LP, CMP and accessory medial portal (AMP).

of the ACL. Surgeon comfort and familiarity dictates the meniscal and cartilage repair and debridement technique. Next, attention is directed toward the ACL.

Tear Identification

Inherent to the principles of anatomic ACL reconstruction, careful identification of both the AM and the PL bundles is achieved, identifying not only the rupture pattern, but also the femoral and tibial footprints. This is usually the most time consuming portion of the operation as it is the most critical for both anatomic single- and double-bundle reconstructive methods. Tears may be classified as femoral, midsubstance, or tibial. In addition, the ACL dysfunction may be categorized as a complete rupture or stretching of an isolated or combined AM and PL bundle. Cautious dissection will occasionally reveal compromise of a single bundle and allow for augmentation or isolated replacement of the affected AM or PL bundle. At some point during the ACL inspection and debridement, it becomes necessary to place the arthroscope within the CMP to visualize the femoral ACL origin. If not performed already, the AMP may now be established with the no. 18G spinal needle and no. 11 blade scalpel. Creation of this portal will allow for further debridement and easier identification of landmarks within the notch. An arthroscopic shaver place through the AMP allows for debridement of the dysfunction ACL remnants, however, contact with the osseous

portion of the notch should be avoided as to preserve the bony landmarks. An arthroscopic low voltage thermal device is used to complete the femoral debridement, leaving a small rim of AM and PL tissue for proprioceptive purposes (13). Bundle identification is easier in the subacute versus the chronic phase as less scarring and resorption has occurred. For chronic cases or when the respective bundles cannot be found, identification of the bony landmarks becomes critical for anatomic reconstruction. The intercondylar ridge represents the superior border of the of femoral ACL footprint on the medial aspect of the lateral femoral condyle. The bifurcate ridge is usually perpendicular to the intercondylar ridge and separates the AM and PL origins (Fig. 71.4). For longstanding ACL ruptures, the loss of ACL stress on the femoral notch may lead to bony loss of the ridges in accordance with Wolff law (14). In this situation, it becomes necessary to rely on a generic formula for determining tunnel placement. With the knee flexed to 90°, the PL tunnel falls within the lower one-third of the notch, 3 mm anterior to the posterior cartilage ridge, and 5 to 7 mm proximal to the articular surface. The AM tunnel is then referenced from the PL origin, occupying the notch space proximally.

SINGLE- VERSUS DOUBLE-BUNDLE RECONSTRUCTION

Once the tibial and femoral footprints have been identified, it is necessary to measure the dimensions. This step is critical because it determines whether or not the patient's native anatomy can accommodate a double-bundle reconstruction or if a single-bundle construct is required. In order to aid surgeons with their decision making whether to perform single- or double-bundle ACL reconstruction, we created an anatomic single- and

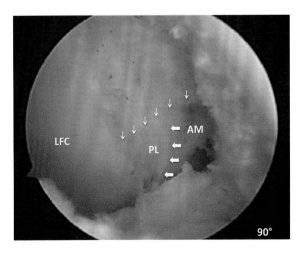

FIGURE 71.4. View of the lateral femoral wall at 90° of flexion through the CMP. *Bold arrows* depict the lateral bifurcate ridge, *thin arrows* depict the lateral intercondylar ridge.

ALGORITHMS

Anatomic Single-and Double-Bundle ACL Reconstruction Flowchart

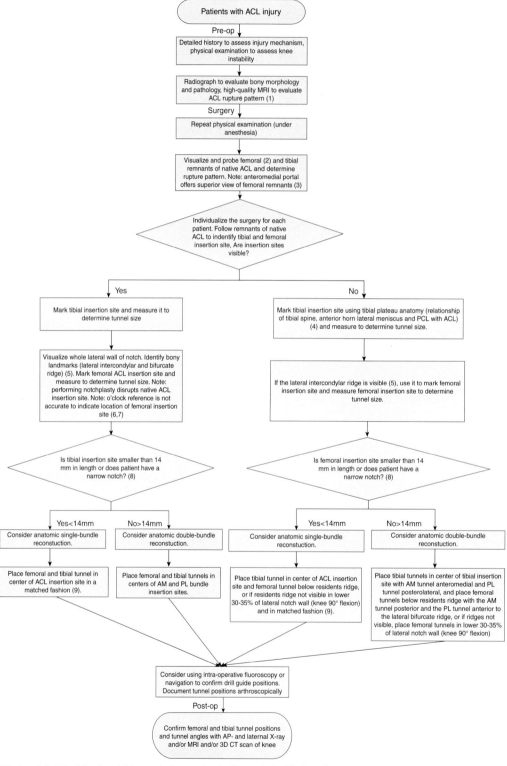

(From van Eck CF, Lesniak BP, Schreiber VM, et al. Anatomic single- and double-bundle anterior cruciate ligament reconstruction flowchart. *Arthroscopy.* 2010;26(2):258–268, with permission)

double-bundle ACL reconstruction flowchart (7). Regardless, preparation of the notch and identification of the patient's unique ACL origin and insertion allows for anatomic reconstruction. The University of Pittsburgh experience with anatomic double-bundle reconstruction has been that femoral notch length (proximal to distal) ≤14 mm precludes four tunnel constructs and requires a single-bundle restoration. Considering that it is necessary to have a 2-mm bone bridge between the tunnels, this limited footprint creates a technically challenging situation that risks tunnel convergence at the aperture. Furthermore, the individual tunnels need to be smaller, subsequently leading to small graft diameters. The femoral tunnel footprint dimensions (length and width) are measured through the LP with visualization through the CMP. If the femoral footprint measures less than 14 mm or the intercondylar notch measures less than 12 mm single-bundle reconstruction is preferred. The tibial footprint is also measured with a ruler through the CMP, but visualization is through the LP (Fig. 71.5). For single-bundle reconstruction, the femoral tunnel is placed 1 to 2 cm proximal to the bifurcate ridge as the AM bundle occupies approximately 60% of the total femoral footprint. The tibial tunnel is centered within the tibial anteroposterior footprint.

Once the femoral and tibial dimensions have been determined, the graft diameters may be sized. Typically, the femoral footprint is 1 to 2 mm smaller than the tibial footprint, therefore, the smaller value is used in order to avoid tunnel convergence and oversized grafts. The PL bundle diameter is usually 5 to 7 mm; the AM bundle typically 6 to 8 mm. For example, a femoral footprint length of 18 mm could easily accommodate an 8-mm AM graft and 6-mm PL graft with a 2-mm bone bridge.

GRAFT SELECTION

The graft choice is made after an open discussion between the patient and the physician. Both autografts and allografts may be considered. Autograft options are bone-patella tendon-bone (BPTB), quadriceps tendon and hamstrings. Examples for allografts used in Pittsburgh are BPTB, Achilles tendon, tensor fascia lata, tibialis anterior

and hamstrings allografts clearly have the added risk of hepatitis, HIV, and other donor-associated contaminants that are avoided with autograft sources. Conversely, autograft adds issues with donor site morbidity and slower short-term recovery (14).

Another variable to consider is the increased failure rate of allograft tissue seen in younger, more athletic populations (15, 16). This 3× increase in failures within this population should be discussed. From our experience, early allograft failure might be contributed to early return to sports, as allograft incorporation takes longer. Therefore, our rehabilitation protocol is rather conservative and we advise our patients to refrain from cutting sports until they reach their 9 to 12 months follow-up. Our practice recognizes these issues and actively offers alternative sources of autograft including quadriceps tendon and hamstrings, as well as allograft sources such as tibialis anterior for reconstruction of the ACL.

TUNNEL PREPARATION

The PL tunnel of the femoral condyle is prepared first. With the arthroscope in the CMP, an awl is used to place a pilot hole centered in the PL origin on the lateral femoral condyle. With the knee flexed to at least 110°, a 3.2-mm guidepin is then place through the AMP into the pilot hole. A 5-mm reamer is passed over the guidepin and drilled. A depth of at least 30 mm should is desired to accommodate a minimum of 25 mm of graft contact within the tunnel and the addition distance to allow for "flipping" of the Endobutton CL (Smith and Nephew, Andover, MA). For the Endobutton CL method, a 4.5-mm reamer is passed through tunnel and the lateral cortex is perforated. The depth is measured and appropriate implant chosen. Occasionally, the depth may be too short for both adequate graft fill and "flipping" distance, and it becomes necessary to use an Endobutton Direct (Smith and Nephew) or substitute fixation such as a screw/post or interference screw to provide fixation. The tunnel should be dilated to match the premeasured footprint diameter. With the tunnel prepared, attention is directed toward the tibial footprint, leaving the creation of the AM tunnel for later.

With arthroscopic visualization through the LP, the ACL guide is placed through the CMP into the PL footprint. Centering of the 45° guide is based on the patient's anatomy rather than a set distance from the PCL. A 3.2-mm guidepin is then placed through a small 3-cm incision placed on the proximal tibial, 2 to 3 cm medial to the tibial tuberosity. A second guidepin is centered on the AM footprint of the tibia and angled at 55°. It is necessary to keep a 2-mm bone bridge between the tunnels. Fluoroscopy may be used to verify pin placement. The two tibial tunnels are then reamed to one size smaller than the measured graft and then dilators are used achieve a tunnel size that approximates that of the graft. The PL tunnel is typically 6 mm and the AM is 8 mm.

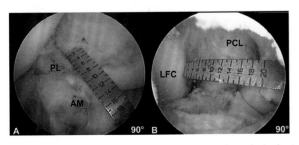

FIGURE 71.5. **A:** View of the tibial insertion site through the lateral portal with a measurement of 18 mm. **B:** View of the intercondylar notch through the CMP with a measurement of 19 mm. Both measurements are taken with the knee in 90° of flexion and allow to perform double bundle reconstruction.

With the tibial tunnels now created, attention is directed toward making the femoral AM tunnel. This is created last as the optimal trajectory occasionally may be transtibial. In 10% of cases, the femoral AM tunnel can be created via the tibial AM tunnel; via the tibial PL tunnel in approximately 60% of cases; and via the accessory CMP in greater than 90% of cases. Again, a 3.2-mm guidepin centered within the AM footprint is used to direct the appropriately sized reamer. Our preference is the Endobutton technique, however, surgeon comfort will dictate the appropriate fixation method.

With all four tunnels created, the focus is now on graft passage. Two individual Beath pins loaded with suture loop are then passed through the AAM into the respective femoral PL and AM tunnels. A suture grabber is the used to load the suture loop into the appropriate tibial AM and PL tunnels. The AM loop should be superficial, or superior, to the PL loop. The PL graft is then advanced, followed by the AM graft. Femoral fixation is achieved, usually by "flipping" the Endobutton, and the knee is then cycled with tension on the graft. The graft within the tibial PL tunnel is then fixed with the knee at full extension. The tibial AM tunnel graft is secured with the knee in 45° of flexion (Fig. 71.6).

CLOSURE

Standard approaches toward wound closure are utilized according to surgeon preference (Fig. 71.7).

COMPLICATIONS

As with any surgical procedure, the patient is faced with potential surgical site infection, arthrofibrosis, deep vein thrombosis or pulmonary embolus, or other complications related to anesthesia including cardiopulmonary events, strokes, permanent nerve damage associated with regional blocks or vascular sequelae related to inadvertent vessel penetration. Concerning allografts, additional risks are involved and include graft rejection, HIV and hepatitis, among other serious infections. Fortunately, these events remain rare but need to be presented as a prerequisite to proper informed consent.

CONTROVERSIES

The double-bundle reconstruction is not without controversy. Perhaps the most important aspect to the procedure is that it is a concept. By appreciating the patient's native anatomy and understanding the function of the ACL and the individual bundles, the surgical intervention can be individualized, and the patient's outcome may be optimized. Not every patient is a candidate for double-bundle reconstruction, and it is here that the anatomic principles can still be instituted. The "o'clock" mentality remains a disservice to the reconstructive process as not every person is an 11 o'clock and "time" actually changes related to portal placement and viewing angle. Furthermore, standard cookbook distances from the PCL oftentimes create a biomechanical mismatch as the tibial tunnel often falls within the PL insertion. Anatomic footprints, however, are reliable and careful dissection in the primary ACL reconstruction can take the guesswork out of the surgical procedure allow for custom tunnel placement.

Inaccurate ACL tunnel placement may lead to notch impingement and subsequently limitations in ranges of motion. Anatomical single- and double-bundle ACL reconstruction have been shown to be impingement free therefore minimizing one of the negative sequelae involved with ACL reconstruction (17).

When comparing the ability of the single- and double-bundle ACL reconstruction to restore knee kinematics and ligament forces, the double-bundle construct has been shown to more closely approximate the graft forces of the native ACL (18).

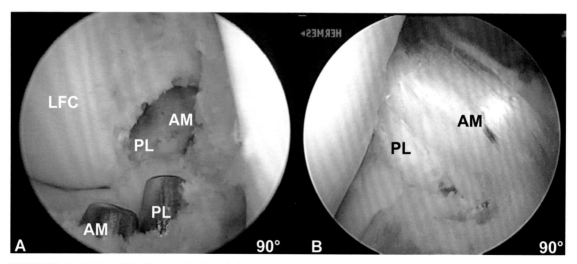

FIGURE 71.6. A: View of the four tunnels through the CMP. **B:** Reconstructed ACL with the AM and PL bundle as seen through the lateral portal.

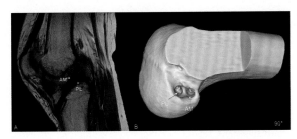

FIGURE 71.7. A: Sagittal MRI status post double bundle ACL reconstruction. **B:** Corresponding 3D CT scan.

The double-bundle technique also has limited outcome data. Short-term results, however, are encouraging and allow for continued offering of the surgical procedure.

Double-bundle ACL reconstruction requires not only appropriate footprint identification but also appropriate tensioning of the AM and PL grafts. The tension patterns of the native ACL have been established (19). There is a paucity of research concerning the ideal knee flexion angles as related to fixation of each bundle, but early cadaveric data suggests that normal knee kinematics are restored with both a 45/15 and a 20/20 (AM/PL) protocol (20).

PEARLS AND PITFALLS

As with any surgical procedure, a learning curve exists. By recognizing the potential pitfalls, the learning curve may be accelerated and complications avoided.

Patient Positioning

In regards to the surgical procedure, patient positioning will influence particular portions of the operation. The surgeon should be able to range the knee from full extension to at least 130° of flexion. Limitations in flexion will interfere with femoral tunnel placement and put the condylar surfaces at risk for iatrogenic damage.

Portal Placement

With improved recognition of the femoral origin of each bundle, it became evident that accurate tunnel creation through the traditional CMP was increasingly difficult, if not impossible. The addition of the accessory CMP has allowed for improved trajectory of both single- and double-bundle methods allowing for more anatomic reconstructions. The AMP should be placed under direct visualization and first trialed with an 18G spinal needle to allow ensure adequate room for guidepin and reamer placement as to avoid the medial femoral condyle upon insertion.

Furthermore, utilization of the LP for visualization of the tibial footprint and for creation of the tibial tunnels has further refined the role of each portal and optimized their use. An additional benefit with appropriate visualization is the negated need for notchplasty.

Reaming

Because the notch comes in various sizes and shapes and is filled with more than the ACL, creation of the femoral tunnel can be challenging even with optimal portal placement. Utilization of flexible reamers has allowed for improved tunnel placement and the surgeon should be comfortable with this technique when difficult tunnel situations arise.

Fixation

Many methods exist for fixation of the graft on both the femoral and the tibial sides. Interference screws with intra-articular aperture fixation potentially alter the coverage of the anatomic footprint. Consideration should be given to methods that allow for graft to fill the footprint. Furthermore, backup methods such as screw/washer fixation allow for a bailout should graft security be an issue.

Return to Activity

A potential pitfall with anatomic reconstruction is that many patients regain their motion earlier and feel better sooner. This perception that the knee is recovering quickly is actually detrimental in that the patient needs to be cautioned about the risk of early graft rupture with earlier return to activity. It is unlikely the biology of healing is in any way accelerated between the techniques.

REHABILITATION

Postoperative rehabilitative therapy for double-bundle ACL reconstruction remains an essential component to toward maximizing the outcome. Based on a five-phase protocol, the total duration usually approaches 9 months. Goals must be reached within each phase before progression to the next is allowed.

Phase I (0 to 6 weeks) begins the day of surgery and initially focuses on modalities to control inflammation, joint effusion, and range of motion while allowing the graft to incorporate. Weight bearing as tolerated with crutch assistance is permitted the day of surgery with a knee immobilizer locked in extension. Continuous passive motion (CPM) may be used for first 2 weeks and initially set at 0° to 45° for 2 hours, twice a day. The range may be increased by 10° daily as tolerated to a maximum of 120°. The patient is weaned from the immobilized as the quadriceps regains strength through quad sets, heel slides, and straight leg raises. Isometric quadriceps activity is performed from 60° to 90°. Full knee extension is expected 1 week after surgery. Most patients crutches for 4 weeks as the extensor mechanism develops and the brace may be removed once the extensor lag has resolved.

Phase II (6 to 8 weeks) centers on gait training and includes the introduction of closed kinetic chain exercises. Patients are encouraged to work on range of motion.

Therapeutic modalities include hamstring curls, wall slides, and stretching. Low impact exercises in a controlled environment are started and include high seat stationary bicycling.

Phase III (8 weeks to 6 months) continues to focus on gait training, proprioception, and encourages full range of motion, and develops strength with advancing closed-kinetic chain exercises. Additional low-impact activities such as treadmill walking and elliptical exercises are added, but light jogging is avoided until quadriceps strength has recovered to greater than 90%.

Phase IV (6 to 9 months) continues the development of flexibility, strength, and endurance. Full speed running is often achieved during this phase and sport specific training started as the patient feels comfortable.

Phase V (>9 months) focuses on sports specific return to play and functional activities. Strength, flexibility, range of motion are still considered. Quadriceps strength is an important criteria (>90%) for return to competitive sports. Objective measurements such as KT-2000 arthrometer testing (MEDmetric Corporation, San Diego, CA) provide a more scientific measure of the outcome, as well as range of motion, strength, and balance in documenting progress. A functional brace may be prescribed but the benefit remains to be validated.

CONCLUSIONS AND FUTURE DIRECTIONS

Anatomic ACL reconstruction remains a concept whose principles can be applied toward both single- and double-bundle constructs. The double-bundle method has been the evolutionary product of an intense focus by orthopedic scientists in understanding the underlying anatomy, biomechanics, and kinematics of the native ACL. Consideration of these principles will allow for anatomic restoration of the each patient's unique footprint and subsequently optimize the outcome of patients with dysfunction of the ACL.

REFERENCES

1. Miyasaka KC, Daniel DM, Stone ML, et al. The incidence of knee ligament injuries in the general population. *Am J Knee Surg.* 1991;4:3–8.
2. Brown CH Jr, Carson EW. Revision anterior cruciate ligament surgery. *Clin Sports Med.* 1999;18:109–171.
3. Palmer I. On the injuries to the ligaments of the knee joint. *Clin Orthop Relat Res.* 2007;454:17–22
4. Chhabra A, Starman JS, Ferretti M, et al. Anatomic, radiographic, biomechanical, and kinematic evaluation of the anterior cruciate ligament and its two functional bundles. *J Bone Joint Surg Am.* 2006;88(suppl 4):2–10.
5. Biau DJ, Tournoux C, Katsahian S, et al. ACL reconstruction: a meta-analysis of functional scores. *Clin Orthop Relat Res.* 2007;458:180–187.
6. Zantop T, Schumacher T, Schanz S, et al. Double-bundle reconstruction cannot restore intact knee kinematics in the ACL/LCL-deficient knee. *Arch Orthop Trauma Surg.* 2010;130(8):1019–1026.
7. van Eck CF, Lesniak BP, Schreiber VM, et al. Anatomic single- and double-bundle anterior cruciate ligament reconstruction flowchart. *Arthroscopy.* 2010;26(2):258–268.
8. Granan LP, Bahr R, Lie SA, et al. Timing of anterior cruciate ligament reconstructive surgery and risk of cartilage lesions and meniscal tears: a cohort study based on the Norwegian National Knee Ligament Registry. *Am J Sports Med.* 2009;37(5):955–961.
9. Sterett WI, Hutton KS, Briggs KK, et al. Decreased range of motion following acute versus chronic anterior cruciate ligament reconstruction. *Orthopedics.* 2003;26:151–154.
10. Shelbourne KD, Wilckens JH, Mollabashy A, et al. Arthrofibrosis in acute anterior cruciate ligament reconstruction: the effect of timing of reconstruction and rehabilitation. *Am J Sports Med.* 1991;19:332–336.
11. Harner CD, Irrgang JJ, Paul J, et al. Loss of motion after anterior cruciate ligament reconstruction. *Am J Sports Med.* 1992;20:499–506.
12. Church S, Keating JF. Reconstruction of the anterior cruciate ligament: timing of surgery and the incidence of meniscal tears and degenerative change. *J Bone Joint Surg Br.* 2005;87(12):1639–1642.
13. Adachi N, Ochi M, Uchio Y, et al. Mechanoreceptors in the anterior cruciate ligament contribute to the joint position sense. *Acta Orthop Scand.* 2002;73(3):330–334.
14. Andersson SM, Nilsson BE. Changes in bone mineral content following ligamentous knee injuries. *Med Sci Sports.* 1979;11(4):351–353
15. Prodromos CC, Joyce BT, Shi K, et al. A metal-analysis of stability of autografts compared to allografts after anterior cruciate ligament reconstructions. *Knee Surg Sports Truamatol Arthrosc.* 2007;15:851–856.
16. Malinin TI, Levitt RL, Bashore C, et al. A study of retrieved allografts used to replace anterior cruciate ligaments. *Arthroscopy.* 2002;18:163–170.
17. Iriuchishima T, Tajima G, Ingham SJ, et al. Impingement pressure in the anatomical and nonanatomical anterior cruciate ligament reconstruction: a cadaver study. *Am J Sports Med.* 2010;38(8):1611–1617.
18. Seon JK, Gadikota HR, Wu JL, et al. Comparison of single- and double-bundle anterior cruciate ligament reconstructions in restoration of knee kinematics and anterior cruciate ligament forces. *Am J Sports Med.* 2010;38(7):1359–1367.
19. Markolf KL, Gorek JF, Kabo JM, et al. Direct measurement of resultant forces in the anterior cruciate ligament. An in vitro study performed with a new experimental technique. *J Bone Joint Surg Am.* 1990;72(4):557–567.
20. Murray PJ, Alexander JW, Gold JE, et al. Anatomic double-bundle anterior cruciate ligament reconstruction: kinematics and knee flexion angle-graft tension relation. *Arthroscopy.* 2010;26(2):202–213.

All-Inside Anterior Cruciate Ligament Reconstruction: Graft-Link

James H. Lubowitz

Understanding "all-inside" (AI) anterior cruciate ligament (ACL) reconstruction or "Graft-Link" requires historical tribute to earlier surgical pioneers.

Historically, surgical treatment of rupture of the ACL has evolved from open repair, to open reconstruction (with or without augmentation), to "2-incision" technique, to arthroscopic or endoscopic "1-incision" technique, and as described in this chapter, to AI ACL technique. AI ACL reconstruction was first described in 1995 by Morgan et al. (1, 2) Unfortunately, the Morgan technique was "often associated with technical difficulties (3)" or, in the words of Morgan himself, "was technically demanding, which limited its popularity (4)." The specific technical challenge involved creating a tibial socket through a high anteromedial (AM) portal, a technique unfamiliar to most practicing arthroscopic surgeons.

The solution, a description of AI ACL using a more familiar transtibial approach, was published by the chapter author in 2006 (5). However, AI ACL technique has continued to evolve, and in 2011, Lubowitz, Ahmad, and Anderson published, "All-inside anterior cruciate ligament Graft-Link technique: second-generation, no-incision anterior cruciate ligament reconstruction (6)."

The reason for the evolution is manifold, but primarily a result of better understanding of ACL anatomy, as well as evolution of surgical instruments and graft fixation implants.

With regard to anatomy, as described by Lubowitz et al. (6), "Transtibial technique for creating the ACL femoral socket is known to be a risk factor for anatomically mismatched posterior tibial tunnel placement and high AM femoral tunnel placement (7–11). Thus . . . some surgeons made the transition to the AM portal technique for creating the ACL femoral tunnel (8, 10, 12–21), yet this technique is associated with potential pitfalls (8, 12, 13, 16–23). Therefore, in 2011, while AM portal technique is anatomic (and may be used as an alternative for AI ACL Graft-Link technique), we recommend as an alternative, creating the ACL femoral socket using outside-in technique (7, 9, 18, 24–27)."

AI ACL ADVANTAGES

Outside-in technique for creating the ACL femoral socket fell out of favor because the requirement for a lateral, distal, femoral, muscle splitting dissection results in a more invasive "2-incision" technique (7, 8, 24, 27). However, new technology, specifically narrow diameter guide pins that may be transformed into retrograde drills,(18, 25) allows "no-incision" outside-in techniques for creating the ACL femoral socket. Advantages of outside-in technique for creating the ACL femoral socket are that it is performed in the comfortable and familiar 90° knee flexion position (unlike AM portal technique); it is unconstrained, allowing independent, anatomic positioning of the femoral socket (unlike transtibial technique for drilling the femoral socket); and it may result in a longer socket (compared with AM portal technique) (18). In addition, outside-in drilling allows measurement of femoral interosseous distance prior to socket creation, using standard, outside-in femoral guides and guide pin sleeves. Premeasurement is a safety feature of the outside-in technique because a short distance may require that less graft tissue is contained within the femoral socket (28).

In addition to retrograde drilling pins, two additional technical developments simplify AI ACL reconstruction. The first development represents an evolution of cortical suspensory fixation button devices. First-generation cortical suspensory fixation buttons have fixed length graft loops, whereas second-generation cortical suspensory fixation buttons have graft loops that are adjustable in length, such that after the button flips and becomes fixed on the cortex, the graft loop may be tightened, pulling the graft in to the socket in a manner that completely fills the socket with graft substance. Furthermore, first-generation cortical suspensory fixation buttons were designed for femoral fixation, whereas second-generation adjustable graft loop buttons are effective for tibial (as well as femoral) fixation. Finally, second-generation adjustable graft loop buttons are unique in that when the graft loop is tightened, graft tension increases. Thus, for the first time, ACL surgeons may increase graft tension after the graft is fixed.

The second technical development that simplifies AI ACL reconstruction is the use of cannulas. Arthroscopic shoulder and hip surgeons have long understood the importance of cannulas for maintaining portals and preventing soft tissue from becoming intertwined in sutures. First, we recommend a cannula in the AM arthroscopic instrumentation portal to prevent soft tissue interposition. Second, we introduce a unique guide pin sleeve, which transforms into a cannula and maintains access to the narrow diameter guide pin tracks used to create AI sockets, allowing suture passage, and later graft passage, after ACL socket retroconstruction (6).

CLINICAL EVALUATION

With regard to patient history, physical evaluation, imaging, classification and decision-making algorithms, AI ACL Graft-Link is not unique. Thus, the focus of this chapter will be on surgical technique, as described below. Of course, with any new surgical technique, patient education and appropriate informed consent with regard to risks, benefits, alternatives, and surgical and nonsurgical treatment options are of particular importance.

TREATMENT

With regard to the indications for nonoperative versus operative treatment of ACL rupture and with regard to the timing of ACL surgery, AI ACL Graft-Link is not unique. Thus, the focus of this chapter will be on the surgical technique, as described below.

SURGICAL TECHNIQUE

No-tunnel, AI socket ACL reconstruction using Graft-Link requires learning new graft preparation, socket creation, and graft fixation techniques. Graft preparation requires consideration of no-incision cosmesis when selecting graft sourceensuring that graft length (GL) is less than the sum of socket lengths (SLs) plus intra-articular graft distance so that the graft will not bottom out in the sockets during final graft tensioning, and learning the graft-link preparation technique. Femoral and tibial socket creation is with second-generation retrodrilling guide pins. Femoral and tibial fixation is with second-generation cortical suspensory fixation devices with pull sutures tensioning an adjustable graft loop.

Special Equipment

Graft Preparation Station and High Strength Suture

High strength sutures (Fiberwire, Arthrex Inc., Naples, FL) secure the graft in a loop.

The loop is sewn in linkage with an ACL femoral tightrope adjustable graft loop (Arthrex) and an ACL tibial reverse tightrope adjustable graft loop (Figs. 72.1 and 72.2).

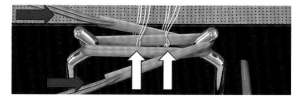

FIGURE 72.1. First, the graft is loaded in linkage with ACL femoral and tibial tightropes *(white arrows)*. Graft free ends are held by hemostats *(red arrows)* and then wrapped around hooks *(silver)* of graft preparation station set to GL (before tensioning) of approximately 65 mm. (Reproduced from Lubowitz JH, Ahmad C, Anderson K. AI ACL Graft-Link technique: second-generation, no-incision ACL reconstruction. *Arthroscopy.* 2011;26:717–727, with permission.)

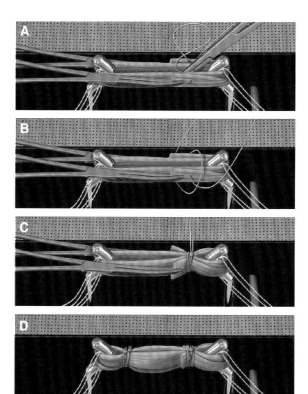

FIGURE 72.2. Graft-link suture technique. **A:** The graft is loaded in linkage with ACL femoral and tibial tightropes (white suture loops at far left and far right of graft loop). Graft ends are held by hemostats and wrapped around hooks *(silver)* of graft preparation station. High-strength suture (no. 2) is passed through the center of each strand of the looped graft. **B:** Suture free ends are crossed, and wrapped around the graft. **C:** First wrapped suture is tied in a wrapped cinch. **D:** A second suture is tied in a similar manner immediately next to the first suture (both shown tied and cut). Two additional sutures are placed cinching the other side of the graft (graft far left). The final construct shown is a graft-linked with ACL femoral tightrope on the left, and ACL tibial tightrope-reverse tension on the right. (Reproduced from Lubowitz JH, Ahmad C, Anderson K. All-inside anterior cruciate ligament Graft-Link technique: second-generation, no-incision anterior cruciate ligament reconstruction. *Arthroscopy.* 2011;26:717–727, with permission.)

A graft preparation station facilitates suturing the graft at a specific length (approximately 65 mm). After suturing, pretensioning of the graft construct results in an ultimate GL of approximately 75 mm (Fig. 72.3).

Flipcutter

Flipcutter (Arthrex) is a second-generation retrograde drill. The Flipcutter guide pin becomes a retrograde drill by flipping a switch on the pin handle. Then, after socket creation with clockwise drilling and retrograde pressure, the Flipcutter retrograde drill is switched back into a guide pin and removed.

The Flipcutter is 3.5 mm in diameter allowing femoral (Figs. 72.4 and 72.5) and tibial socket (Figs. 72.6 and 72.7) creation through portal-sized "stab-incisions" for cosmetic AI technique.

Flipcutter Guide Pin Sleeve

Flipcutter is drilled through a unique graduated-tip guide pin sleeve. The tip of the drill sleeve is "stepped," with a 7-mm length narrow tip. The tip of the cannula is tapped into the distal lateral femoral cortex over the Flipcutter, and subsequently, into the proximal AM tibial metaphysis. When the tip is advanced to the 7-mm mark, it reaches palpable resistance to further tip advancement, because during the retrograde socket formation, the Flipcutter is withdrawn until it stops at the tip of the metal guide pin sleeve. In addition, laser marks on the guide pin sleeve allow observation of the 7-mm tap in distance. The 7-mm sleeve protects and preserves a 7-mm cortical bridge (resulting in sockets, not full tunnels on both the femoral and tibial graft sites). Cortical preservation is required for cortical suspensory fixation using a second-generation adjustable graft loop (Figs. 72.4 to 72.7).

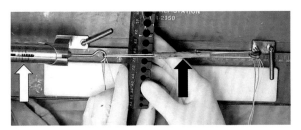

FIGURE 72.3. The final construct is attached to a spring-loaded tensioning device *(white arrow)*. The tension is set to approximately 40 N *(white arrow)*. Graft *(black arrow)* typical ultimate length is 75 mm after tensioning. The construct shown is graft-linked with an ACL femoral tightrope on the hook of the tensioning device **(left)**, and with an ACL tibial tightrope reverse tension on fixed hook of the graft preparation station **(right)**. The surgeon holds the graft diameter sizing block measuring 0.5 mm sizing increments. (Reproduced from Lubowitz JH, Ahmad C, Anderson K. All-inside anterior cruciate ligament Graft-Link technique: second-generation, no-incision anterior cruciate ligament reconstruction. *Arthroscopy.* 2011;26:717–727, with permission.)

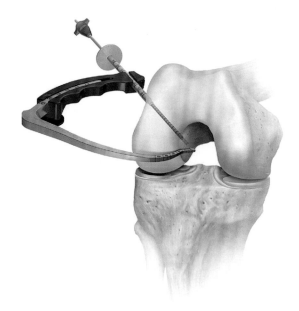

FIGURE 72.4. Right knee. Second-generation retrograde drill (Flipcutter) and ACL femoral guide with marking hook. Guide illustrated in anterolateral portal position. Note that the guide pin sleeve has a 7-mm step-off tip that is impacted over the pin into the bony cortex. Flipping a switch on the handle **(top)** of the Flipcutter will change the guide pin into a retrograde drill. (Reproduced from Lubowitz JH, Ahmad C, Anderson K. All-inside anterior cruciate ligament Graft-Link technique: second-generation, no-incision anterior cruciate ligament reconstruction. *Arthroscopy.* 2011;26:717–727, with permission.)

After the Flipcutter is removed, the sleeve is left in place, facilitating simple and reproducible passage of graft passing sutures, for later graft passage, because the sleeve also serves as a cannula (Fig. 72.8).

PassPort Cannula

The use of a flexible, silicone cannula (PassPort, Arthrex) in the AM arthroscopic portal facilitates AI ACL reconstruction by preventing soft tissue interposition. Inner and outer flanges with dams maintain cannula position and minimize fluid leakage from the larger than usual portal required for AI ACL graft passage, where the graft is passed through the AM portal (Fig. 72.9).

Femoral Fixation with ACL Tightrope

ACL tightrope is a second-generation adjustable graft loop suspensory fixation device. The adjustable graft loop has a four-point, knotless locking mechanism relying on multiple points of friction to create self-reinforcing resistance to slippage under tensioning.

The adjustable graft loop decreases in size under tensioning of the free ends or "pull sutures." The pull suture tensions the graft into the sockets. Because the tightrope loop is adjustable, "one size fits all," reducing inventory and eliminating first-generation calculations required for selecting loop length.

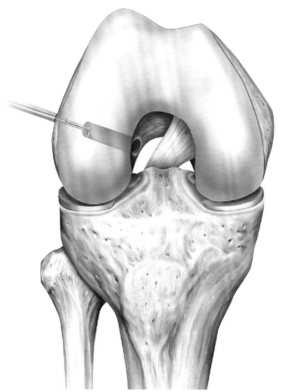

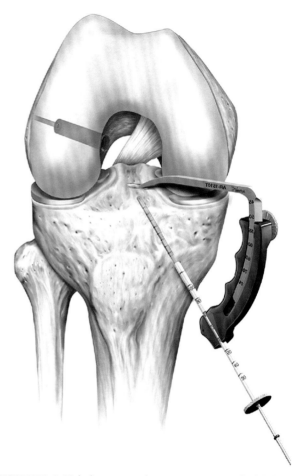

FIGURE 72.5. Right knee. Second generation retrograde drill (Flipcutter) creates ACL femoral socket. Note that the guide pin sleeve has a 7-mm step-off tip impacted over the pin into the bony cortex. Once socket creation is complete, flipping a switch on the handle of the Flipcutter will change the retrograde drill back into a guide pin. (Reproduced from Lubowitz JH, Ahmad C, Anderson K. All-inside anterior cruciate ligament Graft-Link technique: second-generation, no-incision anterior cruciate ligament reconstruction. *Arthroscopy*. 2011;26: 717–727, with permission.)

FIGURE 72.6. Right knee. Second-generation retrograde drill (Flipcutter) and ACL tibial guide with marking hook. Guide is illustrated in AM portal position. Cannulated 7-mm step-off tip guide pin sleeve is impacted over the pin into the bony cortex. Once socket creation is complete, flipping a switch on the handle of the Flipcutter will change the guide pin into a retrograde drill. (Reproduced from Lubowitz JH, Ahmad C, Anderson K. All-inside anterior cruciate ligament Graft-Link technique: second-generation, no-incision anterior cruciate ligament reconstruction. *Arthroscopy*. 2011;26:717–727, with permission.)

Second-generation adjustable loop-length technique allows optimal potential for graft to socket healing, because graft collagen is pulled completely into the socket as the graft loop is tightened.

ACL Tightrope-Reverse Tension

ACL tightrope-reverse tension (ACLTR-RT) is a second-generation adjustable graft loop suspensory fixation device. The tibial tightrope is identical to the femoral tightrope with the exception of reversed "pull sutures." After the tibial tightrope is reverse tensioned using the respective free ends of the pull sutures, the free ends can be tied over the tibial button with an arthroscopic knot pushing device, for backup fixation and protection of the implant when the pull sutures are cut. Figure 72.10 illustrates ACL tightrope and ACLTR-RT.

Graft Length

"AI results in sockets and not full bone tunnels. Therefore, to tension the graft, it must not bottom out in the sockets. Thus, one thing that has not changed in the last 5 years is the principal that GL must be less than the sum of femoral

SL plus intra-articular graft distance plus tibia SL (5). This prevents bottoming out of the graft in the sockets preventing graft tensioning. GL of no more than 75 mm, after tensioning, is a general guideline, and this distance is adjusted by patient size (Fig. 72.3).

Graft Selection

Single Semitendinosis

For autograft, we recommend posterior hamstring harvest technique (29). The technique is cosmetic, in keeping with no-incision philosophy. We recommend sparing of the gracilis, because using GLs as above, the graft generally may be tripled. In cases where the semitendinosis is short or of inadequate diameter when tripled (less than approximately 7.5 mm), the gracilis can be secondarily harvested.

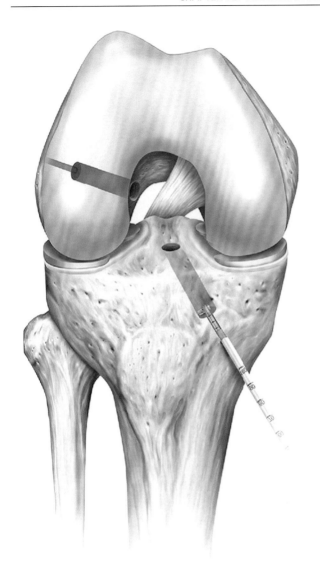

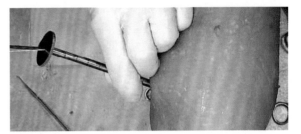

FIGURE 72.8. Right knee. The femoral socket has been retrodrilled, and the Flipcutter has been removed. Note that the Flipcutter guide pin sleeve has been impacted into the femoral cortex and is held in place (surgeon's gloved hand). Fiberstick suture is loaded into the cannula **(left)**. The Fiberstick is passed into the joint and retrieved through the AM arthroscopic portal. The femoral graft passing the Fiberstick is docked, and later retrieved for final ACL femoral graft passage. (Reproduced from Lubowitz JH, Ahmad C, Anderson K. All-inside anterior cruciate ligament Graft-Link technique: second-generation, no-incision anterior cruciate ligament reconstruction. *Arthroscopy.* 2011;26:717–727, with permission.)

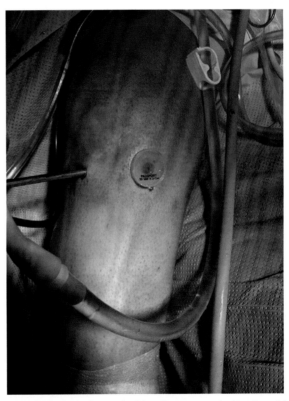

FIGURE 72.7. Right knee. Second generation retrograde drill (Flipcutter) creates ACL tibial socket. Note that the guide pin sleeve has a 7-mm step-off tip impacted over the pin into the bony cortex. Once socket creation is complete, flipping a switch in the handle of the Flipcutter will change the retrograde drill back into a guide pin. (Reproduced from Lubowitz JH, Ahmad C, Anderson K. All-inside anterior cruciate ligament Graft-Link technique: second-generation, no-incision anterior cruciate ligament reconstruction. *Arthroscopy.* 2011;26:717–727, with permission.)

Allograft

Indications for allograft continue to evolve; for proper indications, soft tissue allograft may also be prepared for graft-link, as the cosmetic, "no incision" graft choice with no harvest site morbidity.

Graft Preparation

Graft selection and GL determination are performed as above. The two posts of an ACL graft preparation stand are positioned so that GL equals the planned GL when

FIGURE 72.9. Right knee. Flexible, silicone cannula (PassPort, blue) in the AM arthroscopic portal prevents soft tissue interposition. Inner (not visible) and outer (illustrated) flanges with dams maintain cannula position, and minimize fluid leakage from the larger than usual portal required for AI ACL graft passage through the AM portal. The arthroscope *(silver)* is in the anterolateral portal. (Reproduced from Lubowitz JH, Ahmad C, Anderson K. All-inside anterior cruciate ligament Graft-Link technique: second-generation, no-incision anterior cruciate ligament reconstruction. *Arthroscopy.* 2011;26:717–727, with permission.)

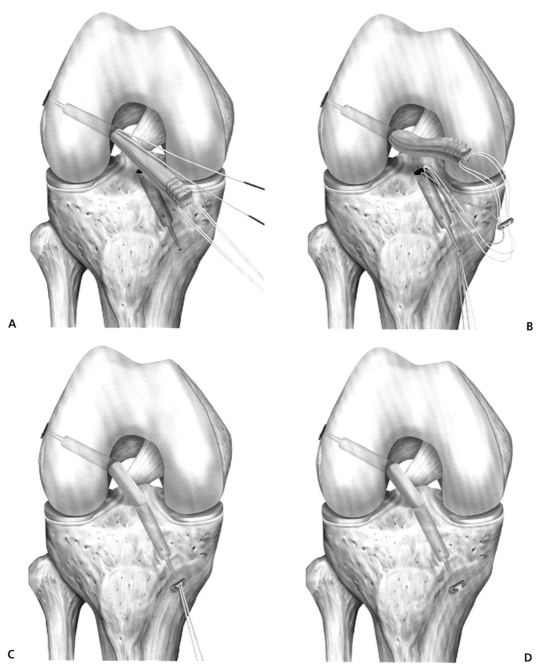

FIGURE 72.10. Right knee. ACL tightrope and ACLTR-RT. In all four illustrations, the lateral femoral cortical suspensory button is flipped. **A:** Graft is illustrated entering the joint through the AM portal position. Tibial side of graft loop is shown linked to ACLTR-RT **(right, white sutures)**. Emerging superior to the graft from the femoral socket is the ACL femoral tightrope "pull sutures" *(white with dark blue ends).* The pull sutures remove the slack from the Tightrope's adjustable graft loop, fully seating the graft in the femoral socket. **B:** Graft is illustrated entering the joint through the AM portal position. Tibial ACLTR-RT passing sutures and "pull sutures" are passed into the tibial socket. **C:** Emerging from the proximal AM tibial metaphysis **(bottom right)** is the ACLTR-RT "pull sutures" *(white).* The pull sutures removed the slack from the ACLTR-RT's adjustable graft loop, tensioning the graft in the tibial socket over the cortical button *(silver,)* which is shown flipped on the metaphysis. **D:** All-inside, graft-link, double-tightrope ACL. The tibial ACLTR-RT pull sutures have been tied and cut. (Reproduced from Lubowitz JH, Ahmad C, Anderson K. All-inside anterior cruciate ligament Graft-Link technique: second-generation, no-incision anterior cruciate ligament reconstruction. *Arthroscopy.* 2011;26:717–727, with permission.)

the graft is tripled in loops around the posts and clamped. The posts should be set to a length of 65 mm (Figs. 72.1 and 72.2), for ultimate GL of 75 mm after pretensioning (Fig. 72.3).

"The graft is baseball stitched into loops using a traditional strand of no. 2 high strength suture (Fig. 72.2). Two sutures are placed on the tibial side of the graft and two on the femoral side. Each stitch must pass through each strand of graft collagen, and the suture limbs are crossed and wrapped once around the collagen bundles, creating a self-reinforcing suture noose when tied.

Graft Linkage

Before the graft loop is clamped and sewn, it must be loaded to create links like a chain (Fig. 72.1). We create a Graft-Link construct, similar to the links in a chain, where a femoral ACL tightrope and tibial ACLTR-RT are linked within each end of the loop (Figs. 72.1 to 72.3).

Socket Diameter

Socket diameter should be a snug fit to ensure graft biologic incorporation. However, if the graft is too large, the graft could get stuck at the socket orifices after the button is flipped, and this represents an intraoperative problem. Bailout solutions include using tunnel dilators or curettes to enlarge the tunnel, or, if the adjustable loop is visible, cutting the loop arthroscopically, which allows the button to be pulled out of the thigh with passing sutures. As a last resort, open button removal by extending the femoral distal lateral stab incision can be considered. If the button is removed, the graft can be retrieved and trimmed, or the socket can be redrilled to a larger size, but prevention is clearly recommended. Therefore, do not undersize the socket diameter. A socket diameter sizing block measuring 0.5 mm sizing increments is illustrated (Fig. 72.3).

Femoral Socket Creation

Soft tissue notchplasty is performed. We perform minimal bony notchplasty and generally only of the notch orifice if stenotic.

It is essential to precisely identify the anatomic ACL footprint centrum on both the femoral and the tibial sides (7–11, 14–18, 27, 30–37). We use radiofrequency through the AM instrumentation portal to mark the ACL footprint centrum, and observe the marks through both portals.

We then switch the scope to the AM arthroscopic portal. AM portal viewing provides an improved perspective for analyzing the ACL femoral footprint anatomy. We assess and adjust our mark to ensure precise identification of the center of the footprint.

Then, the Flipcutter ACL femoral marking hook is locked in the Flipcutter guide ring at an angle of approximately 100° to 110°. The Flipcutter guide pin sleeve is advanced to the level of the skin at a point approximately 1 cm anterior to the posterior border of the iliotibial band, and 2.5 cm proximal to the lateral femoral condyle. A

stab incision is made through the skin and the iliotibial band, and the cannulated guide pin sleeve for the Flipcutter is pushed hard to the bone using a blunt trocar. A laser mark indicates the femoral intraosseous distance. The guide is adjusted to optimize interosseous distance (32-mm distance results in a 25-mm femoral socket with a 7-mm cortical bone bridge). The Flipcutter is advanced with forward drilling into the knee. The Flipcutter handle is loosened, and a handle switch flips the guide pin tip into the retrodrill position.

Next, the Flipcutter cannulated guide pin sleeve with the graduated 7-mm stepped tip is tapped with a mallet and advanced until resistance is felt when the step hits the distal lateral femoral cortex and the laser mark indicates 7 mm.

The guide pin sleeve is firmly held in place at the proper angle and not removed until femoral preparation is complete.

With continued forward drilling but with retrograde force, the femoral socket is retrodrilled until the drill blade stops advancing when it contacts the guide pin sleeve tip. The Flipcutter is pushed back into the knee and flipped back into guide pin mode and removed. The cannulated guide pin sleeve is not removed.

A Fiberstick (Arthrex Inc., Naples, FL) is advanced through the cannulated guide pin sleeve, the arthroscope is placed back in the anterolateral portal, the Fiberstick is retrieved through the AM portal, and the femoral graft passing Fiberstick is docked with a small clamp during tibial surgery. This femoral graft passing suture is later undocked for graft passage, after the tibia is prepared. Femoral socket creation is illustrated in Figs. 72.4, 72.5, and 72.8.

Tibial Socket Creation

With the arthroscope in the anterolateral portal, the Flipcutter ACL tibial marking hook is locked on the Flipcutter guide ring at an angle of approximately 55° to 60°. Guide position and angle are optimized to maximize tibial interosseous distance so that the graft will not bottom out during tensioning. A distance of at least 37 mm will result in a 30-mm socket depth with a 7-mm cortical bone bridge. Distance may be read prior to drilling using laser marks on the Flipcutter guide pin sleeve. As a preventative measure, if the distance is short, readjust the guide before drilling.

The tibial socket creation is completed using Flipcutter following the steps described under femoral socket creation above. Tibial socket creation is illustrated in Figures 72.6 and 72.7.

Marking the Graft

The first distance that should be measured and marked on the Graft-Link construct is the femoral interosseous distance. This distance should be marked on the adjustable graft loop, measuring from the tip of the cortical suspensory button, while the surgeon holds the button in a "preflipped" position. During graft passage, when the mark on the adjustable graft loop reaches the femoral socket orifices, this indicates to the surgeon that the button is in position to flip.

The second distance that should be measured and marked on the graft-link construct is the length of collagen within the femoral socket. The goal is to maximize collagen in the socket but ensure that the graft is not bottoming out during tensioning. A typical amount of collagen in the femoral socket should be 25 mm. This distance is marked on the graft itself, measuring from the femoral graft end. During graft passage, when the mark on the graft itself reaches the femoral socket orifices, this indicates to the surgeon that femoral graft tensioning is complete. This is repeated for the tibial side of the graft.

Graft Passage

A cannula (PassPort, Arthrex, Fig. 72.9) prevents soft tissue interposition and is essential because the graft is passed through the AM arthroscopic portal. Femoral and tibial graft passing sutures are retrieved. A technical pearl is to retrieve the femoral and tibial graft passing sutures from the AM arthroscopic portal at the same time, to avoid suture tangling or soft tissue interposition. To further ensure that the sutures are not tangled, the sliding, open loop suture retriever (Crabclaw, Arthrex) then "runs" the length of the femoral and tibial sutures, independently, from intra-articular to extra-articular through the cannula (Fig. 72.11). Once the sutures are absolutely not tangled, we shuttle femoral tightrope sutures through the AM portal, pass the graft through the AM portal, fix the graft on the femoral side, then shuttle the tibial sutures, and fix the graft on the tibial side (Fig. 72.10).

Grafts up to 9.5-mm diameter can be passed through the AM portal through a 10-mm diameter PassPort cannula. For larger diameter grafts, the cannula should be removed prior to graft passage.

Graft Fixation

First we flip, then we fill.

We first shuttle the femoral graft passing suture through the distal lateral femoral stab incision and pull the femoral adjustable graft loop into the femoral socket through the AM portal until the mark on the graft loop reaches the socket orifice under direct arthroscopic visualization, indicating that the button has exited the femoral cortex proximally and is ready to flip.

Once the button flips, we pull hard on the graft to ensure solid femoral fixation. We next apply tension back and forth on each free end of the femoral "pull suture," tensioning the graft up into the socket until the graft reaches the socket orifice.

An advanced technique is to partially seat the femoral side of the graft, then pass the tibial side, so that graft depth in sockets can be "fine-tuned" during tensioning.

Flip-then-fill technique is repeated on the tibia side. Remember that the tibia ACLTR-RT pull suture free ends are tied over the tibia button at the end of the case. The steps are illustrated in Figure 72.10.

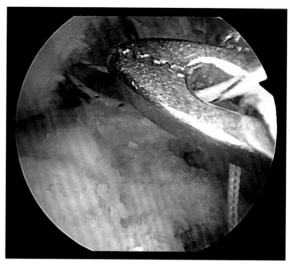

FIGURE 72.11. Right knee. Anterolateral portal arthroscopic view shows open loop suture retriever (Crabclaw, silver) grasping tibial Fiberstick graft passing suture loop *(blue)* and the femoral graft passing suture loop (white with dark stripe, Tigerwire). The technical pearl is that the surgeon must retrieve the femoral and tibial graft passing sutures from the AM arthroscopic portal at the same time, as illustrated, to avoid soft tissue interposition during subsequent graft passage. Next, the open loop suture retriever "runs" the length of the femoral and tibial graft passing sutures, independently, from intra-articular to extra-articular. This doubly ensures that the sutures are not tangled. (Reproduced from Lubowitz JH, Ahmad C, Anderson K. All-inside anterior cruciate ligament Graft-Link technique: second-generation, no-incision anterior cruciate ligament reconstruction. *Arthroscopy.* 2011;26:717–727, with permission.)

Graft Tensioning

The femoral and tibial pull sutures tension the graft so long as the graft is prepared properly to prevent bottoming out. An overly long graft will bottom out on the socket floor and is not acceptable.

The knee is ranged, and additional tension may be applied by pulling the femoral or tibial pull sutures by hand or using a tensioning device on the tibia side. A reverse Lachman maneuver is performed as tensioning is applied.

Cosmesis

Using this technique, the two 4-mm arthroscopic portals and the two 4-mm Flipcutter stab incisions are closed with 3-0 nylon. If autograft is used, posterior hamstring harvest incision is 1 cm in length and hidden on the posterior aspect of the knee, and closed with 3-0 nylon.

Single Bundle Versus Double Bundle

AI ACL Graft-Link technique is versatile. The technique described above is for anatomic single bundle ACL reconstruction, and can be modified for double bundle reconstruction. We hypothesize that fixation using four buttons may be simpler than a first-generation AI × 2 reconstruction technique using cannulated interference screws (21).

In addition, AI technique is bone sparing, and the four-button, Graft-Link technique even more so, and Graft-Link may be an optimal, simple, and reproducible ACL double bundle technique modification as a result of the advantages described above (6).

AUTHOR'S PREFERRED TREATMENT

In older patients, the author prefers AI ACL reconstruction using allograft to allow the no-incision technique. Hamstring autograft is preferred for younger patients.

Outside-in femoral Flipcutter allows socket creation in the comfortable, familiar 90° knee flexion position, and results in a reliable cortical bone bridge of 7 mm, facilitating cortical suspensory button fixation. Outside-in tibial Flipcutter is similar. This is simple and reproducible.

Tightrope adjustable fixation loop length cortical suspensory fixation buttons allow graft tensioning after graft fixation.

COMPLICATIONS, CONTROVERSIES, AND SPECIAL CONSIDERATIONS

By following the surgical technique steps described above, complications unique to AI ACL Graft-Link can be avoided. However, all new techniques have a learning curve. A staged approach to learning AI ACL reconstruction is described as a special consideration immediately below.

With regard to controversy, of greatest importance is the outcome of AI ACL Graft-Link. In the author's experience, excellent 2-year clinical outcomes of AI ACL Graft-Link have been achieved. In addition, patients express satisfaction with the notable cosmesis achieved using no-incision technique. Furthermore, patients have evidence-based less pain than those with endoscopic ACL reconstruction (Lubowitz, Smith, Schwartzberg, in preparation for publication). Anecdotally, many patients do seem to have faster recovery than those having standard ACL reconstruction. Ultimately, however, randomized controlled trials with a minimum of 2-year follow-up are required to produce evidence-based support for AI ACL Graft-Link. Such trials are in preparation for publication as above.

Controversy exists with regard to the biomechanical advantages of aperture fixation of the ACL, in contrast to suspensory fixation, where use of buttons instead of screws allows greater ACL anatomic footprint coverage without displacement of graft material by screws at the aperture. The author's preferred technique is anatomic ACL reconstruction using suspensory fixation buttons (6, 33).

Another current controversy regarding ACL anatomic reconstruction includes double bundle reconstruction. No-tunnel, double bundle ACL retroconstruction: AI × 2 technique has been described (21, 38) and is considered in a subsequent chapter. The chapter author's preferred technique is anatomic single bundle reconstruction, but with regard to double bundle ACL, the author believes that Graft-Link AI × 2 technique, which eliminates the need for screws in favor of TightRope buttons, is a more simple and reproducible method as above.

The special consideration with regard to AI ACL reconstruction is the learning curve. Learning new techniques is often challenging. ACL reconstruction requires experience in performing many steps. AI ACL reconstruction can be learned in stages:

Based on experience, a staged learning approach solution to the AI ACL learning curve challenge is proposed. First, a surgeon should master creation of an anatomic femoral socket, independent of transtibial constraint, using outside-in Flipcutter or AM portal technique. These techniques are independent and unconstrained by the position of the tibial tunnel. Next, mastery of tightrope femoral fixation is required. A third step is to master the nuances of Graft-Link graft preparation. Next, tibial Flipcutter is easy to learn, having mastered the Flipcutter on the femoral side. Once mastered, surgeons may make the transition to AI tibial sockets instead of tunnels. Finally, those emboldened may proceed with AI double bundle retroconstruction. In summary, Graft-Link AI ACL is minimally invasive but anatomic femoral socket creation, Flipcutter, tightrope, and Graft-Link graft preparation present a learning curve. The staged approach outlined above is recommended for making the transition to AI ACL and eliminating bone tunnels in favor of sockets. This staged learning approach was suggested to the author by textbook editor Don Johnson (personal communication, 2008) who must be so credited.

PEARLS AND PITFALLS

AI ACL Reconstruction Pearls

1. The number one pearl is that graft preparation length must be short enough to allow tensioning by not bottoming out in the AI ACL femoral or tibial sockets. Sockets are blind ended; they are cortical sparing, and they are not tunnels. However, the graft must be long enough to achieve adequate graft tissue in the tunnel. Thus, GL should be approximately 5 to 10 mm less than the sum of combined SL plus intra-articular distance (IAD). In summary, GL < SL = IAD.

2. GL of 270 mm or less prior to quadrupling will result in Graft-Link of less than 75 mm.

3. A second top pearl: meticulous focus on preparation of the graft, and Graft-Link construct, may ensure a smooth case.

4. It is necessary to carefully review a series of steps (see text) to prevent soft tissue interposition or graft tangling during AI ACL reconstruction.

5. Flipcutters are designed for forward drilling.

6. A press of a button on the base of the Flipcutter flips and straightens the Flipcutter tip.

7. Outside-in Flipcutter is performed in the comfortable and familiar 90° knee flexion position with optimal viewing of the femoral footprint with the arthroscope in the AM portal. In contrast, knee hyperflexion is essential during ACL femoral socket creation using AM portal technique.
8. Keep the Flipcutter cannula in place after drill pin removal. Insert graft passing suture. Then, remove the cannula.
9. Anatomic tunnel placement is vital.
10. AI ACL sockets (unlike tunnels) do not allow outflow. A large-diameter suction shaver is necessary to remove reaming debris.
11. The graft is passed through the AM portal.
12. AI ACL reconstruction requires new skills and equipment. A staged learning approach is described in the text.

AI ACL Reconstruction Pitfalls

1. Undersized sockets are not permitted because the Tight-Rope fixation button flips prior to graft tensioning.
2. An excessively long graft is not permitted because the graft could bottom out in the sockets prior to graft tensioning.
3. Graft passing sutures may become tangled or soft tissue may become interposed. It is best to retrieve both sutures at the same time, through an AM portal PassPort cannula, and then "run" the individual sutures with a CrabClaw suture retriever to ensure there is no tangle or interposition.

REHABILITATION

AI ACL Graft-Link rehabilitation is not unique. A standard ACL accelerated rehabilitation protocol is the author's preferred technique.

CONCLUSIONS AND FUTURE DIRECTIONS

We describe anatomic single bundle, AI ACL graft-link technique using second generation Flipcutter guide pins that become retrodrills and second generation ACL adjustable graft loop length cortical suspensory fixation devices: femoral tightrope and tibial ACLTR-RT. The technique is minimally invasive using only four 4-mm stab incisions. Graft choice is no-incision allograft or gracilis sparing, posterior semitendinosis harvest. The graft is linked to femoral and tibial adjustable tightrope graft loops and sutured four times through each strand with a wrapped stitch to an ultimate GL of 75 mm after pretensioning. The technique may be modified for double bundle ACL reconstruction (6)."

Randomized controlled trials are required to confirm clinical outcomes compared with standard ACL reconstruction techniques, and are in preparation, with promising results.

In the future, allograft risks and autograft harvest morbidity may both be eliminated by the use of tissue-engineered grafts.

Although the future is unknown, what we do know is that the history of sports medicine in general, and ACL reconstruction in particular, has progressed to less and less invasive techniques. As such, a progression from open to 2-incision to 1-incision to no-incision AI ACL Graft-Link represents a natural progression.

REFERENCES

1. Morgan CD, Kalman VH, Grawl D. Isometry testing for anterior cruciate ligament reconstruction revisited. *Arthroscopy.* 1995;11:647–659.
2. Morgan CD. The all-inside ACL reconstruction. In: *Operative Technique Manual.* Naples, FL: Arthrex Inc.; 1995.
3. Stahelin A, Weiler A. All-inside anterior cruciate ligament reconstruction using a semitendinosus tendon and soft threaded biodegradable interference screw fixation. *Arthroscopy.* 1997;13:773–779.
4. Morgan CD, Stein DA, Leitman EH, et al. Anatomic tibial graft fixation using a retrograde bio-interference screw for endoscopic anterior cruciate ligament reconstruction. *Arthroscopy.* 2002;18:E38.
5. Lubowitz J. No-tunnel anterior cruciate ligament reconstruction: the transtibial all-inside technique. *Arthroscopy.* 2006;22:900.e1–900.e11.
6. Lubowitz J, Ahmad C, Anderson K. All-inside anterior cruciate ligament Graft-Link technique: second-generation, no-incision anterior cruciate ligament reconstruction. *Arthroscopy.* 2011;26:717–727.
7. Abebe ES, Moorman CT III, Dziedzic TS, et al. Femoral tunnel placement during anterior cruciate ligament reconstruction: an in vivo imaging analysis comparing transtibial and 2-incision tibial tunnel-independent techniques. *Am J Sports Med.* 2009;37(10):1904–1911.
8. Bedi A, Musahl V, Steuber V, et al. Transtibial versus anteromedial portal reaming in anterior cruciate ligament reconstruction: an anatomic and biomechanical evaluation of surgical technique. *Arthroscopy.* 2011;27(3):380–390.
9. Marchant BG, Noyes FR, Barber-Westin SD, et al. Prevalence of nonanatomical graft placement in a series of failed anterior cruciate ligament reconstructions. *Am J Sports Med.* 2010;38(10):1987–1996.
10. Steiner M. Independent drilling of tibial and femoral tunnels in anterior cruciate ligament reconstruction. *J Knee Surg.* 2009;22:171–176.
11. Zantop T, Kubo S, Petersen W, et al. Current techniques in anatomic anterior cruciate ligament reconstruction. *Arthroscopy.* 2007;23:938–947.
12. Baer G, Fu F, Shen W, et al. Effect of knee flexion angle on tunnel length and articular cartilage damage during anatomic double-bundle anterior cruciate ligament reconstruction. *Arthroscopy.* 2008;24S:e31.
13. Basdekis G, Abisafi C, Christel P. Influence of knee flexion angle on femoral tunnel characteristics when drilled through the anteromedial portal during anterior cruciate ligament reconstruction. *Arthroscopy.* 2008;24:459–464.

14. Bottoni CR. Anterior cruciate ligament femoral tunnel creation by use of anteromedial portal. *Arthroscopy.* 2008;24:1319.

15. Bottoni CR, Rooney CR, Harpstrite JK, et al. Ensuring accurate femoral guide pin placement in anterior cruciate ligament reconstruction. *Am J Orthop.* 1998;28:764–766.

16. Harner C, Honkamp N, Ranawat A. Anteromedial portal technique for creating the anterior cruciate ligament femoral tunnel. *Arthroscopy.* 2008;24:113–115.

17. Lubowitz J. Anteromedial portal technique for the anterior cruciate ligament femoral socket: pitfalls and solutions. *Arthroscopy.* 2009;25:95–101.

18. Lubowitz JH, Konicek J. Anterior cruciate ligament femoral tunnel length: cadaveric analysis comparing anteromedial portal versus outside-in technique. *Arthroscopy.* 2010;26(10):1357–1362.

19. Neven E, D'Hooghe P, Bellemans J. Double-bundle anterior cruciate ligament reconstruction: a cadaveric study on the posterolateral tunnel position and safety of the lateral structures. *Arthroscopy.* 2008;24:436–440.

20. Smith P. An alternative method for "all-inside" anterior cruciate ligament reconstruction. *Arthroscopy.* 2006;22:451.

21. Smith P, Schwartzberg R, Lubowitz J. All-inside, double-bundle, anterior cruciate ligament reconstruction: a no tunnel, 2-socket, retroconstruction technique. *Arthroscopy.* 2008;24:1184–1189.

22. Golish S, Baumfeld J, Schoderbek R, et al. The effect of femoral tunnel starting position on tunnel length in anterior cruciate ligament reconstruction: a cadaveric study. *Arthroscopy.* 2007;23:1187–1192.

23. Nakamura M, Deie M, Shibuya H, et al. Potential risks of femoral tunnel drilling through the far anteromedial portal: a cadaveric study. *Arthroscopy.* 2009;25:481–487.

24. Harner C, Marks P, Fu F, et al. Anterior cruciate ligament reconstruction: endoscopic versus two-incision technique. *Arthroscopy.* 1994;10:502–512.

25. Kim S, Kurosawa H, Sakuraba K, et al. Development and application of an inside-to-out drill bit for anterior cruciate ligament reconstruction. *Arthroscopy.* 2005;21:1012.e1–1012.e4.

26. Puddu G, Cerullo G. My technique in femoral tunnel preparation: the "Retro-Drill" technique. *Tech Orthop.* 2005;20:224–227.

27. Yu J, Garrett W. Femoral tunnel placement in anterior cruciate ligament reconstruction. *Oper Tech Sports Med.* 2009;14:45–49.

28. Zantop T, Ferretti M, Bell K, et al. Effect of tunnel-graft length on the biomechanics of anterior cruciate ligament-reconstructed knees: intra-articular study in a goat model. *Am J Sports Med.* 2008;36:2158–2166.

29. Prodromos CC, Han YS, Keller BL, et al. Posterior mini-incision technique for hamstring anterior cruciate ligament reconstruction graft harvest. *Arthroscopy.* 2005;21:130–137.

30. Colombet P, Robinson J, Christel P, et al. Morphology of anterior cruciate ligament attachments for anatomic reconstruction: a cadaveric dissection and radiographic study. *Arthroscopy.* 2006;22:984–992.

31. Ho J, Gardiner A, Shah V, et al. Equal kinematics between central anatomic single-bundle and double-bundle anterior cruciate ligament reconstructions. *Arthroscopy.* 2009;25:464–472.

32. Kaz R, Starman JS, Fu FH. Anatomic double-bundle anterior cruciate ligament reconstruction revision surgery. *Arthroscopy.* 2007;23:1250.e1–1250.e3.

33. Lubowitz J, Poehling G. Watch your footprint: anatomic ACL reconstruction. *Arthroscopy.* 2009;25:1059–1060.

34. Petersen W, Zantop T. Anatomy of the anterior cruciate ligament with regard to its two bundles. *Clin Orthop Relat Res.* 2007;454:35–47.

35. Pombo M, Shen W, Fu F. Anatomic double-bundle anterior cruciate ligament reconstruction: where are we today? *Arthroscopy.* 2008;24:1168–1177.

36. Siebold R, Ellert T, Metz S, et al. Tibial insertions of the anteromedial and posterolateral bundles of the anterior cruciate ligament: morphometry, arthroscopic landmarks, and orientation model for bone tunnel placement. *Arthroscopy.* 2008;24:154–161.

37. Siebold R, Ellert T, Metz S, et al. Femoral insertions of the anteromedial and posterolateral bundles of the anterior cruciate ligament: morphometry and arthroscopic orientation models for double-bundle bone tunnel placement—a cadaver study. 2008;24(5):585–592.

38. Smith P, Lubowitz J. No-tunnel double-bundle anterior cruciate ligament retroconstruction: the all-inside X 2 technique. *Oper Tech Sports Med.* 2009;17:62–68.

V. E. The Knee Knee Ligament

All-Inside Double-Bundle Anterior Cruciate Ligament Reconstruction

Patrick A. Smith

All-inside anterior cruciate ligament (ACL) reconstruction refers to a specialized technique where blind sockets as opposed to full tunnels are made for graft placement with the approach on the tibia representing the major change relative to traditional ACL reconstruction. It has been described as a "no-tunnel" procedure (1, 2). Touted patient advantages include less postoperative pain, cosmesis, easier rehabilitation particularly relative to return of motion, and less postoperative supervised physical therapy.

This technique is based on use of the proprietary RetroCutter (Arthrex) for creation of the tibial socket. The femoral socket is generally created through the anteromedial (AM) portal, but can easily be made from a lateral approach through the proprietary FlipCutter (Arthrex). Fixation options are flexible on the femoral side with RetroScrew (Arthrex) aperture fixation classically utilized on the tibia. Initially described for single-bundle ACL reconstruction (1), the all-inside approach is easily adaptable for double-bundle ACL reconstruction with the "all-inside × 2" procedure to be described in this chapter (2). All-inside is also a very useful method for revision ACL reconstruction. The all-inside technique is unique and a valuable surgical skill to have as an ACL surgeon, particularly relative to potential patient advantages due to the very nature of it being such a minimally invasive approach.

CLINICAL EVALUATION

There is never any substitute for a thorough history and physical examination. The classic history of an acute non-contact deceleration or twisting mechanism of injury with or without a "pop" and joint swelling with limitation of knee extension should be considered an ACL tear until proven otherwise, especially in a young female basketball or soccer player. Chronically, patients present with the complaint of giving way instability, typically related to their sports activity usually associated with some joint swelling.

From the examination standpoint, the Lachman test is easy to perform even with an acute injury, and is very sensitive for an ACL tear. However, the key is the presence of the pivot shift diagnostic for rotational instability of the knee, which is the primary indication for surgical reconstruction. Acutely, the Losee test is better tolerated by the patient.

Plain X-rays are very important and represent the simplest and most cost-effective ancillary imaging study to rule out any associated bony pathology. MRI is helpful acutely to assess for significant bone bruising, which would influence the need for protective weight bearing, and also is helpful delineating associated medial and/or lateral ligamentous injury. Meniscal integrity can be assessed on MRI although certainly MRI is far from perfect in that regard. In the chronic setting, MRI is not as important as X-ray.

TREATMENT DECISION MAKING

The decision for ACL reconstruction is made with considerable patient input. First and foremost, if a patient is active in a sport where rotational joint loads are common, reconstruction should be done. If a patient experiences giving way instability with activities of daily living even though they are not active in sports, surgery is appropriate, especially if one has an associated meniscus tear. Surgical rationale is to prevent future instability, and thereby both improve one functionally and prevent abnormal shear stresses on the joint to preserve the menisci and joint surfaces. There really is no age limit for ACL reconstruction, as long as X-rays show no advanced degenerative change. The patient must be committed and motivated for the necessary postoperative rehabilitation program. Plus, the patient needs to also accept the initial restraint necessary before returning to sports activity to minimize stress on their ACL graft until muscle mass is built up sufficiently, and adequate time has passed to allow for biologic graft remodeling and incorporation.

If one has minimal laxity relative to just a pivot glide on examination and does not participate in cutting/pivoting sports activity, conservative treatment emphasizing rehabilitation for muscle strengthening about the involved knee and hip with use of a functional ACL brace for any stressful activity can sometimes be successful. Generally, in this scenario, a partial ACL tear is present, but this is not that common.

Relative to surgical timing, there is no "set" time as individuals react to this injury differently, but rather my decision to proceed with surgery is based on examination criteria of full knee extension with a good quadriceps contraction, minimal effusion, and flexion >120°. In the acute ACL tear setting, initiation of "prehab" with the help of a physical therapist to get the knee ready for surgery can be very helpful.

SURGICAL TECHNIQUES—SINGLE- VERSUS DOUBLE-BUNDLE ACL RECONSTRUCTION

Single-bundle reconstruction drilling the femoral socket transtibially can increase the potential for tunnel mismatch and "vertical graft" placement, which less than optimally controls the pivot shift. Another concern is long-term follow-up studies have shown a rather high incidence of arthritic development after ACL reconstruction (3).

Multiple anatomic dissection studies have shown the presence of distinct anteromedial (AM) and posterolateral (PL) bundles of the ACL, and biomechanical studies have shown different tensioning patterns for these main bundles (4, 5). Experimentally, it has also been shown the double-bundle construct better restores ACL biomechanics, particularly rotational stability compared with single-bundle reconstruction (6). The questions to be answered with the double-bundle approach is whether it will both improve overall joint stability *and* minimize later arthritic development to justify the increased complexity of the procedure. Stability with two grafts should be potentially enhanced by the overall strength of the construct primarily due to increased surface area for tendon to bone healing (7). Theoretically with the inherent different tensioning patterns with the two bundles, there may be load sharing with the double-bundle construct to both optimize knee kinematics and graft healing/incorporation in the process. So far, short-term clinical studies have shown slight improvement over single-bundle comparisons with KT-1000 testing but not with patient outcomes (8, 9). Another variable is the recent change with single-bundle reconstruction actually stimulated by the interest in double bundle moving the femoral socket position more laterally on the femur with a central tibial tunnel to try and "capture" part of both the AM and the PL bundle origins and insertions, which may improve single-bundle outcomes. One of the problems compromising true objective stability evaluation of double versus single bundle is the lack of a rotational stability testing device. Nonetheless, double-bundle ACL reconstruction has merit as a technique to possibly better patient outcomes through restoration of more normal knee anatomy and kinematics.

Double-bundle ACL reconstruction has been described numerous ways. Most commonly it is done through two full tibial tunnels with two femoral sockets sometimes created transtibially. Others have chosen to "manipulate" a single-bundle ACL reconstruction into a double-bundle construct by splitting the graft generally with the fixation device used on the femur or tibia. The all-inside double-bundle technique is uniquely different done through two femoral sockets and two tibial sockets, and has several potential advantages beginning with the patient relative to ease of recovery, as well as for the surgeon from the technical standpoint in performing the procedure, and also possibly biologically in terms of graft healing and incorporation.

ALL-INSIDE RATIONALE/ADVANTAGES

Patient advantages with the all-inside approach relate particularly to it being a minimally invasive "no-tunnel" technique because sockets are also created on the tibial side reaming from inside the joint through use of the RetroCutter (1, 2). Correspondingly, this necessitates just a small tibial incision for placement of the 3-mm RetroCutter guide pin resulting in less dissection over the sensitive periosteum of the proximal tibia helping to minimize postoperative discomfort. Preliminary data from a prospective level one randomized study comparing postoperative pain with a full-tibial tunnel versus an all-inside tibial socket with soft tissue allograft ACL reconstructions has shown significantly less pain with VAS grading from the first postoperative day through two years for the all-inside cohort compared with the endoscopic group. Mean percocet use the first week after surgery was 27.9 for the all-inside patients and 33.2 for the endoscopic patients. (Lubowitz, Smith and Schwartzberg, unpublished study.) Another patient advantage is that clinically, patients with all-inside ACL reconstructions either single or double bundle, seem to get back range of motion much quicker after surgery and need less supervised physical therapy.

From the surgeon perspective, creating tibial sockets with the RetroCutter allows optimal placement on the tibia without any guesswork as to position, compared with any outside-in tunnel technique requiring an aiming guide, which could visually be less precise, and this is particularly important when the tibial footprint is small. More importantly, the retrograde cut tibial socket has been shown by CT analysis to have much less aperture bone disruption than an outside-in antegrade full tunnel, which thereby minimizes the chance for coalescence or fracturing between the two tibial sockets versus two full tunnels (10). This risk is even made less with use of aperture RetroScrew fixation beginning with the PL bundle, which further buttresses the PL tibial socket from the AM tibial socket. Also, the retrograde sockets have smoother walls to enhance fixation stability and possibly graft healing and incorporation. Finally, follow-up X-rays at 1 year following all-inside single-bundle ACL reconstruction have not shown tunnel widening even with use of allografts, which likely is attributable to less synovial egress with the sockets as opposed to traditional full tunnels, especially on the tibial side where RetroScrew aperture fixation also helps to seal the joint (11).

Another surgeon advantage with the all-inside approach relates to drilling the femoral sockets through the AM portal, avoiding the inherent problems with transtibial femoral drilling (12, 13). This serves to optimize femoral socket placement especially critical with double-bundle reconstruction. Furthermore, the versatility of the all-inside technique is exemplified by the ease of performing a "two-incision" equivalent procedure by drilling the femoral sockets from "outside–in." Specifically, the new FlipCutter device, which is a guide pin that converts after placement to a reamer, can easily be drilled from the lateral cortex of the femur into the notch area via an aiming guide to create the either AM or PL femoral sockets, if one prefers that particular approach. Also, the FlipCutter has a tibial guide, so it can be used to drill the tibial sockets as well, comparable to the RetroCutter.

Additionally, the all-inside approach is very versatile relative to the issues of graft choice, femoral and tibial fixation, and graft tensioning, as surgeons have different preferences and beliefs as to what works best for them. Therefore, the all-inside double-bundle procedure can be customized in many ways for the surgeon, but yet still maintain its most important quality relative to being minimally invasive for the patient.

Biologically, there is the theoretic possibility that the all-Inside sockets especially on the tibial side may trap more hematoma and potential growth factors after surgery to help with graft incorporation compared with full tunnels. The analogy would be that of a "potted plant" referring to the graft end surrounded in the dead end bone socket. Plus, the all-inside approach is inherently bone preserving, which is an innate advantage with surgery about the knee joint.

GRAFT CHOICE FOR ALL-INSIDE DOUBLE BUNDLE

All-inside double-bundle ACL reconstruction is very flexible relative to graft choice. One option is for autogenous hamstring autografts harvested through a mini-popliteal incision initially described by Franz and Ulbrich (14). This is a very minimally invasive and cosmetic approach. One advantage of all-inside ACL reconstruction is the grafts are not as long, so if the semitendinosis harvested length is approximately 280 mm, it can be used for both grafts, which are doubled. If the semitendinosis is not that long, then the gracilis is harvested easily through the mini-popliteal approach. Usually the semitendinosis is 6 to 7 mm in diameter doubled, and is used for the AM bundle with the gracilis 5 to 6 mm doubled, for the PL bundle.

My graft choice for the contact athlete is a bit different. Here for the AM bundle, I use a middle third patellar tendon graft harvested with bone only off the tibia, peeling the patellar tendon off the patella for length. The bone plug is 8×20 mm and the tendon width is 10 to 11 mm. A doubled autogenous semitendinosis is used for the PL bundle and usually is 6 to 7 mm in diameter.

Allograft tissue can also be utilized. Two soft tissue grafts generally 6 to 7 mm doubled each work well, or a patellar tendon allograft with one soft tissue allograft is a good combination. I have also done "hybrid" reconstructions where I utilize usually a patellar tendon allograft for the AM bundle with an autogenous semitendinosis for the PL bundle, especially for revision cases.

FIXATION OPTIONS ALL-INSIDE DOUBLE BUNDLE

Fixation options are flexible on the femoral side, and depend in part on graft choice as well as surgeon preference. I favor TightRope (Arthrex) suspensory femoral fixation when I use either autogenous hamstring or soft tissue allografts. The TightRope device consists of a 12×3 mm button with an attached blue # 2 FiberWire (Arthrex) passing suture and a special white # 2 FiberWire shortening suture. The special shortening suture is actually a continuous #2 FiberWire suture spliced on itself creating a loop that tightens around the graft for "fingertrap" fixation providing four points of fixation as the shortening sutures are tightened "hoisting" the graft in the socket against the button on the femoral cortex (Fig. 73.1). I prefer the RT or reverse tension TightRope with the shortening sutures extraarticular on the femoral side where the button is flipped, as opposed to a regular TightRope where the shortening sutures are pulled intraarticularly. Strength of fixation is excellent, and since the length of both the AM and particularly the PL sockets are shorter by drilling them more transversely through the AM portal, the button fixation is closer to the end of the graft. Therefore, the so-called "bungee" effect should be less than would be the case when suspensory ends up far from the joint line well away from the end of the graft. Length of the graft in the femoral socket is not an issue with the AM bundle as this intraosseous distance is always a decent length–approximately 40 to 50 mm. However, the PL intraosseous

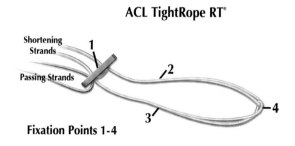

FIGURE 73.1. Schematic of ACL TightRope RT used for suspensory femoral fixation of AM and PL bundle soft tissue grafts, illustrating four points of fixation from the loop.

distance can be short approximately 30 to 35 mm due to its position, which in turn limits how deep the socket can be drilled, and yet still preserve the lateral cortex for TightRope button fixation. Therefore, I always ensure that there is at least 15 mm of graft in the femoral socket with experimental evidence suggesting that should be adequate for bundle strength (15). If though the PL socket is too short to accommodate TightRope fixation relative to potentially not enough graft in the socket, I will then fixate with a bioabsorbable interference screw. Conceivably, one could choose to use interference screw fixation for the both AM and PL bundles on the femoral side with soft tissue grafts. In contact athletes, an absorbable interference screw is used to fix the patellar bone plug on the femur for the AM bundle, and a Tightrope for the semitendinosis for the PL bundle.

On the tibial side, Retroscrew aperture fixation is preferred, but tying the graft sutures over a titanium button here for suspensory fixation can be done with use of a tensioning device.

SURGICAL TECHNIQUE

All-Inside × 2

The procedure is termed "all-inside × 2" to reflect the basic approach of doing an all-inside single-bundle reconstruction for the PL bundle, and then repeating the exact same steps for AM bundle reconstruction. So once one has mastered all-inside single-bundle reconstruction particularly with use of the RetroCutter, "all-inside × 2" is a reasonable progression to a double-bundle construct.

As an overview, both femoral sockets are first prepared drilling through the AM portal in hyperflexion. Next, the PL tibial socket is created with the RetroCutter. The PL bundle is passed and fixed on the femur, and then secured on the tibia with a RetroScrew at the aperture in full extension. Next, the AM tibial socket is created with the RetroCutter. The AM bundle is then passed into the femur and fixed on the tibial side using a RetroScrew at approximately 30° of flexion.

Notably, this sequence of passing and fixing the PL bundle first has been shown recently biomechanically to be superior than creating both tibial sockets, and then passing and fixing the PL bundle (16). This validates what has been done clinically with the "all-inside × 2" approach the past couple of years.

In terms of operative setup, I prefer to use a footholder keeping the table flat. It is very important for AM portal femoral socket drilling to be able to flex the knee to at least 120° of flexion, and then reliably later reproduce that position. Use of a lateral thigh post functions both as a fulcrum to assess and treat medial meniscal pathology, and then to support the thigh with the knee flexed during the case. A tourniquet is not utilized with the fluid pump generally kept at 40 mm.

The following illustrative case is a contact athlete reconstructed using an autogenous patellar graft for the AM bundle with bone only on the tibial side with the tendon

sharply peeled off the patella (Fig. 73.2). An autogenous semitendinosis graft is harvested through a mini-popliteal approach for the PL bundle (Fig. 73.3).

STEP 1—Femoral Preparation

After appropriate meniscal work and treatment for any associated articular cartilage pathology, attention is directed toward femoral socket preparation. Generally, a notchplasty is not done unless notch stenosis is evident. In an acute case, torn ACL fibers are debrided leaving a "footprint" of native tissue both on the femoral and on the tibial side to help with anatomic socket placement. In the chronic setting, without good soft tissue landmarks, socket placement is more challenging especially on the femur, and is based on one's anatomic sense of AM and PL bundle attachment points. Usually on the femur, there is some remnant of the lateral intercondylar ridge or "resident's ridge," and both bundles should be posterior to this bony landmark, and approximately 2 mm from the lateral femoral condyle articular surface posteriorly.

STEP 2—PL Femoral Socket Creation

Both femoral sockets are prepared first through the AM portal drilling in flexion of at least 120°. I prefer to make

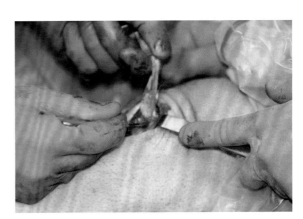

FIGURE 73.2. Harvest of autogenous patellar tendon graft for AM bundle with bone plug only from tibia peeling tendon off patella for adequate length.

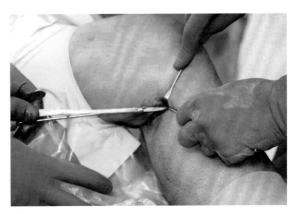

FIGURE 73.3. Harvest of autogenous semitendinosis graft for PL bundle using mini-popliteal approach.

the PL socket first to ensure adequate room for both the PL and the AM socket because in my experience when making the AM socket first, there is a tendency to be too lateral or distal, so that then the PL socket is pushed too distally toward the lateral femoral condyle articular surface. I have not found it necessary to use a so-called accessory medial portal to create the PL femoral socket, but certainly that is a reasonable approach. My concern is the PL socket is short to begin with and the more transverse the starting approach to the femur, the shorter it becomes. One way to make the PL socket is to use a 5-mm transportal guide (Arthrex) positioned under the posterior lateral femoral condyle articular surface with a special measuring guide pin (Arthrex) drilled in hyperflexion across the femur capturing the lateral femoral cortex to measure the intraosseous distance necessary to determine the maximal amount of graft possible in the socket (Fig. 73.4). Specifically, this is calculated by intraosseous distance minus 11 mm for TightRope loop length plus graft radius (usually 3 mm for PL bundle). The key is preserving the lateral femoral cortex to allow for the suspensory button fixation. This is followed by reaming with the appropriate size reamer based on graft diameter to the desired depth of graft in the socket (which is typically less than the calculated maximal socket depth) preserving the lateral femoral cortex. A #2 FiberWire suture is left at the aperture of this PL socket to pull the graft across later.

Alternatively, one can make the PL socket utilizing a low profile reamer with a beath pin to localize the socket visually with the reamer matched to the graft diameter marking the center with the beath pin. Remove both the reamer and the beath pin and then in hyperflexion, drill the measuring guide pin in the beath pin hole across the femur engaging its special tip on the lateral femoral cortex to measure the intraosseous distance, and then ream the graft diameter to the desired depth as outlined above.

PEARL: If you are not hyperflexed enough your exit point laterally will be too low and then the socket depth after reaming will be short. The exit point of the guide pin laterally should be above the lateral epicondyle to give you optimal length of the PL socket to maximize ultimate graft length in the socket.

STEP 3—AM Femoral Socket Creation

The goal is to leave a 2-mm bone bridge between the PL and the AM femoral sockets. A reliable way to do so is to use an appropriate size transportal guide in the proximal aspect of the PL socket to localize the AM center position based on graft radius. For example, if the AM graft diameter is 8 mm for a 4 mm radius, which is the scenario of this illustrated case, using a 6-mm transportal guide in the PL socket positions the AM measuring guide pin so that after reaming with a 6-mm reamer, there will be a 2-mm bone bridge from the PL socket. Another way to create the AM socket is to use a low profile reamer with a beath pin to localize where you want it and mark the center point to then drill across with this pin, which was done in this case for reaming (switch to the special measuring pin if using TightRope fixation for the AM bundle!). I always check the bone bridge by passing the reamer over the femoral pin before I commit and drill it across the femur (Fig. 73.5). If TightRope fixation for the AM bundle is to be utilized, the same steps are followed as with the PL socket measuring the intraosseous distance, and then making the simple calculation for the maximal amount of graft possible in the socket, and ream to desired depth. Again, a #2 FiberWire suture is left at AM socket aperture (Fig. 73.6).

STEP 4—PL Tibial Socket Creation

Generally, a RetroCutter diameter 1 mm larger than the PL graft size is chosen, except in the case of the contact athlete where the patellar tendon width is 10 to 11 mm and where an 8 mm RetroCutter is used for the both PL and

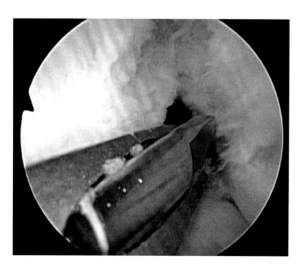

FIGURE 73.4. Five millimeter transportal guide placed to create PL femoral socket using special measuring guide pin.

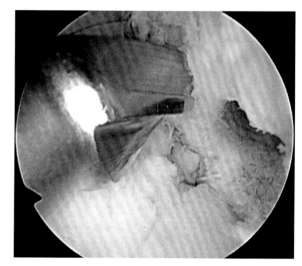

FIGURE 73.5. Eight millimeter reamer with beath pin positioned to create AM femoral socket leaving approximately 2-mm bone bridge from PL femoral socket.

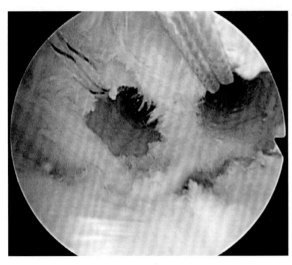

FIGURE 73.6. Final PL and AM femoral sockets with blue FiberWire in PL socket and striped TigerWire in AM socket with approximately 2-mm bone bridge visualized at 90 degrees of flexion.

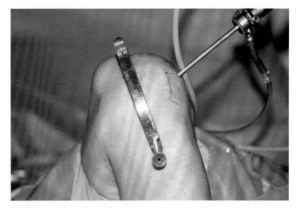

FIGURE 73.8. Necessary orientation of RetroCutter guide to create PL tibial socket starting on media tibia anteriorly close to midline to facilitate later RetroScrew fixation for PL bundle.

AM sockets. It is reverse threaded onto the Constant guide (Arthrex) and then positioned coming through the AM portal right in front of the PCL slightly lateral to the midline. There is almost a sulcus placing the RetroCutter against the lateral spine here just in front of the posterior horn lateral meniscal attachment (Fig. 73.7). The knee is flexed to 90° and the skin is marked anteriorly with the Constant guide sleeve where a 3-mm skin incision is made.

PEARL: If you are not anteriorly positioned with the Constant guide just medial to the tibial tubercle, the drilling angle for the PL tibial socket is such that it will be hard to place the RetroScrew later for graft fixation on the tibia because the RetroScrew has to fit midline in the notch to be able to be passed on the RetroScrewdriver (Arthrex) (Fig. 73.8).

The intraosseous length of tibia available for reaming is read off the guide sleeve held down to bone before reaming so one knows how deep the reaming can be done with

the RetroCutter without violating the tibial cortex. Typically, available length is 60 to 70 mm so there is plenty of room. The RetroCutter guide pin (Arthrex) is drilled across the tibia capturing the RetroCutter off the Constant guide on the joint side keeping the drill in forward. Once the RetroCutter spins freely, it is properly engaged. Pulling back with the drill in forward the tibia socket is then cut 10 mm deeper than the total length needed for the graft, to allow for tensioning of the graft, and to ensure the graft does not "bottom out" by measuring socket depth with the black grommet on the pin (Fig. 73.9). Keeping the drill in forward, the RetroCutter is brought back into the joint until the RetroCutter guide pin engages the Constant guide at which time the drill is reversed so the RetroCutter is threaded back on to the Constant guide off the guide pin, and then removed from the joint leaving the pin in place. The PL socket is circular in the posterior ACL footprint just lateral to midline (Fig. 73.10).

Next, a nitinol wire is passed through the cannulated RetroCutter guide pin and retrieved out the AM portal at which time the RetroCutter guide pin is removed. The special RetroScrewdriver is passed over the nitinol wire to "dilate" the path of the RetroScrewdriver to facilitate

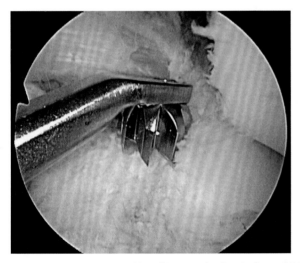

FIGURE 73.7. RetroCutter positioned in natural sulcus in front of PCL and posterior horn lateral meniscus attachment in posterior ACL footprint.

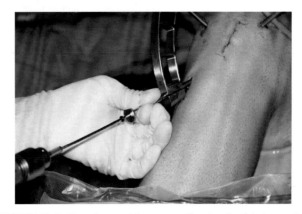

FIGURE 73.9. RetroCutter with grommet showing depth being cut for PL tibial socket (each line is 5 mm).

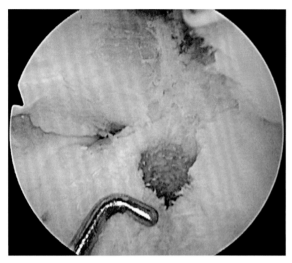

FIGURE 73.10. Final PL tibial socket in posterior ACL footprint slightly lateral to midline.

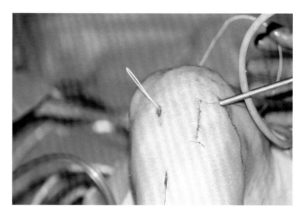

FIGURE 73.12. FiberWire suture with loop tied coming out AM portal to be used to first shuttle grafts in tibial sockets, and then to pull wire in tibial sockets for RetroScrewdriver passage.

when it has to be passed later with the graft already in the tibial socket to secure the aperture RetroScrew (Fig. 73.11). After this dilation step, the nitinol wire is used to shuttle a #2 FiberWire suture with a loop tied in its midportion from the AM portal through the small anterior tibial incision leaving the loop just outside the AM portal (Fig. 73.12). This suture serves two important purposes: it allows for shuttling of the graft in the PL tibial socket, and then it is used to pass the nitinol wire back in the tibial socket anterior to the graft to then allow passage of the RetroScrewdriver anterior to the graft for fixation with the aperture RetroScrew.

STEP 5—PL Graft Preparation

Autogenous hamstring grafts or soft tissue allografts are prepared doubled over TightRope RT loops for femoral fixation with the free ends of the grafts sutured together with #2 FiberLoop (Arthrex) in a speedwhip pattern. For the contact athlete, the semitendinosis is prepared as described above and doubled over a TightRope RT loop usually 6 to 7 mm in diameter for the PL bundle (Fig. 73.13).

Graft length is critical to ensure that the grafts don't "bottom out" in the blind sockets. Graft length calculation = graft in femoral socket + intra-articular distance + tibial socket depth − 10 mm to allow for graft tensioning. As previously described for TightRope fixation, maximal graft length in femoral socket is intraosseous length − 11 mm for the TightRope + graft radius based on that number, desired length of graft in femoral socket is chosen always greater than 15 mm. The intra-articular distance is measured with a special intra-articular measuring device (Fig. 73.14). PL graft length in the femoral socket is usually 15 to 20 mm, and the intra-articular length for the PL bundle is typically 18 to 20 mm, and graft length in the tibial socket is generally 30 mm. Therefore, the PL graft is typically prepared ahead of time to a length of 65 mm.

PEARL: Mark the intraosseous distance on the loop of the Tightrope RT from the closest end of the button with methylene blue to serve as a guide for when the button should flip on the lateral femoral cortex. Also, it is helpful to mark on the tendon graft itself the amount of

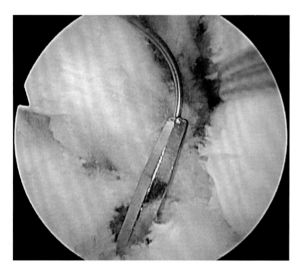

FIGURE 73.11. "Dilation" using RetroScrewdriver over wire in PL tibial socket to widen path for later passage for RetroScrew fixation.

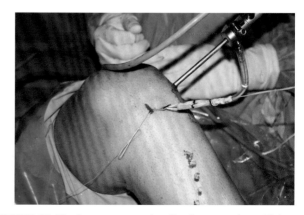

FIGURE 73.13. Autogenous semitendinosis prepared over TightRope RT loop for PL bundle shown prior to insertion.

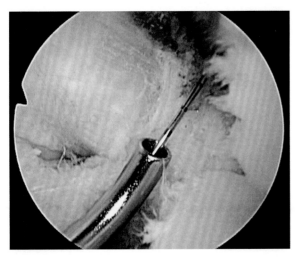

FIGURE 73.14. Intra-articular measuring device for PL intra-articular distance necessary to determine graft length. Each line is 2 mm.

graft expected in the femoral socket to confirm final graft hoisting position (Fig.73.15)

STEP 6—PL Graft Passage and Fixation

The #2 FiberWire suture loop from the aperture of the PL femoral socket is retrieved out the AM portal and used to shuttle the PL graft via the TightRope RT blue passing suture. (Fig. 73.16). The fixation button is pulled further into the femoral socket as the knee is hyperflexed (Fig. 73.17) and just as the mark made on the TightRope loop for the intraosseous distance passes into the socket, the TightRope button flips itself on the lateral cortex for secure fixation with the distinct feeling of a "pop."

PEARL: To easily verify flippage of the button, the arthroscope can be placed in the AM portal for viewing and with the knee flexed, the femoral socket is visualized to watch the button exit out the small pin hole for appropriate flippage (Fig. 73.18). The graft is then "hoisted" (Fig. 73.19) into the femoral socket with alternating pull on the shortening sutures out the skin laterally to the depth of the socket that was reamed (Fig. 73.20).

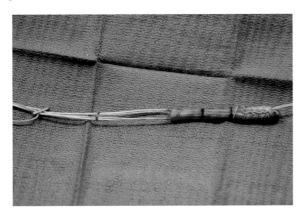

FIGURE 73.15. Prepared PL bundle with intraosseous femoral distance marked from distal end of button to indicate when button should flip on lateral femoral cortex. Note also marks for expected length of graft in femoral socket and intraarticular distance.

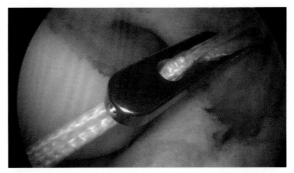

FIGURE 73.16. TightRope RT button for PL bundle pulled into femoral socket by blue passing suture for cortical fixation here.

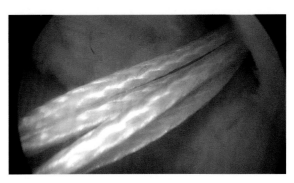

FIGURE 73.17. Shortening sutures only visualized as TightRope RT button has flipped on lateral femoral cortex.

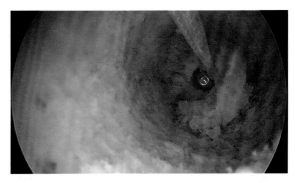

FIGURE 73.18. Arthroscope is in AM portal visualizing TightRope RT button just as it passes out lateral femoral cortex to ensure appropriate flippage.

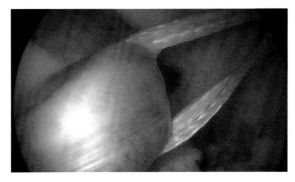

FIGURE 73.19. PL graft being "hoisted" into femoral socket by shortening sutures.

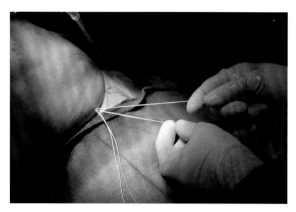

FIGURE 73.20. External view of PL graft "hoisted" into femoral socket by alternating pull on the shortening sutures to desired depth.

The sutured end of the graft is then shuttled through the special #2 FiberWire suture with the loop tied that was left out the AM portal pulling this end of the graft in the tibial socket. Holding the graft sutures taut on the tibial side, the knee is cycled several times to tension the graft.

The graft is fixed on the tibial side with an aperture RetroScrew. First, the nitinol wire is tied to the remaining portion of the no. 2 FiberWire suture left out the AM portal and shuttled back out the anterior tibial incision anterior to the graft. The RetroScrewdriver is then carefully passed over this wire anterior to the graft into the joint made easier by the previous "dilation" step done right after the tibial socket was created (Fig. 73.21). Next, the wire is removed and a #2 FiberStick (Arthrex) suture with the stiff waxed end is passed through the RetroScrewdriver into the joint and retrieved through a shoehorn cannula placed in the AM portal (Fig. 73.22). This suture is then passed through an absorbable Retro-Screw usually 7 mm in diameter, and a mulberry knot is tied on the end to secure it (Fig. 73.23). It is then passed

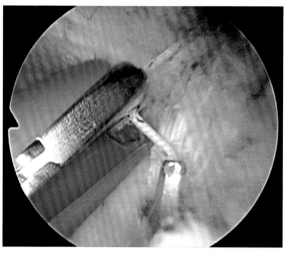

FIGURE 73.22. No. 2 FiberStick suture passed through RetroScrew-driver and retrieved through shoehorn cannula with grasper to pass suture through RetroScrew.

through the shoehorn cannula into the joint and with a hemostat is placed over the RetroScrewdriver, and the suture is pulled taut to make sure the RetroScrew is fully seated on the RetroScrewdriver referenced by a laser mark. The suture is then secured tightly to the anchor cleat on the RetroScrewdriver. Keeping the graft sutures taut, a tamp is brought in through the AM portal over the RetroScrew to apply downward force. The RetroScrew is engaged with the knee somewhat flexed, then the knee is brought into full extension (or hyperextension) as the RetroScrew is tightened with counterclockwise turning down to the aperture of the PL tibial socket for secure fixation (Fig. 73.24). The suture is released off the RetroScrewdriver and removed as is the driver itself. It will be evident watching the PL bundle that it is mildly lax in flexion, but it tightens up in full extension recreating its expected tensioning pattern (Fig. 73.25).

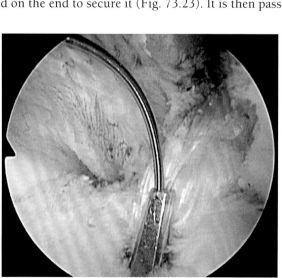

FIGURE 73.21. RetroScrewdriver passed over wire anterior to PL bundle made easier by previous "dilation" step.

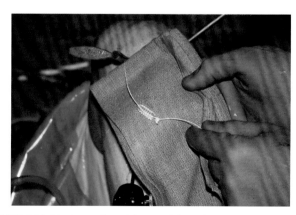

FIGURE 73.23. No. 2 FiberStick passed through RetroScrew with mulberry knot tied at top of screw to then be passed through shoehorn cannula into joint.

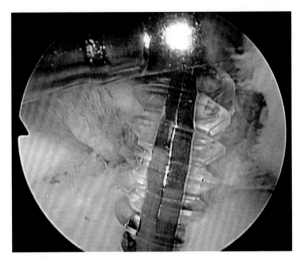

FIGURE 73.24. RetroScrew being secured for PL bundle with tamp in place pushing down on RetroScrew as knee is brought into full extension.

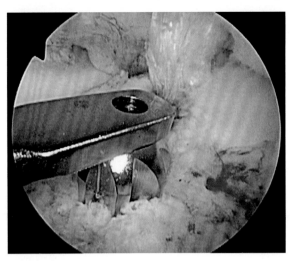

FIGURE 73.26. RetroCutter positioned to create AM tibial socket still within anterior ACL footprint with approximately 2-mm bone bridge from PL aperture RetroScrew.

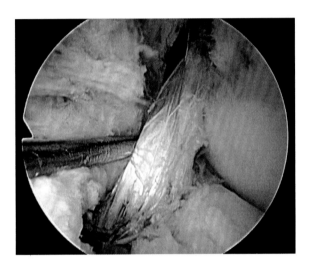

FIGURE 73.25. Completed PL bundle with TightRope RT suspensory fixation on femur and RetroScrew aperture fixation on tibia.

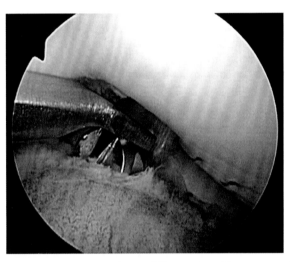

FIGURE 73.27. Knee brought into full extension with RetroCutter in place for creating AM tibial socket in anterior ACL footprint showing no notch impingement tendency.

STEP 7—AM Tibial Socket Creation

Using the same RetroCutter, the AM tibial socket is created with the PL bundle in place. The RetroCutter is positioned anterior and medial to leave a 2-mm bone bridge from the PL tibial RetroScrew, and having this Retro-Screw in place further supports the bone and mitigates the potential for socket coalescence (Fig. 73.26). There is room anteriorly still within the native ACL footprint to position the RetroCutter, and it is easy to rule out notch impingement here by extending the knee with the RetroCutter in position (Fig. 73.27). It should also be appreciated that after passing the AM bundle when it is fixed with its RetroScrew at the aperture, this effectively pushes the graft posteriorly to further help avoid any notch impingement.

With the RetroCutter positioned with the Constant guide, the skin is marked anteromedially and a second 3 mm tibial incision made here to place the sleeve down to bone to stabilize the guide, and measure the tibial intraosseous distance. The AM tibial socket is then retrocut similarly as with the PL, preserving the tibial cortex, but this socket depth is always shorter in the range of 30 to 35 mm. The circular AM tibial socket is still within the anterior ACL footprint with a 2-mm bone bridge from the PL socket/RetroScrew (Fig. 73.28). The same steps are followed with passage of the nitinol wire through the cannulated RetroCutter guide pin followed by "dilation" with the RetroScrewdriver, and then shuttling of the #2 FiberWire suture with the loop tied in it through the AM portal.

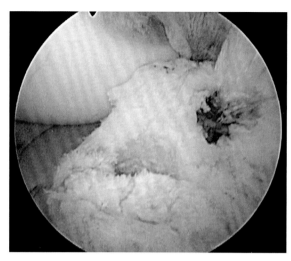

FIGURE 73.28. Final AM tibial socket still within anterior ACL footprint with 2-mm bone bridge from PL aperture RetroScrew.

STEP 8—AM Graft Preparation

The patellar tendon graft for the AM bundle is harvested at a width of 10 to 11 mm with a tibial bone plug 8 mm in diameter and 20 mm long. As previously noted, the tendon is peeled off the patella with no bone attached, and the free end sutured with a #2 FiberLoop in a speedwhip pattern. A FiberWire suture is passed through a drill hole made in the mid portion of the bone plug (Fig. 73.29). As with the PL bundle, overall AM graft length is determined. In the contact athlete construct, the AM socket length in the femur matches the patellar bone plug of 20 mm. The intra-articular distance for the AM is measured generally in the range of 25 to 30 mm. The AM tibial socket depth is shorter usually at 30 to 35 mm. Again, generally10 mm is subtracted from the tibial socket depth for the length of the graft in the tibial socket necessary to make sure the graft does not bottom out and can be tensioned. Usually, the total length of this graft is 75 mm.

If a soft tissue graft is used for the AM bundle with TightRope fixation, then the maximal graft length in the femoral socket is calculated by the previously described formula of intraosseous femoral distance − 11 mm TightRope loop size + graft radius. The femur is then reamed to desired depth, usually 25–30 mm for AM graft length in socket. The graft is folded over the TightRope RT loop, and the two free ends sutured with a #2 FiberLoop suture with the speedwhip method. In this setting, AM graft length is generally 75 to 85 mm and can be precut early in the case.

STEP 9—AM Graft Passage and Fixation

The AM graft is passed retrieving the #2 FiberWire suture loop from the femoral socket out the AM portal to pass the bone plug via its suture into the femoral socket. As with the PL bundle, the sutured end of the graft is shuttled with the #2 FiberWire loop suture from the AM portal into the tibial socket. The graft is first fixed on the femur with an absorbable biocomposite interference screw (Arthrex) after tapping generally 7 × 23 mm in length (Fig. 73.30). Next, the nitinol wire is passed with the other end of the loop suture anterior to the graft out the tibial incision for RetroScrewdriver passage. The knee is cycled and then the same steps for RetroScrew fixation are followed as before with a 7-mm RetroScrew in this case being biocomposite fixing the AM graft at the aperture with the knee at 30° of flexion (Fig. 73.31). If a soft tissue graft is used for the AM bundle, then the #2 FiberWire suture loop from the femoral socket is pulled out the AM portal to pass the TightRope RT sutures across the joint flipping the button laterally for femoral fixation. The graft is then "hoisted" into the socket with the shortening sutures, just like the PL bundle. For "backup" fixation, the # 2 FiberLoop sutures from both grafts are tied together over the anterior tibial cortex, or they could be tied separately to each other over two-hole titanium buttons to increase fixation strength approximately 20% (17). The AM bundle shows better isometry tight in flexion, and almost as tight in full extension (Fig. 73.32).

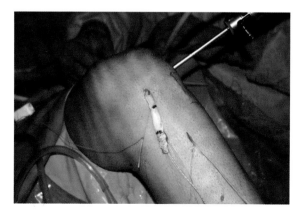

FIGURE 73.29. Autogenous patellar tendon graft with bone only from tibia for AM bundle, seen prior to graft passage. Marks for the intraarticular distance can be seen.

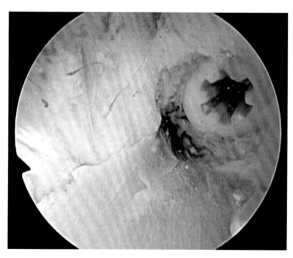

FIGURE 73.30. Biocomposite aperture interference screw in femur for AM bundle bone block.

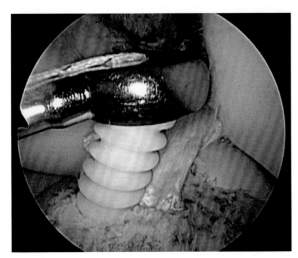

FIGURE 73.31. Biocomposite RetroScrew fixating AM graft on tibia at approximately 30° flexion.

POSTOPERATIVE MANAGEMENT

Early motion is encouraged with use of a continuous passive motion unit in the recovery room. Generally, the patient sees a physical therapist the day after surgery for the first dressing change and institution of quadriceps exercises emphasizing full knee extension, along with active knee flexion. Crutches for weight bearing are used until one has good leg control and a satisfactory gait pattern determined by the therapist—usually 10 to 14 days. A functional ACL brace is fit at the first postoperative visit for additional protection. Closed chain exercises are initiated with the leg press, minisquats, and hamstring curls for weight training. The bicycle and elliptical are preferred for cardiovascular exercise with jogging initiated around 3 months after surgery. Proprioceptive and agility

exercises are added followed by sports-specific exercises, such as jump training for basketball, with return to sports usually 6 months after surgery.

REFERENCES

1. Lubowitz J. No-tunnel anterior cruciate ligament reconstruction: the transtibial all-inside technique. *Arthroscopy.* 2006;22:900.el–900.e11.
2. Smith P, Schwartzberg R, Lubowitz J. All-inside, double-bundle, anterior cruciate ligament reconstruction. *Arthroscopy.* 2008;24:1184–1189.
3. Pinczewski LA, Lyman J, Salmon LJ, et al. A 10-year comparison of anterior cruciate ligament reconstructions with hamstring tendon and patellar tendon autograft. *Am J Sports Med.* 2007;35:564–574.
4. Chhabra A, Starman JS, Ferretti M, et al. Anatomic, radiographic, biomechanical, and kinematic evaluation of the anterior cruciate ligament and its two functional bundles. *J Bone Joint Surg Am.* 2006;88(suppl 4):2–10.
5. Zantop T, Herbort M, Raschke MJ, et al. The role of the anteromedial and posterolateral bundles of the anterior cruciate ligament in anterior tibial translation and internal rotation. *Am J Sports Med.* 2007;35:223–227.
6. Yagi M, Wong EK, Kanamori A, et al. Biomechanical analysis of an anatomic anterior cruciate ligament reconstruction. *Am J Sports Med.* 2002;30:660–666.
7. Lu Y, Markel MD, Nemke B, et al. Comparison of single- versus double-tunnel tendon-to-bone healing in an ovine model: a biomechanical and histological analysis. *Am J Sports Med.* 2009;37:512–517.
8. Muneta T, Koga H, Morito T, et al. A retrospective study of the midterm outcome of two-bundle anterior cruciate ligament reconstruction using quadrupled semitendinosus in comparison with one-bundle reconstruction. *Arthroscopy.* 2006;22:252–258.
9. Siebold R, Dehler C, Ellert T. Prospective randomized comparison of double-bundle versus single-bundle anterior cruciate ligament reconstruction. *Arthroscopy.* 2008;24:137–145.
10. McAdams T, Biswal S, Stevens K, et al. Tibial aperture bone disruption after retrograde versus antegrade tibial tunnel drilling: a cadaveric study. *Knee Surg Sports Traumatol Arthrosc.* 2008;16:818–822.
11. Morgan CD, Stein DA, Leitman EH, et al. Anatomic tibial graft fixation using a retrograde bio-interference screw for endoscopic anterior cruciate ligament reconstruction. *Arthroscopy.* 2002;18:E38.
12. Bottoni CR. Anterior cruciate ligament femoral tunnel creation by use of anteromedial portal. *Arthroscopy.* 2008;24:1319.
13. Harner CD, Honkamp NJ, Ranawat AS. Anteromedial portal technique for creating the anterior cruciate ligament femoral tunnel. *Arthroscopy.* 2008;24:113–115.
14. Franz W, Ulbrich J. A new technique for harvesting the semitendinosus tendon for cruciate ligament reconstruction. *Arthroskopie.* 2004;17:104–107.
15. Zantop T, Ferretti M, Bell KM, et al. Effect of tunnel-graft length on the biomechanics of anterior cruciate ligament-reconstructed knees: intra-articular study in a goat model. *Am J Sports Med.* 2008;36:2158–2166.

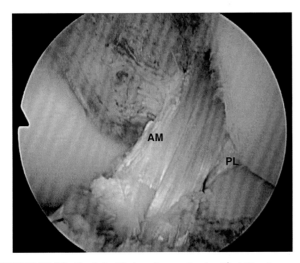

FIGURE 73.32. Final double-bundle construct with AM autogenous patellar tendon graft and PL autogenous doubled semitendinosis graft.

16. Walsh MP, Wijdicks CA, Armitage BM, et al. The 1:1 versus the 2:2 tunnel-drilling technique: optimization of fixation strength and stiffness in an all-inside double-bundle anterior cruciate ligament reconstruction—a biomechanical study. *Am J Sports Med.* 2009;37:1539–1547.

17. Walsh MP, Wijdicks CA, Parker JB, et al. A comparison between a retrograde interference screw, suture button, and combined fixation on the tibial side in an all-inside anterior cruciate ligament reconstruction: a biomechanical study in a porcine model. *Am J Sports Med.* 2009;37:160–167.

Arthroscopic PCL Reconstruction: Transtibial and Arthroscopic Inlay Techniques

Matthew V. Smith • Jon K. Sekiya

Posterior cruciate ligament (PCL) injuries are relatively uncommon compared with anterior cruciate ligament (ACL) injuries. Unlike the ACL, the PCL has the potential to heal (1, 2). However, this does not always result in normal knee kinematics (3–5). Despite this, outcomes after nonoperative treatment for isolated PCL injuries have been favorable (6, 7). Therefore, nonoperative treatment has been advocated for most isolated PCL injuries. However, patients with chronic PCL deficiency can develop pain and disability over time (8). Currently, controversy exists about the surgical indications for the treatment of isolated PCL injuries. Additional controversy exists regarding the appropriate surgical technique to treat PCL-deficient knees. In this chapter, we discuss the evaluation and management of the PCL-deficient knee, highlighting the transtibial single-bundle PCL augmentation technique and the arthroscopic inlay technique.

CLINICAL EVALUATION

Although ACL injuries commonly occur as a result of a noncontact deceleration injury, isolated PCL injuries usually occur from a direct blow to the knee or from a hyperextension injury. A direct blow can occur in motor vehicle accidents when the proximal tibia directly impacts the dashboard with knee in flexion. A PCL injury can also occur during athletic activities when the proximal tibia strikes the ground with the foot in plantar flexion (6). Although PCL injuries can occur with varus, valgus, or twisting forces, these injuries are often associated with collateral ligament injuries. Because of PCL injuries are less common than ACL injuries, PCL injuries are often overlooked during evaluation after a knee injury. Unfortunately, these injuries can be subtle and patients may not know exactly how or when the injury occurred. Despite this, it is important to try and clarify the mechanism of injury to help determine the diagnosis.

In addition to clarifying the mechanism of injury, it is important to determine the timing of injury, as an acute PCL tear may require a different treatment than a chronic tear. It is also important to know if the patient had a previous knee injury that may explain any ligamentous laxity. Age and activity level are key factors in determining treatment options, particularly in patients with partial PCL tears. In addition, it is essential to understand the patient's occupational requirements. When considering surgical treatment in patients with chronic PCL deficiency, it is imperative to determine if pain or instability is the primary complaint. Chronic PCL deficiency has been associated with a higher incidence of medial compartment and patellofemoral chondral damage as well as meniscal tears (9). PCL reconstruction in a painful and degenerative knee may not yield favorable results.

Physical Examination

The physical examination of an injured knee starts with inspection for swelling and ecchymosis. An effusion is likely to develop with an acute PCL injury. Swelling or ecchymosis on the medial or lateral aspect of the knee should heighten concern for a collateral ligament or capsular injury. As with any lower extremity injury, thorough evaluation and clear documentation of the neurovascular status of the affected extremity is critical, especially in multiple ligament knee injuries (10). Peroneal nerve injury has been reported between 13% and 16% in posterolateral corner (PLC) injuries (11, 12).

After evaluating the neurovascular status of the limb, a thorough ligamentous exam should be performed. In patients with a PCL injury, the posterior sag of the tibia reduces with the anterior force applied during a Lachman exam. This may give the examiner the impression that the Lachman's is positive even though the ACL is intact. Prior to performing the Lachman's exam, be sure that the proximal tibia is approximately 1 cm anterior to the medial femoral condyle. Anterior drawer findings and a quadriceps active test (tibia reduces with quad muscle activation) may help to clarify the injury pattern. Evaluation of varus and valgus laxity as well as rotary instability is a critical part of evaluating a PCL-deficient knee since associated ligament injuries are common (13). Rotary instability may result from a PLC injury. PLC deficiency has been shown to increase graft forces after PCL reconstruction (14). The PLC

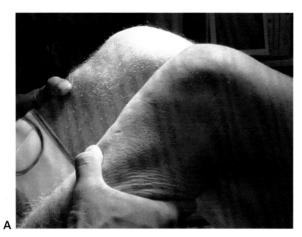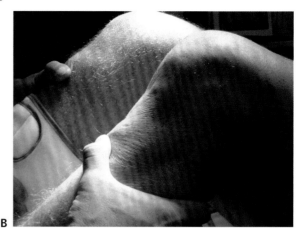

FIGURE 74.1. Photograph of a patient with a PCL injury whose tibia reduces to a normal position with anterior force on the tibia **(A)** and whose tibia sags posteriorly during a posterior drawer examination **(B)**.

is assessed with the Dial test. A patient with an isolated PLC injury will demonstrate 10° to 15° of increased external rotation at 30° of knee flexion compared with the opposite side. PCL- and PLC-deficient knees will also show increased external rotation at 90° of flexion. Lastly, in patients with subacute or chronic injuries, it is important to evaluate the overall static and dynamic limb alignment. A chronic untreated PLC injury may result in a dynamic varus thrust that should be treated with an osteotomy prior to any ligament reconstruction.

PCL injuries are graded by the posterior drawer, which amount of posterior translation of the tibia relative to the femur with knee at 90° of flexion. The posterior drawer is the most accurate test to identify PCL deficiency (15) (Fig. 74.1). This can be evaluated clinically and radiographically. Grade 1 injuries demonstrate less than 5 mm of posterior tibial translation. Posterior tibial translation between 5 and 10 mm is considered a grade 2 injury. Greater than 10 mm of posterior translation is considered a grade 3 injury. In patients with grade 3 PCL injuries, it is important to closely evaluate the PLC as biomechanical studies have shown that PLC sectioning is required to get grade 3 posterior tibial translation in a PCL-deficient knee (16–18). Clinically, if the proximal tibia translates to a level flush with the medial femoral condyle but not farther, it is likely a grade 2 PCL injury. If the proximal tibia drops posterior to the medial femoral condyle, it is likely a grade 3 injury.

Imaging

Radiographic evaluation of an injured knee starts with plain X-rays. Necessary views include an anterior–posterior (AP), a lateral, and an oblique view. Avulsion fractures of the tibial insertion should be evident on these views. A notch view, a Merchant's view, and a weight-bearing 45° flexion posterior–anterior view are additional views that may provide important information in chronic PCL injuries. In patients with chronic PCL deficiency, standing long-leg alignment films are useful to determine the

presence of malalignment. Stress radiographs with TELOS or with 20 lb (9.07 kg) of posterior force applied to the tibia with the knee in 70° to 90° of flexion can provide an objective measure of injury grade compared with the contralateral knee (Fig. 74.2). Gravity lateral views comparing both knees can be used if stress views cannot be performed.

MRI is the imaging modality of choice to evaluate the integrity of the soft tissues in the knee. MRI is especially useful in identifying acute PCL injuries (19) (Fig. 74.3). It can also help define associated ligament injuries, meniscal injuries, and chondral injuries. Chronic PCL injuries may not be evident on MRI as healing may take place over time (1). Therefore, it is important to rely on the clinical exam findings to determine the pattern of injury. In addition to MRI, dynamic ultrasound has been shown to be effective in diagnosing associated PLC injury (20). This may be particularly helpful in subacute or chronic PLC injuries when MRI does not clearly demonstrate injury.

TREATMENT

Treatment for acute PCL injuries continues to evolve. Traditionally, nonoperative management of isolated acute PCL tears has been advocated. Nonoperative treatment of isolated acute PCL tears includes bracing in full knee extension for at least 2 weeks to reduce the posterior sag of the tibia relative to the femur during healing (21, 22). During rehabilitation, emphasis is placed on quadriceps strengthening since patients with good quadriceps strength tend to have better functional outcomes (7). In addition, hamstring strengthening is discouraged during the healing phase to minimize posteriorly directed forces across the knee. While short-term results of nonoperative treatment are favorable, good outcomes can diminish over time (6–8). Keller et al. (8) reported that 90% of patients with PCL deficiency complained of knee pain with activity and 43% complained of problems with walking at an average of 6 years after injury. This has led some to advocate

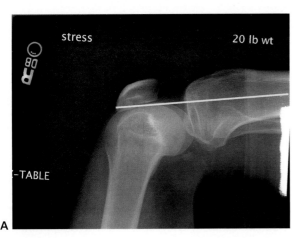
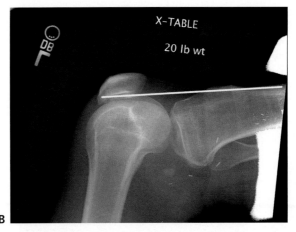

FIGURE 74.2. Radiographs demonstrating the position of the tibia relative to the femur in 90° of flexion with 20 lb (9.07 kg) of applied posterior force in a patient's uninjured knee **(A)** and in the patient's PCL-deficient knee **(B)**.

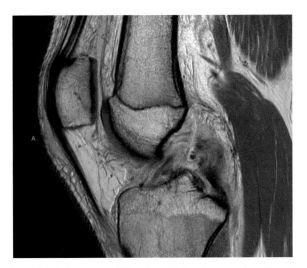

FIGURE 74.3. MRI image (T1-weighted) showing complete disruption of the PCL.

for earlier surgical intervention, especially in patients with higher grade PCL injuries, as surgical outcomes are generally good with up to 90% patient satisfaction (13, 23–25). Current operative interventions have failed to consistently improve posterior laxity to normal (23, 24, 26, 27). However, the degree of PCL laxity does not appear to correlate with outcomes (28). On the other hand, outcomes after acute and subacute (<3 months) surgical intervention for PCL deficiency are better than those after surgical intervention for chronic injuries (23). Nonoperative treatment in patients with multidirectional instability from a combined PCL and associated ligament injury do not fair as well as those with isolated PCL injuries (29).

Operative intervention for acute PCL injuries is clearly indicated in patients with a bony avulsion of the PCL tibial insertion, in combined ligamentous injuries and in knee dislocations unless there is a contraindication to surgery like poor health status or poor functional status. Operative intervention for isolated PCL tears remains controversial. Surgery may be warranted in patients

with persistent symptoms of instability or pain after a trial nonoperative management. Operative treatment options for PCL injuries include PCL repair, PCL augmentation, and PCL reconstruction. Primary PCL repair alone has generally fallen out of favor because of average results (30). There may be a role for passing sutures into the PCL remnant and pulling it into the femoral tunnel with a graft during PCL augmentation (31). Transtibial single-bundle PCL augmentation with autograft or allograft can be used to improve stability in partial PCL tears where the PCL is intact but lax (32). This is particularly helpful in acute injuries when the PCL still has the potential to heal. PCL reconstructions for complete tears can be done with single-bundle or double-bundle grafts using transtibial or inlay techniques.

Single-Versus Double-Bundle PCL Reconstruction

The PCL consists of two main bundles, anterolateral (AL) and posteromedial (PM) (33). The AL bundle originates more anterior on the lateral face of the medial femoral condyle than the PM bundle. The AL bundle inserts more lateral than the PM bundle on the tibial fovea. The AL bundle is tight in flexion, whereas the PM bundle tightens in extension. With the knee in full extension, there is little translation of the tibia relative to the femur in a PCL-deficient knee (34, 35). Therefore, reconstructing the AL bundle is the key component to PCL reconstruction. The addition of a PM bundle reconstruction has been shown to improve stability in biomechanical testing by decreasing posterior tibial translation and enhancing rotational control, especially in a PLC-deficient knee (18). Since PLC injuries commonly accompany PCL injuries, the improved rotational control provided by a double-bundle reconstruction may improve knee kinematics more so than a single-bundle reconstruction (Fig. 74.4). However, there is evidence that a double-bundle PCL reconstruction may over constrain the knee when the PLC is intact (18). The addition of a PM bundle may also increase AL bundle graft

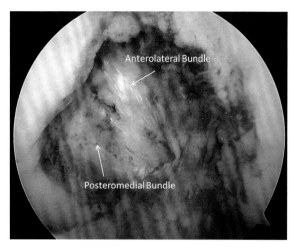

FIGURE 74.4. Arthroscopic image demonstrating the AL and PM-bundle positions after a double-bundle PCL reconstruction.

tension especially if the PM bundle is not placed in the correct position on the femur (36). Currently, there are no clinical studies that demonstrate improved outcomes comparing the two techniques (25, 37–39).

Transtibial Versus Inlay PCL Reconstruction

Traditionally, transtibial and open inlay techniques have been used for PCL reconstruction. The transtibial technique, when compared with the open inlay technique, has the advantage of easier patient positioning and the use of instrumentation that is similar to that used in ACL reconstruction. The transtibial technique may be indicated in patients who have undergone vascular repair or have extensive scarring in the posterior aspect of the knee. The disadvantage of the transtibial technique is the effect of the acute angle taken by the graft as it exits the tibial tunnel and turns toward the femoral tunnel (the killer turn). This angle is between 45° and 75°. Biomechanical studies have shown this acute angle can cause graft elongation, graft thinning, and early failure after graft cycling (40, 41). Drilling a more vertical tibial tunnel can reduce the angle. The open inlay technique solves this problem and may protect the graft from elongation over time. However, the open inlay technique requires a more extensive dissection and presents patient positioning challenges. Some surgeons perform this procedure in a modified lateral position to allow arthroscopic evaluation and femoral tunnel drilling by externally rotating the leg. Others reposition the patient between the prone and the supine positions depending on the part of the procedure being performed. Of note, no studies have proven a difference in clinical outcomes comparing transtibial with open inlay techniques (24, 42).

Recently, arthroscopic inlay techniques have also been described (43, 44). The arthroscopic tibial inlay procedure was developed to gain the advantages of an inlay technique while reducing the difficulties in patient positioning. Like the transtibial technique, an arthroscopic inlay PCL reconstruction may be favored patients who have undergone vascular repair or have extensive scarring in the posterior aspect of the knee (43). A recent clinical study, demonstrated that a double-bundle arthroscopic inlay PCL reconstruction was superior to a single-bundle transtibial and a single-bundle arthroscopic inlay PCL reconstruction in preventing posterior tibial translation (45). However, this study did not show any difference in Lysholm scores between the reconstructive techniques. In addition, human cadaver biomechanical studies have shown equivalent performance between the arthroscopic inlay technique and the open inlay technique regarding mean load to failure, radiographic posterior displacement, graft elongation after cycling, and structural properties after graft cycling (44, 46–48).

AUTHORS' PREFERRED TREATMENT

The senior author's (J.K.S.) preferred technique for the acutely injured knee depends upon the grade of PCL injury. In patients with acute isolated grade 1 or 2 PCL injuries, patients are treated in full extension bracing for 2 weeks followed by a rehabilitation protocol that highlights quadriceps strengthening. If the patient has persistent grade 2 laxity and instability symptoms after immobilization, we consider performing an early transtibial PCL AL-bundle augmentation with tibialis anterior allograft or hamstring autograft while the PCL still has healing potential. PCL augmentation can also be considered in patients with acute multiligament knee injuries as long as there is a significant amount of PCL tissue remaining. In patients with acute isolated grade 3 PCL injuries, we will consider immobilization in extension followed by rehabilitation. However, we are much more assertive about offering surgery to these patients. If acute surgical intervention is decided upon, we perform a transtibial PCL augmentation if there adequate PCL tissue remaining. In patients with acute PCL injuries without adequate PCL tissue remaining or in chronic PCL deficiency without significant degenerative changes, we prefer a double-bundle arthroscopic inlay technique using either Achilles tendon allograft or quadriceps tendon autograft. In acute grade 3 PCL injuries, we are careful to assess for PLC injury and treat it with early repair (within 2 weeks) along with the PCL reconstruction.

SURGICAL TECHNIQUES

Transtibial PCL Reconstruction

A complete examination of the knee is performed with the patient under anesthesia prior to performing any reconstructive procedure. The transtibial technique is performed with the patient in the supine position. A sandbag is secured to the operating table to support the foot so that the knee flexes to 70° and 80°. A lateral thigh post is raised to its maximum height so that a "bump" can be wedged between the thigh and the post (Fig. 74.5). Our preference is to prep the entire leg and foot so that the dorsalis pedis and the posterior tibial pulses can be easily palpated. We cover the toes with an impervious stocking sealed with Ioban (3M). We typically do not use a tourniquet during a PCL reconstruction. Graft choices include hamstring autograft or allograft, bone patellar tendon bone autograft or allograft, tibialis anterior allograft, and quadriceps tendon. Our preference is a tibialis anterior allograft for transtibial single-bundle PCL augmentation.

A thorough arthroscopic evaluation is performed through a standard AL viewing portal. An anteromedial working portal is also created. Care is taken to evaluate the integrity of the ACL. The ACL may appear lax because of the posterior sag of the tibia. It is important to reduce the tibial anteriorly before making a determination

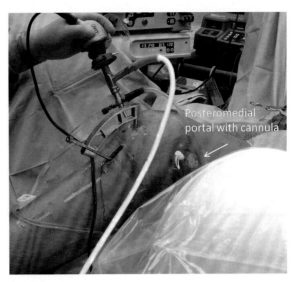

FIGURE 74.7. Photograph showing a threaded arthroscopic cannula placed in a PM portal.

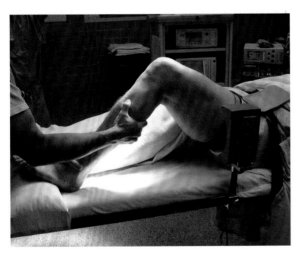

FIGURE 74.5. Photograph demonstrating maximum elevation of the leg postadjacent to the proximal thigh. Note the position of the sandbag secured to a flat radiolucent table. With the foot resting on the sandbag, the knee is flexed to 80°.

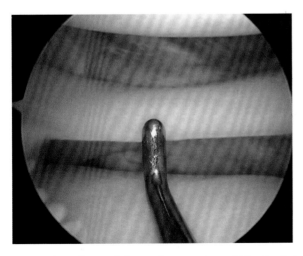

FIGURE 74.6. Arthroscopic image demonstrating a "drive thru" sign with greater than 10 mm of opening. This is indicative of a collateral ligament injury.

regarding the integrity of the ACL. It is also important to assess the continuity of the remaining PCL. During arthroscopic evaluation of the medial and lateral compartments, it is important to assess the amount of opening with valgus and varus stress, respectively. Greater than 10 mm is suggestive of collateral ligament injury (Fig. 74.6). If the presurgical physical examination is equivocal, the so-called drive-thru sign can provide important information to guide treatment of associated injuries.

After a diagnostic arthroscopy is performed, an incision is made over the anteromedial flare of the tibia superior to the pes anserinus and anterior to the superficial MCL. An accessory PM portal is also made under direct arthroscopic visualization using a 70° arthroscope. An arthroscopic-threaded cannula is placed into this portal to facilitate instrument passage during the procedure (Fig. 74.7). For single-bundle transtibial PCL augmentation, the PCL fibers on the tibial footprint are preserved as much as possible. A PCL drill guide is inserted through the anteromedial portal. The guide is passed through notch and positioned on the tibial PCL footprint to reproduce the position of the AL bundle. Care is taken to avoid iatrogenic injury to the ACL while positioning the PCL drill guide. A fluoroscopic image is helpful for confirming the guide placement on the tibia (Fig. 74.8). The PCL drill guide is set at 60° to create a more vertical tunnel that will reduce the angle the graft takes as it exits the tibial tunnel. A guide pin is passed through the PCL drill guide under repeated fluoroscopic imaging so that the pin does not advance posteriorly past the tibial cortex. The appropriate cannulated reamer, based on the size of the graft, is advanced over the guide pin using repeated fluoroscopic guidance to avoid advancing the guide pin while reaming.

A small medial incision is made anterior to the medial femoral epicondyle at the level of the superior pole of the

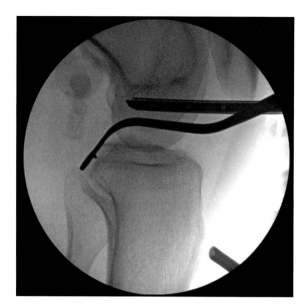

FIGURE 74.8. Fluoroscopic image demonstrating a PCL drill guide placed on the tibial PCL footprint.

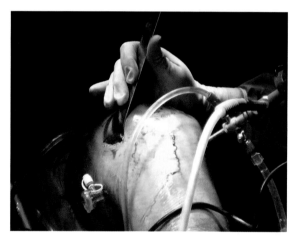

FIGURE 74.9. Photograph demonstrating a medial incision used to expose the medial femoral condyle to facilitate outside-in femoral tunnel drilling.

patella (Fig. 74.9). The distal portion of the vastus medialis is lifted anteriorly. A PCL femoral target drill guide is used to position the guide pin from outside in so that it enters the joint in the 12:30 p.m. position and approximately 5.5 mm off the articular margin on the lateral face of the medial femoral condyle (49). Alternatively, a guide pin can be placed in the 12:30 p.m. position through the anteromedial portal from inside out. However, this creates a more acute graft angle as it enters the femur making it harder to pass and tension the graft (50). Once the guide pin is in the correct position, the appropriately sized cannulated reamer is used to drill the femoral tunnel.

Once the tunnels have been drilled, the anteromedial portal is enlarged to allow the graft to be inserted into the joint. A no. 2 strong-braided suture is passed through the tibial tunnel and taken out of the anteromedial portal with

a grasper. This suture is used to pull the graft into the tibial tunnel. Flexion and extension of the knee can facilitate seating of the graft. The sutures in the femoral portion of the graft are then pulled into the femoral tunnel. The graft is secured first on the femoral side with either an endobutton or by tying the graft sutures over a post. The graft is tensioned with the knee in 90° of flexion with anterior force placed on the tibia. The graft is fixed on the tibial side by tying over a post, using a soft tissue interference screw, or both.

Arthroscopic Tibial Inlay Double-Bundle PCL Reconstruction

The examination, patient positioning, and setup for an arthroscopic tibial inlay double-bundle PCL reconstruction is the same for the transtibial PCL reconstruction. An anteromedial, an AL, and an accessory posterior medial portal are created. The knee is flexed to 80° to 90°. A threaded arthroscopic cannula is placed in the accessory PM portal. A thorough arthroscopic examination of the knee is performed. A radiofrequency probe is inserted into the anteromedial portal to remove the soft tissues from the lateral face of the medial femoral condyle. The radiofrequency probe is then inserted through the accessory PM portal to thoroughly débride the tibial PCL footprint. A PCL tibial drill guide is passed through the anteromedial portal and placed on the tibial PCL footprint. Its position is verified by fluoroscopic imaging. A small incision is made over the anteromedial flare of the tibia where the bullet tip of the drill guide contacts the skin (Fig. 74.10). A 13-mm FlipCutter (Arthrex, Naples, FL) is advanced through the tibia until it makes contact with the posterior tibial cortex (Fig. 74.11). The tip of the FlipCutter is gently advanced through the posterior cortex, a distance of approximately 5 mm under fluoroscopic guidance and direct arthroscopic visualization. The FlipCutter is released and a probe is inserted through the PM portal to flip the blade parallel to the tibial footprint (Fig. 74.12). The bladed handle is turned by hand to gently clear a circular

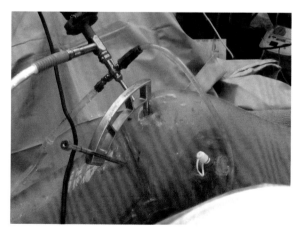

FIGURE 74.10. Photograph showing the PCL drill guide. An incision over the anteromedial flare of the tibia is made where the tip of the guide "bullet" contacts the skin.

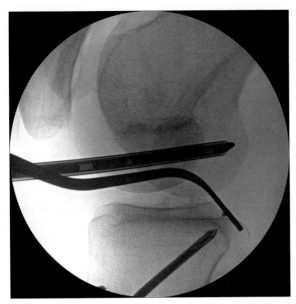

FIGURE 74.11. Lateral fluoroscopic view demonstrating the passage of a drill to the edge of the cortex adjacent to the PCL footprint. Passage of the drill through the cortex is performed by hand to avoid plunging posteriorly into the neurovascular bundle.

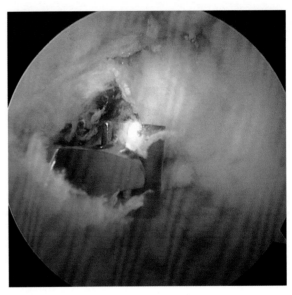

FIGURE 74.12. Arthroscopic image showing the FlipCutter that has been advanced into the joint under direct visualization with the blade flipped so that it is parallel to the tibial PCL footprint.

path for the blade through the surrounding soft tissue. A drill is attached to the FlipCutter distally. A 12-mm deep tunnel is reamed by spinning the FlipCutter and pulling distally using fluoroscopy for guidance (Fig. 74.13). The FlipCutter is advanced back into the joint to reorient the blade back in line with its shaft to remove it from the joint. After reaming, directly visualize the tunnel to verify that it is adequate to accept the graft (Fig. 74.14).

The outside-in technique is used for femoral tunnel drilling similar to that described for the transtibial

single-bundle technique. The AL-bundle tunnel is drilled the same way as the transtibial single-bundle PCL augmentation described above. The PM tunnel is placed in the 3 o'clock position 6 to 7 mm off the articular surface of the medial femoral condyle (Fig. 74.15). The AL and PM tunnels should be divergent. Care should be taken to start the tunnels proximal enough to avoid damaging the subchondral bone as this can lead to avascular necrosis.

Prepare an Achilles tendon allograft by creating a 12-mm circular bone plug on the tibial side. Whipstitch the tendon adjacent to the bone with no. 2 FiberWire (Athrex, Naples, FL) and pull the ends of the suture through the

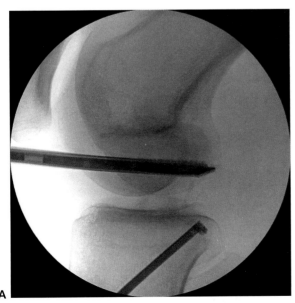
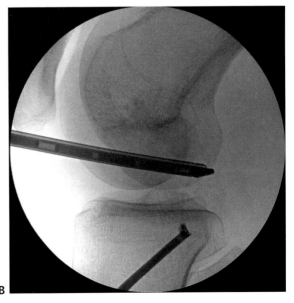

FIGURE 74.13. Lateral fluoroscopic view showing the FlipCutter blade flipped and beginning to ream a tunnel in the tibial PCL footprint (**A**). The FlipCutter is pulled distally a total of 12 mm under fluoroscopic guidance (**B**).

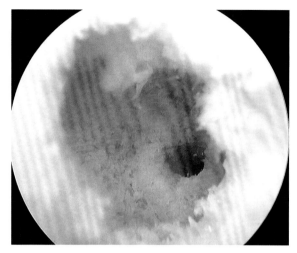

FIGURE 74.14. Arthroscopic image showing the blind tunnel reamed by the FlipCutter.

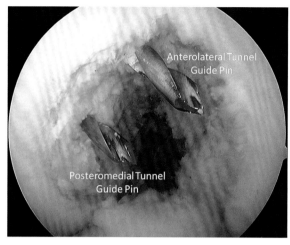

FIGURE 74.15. Arthroscopic image showing the position of the AL and PM femoral tunnel guide pins placed from outside in.

center of the bone plug. Split the Achilles tendon into two limbs. The AL-bundle limb should be the thicker portion of the graft. Whipstitch the free ends with no. 2 FiberWire to facilitate graft passage into the femoral tunnels and to facilitate graft tensioning (Fig. 74.16). Once the tibial and femoral tunnels are drilled, the anteromedial portal is enlarged to facilitate graft passage into the joint. A passing suture is advanced into the tibial tunnel and retrieved out of the anteromedial incision. The sutures in the tibial end of the graft are pulled through the tibial tunnel. The tibial bone plug is seated into the 12-mm deep hole in the tibial footprint. Flexion and extension of the knee may help seat the graft. The bone plug will be visible on a lateral fluoroscopic image. It should appear well seated in the posterior tibia (Fig. 74.17). The sutures on the tibial side are tied over a plastic button while holding firm tension on the sutures. The sutures from the free end of the graft are passed into the femoral tunnels with the larger limb passed into the AL tunnel. The graft limbs in the femoral tunnels are tension in 90° of flexion and secured with soft tissue interference screws. The fixation is reinforced by tying the sutures over postproximally.

SPECIAL CONSIDERATIONS

Multiligament injuries present a challenge to patients and surgeons alike. Multiligament knee injuries may represent spontaneously reduced or unrecognized knee dislocations. Since the popliteal artery is tethered by the adductor canal proximal to the knee and by the soleus arch distal to the knee, vascular injury can occur with knee dislocations. Although arteriography after an acute knee dislocation has been advocated in the past, recent reports demonstrate that patients with an ankle-brachial index (ABI) greater than 0.9 do not have arterial injury (51). Nonetheless, these patients should have their pulses monitored with for 24 hours.

There is controversy about the timing of surgical intervention for multiligament knee injuries. Some advocate

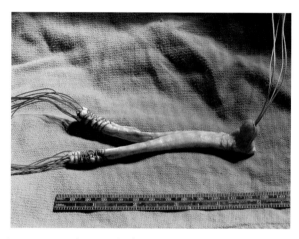

FIGURE 74.16. Photograph of the prepared graft with two free ends whipstitched for graft passage and the bone plug fashioned to fit into the tibial tunnel reamed by the FlipCutter. Note the sutures passed through the center of the bone plug. These are used to pass the graft into the tibial tunnel.

early intervention, especially in patients PLC or PM corner injuries, so that primary repair remains a treatment option. Others advocate early rehabilitation to improve range of motion and swelling and delayed reconstruction to lower the risk of postoperative stiffness. There is no clear evidence that proves that one approach is better than the other. Therefore, the surgeon and patient should weigh the risk and benefits to decide together what is in the patient's best interest.

Return to athletic competition is a reasonable expectation after an isolated PCL injury, however, many do not return to the same level of competition (7). It may prove more difficult in patients with multiligament injuries. To return to sports, patients need to demonstrate a stable ligamentous examination. They need at least 90% quadriceps and hamstring strength compared with the opposite leg. They need to perform jumping and agility drills without a limp. Lastly, they need to be able to perform these

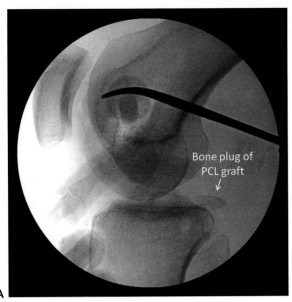
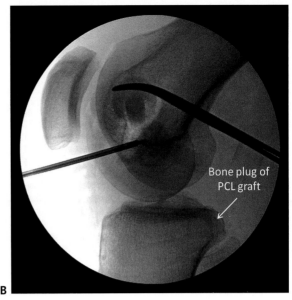

FIGURE 74.17. Lateral fluoroscopic image demonstrating the bone plug of the PCL graft being passed to the back of the knee through the notch **(A)**. The graft is then pulled into the tunnel reamed by the FlipCutter **(B)**. The graft must fall into the tunnel before being tied down over a button anteriorly.

activities without developing an effusion. This may take 9 to 12 months after surgical intervention.

COMPLICATIONS

Like other reconstructive procedure for the knee, complications do arise when treating PCL injuries. Infection is a risk with any surgical procedure but can be particularly troublesome in the face of ligament reconstruction. Also, stiffness is common after both nonoperative and operative intervention for PCL injury. Patients who work diligently with a physical therapist can often avoid this complication. However, stiffness can develop despite appropriate rehabilitation. Patients often have difficulty regaining flexion after PCL reconstruction. We consider arthroscopic scar debridement if patients do not regain more than 90° of flexion by 6 to 8 weeks. Lastly, although good outcomes are expected after PCL reconstruction, many are left with residual laxity (23, 24, 26, 27).

In addition, neurovascular injury, particularly to the popliteal artery and tibial nerve, is another concern when reconstructing the PCL. The neurovascular bundle is approximately 1 cm posterior to the tibial insertion of the PCL (52). It is at risk during all of the reconstructive techniques. The peroneal nerve is at risk when treating the PLC in combined PCL and PLC injuries.

REHABILITATION

Postoperative rehabilitation is directed at protecting the reconstructed PCL. Forces that result in posterior tibial translation are discouraged. Therefore, we typically place the patient in a hinged knee brace locked in full extension immediately after surgery. The patient is allowed to

do quad sets, straight leg raises, and patellar mobilization exercises immediately. Patients also start passive range of motion to regain flexion in the prone position to reduce the posterior force on the tibia during knee flexion. The goal is to regain full flexion by 3 months. After 1 month, patients are allowed to use a stationary bike with minimal resistance. Starting at 4 months closed chain exercises begin to advance quadriceps and hamstring strengthening while promoting cocontraction of the muscles crossing the knee. Light jogging begins at 6 months. Gradual return to sport-specific activities is allowed with hopes that the patient regains enough strength to return to unrestricted activities between 9 and 12 months.

CONCLUSIONS AND FUTURE DIRECTIONS

Isolated PCL injuries are relatively uncommon. They are often accompanied by associated ligament injuries. Careful examination of the knee is critical prior to offering treatment. Isolated grade 1 and 2 PCL injuries respond well to nonoperative treatment in the short term. Persistent PCL laxity may result in patellofemoral and medial compartment degenerative changes long term. Operative intervention is indicated in tibial PCL footprint avulsion fractures, many grade 3 injuries, and combined ligament injuries. Although the clinical outcomes of the transtibial and open tibial inlay PCL reconstruction techniques are similar, biomechanical evidence suggests that transtibial PCL reconstructions may be compromised by graft thinning and elongation at the "killer turn." Open tibial inlay PCL reconstructions are technically more challenging because of the dissection and patient positioning. An arthroscopic tibial inlay PCL reconstruction compares favorably with the open inlay technique in biomechanical studies and makes patient positioning less difficult. Our preference is to perform a transtibial single-bundle PCL augmentation in grade 2 injuries with persistent pain and instability after immobilization or in grade 3 injuries with adequate PCL tissue remaining for healing. We prefer an arthroscopic tibial inlay double-bundle PCL reconstruction in grade 3 injuries without adequate PCL tissue or in chronic PCL-deficient knees without advanced arthrosis. Prospective randomized studies are needed to determine the long-term clinical outcomes comparing operative with nonoperative treatment of PCL injuries. Additional studies are needed to compare the efficacy of the different reconstructive techniques.

PEARLS AND PITFALLS

1. Carefully examine the knee for associated ligament injuries in a PCL-deficient knee.
2. An accessory PM portal with an arthroscopic cannula allows easy instrument passage to the PCL footprint on the tibia.
3. When passing the tibial guide pin for the transtibial or arthroscopic inlay technique, an arthroscopic probe placed in the accessory PM portal can be used to retract the posterior capsule for better visualization as the pin enters the joint.
4. Flexing the knee to 90° during tibial tunnel drilling increases the distance of the neurovascular bundle to the tibial tunnel.
5. When passing the graft into the joint through the anteromedial portal, excising some of the fatpad and using a cannula allows the graft to enter more easily.
6. Flexion and extension of the knee helps the graft to seat in the tibial tunnel.
7. After the graft is secured on the tibial and femoral sides, evaluate the knee range of motion to make sure there is full flexion and extension.

REFERENCES

1. Shelbourne KD, Jennings RW, Vahey TN. Magnetic resonance imaging of posterior cruciate ligament injuries: assessment of healing. *Am J Knee Surg.* 1999;12:209–213.
2. Mariani PP, Margheritini F, Christel P, et al. Evaluation of posterior cruciate ligament healing: a study using magnetic resonance imaging and stress radiography. *Arthroscopy.* 2005;21(11):1354–1361.
3. MacDonald P, Miniaci A, Fowler P, et al. A biomechanical analysis of joint contact forces in the posterior cruciate deficient knee. *Knee Surg Sports Traumatol Arthrosc.* 1996;3(4):252–255.
4. Gill TJ, DeFrate LE, Wang C, et al. The biomechanical effect of posterior cruciate ligament reconstruction on knee joint function. Kinematic response to simulated muscle loads. *Am J Sports Med.* 2003;31(4):530–536.
5. Gill TJ, DeFrate LE, Wang C, et al. The effect of posterior cruciate ligament reconstruction on patellofemoral contact pressures in the knee joint under simulated muscle loads. *Am J Sports Med.* 2004;32(1):109–115.
6. Fowler PJ, Messieh SS. Isolated posterior cruciate ligament injuries in athletes. *Am J Sports Med.* 1987;15(6):553–557.
7. Parolie JM, Bergfeld JA. Long-term results of nonoperative treatment of isolated posterior cruciate ligament injuries in the athlete. *Am J Sports Med.* 1986;14(1):35–38.
8. Keller PM, Shelbourne KD, McCarroll JR, et al. Nonoperatively treated isolated posterior cruciate ligament injuries. *Am J Sports Med.* 1993;21(1):132–136.
9. Geissler WB, Whipple TL. Intraarticular abnormalities in association with posterior cruciate ligament injuries. *Am J Sports Med.* 2004;32:109–115.
10. Wascher DC, Dvirnak PC, DeCoster TA. Knee dislocation: initial assessment and implications for treatment. *J Orthop Trauma.* 1997;11:525–529.
11. DeLee JC, Riley MB, Rockwood CA Jr. Acute posterolateral rotary instability of the knee. *Am J Sports Med.* 1983;11:199–207.
12. LaPrade RF, Terry GC. Injuries to the posterolateral aspect of the knee. Association of anatomic injury patterns with clinical instability. *Am J Sports Med.* 1997;25:433–438.
13. Cooper DE, Stewart D. Posterior cruciate ligament reconstruction using single-bundle patella tendon graft with tibial inlay fixation: 2- to 10-year follow-up. *Am J Sports Med.* 2004;32(2):346–360.
14. Harner CD, Vogrin TM, Hoher J, et al. Biomechanical analysis of a posterior cruciate ligament reconstruction: deficiency of the posterolateral structures as a cause of graft failure. *Am J Sports Med.* 2000;28:32–39.
15. Covey CD, Sapega AA. Injuries of the posterior cruciate ligament. *J Bone Joint Surg Am.* 1993;75:1376–1386.
16. Sekiya JK, Whiddon DR, Zehms CT, et al. A clinically relevant assessment of posterior cruciate ligament and posterolateral corner injuries. Evaluation of isolated and combined deficiency. *J Bone Joint Surg Am.* 2008;90(8):1621–1627.
17. Schulz MS, Steenlage ES, Russe K, et al. Distribution of posterior tibial displacement in knees with posterior cruciate ligament tears. *J Bone Joint Surg Am.* 2007;89(2):332–338.
18. Whiddon DR, Zehms CT, Miller MD, et al. Double compared with single-bundle open inlay posterior cruciate ligament reconstruction in a cadaver model. *J Bone Joint Surg Am.* 2008;90(9):1820–1829.
19. Gross ML, Grover JS, Bassett LW, et al. Magnetic resonance imaging of the posterior cruciate ligament. Clinical use to improve diagnostic accuracy. *Am J Sports Med.* 1992;20(6):732–737.
20. Sekiya JK, Swaringen JC, Wojtys EM, Jacobson JA. Diagnostic ultrasound evaluation of posterolateral corner knee injuries. *Arthroscopy.* 2010 Apr;26(4):494–499. Epub 2010 Feb 11.
21. Swaringen J, Sekiya JK, Wojtys EM, et al. A new diagnostic sonography stress test for posterior lateral corner knee injuries: a clinical comparison with magnetic resonance imaging verified by surgery. Submitted to *Am J Sports Med.*
22. Dowd GS. Reconstruction of the posterior cruciate ligament. Indications and results. *J Bone Joint Surg Br.* 2004;86:480–491.
23. Harner CD, Hoher J. Evaluation and treatment of posterior cruciate ligament injuries. *Am J Sports Med.* 1998;26:471–482.

24. Sekiya JK, West RV, Ong BC, et al. Clinical outcomes after isolated arthroscopic single-bundle posterior cruciate ligament reconstruction. *Arthroscopy*. 2005;21(9):1042–1050.

25. MacGillivray JD, Stein BE, Park M, et al. Comparison of tibial inlay versus transtibial techniques for isolated posterior cruciate ligament reconstruction: minimum 2-year follow-up. *Arthroscopy*. 2006;22(3):320–328.

26. Garofalo R, Jolles BM, Moretti B, et al. Double-bundle transtibial posterior cruciate ligament reconstruction with a tendon-patellar bone-semitendinosus tendon autograft: clinical results with a minimum of 2 years' follow-up. *Arthroscopy*. 2006;22(12):1331–1338.e1.

27. Lipscomb AB Jr, Anderson AF, Norwig ED, et al. Isolated posterior cruciate ligament reconstruction. Long-term results. *Am J Sports Med*. 1993;21(4):490–496.

28. Mariani PP, Adriani E, Santori N, et al. Arthroscopic posterior cruciate ligament reconstruction with bone-tendon-bone patellar graft. *Knee Surg Sports Traumatol Arthrosc*. 1997;5(4):239–244.

29. Shelbourne KD, Muthukaruppan Y. Subjective results of nonoperatively treated, acute, isolated posterior cruciate ligament injuries. *Arthroscopy*. 2005;21(4):457–461.

30. Torg JS, Barton TM, Pavlov H, et al. Natural history of the posterior cruciate ligament-deficient knee. *Clin Orthop Relat Res*. 1989;246:208–216.

31. Richter M, Kiefer H, Hehl G, et al. Primary repair for posterior cruciate ligament injuries. An eight-year followup of fifty-three patients. *Am J Sports Med*. 1996;24(3):298–305.

32. Jung YB, Jung HJ, Tae SK, et al. Tensioning of remnant posterior cruciate ligament and reconstruction of anterolateral bundle in chronic posterior cruciate ligament injury. *Arthroscopy*. 2006;22(3):329–338.

33. Ahn JH, Yang HS, Jeong WK, et al. Arthroscopic transtibial posterior cruciate ligament reconstruction with preservation of posterior cruciate ligament fibers: clinical results of minimum 2-year follow-up. *Am J Sports Med*. 2006;34(2):194–204.

34. Harner CD, Xerogeanes JW, Livesay GA, et al: The human posterior cruciate ligament complex: an interdisciplinary study. Ligament morphology and biomechanical evaluation. *Am J Sports Med*. 1995;23:736–745.

35. Butler DL, Noyes FR, Grood ES. Ligamentous restraints to anteriorposterior drawer in the human knee. A biomechanical study. *J Bone Joint Surg*. 1980;62A:259–270.

36. Fox RJ, Harner CD, Sakane M, et al. Determination of in situ forces in the human posterior cruciate ligament using robotic technology: a cadaveric study. *Am J Sports Med*. 1998;26:395–401.

37. Shearn JT, Grood ES, Noyes FR, et al. Two-bundle posterior cruciate ligament reconstruction: how bundle tension depends on femoral placement. *J Bone Joint Surg Am*. 2004;86A(6):1262–1270.

38. Hatayama K, Higuchi H, Kimura M, et al. A comparison of arthroscopic single- and double-bundle posterior cruciate

ligament reconstruction: review of 20 cases. *Am J Orthop*. 2006;35(12):568–571.

39. Houe T, Jørgensen U. Arthroscopic posterior cruciate ligament reconstruction: one- vs. two-tunnel technique. *Scand J Med Sci Sports*. 2004;14(2):107–111.

40. Wang CJ, Weng LH, Hsu CC, et al. Arthroscopic single- versus double-bundle posterior cruciate ligament reconstructions using hamstring autograft. *Injury*. 2004;35(12):1293–1299.

41. Bergfeld JA, McAllister DR, Parker RD, et al. A biomechanical comparison of posterior cruciate ligament reconstruction techniques. *Am J Sports Med*. 2001;29(2):129–136.

42. Markolf KL, Zemanovic JR, McAllister DR. Cyclic loading of posterior cruciate ligament replacements fixed with tibial tunnel and tibial inlay methods. *J Bone Joint Surg Am*. 2002;84A(4):518–524.

43. Seon JK, Song EK. Reconstruction of isolated posterior cruciate ligament injuries: a clinical comparison of the transtibial and tibial inlay techniques. *Arthroscopy*. 2006;22:27–32.

44. Mariani PP, Margheritini F. Full arthroscopic inlay reconstruction of posterior cruciate ligament. *Knee Surg Sports Traumatol Arthrosc*. 2006;14(11):1038–1044.

45. Campbell RB, Jordan SS, Sekiya JK. Arthroscopic tibial inlay for posterior cruciate ligament reconstruction. *Arthroscopy*. 2007;23(12):1356.e1–1356.e4.

46. Kim SJ, Kim TE, Jo SB, et al. Comparison of the clinical results of three posterior cruciate ligament reconstruction techniques. *J Bone Joint Surg Am*. 2009;91(11):2543–2549.

47. Campbell RB, Torrie A, Hecker A, et al. Comparison of tibial graft fixation between simulated arthroscopic and open inlay techniques for posterior cruciate ligament reconstruction. *Am J Sports Med*. 2007;35(10):1731–1738.

48. Jordan SS, Campbell RB, Sekiya JK. Posterior cruciate ligament reconstruction using a new arthroscopic tibial inlay double-bundle technique [Review]. *Sports Med Arthrosc*. 2007;15(4):176–183.

49. Zehms CT, Whiddon DR, Miller MD, et al. Comparison of a double bundle arthroscopic inlay and open inlay posterior cruciate ligament reconstruction using clinically relevant tools: a cadaveric study. *Arthroscopy*. 2008;24(4):472–480.

50. McAllister DR, Miller MD, Sekiya JK, et al. Posterior cruciate ligament biomechanics and options for surgical treatment. *Instr Course Lect*. 2009;58:377–388.

51. Handy MH, Blessey PB, Kline AJ, et al. The graft/tunnel angles in posterior cruciate ligament reconstruction: a cadaveric comparison of two techniques for femoral tunnel placement. *Arthroscopy*. 2005;21(6):711–714.

52. Mills WJ, Barei DP, McNair P. The value of the ankle-brachial index for diagnosing arterial injury after knee dislocation: a prospective study. *J Trauma*. 2004;56(6):1261–1265.

53. Cosgarea AJ, Jay PR. Posterior cruciate ligament injuries: evaluation and management [Review]. *J Am Acad Orthop Surg*. 2001;9(5):297–307.

PCL Reconstruction Using the Tibial Inlay Technique

Yaw Boachie-Adjei • Mark D. Miller

CLINICAL EVALUATION OF PCL INJURY

History

Patients may report a "dashboard injury" mechanism, in which the patient's bent knee or shin strikes a fixed surface such as a dashboard. Another mechanism of injury is knee hyperflexion, often during athletics when athletes fall on their knee with their foot plantar flexed. This may overload the quadriceps mechanism. These injuries may or may not be accompanied by an audible "pop."

Physical Examination

Effusion: An acute hemarthrosis is often present, but is usually not as remarkable as the effusion seen in an acute anterior cruciate ligament (ACL) injury.

Range of motion: This is often decreased secondary to effusion, pain, and general instability.

Quadriceps tone: This should be noted, as it may be decreased in patients with a chronic tear. This may also be related to posterior tibial subluxation.

Posterior drawer test/tibial station: This is the gold standard test for PCL injury. The point of the anterior tibia should be carefully assessed in relation to medial femoral condyle. This allows grading of PCL injury (Fig. 75.1A–C).

- *Normal*: At 90° of knee flexion, the tibia should lie 1 cm anterior to the femoral condyles
- *Grade I*: Using the normal side for comparison, a 0.5-cm difference in relative posterior translation
- *Grade II*: The anterior surface of the tibia and femoral condyles is flush (>1 cm of relative posterior translation)
- *Grade III*: The tibia can be translated 1 cm posterior to the anterior femoral condyles. Grade III instability usually represents a combined PCL-posterolateral corner (PLC) injury

Quadriceps active test: This test is performed by flexing the patient's knee to 90°, while stabilizing the foot and thigh. The patient then contracts the quadriceps while the examiner evaluates the knee for anterior tibial translation. A positive test is indicative of PCL injury.

External rotation asymmetry: With the patient prone, grasp their heels, flex their knees up (to 30° and then 90°), and externally rotate their feet. If there is more than 15° of asymmetry in tibial external rotation, there may be a PCL and/or PLC injury that needs to be addressed. Tests should be done at both 30° (to assess PLC alone) and 90° (to assess PCL and PLC) of knee flexion. If asymmetry is present at both positions, a combined PCL–PLC injury is likely. A comprehensive ligamentous examination should be performed to rule out other injuries (Fig. 75.2).

Lachmans test: This is an important test to assess ACL injury.

Varus and valgus stress testing: Should also be done to rule out lateral collateral ligament and medial collateral ligament injury. This is particularly concerning if there is an opening in full extension.

Imaging

Plain radiographs: Flexion weight-bearing posteroanterior radiographs allow assessment of arthritis and offer a good view of the intercondylar notch. Look for bony avulsion, tibial plateau fracture, and fibular head fracture, indicative of PLC injury. Chronic PCL injuries may be associated with medial compartment arthrosis. Lateral view to look for relationship between the tibia and the femur (A/P translation, rotation). Patellar sunrise view allows evaluation of patellofemoral arthrosis, which is also associated with a chronic PCL injury. Long-leg cassette view: This is a view taken that images from the hip to the ankle and should be considered if there is any question regarding mechanical alignment. Telos stress radiographs: 15 daN of stress is applied to each tibia and radiographs are taken. The normal side (Fig. 75.3A) is compared with the injured side (Fig. 75.3B). This is a standardized and accurate way to distinguish between different types of PCL lesions and permit grading of posterior knee laxity in the PCL-deficient knee.

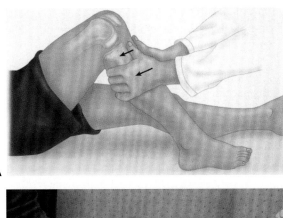

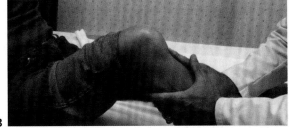

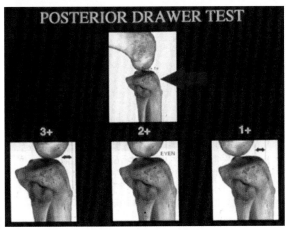

FIGURE 75.1. A–C: Posterior drawer test. (From Miller MD, Cole BJ, Cosgarea A, et al. *Operative Techniques: Sports Knee Surgery.* Philadelphia, PA: Saunders Elsevier; 2008, with permission.)

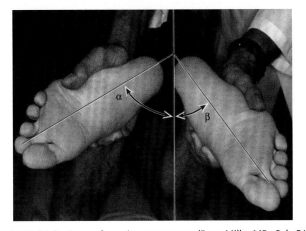

FIGURE 75.2. External rotation asymmetry. (From Miller MD, Cole BJ, Cosgarea A, et al. *Operative Techniques: Sports Knee Surgery.* Philadelphia, PA: Saunders Elsevier; 2008, with permission.)

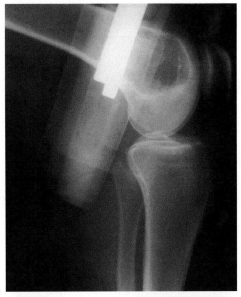

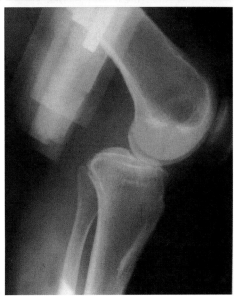

FIGURE 75.3. Telos stress radiographs **(A)** normal side, **(B)** injured side. (From Miller MD, Cole BJ, Cosgarea A, et al. *Operative Techniques: Sports Knee Surgery.* Philadelphia, PA: Saunders Elsevier; 2008, with permission.)

MRI: This is another very useful tool. It aids in evaluation of associated injuries. Other soft-tissue/cartilage/bony injuries about the knee greatly affect the approach to treatment of PCL injuries. It is helpful in imaging (Fig. 75.4); other ligaments, extensor injury, menisci, and articular injury.

Decision Making

Historically, the natural history of the disrupted PCL has been debated. Traditionally, most authors have recommended nonoperative treatment of isolated PCL injuries. Many claim that untreated patients progress with minimal symptoms. Indeed, many patients remain symptom-free despite the lack of a PCL, but it has been shown that

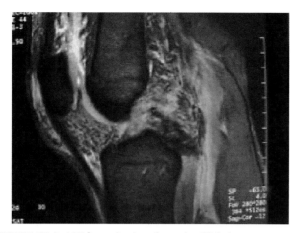

FIGURE 75.4. MRI for evaluation of associated injuries.

articular cartilage degeneration may be accelerated in the patellofemoral compartment and medial compartments. Pain, aching, and effusions may be secondary symptoms, but may not present until several years after PCL injury. Increasing ligamentous laxity does not correlate with severity of any symptoms.

Classification of PCL injury: Based on both chronicity and severity of injury.

Chronicity

* Acute: Injury less than 3 weeks old.
* Chronic: Injury greater than 3 weeks old.

Severity

* Grades I/II/III: This can be obtained from the posterior drawer test and assessing the tibial station.

TREATMENT

Nonoperative Treatment

Indications for nonoperative treatment include chronic injury in older less active patients. Isolated grade I or II injury, PCL tears from a hyperflexion mechanism will often tear only the larger anterolateral band, whereas the posteromedial band remains intact. This type of injury may spare secondary restraints. Nonoperative treatment may be indicated in this case.

Conservative management consists of early brace management followed by a quadriceps strengthening program. It is important to protect the knee from posterior translation. Athletics are typically restricted until 90% of the quadriceps strength is regained.

Operative Treatment

Indications for operative treatment include

* Acute injuries
* Isolated grade III injury
* Active young patients (especially those with symptomatic grade II injuries)

* "Physiologically" young patients
* Symptomatic chronic grade II or III injury that has failed rehabilitation (includes older patients)
* PCL injury combined with any of the following:
  * PLC injury (loss of secondary stabilizer to posterior displacement)
  * ACL injury
  * Grade III MCL injury
  * Bony avulsion injury

Timing

Timing of PCL reconstruction depends on the associated pathology and presence of bony injury. In the presence of a PLC injury, acute (<3 weeks) treatment may not be indicated, as there may still be significant soft-tissue swelling from the injury. If a bony injury is present, this may be fixed acutely, with PLC reconstruction done a few weeks later.

TECHNIQUE

Positioning

The lateral decubitus position is used for the open tibial inlay approach (Figs. 75.5 and 75.6). The contralateral well leg should be padded (Fig. 75.6A). An ankle-foot orthosis type holder may be used to hold the surgical extremity (Fig. 75.5). Position the patient in the lateral decubitus position with the operative leg up (Fig. 75.6B).

Place the tourniquet as high as possible on the operative leg, and in a sterile manner, prep the leg and thigh up to the tourniquet. Now the popliteal fossa can be accessed (Fig. 75.6C). By rotating the hip and placing the foot

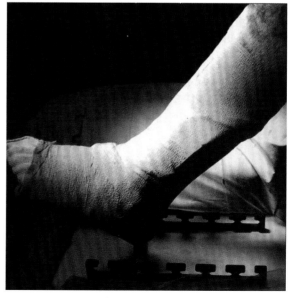

FIGURE 75.5. Supine positioning for use in transtibial tunnel approach. (From Miller MD, Cole BJ, Cosgarea A, et al. *Operative Techniques: Sports Knee Surgery.* Philadelphia, PA: Saunders Elsevier; 2008, with permission.)

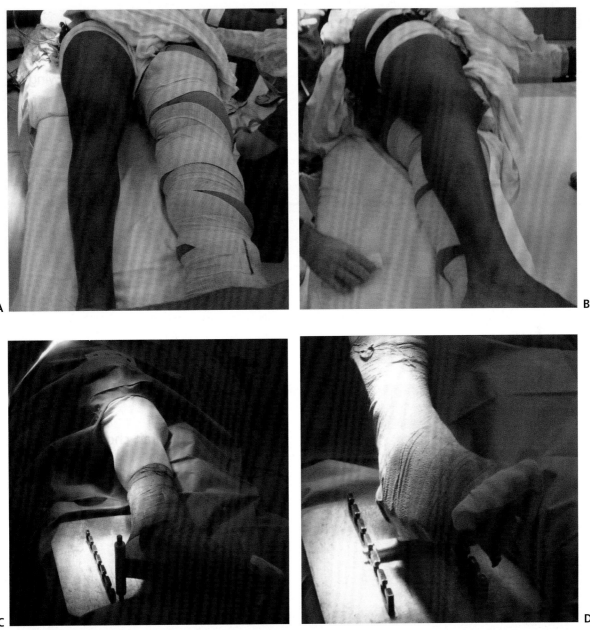

FIGURE 75.6. Lateral decubitus approach for the open tibial inlay approach. (From Miller MD, Cole BJ, Cosgarea A, et al. *Operative Techniques: Sports Knee Surgery.* Philadelphia, PA: Saunders Elsevier; 2008, with permission.)

eccentrically in the foot holder, the leg can be positioned for arthroscopy (Fig. 75.6D).

AUTHORS' PREFERRED TREATMENT

Step 1—Graft Preparation

This step depends on graft chosen and the technique. A bone-patellar tendon-bone (BPTB) allograft can be prepared for single- or double-bundle PCL reconstruction (Fig. 75.7 top). An Achilles tendon allograft can be prepared for either single- or double-bundle PCL reconstruction (Fig. 75.7 bottom).

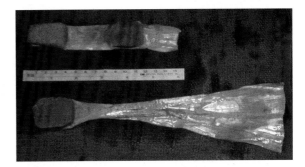

FIGURE 75.7. The BPTB allograft can be prepared for single- or double-bundle PCL reconstruction. (From Miller MD, Cole BJ, Cosgarea A, et al. *Operative Techniques: Sports Knee Surgery.* Philadelphia, PA: Saunders Elsevier; 2008, with permission.)

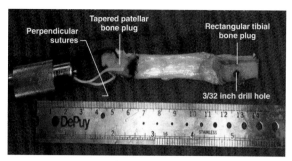

FIGURE 75.8. An patella tendon allograft. (From Miller MD, Cole BJ, Cosgarea A, et al. *Operative Techniques: Sports Knee Surgery*. Philadelphia, PA: Saunders Elsevier; 2008, with permission.)

A quadriceps tendon autograft can be prepared for double-bundle reconstruction. A BPTB autograft can only be prepared for single-bundle reconstruction (Fig. 75.8). Hamstring grafts are typically not used as stand-alone grafts, but can be used for one bundle of double-bundle PCL reconstructions.

Step 2—Debridement and Femoral Tunnel Placement

Debride the PCL stump. The posteromedial bundle and/ or meniscofemoral ligaments can be preserved during this step.

If one tunnel is planned, it should be at the 1 o'clock position (right knee) and 6 to 8 mm posterior to the articular margin (Fig. 75.9A and B).

If two tunnels are planned, the anterolateral tunnel is placed as described above and the posteromedial tunnel is placed inferior and posterior to it (Fig. 75.10). This tunnel should be at approximately the 9:30-o'clock position and 10 mm from the articular surface.

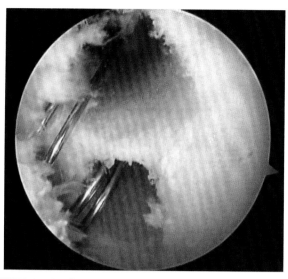

FIGURE 75.10. If two tunnels are planned the posteromedial tunnel is placed inferior and posterior to the anterolateral tunnel. Place at approximately the 9:30 position, 10 mm from the articular surface. (From Miller MD, Cole BJ, Cosgarea A, et al. *Operative Techniques: Sports Knee Surgery*. Philadelphia, PA: Saunders Elsevier; 2008, with permission.)

Tunnels can be drilled from inside out or outside in. Inside-out tunnels are drilled from an inferolateral portal with the knee hyperflexed. Guides are available for guide-wire placement for double-bundle PCL reconstructions.

Outside-in tunnels are drilled from the anteromedial cortex of the femur, deep to the Vastus Medialis Obliquus (VMO). The VMO fibers can be split or a subvastus approach can be made. Once the guidewire placement is confirmed, the tunnels are overdrilled with an appropriately sized drill bit. The posterior portion of the femoral tunnel is rasped in its aperture to prevent graft abrasion.

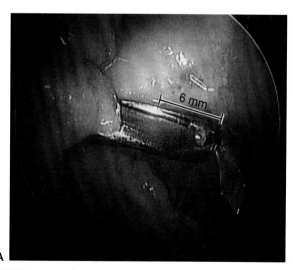
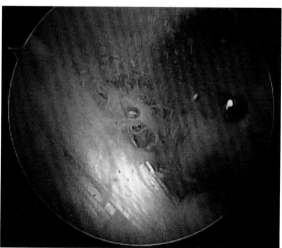

FIGURE 75.9. Place one tunnel at the 1 o'clock position (right knee) 6 to 8 mm posterior to the articular margin. (From Miller MD, Cole BJ, Cosgarea A, et al. *Operative Techniques: Sports Knee Surgery*. Philadelphia, PA: Saunders Elsevier; 2008, with permission.)

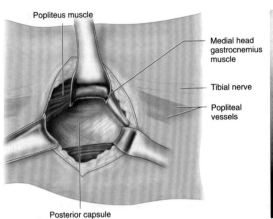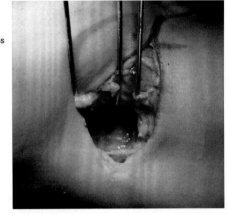

A   **B**

FIGURE 75.11. A, B: The gastrocnemius is retracted laterally and the popliteus muscle belly is exposed. A trought is made in the posterior tibial suculus with an osteotome/curette/burr to allow for the tibial portion of the PCL graft to be inlayed. (From Miller MD, Cole BJ, Cosgarea A, et al. *Operative Techniques: Sports Knee Surgery.* Philadelphia, PA: Saunders Elsevier; 2008, with permission.)

Step 3—Exposures

When performing the tibial inlay technique, a direct posterior approach to the posterior tibia is made. A horizontal incision is made in the popliteal crease and carried down to the subcutaneous tissues. A hockey stick incision is made in the gastrocnemius fascia, extending distally on the medial side.

The interval between the medial head of gastrocnemius and the semimembranosus is developed with blunt dissection, so that the medial head of the gastrocnemius can be mobilized laterally. The gastrocnemius is retracted laterally and the popliteus muscle belly is exposed (Fig. 75.11).

The popliteus is split and the PCL stump is exposed. A posterior arthrotomy is made in the midline, and the posterior aspect of the femoral condyles can be palpated. A trough is made in the posterior tibial sulcus with an osteotome/curette/burr to allow for the tibial portion of the PCL graft to be inlayed (Fig. 75.11).

The position of the inlay trough lies between the posterior eminences. The eminence can be palpated, with the medial eminence being more prominent. The inlay trough should be made between these eminences, or lateral to the medial eminence. Begin with electrocautery and then follow this with a burr to get through the cortical bone on the back of the tibia.

The trough is extended superiorly with electrocautery to create the posterior arthrotomy. Make sure that you can easily pass your index finger through the arthrotomy and into the posterior notch. A looped 18G guidewire is passed through the femoral tunnel(s) and retrieved through the posterior arthrotomy to facilitate graft passage.

Step 4—Graft Passage

The graft is passed from the tibia to the femur. If a double-bundle procedure is planned, the posteromedial bundle is passed first and then the anterolateral is passed (Fig. 75.12).

The graft is first fixed in the tibia. The bone block is fixed with posterior to anterior biocortical screw(s) (Fig. 75.13A). We currently use two cannulated screws with washers (if there is room). This allows the graft to be secured with the guide wires for the screws before drilling. The indirect measuring guide is used to measure screw length prior to placement.

The graft is passed into the femoral tunnel(s) and fixed with interference screws and backed up with a button, a screw and washer, or staple (Fig. 75.13B).

The knee is cycled several times and then placed in 90° of flexion. The sutures from the bone block in the femur are tensioned while an anterior Drawer force is placed on the knee and a 9- × 20-mm interference screw is placed to secure the graft.

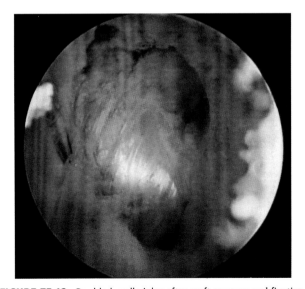

FIGURE 75.12. Double-bundle inlay after graft passage and fixation. (From Miller MD, Cole BJ, Cosgarea A, et al. *Operative Techniques: Sports Knee Surgery.* Philadelphia, PA: Saunders Elsevier; 2008, with permission.)

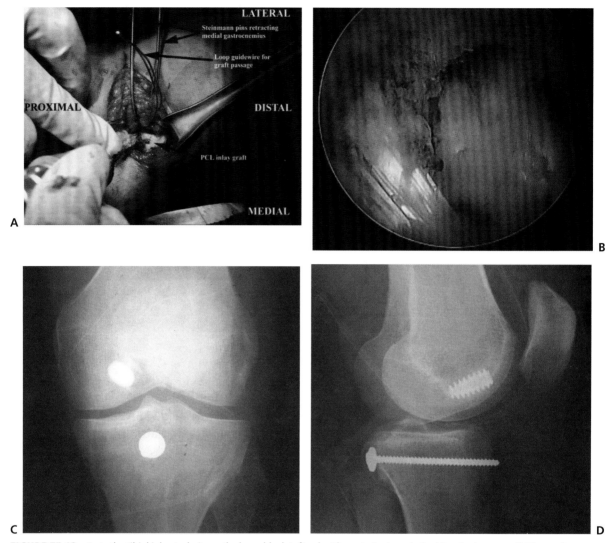

FIGURE 75.13. **A:** In the tibial inlay technique, the bone block is fixed with posterior to anterior bicortical screws. **B:** The graft is passed into the femoral tunnel(s) and fixed with interference screw(s) and vacked up with a button, a screw and washer, or a staple. **C, D:** The final appearance of the PCL reconstruction using the tibial inlay technique is shown in **(C)** AP and **(D)** lateral radiographs. (From Miller MD, Cole BJ, Cosgarea A, et al. *Operative Techniques: Sports Knee Surgery.* Philadelphia, PA: Saunders Elsevier; 2008, with permission.)

The final appearance of the PCL reconstruction using the tibial inlay technique is shown in AP and lateral (Fig. 75.13C and D) radiographs.

REHABILITATION

Immediate Post-op Period

Patients are placed into an extension brace and may ambulate as tolerated. Early passive range of motion can be done in a prone position.

Physical Therapy

Formal physical therapy can begin as early as 2 to 3 days postoperatively. Early therapy involves effusion control and progression of motion and weight bearing.

Quadriceps exercises are encouraged and hamstring exercises are discouraged in the early postoperative period. Quadriceps training is emphasized early, but hamstring training is delayed for 3 months postoperatively.

Most surgeons delay running until 4 to 6 months (longer than for ACL reconstruction). Return to sport is typically 6 to 9 months postoperatively.

COMPLICATIONS, CONTROVERSIES, AND SPECIAL CONSIDERATIONS

Complications

The most severe complication is neurovascular injury. A thorough knowledge of the anatomy of the popliteal fossa is keyed when performing the tibial inlay technique.

Late laxity is the most common complication, but is thought to occur less with tibial inlay reconstruction versus tibial tunnel reconstruction. Loss of motion. Lysis of adhesions and manipulation under anesthesia may be necessary if loss of motion persists at 6 weeks postoperatively. Recurrent instability (most commonly related to not recognizing a PLC injury).

Controversies

The primary controversy is over graft choice, and this tends to be a regional, institutional, or individual surgeon choice. BPTB allograft or autograft (only used for single-bundle reconstruction), Achilles tendon allograft (single- or double-bundle reconstruction), quadriceps tendon autograft (single-bundle reconstruction), and hamstring autograft (usually used as one bundle of a double-bundle reconstruction) are all options.

Which technique should be used, tibial inlay or transtibial/tibial tunnel? Advocates of the tibial inlay technique suggest that the "killer turn" that occurs during the tibial tunnel approach, as the graft exits the tibia and turns toward the femoral tunnel(s) can be eliminated with this technique.

Tibial tunnel advocates suggest that the turn can be minimized if the bone block for the graft is placed at the proximal-most part of the tibial tunnel.

One or two femoral tunnels? Some authors have suggested that two femoral tunnels may be biomechanically superior, but there is a lack of clinical studies to support this.

Inside-out or outside-in drilling? Inside-out femoral tunnels tend to exit more proximally on the femur and therefore may create greater graft-bending angles.

The use of a brace after PCL reconstruction is still debated. This is true for the immediate postoperative period and later with return to activity.

Aggressive versus conservative rehabilitation? Prone ROM is emphasized early, and active motion is encouraged beginning at the 6-week postoperative visit.

What are the return to play criteria? This is surgeon dependent.

Special Considerations

Although unusual, pediatric PCL injuries do occur. In general, initial management should be similar to that in adults, but children may tolerate a PCL-deficient knee less well than adults.

It is possible to do a PCL tibial inlay reconstruction that completely avoids the physes. This technique uses the same approach as in an adult, but uses a quadruple hamstring graft that is looped under the tibial posteroanterior screw and soft-tissue washer and passes through a femoral tunnel below the physis. Figure 75.14A and B shows the AP and LAT radiographs of a pediatric physeal sparing PCL reconstruction.

PEARLS AND PITFALLS

Pearls

Extreme care is taken in padding the contralateral leg, especially if lateral decubitus positioning is used for the "down" leg.

For double bundle reconstructions, make sure the tunnels do not converge.

Use a probe or marked instrument to measure guide pin placement before overdrilling.

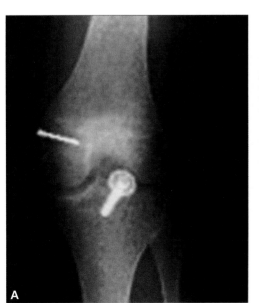
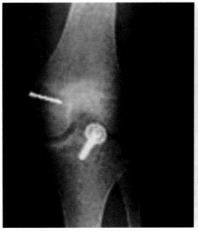
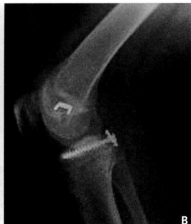

FIGURE 75.14. AP **(A)** and lateral **(B)** radiographs of a pediatric physeal-sparing PCL reconstruction. (From Miller MD, Cole BJ, Cosgarea A, et al. *Operative Techniques: Sports Knee Surgery.* Philadelphia, PA: Saunders Elsevier; 2008, with permission.)

For BPTB autograft, use a fluted drill bit and a sizer to save bone graft for later placement in the patella.

For tibial inlay procedures, the key to the approach is to mobilize the medial head of the gastrocnemius laterally. This muscle can be retracted with Steinmann pins that are drilled from posterior to anterior and bent over (Fig. 75.11).

If the graft hangs up during passage, it is helpful to pull it forward and then direct it into the femoral tunnel.

The knee should be cycled multiple times after graft passage and before fixation to remove any residual laxity.

Tension grafts before fixation.

The knee is cycled several times and then placed in 90° of flexion. The sutures from the bone block in the femur are tensioned while an anterior Drawer force is placed on the knee and a 9- × 20-mm interference screw is placed to secure the graft.

Confirm placement of all fixation devices (arthroscopically and/or fluoroscopically).

Backup all fixation.

Emphasis should be on extension and prone range of motion.

Pitfalls

Tibial inlay technique is contraindicated in patients who have had prior vascular procedures, especially those who have had remote vascular repairs.

Advanced DJD: This is a relative contraindication to knee ligament reconstruction.

Multiple ligament instability (including PLC): This injury may alter the timing and technique of PCL reconstruction. Planning must be done accordingly.

ACL injury: This injury may alter the timing and technique of PCL reconstruction. Planning must be done accordingly.

Extensor tendon injury: This is typically a more severe injury and needs to be addressed first.

For the inlay technique, make sure that you completely mobilize the medial had of the gastrocnemius to protect the popliteal neurovascular structures.

Failure to cycle and tension the graft.

Inadequate fixation.

Failure to regain motion early in the rehabilitation process leads to a poor outcome.

Failure to diagnose a PLC injury.

CONCLUSIONS AND FUTURE DIRECTIONS

PCL injuries are uncommon, but can result in an unstable knee and other unacceptable sequelae if not managed correctly. Early diagnosis of PCL injury is important to achieve an optimal result for the patient. This applies to both operative and nonoperative treatment. Rigorous workup helps in planning and execution of PCL reconstruction. The author believes that the tibial inlay technique produces the most anatomic PCL reconstruction, especially in patients with chronic PCL laxity.

SUGGESTED READINGS

Berg EE. Posterior cruciate ligament tibial inlay reconstruction. *Arthroscopy.* 1995;11:69–76.

Bergfeld JA, Graham SM, Parker RD, et al. A biomechanical comparison of posterior cruciate ligament reconstruction using single- and double-bundle tibial inlay techniques. *Am J Sports Med.* 2005;33:976–981.

Hocher J, Scheffler S, Weiler A. Graft choice and graft fixation in PCL reconstruction. *Knee Surg Sports Traumatol Arthrosc.* 2003;11:297–306.

Johnson DH, Fanelli GC, Miller MD. PCL 2002: indications, double-bundle versus inlay technique and revision surgery. *Arthroscopy.* 2002;18(9)(suppl 2):40–52.

Margheritini F, Mauro CS, Rihn JA, et al. Biomechanical comparison of tibial inlay versus transtibial techniques for posterior cruciate ligament reconstruction. *Am J Sports Med.* 2004;32:587–593

Markoff KL, Zemanovic JR, McAllister DR. Cyclic loading of posterior cruciate ligament replacements fixed with tibial tunnel and tibial inlay methods. *J Bone Joint Surg Am.* 2002;84:518–524.

Miller MD, Kline AJ, Gonzales J, et al. Vascular risk associated with a posterior approach for posterior cruciate ligament reconstruction using the tibial inlay technique. *J Knee Surg.* 2002;15:137–140.

Opening Wedge Tibial Osteotomy

Frank Noyes

INDICATIONS

High tibial osteotomy (HTO) has gained wide acceptance as a treatment option for patients with medial tibiofemoral osteoarthritis and varus deformity of the lower extremity. The recommendations for this procedure are derived from a careful evaluation of subjective symptoms, findings on physical examination, radiographic evidence of malalignment and arthritis, and gait analysis when available. Careful patient selection is the key issue and the surgeon should not overstate or guarantee results of an HTO because the arthritis will eventually progress. The goal is to buy time in younger patients prior to joint replacement.

The author prefers the opening wedge osteotomy technique because it avoids the lateral dissection and fibular osteotomy required in closing wedge osteotomy. The procedure is advantageous in knees that have chronic medial collateral ligament (MCL) deficiency where a distal advancement or reconstruction of the MCL is required. Knees requiring posterolateral reconstruction are candidates for opening wedge osteotomy in order to avoid a proximal fibular osteotomy because a fibular collateral ligament (FCL) graft will be secured to the proximal fibula. Opening wedge osteotomy is advantageous in cases of patella alta or decreased lower limb length, which would be made worse by a closing wedge osteotomy.

The major disadvantage of an opening wedge osteotomy is that an appropriate structural corticocancellous autograft or allograft is required to restore the anteromedial and posteromedial cortex, add fixation strength, and promote osseous union. Autogenous bone grafting of a larger open defect (>10 mm) aids in achieving stability at the osteotomy site, promotes prompt union with less time on crutches, and has a reduced risk of varus collapse due to a delayed union.

The predominant indication for HTO is lower limb varus osseous malalignment (weight-bearing line [WBL] <50% of tibial width) in patients under the age of 50 who have medial tibiofemoral joint pain and wish to maintain an active lifestyle. The patients have mild to moderate symptomatic arthrosis in the medial tibiofemoral compartment and retained articular cartilage. HTO is indicated to achieve normal limb alignment before medial meniscus transplantation, articular cartilage restorative procedures, and ligament reconstructions in double and triple varus knees (Fig. 76.1) (1, 2). The ligament deficiencies most commonly involve the anterior cruciate ligament (ACL) and posterolateral structures, including the FCL, popliteus muscle-tendon-ligament unit, and posterolateral capsule. Correction of the varus alignment decreases the risks of failure of the ligament reconstructive procedures (3, 4).

CONTRAINDICATIONS

HTO is contraindicated in knees in which there is more than a 15 by 15 mm area of exposed bone on both the tibial and the femoral surfaces. There are younger patients in whom the area of exposed bone may be larger and partial knee replacement is not an option. However, as a general rule, articular cartilage should be present over the majority of the medial joint surfaces. The difficult decision is the treatment recommendation for patients between 50 and 60 years of age. With the increasing longevity of unicompartmental knee replacements, patients who have advanced medial compartment damage with major areas of bone exposure will likely experience symptoms after HTO and are better candidates for partial knee replacement.

Major concavity of the medial tibial plateau with loss of bone stock is a contraindication to HTO. Knees that demonstrate (on standing 45° posteroanterior radiographs) no remaining articular cartilage space in the medial compartment are not candidates. Additional contraindications are a limitation of knee flexion (>10°), lateral tibial subluxation (>10 mm), prior lateral meniscectomy, or lateral tibiofemoral joint damage.

An absolute contraindication for a medial opening wedge osteotomy is the use of nicotine products in any form. A relative contraindication is obesity (body mass index >30) because unloading of the medial compartment will not be achieved. Another relative contraindication is increased medial slope to the affected medial tibial plateau

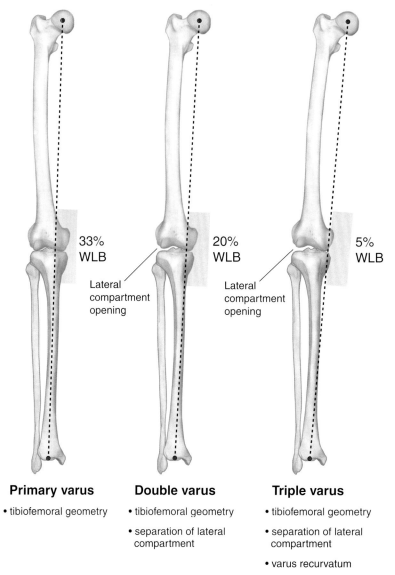

33%
WLB

Lateral
compartment
opening

20%
WLB

Lateral
compartment
opening

5%
WLB

Primary varus

• tibiofemoral geometry

Double varus

• tibiofemoral geometry

• separation of lateral
compartment

Triple varus

• tibiofemoral geometry

• separation of lateral
compartment

• varus recurvatum

FIGURE 76.1. Schematic illustration of primary, double, and triple varus knee angulation. WBL, weight-bearing line. (Reprinted from Noyes FR, Barber-Westin SD. Primary, double, and triple varus knee syndromes: diagnosis, osteotomy techniques, and clinical outcomes. In: Noyes FR, ed. *Noyes Knee Disorders: Surgery, Rehabilitation, Clinical Outcomes.* Philadelphia, PA: Saunders; 2009:821–895.)

in the coronal plane due to advanced medial plateau concavity. This finding indicates that it will not be possible to significantly unload the medial compartment, and a majority of the weight-bearing loads will be confined to the medial compartment. Marked patellofemoral symptoms contraindicate an HTO. Medical contraindications include diabetes, rheumatoid arthritis, autoimmune diseases, and malnutrition states.

CLINICAL EVALUATION

Patients complete questionnaires and are interviewed for the assessment of symptoms, functional limitations, sports and occupational activity levels, and patient perception of

the overall knee condition according to the Cincinnati Knee Rating System (5) or other validated knee rating instruments.

The physical examination of the knee joint to detect all of the abnormalities in the varus-angulated knee includes assessment of (1) the patellofemoral joint, especially extensor mechanism malalignment due to increased external tibial rotation and posterolateral tibial subluxation; (2) medial tibiofemoral crepitus on varus loading, indicative of articular cartilage damage; (3) pain and inflammation of the lateral soft tissues due to tensile overloading; (4) gait abnormalities (excessive hyperextension or varus thrust) during walking and jogging (6); and (5) abnormal knee motion limits and subluxations compared with the contralateral knee (7).

The medial posterior tibiofemoral step-off on the posterior drawer test is done at 90° of flexion. This test is performed first to determine that the tibia is not posteriorly subluxated, indicating a partial or complete posterior cruciate ligament (PCL) tear. The Lachman and pivot-shift tests are performed. FCL insufficiency is determined by the varus stress test at 0° and 30° of knee flexion. An increase in medial joint opening may occur compared with the opposite knee that represents a pseudolaxity, as the increase is actually due to medial tibiofemoral joint narrowing. The true amount of medial and lateral tibiofemoral

compartment opening is later confirmed during the arthroscopic examination with gap tests (Fig. 76.2).

The tibiofemoral rotation dial test (8) is used to estimate the amount of posterior tibial subluxation. A varus recurvatum test in both the supine and the standing positions as well as the reverse pivot shift test are included in the assessment of posterolateral tibial subluxation.

Radiographic assessment of lower limb alignment is based on double-stance, full-length anteroposterior radiographs showing both lower extremities (knee flexed 3° to 5°) from the femoral heads to the ankle joints (9).

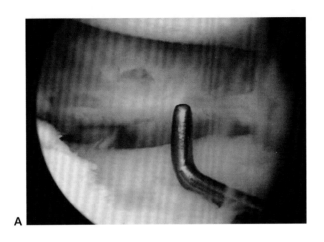

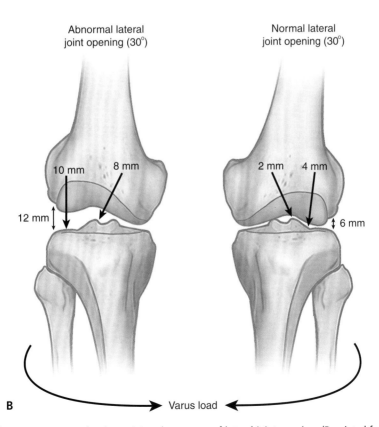

FIGURE 76.2. Arthroscopic gap test for determining the amount of lateral joint opening. (Reprinted from Noyes FR, Barber-Westin SD. Primary, double, and triple varus knee syndromes: diagnosis, osteotomy techniques, and clinical outcomes. In: Noyes FR, ed. *Noyes Knee Disorders: Surgery, Rehabilitation, Clinical Outcomes.* Philadelphia, PA: Saunders; 2009:821–895.)

If separation of the lateral tibiofemoral joint is observed, it is necessary to subtract the lateral compartment opening so that the true tibiofemoral osseous alignment is determined and a valgus overcorrection is avoided. Other radiographs include a lateral at 30° knee flexion, weight-bearing posteroanterior at 45° knee flexion, and patellofemoral axial views. Telos medial or lateral stress radiographs may also be required of both knees. The height of the right and left patella is measured on lateral radiographs to determine if an abnormal patella infera or alta position exists (1).

PREOPERATIVE PLANNING

The preoperative calculations for HTO involve precise measurements to determine the amount of angular correction desired to redistribute tibiofemoral forces, whereas not altering tibial slope and tibiofemoral joint obliquity in the frontal plane (Table 76.1) (1, 9, 10).

An under- or overcorrection in the coronal plane may result if the surgeon fails to recognize the effect of lateral tibiofemoral joint separation on increasing varus angulation that results from slack or deficient lateral soft tissues. Two methods are used to determine the correction wedge on preoperative radiographs, which have been described in detail elsewhere (Figs. 76.3 and 76.4) (9). Lateral radiographs are examined and measurements made of the tibial slope (10, 11).

There are patients who have a distinctly abnormal tibial slope from a prior osteotomy or tibial fracture, or growth abnormality where correction of the tibial

Table 76.1
Preoperative planning

Determine angular correction to achieve redistribution of tibiofemoral forces without altering tibial slope.
Take into account abnormal lateral tibiofemoral joint separation from deficient posterolateral structures.
Measure WBL on bilateral standing hip-knee-ankle radiographs:

— WBL is dependent on femoral and tibial lengths and angular deformity

Measure tibial slope on lateral radiographs.
Increasing tibial slope increases anterior tibial translation; potentially, tensile loads on the ACL.
Decreasing tibial slope increases posterior tibial translation; potentially, tensile loads on PCL.
Do not alter normal tibial slope unless it is markedly abnormal:

— Tibial slope greater than two standard deviations above normal

Do not alter a normal tibal slope in ACL-deficient or PCL-deficient knees.
Maintain normal tibial slope: anterior gap at medial opening wedge should be one-half the posteromedial gap.
  Every 1 mm of anterior gap change = 2° change in tibial slope.
Calculation of millimeters opening posteromedial tibial cortex based on law of triangles for coronal alignment
  correction.
Timing of HTO in knees with ligament deficiencies:

Primary varus knees:

— Cruciate reconstruction with HTO or later (no abnormal lateral joint opening present)

Double varus knees:

— HTO first
— Posterolateral structures may shorten with valgus alignment
— Perform cruciate, posterolateral reconstructions later if required

Triple varus knees:

— HTO first, cruciate and posterolateral reconstruction later

Opening wedge osteotomy advantages:

— Avoids lateral dissection, fibular osteotomy
— Large correction >12°, avoids tibial shortening
— Distal advancement or reconstruction of the MCL in chronic MCL ruptures
— In subsequent posterolateral reconstructions, avoids proximal fibular osteotomy, allows FCL grafts to be fixated securely to proximal fibula

From Noyes FR, Barber-Westin SD. Primary, double, and triple varus knee syndromes: diagnosis, osteotomy techniques, and clinical outcomes. In: Noyes FR, ed. *Noyes Knee Disorders: Surgery, Rehabilitation, Clinical Outcomes.* Philadelphia, PA: Saunders; 2009:821–895.

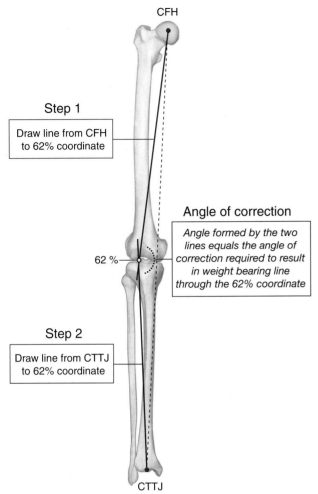

CFH

Step 1

Draw line from CFH to 62% coordinate

Angle of correction

Angle formed by the two lines equals the angle of correction required to result in weight bearing line through the 62% coordinate

62 %

Step 2

Draw line from CTTJ to 62% coordinate

CTTJ

FIGURE 76.3. Graphic depiction of the method used to calculate the correction angle of an HTO using a full-length anteroposterior radiograph of the lower extremity. The lines from the centers of the femoral head (CFH) and tibiotalar joint (CTTJ) converge in this example at the 62% coordinate. (Reprinted from Noyes FR, Barber-Westin SD. Primary, double, and triple varus knee syndromes: diagnosis, osteotomy techniques, and clinical outcomes. In: Noyes FR, ed. *Noyes Knee Disorders: Surgery, Rehabilitation, Clinical Outcomes.* Philadelphia, PA: Saunders; 2009:821–895.)

of triangles (Table 76.2) and confirmed at surgery. The surgeon should determine the proper gap width of the osteotomy opening wedge along the anteromedial cortex to maintain tibial slope and the proper width beneath the tibial plate based on its location along the anteromedial cortex (Table 76.3). The opening wedge gap will always be 3 to 4 mm less where the plate is located.

The timing of HTO and ligament reconstructive procedures is based on several factors discussed elsewhere (Fig. 76.6) (1). The author prefers to perform the HTO first and, after adequate healing of the osteotomy, the required ligament reconstructive procedures. The preferred grafts and operative techniques for ACL (12), PCL (13) and posterolateral ligament (14) reconstructions are described elsewhere.

OPERATIVE TECHNIQUE: OPENING WEDGE TIBIAL OSTEOTOMY

All knee ligament subluxation tests are performed after the induction of anesthesia in both the injured and the contralateral limbs. A thorough arthroscopic examination is conducted, documenting articular cartilage surface abnormalities and the condition of the menisci. The gap test is done during the arthroscopic examination. Knees that have 12 mm or more of joint opening at the periphery of the lateral tibiofemoral compartment will usually require a staged posterolateral reconstructive procedure. Associated meniscus tears are either repaired if possible (15) or partially removal. Appropriate debridement of tissues, inflamed synovium, and notch osteophytes limiting knee extension is performed.

Preoperative calculations are made as previously described. The entire lower extremity is prepped and draped free with the tourniquet placed high on the proximal thigh to assist visual observation of lower limb alignment. If an autogenous iliac crest autograft is to be performed (authors' choice), the ipsilateral anterior iliac crest is prepped and draped for the limited iliac crest bone harvest of the outer cortex.

The technique for the opening wedge osteotomy is summarized in Table 76.4 and has been described in detail elsewhere (1). The iliac crest bone harvest involves a 4-cm incision made over the anterior iliac crest and deepened to the periosteum (Fig. 76.7A and B). In most patients, the graft will be 40 mm in length, 10 mm in width, and 30 mm in depth. However, in smaller patients, the graft may be smaller in width, approximately 8 mm in depth. Patients undergoing large osteotomies may require a longer graft of approximately 45 to 50 mm. The inner iliac cortex is not dissected, the muscle attachments are not disturbed, which reduces postoperative pain, and a spacer of the iliac crest defect is not required.

The operative technique is shown in Figure 76.8. A 5-cm vertical skin incision is made medially midway

slope is required before cruciate ligament surgery or other conditions discussed. Empirically, a tibial slope greater than two standard deviations above normal (e.g., a tibial slope of 15° or greater) usually requires correction.

The rule to remember is that the anterior gap at the medial opening wedge should be one-half of the posteromedial gap to maintain a normal tibial slope (11). For every 1 mm of anterior gap change, an approximate 2° change in tibial slope would be produced (Fig. 76.5). This is based on the angle of the anteromedial tibial cortex, tibial width, and the Anteroposterior (AP) distance where the gap measurement is made. The millimeters of opening of the posteromedial tibial cortex is based on the law

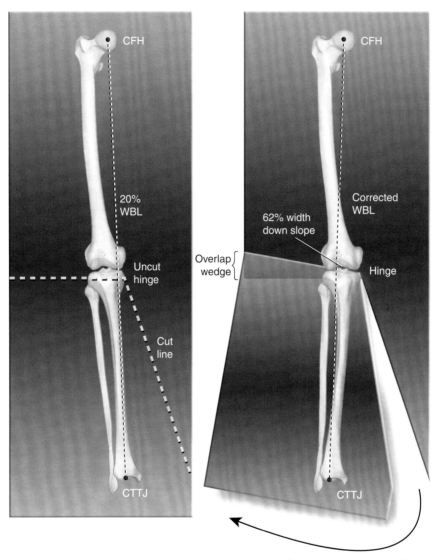

Rotate cut roentgenograph

FIGURE 76.4. Graphic depiction of an alternative method used to calculate the correction angle of an HTO using a full-length anteroposterior radiograph of the lower extremity. The roentgenograph is cut to allow the center of the femoral head (CFH), the 62% coordinate, and the center of the tibiotalar joint (CTTJ) to become colinear. The angle of the resulting wedge of roentgenograph overlap equals the desired angle of correction. The example is provided for a closing wedge osteotomy. The same technique is used for an opening wedge osteotomy where the medial tibial opening wedge is made to obtain the desired correction. (Reprinted from Noyes FR, Barber-Westin SD. Primary, double, and triple varus knee syndromes: diagnosis, osteotomy techniques, and clinical outcomes. In: Noyes FR, ed. *Noyes Knee Disorders: Surgery, Rehabilitation, Clinical Outcomes.* Philadelphia, PA: Saunders; 2009:821–895.)

between the tibial tubercle and the posteromedial tibial cortex, starting 1-cm inferior to the joint line. Once the dissection is complete, a Keith needle is placed in the anteromedial joint just above the tibia, and the distance is marked on the desired point of the osteotomy along the anteromedial cortex. A second Keith needle is placed at the posteromedial tibial joint space, and the same millimeters are marked to provide a measurement of the tibial slope. The two marks are connected to provide the osteotomy line perpendicular to the tibial slope.

A commercial guide system (Arthrex Opening Wedge Osteotomy System, Arthrex Inc., Naples, Florida) may be used to facilitate guide wire placement. The anterior and posterior guide pins are placed at 15° of obliquity to the tibial shaft and verified by intraoperative fluoroscopy or computerized navigation.

The surgeon ensures that the medial osteotomy line (from anterior to posterior) is in line with the tibial slope based on the radiographs and prior anteromedial cortex joint line measurements by the Keith needles. A

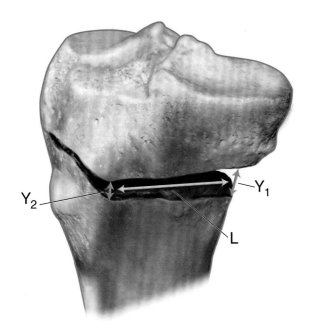

FIGURE 76.5. The opening wedge angle along the anteromedial tibial cortex can be calculated using the three linear measurements along the osteotomy opening wedge. Y_2 = posterior gap, Y_1 = gap anterior to Y_2, L = length between Y_1 and Y_2. (Reprinted from Noyes FR, Barber-Westin SD. Primary, double, and triple varus knee syndromes: diagnosis, osteotomy techniques, and clinical outcomes. In: Noyes FR, ed. *Noyes Knee Disorders: Surgery, Rehabilitation, Clinical Outcomes.* Philadelphia, PA: Saunders; 2009:821–895.)

(medial to lateral cortex) is measured and used following the law of triangles (11) to determine tibial width and the millimeters of osteotomy opening to obtain the desired angular correction.

The osteotomy is initially performed using an oscillating saw for the medial and anterior cortices, followed by a nonflexible thin 3/4- and 1/2-in osteotome, placed in the same orientation and anterior to the guide pin and verified by fluoroscopy. The lateral cortex is osteotomized to Gerdy's tubercle, leaving the posterolateral tibial cortex hinge. A 1/2-in osteotome is used for the posterior cortex, with the osteotome exposed 2 to 3 mm and viewed posterior to the tibia as the osteotome is advanced. The osteotomy is carried to within 10 mm of the posterolateral cortex.

Commercially available calibrated opening wedges are gently inserted into the osteotomy site to achieve the desired angular correction with the opening medial gap hinging on the intact posterolateral cortex. The spreader bars are inserted entirely across the osteotomy site to prevent a fracture extending into the lateral tibial plateau.

The anterior gap of the osteotomy site should be one-half of the posterior gap to maintain the tibial slope (11). The width of the tibial plate along the anteromedial cortex and just anterior to the superficial medial collateral ligament (SMCL) is measured and is always less than the millimeters at the posterior medial gap due to the angular inclination of the anteromedial tibial cortex.

The surgeon verifies by fluoroscopy or by computer navigation techniques that the desired limb alignment has been achieved. Obtaining an alignment correction

measurement of the perpendicular cut from the joint line confirms the distance of each guide pin from the articular surface of the tibia. The length of the posterior pin

Table 76.2

Millimeters of opening at the osteotomy site based on the width of the tibia and the angle of correction

TW[a]	\multicolumn{9}{c}{Degree of angular correction}
	5	6	7	8	9	10	11	12	13
50	4.37	5.25	6.15	7.00	8.00	8.80	9.70	10.85	11.55
55	4.81	5.78	6.77	7.70	8.80	9.68	10.67	11.94	12.71
60	5.25	6.30	7.38	8.40	9.60	10.56	11.64	13.02	13.86
65	5.69	6.83	8.00	9.10	10.40	11.44	12.61	14.11	15.02
70	6.12	7.35	8.61	9.80	11.20	12.32	13.58	15.19	16.17
75	6.56	7.88	9.23	10.50	12.00	13.20	14.55	16.28	17.33
80	7.00	8.40	9.84	11.20	12.80	14.08	15.52	17.36	18.48
85	7.44	8.93	10.46	11.90	13.60	14.96	16.49	18.45	19.64
90	7.87	9.45	11.07	12.60	14.40	15.84	17.46	19.53	20.79
95	8.31	9.98	11.69	13.30	15.20	16.72	18.43	20.62	21.95
100	8.75	10.50	12.30	14.00	16.00	17.60	19.40	21.70	23.10

[a]TW, coronal tibial width at osteotomy site.
From Noyes FR, Goeble SX, West J. Opening wedge tibial osteotomy: the 3-triangle method to correct axial alignment and tibial slope. *Am J Sports Med.* 2005;33:378–387.

Table 76.3

Opening wedge height of Y_2 gap based on tibial width (X_1)^a

Opening at Osteotomy (Y_1), mm	L (mm)	Tibial width at osteotomy (X_1), mm				
		50	55	60	65	70
8	0	8.0	8.0	8.0	8.0	8.0
	20	5.7	5.9	6.1	6.3	6.4
	25	5.2	5.4	5.6	5.8	6.0
	30	4.6	4.9	5.2	5.4	5.6
	35	4.0	4.4	4.7	5.0	5.2
	40	3.5	3.9	4.2	4.5	4.8
	45	2.9	3.4	3.8	4.1	4.4
10	0	10.0	10.0	10.0	10.0	10.0
	20	7.2	7.4	7.6	7.8	8.0
	25	6.5	6.8	7.1	7.3	7.5
	30	5.8	6.1	6.5	6.7	7.0
	35	5.1	5.5	5.9	6.2	6.5
	40	4.3	4.9	5.3	5.6	6.0
	45	3.6	4.2	4.7	5.1	5.5
12	0	12.0	12.0	12.0	12.0	12.0
	20	8.6	8.9	9.2	9.4	9.6
	25	7.8	8.1	8.5	8.7	9.0
	30	6.9	7.4	7.8	8.1	8.4
	35	6.1	6.6	7.1	7.4	7.8
	40	5.2	5.8	6.3	6.8	7.2
	45	4.4	5.1	5.6	6.1	6.5

^{a}By measuring the width of the tibia, the opening wedge height at the most medial point (Y_1), and the distance between vertical measurement points (L), the vertical height at the second measurement point (Y_2) where the plate implant can be found on the table. Calculations based on 45° angle of the anteromedial tibial cortex at osteotomy site.
From Noyes FR, Goeble SX, West J. Opening wedge tibial osteotomy: the 3-triangle method to correct axial alignment and tibial slope. *Am J Sports Med.* 2005;33:378–387.

in which the WBL is transferred to the lateral tibiofemoral compartment within the desired 50% to 62% range is the key to achieving short and long-term decreases in pain in the medial tibiofemoral compartment. The development of computerized navigation techniques to increase the accuracy of obtaining the desired tibial WBL and slope correction is, in the author's opinion, distinctly advantageous. Both fluoroscopy and computerized navigation techniques require defining accurate anatomic landmarks and precision to obtain accurate measurements. As well, it is necessary to perform axial loading at the foot to maintain closure of the medial and lateral tibiofemoral joints with the knee in 5° of flexion.

An appropriate plate is selected and secured. The author uses only a locking plate design (Fig. 76.9). The three corticocancellous bone graft triangular segments are fashioned based on direct measurements of the anterior and posterior widths at the osteotomy site. The three grafts are impacted tightly into the posterior, middle, and anterior portions of the osteotomy site to obliterate the space and

provide added stability, particularly in the sagittal plane. Fluoroscopy is used to confirm the final alignment and tibial slope.

The SMCL fibers are sutured distally and secured to either the plate or to suture anchors to maintain tension. The pes anserine tendons and sartorius fascia are reapproximated. The wound is closed in layers in the usual manner. The neurovascular status is immediately checked in the operating room and over the initial postoperative period. Close observation for lower limb soft tissue swelling is mandatory.

REHABILITATION

Patients receive instructions before surgery regarding the postoperative protocol (Table 76.5) so that they understand what is expected after the procedure (16). The supervised rehabilitation program is supplemented with home exercises that are performed daily. The therapist routinely examines the patient in the clinic postoperatively in order to progress the patient through the

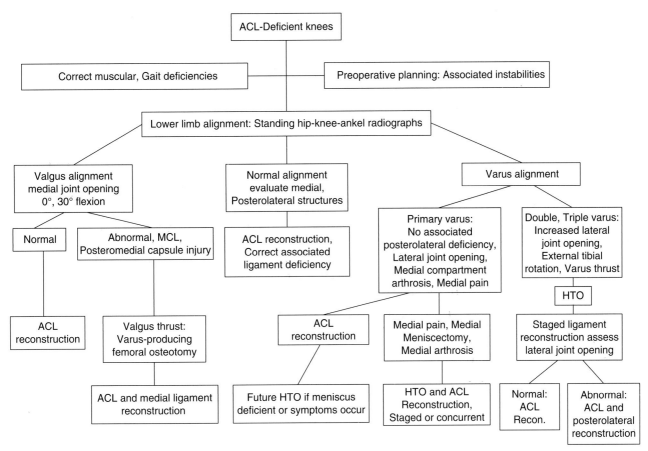

FIGURE 76.6. Timing of HTO and knee ligament reconstructive procedures. (Reprinted from Noyes FR, Barber-Westin SD. Primary, double, and triple varus knee syndromes: diagnosis, osteotomy techniques, and clinical outcomes. In: Noyes FR, ed. *Noyes Knee Disorders: Surgery, Rehabilitation, Clinical Outcomes.* Philadelphia, PA: Saunders; 2009:821–895.)

protocol in a safe and effective manner. Therapeutic procedures and modalities are used as required to achieve a successful outcome.

The overall goals of the osteotomy and rehabilitation are to control joint pain, swelling, and hemarthrosis; regain normal knee flexion and extension; resume a normal gait pattern and neuromuscular stability for ambulation; regain lower extremity muscle strength, proprioception, balance, and coordination for desired activities; and achieve the optimal functional outcome based on orthopedic and patient goals.

Immediately following surgery, the lower limb is wrapped with cotton with additional padding placed posteriorly, followed by a double compression and cotton bandage, postoperative hinged brace, and bilateral ankle-foot compression boots. A commercial ice delivery system is used with the bladder incorporated over the initial cotton wrapping, a few layers from the wound. A calf or foot compression system is used for the first 24 hours to promote venous blood flow. Aspirin is prescribed and, rarely in high-risk patients, Low molecular weight heparin (LMWH) or Coumadin (Bristol-Myers Squibb Company, Plainsboro, JN). During the first

postoperative week, patients are ambulatory for short periods, but are instructed to elevate their limb, remain home, and not resume usual activities.

Prophylaxis for deep venous thrombosis includes intermittent compression foot boots in both extremities, immediate knee motion exercises, antiembolism stockings, ankle pumps performed hourly, and aspirin (600 mg daily for 10 days). Doppler ultrasound is obtained if a patient demonstrates abnormal calf tenderness, a positive Homan's sign, or increased edema.

PREVENTION AND MANAGEMENT OF COMPLICATIONS

Excessive bone loss and concavity on the medial tibial plateau prohibits simultaneous weight-bearing on both plateaus following HTO, and results in an unstable knee in the coronal plane. A teeter effect occurs because tibiofemoral contact shifts, or teeters, from one plateau to the other depending on the relationship of the center of gravity to the center of the knee. Osteotomy is contraindicated when bone loss makes simultaneous contact of both plateaus impossible. Preoperative radiographic evaluation of

Table 76.4

Opening wedge osteotomy technique

Anterior iliac crest autograft harvest: meticulous dissection, remove outer cortex, do not disturb inner cortex or muscle attachments
— Harvest graft 40 mm in length, 10 mm in width, 30 mm in depth to produce three triangular bone grafts

HTO incision: 5-cm vertical medial tibia midway between tibial tubercle and posteromedial tibial cortex, starting 1-cm inferior to joint line

Partially detach gracilis and semitendinosus tendons at their tibial insertion, retract posteriorly exposing SMCL and posterior border of the tibia

Sharp periosteal incision anterior and posteromedial tibial border of the SMCL, meticulous subperiosteal dissection beneath the SMCL fibers. Protect inferior medial geniculate artery beneath the SMCL

Posterior tibial subperiosteal dissection to protect neurovascular structures. Wide dissection not necessary. Surgeon's headlight always used

Small osteotomies ≤5 mm, "pie-crust" procedure using multiple transverse incisions may effectively lengthen SMCL

Transect distal SMCL attachment, carefully elevate to the tibial border, protect and reattach after osteotomy. Prefer to maintain SMCL length rather than cut SMCL at osteotomy site

Keith needle placed anteriorly and posteriorly at the joint space to verify the tibial slope and medial sagittal osteotomy plane

Anterior and posterior guide pins placed at slight obliquity to tibial shaft (approximately 15°), verify position with fluoroscopy, mark osteotomy line along the anteromedial cortex

Ensure guide pins are at least 20 mm distal to the lateral joint line to prevent lateral tibial plateau fracture

Initial osteotomy with oscillating saw for medial and anterior cortices. Follow by nonflexible thin 3/4 in osteotome placed anterior, directly above the guide pin, verified by fluoroscopy. Perform osteotomy through opposite cortex at tibial tubercle

Use 1/2 in osteotome for posterior cortex, with osteotome edge visualized and palpated posterior to the tibia as the osteotome is advanced

Carry osteotomy to within 7–10 mm of the posterolateral cortex, confirm by fluoroscopy

Place thin spreader bars across osteotomy. Initial distraction requires several minutes to prevent fracture of the lateral cortex; if major resistance, place holes in lateral cortex with guide pin. Be careful not to produce fracture into lateral tibial plateau and joint. If resistance, carry osteotomy to lateral cortex (which is always preserved)

Use fluoroscopy to reestablish desired WBL correction of hip-knee-ankle tibial intersection line. Always close tibiofemoral medial and lateral joints by axial compression at foot with knee at 5° flexion

Computerized navigation techniques provide distinct advantage over fluoroscopy

Anterior gap of osteotomy should be 1/2 of the posterior gap to maintain tibial slope. Maintain osteotomy gap, use anterior tibial staple if necessary and posterior wedge, confirm alignment by fluoroscopy

Apply and fixate locking plate with fluoroscopy verification, confirm final coronal and sagittal (slope) alignment

Suture SMCL fibers distally and secure to either plate or by suture anchors to maintain tension. Reapproximate pes anserine tendons and sartorius fascia

Knees with chronic SMCL deficiency may require reconstruction

When the SMCL is advanced distally or reconstructed, incise, reset, and repair medial meniscus attachments

Modified from Noyes FR, Barber-Westin SD. Primary, double, and triple varus knee syndromes: diagnosis, osteotomy techniques, and clinical outcomes. In: Noyes FR, ed. *Noyes Knee Disorders: Surgery, Rehabilitation, Clinical Outcomes.* Philadelphia, PA: Saunders; 2009:821–895.

the bone loss on the tibial plateaus should be performed, specifically evaluating the slope of the plateaus to determine whether loading of both compartments will occur after HTO.

Inadequate or overcorrection of lower limb alignment has been reported after HTO. Loss of the axial alignment obtained at the time of surgery may be attributed to several factors. These include lack of internal fixation or the use of inadequate internal fixation

with collapse of the distal fragments settling into the cancellous bone of the plateau. Late drifting into a varus position may be due to a progressive loss of the medial osteochondral cartilage complex, or to stretching of the posterolateral structures.

Careful preoperative planning is required to avoid inadequate correction, which begins with the calculation of the mechanical or anatomical axis using full-length standing radiographs. During surgery, confirmation of adequate

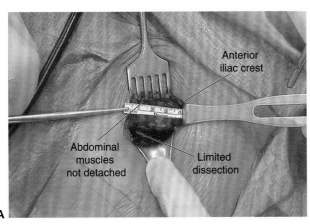
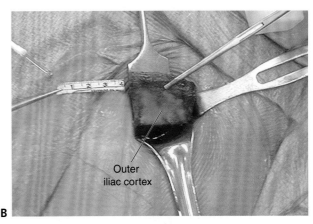

FIGURE 76.7. **A:** A 4-cm incision over the anterior iliac crest is made to harvest the iliac crest bone graft. The graft is comprised of the anterior crest and outer iliac cortex; the inner table is not removed. **B:** The usual iliac crest bone graft dimensions are 40 mm in length, 10 to 12 mm in width, and 30 mm in depth. (Reprinted from Noyes FR, Barber-Westin SD. Primary, double, and triple varus knee syndromes: diagnosis, osteotomy techniques, and clinical outcomes. In: Noyes FR, ed. *Noyes Knee Disorders: Surgery, Rehabilitation, Clinical Outcomes.* Philadelphia, PA: Saunders; 2009:821–895.)

correction that was determined by preoperative measurements is done using fluoroscopy or computer navigation. Even though an ideal position may be verified at surgery, a change in alignment may be detected when postoperative standing radiographs are obtained. The alignment should be verified by the fourth postoperative week under partial weight-bearing conditions.

Delayed union or nonunion has been reported following HTO. In opening wedge osteotomies, a stable construct created by the use of an iliac crest autogenous bone graft (in the anterior, mid, and posterior portions of the osteotomy) and appropriate plate fixation with protection of the lateral tibial buttress (cortex) will sustain postoperative compressive and torsional loads. In summary, the efficacy of allograft or other bone substitute materials for opening wedge osteotomy has not been adequately determined, even though the introduction of commercially available triangular-shaped cortical-cancellous allografts (along with rigid plate designs), has led to their increased usage.

Plates with different designs should be available during surgery. A locking osteotomy plate and screws with an autogenous bone graft and intact lateral cortex pillar provides prompt union without loss of correction. Plate designs that incorporate locking screws provide added stability and are necessary in cases of any violation of the lateral tibial cortex to maintain stability under axial compressive or torsional loads. An alternative fixation method for a lateral tibial cortex fracture at osteotomy is to add a lateral two-hole plate through a separate incision.

The rehabilitation program allows toe-touch weight-bearing during the first 4 weeks and then allows progression over the next 4 weeks to full weight-bearing based on radiographic signs of osteotomy healing. A delayed union

can be treated, if the overall alignment is acceptable, by electric stimulation.

Peroneal nerve palsy may result from several causes; the most common is a cast or bandage, which is applied too tightly after surgery. The use of internal fixation alleviates the need for casting. The nerve may also be directly injured during surgery.

Postoperatively, lateral radiographs are taken to detect any decrease in the patellar vertical height ratio; these are repeated for any patient who shows early signs of developmental patella infera (inability to perform a strong quadriceps contraction after surgery, decreased patellar mobility, decreased palpable tension in the patellar tendon with failure of the patella to displace proximally on quadriceps contraction, or distal malposition of the involved patella compared with the opposite side). Rigid internal fixation should also help to reduce the occurrence of arthrofibrosis and a resultant patella infera.

An immediate knee motion program and exercise protocol of straight leg raises, multiangle isometrics, and electrical muscle stimulation (EMS) are advocated to decrease the incidence of quadriceps weakness and knee motion limitation following HTO. In addition, a phased treatment program is begun for limitations of motion early in the postoperative course when restriction of either extension or flexion is noted.

Most if not all of the complications described in the literature related to iliac crest bone graft harvest may be avoided by the surgical technique described in this chapter. For example, the dissection is limited to include only 10 mm of the superior iliac crest. A meticulous subperiosteal exposure of the outer iliac crest is performed without violating the inner muscle attachments. The inner iliac cortex is never dissected, and the muscle attachments are kept intact. This minimally invasive harvest

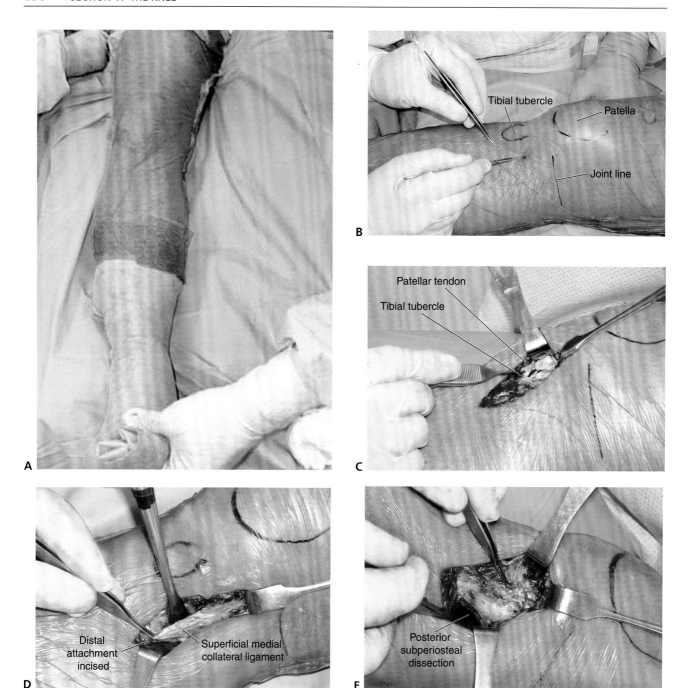

FIGURE 76.8. **A:** Initial draping of varus-aligned lower extremity with right iliac crest draped for bone graft. **B:** Incision location, anterior one-third of medial tibia. **C:** Initial exposure beneath patella tendon under retraction. **D:** Initial subperiosteal dissection SMCL. The distal attachment has been incised. **E:** Posterior subperiosteal exposure to protect neurovascular structures. **F:** Placement of navigation femoral and tibial markers. **G:** A Keith needle placed at the anterior, and later posterior, aspect of the joint line is used to outline the planned osteotomy. **H:** Two guide pins are placed under fluoroscopic control. **I:** A thin osteotomy blade is placed under fluoroscopic control. Different width blades are used to complete the osteotomy within 8 mm of the lateral cortex. **J:** Initial posterior cortex osteotomy using thin power saw under direct visualization. **K:** Completion of posterior cortex osteotomy to within 8 mm of posterolateral cortex. **L:** Initial gentle dislocation of osteotomy. **M:** Guide pin perforation of dense posterolateral tibial cortex to weaken bone due to failure of the osteotomy gap to increase under gentle dislocation. **N:** Further dislocation of osteotomy site. **O:** Use of computerized navigation to monitor valgus alignment. **P:** Staple is placed anterior tibial gap to control tibial slope. **Q:** Initial fixation of osteotomy, maintaining measure osteotomy correction. **R:** Confirmation of anterior and posterior osteotomy gap measurement. **S:** Bicortical iliac crest autografts. **T:** Placement of anterior, central, and posterior iliac crest autografts. **U:** Fixation anterior border SMCL to tibial plate. (Reprinted from Noyes FR, Barber-Westin SD. Primary, double, and triple varus knee syndromes: diagnosis, osteotomy techniques, and clinical outcomes. In: Noyes FR, ed. *Noyes Knee Disorders: Surgery, Rehabilitation, Clinical Outcomes.* Philadelphia, PA: Saunders; 2009:821–895.)

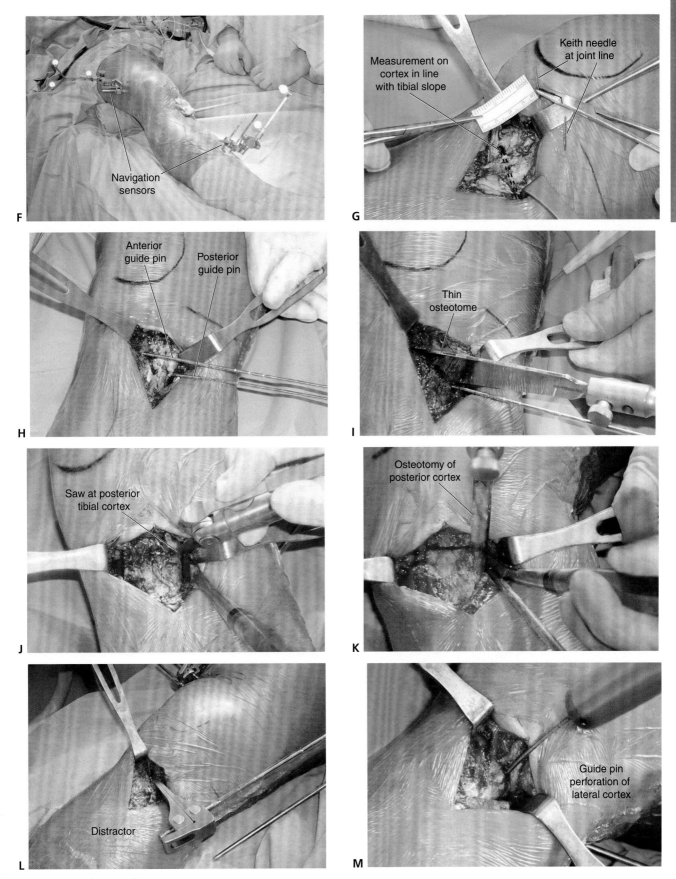

FIGURE 76.8. (continued)

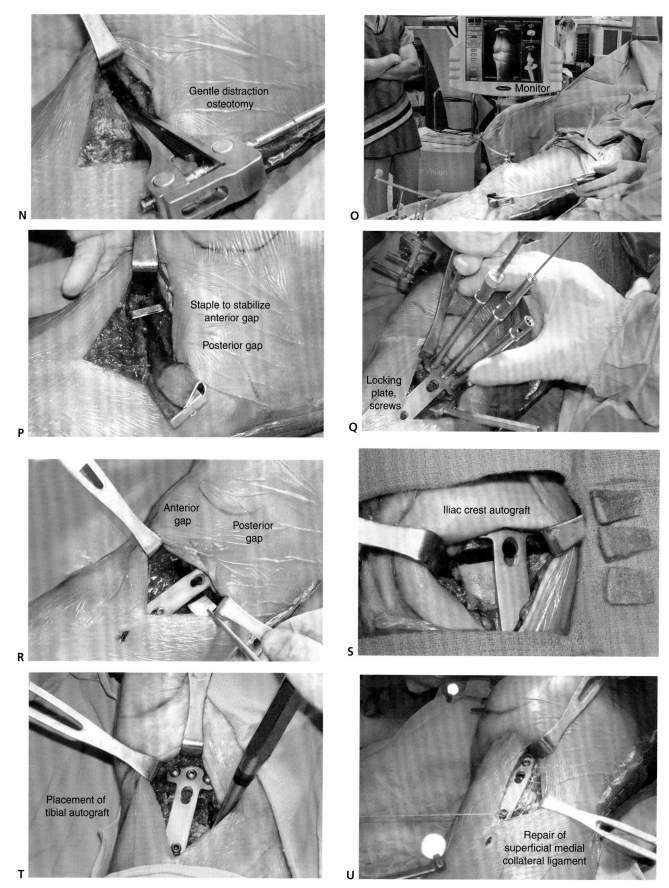

FIGURE 76.8. (continued)

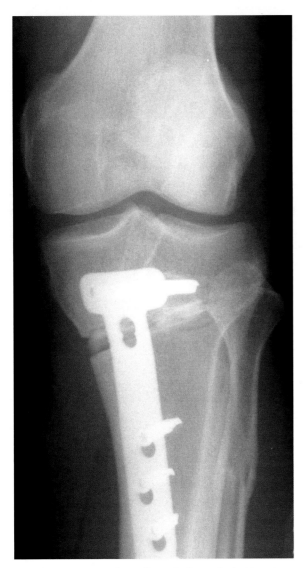

FIGURE 76.9. Postoperative radiograph shows the locking plate and screw fixation with a bone graft within the opening wedge. The lateral tibial cortex at the osteotomy site is intact. Full standing radiographs confirm the desired correction. (Reprinted from Noyes FR, Heckmann T, Barber-Westin SD. Rehabilitation after tibial and femoral osteotomy. In: Noyes FR, ed. *Noyes Knee Disorders: Surgery, Rehabilitation, Clinical Outcomes.* Philadelphia, PA: Saunders; 2009:905–914.)

technique avoids the frequency of complications reported by larger exposures, such as those used for spine fusions.

AUTHOR'S CLINICAL STUDY

A prospective study was conducted of 59 consecutive patients who had a medial opening-wedge proximal tibial osteotomy (10). The patients were followed a mean of 20 months postoperatively (range, 6 to 60 months). Independent physicians examined radiographs pre- and postoperatively for tibial slope and patellar height, and postoperatively for bony union. Postoperative

radiographs were taken at 4 and 8 weeks postoperative, and then as required until bone consolidation was evident. Delayed union was defined as lack of bridging callous and presence of radiolucent areas within the opening wedge defect past a period of 3 months postoperatively. Knee ligament reconstructions were commonly performed.

Healing and union at the osteotomy site was radiographically evident an average of 3 months postoperatively in 52 patients (95%). A delay in union (with no loss of fixation or correction) occurred in three patients (5%). The size of the opening wedge osteotomy in these three patients ranged from 11.0 to 16 mm. In two of these patients, a bone stimulator was applied, and union was achieved by 6 to 8 months postoperatively. The other patient achieved union without intervention by 10 months.

An early postoperative loss of fixation occurred in one patient who admitted to full weight-bearing immediately after surgery. The osteotomy was successfully revised 10 days postoperatively and proceeded uneventfully to union. There were no instances of shortening of the patellar tendon related to a patella infera syndrome. Full weight-bearing was achieved a mean of 8 weeks (range, 4 to 11 weeks) postoperatively.

There was no significant difference between the mean preoperative (9° ± 4°; range, 2° to 16°) and the postoperative (10° ± 3°; range, 3° to 21°) tibial slope measurements. There were no deep infections, loss of knee motion requiring intervention, deep vein thrombosis, nerve or arterial injury, fracture, or complications related to bone grafting.

Additional published studies from the author's Center have reported outcomes in patients undergoing closing wedge HTO for double and triple varus knee syndromes. (2,17) In one study, (2) 18 patients (44%) had severe to moderate pain with activities of daily living before the HTO while at follow-up, only 7 (17%) had such pain. Overall, 29 patients (71%) improved their pain score and 28 (68%) improved their swelling and scores. Giving-way was eliminated in 85%. Twenty-seven patients (66%) were able to return to mostly low-impact athletics without symptoms.

HTO has a beneficial effect if done in properly indicated, younger patients and some authors have reported 85% to 92% 10-year survival rates (18–20). Functional limitations and symptoms with daily activities such as walking and stair climbing are typically reported in most patients before HTO. The majority of studies report pain relief and improvement in these limitations, making patient satisfaction high. In one of the author's studies, 88% of the patients stated they would undergo the operation again, 78% returned to light sports activities, and 78% had significant improvements in the Cincinnati Knee Rating overall rating score.

Table 76.5

Rehabilitation following high tibial or femoral osteotomy

Brace	Postoperative Weeks					Postop Months		
	1–2	3–4	5–6	7–8	9–12	4	5	6
Long-leg postoperative	X	X	X	X	X			
Unloading						(X)	(X)	(X)
Range of motion minimum goals								
0°–110°	X							
0°–130°		X						
0°–135°			X					
Weight-bearing								
None to toe touch	X	X						
1/4 to 1/2 body weight			X					
Full (fracture site healed)				X	(X)			
Patella mobilization	X	X	X	X				
Modalities								
EMS	X	X	X	X				
Pain/edema management (cryotherapy)	X	X	X	X	X	X	X	X
Stretching								
Hamstring, gastrocsoleus, iliotibial band, quadriceps	X	X	X	X	X	X	X	X
Strengthening								
Quad isometrics, straight leg raises, active knee extension	X	X	X	X	X			
Closed chain: gait retraining, toe raises, wall sits, minisquats		(X)	X	X	X	X		
Knee flexion hamstring curls (90°)			X	X	X	X	X	X
Knee extension quads (90°–30°)				X	X	X	X	X
Hip abduction-adduction, multihip				X	X	X	X	X
Leg press (70°–10°)			X	X	X	X	X	X
Balance/proprioceptive training								
Weight-shifting, minitrampoline, BAPS, BBS, plyometrics				X	X	X	X	X
Conditioning								
UBC		X	X	X				
Bike (stationary)			X	X	X	X	X	X
Aquatic program			X	X	X	X	X	X
Swimming (kicking)					X	X	X	X
Walking					X	X	X	X
Stair climbing machine					X	X	X	X
Ski machine					X	X	X	X
Recreational activities								X

BAPS, Biomechanical Ankle Platform System (Camp, Jackson, MI); BBS, Biodex Balance System (Biodex Medical Systems, Inc., Shirley, NY); UBC, upper body cycle (Biodex Medical Systems, Inc., Shirley, NY).
From Noyes FR, Heckmann, T, Barber-Westin SD. Rehabilitation after tibial and femoral osteotomy. In: Noyes FR, ed. *Noyes Knee Disorders: Surgery, Rehabilitation, Clinical Outcomes.* Philadelphia, PA: Saunders; 2009:905–914.

REFERENCES

1. Noyes FR, Barber-Westin SD. Primary, double, and triple varus knee syndromes: diagnosis, osteotomy techniques, and clinical outcomes. In: Noyes FR, ed. *Noyes Knee Disorders: Surgery, Rehabilitation, Clinical Outcomes*. Philadelphia, PA: Saunders; 2009:821–895.

2. Noyes FR, Barber-Westin SD, Hewett TE. High tibial osteotomy and ligament reconstruction for varus angulated anterior cruciate ligament-deficient knees. *Am J Sports Med*. 2000;28(3):282–296.

3. Noyes FR, Barber-Westin SD. Posterior cruciate ligament revision reconstruction, part 1: causes of surgical failure in 52 consecutive operations. *Am J Sports Med*. 2005;33(5):646–654.

4. Noyes FR, Barber-Westin SD. Revision anterior cruciate surgery with use of bone-patellar tendon-bone autogenous grafts. *J Bone Joint Surg Am*. 2001;83-A(8):1131–1143.

5. Barber-Westin SD, Noyes FR, McCloskey JW. Rigorous statistical reliability, validity, and responsiveness testing of the Cincinnati knee rating system in 350 subjects with uninjured, injured, or anterior cruciate ligament-reconstructed knees. *Am J Sports Med*. 1999;27(4):402–416.

6. Noyes FR, Dunworth LA, Andriacchi TP, et al. Knee hyperextension gait abnormalities in unstable knees. Recognition and preoperative gait retraining. *Am J Sports Med*. 1996;24(1):35–45.

7. Noyes FR, Grood ES, Torzilli PA. Current concepts review. The definitions of terms for motion and position of the knee and injuries of the ligaments. *J Bone Joint Surg Am*. 1989;71(3):465–472.

8. Noyes FR, Stowers SF, Grood ES, et al. Posterior subluxations of the medial and lateral tibiofemoral compartments. An in vitro ligament sectioning study in cadaveric knees. *Am J Sports Med*. 1993;21(3):407–414.

9. Dugdale TW, Noyes FR, Styer D. Preoperative planning for high tibial osteotomy: the effect of lateral tibiofemoral separation and tibiofemoral length. *Clin Orthop Relat Res*. 1992;274:248–264.

10. Noyes FR, Mayfield W, Barber-Westin SD, et al. Opening wedge high tibial osteotomy: an operative technique and rehabilitation program to decrease complications and promote early union and function. *Am J Sports Med*. 2006;34(8):1262–1273.

11. Noyes FR, Goebel SX, West J. Opening wedge tibial osteotomy: the 3-triangle method to correct axial alignment and tibial slope. *Am J Sports Med*. 2005;33(3):378–387.

12. Noyes FR, Barber-Westin SD. Anterior cruciate ligament primary and revision reconstruction: diagnosis, operative techniques, and clinical outcomes. In: Noyes FR, ed. *Noyes Knee Disorders: Surgery, Rehabilitation, Clinical Outcomes*. Philadelphia, PA: Saunders; 2009:140–228.

13. Noyes FR, Barber-Westin SD. Posterior cruciate ligament: diagnosis, operative techniques, and clinical outcomes. In: Noyes FR, ed. *Noyes Knee Disorders: Surgery, Rehabilitation, Clinical Outcomes*. Philadelphia, PA: Saunders; 2009:503–576.

14. Noyes FR, Barber-Westin SD. Posterolateral ligament injuries: diagnosis, operative techniques, and clinical outcomes. In: Noyes FR, ed. *Noyes Knee Disorders: Surgery, Rehabilitation, Clinical Outcomes*. Philadelphia, PA: Saunders; 2009:577–630.

15. Rubman MH, Noyes FR, Barber-Westin SD. Technical considerations in the management of complex meniscus tears. *Clin Sports Med*. 1996;15(3):511–530.

16. Noyes FR, Heckmann TP, Barber-Westin SD. Rehabilitation after tibial and femoral osteotomy. In: Noyes FR, ed. *Noyes Knee Disorders: Surgery, Rehabilitation, Clinical Outcomes*. Philadelphia, PA: Saunders; 2009:905–914.

17. Noyes FR, Barber SD, Simon R. High tibial osteotomy and ligament reconstruction in varus angulated, anterior cruciate ligament-deficient knees. A two- to seven-year follow-up study. *Am J Sports Med*. 1993;21(1):2–12.

18. Flecher X, Parratte S, Aubaniac JM, et al. A 12–28-year followup study of closing wedge high tibial osteotomy. *Clin Orthop Relat Res*. 2006;452:91–96.

19. Hernigou P, Ma W. Open wedge tibial osteotomy with acrylic bone cement as bone substitute. *Knee*. 2001;8(2):103–110.

20. Koshino T, Yoshida T, Ara Y, et al. Fifteen to twenty-eight years' follow-up results of high tibial valgus osteotomy for osteoarthritic knee. *Knee*. 2004;11(6):439–444.

Combined Ligament Injuries of the Knee: Anterior Cruciate Ligament/Posterolateral Corner and Medial Collateral Ligament/ Posterior Cruciate Ligament: Diagnosis, Treatment, and Rehabilitation

Mark McCarthy • Lawrence Camarda • Jill Monson • Robert F. LaPrade

Multiligament knee injuries present challenging scenarios for orthopedic surgeons. Advanced physical exam skills are required to focus in on specific ligamentous structures, followed by radiographic imaging that can be complicated to evaluate. The decision to operate or to treat conservatively requires advanced knowledge of classification systems and applying them to tailor to each individual patient. The surgical procedures themselves are technically challenging and demand precision. Finally, the surgeon and patient must be prepared for a long rehabilitation process and treat any complications that may arise. This chapter is designed to be an outline to diagnose and treat two specific patterns of multiligament knee injuries: the anterior cruciate ligament (ACL)/posterolateral corner (PLC) and the medial collateral ligament (MCL)/posterior cruciate ligament (PCL).

ACL/PLC INJURIES

Introduction

PLC injuries are challenging to diagnose and treat. When faced in clinical practice with an acute knee injury, it is vital to keep injuries to the PLC structures in mind throughout the patient encounter. It is well known that injuries to the ACL are common. However, it has also been reported that ACL tears occur, quite commonly, as part of a multiple ligament injury pattern (1, 2). The section of the chapter is dedicated to give hints on the history and physical exam to heighten a clinician's awareness of a possible underlying PLC injury in the setting of an ACL tear, as well as imaging and treatment options of this difficult injury pattern.

Clinical Evaluation

History

Most PLC injuries occur in the setting of other ligament injuries, with the ACL/PLC combination being one of the most common patterns (2). The mechanism of injury is often a hyperextension varus injury (a blow to the anteromedial knee). Patients will often report a sense of instability with everyday activities, especially for positions where the injured knee is in extension. In addition, a thorough history should include questions regarding the functioning of the common peroneal nerve, both for sensation and for motor function, because the literature has reported a 15% incidence of concomitant common peroneal nerve injuries with PLC injuries (2). Any reported numbness, tingling, or weakness with ankle dorsiflexion and/or great toe extension should be dutifully noted.

Physical Exam

After inspecting and palpating the knee for an effusion and tenderness, a focused knee exam to assess its stability should be performed. A straightforward initial test is the external rotation recurvatum test (3). With the patient supine, the clinician lifts the lower extremity by the patient's great toe, with the other hand holding the patient's thigh as needed to assess for knee hyperextension. Increased recurvatum, or hyperextension, often indicates a severe multiligament injury, often involving the ACL, but is also seen when both cruciate ligaments are injured and/or a disruption of the PLC structures exists. In one study of 134 consecutive patients with posterolateral knee injuries, 10 patients demonstrated a positive external rotation recurvatum test. All 10 of these patients had a combined ACL/PLC injury pattern (3). Further, this same study found that 30% of patients with a combined ACL/PLC insufficiency pattern had a positive external recurvatum test. When comparing with the contralateral normal lower extremity, measurements can be taken based on increased heel height differences of the affected leg.

To further specifically assess the PLC, it is helpful to perform the varus stress test, both at 0° and at 30° of knee flexion. To most accurately define the amount of abnormal motion due to injury, the test is best done at 0° by stabilization of the thigh against the examining table and then applying a varus force across the knee by grasping the foot or ankle. At 30°, the leg can be brought over the side of the exam table, with the thigh again stabilized against the table, and a varus force applied (Fig. 77.1). The contralateral knee must be examined to assess for any physiologic varus laxity. The clinician's fingers should be placed at the lateral joint line to estimate the amount of lateral joint space opening. Injuries are graded 1, 2, and 3 based on lateral compartment gapping in millimeters, progressing from lower grades indicating partial tears to higher grades that often indicate complete tears of posterolateral structures. To quantify this more accurately, an *in vitro* study in which PLC structures were sequentially sectioned was performed to simulate isolated PLC injuries and combined cruciate ligament injuries. When an isolated fibular collateral ligament injury was simulated, the average increase in lateral joint space opening with an applied varus stress was 2.7 mm. This increased to 4.0 mm for grade 3 PLC injuries (4). A positive varus stress test at 0° often implies a severe PLC injury in addition to a cruciate ligament injury because the stabilizing effect of the cruciates in full extension is lost.

To assess the integrity of the ACL, the Lachman test is performed with the knee in 15° to 25° of flexion. ACL tears are graded as mild, moderate, and severe based on the approximate displacement found and, again, compared with the contralateral knee. When combined with a PLC injury, the Lachman test becomes more pronounced,

both in reproducible displacement and in relative instability. A pivot shift test can be performed as well, with greater subluxation often indicating a possible combined posterolateral knee injury and ACL tear. Here, the clinician loads the leg with an axial/valgus force. As the knee is brought from extension to flexion, the subluxed knee undergoes reduction due to the stabilizing effect of the iliotibial band at approximately 20° to 30° of knee flexion.

The posterolateral drawer test is helpful to establish the amount of posterolateral rotation of the knee. Like the posterior drawer test, the knee is not only flexed to 90° but also externally rotated approximately 15° to better isolate the popliteus complex. Increased posterolateral rotation compared with the other knee is often seen with popliteus complex injuries. As an adjunct to the posterolateral drawer test, the reverse pivot shift test, which is basically a dynamic posterolateral drawer test, can be performed as well. Here, the knee is flexed to approximately 45°, with a valgus stress applied as the knee is brought out into extension. For a positive test, the knee sits subluxed in flexion and is reduced by the iliotibial band at around 30°.

The dial test, or tibial external rotation test, is done at 30° and 90° of knee flexion with the patient either prone or supine (5). While stabilizing the thigh, the lower leg is externally rotated at both positions (Fig. 77.2). Increased external rotation of at least 15° at 30° of knee flexion compared with the normal contralateral knee indicates a severe PLC injury. If this injury is an isolated PLC injury, the external rotation should decrease to about 5° at 90° of knee flexion. If the amount of external rotation at 90° of knee flexion remains around 15°, a combined PCL/PLC injury pattern is likely.

Imaging

Radiographic images are necessary to precisely define the injury pattern and assist in preoperative planning. Some nonspecific X-ray findings that suggest a PLC injury include a Segond fracture, or bony avulsion of the capsule from the mid-third lateral tibial plateau. Also, an arcuate fracture,

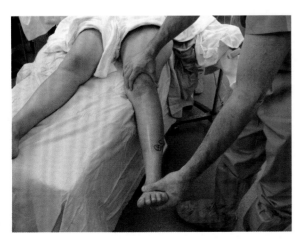

FIGURE 77.1. Varus stress test at 30°: Note the stabilization of the thigh.

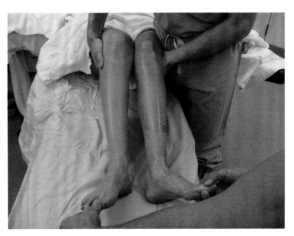

FIGURE 77.2. Dial test at 30°: Excess external rotation observed, indicating severe PLC injury and high likelihood of multiligament involvement.

an avulsion of the fibular head, and styloid at the attachment sites of the PLC structures are best viewed on plain radiographs, whereas the associated ligaments attached to the avulsion fracture, however, are best viewed on coronal and sagittal MRI images (6). Varus stress X-rays at 20° of knee flexion can be performed to more accurately assess lateral joint space gapping (Fig. 77.3). To reiterate, gapping greater than 4 mm has been found to correlate with grade 3 PLC injuries (4). Although X-rays are an appropriate imaging study to begin the radiographic assessment, the preferred imaging modality for acute injuries is an MRI.

MRI has been proven to consistently identify specific PLC structures and also injuries to these structures (6) This is a pivotal aspect of each clinician's diagnostic workup. In an acutely injured knee, it may be challenging, even impossible, to reliably diagnose PLC structure injuries due to patient guarding and other associated injuries. This is critical in operative planning, not only because of the high incidence of concurrent ACL/PLC injuries (1, 2) but also because reconstructing one's ACL without recognition of PLC structure insufficiency is a known cause of ACL graft failure (7).

Decision Making

Once a diagnosis has been made, treatment thereafter is largely based on a few general principles. The severity of the injury, as delineated by the grading system described below, is a major component in deciding to pursue an operative or nonoperative treatment plan. Grade 1 and 2 injuries are typically treated nonoperatively, as described below.

If a surgical intervention is deemed appropriate, the timing of that surgery based on the date of injury becomes important. For injuries less than 3 weeks old (acute injuries), primary repair of the PLC structures is recommended if possible. When injuries have occurred longer than 2 months from the time of surgery (chronic injuries), it is appropriate to perform an anatomic reconstruction. Again, in the setting of a combined ACL/PLC injury, it is necessary to reconstruct the ACL in combination with the PLC for a better functional outcome. Should the chronic PLC injury be present with a combined genu varus malalignment, the patient should undergo a valgus-producing, opening-wedge high-tibial osteotomy prior to PLC reconstruction.

Classification

PLC injuries are typically graded 1, 2, and 3. Grade 1 injuries have minimal disruption of the PLC structures and are not associated with significant increases in abnormal joint movement. Grade 2 injuries have partial tearing and moderate abnormal joint motion. Grade 3 PLC injuries are associated with complete disruption of PLC structures and markedly abnormal joint movement (8). To further quantify ligamentous laxity, some authors describe using 1+, 2+, and 3+ in regard to instability of the PLC, (9) along with varus joint space gapping, described above (3) The treatment of these injuries based on their grade is discussed in the next section.

Treatment

Nonoperative Treatment

It is recommended to treat grade 1 and 2 PLC injuries nonoperatively initially. Studies have found this to yield good results. One study had seven patients diagnosed

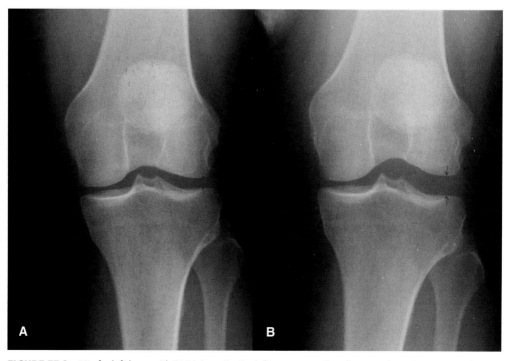

FIGURE 77.3. AP of a left knee with PLC injury: On the left, nonstress view shows no lateral space gapping. On the right, varus stress opens up the lateral space, indicating PLC structural damage.

with 1+ varus instability who were treated nonoperatively. Six of those patients were completely stable on follow-up, with one, treated with a plaster cast, having persistent 1+ varus instability (10). In another study, 11 patients with grade 2 PLC injuries treated nonoperatively were analyzed at an average follow-up of 8 years and had good results (11).

For nonoperative treatment, the patient is placed into a knee immobilizer in full extension for 3 to 4 weeks with no knee motion permitted. The patient is instructed on performing quadriceps sets and straight leg raises in the immobilizer. Further more, strict nonweight-bearing status is kept during this period. Thereafter, the patient begins range of motion (ROM) and weight bearing as tolerated. Once patients can ambulate without a limp, they may be off crutches. For 6 to 10 weeks, patients are not allowed any active hamstring exercises. Closed-chain quadriceps exercises are allowed during this time. It is important to remember that this treatment plan only concerns conservative management of the PLC structures. In cases of concomitant ACL insufficiency, it is recommended to perform a reconstruction to achieve better stability.

Special circumstances arise when treating highly trained athletes with grade 1 or 2 PLC injuries. For these athletes, a medial compartment unloader brace can be used to allow them to return to competition sooner. In these conditions, they are required to wear the unloader brace at all times except to shower. In most cases, athletes are able to return to competition within 2 to 3 weeks. Varus stress radiographs are necessary in following these patients to verify that the partially torn Fibular collated ligament (FCL) does not stretch out with this program.

Operative Treatment

Acute injury operative treatment

Acute primary repair of the PLC should be performed within the first 2 weeks following the injury. Once past 3 weeks from the injurious event, it has been found that significant scar tissue planes develop within the posterolateral knee, tissues become retracted, and tissues no longer hold sutures well (5).

The PLC of the knee can be adequately exposed through a lateral hockey-stick-shaped (Fig. 77.4), straight, or curvilinear incision (12) Major structures such as the biceps femoris (Fig. 77.5), iliotibial band, FCL, Popliteofibular ligament (PFL), and the popliteus tendon should be identified and evaluated. The common peroneal nerve should be identified and a neurolysis should be performed (Fig. 77.6). Repair of the injured structures proceeds from deep to superficial. Anatomic repair of soft-tissue avulsions from bone should be attempted through direct suture, suture anchors, and interference screws. If the severity of the injury precludes a direct repair, the involved structure can be augmented with a hamstring tendon, a portion of the biceps femoris tendon or iliotibial band, or reconstructed with an anatomic FCL or PLC reconstruction (5).

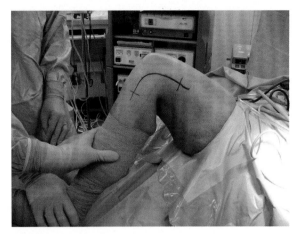

FIGURE 77.4. Lateral incision for approach to posterolateral knee.

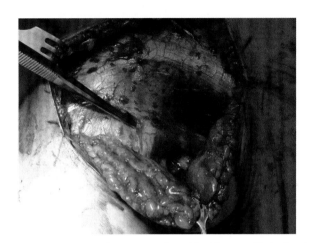

FIGURE 77.5. Biceps femoris insertion with pickups on fibular head.

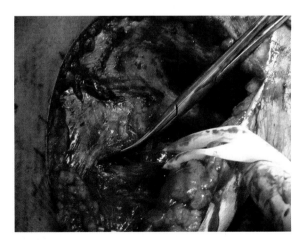

FIGURE 77.6. Common peroneal nerve isolated, protected with Penrose drain.

Chronic injury operative treatment

Chronic injuries of the PLC of the knee are best treated with surgical reconstruction because of extensive pericapsular scar formation and secondary changes to individual structures that make it difficult to perform a direct surgical repair (2, 5).

Varus alignment should be identified and corrected to prevent excessive loads on the lateral structures and to reduce the risk of stretching out with time and failure of the reconstruction. The authors recommend a full-length, weight-bearing AP radiograph to evaluate the overall limb alignment on the affected side. If a varus deformity exists, it should be corrected prior to a PLC reconstruction. Proximal tibial opening wedge osteotomy is preferred to lateral closing wedge tibial osteotomy because it avoids scar tissue formation on the posterolateral aspect of the knee and it has been demonstrated that opening-wedge osteotomy results in increased stability for PLC injuries. The subsequent clinical and functional stability is evaluated, and, if necessary, a second-stage PLC reconstruction should be performed at least 6 months after the osteotomy (13).

The goals of ACL and PLC surgical reconstruction include restoring the AP, lateral, and rotatory knee stability, returning patients to their preinjury activity level, and preventing degenerative articular changes. Several PLC reconstruction procedures have been described in the literature and although general consensus supports improved clinical outcomes after PLC reconstruction for chronic injuries, data on long-term results of PLC reconstruction are limited. Generally, PLC reconstruction can be divided into two main categories: anatomic and nonanatomic techniques. The mean difference between these two types of reconstruction is that the anatomic techniques attempt to restore the normal anatomy of the major PLC structures (FCL, PFL, and Popliteus tendon (PLT)), whereas the nonanatomic techniques, that are the primarily historical procedures, try to stabilize the PLC by tightening specific structures. The anatomic PLC reconstruction requires the use of various grafts, including anterior or posterior tibial tendon allografts, Achilles tendon allograft, or semitendinosus allograft. Native bone-patellar tendon-bone, hamstrings, or the central aspect of the biceps femoris tendon may be also utilized.

Authors' Preferred Operative Treatment

The authors suggest performing stress radiography of both knees to evaluate for any major lateral joint opening. An examination of the affected knee is performed under anesthesia with the patient in the supine position. Furthermore, an arthroscopic evaluation is performed to confirm cruciate ligament injuries and to detect the "drive through sign." Once a grade 3 posterolateral instability is confirmed, with the patient placed supine and the knee flexed approximately at 70°, a lateral hockey stick incision is performed. The superficial layer of the iliotibial band is identified and sharply dissected to allow for the development of a posterior-based tissue flap over the short and long heads of the biceps femoris. Through a blunt dissection, the common peroneal nerve should be identified and released; a neurolysis is important to perform to identify its course and to allow a secure access to all deep structures of the PLC.

One centimeter proximal to the lateral aspect of the fibular head, a small horizontal incision (1.5 cm) is made

through the anterior arm of the long head of the biceps femoris, to access the fibular collateral ligament–biceps bursa (Fig. 77.7). A suture is then placed on the FCL remnant located in this bursa and through a gentle traction the attachment site of the fibular collateral ligament on the femur and on the lateral aspect of the fibular head is identified. A 2-mm guidewire is then drilled through from the insertion of the FCL and directed posteromedially to exit the posteromedial aspect of the fibula at the attachment of the popliteofibular ligament, adjacent to the proximal tibiofibular joint. Then, a 7-mm tunnel is reamed through the fibula over this guidewire. A second guidewire is then drilled in an anteroposterior direction from just distal and medial to Gerdy's tubercle to exit at the posterior tibial popliteal sulcus. During this procedure, the author recommends the use of a large retractor posteriorly to protect the neurovascular bundle. At this point, a 9-mm tunnel is then reamed over the K-wire. Following a horizontal incision of the iliotibial band, the fibular collateral ligament and the popliteus tendon femoral attachments are identified. Two guidewires are then drilled parallel into the popliteus tendon and the

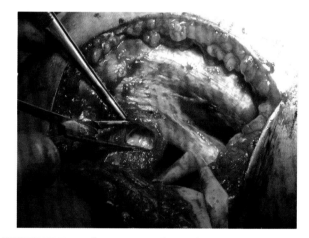

FIGURE 77.7. Small incision over biceps femoris/FCL bursa: Allows for visualization of the FCL insertion (lateral view, left knee).

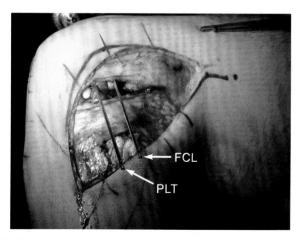

FIGURE 77.8. Guidewires placed into Popliteus tendon and FCL insertions on distal femur. These insertions have been proven to be consistently 18 mm apart (lateral view, left knee).

FCL femoral attachment sites (Fig. 77.8). They have to exit the distal femur proximomedial to the medial epicondyle and adductor tubercle. When the guidewires are aimed to this position, they do not encounter either an ACL or a PCL graft tunnel. At this point, two 9-mm femoral sockets are each reamed to a depth of 25 mm.

Once the PLC tunnels have been created, the ACL reconstruction is performed. Once the ACL tunnels have been reamed, femoral fixation of the ACL graft is then performed with an interference screw. At this point, the authors prefer to reconstruct and fix the PLC grafts before tensioning and permanent fixation of the ACL graft in its tibial tunnel.

For the PLC reconstruction, an Achilles tendon allograft is used and prepared by lengthwise splitting in two the calcaneus and attached Achilles tendon. An Achilles length greater than 22 cm is needed for the graft to exit the anterolateral tibial tunnel and to allow a distal staple fixation. Each femoral bone plug should be sized to fit the 9 × 20 mm femoral tunnels, whereas the tendon graft should be sized to pass through a 7-mm tunnel. At this point, two passing sutures are placed through drill holes placed in each bone plug. The bone block passing sutures are then placed into the eyelet-tipped guide pins and the bone plugs for each graft pulled into their respective femoral

tunnels. Each bone plug is fixed in its femoral tunnel using a 7 × 20 mm cannulated interference screw.

At this point, the graft fixed at the femoral site of the FCL's attachment is passed deep to the superficial layer of the iliotibial band and the anterior arm of the long head of the biceps. The graft is passed through the fibular head from lateral to posteromedial. A 7-mm cannulated bioabsorbable interference screw is used to fix the graft in its fibular tunnel with the knee at 30° flexion, neutral rotation, and a slight valgus stress to reduce any lateral compartment gapping.

The second graft that is used to reconstruct the popliteus tendon is passed from the femoral anatomical attachment through the popliteal hiatus to reach the posterolateral aspect of the lateral tibial plateau and the tibial tunnel. At this point, both grafts are pulled through the tibial tunnel from posterior to anterior. Both grafts are then tightened simultaneously by applying an anterior traction load to the grafts at 60° of flexion and neutral rotation of the leg. The grafts are fixed in the tibia with a 9-mm cannulated bioabsorbable interference screw and a small bone staple (Fig. 77.9). Finally, an anterior load to the tibial ACL graft is performed and it is fixed in the tibia with a 7 × 25 mm interference screw (14).

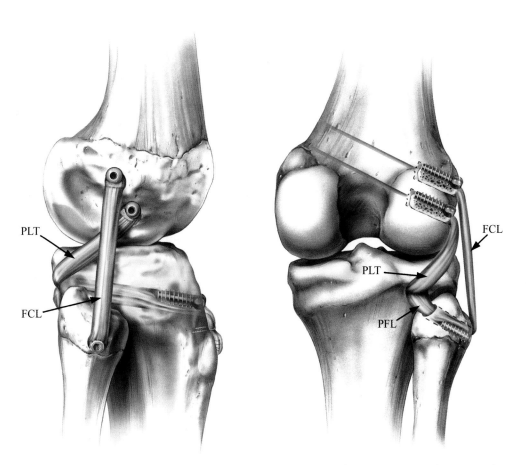

FIGURE 77.9. Illustration of anatomic posterolateral knee reconstruction (permission requested, AJSM 2003).

Complications, Controversies, and Special Considerations

Surgical management of ACL and PLC injuries is not without complications. In addition to ACL surgery complications, the most relevant complication of the PLC surgery is a potential common peroneal nerve injury, especially during the fixation and the drilling of the fibular head. For this reason, we recommend a careful identification, dissection, and protection of the nerve during the PLC surgery. Other complications such as fibular head fractures, vascular injuries, infection, hematoma, Deep venous thrombosis (DVT), hardware irritation, and compartment syndrome are described in literature with a variable rate of incidence.

Pearls and Pitfalls

One of the most frequent errors is to not address the correct anatomical attachments of the FCL and of the popliteus tendon. For this reason, the author recommends to perform a small horizontal incision through the anterior arm of the long head of the biceps femoris to allow for the direct view of the fibular collateral ligament within the biceps bursa. At this point, gentle traction through a suture passed into the FCL remnant assists in the identification of the FCL on the femoral and fibular side.

A special consideration is required for the convergence of femoral ACL and PLC tunnels that could be a possible source of ACL graft failure in multiple ligament reconstruction. For this reason, the author recommends to drill the PLC femoral tunnels to no greater than 25 mm of depth and to be angulated anteromedially in reaming the tunnels across the femur. Once the ACL and PLC femoral tunnels are performed, through the arthroscopy a direct view of the femoral ACL tunnel should be performed to ascertain any tunnel collisions.

The authors recommend following the graft-fixation sequence to reduce the risk of developing a significant external rotation deformity of the knee. The femoral ACL graft fixation should be fixed first followed by the posterolateral reconstruction graft fixation. The tibial ACL graft fixation should be fixed last because it should be less likely to cause a significant amount of tibial external rotation (15)

Rehabilitation

The need for reconstructing the PLC vastly changes the rehabilitation from that of an isolated ACL reconstruction. Instead of early ROM and weight-bearing exercises, many precautions are necessary when the PLC is involved, especially for the first 6 weeks. Caution must be used with varus, external rotation, and posterolateral directed forces to preserve the stability of the reconstruction in the early postoperative period. It is recommended to maintain a non-weight-bearing status, along with wearing a knee immobilizer at all times except for ROM exercises, for the first 6 weeks postoperatively.

When resuming weight bearing, gait training must be supervised by well-versed physical therapists to avoid hyperextension and varus thrusts in these often quadriceps-deficient patients. It is advised to avoid external rotation, squatting below 70° knee flexion and resisted hamstring activities in PLC reconstruction patients to avoid increased forces on the PLC structures that occur with increased knee flexion for the first 4 months. On average, patients are allowed to return to jogging activities at 4 to 6 months postoperatively and can resume cutting or pivoting activities at 6 to 9 months when given clearance following lower extremity functional testing. Although it is recognized that this may increase a patient's chances of arthrofibrosis, it is vital to respect the longer healing time required for multiple graft fixations.

Conclusion/Future Direction

Over the past 15 years, several studies have enabled an increase of cognisance of the anatomy and biomechanics of the PLC. Following these studies, it has been clarified that the fibular collateral ligament, the popliteofibular ligament, and the popliteus tendon play a main role in resisting to external rotation, varus rotation, and posterior tibial translation. For this reason, the surgical treatment for posterolateral knee injuries should be directed to restore the integrity or the function of the three main static restrains of the PLC. Otherwise, more studies of long-term follow-up are needed to assess the outcome of PLC reconstruction surgery.

PCL/MCL INJURIES

Introduction

Injuries to the medial-sided structures of the knee can occur in an isolated pattern with direct valgus stress to the knee. However, MCL injuries are very often seen in combination with tears of the anterior or PCL. In fact, one study found that the risk of concomitant ligament injuries in the setting of a grade 3 MCL injury was nearly 80% (16). This section of the chapter reviews the combination of MCL and PCL injuries from diagnosis to treatment and rehabilitation.

Clinical Evaluation

History

Whether acute or chronic in nature, patients with an MCL/PCL injury pattern will typically describe a history of valgus force injury to the knee joint. With rotation, the posteromedial structure and/or PCL can be concomitantly injured. The patient may describe instability with the knee falling into valgus with weight bearing. Further more, with PCL instability, the addition of instability in knee extension may be reported by patients. Other patients may report an effusion and pain about the affected knee. However, it has been reported that some patients may have complete disruptions of the medial compartment structures without pain or effusion and not have any perceived ambulatory difficulties (17).

Physical Exam

Physical exam of the knee remains the hallmark appropriate diagnosis of MCL and PCL injuries. Beginning with inspection, clinicians may observe effusion or ecchymosis over the femoral attachment of the superficial MCL (sMCL), or tibial collateral ligament, which has been determined to be located in a depression just proximal and posterior to the medial femoral epicondyle (18) This area is helpful in palpation as well in identifying sMCL injuries. It is important to understand the anatomy of the medial knee to appropriate palpate and assess the structures involved. The deep MCL has both meniscofemoral and meniscotibial components. As a thickening of the medial joint capsule, it is most prominent anterior medial joint capsule (18). With the meniscofemoral portion just inferior to the medial epicondyle and meniscotibial just inferior to the medial tibial plateau, palpation of these regions can help delineate their involvement.

Valgus stress applied to the knee at both 0° and 30° of knee flexion can further assist in the diagnosis of the injury pattern involved. For MCL injuries associated with PCL tears, the medial compartment will gap open with an applied valgus stress at both 0° and 30° of knee flexion. If the PCL is intact, the medial compartment should be relatively stable at 0° with gapping open only at 30° of knee flexion.

Imaging

Previously, plain radiographs have not been helpful in assessing the integrity of the medial knee structures. However, a recent study has shown that, with careful measurements in analyzing knee X-rays, the accuracy of anatomic landmarks of major structures can be predicted in a highly reproducible manner (19). Correlating radiographs with known anatomic attachment sites of the sMCL, the posterior oblique ligament and the medial patellofemoral ligament can allow for improved preoperative planning, along with intraoperative and postoperative assessment of reconstructions or repairs (Fig. 77.10). MRI studies of the knee can be used to further assess the integrity of specific structures.

Decision Making

As described in the following sections, the decision to treat nonoperatively versus surgically is dictated by the grade of injury and coexisting injury pattern. A thorough history and focused physical exam, followed by scrutiny of imaging studies obtained, will help delineate the pattern of injury for each individual patient. Once this is accomplished, applying these findings to the guidelines described below can consistently lead to good results for the injured patient.

Classification

Standardization of medial knee injuries has been documented based on the severity of injury (17). Medial knee tears are graded 1, 2, and 3. Grade 1 tears are those with tenderness located over the injured region, typically involving minimal fiber disruption. Grade 2 injuries have

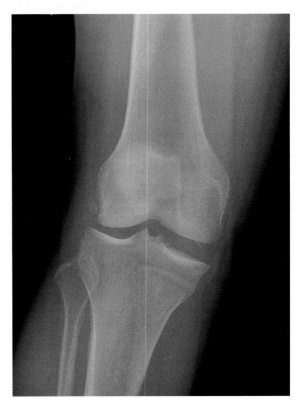

FIGURE 77.10. Valgus stress radiograph: Reveals medial gapping, indicative of medial knee structural damage (right knee).

more generalized tenderness due to more extensive involvement of the ligament, yet no resultant instability. Instability on physical exam indicates a grade 3 tear or complete disruption of the sMCL.

Treatment

Nonoperative Treatment

Although the structures of the medial knee are the most frequently injured knee ligaments, controversy still exists concerning treatment. However, nonoperative treatment should be the first step to treat acute isolated grade 1 or 2 sMCL and the majority of grade 3 injuries. It has been observed that grade 1 and 2 medial knee injuries respond acceptably to nonoperative treatment (20, 21). The clinical outcome of these injuries was generally good; even some residual medial laxity was present. Contrary, grade 3 injuries correlated with worse outcomes, with a high frequency of persisting medial instability, secondary dysfunction of the ACL, muscle weakness, and posttraumatic osteoarthritis of the injured knee (20). Provided the injury pattern does not involve the ACL, it has been found that sMCL injuries can usually be treated conservatively with good to excellent results (21).

Grade 1 and 2 medial knee injuries are best treated nonoperatively and with a functional rehabilitation program. The authors' protocol for the nonoperative treatment includes pain and swelling control and the possible use of a brace for 6 weeks to protect against valgus stress. An immediate knee ROM protocol, early weight bearing, and progressive strength training has been shown to produce excellent results and a high rate of return to sports (22).

Operative Treatment

Acute injury operative treatment

The treatment of acute isolated grade 3 MCL injuries remains controversial. Based on reports that proximal MCL tears heal quicker and with little residual laxity than those that occur distally, acute operative treatment could be considered in specific situation such as valgus instability both in 30° of flexion and in extension. Stener-type lesions of the distal insertion of the torn MCL, which are flipped and unable to heal, tibial plateau fracture, bony avulsion, and complete ligament disruption in a valgus knee alignment, may need to be considered for surgical treatment. In most of the circumstances, a functional rehabilitation program may be initiated and the patient should be possibly brought to surgery if there is no evidence of healing after the first 2 to 3 weeks.

If a primary surgical repair or reconstruction is indicated in the face of a multiple ligament knee injury, it should be performed concurrently with cruciate ligament reconstruction(s) and within 2 weeks after the injury because of the development of scar tissue that could reduce the quality of the remaining tendon and of the potential primary repair. A diagnostic arthroscopy could be helpful after the initial surgical exposure to identify meniscus tears and the site of the deep MCL injury.

The surgical incision chosen depends on the structures that need to be repaired. A straight 10-cm skin incision could be performed over the anteromedial knee, from just anterior to the medial epicondyle to the pes anserine bursal region. Care should be taken to preserve the infrapatellar branch of the saphenous nerve if possible. The dissection is continued through the sartorius fascia and the plane between the sartorius fascia and the gracilis is identified. Through this interval, the femoral and tibial attachments of the sMCL are identified. The posterior oblique ligament is also identified. At this point, all medial structures could be evaluated and repaired or reconstructed starting from the deepest structures (23). Any peripheral meniscus tears should be treated under direct visualization trough an inside-out suture repair. Meniscotibial and meniscofemoral ligament tears of the deep MCL should be treated through a direct suture repair or with a suture anchor fixation. If the posteromedial capsule and/or Posterior oblique ligament are torn, a direct repair through a nonabsorbable suture or through suture anchors is required if the injury is located at the tibial or femoral attachment. If a POL tear is found, a plication or reconstruction has to be performed in extension (23). It is important to not tighten the POL in flexion because this will result in a flexion contracture. The tension of the capsular arm of the semimembranosus should be evaluated by palpation and any laxity should be addressed through interrupted absorbable sutures. At this point, the choice of the treatment of injury to the MCL

depends upon by the surgical findings. Cancellous screws and washers could be easily used for the reduction and the fixation of a large proximal avulsed portion. Complete avulsion of the superficial and deep MCL components from the tibia could be repaired directly using suture anchors. It is important to restore the normal MCL tension and to secure the distal insertion of the MCL to its anatomic insertion for a successful result. Furthermore, an acute repair of midsubstance tears often cannot be performed because of poor quality of the remaining tendon. In this circumstance, an anatomic reconstruction is required with allograft or autologous hamstring grafts.

Chronic injury operative treatment

The operative treatment for chronic medial knee injuries is indicated for patients with symptomatic instability, pain, and excessive medial joint gapping because complete medial knee ruptures may not always heal. Because of contracture of the ligament ends, the formation of scar tissue and the loss of the potential for healing that characterize chronic tears, a reconstruction may be required with hamstring autograft or allograft. However, it should be performed following the complete resolution of acute inflammation and swelling and after full knee motion has been regained to reduce the risk of arthrofibrosis.

An arthroscopic examination can be performed after the initial surgical approach to identify and treat intra-articular pathologies such as chondral or meniscal tears. Different techniques for medial knee injury repair have been described such as tendon transfer, advancement and re-tensioning techniques, and free autograft or allograft tendon reconstructions (24–26) However, in chronic injuries, a complete reconstruction of the sMCL and the POL is required because of extensive pericapsular scar formation.

Authors' Preferred Operative Treatment

Once sMCL and POL tears are confirmed and a decision is made, a surgical reconstruction could be performed. For complete medial knee injuries, the authors' preferred technique is an anatomic reconstruction of the sMCL and the POL (Fig. 77.11). It consists of a reconstruction of the two main structures of the medial side of the knee using two separate grafts with four reconstruction tunnels. A single large medial knee incision or three small knee incisions could be performed to access the anatomic femoral and tibial attachment points of the sMCL and POL. Following the three incision technique, the first incision of 6 cm is performed vertically along the medial knee in line with the distal adductor magnus tendon, ending 1 cm proximal to the joint line. Blunt dissection is performed to expose the femoral anatomic attachments of the sMCL and POL. Once these attachment points are identified, the overlying soft tissues are carefully reflected by sharp dissection. One 5-cm incision is now performed along the anteromedial aspect of the proximal tibia, starting 2 cm distal to the

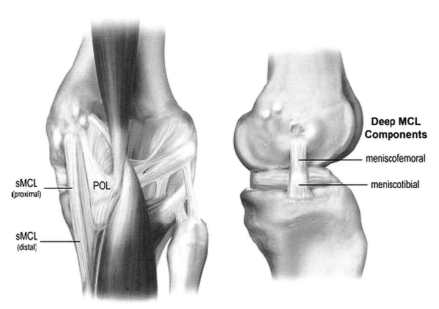

FIGURE 77.11. Illustration depicting medial knee structures (permission requested, AJSM).

joint line. This incision allows access to the tibial insertion of the sMCL. At this point, the gracilis and semitendinosus are exposed following the incision of the sartorius muscle fascia. The semitendinosus is harvested using a hamstring stripper. Alternatively an allograft tendon may be used. The hamstring graft is sectioned into two parts, one measuring 16 cm and the other 12 cm, respectively, for subsequent sMCL and POL reconstructions (Fig. 77.12). Each end of the graft is tubularized using No. 2 nonabsorbable suture to fit into 7-mm tunnels.

The third 5-cm incision is placed along the posteromedial border of the proximal tibia to allow access to the tibial attachment of the POL. This incision is performed 2 cm posterior to the posterior crest of the tibia and located 1 cm proximal to the joint line. Through a careful dissection, the sartorial branch of the saphenous nerve is identified and protected by incising the fascia anterior to the sartorius muscle and retracting the sartorius tendon distally. At this point, the attachment site of the central arm of the POL is identified and a small incision is made parallel to the fibers along the posterior edge of the anterior arm of the semimembranosus tendon to expose this attachment site. Once the anatomic attachments of the sMCL and POL insertions are found, reconstruction tunnels are prepared. Two eyelet pins are drilled, respectively, through the center of the femoral attachment of the sMCL and POL. Then, two 7-mm tunnels are reamed, respectively, to a depth of 30 and 25 mm. At this point, a third eyelet pin is drilled 6 cm distal to the joint line through the center of the distal sMCL anatomic attachment point exiting along the proximal anterolateral lateral compartment of the leg. Then, a 7-mm tunnel is reamed to a depth of 30 mm. Next, an eyelet pin is drilled anterolaterally through the center of the tibial attachment of the central arm of the

POL, exiting just distal and medial to the Gerdy's tubercle. Finally, a 7-mm tunnel is reamed to a depth of 30 mm. Once all four tunnels are reamed, the PCL reconstruction could be performed. For chronic PCL injury, the authors' preferred technique is a double-bundle PCL reconstruction using two femoral sockets. Once, the PCL tunnels are reamed and femoral fixation is performed, the medial side knee reconstruction should be completed. Using an eyelet pin, the 16-cm section of semitendinosus tendon is passed into the femoral MCL tunnel and fixed with a 7-mm cannulated bioabsorbable screw. Similarly, the 12-cm section of the semitendinosus tendon graft is passed into the femoral POL tunnel and fixed with a 7-mm cannulated bioabsorbable screw. After this phase, both tendon fixations are qualitatively evaluated by placing medial traction on the grafts. At this point, the sMCL reconstruction graft

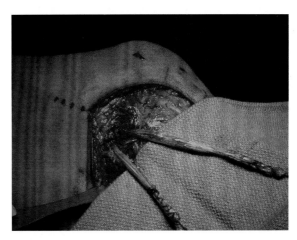

FIGURE 77.12. POL and sMCL hamstring grafts.

is passed through the distal sMCL tunnel. With the knee placed at 20° of flexion, in neutral rotation and applying a knee varus stress force to reduce any potential medial compartment gapping, the graft is then secured in place with a 7-mm bioabsorbable screw. Once proper positioning is verified, the proximal tibial attachment point of the sMCL is recreated by suturing the MCL graft to the anterior arm of the semimembranosus muscle.

The POL graft is then passed in his tibial tunnel. The graft is then secured with a 7-mm bioabsorbable screw with the knee held in extension, in neutral rotation and with a varus force applied to reduce any medial compartment gapping. Finally, the tibial PCL graft is fixed in the tibia.

Complications, Controversies, and Special Considerations

The most common surgical complications of MCL surgery are injury of the saphenous nerve and postoperative arthrofibrosis. For this reason, the authors recommend a careful dissection, especially at the level of the tibial POL attachment site by incising the sartorius fascia anteriorly and retracting it posteriorly. Arthrofibrosis occurs in up to 25% to 30% of acute medial knee surgeries and could be minimized by obtaining a rigid fixation of the grafts that could permit an early knee ROM protocol. Knee motion should be allowed as soon as possible, to achieve a ROM of 0° to 90° at 2 weeks and 0° to 110° at 4 weeks. Other complications such as hardware irritation, infection, bleeding, and DVT could be observed as with any orthopedic surgical procedure.

Pearls and Pitfalls

The authors recommend directing both sMCL and POL femoral tunnels proximally in the axial plane. This should be done to ensure a tunnel separation from the PCL reconstruction tunnels and to avoid a collision that could cause a failure of ligament fixation.

The tibial PCL graft fixation should be performed prior to the sMCL and POL grafts are fixed. This is to make sure that the joint is well reduced prior to medial structure fixation, which could result in residual medial structure laxity.

Rehabilitation

The postoperative course for a reconstructed medial knee and PCL is long and arduous, requiring a strong alliance between patient, surgeon, and physical therapist. When consulting patients with this injury pattern prior to surgery, it is important to inform them that their full return to activity will be, at a minimum, 6 months and, possibly, be up to 9 months after surgical reconstruction.

For the 1st week after reconstruction, it is vital to avoid any ROM exercises. Once motion is allowed, it is important to perform the exercise in the prone position to avoid stress on the PCL graft. At the 2-week postoperative

visit, the patient is placed into a PCL jack brace that is to be worn at all times for the initial 6 months postoperatively to avoid stressors onto the reconstructed PCL graft. The patient must maintain a strict nonweight-bearing status for the 6 weeks following surgery. The patient is instructed, however, to begin simple strengthening exercises within the brace immediately postoperatively. These include quadriceps sets, straight leg raises, and hip extension and abduction exercises.

Once ROM exercises are permitted, extension can be allowed to 0°, but it is essential to avoid any hyperextension and undue tension on the fresh PCL reconstruction. For the initial 6 weeks after surgery, flexion ROM exercises should be done in the prone position with assistance from the nonoperative leg to avoid posterior translation of the tibia which, again, can stress the PCL graft. For the initial 2 weeks, flexion should be limited to 90°, with progression to full ROM thereafter. It is recommended that no resistive/repetitive hamstring exercises be performed for approximately 4 months after reconstruction. When closed kinetic chain exercises are permitted, squatting must be limited to 70°, again, avoiding high stressors on the PCL by minimizing posterior translation.

In regard to the medial knee reconstruction, avoidance of tibial external and internal rotation is advised for the initial 6 months. The patient should be educated on avoiding pivoting motions (cutting, swinging a baseball bat or golf club, etc.) on the operative lower extremity. Provided lower extremity strength and motion are appropriately regained, jogging exercises may be resumed at 5 to 6 months postoperatively. The caveat to this return lies in ascertaining valgus and posterior stress radiographs that are within normal limits. Once the patient has navigated this rehabilitation program without issue, the surgeon can consult the patient on returning to full activity 6 to 9 months after surgery.

Conclusion/Future Direction

Nonsurgical treatment of medial knee tears is usually successful if there is no associated structural damage to the anterior or PCL. However, if a surgical treatment is required, an anatomic reconstruction should be performed. The early knee ROM protocol represents the key to success to reduce the risk of arthrofibrosis and loss of knee motion.

CONCLUSION

This chapter has provided methods to treat specific combinations of multiligament knee injuries. It is necessary to have a high index of suspicion for multiple structure involvement in the evaluation of every knee injury. The practice of appropriate exam techniques and applying decisions for each patient based on their findings, on exam and imaging, will help ensure the most appropriate intervention is recommended to each patient.

REFERENCES

1. LaPrade RF, Wentorf FA, Fritts H, et al. A prospective magnetic resonance imaging study of the incidence of posterolateral and multiple ligament injuries in acute knee injuries presenting with a hemarthrosis. *Arthroscopy.* 2007;23:1341–1347.

2. LaPrade RF, Terry GC. Injuries to the posterolateral aspect of the knee. Association of anatomic injury patterns with clinical instability. *Am J Sports Med.* 1997;25:433–438.

3. LaPrade RF, Ly TV, Griffith C. The external rotation recurvatum test revisited: reevaluation of the sagittal plane tibiofemoral relationship. *Am J Sports Med.* 2008;36:709–712.

4. LaPrade RF, Heikes C, Bakker AJ, et al. The reproducibility and repeatability of varus stress radiographs in the assessment of isolated fibular collateral ligament and grade-III posterolateral knee injuries. An in vitro biomechanical study. *J Bone Joint Surg Am.* 2008;90:2069–2076.

5. LaPrade RF, Wentorf F. Diagnosis and treatment of posterolateral knee injuries. *Clin Orthop Relat Res.* 2002;(402):110–121.

6. LaPrade RF, Gilbert TJ, Bollom TS, et al. The magnetic resonance imaging appearance of individual structures of the posterolateral knee. A prospective study of normal knees and knees with surgically verified grade III injuries. *Am J Sports Med.* 2000;28:191–199.

7. O'Brien SJ, Warren RF, Pavlov H, et al. Reconstruction of the chronically insufficient anterior cruciate ligament with the central third of the patellar ligament. *J Bone Joint Surg Am.* 1991;73:278–286.

8. Noyes FR, Grood ES, Torzilli PA. Current concepts review. The definitions of terms for motion and position of the knee and injuries of the ligaments. *J Bone Joint Surg Am.* 1989;71:465–472.

9. Terry GC, LaPrade RF. The biceps femoris muscle complex at the knee. Its anatomy and injury patterns associated with acute anterolateral-anteromedial rotatory instability. *Am J Sports Med.* 1996;24:2–8.

10. Krukhaug Y, Molster A, Rodt A, et al. Lateral ligament injuries of the knee. *Knee Surg Sports Traumatol Arthrosc.* 1998;6:21–25.

11. Kannus P. Nonoperative treatment of grade II and III sprains of the lateral ligament compartment of the knee. *Am J Sports Med.* 1989;17:83–88.

12. Terry GC, LaPrade RF. The posterolateral aspect of the knee. Anatomy and surgical approach. *Am J Sports Med.* 1996;24:732–739.

13. Laprade RF, Engebretsen L, Johansen S, et al. The effect of a proximal tibial medial opening wedge osteotomy on posterolateral knee instability: a biomechanical study. *Am J Sports Med.* 2008;36:956–960.

14. LaPrade RF, Johansen S, Wentorf FA, et al. An analysis of an anatomical posterolateral knee reconstruction: an in vitro biomechanical study and development of a surgical technique. *Am J Sports Med.* 2004;32:1405–1414.

15. Wentorf FA, LaPrade RF, Lewis JL, et al. The influence of the integrity of posterolateral structures on tibiofemoral orientation when an anterior cruciate ligament graft is tensioned. *Am J Sports Med.* 2002;30:796–799.

16. Fetto JF, Marshall JL. Medial collateral ligament injuries of the knee: a rationale for treatment. *Clin Orthop Relat Res.* 1978;(132):206–218.

17. Hughston JC, Andrews JR, Cross MJ, et al. Classification of knee ligament instabilities. Part I. The medial compartment and cruciate ligaments. *J Bone Joint Surg Am.* 1976;58:159–172.

18. LaPrade RF, Engebretsen AH, Ly TV, et al. The anatomy of the medial part of the knee. *J Bone Joint Surg Am.* 2007;89:2000–2010.

19. Wijdicks CA, Griffith CJ, Laprade RF, et al. Radiographic identification of the primary medial knee structures. *J Bone Joint Surg Am.* 2009;91:521–529.

20. Kannus P. Long-term results of conservatively treated medial collateral ligament injuries of the knee joint. *Clin Orthop Relat Res.* 1988;(226):103–112.

21. Indelicato PA. Non-operative treatment of complete tears of the medial collateral ligament of the knee. *J Bone Joint Surg Am.* 1983;65:323–329.

22. Reider B, Sathy MR, Talkington J, et al. Treatment of isolated medial collateral ligament injuries in athletes with early functional rehabilitation. A five-year follow-up study. *Am J Sports Med.* 1994;22:470–477.

23. Hughston JC, Eilers AF. The role of the posterior oblique ligament in repairs of acute medial (collateral) ligament tears of the knee. *J Bone Joint Surg Am.* 1973;55:923–940.

24. Adachi N, Ochi M, Deie M, et al. New hamstring fixation technique for medial collateral ligament or posterolateral corner reconstruction using the mosaicplasty system. *Arthroscopy.* 2006;22:571.e1–571.e3.

25. Borden PS, Kantaras AT, Caborn DN. Medial collateral ligament reconstruction with allograft using a double-bundle technique. *Arthroscopy.* 2002;18:E19.

26. Fanelli GC, Harris JD. Surgical treatment of acute medial collateral ligament and posteromedial corner injuries of the knee. *Sports Med Arthrosc.* 2006;14:78–83.

The Dislocated Knee

Gregory C. Fanelli • John D. Beck • John T. Riehl • Mark E. McKenna • Craig J. Edson

Knee dislocation occurs when there is complete disruption of the femoral-tibial articulation. These injuries are true orthopedic emergencies. Prompt recognition is essential to avoid catastrophic complications. The incidence of knee dislocation is thought to be around 1 in 100,000 of all hospital admissions (1). Specific studies report varied incidence from low (2, 3) to considerably higher (4). Previous studies on incidence that have been largely based on radiographic or clinical diagnosis in a hospital setting, however, may be under representative of the true incidence as many knee injuries spontaneously reduce in the field. Therefore, any multiligament-injured knee should be treated as a dislocation in the acute setting because the knee may have spontaneously reduced prior to radiographic examination.

Most knee dislocations involve tears of the central pivot, including both the anterior cruciate ligament (ACL) and the posterior cruciate ligament (PCL) along with one or both of the collateral ligaments. Significant capsular injury can further add to instability. In addition to ligamentous and capsular injury, meniscal and cartilaginous lesions may be present as well. Associated fractures, compartment syndrome, and trauma to other parts of the body are not uncommon with these often high-energy mechanisms (2, 5–9).

Neurovascular injury occurs relatively frequently in the multiple ligament-injured knee. Vascular injuries are found in approximately 16% to 64% of these injuries (3, 6, 7, 10, 11). A detailed neurovascular examination is essential, both pre- and postreduction. Any suspected or confirmed arterial injuries warrant prompt attention, as these injuries carry a significant risk of amputation (10–15).

Historically, nonoperative treatment consisting of immobilization was the treatment of choice for multiligament injuries to the knee (16, 17). With advances in arthroscopic techniques of ligament reconstruction, nonoperative treatment is frequently limited to medically unstable patients or those with low functional demands.

ANATOMY AND BIOMECHANICS OF THE KNEE

The primary plane of motion in the knee is in the sagittal plane. Some rotation of the tibia on the femur occurs normally as well. Normal range of motion (ROM) is from 0° of extension (or a few degrees of hyperextension) to approximately 140° of flexion. Internal and external rotations are typically 10° in either direction, and external rotation in full extension leads to the "screw home" mechanism. This allows the knee to "lock" in full extension and reduces the work of the quadriceps during standing. Stability of the knee is maintained in part by the bony articulation between the femoral condyles and the tibial plateau. Medial and lateral menisci increase the contact surfaces and thus increase static stability to the joint.

The osseous anatomy of the knee consists of the articulations of the proximal tibia, the distal femur, and the patella. The tibial plateau has an approximate 10° posterior slope. The medial plateau is slightly concave, whereas the lateral plateau has a more rounded appearance. Although, the tibial plateau is somewhat flattened relative to the curved distal femur, congruency is maintained within the knee as the menisci help to increase conformity within the tibiofemoral articulation. The tibial spines separate the medial and lateral plateaus and serve as attachments for the menisci and cruciate ligaments.

The distal femur is divided into medial and lateral condyles. The size of the condyles are asymmetric with the distal femur, forming a trapezoidal shape (18). The medial condyle projects more distally, whereas the lateral condyle projects more anteriorly. The condyles are separated by the trochlear groove, which contributes to the patellofemoral articulation.

The patella is the largest sesamoid bone in the body and serves as a fulcrum for the extensor mechanism as well as providing a protective surface for the anterior aspect of the knee.

Ligamentous Anatomy

The four major ligamentous stabilizers of the knee include the ACL, the PCL, the medial collateral ligament (MCL), and the lateral collateral ligament (LCL). In addition, the posteromedial corner (PMC) and posterolateral corner (PLC) of the knee are important structures that also contribute to knee stability. If injuries to these two structures are not recognized or addressed at the time of definitive treatment of the four main stabilizers, undue stresses may be placed on repairs/reconstructions and lead to adverse outcomes.

The primary function of the ACL is to resist anterior translation of the tibia relative to the distal femur. In addition, it serves as a secondary adjunct to varus and valgus stability in full extension. The ACL originates on the posteromedial lateral femoral condyle and courses anteriorly and distally to insert in the depression in front of and lateral to the anterior tibial spine (19). Two anatomic bundles make up the ACL. The posterolateral bundle is tight in extension, whereas the anteromedial bundle is tight in flexion (20). The ACL is typically 35 to 40 mm in length and 10 to 12 mm in width (21). It is an intra-articular structure, yet it has its own synovial membrane. It receives its blood supply from the middle geniculate artery and is innervated by the posterior articular nerve, a branch of the tibial nerve (22).

The PCL resists posterior translation of the tibia and is a secondary restraint to tibial external rotation. The PCL has a broad femoral origin on the posterolateral aspect of the medial femoral condyle and it inserts centrally on the posterior tibial plateau. It is an intra-articular structure, but is also encompassed by its own synovial sheath. The posteromedial bundle of the PCL is tight in extension, whereas the anterolateral bundle is under more tension in flexion (23). These bundles are supplemented by the posterior meniscofemoral ligaments. The average length of the PCL is 38 mm and its width is 13 mm (23–25). The vascularity of the PCL is supplied by the middle geniculate artery, and it is innervated by nerve fibers from the popliteal plexus from the tibial and obturator nerves (26).

The MCL and the PMC are the primary restraints to valgus stress in the knee. The medial side of the knee can be divided into thirds from anterior to posterior. The anterior third consists of capsular ligaments covered by the extensor retinaculum. The middle third contains the superficial and deep MCL. The PMC occupies the posterior third and includes the posterior oblique ligament, the posterior horn of the medial meniscus, and the termination of the semimembranosus (27). Alternatively, the anatomy of the medial side of the knee has been described by Warren and Marshall in terms of layers. The most superficial layer is the sartorial fascia. The second layer consists of the superficial MCL. The deep MCL and the medial joint capsule are found in layer three (28).

The superficial MCL is the primary restraint to valgus stress of the knee at 30° of knee flexion. Its origin is on the medial epicondyle of the distal femur, and it inserts just posterior to the insertion of the pes anserinus and just anterior to the adductor tubercle. It inserts on the anteromedial tibia approximately 5 cm below the joint line (29). The posterior oblique ligament, semimembranosus, and oblique popliteal ligament resist valgus stress in full extension as well as providing contribution to anteromedial rotatory stability (30).

The lateral side of the knee has also been divided into layers (31). The biceps femoris and the iliotibial band make up the most superficial layer. The peroneal nerve lies deep to the biceps at the level of the distal femoral condyle. The middle layer consists of the patellar retinaculum anteriorly and the patellofemoral ligaments posteriorly. The deep layer, layer III, consists of the LCL, popliteal tendon, popliteofibular ligament, fabellofibular ligament, arcuate ligament, and lateral joint capsule.

The LCL is the primary restraint to varus stress with the knee in 30° of flexion. In an anatomic study performed by LaPrade et al., the LCL was found to originate on average 1.4 mm proximal and 3.1 mm posterior to the lateral epicondyle of the femur in a bony depression. It attaches on the fibular head, 28.4 mm distal and 8.2 mm posterior to the anterior superior margin of the fibula, again in a bony depression (32). The remaining structures in layer III make up the PLC. The PLC provides static support to resist posterior translation of the tibia as well as external rotation and varus angulation. The popliteus tendon attaches to the femur anterior to the LCL, with an attachment on the posteromedial proximal tibia.

Neurovascular Anatomy

The neurovascular bundle within the popliteal fossa is at significant risk both during and in the period immediately following knee dislocations. The risk of injury to the neurovascular structures in this area can be explained by some of their anatomic features.

The popliteal fossa is bordered by the semimembranosus muscle superomedially, the biceps femoris tendon at its superior lateral border, and the two heads of the gastrocnemius muscle inferiorly. Within the popliteal fossa, the popliteal artery and vein are separated by a thin layer of fat from the underlying posterior joint capsule. Traversing through the popliteal fossa, from deep to superficial, are the popliteal artery, popliteal vein, and posterior tibial nerve. With the knee in full extension, the popliteal fascia is tensioned, making palpation of the popliteal artery difficult. Palpation of the pulse in this region is therefore best performed with the knee in slight flexion. Proximally, the popliteal artery emerges from the adductor hiatus and is tethered to this fibrous tunnel. Distally, the popliteal artery is also relatively immobile as it enters another fibrous canal deep to the soleus. These two somewhat immobile points leave the popliteal artery vulnerable to injury when the knee is dislocated. Superior, inferior, and middle geniculate branches stem from the popliteal artery, but are unable to maintain adequate collateral circulation in the event of a vascular injury.

The sciatic nerve enters the popliteal space from between and deep to the semitendinosus and the long head of the biceps, at a variable level it divides into the tibial and common peroneal nerves. The common peroneal nerve follows the lower edge of the biceps toward the fibula crossing superficially to the lateral head of the gastrocnemius. The tibial nerve continues down the middle of the popliteal fossa and gives off muscular branches to the plantaris and gastrocnemius muscles. The common peroneal nerve then courses distally around the fibular head to innervate the anterior and lateral compartments of the lower leg. The course of the peroneal nerve makes it more susceptible to injury during knee dislocation than the tibial nerve, explaining the significant increase in its observed incidence (14, 17, 33).

CLASSIFICATION OF KNEE DISLOCATIONS

Numerous classification systems exist to describe knee dislocations. The most commonly, the direction of displacement of the proximal tibia relative to the distal femur is used to describe the injury. However, this system does not account for spontaneously reduced dislocations and may fail to recognize other important considerations in the multiple ligament-injured knee. Mechanism of injury, the presence or absence of open wounds, the degree of displacement, and the status of the neurovascular structures are additional aspects of the injury that may be used to help describe knee dislocations. In practice, all of the above characteristics are helpful in the classification of the multiple ligament-injured knee and can assist in determining optimum treatment.

The directional classification of knee dislocations is based on the position of the tibia relative to the distal femur. Anterior dislocations occur after a hyperextension injury greater than 30° (2) and are the most common directional dislocation. Posterior knee dislocations occur in 25% of all knee dislocations and typically result from a posteriorly directed force applied to the proximal tibia. Lateral, medial, and rotatory dislocations have also been described (10). The direction of dislocation may raise the suspicion of the treating physician to certain associated injuries. For example, intimal tears of the popliteal artery are more common with anterior dislocation, whereas popliteal artery transaction is more likely to occur with posterior dislocation.

High-energy dislocations typically occur following motor vehicle collisions and falls from height. Low-energy injuries typically refer to those that occur during athletic activities (34). An ultra-low-energy dislocation has been described in morbidly obese patients that sustain severe ligamentous injury following seemingly trivial trauma (6, 35).

Schenck developed an anatomic classification system that classifies knee dislocations on the basis of the specific structures about the knee that are compromised (Table 78.1) (36). The dislocation is classified in terms of the ligamentous injury pattern, and the letter C designates a circulatory injury, whereas the letter N indicates neurologic injury. It has been used by some authors to direct treatment and predict outcome.

INJURY MECHANISMS

Knee dislocations can occur as the result of high-energy, low-energy, or even "ultra-low-energy" injuries. The

Table 78.1

Modified Schenck classification of knee dislocation

Type	Injury Description
KDI	Dislocation with one cruciate ligament intact (usually PCL intact)
KDII	Bicruciate disruption, collateral ligaments intact
KDIIIL	Bicruciate disruption, LCL–PLC torn (MCL intact)
KDIIIM	Bicruciate disruption, MCL torn (LCL–PLC intact)
KDIV	Bicruciate and both collateral ligaments disrupted
KDV	Dislocation with periarticular fracture
C	Associated vascular injury
N	Associated neurologic injury

direction of the dislocation as well as the injury pattern is dependent upon both the position of the knee at the time of injury and the direction of the force applied. Motor vehicle collisions, falls from height, farm injuries, and industrial accidents make up most of the high-energy knee dislocations. Low-energy knee dislocations typically occur from sports-related injuries and appear to have a lower incidence of associated neurovascular compromise. Ultra-low-energy dislocations have been described as well where seemingly trivial trauma has caused knee dislocations with associated neurovascular injury in morbidly obese patients (35).

Anterior dislocations typically result from a hyperextension mechanism. As Kennedy (2) applied a hyperextension force to the knee in 12 cadaveric specimen, he noted tearing of the posterior capsule of the knee followed by cruciate rupture. This occurred on average at 30° of hyperextension and produced anterior dislocation of the tibia. As hyperextension continued to an average angle of 50°, the popliteal artery was noted to be placed on considerable stretch.

Posterior dislocations are the result of a significant posteriorly directed force applied to the proximal tibia and can be associated with substantial damage to the extensor mechanism (2). This is one possible mechanism in high-energy motor vehicle collisions and may be the result of a dashboard injury. In a low-energy injury, a fall landing on the tibial tubercle with a plantar-flexed ankle may produce a posterior knee dislocation as well.

Lateral and medial dislocations typically result from severe varus and valgus stresses, respectively. Rotational forces produce a rotational type of dislocation. Quinlan and Sharrard (9) described the mechanism for posterolateral dislocation to be a flexed knee with "severe abduction-medial rotation violence to the knee while the limb was not bearing weight."

ASSOCIATED INJURIES

As stated previously, most knee dislocations involve tears of the central pivot, along with one or both of the collateral ligaments. Additional intra-articular pathology such as chondral or meniscal injury is not uncommon. Capsular injuries prevent arthroscopic reconstruction of cruciate ligaments within the first several days postinjury and may also cause swelling to become severe within the first 48 hours.

Swelling and/or vascular injury may lead to compartment syndrome, especially when fractures are present. Injuries to other body regions also are not uncommon. Neurologic and vascular injuries will be covered later in detail.

INITIAL EVALUATION OF THE MULTIPLE LIGAMENT-INJURED KNEE

General Considerations

Initial management of knee dislocations demands a comprehensive and systematic approach to facilitate accurate and efficient diagnosis and treatment. Individuals sustaining high-energy trauma should be treated following standard advanced trauma life support (ATLS) protocols with assessment to screen for orthopedic emergencies including: vascular disruption, open wound, compartment syndrome, or an irreducible joint (37). A secondary survey should include a comprehensive physical examination supplemented by appropriate ancillary studies to formulate a treatment plan.

Patients with obvious deformity or varus/valgus malalignment can be rapidly diagnosed with a knee dislocation. Uncontained heamarthrosis, abrasions or contusions of the knee, gross crepitus, or laxity should alert the examiner to the possibility of a potential knee dislocation (38). These findings are important to recognize as 34% to 50% of knee dislocations present to the emergency department in a reduced position (13, 17). In addition, any patient with two or more ligamentous injuries of the knee should be treated as a potential knee dislocation (2, 6, 39, 40). The importance of accurate and timely diagnosis of knee dislocation lies in the recognition of potential vascular injury as the morbidity associated with delayed revascularization is extremely high (10, 41).

Physical Examination

Following the initiation of ATLS protocols when appropriate, emergency department evaluation should include a thorough, but efficient, history composed of: mechanism of injury, position of limb at time of injury, and manipulation of the limb prior to arrival. This history can provide clues to the direction of dislocation and energy of injury. Physical examination should start with inspection of the extremity to evaluate resting position and gross alignment. Determination of distal vascularity is of foremost concern and should be assessed with palpation/Doppler assessment of dorsalis pedis and posterior tibial pulses, capillary refill, skin color, and skin temperature. Hard signs of vascular injury including active bleeding, distal ischemia, expanding heamatoma, and popliteal bruit warrant emergent vascular surgery consultation. In the setting of knee dislocation with asymmetric or absent pedal pulses, immediate reduction may be required to restore distal blood flow (13). If symmetric pulses are present, orthogonal X-rays of the knee should be obtained emergently prior to manipulation and reduction should be attempted unless a dimple sign is present. Dimpling of the skin on the anterior-medial knee is pathoneumonic for posterolateral dislocation with the medial femoral condyle buttonholing through the anteriomedial joint capsule. Attempted closed reduction of these dislocations is associated with a high rate of skin necrosis and therefore closed reduction should not be attempted if a "dimple sign" is present (42).

Reduction is attempted with longitudinal traction applied to the tibia with manipulation of the proximal tibia according to the direction of the dislocation. Following reduction, a repeat neurovascular examination should be performed and documented. Postreduction examination should include inspection of the skin for abrasions, ecchymosis, swelling, open wounds, and skin dimpling, all of which provide information about underlying pathology. Diffuse swelling with uncontained heamarthrosis on the medial and lateral knee suggest major disruption of the joint capsule and should raise suspension of spontaneously reduced knee dislocation, even in the setting of normal X-rays (38).

A complete neurologic examination is an essential aspect of the initial evaluation and should be performed both prior to and after a closed reduction. Motor and sensory examination of the superficial peroneal, deep peroneal, and tibial nerve distributions should each be evaluated and documented. Sequential neurologic examinations should be performed over the first 48 hours, and repeated at 1 and 2 weeks as motor grades are often acutely reduced after knee dislocation secondary to pain alone (33). On serial examination, the presence of progressive deterioration of neurologic function raises the suspicion of an impending compartment syndrome (43).

In the acute setting, pain and swelling can limit the ability to accurately assess the extent of ligamentous injury in a conscious patient. Examination should be performed in a careful and controlled manner to avoid iatrogenic injury. A stabilized Lachman test in which the examiner's thigh is placed under the injured knee allows for relatively pain-free evaluation of anterior endpoint. The most sensitive test for determining ACL and PCL deficiency are

Lachman test at 20° of flexion and posterior drawer at 90° of flexion, respectively. The collateral ligaments are evaluated at 30° and at full extension by applying varus or valgus stress. Gross laxity at full extension implies disruption of the collateral ligament, one or more of the cruciate ligaments, and associated capsule. A more detailed ligamentous examination typically requires conscious sedation or general anesthesia.

Under anesthesia, a complete examination can be preformed that eliminates confounding variables such as muscular guarding. Evaluation of the PCL includes measurement of tibial step-off compared with contralateral extremity, posterior drawer, and reverse pivot-shift. Lachman, pivot-shift, and anterior drawer are preformed for ACL competence. The posterior lateral and posterior medial corners can be examined with posteriolateal and posteriomedial drawers. The dial test can be used to differentiate PCL and PLC injuries. In addition, the supine heel lift test can evaluate for recurvatum secondary to PLC, PMC, PCL, and posterior capsule deficiency. Finally, varus and valgus stress can be applied to the knee in hyperextension, neutral, and at 30° of flexion.

Imaging Studies

Plain anteroposterior (AP) and lateral radiographs should be obtained in all cases of suspected knee dislocations. Initial X-rays will confirm the direction of dislocation to aid in planning reduction as well as identify associated osseous injuries. Occasionally, tibiofemoral widening on AP X-ray in a swollen knee is the only radiographic sign of a spontaneously reduced knee dislocation. Fracture patterns that suggest ligamentous injury include fibular head avulsion, tibial tubercle avulsion, and Segond fractures. A fibular head fracture can represent disruption of the LCL, popliteofibular ligament, or biceps femoris insertion. A Segond fracture is an avulsion fracture of the lateral tibial plateau associated with a torn ACL (37). Following manipulation, repeat X-rays are mandatory to confirm reduction and evaluate for residual subluxation.

Arteriography remains the gold standard for assessment of vascular injury, following knee dislocation. However, the use of routine angiography for all knee dislocations has come into question. An angiogram and vascular consult is indicated in any patient with signs of vascular compromise including diminished pulses, absent pulses, color or temperature changes of the involved limb or ankle-brachial index (ABI) less than 0.90. Patients with hard signs of vascular injury (active bleeding, distal ischemia following reduction, expanding hematoma, and popliteal bruit) require an emergent vascular surgery consult. In this situation, an angiography should be performed in the OR as angiography in an angiography suite delays the time to repair by an average of 3 hours (44). Recently, the use of MR angiography has been suggested as an alternative to arteriography to evaluate for vascular injury in the acute setting. MRA is less invasive than standard arteriography and avoids potential complications associated with contrast and arterial punctures including renal failure, allergic reaction, and iatrogenic vascular injury. The potential benefits of MRA have been well established in other settings (45, 46). Early data on MRA following knee dislocation have been promising (47), but are still limited in comparison with standard angiography.

Following the acute management of the dislocated knee MRI should be obtained to guide operative management. MRI in the acute setting can determine the presence and extent of ligamentous pathology, avulsion versus intrasubstance tear, as well as concomitant meniscal and articular cartilage injuries. MRI is the gold standard for evaluation of soft tissue injuries about the knee. Numerous studies have evaluated the sensitivity and specificity of MRI in this setting. In 2008, Bui et al. retrospectively reviewed MRI findings of 20 patients with knee dislocations to compare them with operative findings. They had two false negative interpretations, both involving meniscal tears. In their 20 patients, they had four false positive interpretations in which the ligament was reported as a complete tear and was found to be partial or healed at time of injury. This data was confounded by the time of surgery ranging from 26 to 223 days (48). Twaddle et al. (49) found MRI to be 85% to 100% accurate in predicting the extent of soft tissue injury following knee dislocation (49). In addition, abnormalities of the peroneal nerve can also be identified on MRI. In 2002, Potter et al. (47) retrospectively reviewed 21 knee dislocations and correlated MRI findings with operative examination. In their series, all 10 nerve injuries noted on MRI were confirmed at surgery. As MRI and MRA technology continue to improve, the detail and accuracy provided may allow combined MRI/MRA to supplant arteriography as the gold standard.

Vascular Injuries

The popliteal artery is at risk for injury during knee dislocation because of its anatomic location. Proximally, the popliteal artery is tethered at Hunter's canal, and distally it is constrained at the soleal arch (50). This anatomic tethering, combined with the limited collateral circulation of the knee, leads to the high incidence of vascular injury following knee dislocation, ranging from 16% to 64% in the literature (3, 7). The incidence of arterial injury is greatest with anterior and posterior dislocations, 39% and 44%, respectively (10). A full spectrum of vascular injuries can be encountered depending on the mechanism of injury, including transection, contusion, injury to the intimal and medial layers without loss of continuity, and thrombus formation (51). Posterior dislocations typically result in complete transection of the popliteal artery, whereas anterior dislocations produce a traction injury to the artery resulting in extensive intimal injury/tear (10). Initially, it was thought arterial injury was less common with low-velocity knee dislocations (LVKD). Recent studies reported a 58% incidence of arterial injury in obese patients with LVKD. This patient population has a 17% risk of amputation even after repair (35, 52–54). With the epidemic of obesity in America and the difficulty of examination, the evaluation of this patient population must be done carefully to ensure a knee dislocation with a potential arterial injury are not missed.

Regardless of the direction of the dislocation, mechanism of energy, or velocity of injury, vascular injury should always be suspected and evaluated. Delay in diagnosis of vascular injury requiring repair is associated with an extremely high morbidity. Green and Allen (10) reported an 11% amputation rate if vascular repair was undertaken within 8 hours and an 86% amputation rate if delayed for greater than 8 hours. This data was confirmed by the results of the lower extremity assessment project (LEAP) study. They found an average warm ischemia time for patients with amputation following knee dislocation was 7.25 hours; whereas those not requiring amputation averaged 4.7 hours. They concluded that prolonged warm ischemic time was the major factor in determining amputation (41). This reinforces that prompt and accurate diagnosis of vascular trauma is essential in successful management of knee dislocations.

The diagnosis of vascular injury should be made clinically by a detailed history, physical examination, and appropriate ancillary studies. A pointed history should include any manipulation performed prior to arrival and past or present signs of ischemia (pain, paresthesias, paralysis, pallor, and diminished limb temperature). Physical examination should include assessment of pulses by palpation or Doppler compared with the contralateral extremity, signs of active bleeding, distal ischemia, expanding hematoma, and popliteal bruit or thrill. In any patient without obvious vascular injury, ABI should be preformed. Distal perfusion as well as motor and sensory function should be evaluated and documented. Any abnormalities or asymmetry are concerning for vascular injury and should be further investigated. If obvious vascular injury and limb-threatening ischemia are present immediate vascular consultation and repair is necessary.

It is well known that normal pulses, a warm foot, and brisk capillary refill can be present with arterial injury (43). Consequently, vascular injury can be overlooked at time of initial consultation. Collateral circulation through the superior knee arteries, from the profundus femoral and articular branches off the popliteal artery can preserve the vascular supply to the lower extremity in the initial stage of the injury and distal pulses may still be palpable (55). In addition, intimal flap tears initially are undetectable on physical examination because pulses are normal, but may progress to complete arterial occlusion with thrombus. A missed diagnosis of vascular injury and subsequent delay of arterial repair or bypass leads to a significant increase in morbidity with a high rate of amputation. As a result, many authors initially recommended liberal or mandatory angiographic studies in cases of knee dislocations (56–59).

The use of routine angiography has been debated in favor of selective angiograms on the basis of clinical examination and ABI. Proponents of routine angiogram emphasize the high morbidity associated with missed vascular injury (Fig. 78.1). They also note that normal pulses, Doppler signals, and capillary refill after initial closed reduction do not rule out a vascular injury that progresses over time, causing late vascular compromise (2).

Total reliance on physical examination is quite controversial. Miranda et al. prospectively used arteriography to evaluate only those patients with hard signs of potential vascular injury whereas patients without hard signs were followed with serial physical examinations. They reported a 94% positive predictive value (PPV) for vascular injury in patients with hard clinical signs, whereas patients with negative clinical examination had a 100% negative predictive value (NPV) for vascular compromise (60). They concluded that arteriography is unnecessary when physical examination is negative. In a meta-analysis, Barnes et al. (57) found that the presence of an abnormal pedal pulse on initial examination in a patient with a knee dislocation is not sensitive enough to detect a surgical vascular injury. Abnormal pedal pulses had a sensitivity of 79%, specificity of 91%, PPV of 75%, and NPV of 93% to predict surgical vascular injury in this study.

More recent literature has supported the use of selective angiography for patients with knee dislocations. Routine arteriography is criticized for the delay in revascularization that it causes, its potential complications, and its high cost. Most selective angiography protocols suggest angiogram for any patient with abnormal physical examination or an ABI ≤0.9. Mills et al. prospectively studied 38 patients with knee dislocations. All patients with ABI less than 0.9 (determined by Doppler probe and standardized blood pressure cuff) had arteriography, whereas those with ABI greater than 0.9 were admitted for serial observation and delayed arterial duplex examination. All patients with ABI less than 0.9 had vascular lesion requiring vascular surgery intervention. The remaining 27 had no abnormality on serial examination or duplex ultrasound and no vascular complications. The sensitivity and specificity of

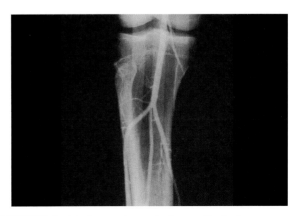

FIGURE 78.1. Arteriogram demonstrating popliteal artery.

an ABI less than 0.9 was 100%. They concluded that ABI is a rapid, reliable, noninvasive tool to diagnose vascular injury (61). Several other retrospective reviews in the literature confirmed that selective angiography is effective in diagnosing vascular lesions requiring surgical repair (62–65). ABI of 0.9 has yielded sensitivities of 95% to 100% and NPV of 99% for detecting flow limiting arterial injury (66).

Duplex ultrasonography has also been proposed as a safer, cheaper, and less invasive method of evaluating the popliteal vasculature. Duplex has been shown to be 98% accurate in detecting vascular trauma to the extremities (67). Proponents stress the benefits of noninvasive examination with great accuracy, whereas opponents argue that ultrasound is operator dependent and cannot account for distorted anatomy surrounding the knee following dislocation (60).

The management of patients with hard signs of limb ischemia is less controversial. These patients require an emergent vascular surgery consult and angiography should be performed in the operating room as angiography in an angiography suite delays time to repair by an average of 3 hours (44). The LEAP study confirmed this data and concluded that patients with obvious signs of vascular injury could be effectively treated without angiography prior to surgery (41). Many authors contend that arteriographic studies in this setting supply little additional information as the location of the lesion is invariably within the popliteal space (10).

Emergent vascular reconstruction with a reverse saphenous vein graft is the treatment of choice for an ischemic limb following a knee dislocation. If there are any signs of increasing compartment pressure or warm ischemia time approaching 6 hours, prophylactic fasciotomies are indicated to prevent reperfusion-induced compartment syndrome (13).

Angiography is absolutely indicated in patients with abnormal or asymmetric pulses without hard evidence of limb ischemia, and those that have developed a change in their vascular status during serial examinations. In conclusion, if there is obvious vascular injury and limb-threatening ischemia, immediate vascular repair is necessary. If there are clinical signs of vascular injury without limb-threatening ischemia, selective arteriography is recommended. If there are no clinical signs of vascular injury, close monitoring without the used of arteriography is recommended (68).

Nerve Injuries

The incidence of nerve palsy following knee dislocation ranges from 10% to 42% in the literature with damage to the common peroneal nerve being more common than the tibial nerve (33). Peroneal nerve palsies are most common in posterolateral dislocations (1, 2). Nerve injury ranges from a stretching of the nerve (neurapraxia), to a more severe injury with axon disruption and an intact endoneurium (axonotomesis), to complete nerve rupture or transaction (neuronotemsis) (33). These injuries carry a poor

prognosis with only 30% to 37% of complete injuries obtaining partial motor recovery. In 2005, Niall et al. evaluated common peroneal nerve injuries following traumatic dislocations of the knee in 55 patients. In their study, all patients with nerve palsy had disruption of the PCL and PLC, whereas 41% of patients with PCL plus PLC had common peroneal nerve palsy. Of these patients, 21% had complete motor recovery, whereas 29% had partial motor recovery. Fifty percent had no useful motor or sensory function return (69, 70). Although common, little consensus has been reached regarding management of these lesions.

The anatomy of the peroneal nerve is directly related to its propensity for injury. There is only 0.5 cm of excursion of the peroneal nerve at the fibular head during knee motion (45). In addition, the thickness of the epineural tissue compared with axonal tissue is low, providing less protection against stretch injuries (71) (Fig. 78.2).

Neurologic evaluation following knee dislocation should include subjective findings of paresthesias, hyperesthesias, and sensory changes as well as objective evaluation of both motor and sensory function of the superficial peroneal, deep peroneal, and tibial nerve distributions. Sequential neurologic evaluation over the first 48 hours, and repeat evaluations 1 and 2 weeks after injury, is imperative, as motor grades are often acutely reduced after dislocation secondary to pain alone (33). In addition, progressive deterioration of neurologic function raises suspicion of impending compartment syndrome (43). Naill et al. (69) found all patients who had functional recovery of the peroneal nerve had a positive Tinel sign distal to the fibular head and objective signs of early recovery by 3 months.

Intraoperative exploration of the peroneal nerve usually reveals that it is in continuity; however, a widespread zone of injury is typically encountered. Poor results have been documented following observation of complete nerve palsies (72, 73). One study found that the best prognosis for recovery was associated with nerves found to be in continuity with a 7 cm or less zone of injury (69).

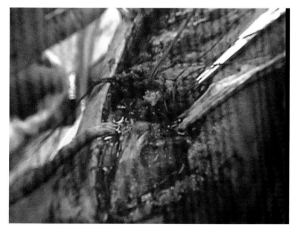

FIGURE 78.2. Peroneal nerve injury in knee dislocation patient.

In the subacute setting of 2 to 3 weeks following nerve injury, needle EMG can provide useful information about the status of the motor axons. EMG changes consistent with axon disruption include fibrillation potentials, positive sharp waves, and absence of activity on voluntary effort or proximal nerve stimulation. The earliest signs of nerve regeneration are noted to occur in the superficial branch of the peroneal nerve supplying the peroneal musculature. This muscle group was noted, in one study, to recover more commonly than any of the muscles of the anterior compartment (69). EMG can also be used to rule out nerve rupture if any voluntary motor unit axon potentials are present. In the subacute time window, neuropraxic lesion can be diagnosed in the setting of a paralyzed muscle without signs of denervation (33). Serial EMGs can be performed to evaluate for signs of reinnervation (polyphasic action potentials and increased amplitude of compound muscle action potentials). There is still no role for EMG in the acute setting.

Current options for the treatment of nerve palsies after knee dislocation include observation, neurolysis, primary repair, or neuroma excision with nerve grafting. Studies demonstrate that patients with incomplete peroneal nerve palsy after knee dislocation have an excellent chance of complete recovery whereas complete palsy have a 37% chance of recovery (33). Limited results are available for primary repair. Kim and Kliine (74) reported 82% of peroneal nerve injuries treated with direct repair regained grade 3 strength. The limited data on nerve grafting shows a direct correlation between length of zone of injury and chance of recovery. Wood (75) reported 100% of nerve grafts recovered grade 4 strength if the nerve graft was less than 6 cm. In a separate study, Sedel and Nizard (76) reported that only 38% of patients regained grade 3 strength if graft length exceeded 7 cm. Kim and Kliine noted 75% of patients regained grade 3 strength if graft was less than 6 cm in length. If the graft was 6 to 12 cm, recovery dropped to 35%, and if graft exceeded 12 cm, recovery was only 14% (74).

Based upon the current literature, the following treatment algorithm was proposed for peroneal nerve injuries (77–80). Observation is the treatment of choice for all incomplete peroneal nerve palsies. If nerve rupture or partial fascicular injury is identified at the time of ligamentous reconstruction, nerve reconstruction should be considered approximately 3 months after the original operation. Acute repairs should be avoided, unless tension free primary repair can be performed. If the nerve is not explored or appears normal at initial exploration, electrical studies should be obtained as a baseline 4 to 6 weeks following injury. If tibialis anterior contraction is absent at 3 months, EMG should be repeated and the patient should be evaluated for surgical treatment. The results of nerve grafts are diminished if surgical intervention is delayed greater than 6 months (74–76, 79). Tibialis posterior transfer can be a useful late reconstructive procedure to restore dorsiflexion.

TREATMENT

Nonsurgical

Indications

Nonsurgical management of a knee dislocation is still a viable option when circumstances dictate. Nonoperative treatment may be appropriate for critically ill patients unable to tolerate a surgical procedure, injuries with significant soft tissue contamination around the prospective surgical site and elderly sedentary patients. Shelbourne et al. (34) found that elderly sedentary patients treated nonoperatively for their knee dislocation had reasonable return to functional level. In the past 40 years, operative versus nonoperative treatment was a source of debate as there were studies supporting both methods (1, 2, 14, 72, 73, 81–84). Over this time period, there has been considerable improvement in surgical techniques, including arthroscopically assisted ligament reconstruction, increased understanding of the ligamentous anatomy, and biomechanics around the knee. This has led to evidence supporting surgical reconstruction and a trend toward surgical fixation (85, 86) Arthroscopic reconstruction has demonstrated improved ligamentous stability of the knee as well as improved function postoperatively.

Methods

A long leg or cylinder cast or a brace locked in extension may be used as the most basic method of nonoperative management. If the cast or brace does not afford enough stability to maintain the knee in a reduced position, a knee spanning external fixator or hinged fixator may be necessary. The knee brace is often helpful in the setting of a critically ill patient by allowing easy access for evaluation of the injured extremity. The external fixator also provides better access to soft tissue injuries if it can be positioned away from contaminated wounds. Regardless of the chosen method of nonsurgical management, frequent radiographs should be obtained to verify continued reduction of the knee.

Surgical Treatment

Early reports of nonoperative treatment of knee dislocation demonstrated reasonable outcomes. However, this data suggested that the surgically stabilized knee dislocations fare better in the long term. Almekinders and Logan retrospectively reviewed their knee dislocations from 1963 to 1988 and compared surgically stabilized knees with those treated conservatively. They concluded that conservative treatment was comparable to surgical treatment. Despite similar outcomes, the conservatively treated knees were grossly unstable compared with surgically stabilized knees (81). Over the time period of their study, the typical surgical treatment was open direct repair of the ligaments. Sisto and Warren (72) found similar results comparing four conservatively treated knees with 16 knees treated with direct suture repair of torn ligaments. Frassica et al. also evaluated direct repair of ligamentous injury within 5 days of injury in 13 of 17 patients. They concluded better results were obtained with early versus late direct repair of torn ligaments. This study supports acute surgical management of the dislocated knee. They found that long-term benefits exist from a ligamentously stable knee (87). Recently, Richter et al. published a similar report with Lysholm scores of 78.3 and 64.8 for operative versus nonoperative treatments, respectively (*P* = .001). On the basis of these improved patient outcomes, the authors concluded surgical treatment is superior to nonsurgical treatment (88). In addition, Plancher and Siliski (17) reported less pain at rest, better knee motion, and return to athletics all improved with operative management.

Within the last decade, the technique of arthroscopically assisted ACL/PCL reconstruction has been refined. Several advancements have made these techniques possible: (1) better procurement, sterilization and storage of allograft tissue, (2) improved arthroscopic surgical instrumentation, (3) better graft fixation methods, (4) improved surgical technique, and (5) improved understanding of the ligamentous anatomy and biomechanics of the knee. Reports of combined ACL/PCL reconstruction are present in the literature, and surgical reconstruction provides superior results to direct repair of the ligaments. Shapiro and Freedman reconstructed seven ACL/PCL injuries with primarily allograft Achilles tendon or bone-patellar tendon-bone. They found that three patients had excellent results, three good results, and one had fair results. Furthermore, average KT-1000 was +3.3 mm side-to-side difference, with very little varus/valgus instability or significant posterior laxity. All seven of their patients were able to return to school or the workplace (86).

Fanelli et al. reported on 20 ACL/PCL arthroscopically assisted ligament reconstructions. The study group included one ACL/PCL tear, 10 ACL/PCL/posterior lateral corner injuries, seven ACL/PCL/MCL tears, and two patients with deficient ACL/PCL/MCL/posterior lateral corners. Achilles tendon allografts and bone-patellar tendon-bone autografts were used in PCL reconstructions, auto and allograft bone-patellar tendon-bone was used in ACL reconstruction (85).

Postoperatively, significant improvement was found utilizing the Lysholm, Tegner, and Hospital for Special Surgery (HSS) knee ligament-rating scales. Postoperatively, 75% of patients had a normal Lachman test, 85% no longer displayed a pivot shift, 45% restored a normal posterior drawer test, whereas 55% displayed grade 1 posterior laxity. All 20 knees were deemed functionally stable, and all patients returned to desired levels of activity. The authors concluded reconstruction can reproducibly produce a stable knee. An additional component of this study, not previously mentioned with any consistency in the literature, was the treatment of associated MCL or posterior lateral corner injuries. It is imperative to address these injuries, or the results of ACL/PCL reconstruction in the setting of a multiligament will be less than optimal.

Noyes and Barber-Westin evaluated 5-year follow-up of surgically reconstructed ACL/PCL tears with additional MCL or LCL/PCL reconstruction. Seven of these knees were acute knee dislocations and four were chronically unstable knees secondary to knee dislocations. Five of the seven acute knee injures had returned to preinjury level of activity. Three of the four chronic knee injuries were asymptomatic with activities of daily living (ADL). Arthrometric measurements at 20° showed less than 3 mm of side-to-side difference with anterior to posterior translation in 10 of the 11 knees; at 70°, there were nine knees that had less than 3 mm side-to-side difference in anterior–posterior translation. These authors concluded that simultaneous bicruciate ligament reconstruction is indicated to restore function to the knee (89). Wong et al. performed a similar retrospective analysis to compare single cruciate reconstruction with bicruciate reconstruction. They found no difference in ROM, but there was a statistically significant difference in AP translation and IKDC scores between groups with patients undergoing bicruciate reconstruction fairing better (90).

AUTHORS' PREFERRED TREATMENT

Indications

In the multiple ligament-injured knee, surgical treatment consisting of ligament repair/reconstruction is indicated in the acute setting in a physically active patient without significant medical comorbidities. With chronic injury, surgical reconstruction is warranted with continued instability without severe arthrosis.

Surgical Timing

Surgical timing of the acute bicruciate multiple ligament-injured knee is dependent upon the vascular status of the involved extremity, the collateral ligament injury severity, the degree of instability, and the postreduction stability. Delayed or staged reconstruction 2 to 3 weeks postinjury has demonstrated a lower incidence of arthrofibrosis (85, 91).

Surgical timing in acute ACL-PCL-medial side injuries is also dependent on the medial side classification. Some medial side injuries will heal with 4 to 6 weeks of brace treatment, provided the tibiofemoral joint is reduced in all planes. Other medial side injuries require surgical intervention. Types A and B medial side injuries are repaired–reconstructed as a single-stage procedure with combined arthroscopic ACL–PCL reconstruction. Type C medial side injuries combined with ACL–PCL tears are often treated with staged reconstruction. The medial posteromedial repair–reconstruction is performed within the first week after injury, followed by arthroscopic combined ACL–PCL reconstruction 3 to 6 weeks later (29, 85, 91–95).

Surgical timing in acute ACL-PCL-lateral side injuries is dependent upon the lateral side classification (96). Arthroscopic combined ACL–PCL reconstruction with lateral side repair and reconstruction can be performed within 2 to 3 weeks postinjury in knees with types A and B lateral posterolateral instability. Type C lateral posterolateral instability combined with ACL–PCL tears is often treated with staged reconstruction. The lateral posterolateral repair–reconstruction is performed within the first week after injury, followed by arthroscopic combined ACL–PCL reconstruction 3 to 6 weeks later.

Staged procedures are required for open multiple ligament knee injuries/dislocations to ensure that ligament grafts are placed into clean tissue. The collateral/capsular structures are repaired/reconstructed after thorough irrigation and debridement, and the combined ACL/PCL reconstruction is performed later after wound healing has occurred. Care must be taken, in all cases of delayed reconstruction, to ensure that reduction is maintained while waiting for definitive.

The surgical timing should always be considered in the context of the individual patient. Multisystem injuries often accompany high-energy knee dislocation, which may lead to surgical delays. Ideal timing protocols may be modified on the basis of the vascular status of the involved extremity, reduction stability, skin condition, open or closed injury, and other orthopedic and systemic injuries. Though some authors have reported less predictable and poorer functional outcomes when reconstruction is delayed greater than 4 weeks, (97–100) reports of excellent results with delayed reconstruction in the multiple ligament-injured knee (85, 101, 102) are present as well.

Chronic bicruciate multiple ligament knee injuries often present to the orthopedic surgeon with progressive functional instability, and possibly, some degree of posttraumatic arthrosis. Considerations for treatment require the definition of all the structural injuries. These may include ligaments injured; meniscus injuries, bony malalignment, articular surface injuries, and gait abnormalities. Surgical procedures under consideration may include proximal tibial or distal femoral osteotomy, ligament reconstruction, meniscus transplant, and osteochondral grafting.

Graft Selection

Our preferred graft for the PCL is the Achilles tendon allograft for single-bundle PCL reconstructions, and an Achilles tendon and tibialis anterior allografts for double-bundle PCL reconstructions. We prefer Achilles tendon allograft or other allograft for the ACL reconstruction. The preferred graft material for the PLC is allograft tissue combined with a primary repair or posterolateral capsular shift procedure. Our preferred method for MCL and posteromedial reconstructions is a primary repair and/or posteromedial capsular advancement with allograft supplementation as needed.

SURGICAL TECHNIQUE

Combined PCL ACL Reconstruction

The principles of reconstruction in the multiple ligament-injured knee are to identify and treat all pathology, accurate tunnel placement, anatomic graft insertion sites, utilize strong graft material, secure graft fixation, and a deliberate postoperative rehabilitation program (103–108).

Allograft tissue is prepared, and arthroscopic instruments are placed with the inflow in the superior lateral portal, arthroscope in the inferior lateral patellar portal, and instruments in the inferior medial patellar portal. An accessory extracapsular extra-articular posteromedial safety incision is used to protect the neurovascular structures, and to confirm the accuracy of tibial tunnel placement.

Notch preparation is performed first and consists of ACL and PCL stump debridement, bone removal, and contouring of the medial wall of the lateral femoral condyle and the intercondylar roof. Specially curved PCL instruments are used to elevate the capsule from the posterior aspect of the tibia (Fig. 78.3).

The arm of the PCL ACL guide is inserted through the inferior medial patellar portal to begin creation of the PCL tibial tunnel. The tip of the guide is positioned at the inferior lateral aspect of the PCL anatomic insertion site. The bullet portion of the guide contacts the anteromedial surface of the proximal tibia at a point midway between the posteromedial border of the tibia and the tibial crest anterior approximately 1 cm below the tibial tubercle. This will provide an angle of graft orientation such that

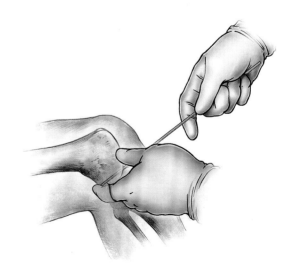

FIGURE 78.3. Posteromedial safety incision protects the neurovascular structures, confirms accurate placement of the PCL tibial tunnel, and facilitates the flow of the surgical procedure. (From Fanelli GC. *Rationale and Surgical Technique for PCL and Multiple Knee Ligament Reconstruction.* 2nd ed. Warsaw, Indiana: Biomet Sports Medicine; 2008.)

the graft will turn two very smooth 45° angles on the posterior aspect of the tibia and will not have an acute 90° angle turn, which may cause pressure necrosis of the graft (Fig. 78.4). The tip of the guide, in the posterior aspect of the tibia is confirmed with the surgeon's finger through the extracapsular extra-articular posteromedial safety incision. Intraoperative AP and lateral X-ray may also be used. The surgeon's finger confirms the position of the guide wire through the posterior medial safety incision. This is a double safety check.

The appropriately sized standard cannulated reamer is used to create the tibial tunnel. The surgeon's finger through the extracapsular extra-articular posteromedial incision is monitoring the position of the guide wire. The drill is advanced until it comes to the posterior cortex of the tibia. The chuck is disengaged from the drill, and completion of the tibial tunnel is performed by hand. This gives an additional margin of safety for completion of the tibial tunnel.

The PCL single-bundle or double-bundle femoral tunnels can be made from inside out (Fig. 78.5). Inserting the appropriately sized double-bundle aimer through a low anterior lateral patellar arthroscopic portal creates the PCL anterior lateral bundle femoral tunnel. The double-bundle aimer is positioned directly on the footprint of the femoral anterior lateral bundle PCL insertion site. The appropriately sized guide wire is drilled through the aimer, through the bone, and out a small skin incision. The double-bundle aimer is removed, and an acorn reamer is used to endoscopically drill from inside out the anterior lateral PCL femoral tunnel. When the surgeon chooses to perform a double-bundle double femoral tunnel PCL reconstruction, the same process is repeated for the posterior medial bundle of the PCL. Care must be taken to ensure that there will be an adequate bone bridge (approximately 5 mm) between the two femoral tunnels prior to drilling.

The ACL tunnels are created using the single-incision technique. The tibial tunnel begins externally at a point

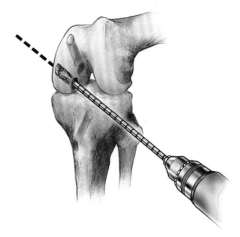

FIGURE 78.5. Creation of double-bundle double-femoral tunnel PCL reconstruction using inside to outside drilling technique. (From Fanelli GC. *Rationale and Surgical Technique for PCL and Multiple Knee Ligament Reconstruction.* 2nd ed. Warsaw, Indiana: Biomet Sports Medicine; 2008.)

1 cm proximal to the tibial tubercle on the anteromedial surface of the proximal tibia to emerge through the center of the stump if the ACL tibial footprint. The femoral tunnel is positioned next to the over the top position on the medial wall of the lateral femoral condyle near the ACL anatomic insertion site. The ACL graft is positioned, and anchored on the femoral side followed by ACL graft tensioning and tibial fixation (Fig. 78.6).

Lateral Posterolateral Reconstruction

One surgical technique for posterolateral reconstruction is the free graft figure-of-eight technique utilizing semitentinosus autograft or allograft, Achilles tendon allograft, or other soft tissue allograft material (92, 93, 103). This technique combined with capsular repair and/or posterolateral capsular shift procedures mimics the function of the popliteofibular ligament and LCL, tightens the posterolateral capsule and provides a post of strong autogenous tissue to reinforce the PLC. When there is a disrupted proximal tibiofibular joint or hyperextension external rotation recurvatum deformity, a two-tailed (fibular head, proximal tibia) posterior lateral reconstruction is used (Fig. 78.7A–C).

A curvilinear incision is made in the lateral aspect of the knee extending from the lateral femoral epicondyle to the interval between Gerdy's tubercle and the fibular head. The peroneal nerve is dissected free and protected throughout the procedure. The fibular head is exposed and a tunnel is created in an anterior to posterior direction at the area of maximal fibular diameter. The tunnel is created by passing a guidepin followed by a cannulated drill usually 7 mm in diameter. The free tendon graft is then passed through the fibular head drill hole. An incision is then made in the iliotibial band in line with the fibers directly overlying the lateral femoral

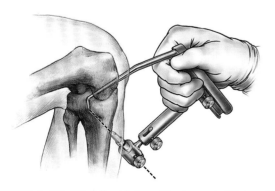

FIGURE 78.4. PCL ACL drill guide in position to create PCL transtibial tunnel. (From Fanelli GC. *Rationale and Surgical Technique for PCL and Multiple Knee Ligament Reconstruction.* 2nd ed. Warsaw, Indiana: Biomet Sports Medicine; 2008.)

The medial meniscus is repaired to the new capsular position, and the shifted capsule is sewn into the MCL. When superficial MCL reconstruction is indicated, this is performed using allograft or autograft tissue. This graft material is attached at the anatomic insertion sites of the superficial MCL on the femur and tibia using a screw and spiked ligament washer or suture anchors. The posteromedial capsular advancement is performed and sewn into the newly reconstructed MCL. The final graft tensioning position is approximately 30° to 40° of knee flexion (Fig. 78.8A and B).

Graft Tensioning and Fixation

The PCL is reconstructed first followed by the anterior cruciate followed by the posterolateral complex and/or medial side. The mechanical tensioning boot (Biomet Sports Medicine, Warsaw, Indiana) is used for tensioning

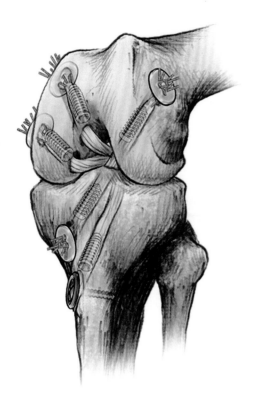

FIGURE 78.6. Completed OCL ACL reconstruction. Note primary and backup fixation of each graft. (From Fanelli GC. *Rationale and Surgical Technique for PCL and Multiple Knee Ligament Reconstruction.* 2nd ed. Warsaw, Indiana: Biomet Sports Medicine; 2008.)

epicondyle. The graft material is passed medial to the iliotibial band, and the limbs of the graft are crossed to form a figure-of-eight. A longitudinal incision is made in the lateral capsule just posterior to the fibular collateral ligament. The graft material is passed medial to the iliotibial band and secured to the lateral femoral epicondylar region with a screw and spiked ligament washer with the allograft insertion sites corresponding to the anatomic insertion sites of the fibular collateral ligament and the popliteus tendon. The posterolateral capsule that had been previously incised is then shifted and sewn into the strut of figure-of-eight graft tissue material to eliminate posterolateral capsular redundancy. The anterior and posterior limbs of the figure-of-eight graft material are sewn to each other to reinforce and tighten the construct. The final graft tensioning position is approximately 30° to 40° of knee flexion.

Medial Posteromedial Reconstruction

Posteromedial and medial reconstructions are performed through a medial hockey stick incision (29, 92–94). The superficial MCL is exposed, and a longitudinal incision is made just posterior to the posterior border of the superficial MCL. The interval between the posteromedial capsule and the medial meniscus is developed. The posteromedial capsule is shifted anterosuperiorly.

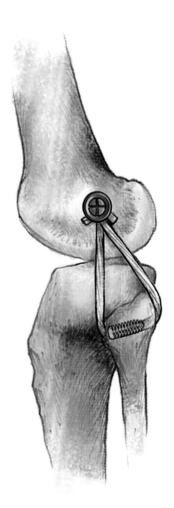

A

FIGURE 78.7. A–C: Posterolateral reconstruction demonstrating figure-of-eight technique **(A)**, and two-tailed technique **(B)**. It is essential to perform a posterolateral capsular repair or shift **(C)** combined with either the figure-of-eight or the two-tailed techniques. (From Fanelli GC. *Rationale and Surgical Technique for PCL and Multiple Knee Ligament Reconstruction.* 2nd ed. Warsaw, Indiana: Biomet Sports Medicine; 2008.)

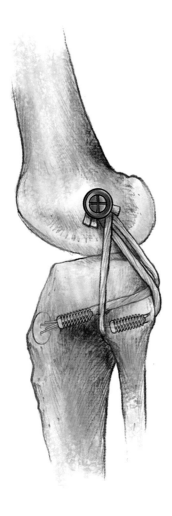

B

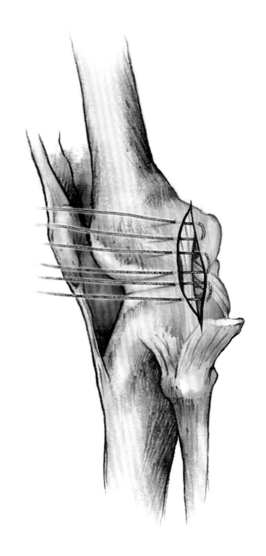

C

FIGURE 78.7. (Continued)

the ACL and PCL reconstructions (Fig. 78.9). The knee is placed in 70° to 90° of flexion, the tensioning boot is tensioned to 20 lb (9.07 kg) to restore the normal tibial step-off, cycled, and fixation is achieved on the tibial side of the PCL graft with a screw and spiked ligament washer and bioabsorable interference screw. The knee is maintained at 70° to 90° of flexion, the tensioning boot is tensioned to 20 lb (9.07 kg) with tension on the ACL graft, cycled, and final fixation is achieved of the ACL graft with an bioabsorable interference screw, and fligament fixation button or spiked ligament washer backup fixation.

POSTOPERATIVE REHABILITATION

Postoperatively, patients are placed in a long leg brace locked in extension nonweight, bearing for postoperative weeks 1 through 5. During postoperative weeks 6 through 10, the brace is unlocked, progressive ROM is performed, and weight bearing is advanced at 20% body weight per week achieving full unassisted weight bearing by the end of postoperative week 10. The long leg hinged knee brace is discontinued at the end of postoperative week 10, and a PCL functional brace is initiated. During postoperative weeks 11 through 24, progressive strength training is started and ROM exercises are continued. Postoperative weeks 25 through 36 include agility drills and continued strength training. Return to unrestricted physically demanding activity occurs during postoperative weeks 37 through 52 provided that strength, ROM, and proprioceptive skills are adequate to support the desired activity level (109). We do not use continuous passive motion machines in our postoperative program.

PEARLS AND PITFALLS

There are certain factors that lead to success with this surgical technique:

1. Identify and treat all pathology (especially posterolateral and posteromedial instability).
2. Accurate tunnel placement.

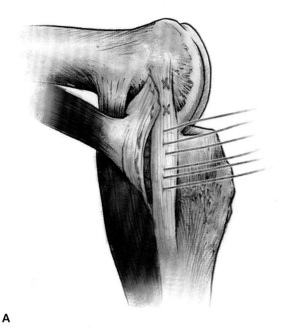

A

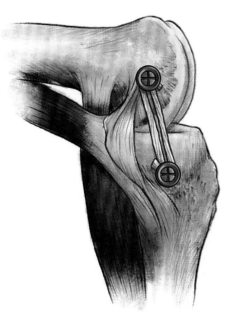

B

FIGURE 78.8. A and B: Medial posteromedial reconstruction with posteromedial capsular shift **(A)**, and free graft reconstruction of the superficial medial collateral ligament **(B)**. (From Fanelli GC. *Rationale and Surgical Technique for PCL and Multiple Knee Ligament Reconstruction.* 2nd ed. Warsaw, Indiana: Biomet Sports Medicine; 2008.)

3. Anatomic graft insertion sites.
4. Strong graft material.
5. Minimize graft bending.
6. Final tensioning at 70´ to 90´ of knee flexion.
7. Graft tensioning.
   a. Biomet mechanical tensioning device.
8. Primary and backup fixation.
9. Appropriate rehabilitation program.

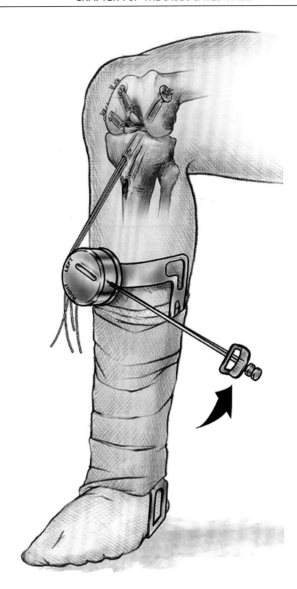

FIGURE 78.9. Biomet Sports Medicine mechanical graft tensioning boot used for PCL and ACL graft tensioning. (From Fanelli GC. *Rationale and Surgical Technique for PCL and Multiple Knee Ligament Reconstruction.* 2nd ed. Warsaw, Indiana: Biomet Sports Medicine; 2008.)

COMPLICATIONS

Complications of the multiple ligament-injured knee can occur immediately, intraoperatively, and postoperatively. Potential complications associated with the initial insult include failure to recognize and treat vascular and nervous injuries. Intraoperative complications include iatrogenic neurovascular injury, iatrogenic tibial plateau fractures at the time of reconstruction, and failure to recognize and treat all components of the instability. Postoperative complications include medial femoral condyle osteonecrosis, knee motion loss, and postoperative anterior knee pain. Stiffness can be a common postoperative complication with ranges from 0% to 18% of knees requiring manipulation and/or lysis of adhesions (99, 110–112).

RESULTS

It has been established that early and accurate diagnosis and treatment of knee dislocations and its associated injuries can improve function and lower morbidity. The majority of recent literature has evaluated the results of ligament reconstruction following knee dislocation. In 2008, Plancher et al. published a retrospective review of 50 knee dislocations followed for an average of 8.3 years. Thirty-one were treated operatively and 19 were treated nonoperatively. Twenty-one percent of their nonoperative group required above knee amputation while 11% required fusion. Average ROM for the remaining 13 patients was 4° to 108°. The operative group had no amputations or fusions with an average ROM of 1.4° to 114.5°. Patients treated nonoperatively had a two times greater chance of having pain with ADLs, pain with rest, grade 2 to 3 arthritis, and subjective instability. Patients treated operatively had better outcomes in HSS scores, Lysholm scores, pain with rest, knee flexion, and return to athletics compared with the nonoperative group. Type of treatment did not alter return to work as both groups measured 80%. When comparing patients treated with ligamentous repair versus reconstruction, patients with ligament repair were twice as likely to fail. In addition, the patients treated with repair had greater than 3 mm of side-to-side difference in 36% of patients compared with 11% in the reconstruction group (17).

In 2008, Ibrahim et al. reported on 20 patients retrospectively reviewed with dislocated knees treated with primary arthroscopic reconstruction with autologous grafting of the ACL, PCL, and collateral ligaments. Average time of follow-up was 43 months. Mean Lysholm score was 91, mean score on the survey of daily activities was 90, and the sports activities score on the knee outcome surgery averaged 86 points. IKDC rating was normal in zero, nearly normal in nine, abnormal in nine, and severely abnormal in two. Mean loss of extension was 0° to 2° and mean loss of flexion was 10° to 15°. Tegner activity score decreased in all patients. Postoperative stiffness was the most common complication (110). Duran et al. retrospectively reviewed 24 arthroscopically assisted ACL and PCL reconstruction with repair of collateral ligaments after knee dislocation at an average of 25 months. 45.8% recovered to normal sports level. The side-to-side difference was less than 5 mm in all 24 patients. Lysholm scores in these patients improved from 41.8 preoperatively to 87 postoperatively, and ROM improved from 87.5 to 125 (113).

Other authors have proposed a two-stage reconstruction for treatment of knee dislocations. In 2007, Bin et al. published results of a two-stage management

of 15 multiple ligament knee reconstructions after knee dislocation with mean follow-up of 88.9 months. Collateral ligaments were repaired or reconstructed within 2 weeks. Once full ROM was obtained ACL and PCL were evaluated. ACL was reconstructed if grade 1+ instability or greater was present on examination and PCL was reconstructed if 1+ laxity was present. By this protocol, 3/15 knees required ACL reconstruction and 7/15 had PCL reconstruction. Thirty-three percent did not require reconstruction. Mean Lysholm and Tegner scores were 87.6 and 3.9, respectively. Final overall IKDC rating was normal in three knees, nearly normal in eight, and abnormal in four. All patients recovered full ROM. They theorize that a two-stage surgical approach shortens operative time and lowers the incidence of arthrofibrosis. They conclude that the two-stage approach results in good outcomes for acute knee dislocation in terms of ROM and stability (112).

Other studies evaluated the results of primary repair of injured ligaments following knee dislocation. In 2007, Owens et al. retrospectively reviewed 28 knee dislocations treated with primary repair of all ligaments coupled with early rehabilitation with a mean follow-up of 48 months. At final follow-up, mean Lysholm score was 89.0. Mean decrease in Tegner activity score was 1.25. Average loss of extension was 1.9° and average loss of flexion was 10.2°, whereas the mean arc of motion was 119.3°. Knees were clinically stable to examination. Patients who underwent surgery within 14 days of injury had a mean Lysholm score of 91.2 compared with 83.6 for those undergoing surgery later than 2 weeks. All patients with unilateral dislocations were able to return to their previous jobs with little or no activity modification. They concluded that primary repair of ligaments coupled with an early rehabilitation program provides comparable outcomes to published results of ligament reconstruction (111).

We have previously published the results of our arthroscopically assisted combined ACL/PCL and PCL/posterolateral complex reconstructions using the reconstructive technique described in this chapter (85, 91, 101, 114). One study reviewed the 2 to 10 year results of 35 arthroscopically assisted combined ACL/PCL reconstructions. All knees had grade 3 preoperative ACL/PCL laxity. Postoperative physical examination results revealed normal posterior drawer/tibial step-off in 46% of knees and normal Lachman and pivot shift tests in 94% of knees. Posterolateral stability was restored to normal in 24% of knees, and tighter than the normal knee in 76% of knees. Thirty-degree varus stress testing was normal in 88% of knees whereas 30° valgus stress testing was normal in 100% of surgically treated MCL tears, and normal in 87.5% of brace treated knees. Postoperative KT 1000 arthrometer testing mean side-to-side difference measurements were 2.7 mm (PCL screen), 2.6 mm (corrected posterior), and 1.0 mm (corrected anterior) measurements, a statistically significant improvement from preoperative status (P = .001). Postoperative Lysholm, Tegner, and HSS knee ligament-rating scale mean values were 91.2, 5.3, and 86.8, respectively, demonstrating a statistically significant improvement from preoperative status (P = .001). This concluded that combined ACL/PCL instabilities could be successfully treated with arthroscopic reconstruction and the appropriate collateral ligament surgery.

A second study presented the 2- to 10-year follow-up of 41 chronic arthroscopically assisted combined PCL/posterolateral reconstructions. Postoperative physical examination revealed normal posterior drawer/tibial step-off in 70% of knees. Posterolateral stability was restored to normal in 27% of knees, and tighter than the normal knee in 71% of knees. Thirty-degree varus stress testing was normal in 40/41 (97%) of knees. Postoperative KT 1000 arthrometer testing mean side-to-side difference measurements were 1.80 mm (PCL screen), 2.11 mm (corrected posterior), and 0.63 mm (corrected anterior) measurements. This is a statistically significant improvement from preoperative status for the PCL screen and the corrected posterior measurements (P = .001). Postoperative Lysholm, Tegner, and HSS knee ligament-rating scale mean values were 91.7, 4.92, and 88.7, respectively, demonstrating a statistically significant improvement from preoperative status (P = .001). This demonstrated that chronic combined PCL/posterolateral instabilities could be successfully treated with arthroscopic PCL reconstruction using fresh frozen Achilles tendon allograft combined with PLC reconstruction using biceps tendon transfer and posterolateral capsular shift procedure (115).

The above reviews show that surgical treatment of multiligament knee injuries and knee dislocations achieved satisfactory stability, ROM, and subjective functional results. However, preinjury activity level may not be regained in most patients. Patients who underwent surgery in the acute phase had overall better functional scores than those with delayed treatment. As a whole, patients treated nonoperatively fared far worse with ROM, subjective scores, pain with rest, and return to athletics compared with operative treatment.

Our PCL double-bundle compared with single-bundle reconstruction results in the PCL-based multiple ligament-injured knee are as follows Fanelli et al. (116). Ninety consecutive arthroscopic transtibial PCL reconstructions were performed by a single surgeon. Forty-five single-bundle and 45 double-bundle reconstructions were performed using fresh frozen Achilles tendon allograft for the anterolateral bundle and tibialis anterior allograft for the posteromedial bundle with all grafts being from the same tissue bank. Postoperative comparative results were assessed using Telos stress radiography, KT 1000, Lysholm, Tegner, and HSS knee ligament-rating scales. Postoperative period ranged from 15 to 72 months in this level 3 retrospective comparative study.

Postoperative KT 1000 arthrometer testing mean side-to-side difference measurements were 1.91 mm (PCL screen, 90°), 2.11 mm (corrected posterior, 70°), and 1.11 mm (30°) in the single-bundle group, and 2.46 mm (PCL screen, 90°), 2.94 mm (corrected posterior, 70°), and 0.44 mm (30°) in the double-bundle group (P = .289694, .231154, and .315546, respectively). The postoperative stress radiographic mean side-to-side difference measurement measured at 90° of knee flexion, and 32 lb (14.5 kg) of posterior directed force applied to the proximal tibia using the Telos device was 2.56 mm in the single-bundle group, and 2.36 mm in the double-bundle group (P = .895792). Postoperative Lysholm, Tegner, and HSS knee ligament-rating scale mean values were 90.3, 5.0, and 86.2, respectively, in the single-bundle group, and 87.6, 4.6, and 83.3 in the double-bundle group, respectively (P = .226327, .308564, and .282588, respectively). All objective parameters demonstrated no statistically significant difference between the single and the double-bundle PCL reconstructions in both acute and chronic cases.

Both the single-bundle and the double-bundle PCL reconstruction surgical techniques using allograft tissue provide successful results in the PCL-based multiple ligament-injured knee when evaluated with stress radiography, arthrometer measurements, and knee ligament-rating scales.

CONCLUSIONS AND FUTURE DIRECTIONS

The multiple ligament-injured knee is a severe injury that may also involve neurovascular injuries and fractures. Surgical treatment offers good functional results documented in the literature by physical examination, arthrometer testing, stress radiography, and knee ligament-rating scales. Mechanical tensioning devices are helpful with cruciate ligament tensioning. Some low-grade MCL complex injuries may be amenable to brace treatment, whereas high-grade medial side injuries require repair–reconstru-ction. Lateral posterolateral injuries are most successfully treated with surgical repair–reconstruction. Surgical timing in acute multiple ligament-injured knee cases depends upon the ligaments injured, injured extremity vascular status, skin condition of the extremity, degree of instability, and the patients' overall health. Allograft tissue is preferred for these complex surgical procedures. Delayed reconstruction of 2 to 3 weeks may decrease the incidence of arthrofibrosis, and it is important to address all components of the instability. Currently, there is no conclusive evidence that double-bundle PCL reconstruction provides superior results to single-bundle PCL reconstruction in the multiple ligament-injured knee. Further research is required for continuous improvement in the treatment of these severe knee injuries.

REFERENCES

1. Shields L, Mital M, Cave EF. Complete dislocation of the knee: experience at the Massachusetts General Hospital. *J Trauma.* 1969;9:192–215.
2. Kennedy JC. Complete dislocation of the knee joint. *J Bone Joint Surg Am.* 1963;45-A:889–904.
3. Hoover NW. Injuries of the popliteal artery associated with fractures and dislocations. *Surg Clin North Am.* 1961;41:1099–1112.
4. Schenck RC Jr. The dislocated knee. *Instr Course Lect.* 1994;43:127–136.
5. Hegyes MS, Richardson MW, Miller MD. Knee dislocation. Complications of nonoperative and operative management. *Clin Sports Med.* 2000;19(3):519–543.
6. Wascher DC, Dvirnak PC, DeCoster TA. Knee dislocation: initial assessment and implications for treatment. *J Orthop Trauma.* 1997;11(7):525–529.
7. Myers MH, Harvey JP. Traumatic dislocation of the knee joint. *J Bone Joint Surg Am.* 1971;53-A:16–29.
8. Lill H, Hepp P, Rose T, et al. Fresh meniscal allograft transplantation and autologous ACL/PCL reconstruction in a patient with complex knee trauma following knee dislocation—a case report. *Scand J Med Sci Sports.* 2004;14:112–115.
9. Quinlan AG, Sharrard WJ. Postero-lateral dislocation of the knee with capsular interposition. *J Bone Joint Surg Br.* 1958;40-B(4):660–663.
10. Green NE, Allen BL. Vascular injuries associated with dislocation of the knee. *J Bone Joint Surg.* 1977;59A:236–239.
11. Jones RE, Smith EC, Bone GE. Vascular and orthopedic complications of knee dislocation. *Surg Gynecol Obstet.* 1979;149:554–558.
12. Welling RE, Kakkasseril J, Cranley JJ. Complete dislocations of the knee with popliteal vascular injury. *J Trauma.* 1981;21(6):450–453.
13. Seroyer ST, Musahl V, Harner CD. Management of the acute knee dislocation: the Pittsburgh experience. *Injury.* 2008;39(7):710–718.
14. Meyers MH, Moore TM, Harvey JP Jr. Traumatic dislocation of the knee joint. *J Bone Joint Surg Am.* 1975;57(3):430–433.
15. Wright DG, Covey DC, Born CT, et al. Open dislocation of the knee. *J Orthop Trauma.* 1995;9(2):135–140.
16. Conwell HE, Alldredge RH. Complete dislocations of the knee joint. *Surg Gynecol Obstet.* 1937;64:94–101.
17. Plancher KD, Siliski J. Long-term functional results and complications in patients with knee dislocations. *J Knee Surg.* 2008;21(4):261–268.
18. Crist BD, Gregory JKR, Murtha YM. Treatment of acute distal femur fractures. *Orthopedics.* 2008;31(7):681–690.
19. Dodds JA, Arnoczky SP. Anatomy of the anterior cruciate ligament: a blueprint for repair and reconstruction. *Arthroscopy.* 1994;10(2):132–139.
20. Arnoczky SP. Anatomy of the anterior cruciate ligament. *Clin Orthop Relat Res.* 1983;172:19–25.
21. Norwood LA, Cross MJ. Anterior cruciate ligament: functional anatomy of its bundles in rotatory instabilities. *Am J Sports Med.* 1979;7:23–26.
22. Kennedy JC, Weinberg HW, Wilson AS. The anatomy and functions of the anterior cruciate ligament. *J Bone Joint Surg.* 1974;56:223–235.
23. Girgis FG, Marshall JL, Monajem A. The cruciate ligaments of the knee joint. Anatomical, functional and experimental analysis. *Clin Orthop Relat Res.* 1975;(106):216–231.
24. Harner CD, Xerogeans JW, Livesay GA, et al. The human posterior cruciate ligament complex: an interdisciplinary study. Ligament morphology and biomechanical evaluation. *Am J Sports Med.* 1995;23(6):736–745.
25. Johnson CJ, Bach BR. Current concepts review. Posterior cruciate ligament. *Am J Knee Surg.* 1990;3:143–153.
26. Kennedy JC, Alexander IJ, Hayes KC. Nerve supply of the human knee and its functional importance. *Am J Sports Med.* 1982;10:329–335.
27. Cole BJ, Sekiya JK. *Surgical Techniques of the Shoulder, Elbow, and Knee in Sports Medicine.* Philadelphia, PA: Saunders; 2008.
28. Warren LF, Marshall JL. The supporting structures and layers on the medial side of the knee: an anatomical analysis. *J Bone joint Surg Am.* 1979;61-A:56–62.
29. Fanelli GC, Harris JD. Surgical treatment of acute medial collateral ligament and posteromedial corner injuries of the knee. *Sports Med Arthrosc.* 2006;14(2):78–83.
30. Robinson JR, Sanchez-Ballester J, Bull AM, et al. The posteromedial corner revisited. An anatomical description of the passive restraining structures of the medial aspect of the human knee. *J Bone Joint Surg Br.* 2004;86:647–681.
31. Seebacher JR, Ingilis AE, Marshall JL, et al. The structure of the posterolateral aspect of the knee. *J Bone Joint Surg Am.* 1932;64(4):536–541.
32. LaPrade, RF, Ly TV, Wentorf FA, et al. The posterolateral attachments of the knee. *Am J Sports Med.* 2003;31(6):854–860.
33. Goitz RJ, Tomaino MM. Management of peroneal nerve injuries associated with knee dislocations. *Am J Orthop.* 2003;32(1):14–16.
34. Shelbourne KD, Porter DA, Clingman JA, et al. Low velocity knee dislocation. *Orthop Rev.* 1991;20:995–1004.
35. Hagino RT, Decaprio JD, Valentine RJ, et al. Spontaneous popliteal vascular injury in the morbidly obese. *J Vasc Surg.* 1998;28(3):458–463.
36. Wascher DC. High-velocity knee dislocation with vascular injury. Treatment principles. *Clin Sports Med.* 2000;19(3):457–477.
37. Helgeson MD, Lehman RA Jr, Murphy: initial evaluation of the acute and chronic multiple ligament injured knee. *J Knee Surg.* 2005;18(3):213–219.
38. Robertson A, Nutton RW, Keating JF. Dislocation of the knee. *J Bone Joint Surg Br.* 2006;88(6):706–711.
39. Brautigan B, Johnson DL. The epidemiology of knee dislocations. *Clin Sports Med.* 2000;19:387–397.
40. Henshaw RM, Shapiro MS, Oppenheim WL. Delayed reduction of traumatic knee dislocation. A case report and literature review. *Clin Orthop.* 1996;330:152–156.
41. Patterson BM, Agel J, Swiontkowski MF, et al; LEAP Study Group. Knee dislocations with vascular injury: outcomes in the Lower Extremity Assessment Project (LEAP) Study. *J Trauma.* 2007;63(4):855–858.
42. Hill JA, Rana NA. Complications of posterolateral dislocation of the knee: case report and literature review. *Clin Orthop Relat Res.* 1981;154:212–215.
43. Rihn JA, Groff YJ, Harner CD, et al. The acutely dislocated knee: evaluation and management. *J Am Acad Orthop Surg.* 2004;12(5):334–346.

44. Treiman GS, Yellin AE, Weaver FA, et al. Examination of the patient with a knee dislocation. The case for selective arteriography. *Arch Surg.* 1992;127:1056–1063.

45. Bok AP, Peter JC. Carotid and vertebral artery occlusion after blunt cervical injury: the role of MR angiography in early diagnosis. *J Trauma.* 1996;40:968–972.

46. Friedman D, Flanders A, Thomas C, et al. Vertebral artery injury after acute cervical spine trauma: rate of occurrence as detected by MR angiography and assessment of clinical consequences. *AJR Am J Roentgenol.* 1995;164:443–447.

47. Potter HG, Weinstein M, Allen AA. Magnetic resonance imaging of the multiple-ligament injured knee. *J Orthop Trauma.* 2002;16:330–339.

48. Bui KL, Ilaslan H, Parker RD, et al. Knee dislocations: a magnetic resonance imaging study correlated with clinical and operative findings. *Skeletal Radiol.* 2008;37(7):653–661.

49. Twaddle BC, Hunter JC, Chapman JR, et al. MRI in acute knee dislocations: a prospective study of clinical, MRI, and surgical findings. *J Bone Joint Surg Br.* 1996;78:573–579.

50. McDonough EB Jr, Wojtys EM. Multiligamentous injuries of the knee and associated vascular injuries. *Am J Sports Med.* 2009;37(1):156–159.

51. Reckling FW, Peltier LF. Acute knee dislocations and their complications. *Clin Orthop Relat Res.* 2004;422:135–141.

52. Axar FM, Brandt JC, Phillips BB, et al. Ultra-low velocity knee dislocation. *J Orthop Trauma.* 2000;14:153–154.

53. Marin EL, Bifulco SS, Fast A. Obesity. A risk factor for knee dislocation. *Am J Phys Med Rehabil.* 1990;69:132–134.

54. Najem M, Kambal A, Hussain TS. Popliteal artery reconstruction secondary to minor trauma in a 19-year-old morbidly obese woman. *Obes Surg.* 2004;14:1435–1436.

55. Papadopoulos AX, Panagopoulos A, Kouzelis A, et al. Delayed diagnosis of a popliteal artery rupture after a posteromedial tibial plateau fracture-dislocation. *J Knee Surg.* 2006;19(2):125–127.

56. Alberty RE, Goodfried G, Boyden AM. Popliteal artery injury with fractural dislocation of the knee. *Am J Surg.* 1981;142:36–40.

57. Barnes CJ, Pietrobon R, Higgins LD. Does the pulse examination in patients with traumatic knee dislocation predict a surgical arterial injury? A meta-analysis. *J Trauma.* 2002;53:1109–1114.

58. Cone JC. Vascular injury associated with fracture-dislocations of the lower extremity. *Clin Orthop Relat Res.* 1989;243:30–35.

59. McCoy GF, Hannon DG, Barr RJ, et al. Vascular injury associated with low-velocity dislocations of the knee. *J Bone Joint Surg.* 1987;69B:285–287.

60. Miranda FE, Dennis JW, Veldenz HC, et al. Confirmation of the safety and accuracy of physical examination in the evaluation of knee dislocation for injury of the popliteal artery: a prospective study. *J Trauma.* 2002;52:247–252.

61. Mills WJ, Barei DP, McNair P. The value of the ankle-brachial index for diagnosing arterial injury after knee dislocation: a prospective study. *J Trauma.* 2004;56(6):1261–1265.

62. Abou-Sayed H, Berger DL. Blunt lower-extremity trauma and popliteal artery injuries: revisiting the case for selective arteriography. *Arch Surg.* 2002; 137:585–589.

63. Kendall RW, Taylor DC, Salvian AJ, et al. The role of arteriography in assessing vascular injuries associated with dislocations of the knee. *J Trauma.* 1993;35:875–878.

64. Martinez D, Sweatman K, Thompson EC. Popliteal artery injury associated with knee dislocations. *Am Surg.* 2001;67:165–167.

65. Stannard JP, Sheils TM, Lopez-Ben RR, et al. Vascular injuries in knee dislocations: the role of physical examination in determining the need for arteriography. *J Bone Joint Surg Am.* 2004;86:910–915.

66. Johansen K, Lynch K, Paun M, et al. Non-invasive vascular tests reliably exclude occult arterial trauma in injured extremities. *J Trauma.* 1991;31:515–522.

67. Bynoe RP, Miles WS, Bell RM, et al. Noninvasive diagnosis of vascular trauma by duplex ultrasonography. *J Vasc Surg.* 1991;14:346–352.

68. Schenck RC Jr, Hunter RE, Ostrum RF, et al. Knee dislocations. *Instr Course Lect.* 1999;48:515–522.

69. Niall DM, Nutton RW, Keating JF. Palsy of the common peroneal nerve after traumatic dislocation of the knee. *J Bone Joint Surg Br.* 2005;87(5):664–667.

70. Berry H, Richardson PM. Common peroneal nerve palsy: a clinical electrophysiological review. *J Neurol Neurosurg Psychiatry.* 1976;39:1162–1171.

71. Haftek J. Stretch injury of peripheral nerve. *J Bone Joint Surg Br.* 1970;52:354–365.

72. Sisto DJ, Warren RF. Complete knee dislocation: a follow-up study of operative treatment. *Clin Orthop Relat Res.* 1985;198:94–101.

73. Taylor AR, Arden GP, Rainey HA. Traumatic dislocation of the knee: a report of forty-three cases with special reference to conservative treatment. *J Bone Joint Surg.* 1972;54B:96–102.

74. Kim DH, Kliine DG. Management and results of peroneal nerve lesions. *Neurosurgery.* 1996;39:312–320.

75. Wood MB. Peroneal nerve repair: surgical results. *Clin Orthop.* 1991;267:206–210.

76. Sedel L, Nizard RS. Nerve grafting for traction injuries of the common peroneal nerve: a report of 17 cases. *J Bone Joint Surg Br.* 1993;75:772–774.

77. McMahon MS, Craig SM. Interfascicular reconstruction of the peroneal nerve after knee ligament injury. *Ann Plast Surg.* 1994;32:642–664.

78. Kline DG. Surgical repair of peripheral nerve injury. *Muscle Nerve.* 1990;13:843–852.

79. Tomaino M, Day C, Papageorgiou C, et al. Peroneal nerve palsy following knee dislocation: pathoanatomy and implications for treatment. *Knee Surg Sports Traumatol Arthrosc.* 2000;8:163–165.

80. Kline DG, Tiel R, Kim D, et al. Lower extremity nerve injuries. In: Omer GE Jr, Spinner M, Van Beck AL, eds. *Management of Peripheral Nerve Problems.* 2nd ed. Philadelphia, PA: Saunders; 1998:420–427.

81. Almekinders LC, Logan TC. Results following treatment of traumatic dislocation of the knee. *Clin Orthop Relat Res.* 1991;284:203–207.

82. Meyers MH, Harvey JP Jr. Traumatic dislocation of the knee joint: a study of eighteen cases. *J Bone Joint Surg.* 1971;53A:16–29.

83. Reckling FW, Peltier LF. Acute knee dislocations and their complications. *J Trauma.* 1969;9:181–191.

84. Myles JW. Seven cases of traumatic dislocation of the knee. *Proc R Soc Med.* 1967;60:279–281.

85. Fanelli GC, Gianotti BF, Edson CJ. Arthroscopically assisted combined anterior and posterior cruciate ligament reconstruction. *Arthroscopy.* 1996;12(1):5–14.

86. Shapiro MS, Freedman EL. Allograft reconstruction of the anterior and posterior cruciate ligaments after traumatic knee dislocation. *Am J Sports Med.* 1995;23(5):580–587.

87. Frassica FJ, Sim FH, Staeheli JW, et al. Dislocation of the knee. *Clin Orthop Relat Res.* 1991;263:200–205.

88. Richter M, Bosch U, Wippermann B, et al. Comparison of surgical repair or reconstruction of the cruciate ligaments versus nonsurgical treatment in patients with traumatic knee dislocation. *Am J Sports Med.* 2002;30(5):718–727.

89. Noyes FR, Barber-Westin SD. Reconstruction of the anterior and posterior cruciate ligaments after knee dislocation. *Am J Sports Med.* 1997;25(6):769–778.

90. Wong CH, Tan JL, Chang HC, et al. Knee dislocations-a retrospective study comparing operative versus closed immobilization treatment outcomes. *Knee Surg Sports Traumatol Arthrosc.* 2004;14(2):112–115.

91. Fanelli GC, Edson CJ. Arthroscopically assisted combined ACL/PCL reconstruction. 2–10 year follow-up. *Arthroscopy.* 2002;18(7):703–714.

92. Fanelli GC, Orcutt DR, Edson CJ. The multiple-ligament injured knee: evaluation, treatment, and results. *Arthroscopy.* 2005;21(4):471–486.

93. Fanelli GC, Edson CJ, Orcutt DR, et al. Treatment of combined anterior cruciate-posterior cruciate ligament-medial-lateral side knee injuries. *J Knee Surg.* 2005;18(3):240–248.

94. Fanelli GC, Harris JD. Late MCL (medial collateral ligament) reconstruction. *Tech Knee Surg.* 2007;6(2):99–105.

95. Miyamoto RG, Bosco JA, Sherman OH. Treatment of medial collateral ligament injuries. *J Am Acad Orthop Surg.* 2009;17(3):152–161.

96. Fanelli GC, Feldmann DD. Management of combined anterior cruciate ligament/posterior cruciate ligament/posterolateral complex injuries of the knee. *Oper Tech Sports Med.* 1999;7(3):143–149.

97. Shelbourne KD, Haro MS, Gray T. Knee dislocation with lateral side injury: results of an en masse surgical repair technique of the lateral side. *Am J Sports Med.* 2007;35(7):1105–1116.

98. Kurtz CA, Sekiya JK. Treatment of acute and chronic anterior cruciate ligament-posterior cruciate ligament-lateral side knee injuries. *J Knee Surg.* 2005; 18(3):228–239.

99. Chhabra A, Cha PS, Rihn JA, et al. Surgical management of knee dislocations. Surgical technique. *J Bone Joint Surg Am.* 2005;87(pt 1)(suppl 1):1–21.

100. Liow RY, McNicholas MJ, Keating JF, et al. Ligament repair and reconstruction in traumatic dislocation of the knee. *J Bone Joint Surg Br.* 2003;85(6):845–851.

101. Fanelli GC, Gianotti BF, Edson CJ. Arthroscopically assisted combined posterior cruciate ligament/posterior lateral complex reconstruction. *Arthroscopy.* 1996;12(5):521–530.

102. Tzurbakis M, Diamantopoulos A, Xenakis T, et al. Surgical treatment of multiple knee ligament injuries in 44 patients: 2–8 years follow-up results. *Knee Surg Sports Traumatol Arthrosc.* 2006;14(8):739–749.

103. Fanelli GC, Edson CJ, Reinheimer KN, et al. Posterior cruciate ligament and posterolateral corner reconstruction. *Sports Med Arthrosc Rev.* 2007;15(4):168–175.

104. Gregory C. Fanelli, ed. *Posterior Cruciate Ligament Injuries: A Practical Guide to Management.* New York, NY: Springer-Verlag; 2001.

105. Gregory C. Fanelli, ed. *The Multiple Ligament Injured Knee. A Practical Guide to Management.* New York, NY: Springer-Verlag; 2004.

106. Fanelli GC. *Rationale and Surgical Technique for PCL and Multiple Knee Ligament Reconstruction.* 2nd ed. Warsaw, Indiana: Biomet Sports Medicine; 2008.

107. Giannoulias CS, Freedman KB. Knee dislocations: management of the multiligament-injured knee. *Am J Orthop.* 2004;33(11):553–559.

108. Harner CD, Waltrip RL, Bennett CH, et al. Surgical management of knee dislocations. *J Bone Joint Surg Am.* 2004;86-A(2):262–273.

109. Fanelli GC. Posterior cruciate ligament rehabilitation: how slow should we go? *Arthroscopy.* 2008;24(2):234–235.

110. Ibrahim SA, Ahmad FH, Salah M, et al. Surgical management of traumatic knee dislocation. *Arthroscopy.* 2008;24(2):178–187.

111. Owens BD, Neault M, Benson E, et al. Primary repair of knee dislocations: results in 25 patients (28 knees) at a mean follow-up of four years. *J Orthop Trauma.* 2007;21(2):92–96.

112. Bin SI, Nam TS. Surgical outcome of 2-stage management of multiple knee ligament injuries after knee dislocation. *Arthroscopy.* 2007;23(10):1066–1072.

113. Duran X, Yang Y, Xiao G, et al. Clinical effect of arthroscopically assisted repair and reconstruction for dislocation of the knee with multiple ligament injuries [Chinese]. *Zhongguo Xiu Fu Chong Jian Wai Ke Za Zhi.* 2008;22(6):673–675.

114. Fanelli GC, Gianotti BF, Edson CJ. The posterior cruciate ligament arthroscopic evaluation and treatment. *Arthroscopy.* 1994;10(6):673–688.

115. Fanelli GC, Edson CJ. Arthroscopically assisted combined PCL-posterolateral reconstruction. 2–10 year follow-up. *Arthroscopy.* 2004;20:339–345.

116. Fanelli GC, Beck JD, Edson CJ. Single compared to double bundle PCL reconstruction using allograft tissue. *J Knee Surg.* 2012;25(1):59–64

Revision ACL and PCL Reconstruction

Daniel R. Stephenson • Darren L. Johnson

Anterior cruciate ligament (ACL) injuries are one of the most common sports injuries in the United States. In fact, it is estimated that there are over 200,000 ACL injuries each year (1). As they are such common injuries, ACL reconstruction is one of the most common procedures performed by orthopedic surgeons, at a near similar rate. Injuries to the posterior cruciate ligament (PCL) are considerably less common, with reports that they account for 1% to 30% of all acute knee injuries. They are more often seen in trauma patients than in athletes, but nonetheless pose a risk to knee stability and late degenerative arthritis is left untreated. Of concern with ACL reconstruction is that it is estimated that 85% of ACL reconstructions performed in the United States are done by surgeons that do fewer than 10 ACL surgeries a year (2). Despite this ACL reconstruction is generally considered a good procedure to restore normal or near normal knee stability and kinematics. With this high number of injuries and surgery, there are also a relatively high number of failures that require revision. On the other hand, PCL injuries are less common, less commonly recognized and therefore treated operatively and thus much less frequently revised.

Any surgery can fail for a myriad of reasons, and ACL and PCL reconstructions are no different. One must generally ascertain the reason of failure in order to succeed in the designing a treatment algorithm for operative revision reconstruction. The goal of a revision surgery of either cruciate is to provide a stable and functional knee that will recreate the normal kinematics of the knee. In order to restore normal knee kinematics, our belief is that the ligaments must be reconstructed anatomically, just as one attempts to achieve in fracture management. Increasing research in the past decade has focused on the detailed three-dimensional (3D) and insertional anatomy of the cruciate ligaments. The ACL is now known to have two functional bundles—the anteromedial (AM) bundle and posterolateral (PL) bundle. Likewise, the PCL is also recognized to have two functional bundles—the anterolateral (AL) bundle and posteromedial (PM) bundle. This knowledge and detailed studies as to the exact locations of the femoral origins and tibial footprints of the cruciate

ligaments are transforming the approach to the operative reconstruction of these ligaments (3, 4).

How we assess a failure remains somewhat controversial. Some clinical failures are a failure to the patient but may not be to the clinician. An elite athlete who does not return to the same level of performance after surgery, may consider that a failure, whereas a surgeon may feel the kinematics and stability to be acceptable. There are subjective complaints following an ACL or PCL injury such as pain, stiffness, or recurrent instability. These require further investigation as to the source of the problem. Objectively, these complaints may be seen with laxity, degenerative joint disease, and decreased range of motion.

This chapter will discuss the evaluation and treatment of failures of both ACL and PCL reconstruction. Our philosophy is that the restoration of the true anatomic location of the ACL and PCL is critical to restore the function of the knee. We utilize an anatomic double-bundle technique in a majority of our ACL revisions to achieve this. In the setting of a revision PCL reconstruction, the rate of recurrence and rate of reoperation are both low. As such, there is much less known and published in regard to revision PCL surgery. Decisions about graft selection and single-versus double-bundle reconstructions are often individually based on the patholaxity of the involved knee as well as the patients own unique anatomy.

ACL REVISION

Etiology

ACL failures are attributed to an array of causes. To best understand these, we must begin by defining what constitutes a "failure." Nearly all would agree that a rerupture with patholaxity is a failure. Most would then consider the realm of "clinical failures" as any situation where there is either recurrent instability or significant arthrofibrosis with limitations in range of motion. We would also consider most situations that result in significant pain, which precludes the participation in activities of daily living (ADLs) or the inability to return to level 1 sports as failures. There are also the failures that some would consider significant, but many would exclude the athlete that returns to their chosen sport but remains at a suboptimal performance level. This group is estimated at nearly 40% of elite athletes and those who participate in level 1 sports year round. These are the outcomes that are most difficult to quantify or even achieve agreement that they are in fact failures. The literature reports failure rates from 3% to 52%, a large range likely due in part to the poor consensus on what constitutes failure (5).

We generally think of failures in broad categories: (1) recurrent pathologic laxity or instability (including traumatic rerupture), (2) decreased motion or arthrofibrosis, (3) persistent pain, and (4) extensor mechanism dysfunction. There are multiple reasons that a failure can result in any of the above situations. In order to best approach the failed primary surgery, you must begin by knowing which of the etiologic mechanisms caused the particular problem. Armed with this knowledge you can begin to determine the underlying cause, and design a treatment algorithm for that particular patient.

When examining recurrent instability, there are four major reasons for failure. The most likely cause of failure is technical error—most commonly nonanatomic tunnel placement. Battaglia et al. (6) estimate that 70% to 80% of failures are a result of nonanatomic tunnels. There are various forms of tunnel malpositioning; the most common being vertical tunnels (Fig. 79.1). This occurs when the tibial tunnel is too posterior and the femoral tunnel is more central in the roof of the intercondylar notch often from transtibial single incision ACL surgery. The resulting complaint tends to be related more toward rotational instability, rather than complaints of anterior posterior instability. On physical examination, this patient may have a positive pivot-shift in light of a negative Lachman's or Anterior Drawer test (7, 8). We find this error is most commonly seen in ACL reconstructions performed via a transtibial technique versus creating femoral tunnels through the accessory anteromedial (AAM) portal or two-incision technique. Error in tunnel placement can also be attributed to inadequate visualization due to portal placement. While a large notchplasty may not be required in all patients, enough must be removed to allow adequate visualization of native anatomic bony landmarks.

A second cause of recurrent instability that is commonly encountered is the failure to address other injuries, such as meniscal injuries, injury to the medial collateral ligament (MCL), posterior oblique ligament (POL), or posterolateral corner (PLC) including the popliteal fibular ligament, and the fibular collateral ligament. It is estimated that 15% of ACL failures occur because of the failure to recognize or treat concomitant injuries (9). This will cause nonphysiologic strain on the graft and ultimately end in graft attrition and surgical failure in the relative short term. Third, there are failures associated with fixation. This can be frank failure, or error in the tensioning of the graft, these are much less common but may occur.

Graft-tunnel mismatch and interference screw divergence are the most common technical errors. Finally, there is the true traumatic rerupture. This is perhaps the hardest to prevent, as often times it is a result of the player in the wrong place at the wrong time. The caveat to this would be the use of bracing in downhill skiers. This has shown to be protective of further injury. The use of bracing has not shown to be beneficial in the prevention or recurrence of ACL injuries in the majority of athletes.

The next major category to examine is that of stiffness or decreased range of motion. One of the most difficult problems to address after ACL reconstruction is the loss of terminal extension. Patients that are unable to fully extend their knee (even 5° from full extension) often complain of significant discomfort and functional disability. This is one area where being aggressive with range of motion therapy in the 1st month after surgery is crucial. Difficulty with flexion is much less commonly seen and more functionally tolerated. Flexion deficits tend to achieve better resolution with manipulation and lysis of adhesions. Aside from these issues, there are other reasons that range of motion may be affected. Certainly, the "cyclops lesion" is of concern. This is created by scarring of the tibial stump in the intercondylar notch if the athlete does not get full extension within the first 2 weeks, which may then prevent full extension. This, however, is easily treated with arthroscopic debridement. Nonanatomic tunnels may also contribute to decreased range of motion. The phenomenon of a "captured knee" is generally associated with a femoral tunnel that is too far anterior—thus creating what is effectively a shortened graft. The third major cause of loss of motion is arthrofibrosis. These patients have generally lost greater than 10° of knee extension and more than 25° of knee flexion, with decreased patellar mobility. Failure to recognize this condition, and its associated swelling and inflammation can result in infrapatellar contracture and patella baja. It is also important to distinguish between primary or iatrogenic arthrofibrosis and secondary arthrofibrosis (acute surgery, technical errors, delayed rehabilitation) (10). Primary arthrofibrosis is a diagnosis of exclusion, and other causes must be ruled out. Management focuses on therapeutic exercises and modalities to regain patellar mobility and passive stretching. Secondary arthrofibrosis is generally preventable by performing surgery at the proper time, with proper technique and adequate, early rehabilitation. Primary surgery should generally be delayed at least 3 weeks from injury, with adequate decrease in swelling and inflammation. Surgery performed in this period of acute inflammation may actually accelerate the healing process, resulting in increased fibrotic scar formation. In regard to arthrofibrosis, it is important to distinguish between primary or iatrogenic arthrofibrosis and secondary arthrofibrosis (acute surgery, technical errors, delayed rehabilitation).(10) Primary arthrofibrosis is a diagnosis of exclusion, and other causes must be ruled out. Management focuses on therapeutic exercises and

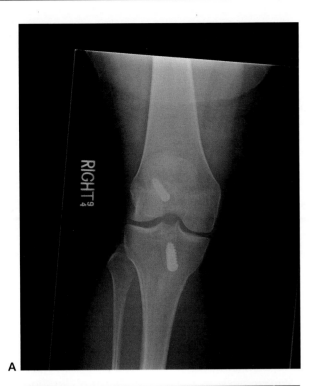

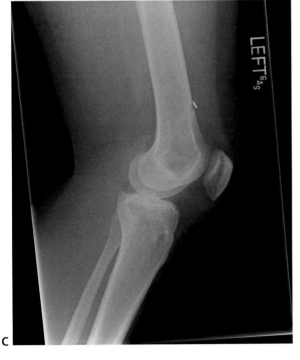

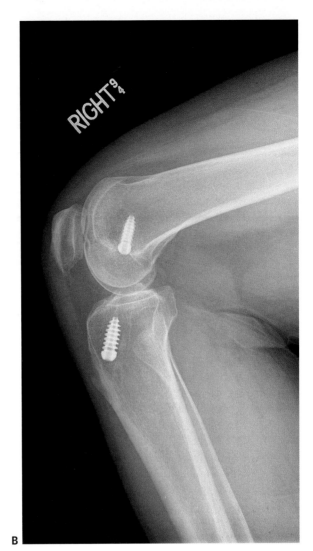

FIGURE 79.1. AP and lateral radiographs demonstrating a vertical ACL reconstruction with interference screws **(A and B)**, and with a soft-tissue graft and endobutton **(C)**. Note that the endobutton is exiting very distal from the joint.

modalities to regain patellar mobility and passive stretching. Secondary arthrofibrosis is generally preventable by performing surgery at the proper time, with proper technique and adequate early rehabilitation. Primary surgery should generally be delayed at least 3 weeks from injury, with adequate decrease in swelling and inflammation. Surgery performed in this period of acute inflammation may actually accelerate the healing process, resulting in increased fibrotic scar formation. Less common causes of decreased range of motion include simultaneous additional

ligament surgery, complex regional pain syndrome, poor rehabilitation compliance, and prolonged immobilization.

The third major cause of failure of ACL reconstructions is extensor mechanism dysfunction. There are a variety of problems that can affect the function of the extensor mechanism; the most catastrophic is a patellar fracture. This can be seen most often with technical error associated with bone-patellar tendon-bone (BTB) and quadriceps autografts. Another problem that can arise with ACL reconstructions is anterior knee pain, which is most often associated with BTB autograft. This complication can often be prevented by getting the patient into aggressive postoperative rehabilitation immediately after surgery. The rehabilitation program should focus on the restoration of patellar mobility including maintenance of patellar glide and patellar tilt symmetric to the uninvolved knee. Finally, there can be problems that occur due to general quadriceps weakness. Specifically, weakness in the vastus medialis (VMO) can result in patellar maltracking and be problematic in the first 2 months of rehabilitation. Fortunately, this is a problem that is treated with reassurance and continued work in therapy.

The fourth and final major source of failure is degenerative joint disease. This is an issue that can arise in the 1st year (most often if there is an isolated chondral defect or meniscectomy) or with time. Chondral injuries generally will require a second operative intervention to help restore the cartilage surface, which is beyond the scope of this chapter. Several studies have shown that ACL deficient knees can have radiographic evidence of osteoarthritis in greater than 50% of patients in 5 to 15 years after injury, but many of these are poorly designed studies, and the natural history has not been well studied particularly with current anatomic ACL techniques. Neuman et al. (11) found that there was a 16% incidence of radiographic knee OA 15 years after injury, with that number decreasing to 14% in patients less than 30 years of age. More indicative is the presence or absence of meniscal injury, where rates approach 44% after meniscectomy 10 years after reconstruction (12). Graft selection has not been shown to be associated with development of osteoarthritis (13). Patients may also present with unicompartmental arthritis (most often in the medial compartment), or tricompartmental arthritis, generally several years down the road. This patient population presents a unique challenge based on the age of the patient, as options may range from conservative measures to a partial or total joint arthroplasty.

Preoperative Evaluation and Planning

As with most evaluations, it is crucial to begin with a thorough history and physical examination. Begin with discussing the initial injury, surgery, and rehabilitation. When discussing the issues with your patient, it is important to discern the following: What was chronicity of the problem? Was there or was there not a traumatic event? Did the onset of symptoms develope late after ACL reconstruction or in the immediate postoperative period? It is important to know whether the patient ever made it back successfully to level 1 ACL dependent sports and if so, for how long? Often times this will let you start focusing on whether you are looking at a technical error, biologic problem, or at simply bad luck. It is also important to discuss what the patient is or is not able to do, and their expectations of the activities they would like to return to. Are the patients complaints related more to pain or to instability or a combination of both? This will help to assess

if a revision is the correct treatment, as patients with pain may not have a problem that can be addressed by a revision surgery. In regard to instability, we have found that patients with instability will often describe the "double fist" sign. This is when they make a fist with both hands and show the knee feels like the two fists rotating against each other. This is almost always indicative of rotatory instability or a knee that will have a remarkable pivot-shift in surgery. It is also important to try to obtain any operative notes and intraoperative photographs to determine the plan of action. The Multicenter ACL Revision Study group recently reported that a mere 10% of patients will have normal articular cartilage or menisci when they undergo revision surgery (14). Armed with this information, the surgeon can begin to effectively plan for revision surgery treatment alternatives. This includes equipment, potential pitfalls (fixation, grafts, bone loss), and the expectation of the surgeon and the patient in regard to the outcome if surgical treatment is considered.

Physical Examination

For revision ACL reconstructions, it is crucial to perform a complete physical examination. Initial observation will allow the surgeon to see prior incisions, generally alignment and any gait abnormalities, which may show a varus or valgus thrust. The range of motion and tests for extensor mechanism dysfunction should be performed to assess for any potential adversity they may cause in regards to revision surgery and graft selection. The range of motion is best objectively measured with the patient in the prone position, and patellar mobility (glide and tilt) is compared with the uninvolved extremity. Furthermore, one needs to not only assess the stability of the ACL, but also any laxity relating to the MCL, PLC, PM corner, and the menisci. Having an idea of concomitant injuries will help assessment of additional procedures that may need to be addressed. This is the time to begin explaining the current understanding of the involved injuries to the patient. But it is also important to stress that during the examination under anesthesia, in the operating room, other injuries may be detected that should be addressed, for example, most patients will not permit a good pivot-shift exam in the office setting, which would help in determining the degree rotatory instability, which may influence your specific anatomic technique.

Imaging Studies

The work-up of the knee after previous ACL reconstruction also includes a return to basic imaging studies. Getting an anteroposterior (AP), lateral, Merchant or sunrise, and posteroanterior weight-bearing view with 45° of flexion (Rosenberg view) are routine. This will help to identify the majority of concerns. One can assess tunnel placement, location and type of hardware, degenerative joint disease, tunnel lysis, and notch geometry (15). By beginning with plain films, much needed information can be obtained, and may help exclude the need for advanced imaging. If there is a high index of suspicion of additional pathology or significant tunnel widening, MRI or CT may be indicated. A CT is generally more useful when there may appear to be significant tunnel lysis to aid in determining the degree of bone loss. The use of newer technology, such as 3D reconstructions, may be of the greatest value when there is a concern for lysis or tunnel positioning. When there is more a suspicion of missed on new injury to the menisci, articular cartilage, or other ligaments in the knee, MRI tends to be of greater value. MRI should not be used to diagnose an ACL failure but can be used to confirm the clinical diagnosis. Based on the plain films, MRI and CT scans, one can usually determine if anatomic graft placement is possible or whether a staged surgery is required. On occasion, it may also be required to get full-length hip-to-ankle standing films if there is concern that limb malalignment may have contributed to the graft failure. Once all the appropriate studies have been gathered and analyzed, focus can turn to the surgery.

Staging

At times, there are limitations that will preclude single-stage ACL revision. Patients must be told in their preoperative appointment that this is a possibility as despite a thorough preoperative work-up, intraoperative findings may eliminate the possibility of a single-stage revision. If the patient has any of the following, the procedure should be staged: inability to create anatomic tunnels, inability to achieve stable graft fixation, which allows for unlimited range of motion immediately after surgery, or significant limb malalignment. Often with extensive osteolysis, it is impossible to achieve stable fixation in an anatomic position, this will require bone grafting prior to revision ACL reconstruction. Likewise, if the patient has significant stiffness with arthrofibrosis, the patient should undergo manipulation, lysis of adhesions, and therapy to regain full tibiofemoral and patellar motion prior to considering revision of surgery. The down side to a staged procedure is the risks of a repeat exposure to anesthesia and further delay in the ultimate return to sports. In the majority of patients, return to level 1 sports is delayed 9 to 12 months.

Equipment

When planning revision surgery, one must have the proper tools, physically and mentally going in. In situations where there is potential hardware to remove, ensure that you have the correct screwdriver, as well as a universal screw removal system, trephines, curettes, picks, and end-cutting reamers. It is also useful to have a variety of instruments to address nonanatomic tunnels. Dilators, half-sized reamers, single-fluted acorn drill bits, and a soft-tissue fixation device such as an endobutton all must be available. In patients with poor bone quality, half-sized dilators help expand the tunnels without creating additional bone loss and may also help with impaction of the bone graft. It may

also require an alternate technique such as an over-the-top reconstruction or two-incision technique. If it appears significant bone grafting may be required, you may also need a bone tamp and allograft bone, which preoperatively you should have ordered. The allograft used will depend on the size of defect, some defects can be treated with cancellous chips, while others will require bone plugs taken from a femoral head allograft. In patients with poor bone quality, you may be required to use a screw or staple to secure the bone graft on the lateral border of the femur, while avoiding the path of future tunnel placement.

Graft Selection

The decision of when to harvest the graft or prepare the graft is dependent on what is found in the preoperative planning phase. Our graft selection is individualized to the patient and is often dictated by the graft used in previous reconstruction(s). For young athletes that would like to continue their high-demand athletic endeavors (collegiate or high school), our graft of choice is autogenous tissue if it is still available. An anatomic double-bundle ACL revision reconstruction is contraindicated in patients with a small notch, limited bone, multiligamentous knee injury, and skeletally immature patients. If we are to perform an anatomic double-bundle reconstruction, we prefer the central third BTB autograft for the AM bundle and a gracilis or semitendinosis for the PL bundle. For patients who are low-demand recreational athletes, above the age of 25, or failed previous autograft procedures, we like to use Achilles tendon allograft with calcaneus bone block in revision ACL reconstructions. This tends to be a large graft that can be used for the reconstruction of both bundles and limits the costs to both the patient and the hospital or surgery center. The bone block is also useful when there are bony defects that need either a grafting or a large bone plug in order to fit a large tunnel.

Procedure

We always begin our procedures with an examination under anesthesia, as the office exam is often be unreliable and underestimates the degree of patholaxity. We like to examine the knee by performing a Lachman's and pivot-shift test. This can give us valuable information about AP versus rotational instability. If the Lachman's is intact but there is a positive pivot-shift, our preference may be to augment the intact AM graft with a PL bundle if possible rather than performing a complete reconstruction (Fig. 79.2). We also will examine the knee's stability to varus and valgus stress at both 0° and 30° and a dial test. This will aid in determining if there are secondary stabilizers that are deficient and need reconstruction.

Following the examination under anesthesia, the patient is positioned such that the gluteal folds are at the distal break in the table. We then place a nonsterile tourniquet on the operative extremity and then place the leg in an arthroscopic leg holder. The leg holder is placed

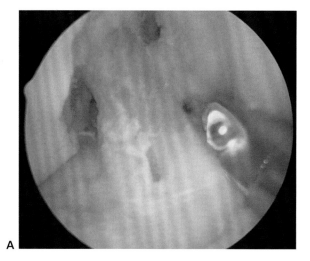

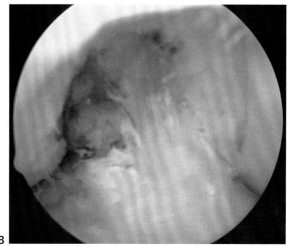

FIGURE 79.2. Arthroscopic view of an intact vertical graft **(A)** and the subsequent augmentation of the PL bundle **(B)**.

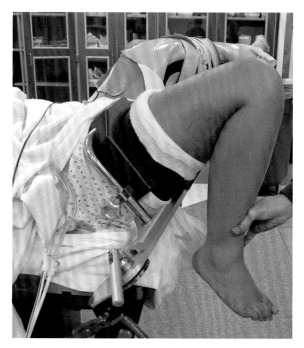

FIGURE 79.3. Patient setup in arthroscopic leg holder with leg in a hyperflexed position.

such that there is enough hip flexion to allow for the knee to be flexed to 130°, the position for drilling either an anatomic single bundle or the AM tunnel through an AAM portal (Fig. 79.3). The nonoperative extremity is then placed in a well-padded, well leg holder in a hemi-lithotomy position with the hip flexed and externally rotated. The leg is then prepped and draped, and we begin the procedure.

When performing diagnostic arthroscopy, careful portal placement cannot be overemphasized. Previous portals may not have been ideal, so we begin with new portals that will allow us to perform the required procedure. We begin with a "high and tight" lateral portal, adjacent to the patella, but proximal to the inferior pole. We then create a "low and tight" medial portal again adjacent to the patellar tendon under direct visualization of a spinal needle. The needle should be in line with the ACL fibers at the attachment site on the tibia just above the intermeniscal ligament. This will allow for spacing and visualization as we perform the surgery. We find that the high lateral portal provides an excellent viewing portal of the tibial footprint

and associated landmarks. Besides the obvious assessment of the previous graft, the diagnostic arthroscopy will help in assessing the articular cartilage, menisci, and associated injuries. The "drive through" sign (opening of the joint space >10 mm) can be an indicator of injury to the collateral ligaments. If the diastasis is greater above or below the meniscus also aids in determination of whether the injury is tibial or femoral based (16). We may also need to debride the fat pad at this time to allow adequate visualization of the anatomic tibial footprint.

At the conclusion of the diagnostic arthroscopy, a notchplasty can be performed as indicated for visualization of the normal osseous insertion site on the femur. If there is complete graft failure, the graft is debrided from the medial wall of the lateral femoral condyle. We attempt to identify the anatomic landmarks of the femoral origin of the ACL (lateral intercondylar ridge and bifurcate ridge) and the previous tunnels. If there is a screw in place, we will assess whether it needs to be removed or if we are able to place our anatomic tunnels while leaving the screw in place. If the screw is to be removed, one must also try to determine whether the screw can be removed from the medial portal, transtibial or via an AAM portal. The determination can often be made at this time as to whether bone grafting will be required. If it is possible to leave the hardware in place, this can obviate the need for bone grafting (Fig. 79.4). If there is a large defect, it can often be filled with a portion of bone from the calcaneal bone block. This is generally the point where we proceed with creating our AAM portal under direct visualization with a spinal needle just superior to the superior border of the medial meniscus, as far medial as possible (Fig. 79.5).

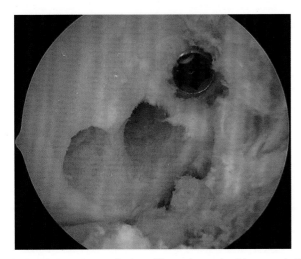

FIGURE 79.4. Arthroscopic view of femoral tunnels with anatomic DB ACL reconstruction. Note the retained hardware from previous nonanatomic ACL reconstruction.

We then make the incision horizontally to allow for less traumatic passage of instruments.

This is the point where we move the scope to the middle portal (immediately adjacent to the patellar tendon) to provide the best visualization of the medial wall of the lateral femoral condyle. The knee is flexed to 90° to allow the best visualization of the anatomic location of the femoral tunnel(s). A microfracture awl is introduced from the AAM and used to mark the anatomic position between the AM and the PL bundles (single-bundle reconstruction) or the origin of both the AM and the PL bundles (double-bundle reconstruction) (17). We generally try to use an anatomic double-bundle reconstruction for the majority of our revision cases; we will use the single bundle, however, if it is felt that the patient's unique anatomy would prohibit an anatomic double-bundle reconstruction (usually small femoral condyles).

Once the starting point has been identified, the knee is flexed to 110° and a guide pin is placed into the PL starting point. This is then reamed with a single-fluted acorn reamer to 5 or 6 mm (based on graft size) and the pin is removed. We use the single-fluted acorn reamers to decrease the risk of injury to the articular cartilage. The anterior and inferior edges of the tunnel are then smoothed with an arthroscopic shaver, as well as to help remove any bony debris. The knee is then flexed to 130° and a guide pin is inserted in the AM bundle's starting point. This is reamed to a diameter of 7 to 9 mm, again based on the graft size. The guide pin and reamer are removed and again the arthroscopic shaver is used to smooth the anterior and inferior edges of the tunnel and remove any bony debris (Fig. 79.6). Hyperflexion of the knee allows for tunnel divergence, increased tunnel length, and decreases the risk of posterior wall blowout. It also reliably produces tunnels of near 32 and 34 mm for the PL and AM bundles. A tunnel length of less than 25 mm is caused by lack of

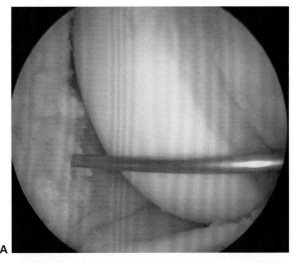

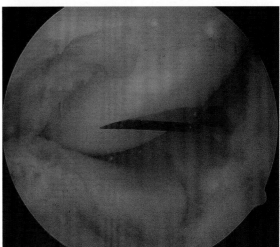

FIGURE 79.5. Arthroscopic view establishing AAM portal with a spinal needle **(A)**. Note the far lateral entry and proximity to femoral condyle. We make this incision horizontal to allow for instrument passage **(B)**.

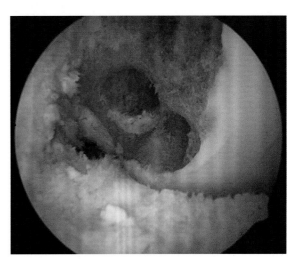

FIGURE 79.6. Arthroscopic view of the AM (posterior) and PL (anterior) bundles of the femur after reaming.

flexion and/or not creating a far medial enough AAM portal. In situations where it appears that the previous tunnel is going to cause interference or overlap, we will try to divergently overream this tunnel. This tunnel generally will involve the AM bundle and will be used as such. If there is significant difficulty to achieve the AM bundle tunnel, then a two-incision technique may be used.

Following the creation of the femoral tunnels, attention is then turned to the tibial tunnel preparations. First, we return the scope to the lateral portal. This should give a view of the tibial footprint of the ACL (Fig. 79.7). Generally the tibial hardware is in a location that will likely interfere with tibial tunnel placement for double-bundle revisions, and thus must be removed. After removal of the hardware, soft tissue should be debrided from the tunnel, and the tibial guide should be placed in the middle portal set at 60° for the AM tunnel. This tunnel starts on the tibial cortex more laterally relative to standard tibial tunnels. A guide pin should be placed into the tibia and should be anteriorized if it falls within the previous tibial tunnel. It can be held in the proper trajectory by driving the pin into the femur. The PL tibial tunnel may require switching the guide to the AAM portal to allow access medial enough to not cause difficulty. The angle of the guide should be set at 45°. The starting point on the tibial cortex should be medial to the AM tunnel and just anterior to the superficial MCL. The tibial guide pin should enter the joint just posterior and lateral to the AM tunnel (Fig. 79.8). Again the pin can be placed into the femur for stabilizing the pin. Once proper placement of the pins has been achieved and confirmed, the AM tunnel should expanded as needed using dilators or cannulated drills. The PL tunnel should be created in a similar manner. If the tunnels converge at the level of the joint, this is generally acceptable and will not compromise the grafts, tensioning, or fixation. When initially performing double-bundle reconstructions, the use of intraoperative imaging can help in the assessment

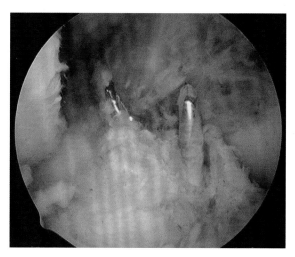

FIGURE 79.8. Arthroscopic view of the guide pins for AM (anterior) and PL (posterior) bundles prior to reaming.

of anatomic tunnel placement, which may accelerate your personal learning curve.

At this point, it is time to prepare for graft passage. The scope is moved back to the medial portal; a passing pin is loaded with a suture and placed through the AAM portal. The knee is flexed to 110° and the nonlooped end of the suture is pulled through the PL femoral tunnel. The looped end is then slowly pulled into the joint and grasped with a pituitary rongeur through the PL tibial tunnel and pulled out this tunnel. This should be repeated for the AM bundle, ensuring that the AM-bundle loop passes over the PL loop. The femoral tunnel placement is also confirmed at this point as the pins should exit the skin about 2 to 3 cm apart in line with the iliotibial band (PL should be distal) (Fig. 79.9). Each graft is then pulled into the appropriate tunnel, beginning with the PL bundle. The femoral side should be fixed for the PL bundle, prior to the fixation of the AM bundle. The PL bundle is generally fixed with a 15-mm endobutton type device, whereas the AM bundle has variable fixation depending on graft selection.

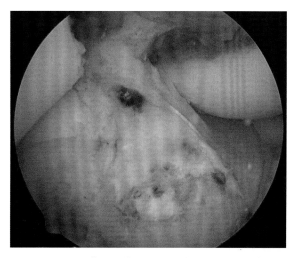

FIGURE 79.7. View from a "high and tight" lateral portal showing anatomy of the ACL's tibial footprint. Note the relationship to the anterior horn of the lateral meniscus.

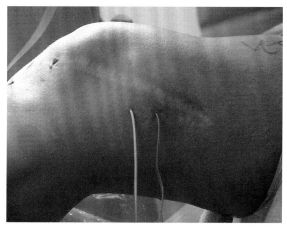

FIGURE 79.9. Lateral exit point of the AM (proximal) and PL (distal) bundles through the skin. Note that they exit parallel to the floor.

If the AM bundle is a soft-tissue graft, it should be fixed with an endobutton type device; if it has a bone block, we prefer the use of a cannulated interference screw. Once both grafts are fixed on the femoral side, they are cycled individually to assess for isometry and allow for pretensioning, which is important for soft-tissue grafts.

Tibial fixation is generally performed with the leg in extension for the PL bundle and at 45° for the AM bundle as described by Gabriel et al (18). The grafts are then fixed with either a staple fixation or a screw and washer on the tibia. Final arthroscopic visualization is then performed to ensure the grafts are properly tensioned and there is no evidence of impingement in the notch (Fig. 79.10).

Postoperative Care

After revision ACL reconstruction, the rehabilitation may sometimes be considered more conservative, but generally, we are able to follow our same protocol as for primary ACL reconstructions. We will place our revision patients into a hinged knee brace for the first 8 weeks after surgery, allowing full weight-bearing with the brace locked in extension immediately after surgery. A conservative protocol is more likely to benefit a revision that is considered a salvage procedure, with a goal more toward a stable knee that can be effective for ADLs.

In the 1st month, the patient must keep the brace locked when ambulating, but it can otherwise be unlocked. The focus needs to be on maintaining full extension and working on range of motion for the first 6 to 8 weeks. At the end of this time, the patient should have full range of motion. In revision surgery, it is important to allow adequate time for healing, as well as to ensure there is adequate strength to help protect the graft. As such, return to play is generally more on the magnitude of 9 to 12 months, and depending on the sport or level of play, may require a functional evaluation before hand. We generally obtain a postoperative radiograph, AP and lateral in full extension at the 1-year postoperative visit (Fig. 79.11).

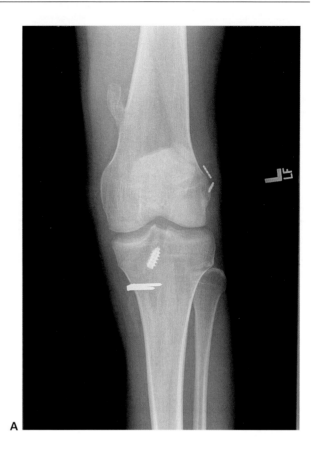

A

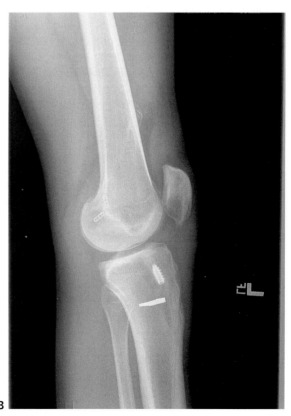

B

FIGURE 79.11. Radiographs (AP and lateral) demonstrating hardware and tunnel position at 1-year follow-up.

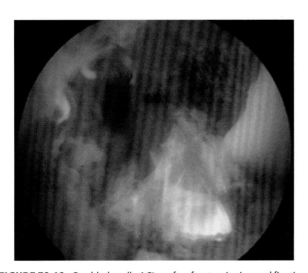

FIGURE 79.10. Double-bundle ACL grafts after tensioning and fixation.

PCL REVISION

Etiology

As PCL injuries are considerably less common, so too are the treatments less studied. Similar to ACL injuries, one must identify the source of failure. It is also important to try to discern whether the complaint is one of pain or instability. Potential causes of failure are continued instability or patholaxity, decreased motion or arthrofibrosis, and persistent pain. Persistent or recurrent laxity is most often from technical errors such as improper tunnel placement, inadequate tensioning, or undiagnosed or undertreated secondary pathology. In a study of 52 patients with failed PCL reconstruction, there was 40% incidence of untreated PLC injury, 33% had improper tunnel placement, and 31% had untreated varus malalignment (19). Just as with ACL surgery, tunnel malpositioning, may also lead to limitations in motion. We have seen the central PCL tunnels, may also lead to a "captured knee" (Fig. 79.12A). Secondary failure may also occur due to issues with fixation, biologic healing, aggressive rehabilitation, and patient noncompliance.

Preoperative Planning

Much like with ACL reconstruction the planning involves a comprehensive history and physical examination. Of particular note is to attempt to discover any concomitant pathology that may have been missed previously. Again, it is imperative to attempt to review all the prior notes and operative reports and images. The physical examination should evaluate previous incisions, range of motion, gait analysis, collateral ligament integrity, and neurovascular assessment. Special tests such as the posterior drawer, Godfrey's, and dial test should all be performed. Posterior translation of the tibia greater than 10 mm (grade 3) on posterior drawer testing should heighten suspicion of a PLC injury as well (20).

Radiographic assessment should also include AP, lateral, Merchant or sunrise, and Rosenberg views. Radiographs allow assessment of previous hardware, tunnel size and location, subluxation, and the presence of tibial translation (Fig. 79.12B and C). As with ACL injuries, degenerative joint disease is seen most commonly in the medial compartment (21). If there is a concern with alignment, long leg standing alignment films should be obtained. MRI can be used for suspected meniscal, cartilaginous, of collateral ligament injury.

When determining the proper operative candidates, one must consider the indications and contraindications for revision PCL reconstruction. Indications for revision are patients with persistent pain and/or instability following a previous PCL reconstruction. Absolute contraindications to revision surgery are active infection and severe degenerative joint disease. In between these lie patients that may have relative contraindications to surgery. These include significant loss of range of motion and a fixed posterior drawer. It is also important to consider the reliability and compliance of a patient, as noncompliance will likely assure a subpar outcome, as revision surgeries often do not do as well as a primary surgery.

The equipment required for a revision PCL is the same as for a revision ACL, with a few exceptions. We use two translucent 8.5 mm cannulas, a 70° scope, and a looped wire (for graft passage). The graft choices for a revision PCL are slightly different. We tend to use allograft more often in PCL reconstructions, most commonly Achilles with a bone block. This allows for a long graft with a bony interface for femoral fixation. We tend to use a biointerference screw on the femoral side and a variety of fixation devices on the tibial side. Other options include using an all soft-tissue graft such as a semi-tendinosis allograft.

Procedure

We always begin our procedures with an examination under anesthesia, as the office examination can often be unreliable. We like to examine the knee by performing a Lachman's and posterior drawer and dial test. This can give us valuable information about AP versus rotational instability. We also will examine the knee's stability to varus and valgus stress at both 0° and 30°. This will aid in concerns with injuries to secondary stabilizers that may need to be addressed.

Following the examination under anesthesia, the patient is positioned such that the gluteal folds are at the distal break in the table. We then place a nonsterile tourniquet on the operative extremity and then place the leg in an arthroscopic leg holder. The nonoperative extremity is then placed in a well-padded, well-leg holder in a hemilithotomy position with the hip flexed and externally rotated. The leg is then prepped and draped, and we begin the procedure.

When performing diagnostic arthroscopy, portal placement cannot be overemphasized. Previous portals may not have been ideal, so we begin with new portals that will allow us to perform the required procedure. We begin with a "high and tight" lateral portal, adjacent to the patella, but at or just distal to the inferior pole (unlike with ACL reconstructions). We then create a "low and tight" medial portal again adjacent to the patellar tendon under direct visualization of a spinal needle. The needle should be in line with the ACL and just above the intermeniscal ligament. This will allow for spacing and visualization as we perform the surgery. Besides the obvious assessment of the previous graft, the diagnostic arthroscopy will help in assessing the articular cartilage, menisci, and associated injuries. We also will debride the fat pad at this time to allow adequate visualization.

With PCL reconstruction, we perform our notchplasty on the inferior portion of the medial wall below PCL insertion. This will allow for the scope and the graft to reach the posterior portion of knee. It is important to remove enough bone, as well as the old graft, to allow for new graft to be easily passed. This is the point when it is

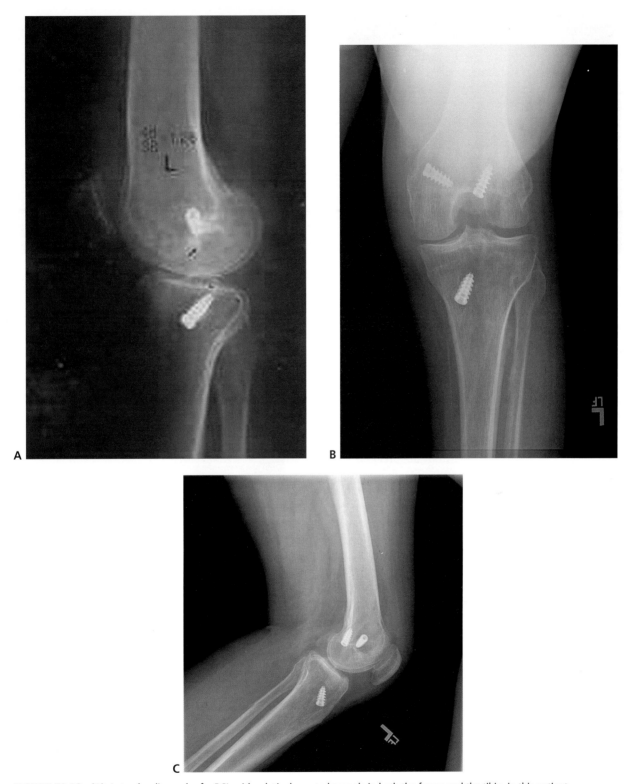

FIGURE 79.12. **(A)**. Lateral radiograph of a PCL with relatively central tunnels in both the femur and the tibia, in this patient, they actually experienced the captured knee phenomenon. Separate patient with AP **(B)** and lateral **(C)** radiographs of a PCL with a central tunnel on both the femur and the tibial.

also beneficial to look for old hardware, if it is going to interfere with the revision surgery. After the notchplasty has been completed, the 30° scope should be exchanged for a 70° scope. With this scope, we can begin with tibial

preparation. We generally begin by looking medially behind the medial femoral condyle to make our PM portal (Fig. 79.13). Using a spinal needle, attempts should be made to the portal entering superior and posterior as

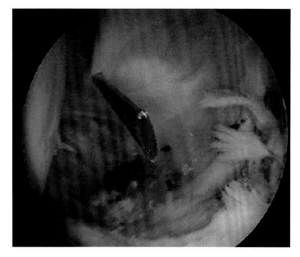

FIGURE 79.13. Spinal needle used to establish PM portal.

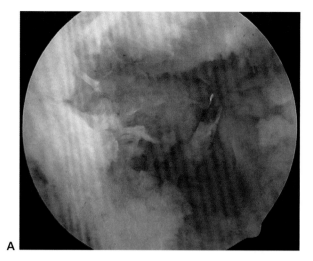

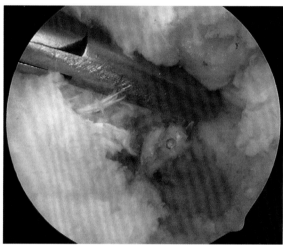

FIGURE 79.14. Guide pin entering the posterior tibia **(A)**. Note the poor visualization of standard landmarks such as the posterior horn of the medial meniscus. A pituitary is used to grasp the guide pin and protect the posterior neurovascular structures **(B)**.

viewed from the scope. This portal is then maintained with a threaded 8.5-mm cannula. This allows easy passage of instruments into the posterior compartment of the knee.

Tibial preparation begins by gaining orientation, to find insertion of PCL, look just posterior to the root of medial meniscus and carefully debride tissue between the meniscal root and the tibial insertion of the PCL (safe interval) (22). The challenge in revision cases is that you may be reliant on altered anatomy from the previous surgery (Fig. 79.14). Once the bone of the tibial footprint has been exposed, the tibial PCL guide can be used to create the tibial tunnel. The tibial guide should be adjusted to be as vertical as possible, in order to decrease the angle of turn the graft will take from the tibial tunnel toward the anterior femur, also known as "the killer turn." Once the guide is in place, the pin is run until it is near the cortex, and then it is gently tapped into the joint under direct visualization. It is then grasped with a pituitary and stabilized from the PM portal. If uncertain of pin location, the trajectory and exit point can be confirmed at this point using intraoperative fluoroscopy. We then proceed to ream or dilate the tibial tunnel to the diameter of the graft. This should be done with power until fat droplets are seen. Then the tunnel should be completed by hand. The anterior edge of the tunnel should be smoothed with the arthroscopic shaver, and then plug the tibial tunnel.

For preparation of the femoral tunnel, we make an accessory anterolateral (AAL) portal inferior to lateral portal. This is made under direct visualization with a spinal needle to ensure the portal allows for the proper angle to drill the femoral tunnel. After placing a second threaded cannula in the AAL portal, a Steinman pin is drilled into femoral origin of the PCL. The lateral wall of the medial femoral condyle is then reamed or dilated over the pin with appropriately sized reamer, and again the edges of the tunnel are smoothed. One must also assess if there is an issue with the hardware from the

previous surgery, or if you can proceed with the hardware in place (Fig. 79.15).

To pass the graft, a looped wire is inserted into AAL portal and fed posteriorly to the articular entrance of tibial tunnel. A pituitary is then inserted through the tibial tunnel to grasp the wire loop and pull it out through the tibial tunnel. If there is difficulty getting the wire to the pituitary, a blunt trochar from the PM portal can be utilized to push wire. The graft sutures are then placed in the loop, and they are pulled out through the AAL portal. The graft is carefully pulled into the joint, we will often pull this over the trochar to aid in mechanical advantage as described by Mariani and colleagues (23).

The graft sutures can then be pulled out the AAL portal and feed through a passing pin. This is then passed through the femoral tunnel, exiting medially. The graft is secured in the femoral tunnel with an interference screw. To achieve tibial fixation, we place the leg at 90° with normal tibial step-off, which can be confirmed arthroscopically

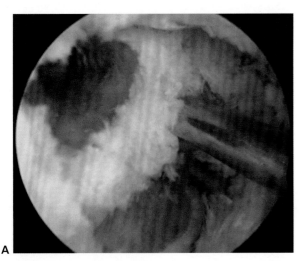 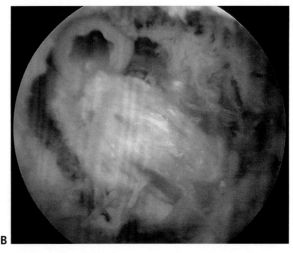

FIGURE 79.15. The new femoral tunnel is seen, anterior to the previous central tunnel **(A)**. You can also see the previous interference screw within the tunnel. In this situation, the graft has been passed and secured with a biointerference screw without the removal of the old hardware **(B)**.

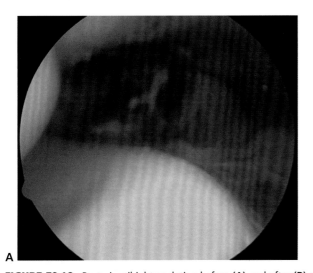 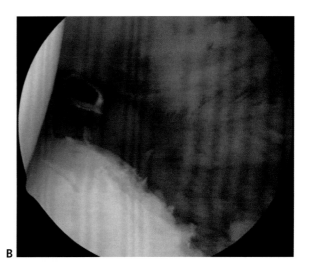

FIGURE 79.16. Posterior tibial translation before **(A)** and after **(B)** graft fixation and while performing a posterior drawer as seen from the Gillquist view.

(Fig. 79.16). The graft can then be secured with a screw and spiked washer or with staples.

Postoperative Management

After PCL fixation, the patient is kept non-weight-bearing for 6 weeks, with a brace locked at 30° when up right. We initially promote motion from 15° to 60° and at 1 to 2 weeks start trying to obtain a range of motion from 0° to 90° by 1 month. After a month, range of motion is then advanced to as tolerated, with the caveat that the patient is not to perform active hamstring exercises for 12 weeks. The brace will remain in use for 3 months. Again we generally obtain AP and lateral radiographs at the 1-year

anniversary from surgery to assess hardware, arthritic change, and tunnel lysis (Fig. 79.17).

SUMMARY

It is important to remember that as the number of primary surgeries is rising, so too are the number of revisions. And in general, the revision is not the same as a primary surgery. It is crucial to analyze why the grafts failed and have a plan of how to approach the revision. One must take into account additional equipment or alternate techniques to be able to perform an anatomic revision surgery.

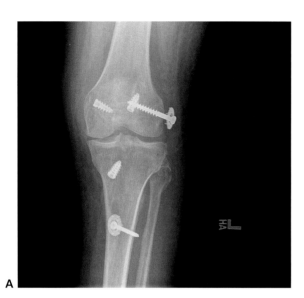 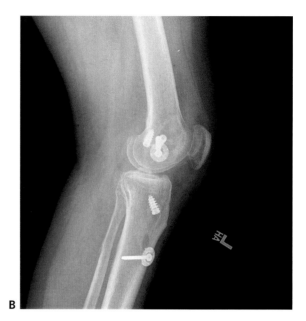

FIGURE 79.17. Postoperative radiographs (AP and lateral) after revision PCL reconstruction with LCL reconstruction as well.

REFERENCES

1. Miyasaka K, Daniel D, Stone M. The incidence of knee ligament injuries in the general population. *Am J Knee Surg.* 1991;4:43–48.
2. Fu F, Christel P, Miller MD, et al. Graft selection for anterior cruciate ligament reconstruction. *Instr Course Lect.* 2009;58: 337–354.
3. Fu FH, Jordan SS. The lateral intercondylar ridge—a key to anatomic anterior cruciate ligament reconstruction. *J Bone Joint Surg Am.* 2007;89:2103–2104.
4. Harner CD, Baek GH, Vogrin TM, et al. Quantitative analysis of human cruciate ligament insertions. *Arthroscopy.* 1999;15:741–749.
5. Diamantopoulos AP, Lorbach O, Paessler HH. Anterior cruciate ligament revision reconstruction: results in 107 patients. *Am J Sports Med.* 2008;36:851–860.
6. Battaglia MJ II, Cordasco FA, Hannafin JA, et al. Results of revision anterior cruciate ligament surgery. *Am J Sports Med.* 2007;35:2057–2066.
7. Bach BR Jr. Revision anterior cruciate ligament surgery. *Arthroscopy.* 2003;19(suppl 1):14–29.
8. Stevenson WW III, Johnson DL. "Vertical grafts": a common reason for functional failure after ACL reconstruction. *Orthopedics.* 2007;30:206–209.
9. Getelman MH, Friedman MJ. Revision anterior cruciate ligament reconstruction surgery. *J Am Acad Orthop Surg.* 1999;7:189–198.
10. Johnson DL, Fu FH. Anterior cruciate ligament reconstruction: why do failures occur? *Instr Course Lect.* 1995;44:391–406.
11. Neuman P, Englund M, Kostogiannis I, et al. Prevalence of tibiofemoral osteoarthritis 15 years after nonoperative treatment of anterior cruciate ligament injury: a prospective cohort study. *Am J Sports Med.* 2008;36:1717–1725.
12. Hart AJ, Buscombe J, Malone A, et al. Assessment of osteoarthritis after reconstruction of the anterior cruciate ligament: a study using single-photon emission computed tomography at ten years. *J Bone Joint Surg Br.* 2005;87:1483–1487.
13. Liden M, Sernert N, Rostgard-Christensen L, et al. Osteoarthritic changes after anterior cruciate ligament reconstruction using bone-patellar tendon-bone or hamstring tendon autografts: a retrospective, 7-year radiographic and clinical follow-up study. *Arthroscopy.* 2008;24:899–908.
14. Cheatham SA, Johnson DL. Anatomic revision ACL reconstruction. *Sports Med Arthrosc.* 2010;18:33–39.
15. Shulte K, Majewski M, Irrgang J. Radiographic tunnel changes following arthroscopic ACL reconstruction: autograft vs. allograft. *Arthroscopy.* 1995;11:372–373.
16. Stephenson DR, Rueff D, Johnson DL. MRI and arthroscopic analysis of collateral knee ligament injuries in combined knee ligament injuries. *Orthopedics.* 2010;33:187–189.
17. Edwards A, Bull AM, Amis AA. The attachments of the anteromedial and posterolateral fibre bundles of the anterior cruciate ligament. Part 2: femoral attachment. *Knee Surg Sports Traumatol Arthrosc.* 2008;16:29–36.
18. Gabriel MT, Wong EK, Woo SL, et al. Distribution of in situ forces in the anterior cruciate ligament in response to rotatory loads. *J Orthop Res.* 2004;22:85–89.
19. Noyes FR, Barber-Westin SD. Posterior cruciate ligament revision reconstruction, part 1: causes of surgical failure in 52 consecutive operations. *Am J Sports Med.* 2005; 33:646–654.
20. Johnson DH, Fanelli GC, Miller, MD. PCL 2002: indications, double-bundle versus inlay technique and revision surgery. *Arthroscopy.* 2002;18:40–52.
21. Clancy WG Jr, Shelbourne KD, Zoellner GB, et al. Treatment of knee joint instability secondary to rupture of the posterior cruciate ligament. Report of a new procedure. *J Bone Joint Surg Am.* 1983;65:310–322.
22. Kantaras AT, Johnson DL. The medial meniscal root as a landmark for tibial tunnel position in posterior cruciate ligament reconstruction. *Arthroscopy.* 2002;18:99–101.
23. Mariani PP, Adriani E, Maresca G. Arthroscopic-assisted posterior cruciate ligament reconstruction using patellar tendon autograft: a technique for graft passage. *Arthroscopy.* 1996;12:510–512.

Anterior Cruciate Ligament Reconstruction in the Pediatric Patient

Craig Finlayson • Adam Nasreddine • Mininder S. Kocher

The knee is the most common site of injury in the skeletally immature athlete (1). The incidence of anterior cruciate ligament (ACL) tears appears to be on the rise. The treatment of these injuries is controversial. Nonoperative management can lead to functional instability and difficulty with cutting and pivoting sports. In addition, the pathologic shear forces are associated with meniscal and chondral damage over time. ACL reconstruction in children and adolescents risks iatrogenic injury to the physis. This chapter reviews the historic perspective of ACL injuries in the young patient, clinical and diagnostic findings in children, treatment options, and results of treatment.

HISTORICAL NOTE

The ACL is the principal intraarticular stabilizer of the knee. As in adults, an ACL injury in a child or adolescent is usually a noncontact valgus injury. Before the 1980s, these injuries were thought to be rare in the pediatric athlete. Advances in diagnostic imaging and improved clinical acumen have allowed physicians to identify midsubstance ACL tears in patients with open physis (2–4).

The results of nonoperative management in children are consistently associated with poor outcomes (5, 6). Aichroth et al. reported on 23 children that were treated nonoperatively between 1980 and 1990. At final follow-up, meniscal tears were present in 15 knees, three osteochondral fractures occurred, and osteoarthritic changes developed in 10 knees. From 1980 to 1985, McCarroll followed 16 patients younger than 14 years with open physes and midsubstance tears of the ACL treated without reconstruction. Six patients underwent arthroscopy for meniscal tears. Only seven patients returned to sports, all experiencing recurrent episodes of giving way, effusions, and pain.

Attempts at primary repair of the ligament in children have resulted in poor outcomes (7). Engebretsen et al. presented eight adolescents that were followed 3 to 8 years after primary suture of a midsubstance rupture of the ACL. Only three patients had good function, and five were functionally unstable. Failure of primary repair has led to the development of various procedures to stabilize the knee. Surgical options include transphyseal, partial transphyseal, and physeal-sparing reconstructions.

TIBIAL SPINE FRACTURES AND PARTIAL ACL TEARS

It is important to understand the different types of injuries that can occur in the skeletally immature patient. Partial ACL tears and avulsion fractures of the tibial spine are more common in the pediatric population (8). Excellent functional results have been reported following arthroscopic reduction and internal fixation of tibial spine fractures, although long-term follow-up does demonstrate some residual laxity, indicative of associated intrasubstance injury to the ACL (2). Many partial tears can be treated nonoperatively (9). On the basis of a prospective study of arthroscopically confirmed partial ACL tears, failure of nonreconstructive treatment has been associated with tears greater than 50%, tears of the posterolateral bundle, older skeletal age, and presence of a pivot shift.

CLINICAL EVALUATION

History and Physical Examination

Important history questions are as follows:

1. How did the injury occur?
   a. Was there contact with another athlete?
   b. Was there a fixed position of the foot and rotation or twisting movement?
2. Were you able to continue to compete?
3. Was there significant swelling directly after the injury?
4. Have there been previous injuries to the knee?

Our understanding of ACL tears in the setting of younger athletes has changed considerably. The tibial spine fracture was once thought to be the pediatric equivalent of an ACL tear. Midsubstance ACL ruptures are now diagnosed more frequently in pediatric athletes participating in cutting and contact sports. The typical presentation is a young athlete who has a decelerating, twisting injury. Approximately two-thirds of ACL injuries occur by noncontact mechanisms (10). The patient will often report a "pop" and the inability to return to the field. A large amount of swelling due to hemarthrosis is expected. The presentation is less dramatic in athletes who have had a prior partial tear of the ACL.

The findings on physical examination are dependent on the timing in relation to the injury. Directly after the injury, the stability of the knee can be tested on the sideline. The Lachman and pivot shift tests are positive before swelling and guarding occurs. When the patient presents for evaluation in the emergency department or clinic, the knee is typically swollen, compromising the ability to perform an accurate physical examination. Rates of ACL injury are reported between 10% and 65% in pediatric patients presenting with traumatic hemarthrosis of the knee; therefore, young athletes presenting with a hemarthrosis of the knee should raise suspicion for an ACL tear (11, 12). The differential diagnosis of hemarthrosis of the knee includes patellar dislocation, meniscal tear, osteochondral fracture, tibial spine fracture, and epiphyseal fracture of the femur or tibia.

A thorough examination of the knee must be performed to rule out concomitant injuries. Associated injuries include meniscal tears, posterior cruciate and/or collateral ligament tears, osteochondral fractures, and physeal fractures of the distal femur or proximal tibia. Given the higher prevalence of generalized ligamentous laxity in skeletally immature patients, a direct comparison to the contralateral knee should also be made. The Lachman and pivot shift maneuvers are used to test for ACL insufficiency.

Imaging

Evaluation of the knee by MRI is an important part of the assessment, particularly in children. The MRI is useful to distinguish between partial tears, avulsions, and midsubstance tears of the ACL. Secondary findings in an acute injury include hemarthrosis and the presence of a bone contusion at the posterior lateral tibial plateau and anterior lateral femoral condyle. The MRI is useful for confirming the diagnosis of ACL tear, ruling out associated injuries, and assisting in preoperative planning (Fig. 80.1).

INDICATIONS AND TIMING OF SURGERY

Indications for ACL reconstruction in a skeletally immature patient include complete ACL tear with functional instability, partial ACL tear that has failed nonoperative treatment, and ACL injury with associated repairable meniscal or chondral injury. Owing to higher rates of postoperative stiffness, acute ACL reconstruction is not

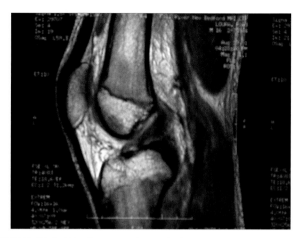

FIGURE 80.1. MRI demonstrating midsubstance ACL tear.

recommended for isolated ACL tears (13). Surgery is typically delayed at least 3 weeks from the time of injury until adequate range of motion has been achieved and joint effusion minimized. Patients must be mature enough to participate in the extensive rehabilitation process following ACL reconstruction.

TREATMENT OPTIONS

The choice of surgical technique is dependent on the physiologic age of the patient and the amount of growth remaining. For prepubescent children, violation of the tibial and femoral physis presents a risk of significant growth disturbance that would require limb lengthening or osteotomy. Animal studies have demonstrated a risk of physeal arrest with transphyseal ACL reconstruction(14, 15). A number of growth disturbances following ACL reconstruction in this age group have been documented (16). Radiographs and developmental findings are used to determine the physiologic age. Referencing radiographs of the left wrist to the atlas of Greulich and Pyle (17) provides an efficient means to determine skeletal age. The physiologic age is based on the Tanner staging system (Fig. 80.2 and Table 80.1) (18).

The prepubescent child (Tanner stage I or II) with a midsubstance ACL tear presents a difficult problem. Because of the large amount of growth remaining, the consequences of iatrogenic physeal arrest are severe. Unfortunately, activity modification such as refraining from cutting sports is difficult in this age group, and nonreconstructive treatment has been associated with meniscal and chondral injury (19–22).

Surgical techniques include physeal-sparing, transphyseal, and partial transphyseal reconstructions. In theory the extraarticular reconstruction provides a method to restore stability and avoid risk of growth disturbance. At our institution, we use a modification of the MacIntosh ACL reconstruction to perform a physeal-sparing reconstruction with an extra- and intraarticular component that is described in detail later in the chapter.

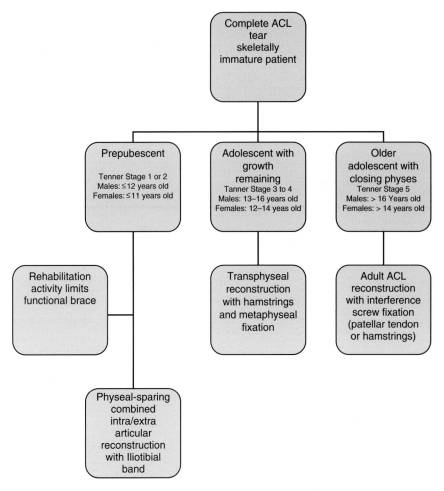

FIGURE 80.2. Algorithm for management of complete ACL injuries in skeletally immature patients.

Table 80.1

Tanner staging classification of secondary sexual characteristics

Tanner Stage		Male	Female
Stage I (prepubertal)	Growth development	5–6 cm/y Testes <4 mL or <2.5 cm No pubic hair	5–6 cm/y No breast development No pubic hair

Stage II	Growth development	5–6 cm/y
		Testes 4 mL or
		  2.5–3.2 cm
		Minimal pubic hair
		  at base of penis
			7–8 cm/y
			Breast buds
			Minimal pubic hair
			  on labia

Stage III	Growth development	7–8 cm/y
		Testes 12 mL
		  or 3.6 cm
			8 cm/y
			Elevation of breast;
			  areolae enlarge

(Continued)

Table 80.1

Tanner staging classification of secondary sexual characteristics (continued)

Tanner Stage		Male	Female
		Pubic hair over pubis Voice changes Muscle mass increases	Pubic hair of mons pubis Axillary hair Acne
Stage IV	Growth development	10 cm/y Testes 4.1–4.5 cm Pubic hair as adult Axillary hair Acne	7 cm/y Areolae enlarge Pubic hair as adult
Stage V	Growth development	No growth Testes as adult Pubic hair as adult Facial hair as adult Mature physique	No growth Adult breast contour Pubic hair as adult
Other		Peak height velocity: 13.5 y	Adrenarche: 6–8 y Menarche 12.7 y Peak height velocity: 11.5 y

The results of 44 patients with a mean follow-up of 5.3 years after this combined intra- and extraarticular ACL reconstruction were examined. There were two failures at 4.7 and 8.3 years, and no episodes of growth disturbance. The mean International knee documentation commitee subjective knee score and Lysholm score were 96.7 and 95.7, respectively (26).

Surgical treatment with conventional transphyseal tunnels has been described (23, 24). Liddle et al. describe the results of 17 patients treated with transphyseal ACL reconstruction with four-strand hamstring autograft. Eight Tanner stage I and nine Tanner stage II patients were followed for a mean of 44 months. The mean Lysholm score at follow-up was 97.5. There was one failure because of an additional injury. One child was noted to have a 5° valgus deformity.

An alternative physeal-sparing technique using epiphyseal tunnels has been described by Anderson (24) (Fig. 80.3). A transepiphyseal technique using fluoroscopy was performed in 12 patients. The mean IKDC subjective score was 96.4 at 4.1 years with no graft failures or growth arrests noted.

For adolescents with significant growth remaining (Tanner stage III and IV), we perform transphyseal ACL reconstruction with autogenous hamstrings. Sixty-one ACL reconstructions were reviewed in skeletally immature pubescent adolescents. Two patients underwent revision ACL reconstruction because of graft failure at 14 and 21 months postoperatively. For the remaining 59 knees, the mean IKDC subjective knee score was 89.5 and the mean Lysholm knee score was 91.2 (25).

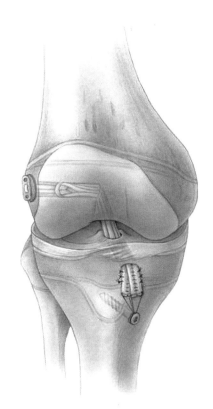

FIGURE 80.3. Physeal-sparing intraarticular ACL reconstruction with epiphyseal tunnels.

SURGICAL TECHNIQUE

ACL Reconstruction with the Iliotibial Band

For prepubescent children, Tanner stage I or II, a physeal-sparing reconstruction is recommended (26). Skeletal age is usually less than 14 in males and less than 13 in females. The patient is placed supine on the operating room table. Examination under anesthesia is performed to confirm Tanner staging and verify ACL insufficiency. The operative extremity is prepped and draped from the level of the foot to the level of a tourniquet placed at the thigh. It is important to place the tourniquet as proximally as possible in case a counter incision is necessary to assist in harvesting the ilio-tibial (IT) band proximally. The insertion of the IT band on the tibia is palpated at Gerdy's tubercle. The incision runs obliquely from the lateral joint line to the superior border of the IT band. The tourniquet is not routinely inflated to prevent tethering of the IT band. The incision is then made, and self-retaining retractors are placed. Dissection is carried down to the level of the IT band. In young, thin patients the IT band may be quite superficial. The anterior and posterior borders of the IT band are defined (Fig. 80.4A). Posteriorly the IT band blends with the lateral hamstrings, and harvesting too far posteriorly risks injury to the common peroneal nerve. A Cobb elevator is used to dissect the subcutaneous tissue away from the IT band along its course.

A no. 15 blade is used to make an incision at the anterior border of the IT band, starting 2 cm above Gerdy's tubercle. A Kelly clamp is placed in this incision and pushed posteriorly along the deep surface of the IT band until the intramuscular septum is palpated. The clamp is then passed through the posterior border of the IT band just above the intramuscular septum. The clamp is then spread in line with the fibers of the tendon to start the posterior split in the tendon. Adhesions to the underlying tissue are often present and should be released. A meniscotome is used to extend the two parallel incisions proximally in line with the fibers of the tendon. The incisions should be continued as proximally as possible to maximize graft length. The angled meniscotome is then used to amputate the graft proximally (Fig. 80.4B). If there is difficulty releasing the graft with the curved meniscotome, a counter incision is made near the tourniquet.

The graft is tubularized, and a whipstitch is placed at its proximal end with no. 5 ethibond. The tendon is separated from the underlying joint capsule and lateral femoral condyle. The capsule in this area is thin, but an effort should be made to maintain the integrity of the capsule to prevent fluid extravasation during later arthroscopy. The graft is left attached to Gerdy's tubercle distally and tucked under the skin for the arthroscopic portion of the case.

The leg is elevated and the tourniquet is inflated. The anterolateral viewing portal is established, and the arthroscope is inserted. An anteromedial portal is established under arthroscopic visualization. Diagnostic arthroscopy is performed and any associated injuries are treated. A limited notchplasty is performed to aid in visualization

and identification of the over-the-top position on the distal femur. Excessive dissection should be avoided to prevent injury to the perichondral ring of the distal femoral physis during notchplasty. The distance from the femoral footprint of the ACL to the physis is typically 3 to 5 mm (16). Because there is no femoral tunnel, retaining a portion of the native ACL can help to maintain the position of the graft in the over-the-top position by acting as a sling.

Now it is necessary to pass the IT band into the over-the-top position. A full-length clamp is placed through the anteromedial portal and into the over-the-top position. The clamp is then passed through the joint capsule along the posterolateral femur and into the site of the IT band harvest (Fig. 80.4C). The clamp is then spread open to dilate a passage for the graft. The ethibond sutures at the free end of the graft are placed into the clamp, and the graft is passed into the knee joint (Fig. 80.4D).

The distal insertion of the graft is then prepared. An additional 3-cm incision is made on the anteromedial aspect of the proximal tibial. The incision must be distal to the tibial physis and medial to the tibial tubercle apophysis. Fluoroscopy can be used to confirm the location of the metaphyseal incision. Dissection is carried down to the periosteum. Under arthroscopic visualization, a rasp is then passed along the periosteum and into the knee joint proximally. The rasp must enter the joint underneath the intermeniscal ligament. Using the rasp, a groove is then made in the tibial epiphysis to facilitate graft passage under the ligament and to translate the graft posteriorly to achieve a more anatomic position of the graft. The graft pulled is under the intermeniscal ligament with a clamp and delivered into the distal incision (Fig. 80.4E).

Graft fixation proceeds from proximal to distal. With the knee in 90° of flexion, tension is applied to the graft and the proximal aspect of the graft is sutured to the periosteum of lateral femoral condyle. This forms the extraarticular component of the reconstruction and helps to limit rotation of the tibia. Distally, an incision is made in the periosteum of the tibia. Periosteal flaps are raised medially and laterally to accommodate the diameter of the graft. Care is taken to avoid excessive dissection laterally, as this risks injury to the tibial tubercle apophysis. Again, the location of this groove can be verified using fluoroscopy. A trough is then created in the tibia using a burr. With the knee in 20° to 30° of flexion, distal tension is applied to the graft. No. 5 ethibond sutures are then placed through the medial periosteum, the graft, and then the lateral periosteum. At least three sutures should be placed proximally in the femur and distally in the tibia (Fig. 80.5). Tibial fixation may be supplemented with a post if necessary. Wounds are closed in layered fashion with absorbable suture. A sterile dressing and a cryotherapy unit are applied to the knee. A hinged knee brace is placed over the cryotherapy unit.

Postoperative range of motion is limited from 0° to 30° for 2 weeks. A continuous passive motion unit is used for 2 weeks. Flexion is gradually increased to 90° from

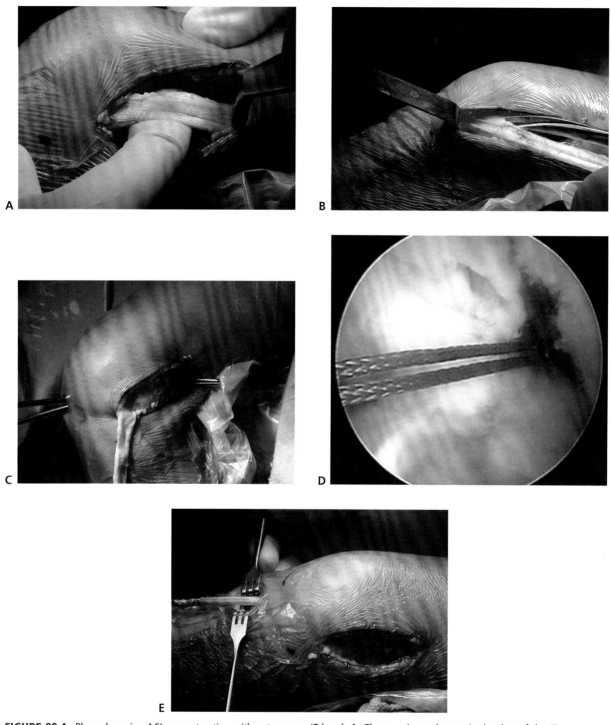

FIGURE 80.4. Physeal-sparing ACL reconstruction with autogenous IT band. **A:** The anterior and posterior borders of the IT band are identified through a lateral incision. **B:** The IT band graft is amputated proximally and released from the lateral condyle. **C:** A full-length clamp is placed into the over-the-top position arthroscopically and pushed through the posterior capsule. **D:** The graft is pulled into the over-the-top position. **E:** The graft is pulled under the intermeniscal ligament and delivered into the distal incision.

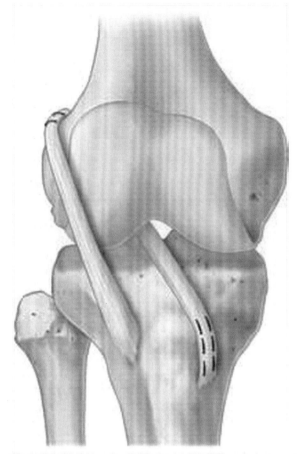

FIGURE 80.5. Combined intraarticular/extraarticular physeal-sparing ACL reconstruction.

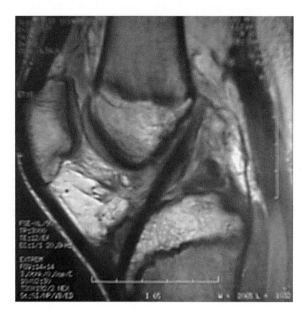

FIGURE 80.6. MRI s/p physeal-sparing ACL reconstruction.

week 2 to 6, after which motion is unrestricted. Touch-down weight-bearing in full extension is recommended for 6 weeks postoperatively. The patient may be placed into a simple hinge brace at 6 weeks. Jogging is instituted at 3 months with return to cutting sports at 6 months pending clearance. An ACL brace is worn for high-risk activities for the first 1 to 2 years after return to sport. Radiographs are obtained at 6 months to evaluate for growth arrest (Fig. 80.6). Clinical follow-up with assessment for leg length discrepancy or angular deformity is done yearly for at least 2 years. Additional radiographs are obtained as indicated by clinical examination.

Modified Transphyseal ACL Reconstruction with Hamstrings Autograft

The modified ACL reconstruction is indicated in the adolescent with significant growth remaining. These patients are typically Tanner stage III with pigmented axilla and pubic hair for boys. The females at this stage are typically postmenarchal. For males, the bone age is from 14 years until skeletal maturity; for females, 13 years until skeletal maturity. Adolescents nearing skeletal maturity (Tanner V) can be treated as adults with conventional tunnels and bone plugs if desired.

Factors associated with growth arrest in transphyseal ACL reconstruction include hardware placement across the lateral distal femoral physis/tibial tubercle apophysis, bone plugs placement across the physis/large tunnels, and vigorous over-the-top dissection.

The patient is placed supine on the operating table. It can be useful to palpate the insertion of the hamstrings before prepping and draping the patient. A tourniquet is placed at the proximal thigh. The examination under anesthesia is performed. If the pivot shift is present, the hamstrings autograft is harvested initially. If the diagnosis is in doubt, diagnostic arthroscopy is performed first.

The leg is prepped and draped sterilely. The limb is exsanguinated and tourniquet inflated. The leg is placed in the figure-of-four position. Typically, the superior border of the medial hamstrings is 3 cm below the joint line. The superior and inferior borders of the hamstrings are marked 3 cm medial to the tibial tubercle (Fig. 80.7).

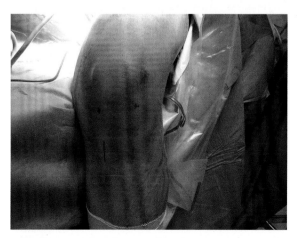

FIGURE 80.7. Incisions for transphyseal ACL reconstruction with hamstrings.

A vertical incision is made, and dissection is carried down to the sartorius fascia. Blunt dissection is used to separate the sartorius fascia from the subcutaneous tissue. The gracilis and semitendinosus should be palpated just below the sartorius fascia. The thin layer of sartorius fascia is carefully incised. A right-angled clamp or Metzenbaum scissors are used to define the superior and inferior borders of the hamstrings tendons. The gracilis and semitendinosus are then isolated individually with vessel loops placed around each tendon (Fig. 80.8). A clamp may be passed deep to the tendons to apply distal traction on the tendons, and this will help free the tendons from the sartorius fascia. The gracilis tendon is then dissected distally and released from its insertion on the tibia. Care should be taken to maintain a pick up or clamp on the tendon to prevent proximal retraction after release. A whipstitch is then placed at the free end of the tendon with no. 5 ethibond suture. This is repeated for the semitendinosus (Fig. 80.9). Distal traction is again applied to the tendons individually, and any adhesions are released. Special attention should be paid to adhesions from the semitendinosus to the medial head of the gastrocnemius. Such adhesions can be quite fibrous and risk diverting the tendon stripper,

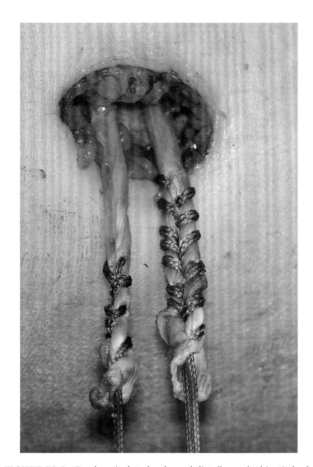

FIGURE 80.9. Tendons isolated, released distally, and whipstitched.

which will result in premature graft amputation. The tendons are then harvested with a closed-loop tendon stripper and taken to the back table for preparation (Fig. 80.10).

Excess muscle is removed from the proximal ends of the tendons, and whipstitches are placed. The tendons are then folded over a closed-loop endobutton to form a quadrupled graft, placed under tension, and covered with a moist sponge. Graft diameter is measured at this time.

A diagnostic arthroscopy is performed using standard anteromedial and anterolateral portals. The menisci are carefully evaluated, as there should be a low threshold for meniscal repair in this patient population. The soft tissue is cleared from the notch with a shaver. A limited notchplasty is performed if necessary for visualization or to avoid impingement (Fig. 80.11). The tibial guide is set at 55°. With the leg hanging over the side of the table, the tibial guide is placed through the anterior medial portal. To avoid the tibial tubercle apophysis, the guide wire entry point on the tibia should be medial through the same incision used to harvest the hamstrings. The guide is typically at 20° to the knee in the sagittal plane. The entrance for the tip of the guide wire is 5 mm in front of the PCL. It should be in line with the posterior portion of the anterior horn of the lateral meniscus and slightly more medial than lateral in the joint. The tibial tunnel

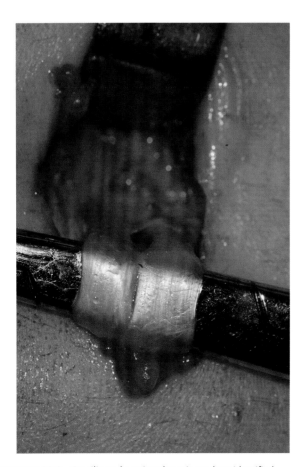

FIGURE 80.8. Gracilis and semitendonosis tendons identified.

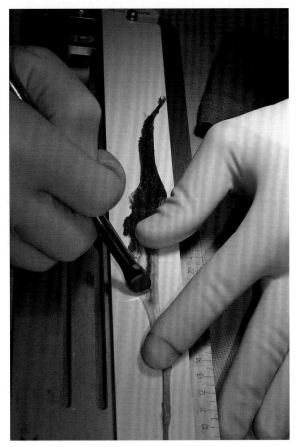

FIGURE 80.10. Graft preparation with removal of excess muscle.

is then drilled based on the width of the harvested graft (Figs. 80.12 and 80.13).

A bump is placed under the thigh to keep the knee at 90°. A long guide pin is placed through the tibial tunnel to the over-the-top position on the femur. The pin is drilled through the proximal femur. The 4.5-mm endobutton

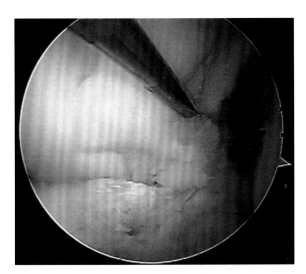

FIGURE 80.11. The ACL stump is debrided and the over-the-top position is visualized.

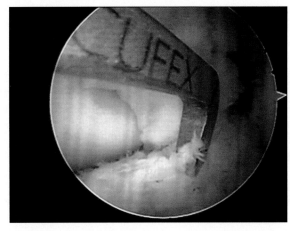

FIGURE 80.12. A tibial guide is used to make the tibial tunnel.

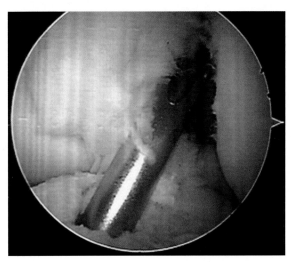

FIGURE 80.13. A transtibial femoral offset guide is used to make the femoral tunnel. Alternatively, the femoral tunnel can be drilled through a medial portal.

drill is then advanced through the lateral cortex. The pin and drill are then removed from the knee. A depth gauge is used to determine the total tunnel length. The depth of the femoral tunnel is determined by subtracting the length of the endobutton loop from the total length. An additional 8 mm is required to flip the endobutton. For example, if the total tunnel length is 60 mm and a standard endobutton length of 15 mm is used, the necessary femoral tunnel depth would be 45 mm. An additional 8 mm is added to flip the endobutton, making the total drill depth 53 mm.

The pin is then placed back into the femoral tunnel transtibially. The acorn drill corresponding to the width of the graft is then used to ream to the calculated femoral depth. Excess bone should be removed with the shaver. If there is any question regarding the adequacy of the tunnels, the arthroscope can be placed through the tibial tunnel to visualize the femoral tunnel.

A looped no. 5 ethibond suture is then placed at the end of the guide pin and pulled through the knee for use as a passing suture. The loop should remain visible through the distal incision with the two free ends exiting proximally through the femoral tunnel and skin. The two passing endobutton sutures of the endobutton are then passed through the looped no. 5 ethibond, and the loop is pulled through the tibial and femoral tunnels (Fig. 80.14). The two endobutton sutures are then used to pass the graft through the tibial and femoral tunnels. The endobutton is flipped on the femoral cortex and fixation confirmed by pulling distally on the graft (Fig. 80.15). The arthroscope is placed back into the knee to evaluate the ACL graft. Additional notchplasty may be performed if there is evidence of graft impingement in extension. The length of the tibial tunnel should also be evaluated. The tibial physis can be visualized by placing the scope into the tibial tunnel. A gross measurement of the metaphyseal portion of the tibial tunnel can be made by bringing the scope up to the level of the physis and measuring the length of the scope within the tunnel. If this distance is less than 25 mm, an interference screw should not be used for fixation. A post, spike washer or staple may be used alternatively (Fig. 80.16).

If the tibial tunnel is of sufficient length, the graft is then fixed on the tibial side with a bioabsorbable

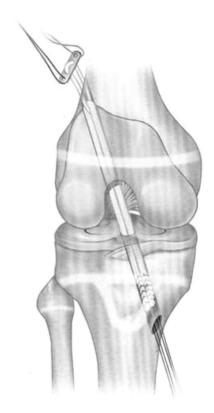

FIGURE 80.15. The graft is passed, and the endobutton is flipped on the femoral cortex.

interference crew (Fig. 80.17). Tension is applied to the graft at all times, and the knee is held in 20° to 30° of flexion. Generally, the screw size matches the tibial tunnel diameter. The endobutton sutures are cut and removed from the femur. The wounds are irrigated and closed in layered fashion with absorbable suture.

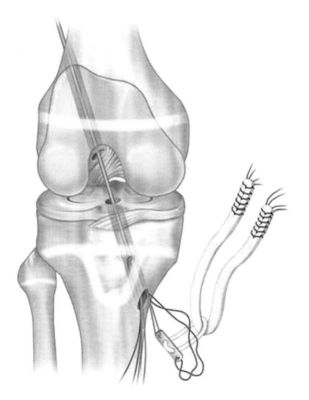

FIGURE 80.14. The leading sutures of the endobutton are passed through the tibial and femoral tunnels.

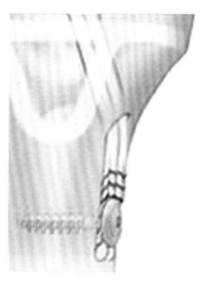

FIGURE 80.16. Alternative tibial fixation with a post.

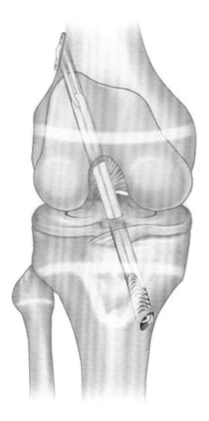

FIGURE 80.17. The graft is fixed distally using an absorbable interference screw.

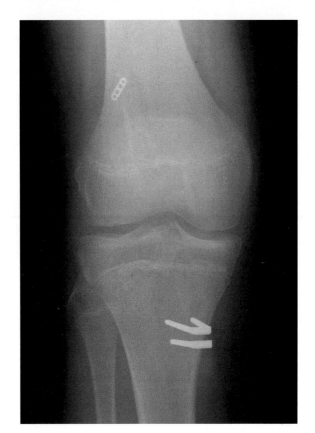

FIGURE 80.19. One month postoperative X-ray.

Sterile dressings, a cryotherapy unit, and a hinged knee brace are applied. Range of motion is limited from 0° to 90° for the first 6 weeks postoperatively. Touchdown weight-bearing with the knee in extension is maintained for 2 weeks. Home CPM is used for 2 weeks starting at 0° to 30° immediately after surgery and advancing up to 90°. After 6 weeks, rehabilitation and clinical follow-up are identical to physeal-sparing reconstruction (Figs. 80.18 to 80.20).

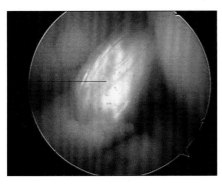

FIGURE 80.18. ACL reconstruction.

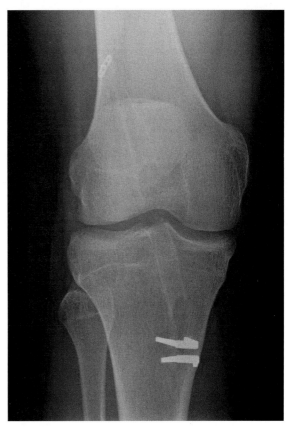

FIGURE 80.20. Four years post-op X-ray.

REFERENCES

1. Smith AD, Tao SS. Knee injuries in young athletes. *Clin Sports Med.* 1995;14:629–650.
2. Kocher MS, Foreman ES, Micheli LJ. Laxity and functional outcome after arthroscopic reduction and internal fixation of displaced tibial spine fractures in children. *Arthroscopy.* 2003;19:1085–1090.
3. Kocher MS, Micheli LJ, Gerbino P, et al. Tibial eminence fractures in children: prevalence of meniscal entrapment. *Am J Sports Med.* 2003;31:404–407.
4. Rang M, Pring ME, Wenger DR. *Rang's Children's Fractures.* Lippincott Williams & Wilkins; 2006.
5. Aichroth PM, Patel DV, Zorrilla P. The natural history and treatment of rupture of the anterior cruciate ligament in children and adolescents. A prospective review. *J Bone Joint Surg Br.* 2002;84:38–41.
6. McCarroll JR, Rettig AC, Shelbourne KD. Anterior cruciate ligament injuries in the young athlete with open physes. *Am J Sports Med.* 1988;16:44–47.
7. Engebretsen L, Svenningsen S, Benum P. Poor results of anterior cruciate ligament repair in adolescence. *Acta Orthop Scand.* 1988;59:684–686.
8. Stanitski CL, Harvell JC, Fu F. Observations on acute knee hemarthrosis in children and adolescents. *J Pediatr Orthop.* 1993;13:506–510.
9. Kocher MS, Micheli LJ, Zurakowski D, et al. Partial tears of the anterior cruciate ligament in children and adolescents. *Am J Sports Med.* 2002;30:697–703.
10. Noyes FR, Bassett RW, Grood ES, et al. Arthroscopy in acute traumatic hemarthrosis of the knee. Incidence of anterior cruciate tears and other injuries. *J Bone Joint Surg Am.* 1980;62:687–695, 757.
11. Eiskjaer S, Larsen ST, Schmidt MB. The significance of hemarthrosis of the knee in children. *Arch Orthop Trauma Surg.* 1988;107:96–98.
12. Vahasarja V, Kinnuen P, Serlo W. Arthroscopy of the acute traumatic knee in children. Prospective study of 138 cases. *Acta Orthop Scand.* 1993;64:580–582.
13. Shelbourne KD, Wilckens JH, Mollabashy A, et al. Arthrofibrosis in acute anterior cruciate ligament reconstruction. The effect of timing of reconstruction and rehabilitation. *Am J Sports Med.* 1991;19:332–336.
14. Guzzanti V, Falciglia F, Gigante A, et al. The effect of intra-articular ACL reconstruction on the growth plates of rabbits. *J Bone Joint Surg Br.* 1994;76:960–963.
15. Houle JB, Letts M, Yang J. Effects of a tensioned tendon graft in a bone tunnel across the rabbit physis. *Clin Orthop Relat Res.* 2001;(391):275–281.
16. Kocher MS, Saxon HS, Hovis WD, et al. Management and complications of anterior cruciate ligament injuries in skeletally immature patients: survey of the Herodicus Society and The ACL Study Group. *J Pediatr Orthop.* 2002; 22:452–457.
17. Greulich WW, Pule SI. *Radiographic Atlas of Skeletal Development of the Hand and Wrist.* Stanford, CA: Stanford University Press; 1959.
18. Tanner JM, Whitehouse RH. Clinical longitudinal standards for height, weight, height velocity, weight velocity, and stages of puberty. *Arch Dis Child.* 1976;51:170–179.
19. Andersson C, Odensten M, Good L, et al. Surgical or non-surgical treatment of acute rupture of the anterior cruciate ligament. A randomized study with long-term follow-up. *J Bone Joint Surg Am.* 1989;71:965–974.
20. Giove TP, Miller SJ III, Kent BE, et al. Non-operative treatment of the torn anterior cruciate ligament. *J Bone Joint Surg Am.* 1983;65:184–192.
21. McDaniel WJ Jr, Dameron TB Jr. The untreated anterior cruciate ligament rupture. *Clin Orthop Relat Res.* 1983;(172):158–163.
22. McDaniel WJ Jr, Dameron TB Jr. Untreated ruptures of the anterior cruciate ligament. A follow-up study. *J Bone Joint Surg Am.* 1980;62:696–705.
23. Liddle AD, Imbuldeniya AM, Hunt DM, et al. Transphyseal reconstruction of the anterior cruciate ligament in prepubescent children. Transepiphyseal replacement of the anterior cruciate ligament using quadruple hamstring grafts in skeletally immature patients. *J Bone Joint Surg Br.* 2008;90:1317–1322.
24. Anderson AF. Transepiphyseal replacement of the anterior cruciate ligament in skeletally immature patients. A preliminary report. *J Bone Joint Surg Am.* 2003;85-A:1255–1263.
25. Kocher MS, Smith JT, Zoric BJ, et al. Transphyseal anterior cruciate ligament reconstruction in skeletally immature pubescent adolescents. *J Bone Joint Surg Am.* 2007;89: 2632–2639.
26. Kocher MS, Garg S, Micheli LJ. Physeal sparing reconstruction of the anterior cruciate ligament in skeletally immature prepubescent children and adolescents. *J Bone Joint Surg Am.* 2005;87:2371–2379.

Miscellaneous

Arthroscopic Approaches to Arthrofibrosis

Benjamin I. Chu • David S. Ryan • William R. Beach

INTRODUCTION

Motion loss in the knee can range widely, from slight loss of extension to significantly restricted motion. Historically, the term arthrofibrosis has been used to describe any loss of knee motion, in flexion, extension, or both. Most commonly, extension loss after anterior cruciate ligament (ACL) reconstruction, such as from a cyclops lesion or notch impingement, has been incorrectly referred to as arthrofibrosis.

For the purposes of this chapter, we define arthrofibrosis of the knee as a condition of diffuse, proliferative scar tissue formation that results in progressive loss of motion in both flexion and extension. The scar tissue associated with arthrofibrosis may form intra-articular and/or extra-articular. A key characteristic of arthrofibrosis is the progressive decrease in the total arc of knee motion. In contrast, motion loss from a focal lesion reaches a certain limit and then plateaus.

Normal Knee Motion

Normal arc of knee motion has been reported from hyperextension of 5° and 6° to flexion of 140° and 143°, for men and women, respectively (1). Passive flexion to 165° is seen in societies that require kneeling and squatting, as in Japan, India, or the Middle East. The functional arc of knee motion required for most daily activities is 10° to 125°.

Hyperextension is required for two important knee motions to occur. First, it permits the screw home mechanism to occur for normal tibiofemoral kinematics. Second, it enables the knee to lock out, allowing the quadriceps muscle to relax during the stance phase. Loss of 5° or greater of extension can cause patellofemoral pain and limping (2). With increasing degrees of knee flexion, greater quadriceps muscle force is required to stabilize the knee (3). Greater quadriceps muscle force results in increased compressive forces at the tibiofemoral and patellofemoral articulations.

Knee flexion of at least 125° is required for sitting and stair climbing. Loss of flexion beyond 125° may make squatting and kneeling difficult. In general, flexion loss is better tolerated than extension loss. However, athletes involved in running and jumping sports may not tolerate any loss of flexion, even less than 10°.

Pathophysiology

The exact pathogenesis of arthrofibrosis is not clearly understood, and the etiology is most likely multifactorial. Primary arthrofibrosis, which develops without an inciting event, has been reported although this is rare. The majority of cases of arthrofibrosis are secondary, following a knee injury, surgery, or prolonged immobilization.

After any trauma there is a normal inflammatory healing response. Arthrofibrosis may result from exaggerated inflammation. Microscopic examination of tissue from arthrofibrotic knees demonstrates a dense fibrous or fibrovascular tissue associated with inflammatory reaction (4, 5). Immunohistologic analysis of the infrapatellar fat pad after ACL injury demonstrates increased expression of fibrogenic cytokines, platelet-derived growth factor, and transforming growth factor-ß, which may promote an arthrofibrotic reaction (6).

Other studies have shown 10 times the amount of ∝-smooth muscle actin-containing myofibroblasts in the infrapatellar fat pad of arthrofibrotic knees (7). Myofibroblasts—highly differentiated fibroblastic cells—play a role in tissue contraction during wound healing as well as pathologic states such as Dupuytren's contracture. Alman et al. (8) demonstrated proliferation of the abnormal fibroblasts in Dupuytren's contracture with cyclic repetitive strain, which may explain the paradoxical decrease in range of motion with increased therapy. Increased levels of collagen type VI, which is upregulated in keloid formation and lung fibrosis, has also been implicated in the development of arthrofibrosis (9).

Incidence

The reported rate of loss of knee motion following trauma or surgery ranges from 2% to 35%. The true incidence of arthrofibrosis is more difficult to determine because of varying definitions of arthrofibrosis and mixed patient populations and varying tolerances for loss of motion. There are many potential causes of limited knee motion that must be ruled out before making the diagnosis of arthrofibrosis. These include mechanical block (incongruent articular surface, displaced bucket handle meniscus tear, and loose body), effusion, quadriceps inhibition, or neurologic deficit.

915

Risk Factors

Numerous risk factors have been associated with knee motion loss. In general, the magnitude of injury or surgery is correlated with the risk of knee stiffness. Loss of motion may also result from prolonged immobilization, infection, or complex regional pain syndrome.

Recent research suggests that some patients may have a genetic predisposition for developing arthrofibrosis. Skutek et al. (10) demonstrated a link between various human leukocyte antigen loci and the development of primary arthrofibrosis.

CLINICAL EVALUATION

Pertinent History

The primary symptom of arthrofibrosis is stiffness, which is often worse in the morning. As described earlier, the patients may report a progressive loss of knee motion, despite attempts at range of motion as part of a home exercise program or formal physical therapy. Patients will often experience significant pain, which may make arthrofibrosis difficult to differentiate from complex regional pain syndrome. Patients will also complain of warmth and swelling in the knee that is exacerbated by attempted motion or activity. These symptoms are often associated with complaints of weakness. The combination of limited motion, pain, and quadriceps weakness can significantly limit activities of daily living.

Physical Examination

Patients will present with a diffusely swollen knee that is warm and tender to touch. An effusion may or may not be present. Swelling is because of inflamed and thickened tissues that often make visualization and palpation of surface landmarks difficult (Fig. 81.1). The skin incision may demonstrate advanced healing or contracture compared with what is normally seen at that point postoperatively.

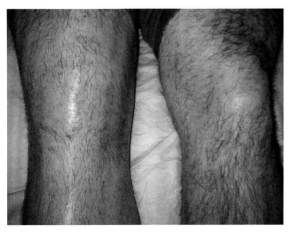

FIGURE 81.1. Diffuse swelling of the arthrofibrotic knee makes visualization and palpation of landmarks difficult.

The knee is often held in a slightly flexed position. The quadriceps muscle will be weak and atrophic, and the patient will walk with an antalgic, bent knee gait.

Active and passive ranges of motion of the knee will be restricted. With passive range of motion, there may be a spring-like endpoint owing to the inflamed and thickened tissues. Patellar mobility is reduced as well, reflecting the diffuse nature of the scar tissue formation.

Imaging

Arthrofibrosis is typically diagnosed based on history and physical examination. Plain radiographs may demonstrate calcification in the soft tissues but often require more than 6 weeks following the injury to develop. Radiographs can be useful in identifying patella infera (baja) in cases of infrapatellar contracture syndrome (IPCS). In cases of stiffness following ACL reconstruction, radiographs to assess tunnel placement are helpful. MRI may be helpful in ruling out other causes of motion loss such as loose body, cyclops lesion, scarring of the fat pad, or graft impingement. One specific advantage of MRI is the ability to evaluate the articular cartilage surfaces, which may provide valuable information when counseling patients regarding their long-term expectations.

Classification

There are multiple classification systems for arthrofibrosis. The first classification system for arthrofibrosis was developed by Sprague et al. (11) and was based on pathoanatomy (Table 81.1).

Shelbourne et al. (12) more recently introduced a system of classification based on motion loss in comparison to the normal, contralateral side (Table 81.2). Paulos et al. (4) described IPCS, an extreme subset of arthrofibrosis. IPCS is characterized by restricted knee flexion, extension, and patellar entrapment, which progresses to patella infera.

We have found that classification is not critical as many patients will not fit into a single group. It is more

Table 81.1	
Sprague et al. (11) arthrofibrosis classification system	
Group	Pathoanatomy Present at Arthroscopy
1	Discrete bands or single sheet of adhesions traversing suprapatellar pouch
2	Complete obliteration of suprapatellar pouch and peripatellar gutters
3	Group 2 combined with extracapsular involvement (bands of tissue from proximal patella to anterior femur)

Table 81.2

Shelbourne et al. (12) arthrofibrosis classification system

Type	Range of Motion Compared with the Normal Contralateral Side
1	Normal flexion, extension loss <10°
2	Normal flexion, extension loss >10°
3	Flexion loss >25°, extension loss >10°
4	Flexion loss >30°, extension loss >10° with patella infera

important to accurately identify the extent of motion loss in flexion, extension, and patellar mobility as this will influence management decisions.

Decision-Making Algorithm

Figure 81.2 depicts the authors' decision-making algorithm.

TREATMENT

Prevention

As the treatment of severe arthrofibrosis is very challenging, early recognition and intervention is critical. Surgeons and therapists must be concerned that any patient not regaining knee motion at an acceptable rate may be developing arthrofibrosis. If surgical treatment is indicated after a knee injury, delaying surgery to allow recovery of range of motion and healing of soft tissues is recommended. Preoperative initiation of nonoperative treatment, as described below, should be considered.

In situations where surgery is not indicated or delaying surgery is not an option, close monitoring of patients in the postoperative period will allow early recognition and intervention. As previously described in the clinical evaluation section, patients with greater than expected pain, redness, or swelling and limited motion may be developing arthrofibrosis. Millett et al. (13) recommend a 2-week goal of obtaining full extension and 120° of flexion.

Nonoperative Treatment

When arthrofibrosis is recognized early, the knee will be undergoing an active inflammatory process. The key during this stage is to avoid further irritation. Forceful attempts to regain range of motion through physical therapy or bracing will exacerbate the inflammation, resulting in further motion loss. A nonforceful mobilization program performed by the patient, including active range of motion within a painless arc of flexion and extension and patellar mobilization, is beneficial. Quad sets and straight leg raise exercises may be performed to maintain quadriceps strength as long as this does not result in further irritation. Treatment should include ice, elevation, and oral nonsteroidal anti-inflammatories (NSAIDs) or a short course of oral corticosteroids. There is paucity of literature regarding intra-articular corticosteroid injection for postoperative treatment of the arthrofibrotic knee following arthroscopic surgery. However, extrapolating from some studies concerning postoperative stiffness following total knee arthroplasty, the literature would suggest that intra-articular steroid injections may be of some benefit (14, 15). Formal physical therapy for modalities such as electrical stimulation and ultrasound may be helpful as well.

As the inflammatory process subsides, more aggressive physical therapy to increase the endpoints of flexion, extension, and patellar mobility may begin. Use of a

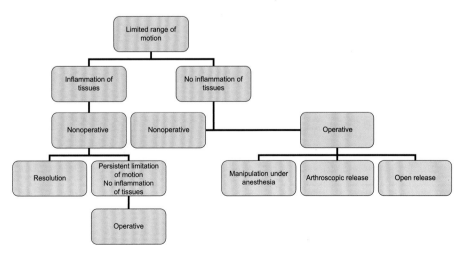

FIGURE 81.2. The authors' decision-making algorithm. MUA, Manipulation under anesthesia; Nonop, nonoperative; Op, operative.

continuous passive motion (CPM) machine may be beneficial in regaining flexion but not extension. Extension may be increased with use of extension board, serial extension casting, or hanging weights. Careful attention should be paid to avoid reinitiation of the inflammatory process. If therapy increases pain, swelling, or inflammation attempts to regain motion must be reduced.

OPERATIVE INDICATIONS, TIMING, AND TECHNIQUE

The indications for operative treatment in arthrofibrosis are failure to progress with physical therapy or persistent limitation in range of motion, 4 months or more following the index injury or surgery. Contraindications to surgical intervention are an active inflammatory process, infection, or chronic regional pain syndrome.

General or regional anesthesia, either alone or in combination, is appropriate for patients undergoing surgical intervention. Use of an indwelling epidural catheter allows for patient-controlled analgesia postoperatively but requires hospitalization. Regional blocks also provide excellent pain control in the immediate postoperative period.

The first step of operative treatment is to perform a thorough evaluation under anesthesia. Careful assessment of range of motion with gravity flexion, passive extension,

and patellar mobility provides insight on where scar tissue has formed. Adhesions in the suprapatellar pouch will limit knee flexion as well as patellar mobility. Knee flexion loss may also result from scarring of the medial and lateral gutters or the anterior interval. The anterior interval consists of the infrapatellar fat pad and tissue in the pretibial recess. Loss of knee extension may be because of scar tissue formation within the intercondylar notch or contracture of the posterior capsule; Table 81.3 lists other common causes of loss of extension and flexion (13).

Manipulation under anesthesia (MUA) may be performed, although it should be done only in conjunction with an arthroscopic or open procedure. Forced manipulation of an arthrofibrotic knee may result in fracture, disruption of the patellar or quadriceps tendons, or intra-articular tissue damage. After prolonged knee stiffness, the articular cartilage is at risk for injury from the contact forces generated during MUA or possible avulsion by mature adhesions.

Arthroscopic treatment has become the first-line approach to arthrofibrosis given the significant morbidity associated with open procedures. Prior to creating the standard inferolateral and inferomedial portals, consider distending the capsule with 120 to 180 mL of solution to reestablish the effective joint space (16). Capsular distention facilitates insertion of arthroscopic instruments, tamponades vessels, and safely stretches the entire capsule,

Table 81.3	
Causes of motion loss (13)	
Loss of Extension	**Loss of Flexion**
Malpositioned or nonisometric graft (anterior tibial tunnel, anterior femoral tunnel)	Suprapatellar adhesions
Notch impingement	Patellar entrapment
ACL nodule	Medial and lateral gutter adhesions or fibrosis
IPCS	Improper graft position
Captured joint capsule after meniscal repair	IPCS
Posterior capsular scarring	Reflex sympathetic dystrophy
Hamstring tightness	Soft tissue calcifications of capsule or MCL
MCL calcification	Postinfection
Postoperative infection	Quadriceps contracture or myositis
Reflex sympathetic dystrophy	—

MCL, medial collateral ligament.
Reprinted from Millett PJ, Wickiewicz TL, Warren RF. Motion loss after ligament injuries to the knee: Part II: Prevention and treatment. *Am J Sports Med.* 2001;29(6):822–828, by Permission of SAGE Publications.

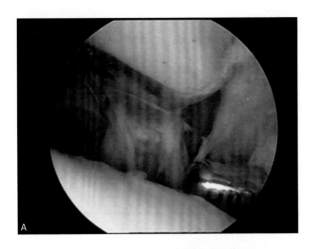

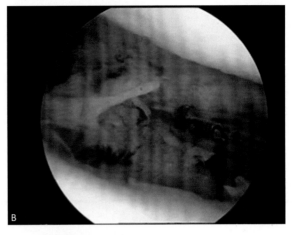

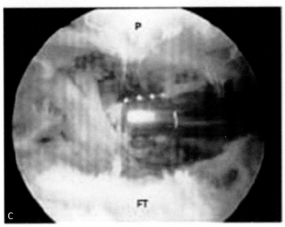

FIGURE 81.3. Suprapatellar adhesions. **A, B:** Adhesions formed between the capsule and femur are removed with an arthroscopic shaver to reestablish the suprapatellar pouch. **C:** The suprapatellar pouch normally extends 3 to 4 cm proximal to the patella. P, patella; FT, femoral trochlea.

including areas that are difficult to reach arthroscopically, such as the posterior capsule.

Millett et al. (13, 17) describe a systematic arthroscopic approach to arthrofibrosis of the knee. The first step is to reestablish the suprapatellar pouch, which normally extends 3 to 4 cm proximal to the patella (Fig. 81.3A–C). Next, the medial and lateral gutters are reestablished. Electrocautery, arthroscopic shaver, and/or meniscal punch can be used to lyse the adhesions formed between the capsule and the femur.

The anterior interval release is then performed. Electrocautery is used to release the infrapatellar fat pad and scar tissue in the anterior interval (Fig. 81.4A, B). Release should begin proximally at a level just anterior to the peripheral rim of the anterior horn of each meniscus and proceed to approximately 1 cm distal along the anterior tibial cortex (Fig. 4C).

The lateral and medial retinacular structures are then assessed. If there is tightness of the retinaculum causing patellofemoral compression or limited patellar mobility, then selective releases may be performed (Fig. 81.5). The intercondylar notch is then examined. Notchplasty should be performed if there is evidence of impingement. Scar

tissue or osteophytes within the notch may impinge as well and should be removed.

After evaluation of the intercondylar notch, knee range of motion should be reassessed. If a tourniquet is used, it should be deflated to allow excursion of the quadriceps. If limitation of extension remains, the posterior capsule must be addressed. Arthroscopic release of the posteromedial capsule has been described (18) as well as various versions of open approaches (19).

During arthroscopy it is important to maintain meticulous hemostasis. Consider placing a drain following arthroscopy, particularly if a lateral release was performed. Postoperatively, a CPM machine may be used to maintain the range of motion obtained in the operating room. Physical therapy, beginning on the first postoperative day, is necessary to obtain the terminal ranges of motion. The focus of therapy is on end range stretching, both passive and active.

AUTHORS' PREFERRED TREATMENT

Although the soft tissues are inflamed, we recommend that patients perform a home program of gentle active range of motion and patellar mobilization. Quadriceps

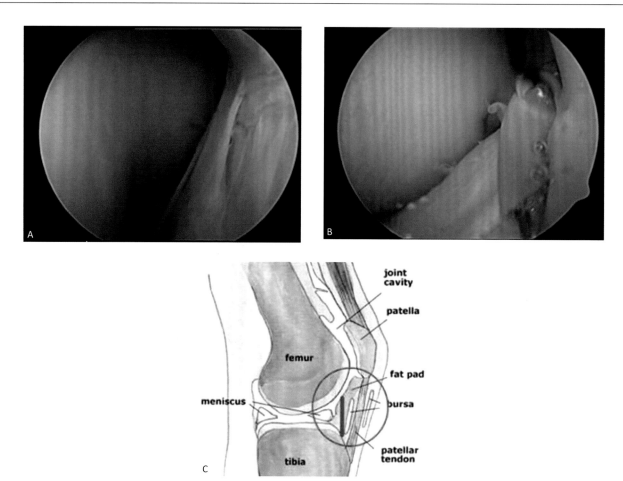

FIGURE 81.4. Anterior interval release. **A:** Fibrosis of the infrapatellar fat pad and scar tissue in the anterior interval. **B:** Electrocautery is used to release scar tissue in the anterior interval, beginning anterior to the peripheral rim of the anterior horn of the medial meniscus and extending approximately 1 cm distal along the anterior tibial cortex. **C:** Illustration demonstrating line of anterior interval release.

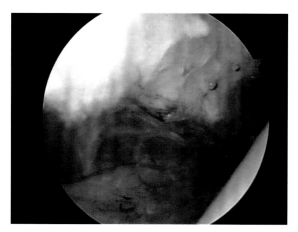

FIGURE 81.5. Lateral release.

strengthening exercises may be included as well. We reassure patients that forceful attempts to increase range of motion at this time will be counterproductive. Ice, elevation, and anti-inflammatory agents are integral components of the treatment. We discuss with the patient that intra-articular corticosteroids may be helpful, particularly early in the course of the arthrofibrotic knee. However, if the patient does not want an injection, we are not forceful in our recommendation.

As the warmth and swelling resolve, formal physical therapy is initiated. We recommend that therapy be performed two times per week with at least 2 days in between sessions to allow the soft tissues to recover. In between sessions, the patient can maintain motion gains with active range of motion exercises. It is important to closely monitor for return of inflammation with increasing therapy. If inflammation returns, forceful attempts to regain motion are discontinued until the inflammation resolves.

We continue nonoperative management as long as the patient continues to experience improvements in range of motion. Our indication for operative treatment is failure to improve with nonoperative management or persistent limitation of range of motion more than 4 months. In our experience, the majority of patients can be treated arthroscopically.

When surgery is indicated, we recommend the use of general anesthetic as well as regional technique. If surgery is performed on an outpatient basis, we have found that a femoral and sciatic nerve block is an effective way to control pain postoperatively. If an inpatient stay is required, an indwelling epidural catheter is recommended.

Intraoperatively, the patient is positioned supine so that the hip is able to be flexed. Careful examination under anesthesia is performed first. We do not perform manipulation prior to arthroscopic release. Following examination under anesthesia, a tourniquet is placed, and the knee is positioned in a standard arthroscopic leg holder. Systematic arthroscopic examination as described by Millett et al. is performed. We use the arthroscopic shaver to lyse the adhesions in the suprapatellar pouch and gutters. To re-establish the anterior interval, our preference is to use electrocautery. This allows us to divide the scar tissue while avoiding damage to the anterior horns of the menisci. The arthroscopic shaver is then used to debride the excessive scar tissue after it is divided.

The knee is then taken out of the leg holder, the tourniquet deflated, and range of motion is reexamined. Gentle manipulation may be performed at this time. It has been our experience that this is usually all the release that is necessary. However, there have been times where full extension is still not achieved despite adequate anterior release. If this is the case, the posterior capsule may have to be released as well. It should be emphasized, however, that this is done very infrequently in our experience and the adequacy of anterior release (particularly removal of scar tissue built up in the notch and anterior interval) needs to be confirmed prior to addressing the posterior capsule. If a posterior capsulotomy needs to be performed, we prefer to do this through medial and lateral open incisions. The tourniquet is inflated and the knee is placed in 90° of flexion. The incisions on either side, and the approach to the posterior capsule, are the same as that used for meniscus repair. Once these are established, blunt finger dissection is used to complete the plane between the posterior musculature and capsule in the midline of the joint so that there is a continuous plane from medial to lateral between the posterior musculature/neurovascular structures and the posterior capsule. Then, while protecting the posterior soft tissues, the capsule is divided. It is important to remember that no matter how extensive a release is done, postoperative range of motion will not improve from that obtained in the operating room.

Our postoperative protocol includes formal physical therapy two times per week with active range to the endpoints of motion and nonforceful passive end range stretching. Patients are instructed to perform their gentle home program in between sessions. We do not routinely include use of CPM. Prescriptions for NSAIDs and analgesics are provided. When a posterior release is performed, dynamic or static extension splinting will help to maintain extension gains.

COMPLICATIONS, CONTROVERSIES, AND SPECIAL CONSIDERATIONS

Motion Loss after ACL Reconstruction

A significant amount of literature has investigated the relationship of arthrofibrosis and ACL reconstruction. The pathophysiology behind idiopathic arthrofibrosis of the knee and postoperative stiffness following surgery is likely different, although this has not been proven yet, to our knowledge. The former is an inflammatory process that leads to capsular thickening and progressive loss of motion with no obvious insult (i.e., surgery).

Risk factors for loss of motion specific to ACL reconstruction include timing of surgery, technical factors (graft choice, graft tensioning, and tunnel placement), concomitant procedures, and postoperative rehabilitation protocols. However, as surgical techniques and rehabilitation protocols improve, the reported rate of knee motion loss following ACL reconstruction has improved significantly.

Salvage Procedures

If knee range of motion is limited despite thorough arthroscopic lysis of adhesions, open surgical treatment may be required. This will usually require an anterior as well as posterior open full capsulectomy, which can be associated with significant morbidity. In addition, certain operative techniques may have to be considered when treating a chronically stiff knee such as quadriceplasty for exposure and proximal sliding tibial tubercle osteotomy for patella infera (baja). Arthrodesis is the salvage treatment when all other treatments fail.

PEARLS AND PITFALLS

1. Arthrofibrosis is an inflammatory process, but the exact etiology is unknown.
2. Key characteristic is progressive motion loss.
3. Early recognition and prevention are important.
4. When inflammation is present, do not make it worse.
5. Do not manipulate prior to arthroscopic release.
6. Use a systematic approach during arthroscopic release.

REHABILITATION

Basic rehabilitation protocols have been addressed in prior sections.

CONCLUSIONS AND FUTURE DIRECTIONS

The progressive loss of motion from arthrofibrosis can have devastating consequences. Prevention and early recognition by physicians and therapists are critical. When motion loss is identified early, nonoperative treatment is often successful. When the inflammatory process is ongoing, forced manipulation may be counterproductive. Anti-inflammatory agents are useful adjuncts to reduce inflammation before initiating more aggressive intervention. Surgical treatment is indicated when there is a failure to progress with physical therapy or persistent limitation in motion, 4 months or more following the index injury. Manipulation should not be performed prior to lysis of adhesions owing to the risk of injury to the articular cartilage surfaces. Arthroscopic treatment is the first line treatment given the significant morbidity associated with open procedures. A systematic approach to release of the scar tissue should be followed, as failure to address all areas of possible adhesion may result in persistent limitation of knee motion. Postoperative rehabilitation protocols should emphasize early motion while closely monitoring for return of the inflammatory process. In the future, better understanding of the molecular pathways in the development of arthrofibrosis may allow identification of high risk patients and intervention through manipulation of the grown factors responsible for the arthrofibrotic reaction.

REFERENCES

1. DeCarlo MS, Sell K. Normative data for range of motion and single leg hop in high school athletes. *J Sport Rehabil.* 1997;6:246–255.
2. Sachs RA, Daniel DM, Stone ML, et al. Patellofemoral problems after anterior cruciate ligament reconstruction. *Am J Sports Med.* 1989;17:760–765.
3. Perry J, Antonelli D, Ford W. Analysis of knee-joint forces during flexed-knee stance. *J Bone Joint Surg Am.* 1975;57:961–967.
4. Paulos LE, Rosenberg TD, Drawbert J, et al. Infrapatellar contracture syndrome: an unrecognized cause of knee stiffness with patella entrapment and patella infera. *Am J Sports Med.* 1987;15:331–341.
5. Cosgarea AJ, DeHaven KE, Lovelock JE. The surgical treatment of arthrofibrosis of the knee. *Am J Sports Med.* 1994;22:184–191.
6. Murakami S, Muneta T, Furuya K, et al. Immunohistologic analysis of synovium in infrapatellar fat pad after anterior cruciate ligament injury. *Am J Sports Med.* 1995;23:763–768.
7. Unterhauser FN, Bosch U, Zeichen J, et al. Alpha-smooth muscle actin containing contractile fibroblastic cells in human knee arthrofibrosis tissue. *Arch Orthop Trauma Surg.* 2004;124:585–591.
8. Alman BA, Greel DA, Ruby LK, et al. Regulation of proliferation and platelet-derived growth factor expression in palmar fibromatosis (Dupuytren contracture) by mechanical strain. *J Orthop Res.* 1996;14:722–728.
9. Zeichen J, van Griensven M, Albers I, et al. Immunohistochemical localization of collagen VI in arthrofibrosis. *Arch Orthop Trauma Surg.* 1999;119:315–318.
10. Skutek M, Elsner HA, Slateva K, et al. Screening for arthrofibrosis after anterior cruciate ligament reconstruction: analysis of association with human leukocyte antigen. *Arthroscopy.* 2004;20:469–473.
11. Sprague NF III, O'Connor RL, Fox JM. Arthroscopic treatment of postoperative knee fibroarthrosis. *Clin Orthop Relat Res.* 1982;166:165–172.
12. Shelbourne KD, Patel DV, Martini DJ. Classification and management of arthrofibrosis of the knee after anterior cruciate ligament reconstruction. *Am J Sports Med.* 1996;24:857–862.
13. Millett PJ, Wickiewicz TL, Warren RF. Motion loss after ligament injuries to the knee: part II: prevention and treatment. *Am J Sports Med.* 2001;29:822–828.
14. Sharma V, Maheshwari AV, Tsailas PG, et al. The results of knee manipulation for stiffness after total knee arthroplasty with or without an intra-articular steroid injection. *Indian J Orthop.* 2008;42:314–318.
15. Bong MR, Di Cesare PE. Stiffness after total knee arthroplasty. *J Am Acad Orthop Surg.* 2004;12:164–171.
16. Millett PJ, Steadman JR. The role of capsular distention in the arthroscopic management of arthrofibrosis of the knee: a technical consideration. *Arthroscopy.* 2001;17:e31–e32.
17. Kim DH, Gill TJ, Millett PJ. Arthroscopic treatment of the arthrofibrotic knee. *Arthroscopy.* 2004;20:187–194.
18. LaPrade RF, Pedtke AC, Roethle ST. Arthroscopic posteromedial capsular release for knee flexion contractures. *Knee Surg Sports Traumatol Arthrosc.* 2008;16:469–475.
19. Steadman JR, Burns TP, Peloza J. Surgical treatment of arthrofibrosis of the knee. *J Orthop Tech.* 1993;1:119–127.

Arthroscopic Approaches to Synovial Pathology

Keith Monchik • Paul Fadale

The synovial membrane of the knee is the largest and most extensive in the body. The synovium of the knee is the deepest layer of the joint capsule and frequently has several embryologic invaginations, called plica. The synovium starts at the superior pole of the patella, where it forms a large pocket beneath the quadriceps femoris. On both the medial and the lateral sides of the knee, the synovium lies on the inner surface of the capsule, except at the attachments of the meniscus to the capsule itself. On the lateral side, it is separated from the capsule by the popliteus. Anteriorly, the synovium covers the deep surface of the patella tendon, as well as attaching to the articular margins of the patella. Below the patella it lines the deep surface of the infrapatella fat pad, and a horizontal ala fold can be identified on each side of the fat pad; below, these folds converge and are continued as a single band, the patella fold (ligamentum mucosum). On either side of the patella, the synovial membrane extends beneath the aponeuroses of the vasti, and more beneath the Vastus medialis. The synovium continues along the capsule distally from the femur to the tibia. It is reflected anterior to the cruciate ligaments, which are therefore considered outside the synovial cavity. Both benign and malignant processes can involve the synovial membrane. For most conditions that require surgical treatment, arthroscopic synovectomy is a safe and effective method.

BENIGN CONDITONS

Plica Syndrome

The medial plica, normally found in approximately 70% of patients, may become hypersensitive with direct trauma to a flexed knee. The medial plica is also prone to injury due to overuse. The lateral fold is rarely symptomatic (1). Clinical presentation is similar to that of medial meniscal tears and patella tendonitis as well as other conditions of the knee. There may also be a snapping sensation along the medial aspect of the flexed knee. Therefore, one should exclude other more common pathologies before making a diagnosis of plica syndrome. In 2007,

demonstrated that MRI is of limited value in detecting normal or pathologic plicae in the knee. Arthroscopic resection is considered after a failed course of anti-inflammatories, steroids, and physical therapy. Arthroscopic evaluation usually reveals an inflamed or hypertrophied medial plica. Postoperative physical therapy begins immediately, and the outcome of resection in well-selected patients is very good, approaching a success rate of higher than 80% in one study.

Pigmented Villonodular Synovitis

Pigmented villonodular synovitis (PVNS) is a slow growing, benign, locally invasive tumor characterized by the presence of inflammation and hemosiderin deposits within the synovium. It is typically a monoarticular process, most often affecting the knee joint with an incidence of 1.8 per million population. PVNS is subdivided into two entities: Diffuse PVNS (DPVNS) and localized PVNS (LPVNS). In the knee, the diffuse form is more common than the localized disease. The lobular, pedunculated LPVNS lesions most frequently present in the anterior compartment of the knee, with most arising at the meniscocapsular junction. As the synovium in the area of the anterior horn is most often affected, patients commonly present with clinical symptoms similar to meniscal pathology. However, other areas of the knee including the suprapatella fat pad, intercondylar notch, suprapatella pouch, both the medial and the lateral recesses, and the anterior horn of the lateral meniscus have been reported. Due to its localized nature, symptoms most commonly include pain, locking, catching, and instability (2). In addition, this is usually, but not always, accompanied by swelling and pain.

In contrast, DPVNS has an insidious, slow onset of pain with swelling and stiffness. In less than 30% of patients, plain radiographs may show nonspecific findings of soft tissue swelling or signs of joint effusion, which are not specific enough to establish the correct diagnosis. While synovial fluid aspiration may reveal a brownish-stained bloody fluid, this may indicate any one of a variety of knee pathologies and is not sensitive or specific to PVNS. CT examination may demonstrate a soft tissue mass of high density relative to skeletal muscle and in long standing cases, bone erosions and subchondral cysts. MRI is the most useful diagnostic tool. The iron in hemosiderin shortens T2 relaxation times on spin echo sequences and causes susceptibility effects on T2* gradient echo sequences resulting in low signal intensity on both types of images, but more so on the gradient echo images, which are more sensitive the presence of hemosiderin (Fig. 82.1). High signal intensity regions may be present on T1 images (fat deposition or hemorrhage) or T2 images (joint effusions or synovial inflammation). MRI is also useful in gauging the extent of the lesion, especially in areas less easily accessible with an arthroscope. Surgery is the definitive treatment for both the localized and the diffuse forms of the disease. Corticosteroids may provide temporary pain relief. In most series, recurrence following excision of LPVNS is rare. Recurrence after total synovectomy of DPVS can be as low as 9% (3). There have been rare reports of malignant transformation and metastasis in patients diagnosed with PVNS (4). In this series, the mortality rate was 50%. Arthroscopic synovectomy lends itself particularly well to the treatment of PVNS, especially the localized form. Arthroscopy has been associated with better functional results and lower rates of postoperative stiffness; however, improper use of this technique has may result in unacceptable recurrence rates. Arthroscopy allows for excellent visualization of lesions, especially in some areas not easily accessible through open treatment such as the posterior compartment. Complete synovectomy in DPVNS results in a substantially lower rate of recurrence than partial excision, but is technically very challenging. Because the posterior compartment is almost always involved in the diffuse form, the surgeon must be comfortable working with both the posteromedial (PM) and the posterolateral portals. Arthroscopic treatment carries a risk of incomplete resection in the diffuse form, as well as the theoretical risk of portal/joint seeding. However, when compared with open synovectomy, arthroscopy is associated with a shorter hospital stay and a shorter rehabilitation period. In a study by Flandry et al., rates of postoperative stiffness following open synovectomy were as high as 24% with the need for further manipulation. The combination of arthroscopic treatment with open synovectomy has not been well described, and thus its effectiveness remains unclear. Poor prognosis has been reported (both open and arthroscopically treated) with invasion of subchondral bone. Radiation therapy has been used as an alternative to surgical treatment, but the results of radiation synovectomy have been mixed.

Chondromatosis/Osteochondromatosis

Synovial chondromatosis is a benign and rare metaplasia of the synovial membrane resulting in the formation of multiple intra-articular cartilaginous or osteocartilagenous bodies. This is most often a monoarticular condition occurring most commonly in middle-age men with over half the cases presenting in the knee. Synovial chondromatosis occurs as either a primary or a secondary form. In primary synovial chondromatosis occurs without an identifiable joint pathology, whereas the secondary form is present in the setting of preexistent disease (osteoarthritis, rheumatoid arthritis [RA], osteochondritis dissecans, etc.). Typically, patients present with pain and swelling, with or without mechanical symptoms. In the absence of calcification, plain radiographs will not reveal

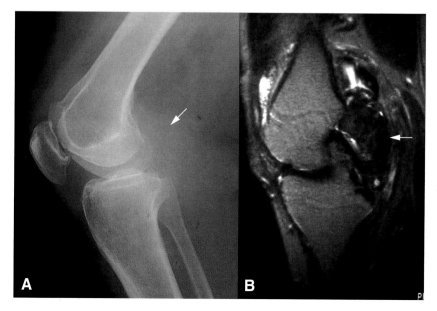

FIGURE 82.1. A: Diffuse PVNS showing increased density on plane films in the posterior knee soft tissues (arrow). **B:** T2 images in patient with diffuse PVNS showing low signal focus of PVNS (white arrow) in posterior joint recess adjacent to posterior cruciate ligament. **C:** Gradient echo images of same patient showing posterior low signal focus of PVNS (black arrow). Note that suprapatella joint recess and anterior juxtameniscal disease is seen well only on the gradient echo image (white arrows). (Photo courtesy of Dr. Jeffery Brody.)

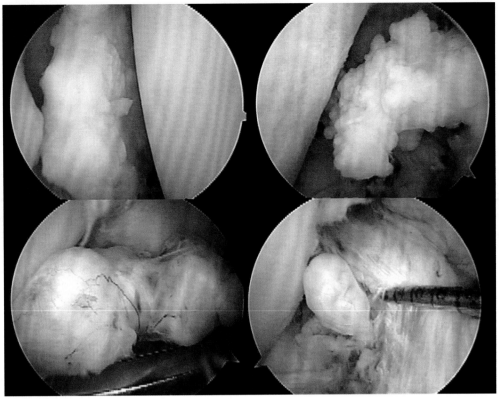

FIGURE 82.2. Osteocartilagenous bodies seen in various compartments of the knee. (Photo courtesy of Dr. Michael Hulstyn.)

loose bodies. CT examination is useful for identifying calcified loose bodies only. MRI is useful depending on the amount of synovial proliferation and amount of calcification within the nodules. Cartilaginous nodules have intermediate signal intensity on T1-weighted images, and high signal intensity on T2-weighted images. Intra-articular gadolinium contrast increases the sensitivity for detecting lesions. Patients with recurrent painful effusions or mechanical symptoms are candidates for surgical treatment (Fig. 82.2). Arthroscopic loose body removal and synovectomy are a safe and effective treatment for this disease (5). Recurrence rates between arthroscopic and open synovectomy are equivalent (0% to 31%), with open treatment having a higher incidence of prolonged rehabilitation and decreased range of motion. Postoperatively, the prognosis is generally good with low rates of recurrence and malignant transformation. Osteoarthritis remains a significant long-term complication, sometimes requiring joint arthroplasty.

Lipoma Arborescens

Lipoma arborescens is a rare intra-articular lesion, characterized by diffuse replacement of the subsynovial tissue by mature fat cells, producing prominent villous transformation of the synovium (6). This condition is sometimes referred to as villous lipomatous proliferation of the synovial membrane. Macroscopically, it is a bulky mass of tissue with a frond-like appearance of numerous broad-based villi composed of fatty yellow tissue. Lipoma arborescens is typically located in the suprapatella pouch, affects males and females equally in the fifth through seventh decade, and is uncommon with less than 100 reported cases. A rare case of an affected pediatric patient has been reported (7). Patients typically present with a joint effusion, enlarged suprapatella pouch, decreased range of motion, stiffness, and occasionally mechanical symptoms. The lesion may arise de novo or develop in patients with degenerative joint disease, RA, or trauma. Plain radiographs may reveal soft tissue swelling in the suprapatella pouch. MRI shows villous lipomatous proliferation with signal intensity similar to that of fat on T1- and T2-weighed images, and a joint effusion. Other findings less commonly seen are a mass-like subsynovial fat deposition, associated synovial cysts, and degenerative changes. Temporary relief of symptoms has been proven with intra-articular injection of steroids or radioisotope (e.g., Y-90). Definitive treatment is complete synovectomy associated with a very low recurrence rate. Successful management by arthroscopic synovectomy has been reported.

Synovial Hemangioma

This is a benign, vascular tumor that occurs mainly in the knee as recurrent painful monoarticular hemarthrosis. It is more frequent in children and young adults and is rare with less than 200 reported cases. Patients usually present in the second decade with pain, limited range of motion, and stiffness in the absence of trauma. Forty percent of patients may have an associated cutaneous hemangioma. A palpable, spongy, compressible mass may be present. Hemangiomas of the knee are described as synovial, juxta-articular or intermediate, where both synovial and juxta-articular component. The intermediate form is often diffuse and unresectable. Radiographs may reveal soft tissue masses, calcified phleboliths, and a hemophilia-like arthropathy with epiphyseal enlargement. MRI findings are more specific consisting of a lobulated intra-articular mass. The mass has an intermediate signal intensity on T1-weighted images. T2 images show area of hypersensitivity (pooling of blood within vascular spaces) and low signal intensity areas (fibrous septa or vascular channels). More importantly, MRI localizes the area and extent of the lesion, which aids in preoperative planning (8). Surgical excision is the definitive treatment. Preoperatively, embolization of the lesion may be useful in decreasing bleeding. Use of a coagulation/ablater during much of the resection will aid in reduced surgical bleeding (9), but no studies exist as to whether resection with a standard rotary shaver versus coagulation has improved outcomes. For localized lesions, partial arthroscopic synovectomy is effective. For diffuse lesions, a complete synovectomy is required.

Popliteal (Baker's) Cyst

Lindgren described a continuous unidirectional flow between the capsular fold on the PM capsule and the gastrocnemius-semimembranosus bursa (GSB) as a result of a valvular mechanism (10), which gives rise to repeated bursal effusions or "Baker's cyst." The predominance of popliteal cysts are treated conservatively. Some are amenable to drainage under ultrasound guidance. However, due to a significant association of intra-articular pathology with recurrent cysts, concurrent treatment of the cyst is warranted at initial arthroscopy as recurrence rates seem to be high after simple open resection (11). Treatment of the cyst involves the obliteration of the slit-like valve, which acts as the gateway between the knee joint and the bursa. Described methods of treatment include an arthroscopic approach through an anteromedial portal (12), cystectomy through a PM cystic portal, and an arthroscopic all-inside suturing of the valve-like structure (13). Regardless of the method chosen, any other associated joint disorder must be addressed in order to minimize the risk of recurrent effusions.

MALIGNANT CONDITIONS

Synovial Sarcoma

This is a malignant condition accounting for between 5% and 10% of the approximately 10,000 new soft tissue tumors diagnosed annually (fourth most commonly occurring sarcoma). It affects mostly young adults with a median age of 26.5 with approximately 30% of patients younger than 30 years old (14). Men are more affected than women. Because synovial sarcomas are usually slow

growing, onset of symptoms is insidious. The most common symptoms are swelling or a mass that may be tender or painful. Range of motion may be decreased. Grossly, the tumor appears as a well demarcated, pink, fleshy mass with a heterogeneous appearance. Calcification foci are sometimes noted with heavy calcification, tending to indicate less aggressive lesions and a more favorable prognosis. Histologically, these tumors have large polygonal cells (epithelioid), which secrete hyaluronic and are surrounded by spindle cells. More than 90% of patients have a t(X:18) translocation mutation specific to synovial sarcoma. Overall, survival rates are 36% to 76% at 5 years and 20% to 63% at 10 years because of the treatment with primary radical surgery, along with chemotherapy and radiation (15). MRI is the imaging modality of choice as 50% of plain radiographs of patients with synovial sarcoma are interpreted as normal. Thirty-percent of patients, however, will have detectable calcifications on plain radiograph. Most synovial sarcomas tend to be large (>8 cm) and appear as a heterogeneous intermediate signal intensity on T1-weighted MRIs and hyperintense on T2-weighted images. Chemotherapy has not proved to provide significant benefit in survival rates in all series; thus, this treatment remains controversial. Surgical excision is the cornerstone of treatment with a recommended tumor-free margin of 1 to 3 cm (16). There is no indication for arthroscopic resection of the tumor. Surgery must include a radical or wide excision, with the possibility of amputation (primarily in 20% of patients), depending on the location of the tumor. Postoperatively, most patients are treated with local radiation.

Hemangiopericytoma

These are typically malignant tumors of mesenchymal origin that occurs in the extremities. They typically occur in adults with an equal male to female ratio. They are extremely rare accounting for less than 1% of all soft tissue sarcomas. Histologically, these tumors consist of pericytes that form solid sheets and nests around irregularly formed vascular channels. A histologic diagnosis is made based on architectural patterns. Grossly, the tumor appears hypervascular, asymmetric with large vascular cavities. MRI is the imaging modality of choice, as findings on plain film are usually nonspecific. Treatment is based on the grade of the sarcoma. Depending on the extent of involvement, surgical treatment may range from local excision to amputation. High-grade tumors may be treated with chemotherapy, but the direct benefit of treatment is unknown. Radiation therapy usually follows surgical resection to reduce local occurrence.

SEROPOSITIVE ARTHRITIS

Rheumatoid Arthritis

Approximately 1.3 million people in the United States have RA. It is most likely to affect people of all races 35 to 50 years of age, with a 75% female predominance. The inflammation associated with the disease causes pain and stiffness within the joint. Exacerbations of the disease may result in hemorrhage and effusion, leading to progressive joint deterioration. MRI will show a low/intermediate signal intensity on T1-weighted images and a high signal intensity on T2-weighted images (active form). Both erosions and loss of cartilage show enhancement. Diagnosis is confirmed by the presence of four out of seven American College of Rheumatology criteria including (1) Morning stiffness around the joint that lasts at least 1 hour; (2) Arthritis of three or more joints for at least 6 weeks; (3) Arthritis of the hand joints for at least 6 weeks; (4) Arthritis on both sides of the body for at least 6 weeks; (5) Rheumatoid nodules under the skin; (6) Rheumatoid factor present in blood testing; and (7) Evidence of RA on X-rays. Histologically, a villous pattern with lymphocytic nodules and a hypervascular synovium is identified. New disease-modifying antirheumatic drugs (DMARDs) are available and are successful in treating most RA patients. For those who have suffered complete destruction of the knee joint, arthroplasty remains a definitive procedure for the older patients. However, for the subset of younger patients who do not have an adequate response to DMARDS, arthroscopic synovectomy can be an effective treatment in reducing joint destruction (17). In theory, synovectomy is useful in eliminating the synovium as a major source of cytokines and chemokines. Historically, open synovectomy was the procedure of choice for removal of the synovium. However, given the advances in arthroscopy, the fragility of the skin in RA patients, and propensity toward infection, complete arthroscopic synovectomy is a viable alternative but is technically demanding (18). Arthroscopic synovectomy has been shown to reduce blood loss, shorten hospitalization, and permit faster recovery when compared with open procedures in rheumatoid patients (19).

SERONEGATIVE ARTHRITIS

Seronegative arthritis refers to a diverse group of musculoskeletal syndromes linked by common clinical and immunopathologic mechanisms. This group includes Reiter's syndrome, psoriatic arthritis, ankylosing spondylitis, and juvenile idiopathic arthritis. In contrast to seropositive arthritis, male patients are predominant. The age of onset is variable, but tends to start in the teens or early twenties. The disease frequently runs in families where it is linked to HLA genes, including but not limited to, HLA-B27. Frequency is estimates at 3.5 cases per 100,000. Patients may present with myalgias early in the course of the disease followed by asymmetric joint stiffness, low back pain, and symptoms worsening with rest or inactivity. In addition to the musculoskeletal symptoms, patient may experience ophthalmologic problems, urethritis, constitutional symptoms, and mild recurrent abdominal complaints after precipitating episodes of diarrhea. Plain radiographs may show no abnormalities early in the disease, followed by progressive asymmetric oligoarticular join involvement, juxta-articular

osteoporosis, and a distinctive spinal pattern in the case of sacroiliitis and ankylosing spondylitis. Like seropositive arthritis, medication and physiotherapy are the mainstay of treatment. However, in the growing child, joint replacement is rare and surgery is limited to prophylactic therapy. Arthroscopic synovectomy has been shown to maintain range of motion of the joint, allow earlier mobilization than open synovectomy and shorten hospitalization (20).

HEMOPHILIA

Hemophilia is a bleeding disorder characterized by a lack of function of factor IX or coagulation factor VIII. Hemarthrosis is the most common and most disabling musculoskeletal manifestation of the disease leading to an arthropathy, capsular fibrosis, and joint contracture. Arthroscopic synovectomy has been shown to decrease the episodes of hemarthrosis, decrease pain, improve range of motion, and decrease the need for factor replacement (21, 22). However, bony deformities, presence of osteophytes, joint space narrowing, and destruction makes this a technically demanding procedure. The primary indication for this procedure is recurrent hemarthrosis that has failed to respond to conservative treatment for a period of 6 months. Perioperative considerations focus on the reduction of unnecessary bleeding through maximizing factor replacement. The minimal circulating concentration of factors VIII and IX to control bleeding is around 20% to 40%. Due to the stress of surgery, inflammatory changes that occur, and the risk of intraoperative bleeding, suggested circulating levels at the time of surgery is thought to approach 200% to 400%. Careful coordination with hematology is essential for preoperative levels, intraoperative required testing, and postoperative follow-up and management of factor levels. If excessive bleeding is experienced during surgery, the patient may require an additional intraoperative bolus of factor replacement based on circulating levels, and this should be available. The use of a drain postoperatively along with a compression wrap is suggested. All patients are admitted to the hospital for at least 3 days of monitoring and factor replacement as well as immediate physical therapy. The drain remains until output has leveled off and factor levels have returned to and stay at 100%. Patients are made weight-bearing as tolerated, and the use of a locked knee brace helps to maintain terminal extension. Some surgeons advocate the use of cold therapy to reduce swelling and improve pain, and the use of a continuous passive motion (CPM) to facilitate early motion. Outcome is usually closely related to the degree of joint destruction evident on X-ray and evident at arthroscopy.

ARTHROSCOPIC SYNOVECTOMY

Removal of the synovium of the knee arthroscopically has major advantages over open surgical techniques including decreased postoperative knee stiffness, better complete synovectomy, decreased hospitalization, better visualization of all knee joint surfaces, decreased pain, decreased hemarthrosis, division of the quadriceps is unnecessary, easier preservation of the menesci, and easier revision surgery if required. The major disadvantage is that it is a technically challenging operation to perform.

Equipment

Typically, a 30° arthroscope is used for most of the procedures; however, a 70° arthroscope is particularly useful for visualizing the posterior compartment and should be available intraoperatively. While knee distention has been described through the use of gravity flow systems, in our experience a pump with an initial low pressure setting is essential in keeping the field clear at all times. The use of a proximal thigh tourniquet after exsanguination of the extremity is also essential. Choice of shavers will to some degree be dependent on the patient's anatomy, but in general, a 5.5-mm full radius synovectomy blade works well in the anterior compartment and will be the workhorse for most of the resections. A 3.5-mm full radius synovectomy blade or 4.5 curved synovial resector can be used in restricted areas such as under the mensci, in the posterior compartment, or in patients with smaller knees.

Preoperative Planning

General indications for arthroscopic synovectomy are patients who have been disabled for at least 6 months by pain and swelling, and have not responded to conservative treatment. An established diagnosis of a synovial disorder is essential, especially in the case of PVNS where a histologic diagnosis should be made preoperatively. Informed consent should include a full discussion of the risks associated with arthroscopy of the posterior compartment including damage to the neurovascular bundle. We recommend the use of a general or spinal anesthetic. In addition, the use of a femoral nerve block aids in decreased postoperative pain.

Technique

The basis of arthroscopic synovectomy of the knee is the use of six portals (anterolateral [AL], lateral suprapatellar [LS], anteromedial [AM], medial suprapatellar [MS], posteromedial [PM], and posterolateral [PL]) to visualize and resect all areas of the synovium (Fig. 82.3). Synovial resection is carried out until the shiny capsular surface below it is seen. A thorough history and physical exam is required preoperatively including documentation of the limb's neurovascular status. Intraoperatively, after the induction of general anesthesia, an examination under anesthesia is performed assessing both range of motion and stability of the joint. After, the patient's operative leg is placed into a thigh holding device, the table is flexed, and the leg is allowed to hang free off the end of the table. The well leg is placed into a well leg holder. Alternatively, the procedure

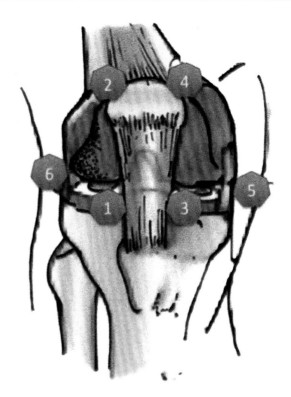

FIGURE 82.3. Six arthroscopic portals used in synovectomy. (Illustration by Dr. Robert Villareal.)

may be performed supine with the use of a lateral post and the well leg placed supine on the flattened operative table. Sterile prepping and draping is then performed. Appropriate antibiotics are given approximately 30 minutes prior to incision. The tourniquet is then inflated after eschmarch or gravity exsanguination if the extremity.

A standard AL portal is then created and the 30° arthroscope is inserted into the suprapatellar pouch and a routine diagnostic arthroscopy is performed of the suprapatellar pouch, medial and lateral gutters, trochlear groove, and undersurface of the patella, medial and lateral compartments including both mensci, intercondylar notch, and cruciate ligaments (Fig. 82.4). Concurrent pathology such as meniscal or chondral injury is addressed at this time. An AM portal is made to aid in the diagnostic arthroscopy and to use to pass a probe into the knee joint (Fig. 82.5). A biter may be used through the AM portal to obtain a sample of synovial of tissue from an area of significant pathology. With the camera still in the AL portal and in the suprapatellar pouch, an LS portal is made approximately 1 cm above and 1 cm lateral to the corner of the patella, followed by an MS portal directly opposite the LS portal (Fig. 82.6). The 5.5-mm or 4.5-mm full radius synovectomy blade is inserted through these portals, and the synovium of the suprapatellar pouch and upper gutters are resected. Access to any portion of a hypertrophic fat pad can also be achieved through these two portals. To reach the lower portions of the gutters, the instrumentation is reversed with the camera alternating between the LS and the

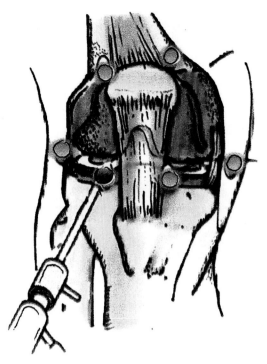

FIGURE 82.4. Diagnostic arthroscopy with a 30° arthroscope in the AL portal. (Illustration by Dr. Robert Villareal.)

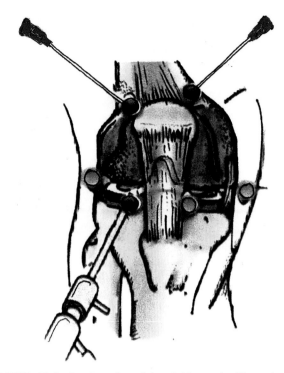

FIGURE 82.6. Creation of medial and LS portals. (Illustration by Dr. Robert Villareal.)

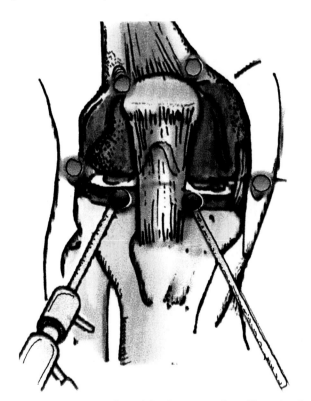

FIGURE 82.5. AM portal used for instrumentation. (Illustration by Dr. Robert Villareal.)

MS portals and the shaver introduced through the AM and AL portals. Next, synovectomy of the anterior compartment and intercondylar notch is achieved through triangulation through the AM and AL portals. The lower ends of the

gutters can also be visualized and resected through these two portals. We then excise any perimeniscal synovium with the use of a 3.5-mm or curved 4.5 mm shaver through the AM or AL portal while viewing the opposite anterior portal. Submeniscal pathology is more easily addressed arthroscopically than with open procedures and spares sacrificing any meniscal tissue. A 70° arthroscope is then selected to gain access to the posterior compartment. The knee is flexed and held at 70° to 90°, aiding access to the posterior compartment by widening the intercondylar notch and allowing the posterior neurovascular bundle to fall posteriorly. Using a modified Gilquist maneuver with the arthroscope in the AL portal, and advanced under the posterior cruciate ligament, a PM portal can be made. A spinal needle is introduced into the PM knee at the PM corner of the joint and aiming anteriorly (Fig. 82.7). Palpation of this area is evident intra-articularly through visualization using the arthroscope. Dimming of the operative lights and transillumination may also aid in introduction of the spinal needle. The portal is then made with a no. 11 blade, and a blunt metal or disposable cannula is then introduced into the joint. We routinely introduce the cannula over a switching stick as we believe the switching stick aids in a more accurate placement of the cannula (Fig. 82.8). Passage of any instrument or cannula into the knee joint at this anatomic location must be aimed slightly anterior to avoid placement into the posterior neurovascular bundle. Resection of the PM compartment is then carried out using a 4.5-mm shaver working systematically from the periphery to the center of the posterior

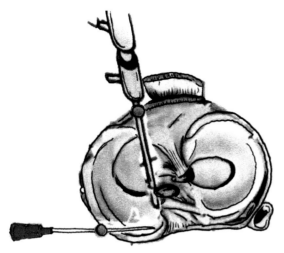

FIGURE 82.7. An anteriorly directed spinal needle is used to establish the location for the PM portal. (Illustration by Dr. Robert Villareal.)

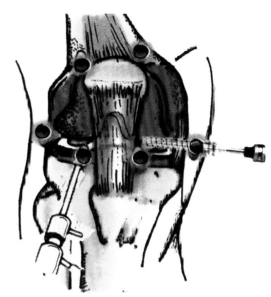

FIGURE 82.9. Resection of the PM compartment using a 4.5-mm shaver and a 70° arthroscope. (Illustration by Dr. Robert Villareal.)

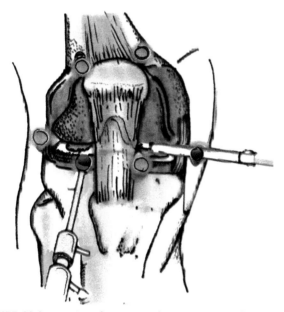

FIGURE 82.8. Creation of a PM portal. A 5.5-mm cannula is introduced over a switching stick. (Illustration by Dr. Robert Villareal.)

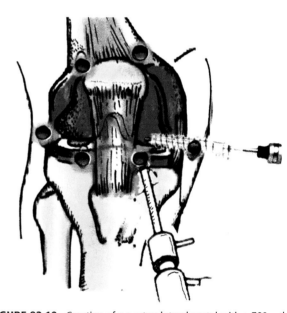

FIGURE 82.10. Creation of a posterolateral portal with a 70° arthroscope in the AM portal. (Illustration by Dr. Robert Villareal.)

compartment (Fig. 82.9). Careful use of suction will prevent the capsule from being drawn into the shaver, thereby increasing the risk of accidental damage to vital posterior structures. The posterolateral area of the posterior compartment is then addressed in a similar fashion by switching the arthroscope to the AM portal (Fig. 82.10). With the knee in 90° of flexion, the common peroneal nerve should fall well posterior to the field, hidden by the biceps tendon. A spinal needle is introduced 1 cm posterior to the femoral condyle and 1 cm above the joint line, always anterior to the biceps tendon. Like the PM portal,

the PL portal is widened with a cannula over a switching stick after incision with a no. 11 blade. The posterolateral synovium is then resected similar to the opposite side (Fig. 82.11).

Postoperative Management

A drain is frequently used for at least 1 day; however, the surgeon may elect to forgo this if bleeding does not appear to be significant. A compression dressing is applied over the drain. Patients are usually discharged home the same day with crutches and partial weight-bearing. Some form

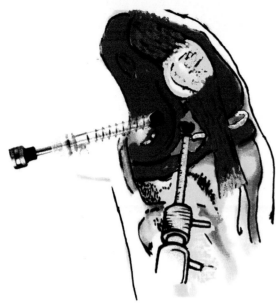

FIGURE 82.11. Resection of the posterolateral synovium with a 4.5-mm shaver. (Illustration by Dr. Robert Villareal.)

of cold therapy may be useful in aiding postoperative discomfort and swelling. Oral pain medication is prescribed. All patients are scheduled for early physical therapy, and are given an instruction booklet to begin immediate postoperative home therapy until their first appointment. This includes active range of motion exercises and quadriceps strengthening. The use of a CPM machine is to aid in early motion is also certainly acceptable. Most patients are ready for near normal activity by the fourth postoperative week.

Complications

In general, the complications of arthroscopic synovectomy are those of any arthroscopic procedures. Specifically, inadvertent damage to the posterior neurovascular bundle, saphenous vein or nerve, or common peroneal nerve when working through both the PL and the PM portals is certainly the most devastating. Other complications specific to this procedure include recurrence or subtotal resection of the synovial pathology requiring additional surgery, reflex sympathetic dystrophy, postoperative stiffness requiring manipulation, or arthroscopic lyses of adhesions and hemarthrosis.

REFERENCES

1. Shetty VD, Vowler SL, Krishnamurthy S, et al. Clinical diagnosis of medial plica syndrome of the knee: a prospective study. *J Knee Surg.* 2007;20(4):277–280.
2. Dines JS, Bernadino TM, Wells JL, et al. Long-term follow-up of surgically treated pigmented villonodular synnovitis of the knee. *Arthroscopy.* 2007;23;9:930–937.
3. Flandry FC, Hughston JC, Jacobson KE, et al. Surgical treatment of diffuse pigmented villonodular synovitis of the knee. *Clin Orthop Relat Res.* 1994;300:183–192.
4. Bertoni F, Unni K, Beabout JW, et al. Malignant giant cell tumor of the tendon sheaths and joints (malignant pigmented vilonodular synovitis). *Am J Surg Pathol.* 1997;21:153–163.
5. Samson L, Mazurkiewicz S, Treder M, et al. Outcome in the arthroscopic treatment of synovial condromatosis of the knee. *Orthop raumatol Rehabil.* 2005;7(4):391–396.
6. Davies AP, Blewitt N. Lipoma arborescens of the knee. *Knee.* 2005;12:394–396.
7. Bansal M, Changulani M, Shukla R, et al. Synovial lipomatosis of the knee in an adolescent girl. *Orthopedics.* 2008;31(2):185.
8. Winzenberg T, Ma D, Taplin P, et al. Synovial haemangioma of the knee. *Clin Rheumatol.* 2006;25:753–755.
9. Barakat MJ, Hirehal K, Hopkins JR, et al. Synovial hemangioma of the knee—Case report. *J Knee Surg.* 2007;20:296–298.
10. Lindgren PG. Gastrocnemio-semimembranosus bursa and its relation to the knee joint. III. Pressure measurements in joint and bursa. *Acta Radiol Diagn (Stockh).* 1978;19:377–388.
11. Takahashi M, Nagano A. Arthroscopic treatment of popliteal cysts and visualization of its cavity through the posterior portal of the knee. *Arthroscopy.* 2005:21:638.e1–638.e4.
12. Sansone V, DePonti A. Arthroscopic treatment of popliteal cyst and associated intra-articular knee disorders in adults. *Arthroscopy.* 1999;15:368–372.
13. Calvisi V, Lupparelli S, Giuliani P. Arthroscopic all-inside suture of symptomatic baker's cysts: a technical option for surgical treatment in adults. *Knee Surg Sports Traumatol Arthrosc.* 2007;15:1452–1460.
14. Zeitouni N, Cheney RT, Oseroff AR. Unusual cutaneous malignancies. In: Williams CJ, Krikorian JG, Green MR, Raghavan D, eds. *Textbook of Uncommon Cancers.* 2nd ed. New York, NY: John Wiley & Sons; 1999.
15. Eilber FC, Dry SM. Diagnosis and management of synovial sarcoma. *J Surg Oncol.* 2008;15;97(4):314–320.
16. Zagard G. Ballo M, Pisters P, et al. Prognostic factors for patients with localized soft tissue sarcoma treated with conservation surgery and radiation therapy. *Cancer.* 2003;97(10):2530–2543.
17. Ogawa H, Itokazu I, Ito Y, et al. The therapeutic outcome of minimally invasive synovectomy assisted with arthroscopy in the rheumatoid knee. *Mod Rheumatol.* 2006;16:360–363.
18. Kim S, Jung K, Kwun D, et al. Arthroscopic synovectomy of the knee joint in rheumatoid arthritis: surgical steps for complete synovectomy. *Arhroscopy.* 2006;22(4)461.e1–461.e4.
19. Monabang CZ, De Maeseneer M, Shahabpour M, Lenchik L, Pouliart N. MR imaging findings in patients with a surgically significant mediopatellar plica. *JBR-BTR.* Sep-Oct 2007;90(5):384-7
20. Maston A, Witonski D, Pieszynski I, et al. Early clinical results of open and arthroscopic synovectomy in knee inflammation. *Orthop Traumatol Rehabil.* 2007;9(5):520–526.
21. Dell'Era L, Facchini R, Corona F. Knee synovectomy in children with juvenile idiopathic arthritis. *J Pedi Orthop B.* 2008;17:128–130.
22. Verma N, Valentino A, Chawla A. Arthroscopic synovectomy in haemophilia: indications, technique and results. *Haemophilia.* 2007;13(suppl 3):38–44.
23. Yoon KH, Bae DK, Kim HS, et al. Arthroscopic synovectomy in haemophilic arthropathy of the knee. *Int Orthop.* 2005;29:296–300

Complications of Knee Arthroscopy

Orrin Sherman • David Hergan • David Thut

The adoption of arthroscopic techniques has led to an overall decrease in many complications associated with knee surgery. Arthroscopic meniscectomies, in fact, have become so routine that both patients and surgeons often view it as nearly risk free. Multiple series have been published over the years showing that this view is overly optimistic. The results of a survey performed by the Arthroscopy Association of North America (AANA) were published in 1985 and reported an overall complication rate of 0.3% (1). In 1986, Sherman et al (2). reported an 8.2% complication rate in a retrospective review of 2,640 patients, having routine arthroscopic knee procedures not involving ligament reconstruction. Small published several reports culminating in the 1988 review of a registry of cases performed by 21 experienced arthroscopists over a 19-month period compiled by the Complications Committee of AANA. The complication rate for knee arthroscopy was 1.8% (3). More recently, Reigstad and Grimsgaard (4) reported a 5% complication rate in 876 simple knee arthroscopies performed between 1999 and 2001. The rate of complications requiring intervention was 0.68%. When the full range of arthroscopic procedures in the knee is taken into consideration, the rate of complications is significantly higher. The goal of this chapter is to give an overview of the most significant and most common complications associated with common arthroscopic procedures of the knee and to offer guidance on the prevention, identification, and treatment of those complications.

INFECTION

Postoperative infection after knee arthroscopy is fortunately quite rare. Deep infection rates have been reported as being less than 0.3% (1–4). Superficial wound healing problems are somewhat more common. The infection rate for ACL reconstruction, however, has been reported to be as high as 1.74%, with a mean incidence in the literature of 0.52% (5, 6). Most infections are felt to be due to inoculation at the time of surgery, but concomitant infection at the tibial tunnel site is common, suggesting communication to the joint from an infected superficial wound was

possible (7, 8). Rapid diagnosis and treatment of intra-articular infection is important, as the loss of glycosaminoglycan in cartilage begins within 8 hours and can progress to cartilage loss and degenerative changes, full-thickness cartilage defects, and osteomyelitis (5, 8–11). With prompt treatment, postoperative infections can be eradicated.

Most patients with postoperative knee infections present in the acute (<2 weeks) or subacute (<2 months) periods (12). It has been noted that presenting symptoms of postoperative infection can be confused with postoperative changes. In fact, Schollin-Borg et al. (5) reported that 60% of the time there was a failure to appreciate an infection at the first visit. The classic presentation is an acutely swollen painful knee with limited range of motion (12). Increased pulsatile pain, painful range of motion, rapidly increased and persistent effusion, incision drainage, local erythema, and warmth with intermittent fever are common symptoms as well. A subtle increase in pain and difficulty in physical therapy should be seen as ominous signs (8, 13). If there is clinical suspicion of a joint infection, the knee should be aspirated and the fluid sent for cell count, Gram stain, and cultures. Fluid analysis for glucose, protein, and LDH may be helpful as well. The sensitivity and specificity of each test is shown in Table 83.1. Given the relatively low specificities of most tests, the data should be viewed as a whole. The most common organism found in culture is *Staphylococcus aureus*, which is present in 48.5% of positive cultures. The second most common is *Staphylococcus epidermidis*, which is present in 39.5% of positive cultures. Gram-negative bacteria were present in 7% of cases and anaerobes in 11.5% cases (6). Infection after allograft reconstruction should raise concern for allograft contamination, particularly when the cultured organisms are atypical (15).

The primary goal in treating an infection after ligament reconstruction is protection of the articular surface (16). Arthroscopic debridement with extensive synovectomy using accessory portals has been shown to decrease the bacterial load in the joint (7). Although some authors have advocated graft removal and early reimplantation, most surgeons prefer to save the graft if possible (13, 17).

Table 83.1

Laboratory analysis of serum and joint aspirate sensitivities and specificities for joint infection (14)

Laboratory Analysis	Laboratory Value	Sensitivity (%)	Specificity (%)
Joint aspirate	WBC > 100,000/µL	29	99
Joint aspirate	WBC > 50,000/µL	62	92
Joint aspirate	WBC > 25,000/µL	77	73
Joint aspirate	Polymorphonuclear cells ≥ 90%	73	79
Joint aspirate	Synovial fluid glucose < 1.5 mmol/mL	51	85
Joint aspirate	Protein > 3.0 g/dL	48	46
Joint aspirate	LDH > 250 U/L	100	51
Serum lab values	WBC > 10,000/µL	90	36
Serum lab values	Erythrocyte sedimentation rate > 30 mm/h	95	29
Serum lab values	C-reactive protein	77	53

In their systematic review, Mouzopoulos et al. (12) suggested a protocol for treatment after ligament reconstruction. The graft should be removed only if it is unstable, if it is impregnated by thick purulent exudates, or if cultures have shown *S. aureus* and antibiotic treatment was significantly delayed. Empirical IV antibiotic therapy should be broad. A thorough arthroscopic synovectomy should be carried out using 10 to 15 L of fluid and accessory wounds should be opened if they are at all suspicious. If there is any exudate on the graft, it should be removed. They recommend leaving wounds open and using continuous irrigation drains if felt necessary. Repeat arthroscopy should be performed every 2 to 3 days as needed. Parenteral antibiotic therapy should be narrowed per culture results and continued for 6 weeks. Oral antibiotics should follow for another month. With careful treatment, the graft can be retained and the patient can expect a good outcome (18).

Intraoperative Graft Contamination

Studies have shown culture evidence of autograft contamination in 13% of uncomplicated ACL reconstructions despite no clinical evidence of postoperative infection (19, 20). Although rare, intraoperative graft contamination due to a break in sterile technique is possible. Izquierdo et al. (21) surveyed sports medicine specialists and found that 25% of 196 respondents had experienced a total of 57 intraoperative graft contaminations. In 75% of those cases, the graft was cleansed and implanted. There were no reported postoperative infections. The most common cleansing technique was soaking the graft in Chlorhexidine solution, and the paper concluded that this represented the standard of care. The efficacy of Chlorhexidine soaks has been supported by basic science papers as well (22, 23). In reporting his experience with three contaminated ACL grafts, Pasque notes that the risk appears to

be higher when there is turnover in the surgical team. He noted no postoperative infections after rinsing the grafts in Chlorhexidine followed by a triple antibiotic bath (24). Authors have noted that Chlorhexidine is potentially chondrotoxic, so a subsequent antibiotic soak serves the dual purpose of completion of graft sterilization and as a rinse. The use of antibiotic soaks alone, however, is not recommended (25).

ARTHROFIBROSIS

Localized Arthrofibrosis

Infrapatellar contracture syndrome is a pathologic fibrous hyperplasia of the infrapatellar fat pad. It has been described as having three stages beginning with periarticular inflammation, edema, and quadriceps weakness. After 6 weeks, this progresses to limited patellar mobility, inferior patellar tilt, and a flexed knee gait. After 8 months, patellar mobility improves, but the patella baja remains and patellofemoral degenerative changes begin (26, 27). Scarring in the anterior interval leads to tethering of the patellar tendon, pain, and loss of extension (28). The fat pad itself appears to be important in the pathogenesis, and the syndrome has been associated with acute surgery, patellar tendon autograft, and multiple surgical procedures (27). Prevention consists of minimizing injury to the fat pad at the time of procedure and starting aggressive rehabilitation in the early postoperative period. Treatment should focus on allowing the inflammation to decrease by backing off on physical therapy, performing passive patellar mobilization. Nonsteroidal anti-inflammatory drugs (NSAIDs) and oral corticosteroids may be useful as well. In chronic cases, a low signal area of scar coursing from the fat pad to the anterior tibia can be seen on MRI (Fig. 83.1).

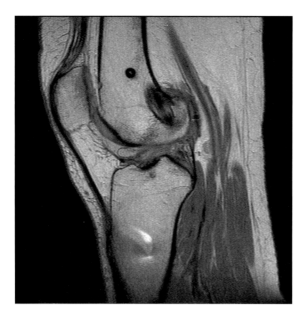

FIGURE 83.1. Scar tissue interposed between fat pad and tibia.

Patients often have a positive Hoffa test, defined as pain in the anterior knee with pressure near the patellar tendon with knee extension. Good results have been seen with arthroscopic debridement using a high-viewing portal (Fig. 83.2) (28).

Generalized Arthrofibrosis

There appears to be a genetic predisposition to excessive scarring after trauma or surgery. Skutek et al. (29) have reported that certain HLA types are at increased risk. Studies have shown that the fat pad is capable of releasing proinflammatory cytokines, which may contribute to the inflammatory response in the joint (27, 30–32). Given this association with fat pad injury, authors have suggested that minimizing trauma to the fat pad at the time of surgery may help limit the risk or generalized arthrofibrosis (26, 33).

There is a clear association between multiple ligament injuries and arthrofibrosis. Injury to the MCL and ACL together is a particular problem. Bracing the MCL and allowing it to heal before reconstructing the ACL may minimize the risk. In cases of grade 3 MCL injury, a tear above the joint line increased arthrofibrosis risk (34). In repairing the MCL, surgeons must take care not to tie the MCL down too close to the joint line.

In addition to taking meticulous care at the time of surgery to minimize trauma to the joint, injury to the fat pad, and postoperative hemarthrosis, surgeons can limit the risk of arthrofibrosis by encouraging aggressive rehabilitation. Special attention should be paid to regaining full extension early. Some authors have recommended the use of bracing to help with extension, but a recent systematic review of bracing found no benefit (35). There is evidence that acute ACL reconstructions are associated with increased risk of arthrofibrosis. The consensus appears to be that surgery should be delayed until the knee has become less swollen and inflamed and full extension is restored (33, 36–38).

Early treatment for motion loss consists of carefully managed rehabilitation. If there is evidence of significant joint inflammation, it is important not to push the knee too hard to allow it to settle down. If no inflammation is appreciated, an aggressive phased physical therapy program is warranted, focusing on full knee extension. Authors have differed on the usefulness of manipulation under anesthesia (35, 39–41). There appears to be agreement that manipulation is best in cases of mild arthrofibrosis with problems in flexion. If conservative treatments fail, aggressive arthroscopic treatment has been advocated (Fig. 83.3). Millett and colleagues (35) have outlined a nine-point arthroscopic release that ensures careful assessment of all areas in the joint that could contribute to the problem. If arthroscopic treatment fails, an aggressive open surgical salvage treatment that has offered good results (42).

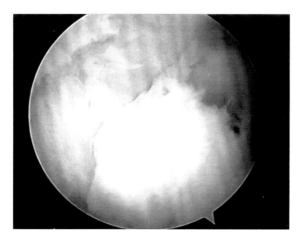

FIGURE 83.2. Arthroscopic view of anterior compartment scar tissue.

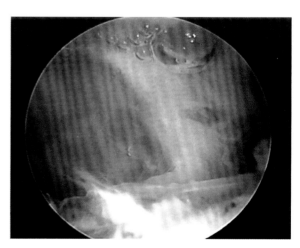

FIGURE 83.3. Arthroscopic view of adhesions in the suprapatellar pouch.

DEEP VENOUS THROMBOSIS AND VENOUS THROMBOEMBOLISM

The incidence of deep venous thrombosis (DVT) after arthroscopic surgery has been reported to be as low as 0.6% when purely clinical diagnostic criteria are used and as high as 41% diagnosed using MR venogram (43, 44). Most clots after knee arthroscopy appear to be below the knee, and reports of fatal PE after knee arthroscopy are rare (45–49). Two papers specifically looking for surgical and patient factors associated with increased DVT risk showed that tourniquet time longer than 60 minutes and prior history of DVT are the only significant factors (50, 51).

In their Cochrane Database Review, Ramos et al. (49) found that treatment with low molecular weight heparin offered a relative risk of 0.16 for DVT when compared with control. This was balanced by a relative risk of 2.04 for minor complications such as hemarthrosis and gastric bleeding. The only patient with a PE in their pooled data was in the treatment group. They concluded that "no strong evidence was found to conclude thromboprophylaxis is effective in preventing thromboembolic events."

The American College of Chest Physicians released their recommendations on thromboprophylaxis after the Eighth ACCP Conference on Antithrombotic and Thrombolytic Therapy in 2008. After their review of the literature, they concluded that the risk of VTE appears to be low in arthroscopic procedures when compared with major orthopedic procedures. They note that the results of three studies have shown a decrease in the rate of asymptomatic DVT through LMWH use, but that adverse bleeding events were increased. They felt that patients should be encouraged to mobilize as soon as possible after surgery. The formal recommendations were that no routine thromboprophylaxis other than early mobilization be used in patients with no thromboembolic risk factors. They did, however, recommend LMWH thromboprophylaxis of an unspecified duration if the patient has any of the risk factors in Table 83.2 or if the procedure is unusually long or complicated (52).

VASCULAR COMPLICATIONS

Vascular injury associated with arthroscopy is rare. In two reports by Small (3, 53), there were no vascular injuries in 9,791 knee arthroscopies. Sherman et al. (2) reported no vascular complications in 2,640 cases. DeLee (1), however, reported nine cases of penetrating artery injuries in 118,590 arthroscopies. Six were popliteal artery injuries, resulting in four amputations. Popliteal artery injuries are typically associated with PCL reconstruction and repairs of the posterior horn of the meniscus (54, 55). There are two reports, however, of popliteal injury associated with ACL reconstruction (56, 57). With the knee in flexion, the popliteal artery lies an average of 29.13 mm posterior to the PCL at its midpoint, and only 9.69 mm from its tibial insertion (58).

Table 83.2

Risk factors for VTE Geerts et al. (52)

Surgery

Trauma (major trauma or lower extremity injury)
Immobility, lower extremity paresis
Cancer (active or occult)
Cancer therapy (hormonal, chemotherapy, angiogenesis inhibitors, radiotherapy)
Venous compression (tumor, hematoma, arterial abnormality)
Previous VTE
Increasing age
Pregnancy and postpartum period
Estrogen containing oral contraceptives or hormone replacement therapy
Selective estrogen receptor modulators
Erythropoiesis-stimulating agents
Acute medical illness
Inflammatory bowel disease
Nephrotic syndrome
Myeloproliferative disorders
Paroxysmal nocturnal hemoglobinuria Obesity
Central venous catheterization
Inherited or acquired thrombophilia

The artery has been shown to be farther from the PCL in 100° of knee flexion than it is in lesser angles (59). It has also been noted that with the leg in external rotation the artery is brought into proximity to the posterior horn of the lateral meniscus (60). Penetrating injury to the popliteal artery can cause a pseudoaneurysm. About 30% of these are asymptomatic. Symptoms generally become apparent 2 to 3 weeks after surgery and can include a popliteal mass, claudication, venous stasis, neurologic changes, ischemia, and thrombotic events. The amputation rate has been reported to be over 20%. Vascular imaging and rapid referral to a vascular surgeon are essential (57, 61).

Given the proximity of the popliteal artery to the PCL, care must be exercised in PCL reconstructions. Guides that capture the pin as it exits the posterior tibia are advisable to avoid overpenetration (55). Surgeons would be wise to perform their posterior notch work for both PCL and ACL reconstruction with the knee at a high flexion angle to minimize risk to posterior structures. Care must be taken in creating posterior portals, as there is risk to the popliteal artery from both the spinal needle and the cannula (62). Injury to the popliteal artery has been described after both medial and lateral posterior horn meniscectomies (60, 63).

Use of bicortical screw fixation like a post and washer for ACL graft fixation puts the popliteal artery at risk below the joint line (56). This risk is minimized by aiming toward the fibula when drilling through the posterior tibial cortex. With appropriate trajectory, the popliteal artery and vein were on average 11.4 mm from the drill hole, although in one specimen, the distance was only 3.5 mm (64).

The popliteal artery is also at risk during meniscal repair. When an inside-out technique is used, retractors should be placed to capture the needles and they should be passed under direct visualization (65). Needles should be directed away from the posterior midline. With all inside meniscal repair systems, the surgeon must be careful to avoid overpenetration as well, particularly in the posterior horn of the lateral meniscus, which is closest to the popliteal artery (66). Depth limiters should be used, as studies have shown that some devices can come within 3 mm of the artery (67).

Injury to the medial inferior geniculate artery has been associated with hamstring tendon harvest and medial periosteal stripping in the area of the tibial tunnel entrance (68, 69). The medial and lateral inferior geniculate, descending geniculate, and sural arteries have all been injured during meniscectomies as well (68, 70–72). Recognition of these injuries, which can cause heavy bleeding and hematoma, may allow ligation of the artery. Saphenous vein injury has been reported with all-inside meniscal repair techniques causing persistent hematoma (73).

NEUROLOGIC COMPLICATIONS

Neurologic complications after knee arthroscopy are rare. Large reviews have placed the incidence at between 0.01% and 0.6% (1, 3, 53, 74, 75). Lesions of the common peroneal nerve have been reported after routine knee arthroscopy through both traction and direct injury during lateral meniscectomy (76, 77). Peroneal injuries are most commonly associated with needle injury or suture entrapment during lateral meniscal repair (53, 78–81). When performing an inside-out meniscal repair, a posterolateral incision made at the joint line behind the lateral collateral ligament should be used. With the knee flexed 90°, dissection is carried between the biceps femoris tendon and the iliotibial band to allow placement of a retractor under the lateral head of the gastrocnemius on the posterolateral joint capsule. The needles can be retrieved and tied under direct visualization (82). If the nerve function is decreased after a repair, release of the sutures has been reported to result in complete recovery (81, 83). Two studies have shown that the peroneal nerve is at a small risk of injury when drilling the posterolateral femoral tunnel during double-bundle ACL reconstruction. Higher knee flexion angles of 110° to 120° minimize that risk (84, 85).

The neurologic structures most at risk with ACL reconstruction are the superior and inferior trunks of the infrapatellar branch of the saphenous nerve (86). Laceration of the nerves causes numbness and dysesthesia lateral and distal to the incision and can lead to painful neuromas (87). This can lead to bothersome anterior knee pain and possible complex regional pain syndrome (CRPS). The nerve is at risk at the time of skin incision from hamstring and patellar tendon harvest, tendon stripping, and drilling of the tibial tunnel. Risk of injury during patellar tendon harvest can be lowered by using horizontal incisions or two spaced vertical incisions (88, 89). A traditional longitudinal incision is less likely to injure the braches if it is made with the knee in full flexion as this moves the branches distally (86). If the branches can be identified at the time of surgery, an effort should be made to protect them. Injury can occur during hamstring harvest as well (90). The nerve lies just superficial to the gracilis tendon. With a traditional vertical incision for hamstring harvest, 68% of patients have been shown to have sensory disturbances affecting an average surface area of 48 cm^2. By making an oblique incision that follows the path of the tendons, only 24% of patients have sensory disturbance over a much smaller 8.4 cm^2 (91). It has been suggested that the tendons should be harvested with the knee flexed and hip externally rotated in order to minimize tension on the nerve during harvesting (92). Management of symptomatic injury to the infrapatellar branch includes padding, physical therapy, and direct skin desensitization. It is important to continue aggressive mobilization to minimize risk of CRPS.

The saphenous nerve is also at risk during inside-out meniscal repair. A retractor should be placed on the posterior capsule through an incision made just above the joint line behind the medial collateral ligament. With the knee at 90° of flexion to keep the infrapatellar branch 1 cm proximal to the joint line, the sartorius fascia is opened and the interval between the fascia and the capsule can be exploited. Care should be taken to avoid the sartorial branch of the saphenous nerve, as it can often be encountered in this incision (93). Transillumination may help identify the location of the saphenous vein that runs with the nerve (94). Needles in inside-out repairs can be passed under direct visualization (82, 87).

The tibial nerve is at small risk in repair of the posterior horns of both the medial and the lateral menisci. Placement of retractors as described and directly inside-out needles away from the center of the popliteal fossa should minimize the risk. Because the tibial nerve lies in proximity to the popliteal artery behind the knee, techniques described to minimize vascular complications during PCL reconstruction should also protect the tibial nerve.

Modern suture-based all-inside meniscal repair devices appear to decrease risk of neurologic injury (95, 96). The manufacturer's instructions should be followed to avoid posterior overpenetration. Implants should be directed away from the central portion of the knee posteriorly. Clinical reports of meniscal repair success have not noted any neurologic complications associated with the devices (97–101).

PUMP/TOURNIQUET/COMPARTMENT SYNDROME

During arthroscopy, fluid is instilled into the knee under pressure by either a gravity fed inflow or an infusion pump. The infusion pump allows control of both fluid pressure and flow, which is helpful in maintaining hemostasis during the procedure. Under normal circumstances, the use of a pump is not associated with a significant increase in leg compartment pressures (102, 103). Complications are associated with extravasation of fluid. Femoral nerve palsies have been reported after fluid tracked into the thigh with pump pressures between 150 and 300 mm Hg (104). Extravasation leading to thigh and leg compartment syndrome has been associated with pressures as low as 30 mm Hg (105). When the pressure sensor failed, Romero et al. (106) reported extravasation into the scrotum and peritoneum. Fluid has been shown to flow into the thigh through a defect in the suprapatellar pouch and into the leg through a defect in the bursa between the semimembranosis and the gastrocnemius muscles caused by increased pressure (107). The risk is increased in patients with capsular rents associated with tibial plateau fractures or combined ligament reconstruction and high tibial osteotomy procedures (108, 109). If there are no fascial defects in the leg, it has been shown in swine that extravasated fluid dissipates from the compartments quickly and is unlikely to cause ongoing muscle damage (110, 111). Surgeons should be aware of the possibility of fluid extravasation and watch for it. If the compartments are noted to be tense, a brief period of watchful waiting may be warranted before definitive fasciotomy.

The tourniquet is another common means of maintaining hemostasis during knee arthroscopy. Although generally accepted as safe, tourniquet use is associated with a reversible decrease in both muscle and nerve function (112–115). Leg compartment syndromes have been attributed to tourniquet use as well (116, 117). Curved and wide cuffs appear to be better tolerated (74). Surgeons are advised to follow the generally accepted advice of limiting tourniquet time to less than 2 hours (77).

COMPLEX REGIONAL PAIN SYNDROME

Schutzer and Gossling (118) provided a comprehensive definition of reflex sympathetic dystrophy (RSD) as an exaggerated response to injury of a limb manifested by intense prolonged pain, vasomotor disturbances, delayed functional recovery, and trophic changes. Multiple terminologies have been used for this condition, but the International Association for the Study of Pain has recommended the term CRPS types I and II (119). CRPS can be a multisystem disorder, but is usually confined to one extremity. The exact etiology is unknown, but multiple investigations have confirmed that it is mediated by a disorder of the autonomic nervous system (120, 121). The syndrome presents when a noxious stimulus, which often is minor, causes an excessive response with sensory findings associated with a sympathetic disorder manifested by temperature changes, skin discoloration, and swelling (122, 123). Trophic changes occur in the skin, nails, and bone (Fig. 83.4). Motor changes may present as impaired voluntary movements, tremors, and dystonic posturing (124).

The initiating stimulus to the knee ranges from a simple traumatic blow to the knee to a surgical procedure. Arthroscopic surgical procedures of the knee seem to be a common precipitating event (124, 125–127). For this reason, an arthroscopic procedure of the knee for diagnostic purposes alone, or solely for evaluation of pain, can either be a cause of CRPS or exacerbate a preexisting, undiagnosed CRPS (128). Injury to the saphenous nerve during meniscal repair and minor injury to a collateral ligament from positioning of the leg during knee arthroscopy have both been implicated as initiators of CRPS of the knee (123). A particularly common trigger in the knee seems to be pathology and/or injury to the patellofemoral joint, which some authors believe is always involved in cases of CRPS of the knee (126, 129).

CRPS occurs in less than 1% of patients after arthroscopic knee procedures, but the exact incidence and prevalence are not known. CRPS occurs in children and adults, but seems to favor the lower limb in children and the upper limb in adults (130). In the knee, the overall

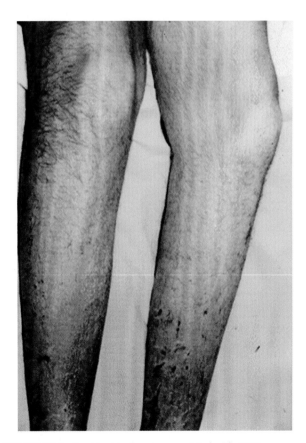

FIGURE 83.4. Trophic skin changes associated with CRPS.

incidence is higher in adults, affecting females predominantly (126, 131). Although the incidence of severe CRPS is quite low, some authors have proposed that knee stiffness as a long-term postarthroscopic sequel could be due to a mild form of CRPS (132). CRPS has traditionally been divided into three stages describing clinical features over a 0- to 12-month time course (Table 83.3). The classic clinical presentation and disease progression are often absent in CRPS of the knee, making the diagnosis difficult (126).

CRPS is predominantly a clinical diagnosis and a diagnosis of exclusion. Complete blood count, erythrocyte sedimentation rate, calcium levels, fasting blood glucose, and thyroid levels should be checked in order to exclude systemic causes of pain. One hallmark symptom of CRPS is pain out of proportion to the injury, but the clinical diagnosis can encompass a wide variety of signs and symptoms, with varying degrees of expression. The pain is classically nonanatomical in distribution and involves a burning sensation along with intolerance to cold. Any test that relieves the symptoms of CRPS by blocking the sympathetic nervous system is considered diagnostic.

CRPS is difficult to treat effectively. The symptoms of CRPS in the lower extremity are frequently more refractory to intervention than those in the upper extremity (133). Because of the many physiologic and psychological factors involved in pain, a multidisciplinary approach should be implemented for each patient. However, no consensus currently exists regarding the most effective treatment for CRPS of the lower extremity. Ghai and Dureja (134) named five important goals in treating a patient with CRPS: (1) perform a comprehensive diagnostic evaluation (2), be prompt and aggressive in treatment interventions (3), assess the patient's clinical and psychological status (4), consistently be supportive, and (5) strive for maximal pain relief and functional improvement.

Table 83.3
Clinical presentation of the different stages of CRPS

Stage I (lasts 1–3 mo)	Increased nail and hair growth, pain that travels along affected limb, severe burning/aching pain, dry skin that changes color, swelling with warmth or coolness
Stage II (lasts 3–6 mo)	Decreased hair growth, noticeable changes in skin texture/color, stiff muscles and joints
Stage III (irreversible changes can be seen)	Contractions involving muscles and tendons, limited movement in limb, pain in entire limb, muscle wasting

Physical therapy is crucial in the treatment of CRPS and should be the first line of treatment. Aggressive therapy should be avoided, but gentle physiotherapy is effective and should be directed at edema control, preventing contractures, and reestablishing voluntary motor control. In the knee, this should include gentle patellar mobilization, progressive range of motion exercises, and eventually strengthening. Psychological support and counseling are also both effective for recovery (131). Avoidance of painful stimuli, prolonged splinting, cryotherapy, and patient confrontation are all important (120, 123).

Pharmacologic agents to treat CRPS include simple analgesics, NSAIDs, steroids, narcotics, antineuropathics (gabapentin), calcium metabolism modulators (bisphosphonates, calcitonin), propanolol, and nifedipine (135). Pain control is essential in the treatment algorithm, and often multiple drug combinations are necessary. Early evaluation by a pain management specialist is therefore imperative as early treatment has been shown to result in a more favorable outcome (120, 136).

If the CRPS patient fails to respond to noninvasive methods, sympathetic blockade becomes the mainstay of treatment. Cooper and DeLee (126) suggested resorting to a sympathetic block if after 6 weeks of noninvasive treatment, symptoms continue to progress. Lumbar sympathetic blocks can be performed in an outpatient setting and combined with physical therapy and other modalities (128). Indwelling epidural blocks with bupivacaine combined with oral medications avoid the need for repeated procedures and can also assist with a rehabilitation program (137). Although a few published reports exist concerning the efficacy of spinal stimulators and spinal pumps, these have been used for patients with CRPS of the knee (138), and there is some evidence showing improved health status with this treatment for patients with CRPS type I (139, 140). When lumbar sympathetic blocks temporarily relieve pain but symptoms predictably recur, sympathectomy is a drastic treatment option. Treatment results of sympathectomy can vary and complications can occur; therefore it is reserved for severely afflicted patients with few other options.

Most authors agree that when early diagnosis and treatment of CRPS of the knee are implemented, within 6 to 12 months, an overall good outcome can be expected (129, 136). Chronic syndromes, however, can be extremely difficult to manage and lead to restricted movement and patellofemoral pain. Patella baja with changes in the tibiofemoral mechanics leading to chondral degeneration can ultimately be the result (123).

Although surgery is strongly discouraged in the presence of CRPS, if it is necessary, an attempt at resolution of most if not all the pain in the knee preoperatively is crucial. Preoperative physical therapy and continuous epidural anesthetic sufficient to cause sympathetic blockade for several days perioperatively are also recommended.

SECONDARY OSTEONECROSIS

Secondary osteonecrosis has been seen in the postoperative knee after arthroscopic interventions such as meniscectomy (141, 142), cartilage debridement (143), and anterior cruciate ligament reconstructions (144). Secondary osteonecrosis has been associated with other factors, such as systemic lupus erythematosus, corticosteroid therapy, alcoholism, and renal transplantation; however, due to the nature of this text, we will be focusing only on postarthroscopic osteonecrosis of the knee. Unlike spontaneous osteonecrosis of the knee, which predominantly affects females older than 60 years, postoperative osteonecrosis of the knee affects both genders equally, with a mean age of 58 years (145). There are currently a total of 47 patients reported in the literature who have developed secondary osteonecrosis after arthroscopic meniscectomy. Most commonly affected was the medial femoral condyle (82% of cases), followed by the lateral femoral condyle (8.5%) and the lateral and medial tibial plateaus (2.1% each) (Fig. 83.5). Pape suggests that it is possible that as many as 59% of the reported postoperative osteonecrosis lesions reported in the literature could actually represent an undiagnosed preexisting case of spontaneous osteonecrosis of the knee. The following two prerequisites must be fulfilled to establish the diagnosis of postoperative osteonecrosis: (1) absence of osteonecrosis on preoperative imaging and (2) timely association between knee arthroscopy and a suspicious bone marrow edema pattern on postoperative MRI (146).

There seems to be a higher incidence of postoperative osteonecrosis in elderly patients undergoing arthroscopy for meniscal tears or chondral lesions; although in relation to the number of knee arthroscopies performed, the incidence is still rare. Patients with postoperative osteonecrosis present with knee pain of sudden onset, a mild effusion, and a tender joint line. The diagnosis must be distinguished from a meniscal tear or re-tear. Symptoms usually lag behind bone edema changes on MRI by about 2.2 months (142).

In the mid-1990s, multiple articles demonstrated that arthroscopic meniscectomies performed with lasers resulted in a particularly high incidence of postoperative osteonecrosis (142, 147, 148). The exact etiology of postoperative osteonecrosis is unknown. Vascular interruption to subchondral bone is a leading theoretical cause.

Although secondary osteonecrotic lesions of the knee have the potential to progress to irreversible stages, the progression can also stop at any time. Complete resolution of the lesion, however, seems to be restricted to the early stages of osteonecrosis, and thus stage-dependent therapy is recommended (Table 83.4) (149–151).

Nonoperative treatment consists of protected weight-bearing, anti-inflammatory medications, and analgesics, followed by a second postoperative MRI for follow-up evaluation of the bone marrow edema. Normally, the bone marrow edema progresses, and when it does, and symptoms worsen, a second surgical procedure is indicated.

ANTERIOR CRUCIATE LIGAMENT RECONSTRUCTION

Motion Loss

The incidence of motion loss after ACL reconstruction has been reported between 2% and 11% in isolated ACL reconstruction and as high as 35% when the ligament was repaired or reconstructed acutely (38, 152, 153). Although athletes are adversely affected in jumping and running abilities with minimal losses of flexion, small losses of extension are particularly poorly tolerated due to constant quadriceps activity (154). Shelbourne and Gray (155) reported that at a 10-year follow-up after ACL reconstruction, extension loss compounded degeneration associated with meniscal or chondral pathology. The goal of ACL reconstruction is to restore knee stability while maintaining full knee motion. Causes of motion loss are most commonly attributed either to technical problems with tunnel positioning or graft tensioning or to localized or generalized arthrofibrosis. Technique-specific issues are discussed here.

Tunnel Malposition

The goal of the commonly performed single-bundle technique is to place the femoral and tibial tunnels in positions that allow the graft to be isometric with knee motion while not impinging on the roof of the notch, the lateral femoral condyle, or the PCL. Graft isometry is most affected by femoral tunnel placement (Fig. 83.6) (156). Ideal

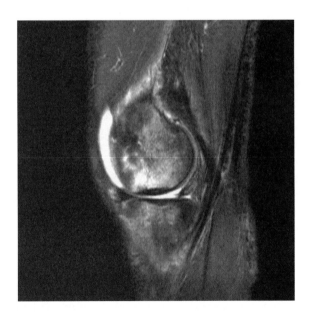

FIGURE 83.5. MRI demonstrating osteonecrosis involving medial femoral condyle.

Table 83.4

Classification of idiopathic osteonecrosis and treatment as described by Soucacos et al. (151)

Stage	Findings	Imaging Method to Establish Dx	Additional Imaging	Time Interval Since Onset of Symptoms	Progression to Further Stages	Treatment Recommended
I	Incipient	MRI/bone scan	Bone scan/MRI	1–2 mo	Likely but potentially reversible	Conservative
II	Flattening of condyle	MRI	Bone scan, plain radiography	2–4 mo	Likely but potentially reversible	Dependent on size
III	Crescent sign	Plain radiographs	—	3–6 mo	Irreversible	Surgical
IV	Collapse of subchondral bone and cartilage	Plain radiographs	—	9–12 mo	Irreversible	Surgical

placement is at the 10 or 2 o'clock position in the notch (with the knee flexed 90°) just anterior to the back wall of the femur. This is where the zone described by Hefzy et al. is the widest. Tibial tunnel placement has less effect on graft isometry, but is equally important. Hutchinson and Bae (157) determined that the PCL is the most predictable landmark for guiding the position of the ACL, and most tibial drill guides reference off it. Ramification of targeting errors are shown in Table 83.5.

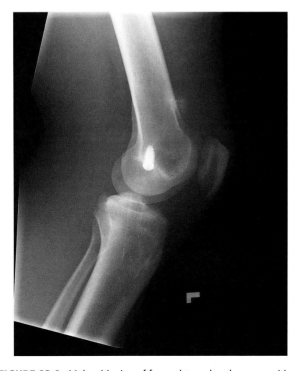

FIGURE 83.6. Malpositioning of femoral tunnel and screw position.

Graft Tension and Knee Capture

After a cadaveric study by Melby et al. (158), there has been concern that overly tensioned grafts could lead to motion loss. Other studies have shown no impact of excessive graft tension in vivo (159–162). In a systematic review, Arneja et al. (163) were unable to find support in the literature for any specific tensioning recommendations. It appears that as long as the tunnels are appropriately placed, graft tension is not likely to capture the knee. Because most grafts are slightly anisometric, however, fixing the graft at excessive flexion angle can limit extension because the graft is too tight as the knee extends. Fixation of the graft in slight flexion appears to be the safest strategy (33, 35, 154).

Cyclops Lesion

Multiple authors have described lesions of fibroproliferative scar anterolateral to the tibial tunnel (164–167). This nodule causes pain and crepitance and can block full knee extension. Histologic and electron microscopic evaluation has suggested that repeated microtrauma that damages and exposes the collagen within the graft leads to neovascularization and hyperplasia (168, 169). Avoiding anterior placement of the tibial tunnel and subsequent notch impingement is felt to be important in prevention. It has been postulated that ensuring full knee extension will help block nodule formation (170). Clinically, patients often present within the first 4 months, but delayed presentation has been reported 4 years after reconstruction (171). The lesion is often visible on MRI scanning. Treatment consisting of arthroscopic excision of the lesion and roofplasty if needed for impingement predictably returns full extension and relieves symptoms (Fig. 83.7).

Table 83.5

Effect of ACL graft malposition

Tunnel	Malposition	Consequence
Femoral	Posterior	Graft tight in extension with risk of capture and limitation of extension
Femoral	Anterior	Graft tight in flexion resulting in capture and early failure
Femoral	High	Graft high in notch has limited ability to control rotation
Tibial	Posterior	Vertical graft with limited ability to control rotation or translation
Tibial	Anterior	Impingement on notch roof limiting extension and leading to failure
Tibial	Lateral	Impingement on lateral wall of notch leading to abrasion
Tibial	Medial	Impingement on the PCL in flexion leading to graft stretch

Patella Fracture

After patellar tendon harvest, a bony defect is left in the patella that is at risk for fracture. Although intraoperative patella fracture is possible with especially deep saw cuts or aggressive use of the osteotome, it is fortunately rare. Retrospective studies have reported a postoperative fracture incidence between 0.1% and 2.3% (146, 172–175). Fractures tend to be transverse in nature and are typically caused by muscle loading although traumatic stellate fractures are described (Fig. 83.8) (176, 177). Patients present at an average of 8 weeks after surgery. The surgeon should minimize stress risers in the anterior patellar cortex, particularly with the superior transverse cut (178). The use of a 7-mm rather than a 9-mm saw may be beneficial. Bone blocks should not be larger than necessary and should be less than two-third of the patellar length (172). It has been shown that filling of the defect returns patellar strength to normal and so authors have suggested bone grafting of the patellar defect to encourage healing (177, 179–181). If a displaced patellar fracture develops, surgical intervention is warranted to allow continued knee rehabilitation. Good outcomes can be expected despite this significant complication (174).

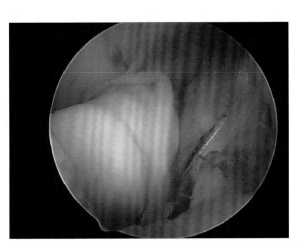

FIGURE 83.7. Arthroscopic view of cyclops lesion anterior to ACL graft.

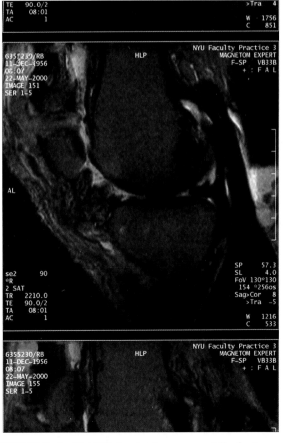

FIGURE 83.8. Sagittal MRI showing transverse patellar fracture.

Intraoperative Issues

Anterior cruciate ligament reconstruction is a technically demanding procedure that requires successful completion of many steps for optimal outcome. There are a number of common intraoperative pitfalls that are worth reviewing.

Bone–Tendon–Bone

Posterior wall blowout: The goal of femoral tunnel positioning is to have a millimeter or two of bone posterior to the tunnel. This rim of bone allows for interference screw fixation in the femoral tunnel. If the tunnel blowout occurs during screw placement, it is best to remove the screw and assess the tunnel. If it is just the tunnel entrance that is fractured, then the wire can be replaced and the tunnel drilled a few millimeters deeper to allow adequate fixation (181). If the fracture is more extensive, the technique can be adjusted to use a suture button or cross-pin construct.

Insufficient or fractured bone plugs: The bone plug can occasionally be harvested too small, or fracture can occur during graft preparation. If the plug is too injured to use, a locked suture can be placed into the tendon and soft tissue fixation at the tibial joint aperture may be used. Alternatively, a post or staple can be used at the tibial tunnel entrance. The intact bone plug is best used in the femur. If the bone plug is intact but much smaller than the tunnel, bone graft wafers can be placed in the tibial tunnel to improve the press fit (182).

Graft tunnel mismatch: Graft-tunnel mismatch is most problematic when the tibial tunnel is too short causing the graft to hang out of the tunnel entrance, compromising interference fixation. This complication is best prevented through careful attention to tunnel length when drilling the guide pin. Briefly, the surgeon should assume that the entirety of the femoral bone plug will be in the tunnel. Total length of the tibial bone plug and graft tendon dictates tibial tunnel length. We assume that there is, on average, 3 cm of intra-articular tendon. The plug/tendon length minus 3 cm therefore is the needed tibial tunnel length. Using the graduated bullet on the tibial drill guide, the surgeon should ensure adequate tunnel length prior to drilling the guide pin (180).

If it is determined that the tunnel is too short after it is already drilled, one option is reversing the tibial bone plug on the graft to shorten overall graft length (Barber 2000). One might cut a trough in the anterior tibia for the plug to lie in and then fixing with a screw or staple. Finally, one could remove the graft and cut the tibial bone plug off. After whipping a suture through the graft, the graft can be reinserted and the tibial side fixed with a soft tissue interference screw, a tibial post, or a staple. Finally, if the mismatch is not too severe, one could remove the graft and drill a deeper femoral hole in order to sink the graft deeper in the femur.

Other: When there is difficulty in starting the femoral interference screw, we have seen instances of the screw shearing the graft off the femoral bone plug. This complication is best prevented by ensuring an adequate starting hole for the femoral screw, using a sheath during screw insertion and ensuring that the screw is being driven colinear with the hole. If the graft shears off, the graft can usually be removed and flipped. A suture can be woven through the graft and soft tissue fixation used in the tibia. It is also possible to convert to a two-incision technique and use soft tissue fixation on the femoral side (183).

Hamstring: The most common difficulty specific to hamstring ACL reconstruction is insufficient graft. Amputation with the tendon stripper can lead to one limb being too short. Often the amputation occurs proximal enough that there is still sufficient graft to use near aperture interference fixation on the tibial side. Otherwise, unfortunately, the surgeon is left with the options of using a three-stranded graft or adding allograft to bring the graft backup to size.

Posterior wall blowout on the femur is less of an issue with hamstring than patellar tendon grafts. Suspensory fixation such as a suture button or cross-pin can be used easily and should be on hand as a bailout. These forms of fixation do not rely on an intact posterior wall.

Tibial fixation with hamstring grafts can be poor, particularly in women. It has been shown that backup fixation with a staple on the anterior cortex provides better KT scores than interference screw alone in women (184). A push in suture anchor can be used on the anterior tibia as well.

LATERAL RELEASE

Arthroscopic lateral release (LR) is a procedure for which numerous complications have been reported. The indications for an isolated LR have evolved over the past 20 years. Some of the complications are due to an error in patient selection. In a review of 446 lateral retinacular releases performed by 21 surgeons at different centers, Small (185) found the overall complication of the isolated procedure to be 7.2%. A higher complication rate was noted with tourniquet use and with the use of a postoperative suction drain for 24 hours or longer (185).

Hemarthrosis is the most commonly cited complication after lateral retinacular release. Although a hemarthrosis is usually not associated with a poor long-term outcome, it can lead to significant disability in the short term. Loss of motion, arthrofibrosis, and even patellar entrapment syndrome or CRPS can result from a significant postoperative hemarthrosis. The incidence of hemarthrosis after arthroscopic LR ranges from 15% to 42% (186, 187). Careful attention to hemostasis, particularly attempting to avoid the lateral superior geniculate vessels is crucial (Fig. 83.9).

Incomplete LR or postoperative scarring can result in persistence of symptoms or even exacerbation of preoperative symptoms. A typical clinical scenario after an incomplete release is a patient who only has several months of

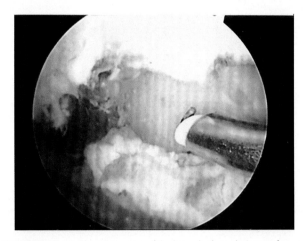

FIGURE 83.9. Arthroscopic view of the lateral release being performed.

pain improvement. It is important both before and after the LR to arthroscopically confirm that the patella centralizes in the trochlea at 30° of flexion. Failure to release the patella-tibial ligament produces a significant decrease in the ability to translate the patella medially when compared with a complete release down to the tibial tubercle (188). Careful physical examination with pain localized at the inferior aspect of the ligament is necessary to make this diagnosis.

Multiple studies have shown that performing a LR for patellar instability is unsuccessful (189). LR has led to recurrent patellar dislocations (190) and significant drops in patient satisfaction after 4 years when performed for patellar instability (191). A recent systematic review showed that lateral retinacular release results in significantly inferior long-term results with respect to symptoms of recurrent patellar instability when compared with LR with medial plication (192).

Medial patellar subluxation or instability is another reported complication of LR (193). This can result if a LR is performed without a malalignment of the extremity or if an overly aggressive release extends into and detaches the vastus lateralis obliquus (191). Medial patellar subluxation can result from a lateral retinacular release, particularly if a subtle medial patellar subluxation or gross patellar hypermobility was missed preoperatively. In a group of 40 patients with persistent symptoms after a LR, Shellock et al. (194) found that 63% of the patients had medial subluxation of the patella on the operative side. Treatment of iatrogenic medial patellar instability includes bracing and eventual repair or reconstruction of the lateral retinacular restraints.

Overrelease into the vastus lateralis may also lead to permanent quadriceps insufficiency. A patient presents with vague anterior knee pain, episodes of the knee giving way, and persistent weakness.

MENISCECTOMY AND MENISCAL REPAIR

Other than neurologic and vascular complications associated with arthroscopic meniscectomy and meniscal repair (see Neurologic Complications and Vascular

Complications), other potential complications related to patient positioning and implant devices are worthy of attention.

Prolonged surgery in any one position may increase the risks of neuropathy (195). Warner et al. (196) reported that the most common perioperative neuropathies to be common peroneal (81%), sciatic (15%), and femoral (4%). The use of leg holders to maintain the position of the unoperated leg may also place these nerves at risk (197). Peroneal nerve injury can be caused by direct compression as it wraps around the fibular neck or a traction injury secondary to prolonged varus stress. Although rare, there have been case reports of common peroneal nerve palsies due to traction injuries related to patient positioning during arthroscopic lateral meniscectomy (76). Extreme hyperextension of the hip places the femoral nerve at risk of a stretch injury, a concern when placing the nonoperated leg in a holder (81).

Certain risks are associated with the use of a circumferential leg holder. When the holder is overtightened, a venous tourniquet is created (198). The most common complication associated with manipulating a leg secured in a holder is rupture of the medial collateral ligament (199). Even greater valgus stress has rarely been associated with femur fracture (199). Injury to the lateral femoral cutaneous nerve has also been reported with inappropriate placement of the circumferential leg holder (74).

Patient-specific factors such as very thin body habitus and smoking in the perioperative period are associated with a higher risk of development of these neuropaties (196). Attention must be paid to padding bony prominences and avoiding lengthy operative times, particularly when the lower extremities are in a precarious position.

All-inside meniscus repair was introduced in 1991 in an attempt to eliminate extra incisions, as well as to decrease technical difficulty, surgical time, and risk to neurovascular structures (200). An intact rim of meniscus is required to anchor the device for all generations of repair devices. Therefore, the all-inside repair device is not indicated for meniscocapsular separations (96). Anterior horn meniscus tears are also a relative contraindication and are preferentially repaired with an alternate technique (96). The third generation of all-inside meniscal repairs attempted to produce a more rigid, simpler device to improve compression and resulted in the creation of arrows, screws, tacks, darts, and staples. The most popular of these devices was the Meniscal Arrow (Linvatec, Largo, FL) because of its ease of insertion and early success rates. However, as longer-term data became available, failure rates of up to 42% have been reported (201, 202). These devices were made of poly-l-lactic acid (PLLA), and it is thought that symptoms return at 2 to 3 years when the device dissolves. Numerous complications became apparent, including transient synovitis, device failure, device migration, cyst formation, and chondral damage (73, 203–207). If the rigid third-generation devices are placed too proud, loosen, or migrate prior to dissolving, significant chondral damage can occur, usually by abrasion of the adjacent femoral condyle (202). With the development of fourth-generation repair devices, the flexibility and lower profile minimize some of the complications seen with the earlier designs (208). However, concerns about the defect created in the meniscus by the suture anchor, and how it effects healing remain.

ARTHROSCOPIC CARTILAGE RESTORATION PROCEDURES

Autologous Osteochondral Grafting

More complications are seen with autologous osteochondral grafting when implanting larger plugs and a greater number of plugs (209). Increasing the number of osteochondral plugs results in more area in between plugs in which fibrocartilage must grow. Increasing the number and the size of the plugs results in greater donor site morbidity, as well and greater difficulty matching the contour of the defect. The ideal defect size to treat with autologous osteochondral grafting is 1 to 4 cm^2.

Concerns regarding donor site morbidity are legitimized by studies demonstrating continued pain and/or crepitation in the knee after graft is harvested (210). There is no current evidence showing that graft harvest results in further degenerative changes; however, a biomechanical study performed by Simonian et al. (211) demonstrated that there is relatively high loading forces in the donor site area. Another potential complication is bleeding from donor sites, leading to painful postoperative hemarthroses (212).

The recreation of joint congruity with osteochondral autologous grafting can be technically challenging. Graft harvesting and insertion should be perpendicular to the articular surface. A wrong angle will compromise the end result by creating a step off. Koh et al. (213) have found that a plug that is inserted flush normalizes the contact pressure; however, a plug left 0.5 mm proud increases the contact pressure by 40% and a plug that is countersunk increases contact pressure by approximately 10%. Articular incongruence seen at second-look arthroscopy was noted in 17% in a series by Hangody and Fules (214) and 22% in a series by Chow et al. (212) Graft loosening and graft migration are other potential complications. Delivering the graft flush with the joint surface will allow rapid graft incorporation and limit graft micromotion (215). Using a porcine model, Duchow et al. (216) have shown the stability of press-fit osteochondral autografts to be better with 10-mm long grafts rather than with 15-mm long grafts and 8 mm diameter versus 11 mm diameter.

Finally, osteointegration of the osteochondral plug is also a concern. Reports of disintegration and cystic changes of the plugs exist, as it is resorbed. It is not yet known how to prevent this subchondral resorption of the graft (Fig. 83.10).

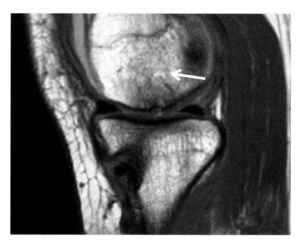

FIGURE 83.10. Sagittal MRI demonstrating cystic changes in femoral osteochondral autografts.

Microfracture

On the basis of animal studies, complete removal of the calcified cartilage layer at the base of a chondral defect is crucial for optimization of microfracture results (217). However, in order to preserve the subchondral plate, care must be taken not to debride too deeply, as this is what holds the marrow clot in place. Another potential way to damage the subchondral plate is with coalescence of the microfracture holes. The holes should be made as close together as possible, but not so close that they break into one another and damage the subchondral plate between them.

Some patients have transient pain after microfracture in the postoperative period, particularly after microfracture in the patellofemoral joint. Often, when a patient begins full range of motion and weight bearing, they can experience an unsettling sensation underneath their patella, which usually resolves spontaneously within weeks. Recurrent effusions can also occur, particularly after the patient starts to bear weight after having had microfracture performed on a femoral condyle. The effusion normally occurs 6 to 8 weeks postoperatively and resolves within several weeks. A second arthroscopy is rarely necessary for this type of effusion.

SUMMARY

Although arthroscopy of the knee is a relatively low-risk surgical procedure, complications do occur. General complications of arthroscopy include neurologic problems related to patient positioning or tourniquet use as well as compartment syndrome related to infusion pumps. As in any other surgical procedure of the knee, postoperative complications include infection, venous thrombosis, and arthrofibrosis. Technical complications related to specific arthroscopic procedures also exist, and as the complexity of the arthroscopic procedure rises, so does the incidence and complexity of the complications. Arthroscopic anterior cruciate and posterior cruciate ligament reconstructions can be associated with a myriad of complications related to tunnel placement, graft harvesting, graft tensioning, and neurovascular injury. Cartilage restorative procedures performed arthroscopically can also be technically demanding and can result in harmful complications. Although complications occur even in the hands of the most experienced arthroscopic surgeons, a certain level of arthroscopic expertise should be reached before attempting certain procedures arthroscopically. Even low complexity arthroscopic procedures of the knee can result in devastating complications, regardless of technical expertise. CRPS, arthrofibrosis, and secondary osteonecrosis occur at times without a specific cause. Although they occur relatively infrequently, complications of knee arthroscopy do occur, and it is important to recognize how to avoid these complications and how to manage them when they arise.

REFERENCES

1. DeLee JC. Complications of arthroscopy and arthroscopic surgery: results of a national survey. Committee on Complications of Arthroscopy Association of North America. *Arthroscopy.* 1985;1(4):214–220.
2. Sherman OH, Fox JM, Snyder SJ, et al. Arthroscopy—"no-problem surgery." An analysis of complications in two thousand six hundred and forty cases. *J Bone Joint Surg Am.* 1986;68(2):256–265.
3. Small NC. Complications in arthroscopic surgery performed by experienced arthroscopists. *Arthroscopy.* 1988;4(3):215–221.
4. Reigstad O, Grimsgaard C. Complications in knee arthroscopy. *Knee Surg Sports Traumatol Arthrosc.* 2006;14(5):473–477.
5. Schollin-Borg M, Michaelsson K, Rahme H. Presentation, outcome, and cause of septic arthritis after anterior cruciate ligament reconstruction: a case control study. *Arthroscopy.* 2003;19(9):941–947.
6. Zalavras CG, Patzakis MJ. Infections in anterior cruciate ligament surgery. In: Prodromos CC, ed. *The Anterior Cruciate Ligament: Reconstruction and Basic Science.* Philadelphia, PA: Saunders Elsevier; 2008:551–560.
7. Binnet MS, Basarir K. Risk and outcome of infection after different arthroscopic anterior cruciate ligament reconstruction techniques. *Arthroscopy.* 2007;23(8):862–868.
8. Judd D, Bottoni C, Kim D, et al. Infections following arthroscopic anterior cruciate ligament reconstruction. *Arthroscopy.* 2006;22(4):375–384.
9. Smith RL, Schurman DJ, Kajiyama G, et al. The effect of antibiotics on the destruction of cartilage in experimental infectious arthritis. *J Bone Joint Surg Am.* 1987;69(7):1063–1068.
10. Van Tongel A, Stuyck J, Bellemans J, et al. Septic arthritis after arthroscopic anterior cruciate ligament reconstruction: a retrospective analysis of incidence, management and outcome. *Am J Sports Med.* 2007;35(7):1059–1063.
11. Wind WM, McGrath BE, Mindell ER. Infection following knee arthroscopy. *Arthroscopy.* 2001;17(8):878–883.
12. Mouzopoulos G, Fotopoulos VC, Tzurbakis M. Septic knee arthritis following ACL reconstruction: a systematic review. *Knee Surg Sports Traumatol Arthrosc.* 2009;17(9):1033–1042.
13. Burks RT, Friederichs MG, Fink B, et al. Treatment of postoperative anterior cruciate ligament infections with graft removal and early reimplantation. *Am J Sports Med.* 2003;31(3):414–418.
14. Margaretten ME, Kohlwes J, Moore D, et al. Does this adult patient have septic arthritis? *JAMA.* 2007;297(13):1478–1488.
15. Centers for Disease Control and Prevention. Septic arthritis following anterior cruciate ligament reconstruction using tendon allografts—Florida and Louisiana, 2000. *MMWR Morb Mortal Wkly Rep.* 2001;50(48):1081–1083.
16. McAllister DR, Parker RD, Cooper AE, et al. Outcomes of postoperative septic arthritis after anterior cruciate ligament reconstruction. *Am J Sports Med.* 1999;27(5):562–570.
17. Matava MJ, Evans TA, Wright RW, et al. Septic arthritis of the knee following anterior cruciate ligament reconstruction: results of a survey of sports medicine fellowship directors. *Arthroscopy.* 1998;14(7):717–725.
18. Wang C, Ao Y, Wang J, et al. Septic arthritis after arthroscopic anterior cruciate ligament reconstruction: a retrospective analysis of incidence, presentation, treatment, and cause. *Arthroscopy.* 2009;25(3):243–249.
19. Gavriilidis I, Pakos EE, Wipfler B, et al. Intra-operative hamstring tendon graft contamination in anterior cruciate ligament reconstruction. *Knee Surg Sports Traumatol Arthrosc.* 2009;17(9):1043–1047.
20. Hantes ME, Dimitroulias AP. Anterior knee problems after anterior cruciate ligament reconstruction. In: Prodromos CC, ed. *The Anterior Cruciate Ligament: Reconstruction and Basic Science.* Philadelphia, PA: Saunder Elsevier; 2008:607–614.
21. Izquierdo R Jr, Cadet ER, Bauer R, et al. A survey of sports medicine specialists investigating the preferred management of contaminated anterior cruciate ligament grafts. *Arthroscopy.* 2005;21(11):1348–1353.
22. Goebel ME, Drez D Jr, Heck SB, et al. Contaminated rabbit patellar tendon grafts. In vivo analysis of disinfecting methods. *Am J Sports Med.* 1994;22(3):387–391.
23. Molina ME, Nonweiller DE, Evans JA, et al. Contaminated anterior cruciate ligament grafts: the efficacy of 3 sterilization agents. *Arthroscopy.* 2000;16(4):373–378.
24. Pasque CB, Geib TM. Intraoperative anterior cruciate ligament graft contamination. *Arthroscopy.* 2007;23(3):329–331.
25. Cooper DE, Arnoczky SP, Warren RF. Contaminated patellar tendon grafts: incidence of positive cultures and efficacy of an antibiotic solution soak—an in vitro study. *Arthroscopy.* 1991;7(3):272–274.
26. Paulos LE, Rosenberg TD, Drawbert J, et al. Infrapatellar contracture syndrome. An unrecognized cause of knee stiffness with patella entrapment and patella infera. *Am J Sports Med.* 1987;15(4):331–341.
27. Paulos LE, Wnorowski DC, Greenwald AE. Infrapatellar contracture syndrome. Diagnosis, treatment, and long-term followup. *Am J Sports Med.* 1994;22(4):440–449.
28. Steadman JR, Dragoo JL, Hines SL, et al. Arthroscopic release for symptomatic scarring of the anterior interval of the knee. *Am J Sports Med.* 2008;36(9):1763–1769.
29. Skutek M, Elsner HA, Slateva K, et al. Screening for arthrofibrosis after anterior cruciate ligament reconstruction: analysis of association with human leukocyte antigen. *Arthroscopy.* 2004;20(5):469–473.
30. Murakami S, Muneta T, Ezura Y, et al. Quantitative analysis of synovial fibrosis in the infrapatellar fat pad before and after anterior cruciate ligament reconstruction. *Am J Sports Med.* 1997;25(1):29–34.

31. Ushiyama T, Chano T, Inoue K, et al. Cytokine production in the infrapatellar fat pad: another source of cytokines in knee synovial fluids. *Ann Rheum Dis.* 2003;62(2):108–112.

32. Wahl SM. Transforming growth factor beta: the good, the bad, and the ugly. *J Exp Med.* 1994;180(5):1587–1590.

33. Karistinos A, Paulos LE. Stiffness: prevention and treatment. In: Prodromos CC, ed. *The Anterior Cruciate Ligament: Reconstruction and Basic Science.* Philadelphia, PA: Saunders Elsevier; 2008:565–571.

34. Robins AJ, Newman AP, Burks RT. Postoperative return of motion in anterior cruciate ligament and medial collateral ligament injuries. The effect of medial collateral ligament rupture location. *Am J Sports Med.* 1993;21(1):20–25.

35. Millett PJ, Wickiewicz TL, Warren RF. Motion loss after ligament injuries to the knee. Part II: prevention and treatment. *Am J Sports Med.* 2001;29(6):822–828.

36. Meighan AA, Keating JF, Will E. Outcome after reconstruction of the anterior cruciate ligament in athletic patients. A comparison of early versus delayed surgery. *J Bone Joint Surg Br.* 2003;85(4):521–524.

37. Shelbourne KD, Wilckens JH, Mollabashy A, et al. Arthrofibrosis in acute anterior cruciate ligament reconstruction. The effect of timing of reconstruction and rehabilitation. *Am J Sports Med.* 1991;19(4):332–336.

38. Strum GM, Friedman MJ, Fox JM, et al. Acute anterior cruciate ligament reconstruction. Analysis of complications. *Clin Orthop Relat Res.* 1990;(253):184–189.

39. DeHaven KE, Cosagarea AJ, Sebastianelli WJ. Arthrofibrosis of the knee following ligament surgery. In: Ferlic DC, ed. *Instructional Course Lectures.* Vol 52. Rosemont, IL: American Academy of Orthopaedic Surgeons; 2003:369–381.

40. Dodds JA, Keene JS, Graf BK, et al. Results of knee manipulations after anterior cruciate ligament reconstructions. *Am J Sports Med.* 1991;19(3):283–287.

41. Noyes FR, Wojtys EM, Marshall MT. The early diagnosis and treatment of developmental patella infera syndrome. *Clin Orthop Relat Res.* 1991;(265):241–252.

42. Millett PJ, Williams RJ 3rd, Wickiewicz TL. Open debridement and soft tissue release as a salvage procedure for the severely arthrofibrotic knee. *Am J Sports Med.* 1999;27(5):552–561.

43. Dahl OE, Gudmundsen TE, Haukeland L. Late occurring clinical deep vein thrombosis in joint-operated patients. *Acta Orthop Scand.* 2000;71(1):47–50.

44. Marlovits S, Striessnig G, Schuster R, et al. Extended-duration thromboprophylaxis with enoxaparin after arthroscopic surgery of the anterior cruciate ligament: a prospective, randomized, placebo-controlled study. *Arthroscopy.* 2007;23(7):696–702.

45. Bushnell BD, Anz AW, Bert JM. Venous thromboembolism in lower extremity arthroscopy. *Arthroscopy.* 2008;24(5):604–611.

46. Eynon AM, James S, Leach P. Thromboembolic events after arthroscopic knee surgery. *Arthroscopy.* 2004;20(suppl 2):23–24.

47. Janssen RP, Sala HA. Fatal pulmonary embolism after anterior cruciate ligament reconstruction. *Am J Sports Med.* 2007;35(6):1000–1002.

48. Navarro-Sanz A, Fernandez-Ortega JF. Fatal pulmonary embolism after knee arthroscopy. *Am J Sports Med.* 2004;32(2):525–528.

49. Ramos J, Perrotta C, Badariotti G, et al. Interventions for preventing venous thromboembolism in adults undergoing knee arthroscopy. *Cochrane Database Syst Rev.* 2008;(4):CD005259.

50. Delis KT, Hunt N, Strachan RK, et al. Incidence, natural history and risk factors of deep vein thrombosis in elective knee arthroscopy. *Thromb Haemost.* 2001;86(3):817–821.

51. Demers C, Marcoux S, Ginsberg JS, et al. Incidence of venographically proved deep vein thrombosis after knee arthroscopy. *Arch Intern Med.* 1998;158(1):47–50.

52. Geerts WH, Bergqvist D, Pineo GF, et al. Prevention of venous thromboembolism: American College of Chest Physicians Evidence-Based Clinical Practice Guidelines (8th Edition). *Chest.* 2008;133(6)(suppl):381S–453S.

53. Small NC. Complications in arthroscopic surgery of the knee and shoulder. *Orthopedics.* 1993;16(9):985–988.

54. Jeffries JT, Gainor BJ, Allen WC, et al. Injury to the popliteal artery as a complication of arthroscopic surgery. A report of two cases. *J Bone Joint Surg Am.* 1987;69(5):783–785.

55. Makino A, Costa-Paz M, Aponte-Tinao L, et al. Popliteal artery laceration during arthroscopic posterior cruciate ligament reconstruction. *Arthroscopy.* 2005;21(11):1396.

56. Janssen RP, Scheltinga MR, Sala HA. Pseudoaneurysm of the popliteal artery after anterior cruciate ligament reconstruction with bicortical tibial screw fixation. *Arthroscopy.* 2004;20(1):E4–E6.

57. Kanko M, Buluc L, Yavuz S, et al. Very rare aetiology of giant popliteal pseudoaneurysm: anterior cruciate ligament surgery. *Postgrad Med J.* 2008;84(989):158–159.

58. Cosgarea AJ, Kramer DE, Bahk MS, et al. Proximity of the popliteal artery to the PCL during simulated knee arthroscopy: implications for establishing the posterior trans-septal portal. *J Knee Surg.* 2006;19(3):181–185.

59. Matava MJ, Sethi NS, Totty WG. Proximity of the posterior cruciate ligament insertion to the popliteal artery as a function of the knee flexion angle: implications for posterior cruciate ligament reconstruction. *Arthroscopy.* 2000;16(8):796–804.

60. Bernard M, Grothues-Spork M, Georgoulis A, et al. Neural and vascular complications of arthroscopic meniscal surgery. *Knee Surg Sports Traumatol Arthrosc.* 1994;2(1):14–18.

61. Gouny P, Bertrand P, Duedal V, et al. Limb salvage and popliteal aneurysms: advantages of preventive surgery. *Eur J Vasc Endovasc Surg.* 2000;19(5):496–500.

62. Kramer DE, Bahk MS, Cascio BM, et al. Posterior knee arthroscopy: anatomy, technique, application. *J Bone Joint Surg Am.* 2006;88(suppl 4):110–121.

63. Potter D, Morris-Jones W. Popliteal artery injury complicating arthroscopic meniscectomy. *Arthroscopy.* 1995;11(6):723–726.

64. Post WR, King SS. Neurovascular risk of bicortical tibial drilling for screw and spiked washer fixation of soft-tissue anterior cruciate ligament graft. *Arthroscopy.* 2001;17(3):244–247.

65. Kale AA, Vangsness CT Jr. Technical pitfalls of meniscal surgery. *Clin Sports Med.* 1999;18(4):883–896.

66. Miller MD, Kline AJ, Gonzales J, et al. Pitfalls associated with FasT-Fix meniscal repair. *Arthroscopy.* 2002;18(8):939–943.

67. Cohen SB, Boyd L, Miller MD. Vascular risk associated with meniscal repair using Rapidloc versus FasT-Fix: comparison of two all-inside meniscal devices. *J Knee Surg.* 2007;20(3):235–240.

68. Evans JD, de Boer MT, Mayor P, et al. Pseudoaneurysm of the medial inferior genicular artery following anterior cruciate ligament reconstruction. *Ann R Coll Surg Engl.* 2000;82(3):182–184.

69. Milankov M, Miljkovic N, Stankovic M. Pseudoaneurysm of the medial inferior genicular artery following anterior cruciate ligament reconstruction with hamstring tendon autograft. *Knee.* 2006;13(2):170–171.

70. Carlin RE, Papenhausen M, Farber MA, et al. Sural artery pseudoaneurysms after knee arthroscopy: treatment with transcatheter embolization. *J Vasc Surg.* 2001;33(1):170–173.

71. Puig J, Perendreu J, Fortuno JR, et al. Transarterial embolization of an inferior genicular artery pseudoaneurysm with arteriovenous fistula after arthroscopy. *Korean J Radiol.* 2007;8(2):173–175.

72. Tozzi A, Ferri E, Serrao E, et al. Pseudoaneurysm of the descending genicular artery after arthroscopic meniscectomy: report of a case. *J Trauma.* 1996;41(2):340–341.

73. Hechtman KS, Uribe JW. Cystic hematoma formation following use of a biodegradable arrow for meniscal repair. *Arthroscopy.* 1999;15(2):207–210.

74. Kim TK, Savino RM, McFarland EG, et al. Neurovascular complications of knee arthroscopy. *Am J Sports Med.* 2002;30(4):619–629.

75. Small NC. Complications in arthroscopy: the knee and other joints. Committee on Complications of the Arthroscopy Association of North America. *Arthroscopy.* 1986;2(4):253–258.

76. Johnson DS, Sharma DP, Bangash IH. Common peroneal nerve palsy following knee arthroscopy. *Arthroscopy.* 1999;15(7):773–774.

77. Rodeo SA, Forster RA, Weiland AJ. Neurological complications due to arthroscopy. *J Bone Joint Surg Am.* 1993;75(6):917–926.

78. Deutsch A, Wyzykowski RJ, Victoroff BN. Evaluation of the anatomy of the common peroneal nerve. Defining nerve-at-risk in arthroscopically assisted lateral meniscus repair. *Am J Sports Med.* 1999;27(1):10–15.

79. Jurist KA, Greene PW 3rd, Shirkhoda A. Peroneal nerve dysfunction as a complication of lateral meniscus repair: a case report and anatomic dissection. *Arthroscopy.* 1989;5(2):141–147.

80. Krivic A, Stanec S, Zic R, et al. Lesion of the common peroneal nerve during arthroscopy. *Arthroscopy.* 2003;19(9):1015–1018.

81. Miller DB Jr. Arthroscopic meniscus repair. *Am J Sports Med.* 1988;16(4):315–320.

82. Greis PE, Holmstrom MC, Bardana DD, et al. Meniscal injury: II. Management. *J Am Acad Orthop Surg.* 2002;10(3):177–187.

83. Anderson AW, LaPrade RF. Common peroneal nerve neuropraxia after arthroscopic inside-out lateral meniscus repair. *J Knee Surg.* 2009;22(1):27–29.

84. Hall MP, Ryzewicz M, Walsh PJ, et al. Risk of iatrogenic injury to the peroneal nerve during posterolateral femoral tunnel placement in double-bundle anterior cruciate ligament reconstruction. *Am J Sports Med.* 2009;37(1):109–113.

85. Nakamura M, Deie M, Shibuya H, et al. Potential risks of femoral tunnel drilling through the far anteromedial portal: a cadaveric study. *Arthroscopy.* 2009;25(5):481–487.

86. Tifford CD, Spero L, Luke T, et al. The relationship of the infrapatellar branches of the saphenous nerve to arthroscopy portals and incisions for anterior cruciate ligament surgery. An anatomic study. *Am J Sports Med.* 2000;28(4):562–567.

87. Mochida H, Kikuchi S. Injury to infrapatellar branch of saphenous nerve in arthroscopic knee surgery. *Clin Orthop Relat Res.* 1995;(320):88–94.

88. Kartus J, Ejerhed L, Eriksson BI, et al. The localization of the infrapatellar nerves in the anterior knee region with special emphasis on central third patellar tendon harvest: a dissection study on cadaver and amputated specimens. *Arthroscopy.* 1999;15(6):577–586.

89. Mishra AK, Fanton GS, Dillingham MF, et al. Patellar tendon graft harvesting using horizontal incisions for anterior cruciate ligament reconstruction. *Arthroscopy.* 1995;11(6):749–752.

90. Jameson S, Emmerson K. Altered sensation over the lower leg following hamstring graft anterior cruciate ligament reconstruction with transverse femoral fixation. *Knee.* 2007;14(4):314–320.

91. Luo H, Yu JK, Ao YF, et al. Relationship between different skin incisions and the injury of the infrapatellar branch of the saphenous nerve during anterior cruciate ligament reconstruction. *Chin Med J (Engl).* 2007;120(13):1127–1130.

92. Bertram C, Porsch M, Hackenbroch MH, et al. Saphenous neuralgia after arthroscopically assisted anterior cruciate ligament reconstruction with a semitendinosus and gracilis tendon graft. *Arthroscopy.* 2000;16(7):763–766.

93. Dunaway DJ, Steensen RN, Wiand W, et al. The sartorial branch of the saphenous nerve: its anatomy at the joint line of the knee. *Arthroscopy.* 2005;21(5):547–551.

94. Kelly M, Macnicol MF. Identification of the saphenous nerve at arthroscopy. *Arthroscopy.* 2003;19(5):E46.

95. Barber FA, McGarry JE. Meniscal repair techniques. *Sports Med Arthrosc.* 2007;15(4):199–207.

96. Turman KA, Diduch DR. Meniscal repair: indications and techniques. *J Knee Surg.* 2008;21(2):154–162.

97. Albrecht-Olsen P, Kristensen G, Burgaard P, et al. The arrow versus horizontal suture in arthroscopic meniscus repair. A prospective randomized study with arthroscopic evaluation. *Knee Surg Sports Traumatol Arthrosc.* 1999;7(5):268–273.

98. Barber FA, Schroeder FA, Oro FB, et al. FasT-Fix meniscal repair: mid-term results. *Arthroscopy.* 2008;24(12):1342–1348.

99. Haas AL, Schepsis AA, Hornstein J, et al. Meniscal repair using the FasT-Fix all-inside meniscal repair device. *Arthroscopy.* 2005;21(2):167–175.

100. Hurel C, Mertens F, Verdonk R. Biofix resorbable meniscus arrow for meniscal ruptures: results of a 1-year follow-up. *Knee Surg Sports Traumatol Arthrosc.* 2000;8(1):46–52.

101. Steenbrugge F, Verdonk R, Hurel C, et al. Arthroscopic meniscus repair: inside-out technique vs. Biofix meniscus arrow. *Knee Surg Sports Traumatol Arthrosc.* 2004;12(1):43–49.

102. Amendola A, Faber K, Willits K, et al. Compartment pressure monitoring during anterior cruciate ligament reconstruction. *Arthroscopy.* 1999;15(6):607–612.

103. Jerosch J, Castro WH, Geske B. Intracompartmental pressure in the lower extremity after arthroscopic surgery. *Acta Orthop Belg.* 1991;57(2):97–101.

104. DiStefano VJ, Kalman VR, O'Malley JS. Femoral nerve palsy after arthroscopic surgery with an infusion pump irrigation system. A report of three cases. *Am J Orthop.* 1996;25(2):145–148.

105. Bomberg BC, Hurley PE, Clark CA, et al. Complications associated with the use of an infusion pump during knee arthroscopy. *Arthroscopy.* 1992;8(2):224–228.

106. Romero J, Smit CM, Zanetti M. Massive intraperitoneal and extraperitoneal accumulation of irrigation fluid as a complication during knee arthroscopy. *Arthroscopy.* 1998;14(4):401–404.

107. Noyes FR, Spievack ES. Extraarticular fluid dissection in tissues during arthroscopy. A report of clinical cases and a study of intraarticular and thigh pressures in cadavers. *Am J Sports Med.* 1982;10(6):346–351.

108. Belanger M, Fadale P. Compartment syndrome of the leg after arthroscopic examination of a tibial plateau fracture. Case report and review of the literature. *Arthroscopy.* 1997;13(5):646–651.

109. Marti CB, Jakob RP. Accumulation of irrigation fluid in the calf as a complication during high tibial osteotomy combined with simultaneous arthroscopic anterior cruciate ligament reconstruction. *Arthroscopy.* 1999;15(8):864–866.

110. Ekman EF, Poehling GG. An experimental assessment of the risk of compartment syndrome during knee arthroscopy. *Arthroscopy.* 1996;12(2):193–199.

111. Peek RD, Haynes DW. Compartment syndrome as a complication of arthroscopy. A case report and a study of interstitial pressures. *Am J Sports Med.* 1984;12(6):464–468.

112. Benzon HT, Toleikis JR, Meagher LL, et al. Changes in venous blood lactate, venous blood gases, and somatosensory evoked potentials after tourniquet application. *Anesthesiology.* 1988;69(5):677–682.

113. Fowler TJ, Danta G, Gilliatt RW. Recovery of nerve conduction after a pneumatic tourniquet: observations on the hind-limb of the baboon. *J Neurol Neurosurg Psychiatry.* 1972;35(5):638–647.

114. Jacobson MD, Pedowitz RA, Oyama BK, et al. Muscle functional deficits after tourniquet ischemia. *Am J Sports Med.* 1994;22(3):372–377.

115. Kornbluth ID, Freedman MK, Sher L, et al. Femoral, saphenous nerve palsy after tourniquet use: a case report. *Arch Phys Med Rehabil.* 2003;84(6):909–911.

116. Hirvensalo E, Tuominen H, Lapinsuo M, et al. Compartment syndrome of the lower limb caused by a tourniquet: a report of two cases. *J Orthop Trauma.* 1992;6(4):469–472.

117. Luk KD, Pun WK. Unrecognised compartment syndrome in a patient with tourniquet palsy. *J Bone Joint Surg Br.* 1987;69(1):97–99.

118. Schutzer SF, Gossling HR. The treatment of reflex sympathetic dystrophy syndrome. *J Bone Joint Surg Am.* 1984;66(4):625–629.

119. Justins D. Reflex sympathetic dystrophy. Has been renamed complex regional pain syndrome. *BMJ.* 1995;311(7008):812.

120. Hogan CJ, Hurwitz SR. Treatment of complex regional pain syndrome of the lower extremity. *J Am Acad Orthop Surg.* 2002;10(4):281–289.

121. Miller RL. Reflex sympathetic dystrophy. *Orthop Nurs.* 2003;22(2):91–99; quiz 100–101.

122. Bach BR Jr, Wojtys EM, Lindenfeld TN. Reflex sympathetic dystrophy, patella infera contracture syndrome, and loss of motion following anterior cruciate ligament surgery. *Instr Course Lect.* 1997;46:251–260.

123. Lindenfeld TN, Bach BR Jr, Wojtys EM. Reflex sympathetic dystrophy and pain dysfunction in the lower extremity. *Instr Course Lect.* 1997;46:261–268.

124. Dowd GS, Hussein R, Khanduja V, et al. Complex regional pain syndrome with special emphasis on the knee. *J Bone Joint Surg Br.* 2007;89(3):285–290.

125. Cooper C. A review of the autonomic nervous system and exploration of diagnoses associated with reflex sympathetic dystrophy. *J Hand Ther.* 1994;7(4):245–250.

126. Cooper DE, DeLee JC. Reflex sympathetic dystrophy of the knee. *J Am Acad Orthop Surg.* 1994;2(2):79–86.

127. Poehling GG, Pollock FE Jr, Koman LA. Reflex sympathetic dystrophy of the knee after sensory nerve injury. *Arthroscopy.* 1988;4(1):31–35.

128. O'Brien SJ, Ngeow J, Gibney MA, et al. Reflex sympathetic dystrophy of the knee. Causes, diagnosis, and treatment. *Am J Sports Med.* 1995;23(6):655–659.

129. Katz MM, Hungerford DS. Reflex sympathetic dystrophy affecting the knee. *J Bone Joint Surg Br.* 1987;69(5):797–803.

130. Wilder RT, Berde CB, Wolohan M, et al. Reflex sympathetic dystrophy in children. Clinical characteristics and follow-up of seventy patients. *J Bone Joint Surg Am.* 1992;74(6):910–919.

131. Tietjen R. Reflex sympathetic dystrophy of the knee. *Clin Orthop Relat Res.* 1986;(209):234–243.

132. Atkins RM. Complex regional pain syndrome. *J Bone Joint Surg Br.* 2003;85(8):1100–1106.

133. Poplawski ZJ, Wiley AM, Murray JF. Post-traumatic dystrophy of the extremities. *J Bone Joint Surg Am.* 1983;65(5):642–655.

134. Ghai B, Dureja GP. Complex regional pain syndrome: a review. *J Postgrad Med.* 2004;50(4):300–307.

135. Hamamci N, Dursun E, Ural C, et al. Calcitonin treatment in reflex sympathetic dystrophy: a preliminary study. *Br J Clin Pract.* 1996;50(7):373–375.

136. Ogilvie-Harris DJ, Roscoe M. Reflex sympathetic dystrophy of the knee. *J Bone Joint Surg Br.* 1987;69(5):804–806.

137. Galer BS, Harle J, Rowbotham MC. Response to intravenous lidocaine infusion predicts subsequent response to oral mexiletine: a prospective study. *J Pain Symptom Manage.* 1996;12(3):161–167.

138. Goodman RR, Brisman R. Treatment of lower extremity reflex sympathetic dystrophy with continuous intrathecal morphine infusion. *Appl Neurophysiol.* 1987;50(1–6):425–426.

139. Forouzanfar T, Kemler MA, Weber WEJ, et al. Spinal cord stimulation in complex regional pain syndrome: cervical and lumbar devices are comparably effective. *Br J Anaesth.* 2004;92(3):348–353.

140. Kemler MA, De Vet HCW, Barendse GAM, et al. The effect of spinal cord stimulation in patients with chronic reflex sympathetic dystrophy: two years' follow-up of the randomized controlled trial. *Ann Neurol.* 2004;55(1):13–18.

141. Faletti C, Robba T, de Petro P. Postmeniscectomy osteonecrosis. *Arthroscopy.* 2002;18(1):91–94.

142. Muscolo DL, Costa-Paz M, Makino A, et al. Osteonecrosis of the knee following arthroscopic meniscectomy in patients over 50-years old. *Arthroscopy.* 1996;12(3):273–279.

143. Herber S, Runkel M, Pitton MB, et al. Indirect MR-arthrography in the follow up of autologous osteochondral transplantation [in German]. *Rofo.* 2003;175(2):226–233.

144. Athanasian EA, Wickiewicz TL, Warren RF. Osteonecrosis of the femoral condyle after arthroscopic reconstruction of a cruciate ligament. Report of two cases. *J Bone Joint Surg Am.* 1995;77(9):1418–1422.

145. Pape D, Seil R, Anagnostakos K, et al. Postarthroscopic osteonecrosis of the knee. *Arthroscopy.* 2007;23(4):428–438.

146. Papageorgiou CD, Kostopoulos VK, Moebius UG, et al. Patellar fractures associated with medial-third bone-patellar

tendon-bone autograft ACL reconstruction. *Knee Surg Sports Traumatol Arthrosc.* 2001;9(3):151–154.

147. Brahme SK, Fox JM, Ferkel RD, et al. Osteonecrosis of the knee after arthroscopic surgery: diagnosis with MR imaging. *Radiology.* 1991;178(3):851–853.

148. Fink B, Schneider T, Braunstein S, et al. Holmium: YAG laser-induced aseptic bone necroses of the femoral condyle. *Arthroscopy.* 1996;12(2):217–223.

149. Johnson TC, Evans JA, Gilley JA, et al. Osteonecrosis of the knee after arthroscopic surgery for meniscal tears and chondral lesions. *Arthroscopy.* 2000;16(3):254–261.

150. Santori N, Condello V, Adriani E, et al. Osteonecrosis after arthroscopic medial meniscectomy. *Arthroscopy.* 1995;11(2):220–224.

151. Soucacos PN, Xenakis TH, Beris AE, et al. Idiopathic osteonecrosis of the medial femoral condyle. Classification and treatment. *Clin Orthop Relat Res.* 1997;(341):82–89.

152. Harner CD, Irrgang JJ, Paul J, et al. Loss of motion after anterior cruciate ligament reconstruction. *Am J Sports Med.* 1992;20(5):499–506.

153. Shelbourne KD, Patel DV. Prevention of complications after autogenous bone-patellar tendon-bone ACL reconstruction. In: Pritchard DJ, ed. *Instructional Course Lectures.* Vol 45. Rosemont, IL: American Academy of Orthopaedic Surgeons; 1996:253–262.

154. Millett PJ, Wickiewicz TL, Warren RF. Motion loss after ligament injuries to the knee. Part I: causes. *Am J Sports Med.* 2001;29(5):664–675.

155. Shelbourne KD, Gray T. Minimum 10-year results after anterior cruciate ligament reconstruction: how the loss of normal knee motion compounds other factors related to the development of osteoarthritis after surgery. *Am J Sports Med.* 2009;37(3):471–480.

156. Hefzy MS, Grood ES, Noyes FR. Factors affecting the region of most isometric femoral attachments. Part II: the anterior cruciate ligament. *Am J Sports Med.* 1989;17(2):208–216.

157. Hutchinson MR, Bae TS. Reproducibility of anatomic tibial landmarks for anterior cruciate ligament reconstructions. *Am J Sports Med.* 2001;29(6):777–780.

158. Melby A 3rd, Noble JS, Askew MJ, et al. The effects of graft tensioning on the laxity and kinematics of the anterior cruciate ligament reconstructed knee. *Arthroscopy.* 1991;7(3):257–266.

159. Kim SG, Kurosawa H, Sakuraba K, et al. The effect of initial graft tension on postoperative clinical outcome in anterior cruciate ligament reconstruction with semitendinosus tendon. *Arch Orthop Trauma Surg.* 2006;126(4):260–264.

160. Nicholas SJ, D'Amato MJ, Mullaney MJ, et al. A prospectively randomized double-blind study on the effect of initial graft tension on knee stability after anterior cruciate ligament reconstruction. *Am J Sports Med.* 2004;32(8):1881–1886.

161. Van Kampen A, Wymenga AB, van der Heide HJ, et al. The effect of different graft tensioning in anterior cruciate ligament reconstruction: a prospective randomized study. *Arthroscopy.* 1998;14(8):845–850.

162. Yoshiya S, Kurosaka M, Ouchi K, et al. Graft tension and knee stability after anterior cruciate ligament reconstruction. *Clin Orthop Relat Res.* 2002;(394):154–160.

163. Arneja S, McConkey MO, Mulpuri K, et al. Graft tensioning in anterior cruciate ligament reconstruction: a systematic review of randomized controlled trials. *Arthroscopy.* 2009;25(2):200–207.

164. Fullerton LR Jr, Andrews JR. Mechanical block to extension following augmentation of the anterior cruciate ligament. A case report. *Am J Sports Med.* 1984;12(2):166–168.

165. Jackson DW, Schaefer RK. Cyclops syndrome: loss of extension following intra-articular anterior cruciate ligament reconstruction. *Arthroscopy.* 1990;6(3):171–178.

166. Marzo JM, Bowen MK, Warren RF, et al. Intraarticular fibrous nodule as a cause of loss of extension following anterior cruciate ligament reconstruction. *Arthroscopy.* 1992;8(1):10–18.

167. Recht MP, Piraino DW, Cohen MA, et al. Localized anterior arthrofibrosis (cyclops lesion) after reconstruction of the anterior cruciate ligament: MR imaging findings. *AJR Am J Roentgenol.* 1995;165(2):383–385.

168. Delcogliano A, Franzese S, Branca A, et al. Light and scan electron microscopic analysis of cyclops syndrome: etiopathogenic hypothesis and technical solutions. *Knee Surg Sports Traumatol Arthrosc.* 1996;4(4):194–199.

169. Delince P, Krallis P, Descamps PY, et al. Different aspects of the cyclops lesion following anterior cruciate ligament reconstruction: a multifactorial etiopathogenesis. *Arthroscopy.* 1998;14(8):869–876.

170. Shelbourne KD, Trumper RV. Preventing anterior knee pain after anterior cruciate ligament reconstruction. *Am J Sports Med.* 1997;25(1):41–47.

171. Balcarek P, Sawallich T, Losch A, et al. Delayed cyclops syndrome: symptomatic extension block four years after anterior cruciate ligament reconstruction. *Acta Orthop Belg.* 2008;74(2):261–265.

172. Christen B, Jakob RP. Fractures associated with patellar ligament grafts in cruciate ligament surgery. *J Bone Joint Surg Br.* 1992;74(4):617–619.

173. Lee GH, McCulloch P, Cole BJ, et al. The incidence of acute patellar tendon harvest complications for anterior cruciate ligament reconstruction. *Arthroscopy.* 2008;24(2):162–166.

174. Stein DA, Hunt SA, Rosen JE, et al. The incidence and outcome of patella fractures after anterior cruciate ligament reconstruction. *Arthroscopy.* 2002;18(6):578–583.

175. Viola R, Vianello R. Three cases of patella fracture in 1,320 anterior cruciate ligament reconstructions with bone-patellar tendon-bone autograft. *Arthroscopy.* 1999;15(1):93–97.

176. Sharkey NA, Donahue SW, Smith TS, et al. Patellar strain and patellofemoral contact after bone-patellar tendon-bone harvest for anterior cruciate ligament reconstruction. *Arch Phys Med Rehabil.* 1997;78(3):256–263.

177. Steen H, Tseng KF, Goldstein SA, et al. Harvest of patellar tendon (bone-tendon-bone) autograft for ACL reconstruction significantly alters surface strain in the human patella. *J Biomech Eng.* 1999;121(2):229–233.

178. Mithofer K, Gill TJ. Fracture complications after anterior cruciate ligament reconstruction. In: Prodromos CC, ed. *The Anterior Cruciate Ligament: Reconstruction and Basic Science.* Philadelphia, PA: Saunders Elsevier; 2008:598–606.

179. Daluga D, Johnson C, Bach BR Jr. Primary bone grafting following graft procurement for anterior cruciate ligament insufficiency. *Arthroscopy.* 1990;6(3):205–208.

180. Fineberg MS, Zarins B, Sherman OH. Practical considerations in anterior cruciate ligament replacement surgery. *Arthroscopy.* 2000;16(7):715–724.

181. Malek MM, Kunkle KL, Knable KR. Intraoperative complications of arthroscopically assisted ACL reconstruction using patellar tendon autograft. In: Pritchard DJ, ed. *Instructional Course Lectures*. Vol 45. Rosemont, IL: American Academy of Orthopaedic Surgeons; 1996:297–302.

182. Sgaglione NA, Douglas JA. Allograft bone augmentation in anterior cruciate ligament reconstruction. *Arthroscopy*. 2004;20(suppl 2):171–177.

183. Arciero RA. Endoscopic anterior cruciate ligament reconstruction: complication of graft rupture and a method of salvage. *Am J Knee Surg*. 1996;9(1):27–31.

184. Hill PF, Russell VJ, Salmon LJ, et al. The influence of supplementary tibial fixation on laxity measurements after anterior cruciate ligament reconstruction with hamstring tendons in female patients. *Am J Sports Med*. 2005;33(1):94–101.

185. Small NC. An analysis of complications in lateral retinacular release procedures. *Arthroscopy*. 1989;5(4):282–286.

186. Schneider T, Fink B, Abel R, et al. Hemarthrosis as a major complication after arthroscopic subcutaneous lateral retinacular release: a prospective study. *Am J Knee Surg*. 1998;11(2):95–100.

187. Sherman OH, Fox JM, Sperling H, et al. Patellar instability: treatment by arthroscopic electrosurgical lateral release. *Arthroscopy*. 1987;3(3):152–160.

188. Marumoto JM, Jordan C, Akins R. A biomechanical comparison of lateral retinacular releases. *Am J Sports Med*. 1995;23(2):151–155.

189. Colvin AC, West RV. Patellar instability. *J Bone Joint Surg Am*. 2008;90(12):2751–2762.

190. Kolowich PA, Paulos LE, Rosenberg TD, et al. Lateral release of the patella: indications and contraindications. *Am J Sports Med*. 1990;18(4):359–365.

191. Lattermann C, Toth J, Bach BR Jr. The role of lateral retinacular release in the treatment of patellar instability. *Sports Med Arthrosc*. 2007;15(2):57–60.

192. Ricchetti ET, Mehta S, Sennett BJ, et al. Comparison of lateral release versus lateral release with medial soft-tissue realignment for the treatment of recurrent patellar instability: a systematic review. *Arthroscopy*. 2007;23(5): 463–468.

193. Hughston JC, Deese M. Medial subluxation of the patella as a complication of lateral retinacular release. *Am J Sports Med*. 1988;16(4):383–388.

194. Shellock FG, Mink JH, Deutsch A, et al. Evaluation of patients with persistent symptoms after lateral retinacular release by kinematic magnetic resonance imaging of the patellofemoral joint. *Arthroscopy*. 1990;6(3): 226–234.

195. Alvine FG, Schurrer ME. Postoperative ulnar-nerve palsy. Are there predisposing factors? *J Bone Joint Surg Am*. 1987;69(2):255–259.

196. Warner MA, Martin JT, Schroeder DR, et al. Lower-extremity motor neuropathy associated with surgery performed on patients in a lithotomy position. *Anesthesiology*. 1994;81(1):6–12.

197. Sawyer RJ, Richmond MN, Hickey JD, et al. Peripheral nerve injuries associated with anaesthesia. *Anaesthesia*. 2000;55(10):980–991.

198. Sperber A, Jogestrand T, Wredmark T. Knee arthroscopy and venous blood flow in the lower leg. *Acta Orthop Scand*. 1996;67(6):553–556.

199. Cautilli R Jr. Introduction to the basics of arthroscopy of the knee. *Clin Sports Med*. 1997;16(1):1–16.

200. Morgan CD. The "all-inside" meniscus repair. *Arthroscopy*. 1991;7(1):120–125.

201. Gifstad T, Grontvedt T, Drogset JO. Meniscal repair with biofix arrows: results after 4.7 years' follow-up. *Am J Sports Med*. 2007;35(1):71–74.

202. Kurzweil PR, Tifford CD, Ignacio EM. Unsatisfactory clinical results of meniscal repair using the meniscus arrow. *Arthroscopy*. 2005;21(8):905.

203. Anderson K, Marx RG, Hannafin J, et al. Chondral injury following meniscal repair with a biodegradable implant. *Arthroscopy*. 2000;16(7):749–753.

204. Hutchinson MR, Ash SA. Failure of a biodegradable meniscal arrow. A case report. *Am J Sports Med*. 1999;27(1): 101–103.

205. Menche DS, Phillips GI, Pitman MI, et al. Inflammatory foreign-body reaction to an arthroscopic bioabsorbable meniscal arrow repair. *Arthroscopy*. 1999;15(7):770–772.

206. Sgaglione NA, Steadman JR, Shaffer B, et al. Current concepts in meniscus surgery: resection to replacement. *Arthroscopy*. 2003;19(suppl 1):161–188.

207. Song EK, Lee KB, Yoon TR. Aseptic synovitis after meniscal repair using the biodegradable meniscus arrow. *Arthroscopy*. 2001;17(1):77–80.

208. Hospodar SJ, Schmitz MR, Golish SR, et al. FasT-Fix versus inside-out suture meniscal repair in the goat model. *Am J Sports Med*. 2009;37(2):330–333.

209. Marcacci M, Kon E, Delcogliano M, et al. Arthroscopic autologous osteochondral grafting for cartilage defects of the knee: prospective study results at a minimum 7-year follow-up. *Am J Sports Med*. 2007;35(12):2014–2021.

210. Jakob RP, Franz T, Gautier E, et al. Autologous osteochondral grafting in the knee: indication, results, and reflections. *Clin Orthop Relat Res*. 2002;(401):170–184.

211. Simonian PT, Sussmann PS, Wickiewicz TL, et al. Contact pressures at osteochondral donor sites in the knee. *Am J Sports Med*. 1998;26(4):491–494.

212. Chow JC, Hantes ME, Houle JB, et al. Arthroscopic autogenous osteochondral transplantation for treating knee cartilage defects: a 2- to 5-year follow-up study. *Arthroscopy*. 2004;20(7):681–690.

213. Koh JL, Wirsing K, Lautenschlager E, et al. The effect of graft height mismatch on contact pressure following osteochondral grafting: a biomechanical study. *Am J Sports Med*. 2004;32(2):317–320.

214. Hangody L, Fules P. Autologous osteochondral mosaicplasty for the treatment of full-thickness defects of weight-bearing joints: ten years of experimental and clinical experience. *J Bone Joint Surg Am*. 2003;85-A(suppl 2):25–32.

215. Pearce SG, Hurtig MB, Clarnette R, et al. An investigation of 2 techniques for optimizing joint surface congruency using multiple cylindrical osteochondral autografts. *Arthroscopy*. 2001;17(1):50–55.

216. Duchow J, Hess T, Kohn D. Primary stability of press-fit-implanted osteochondral grafts. Influence of graft size, repeated insertion, and harvesting technique. *Am J Sports Med*. 2000;28(1):24–27.

217. Frisbie DD, Oxford JT, Southwood L, et al. Early events in cartilage repair after subchondral bone microfracture. *Clin Orthop Relat Res*. 2003;(407):215–227.

218. Barber FA, Flipped patellar tendon autograft anterior cruciate reconstruction. *Arthroscopy*. 2000;16(5):483–490.

Arthroscopic Management of Fractures Around the Knee

Roberto Rossi • Davide Edoardo Bonasia • Filippo Castoldi

The use of arthroscopic and arthroscopic-assisted techniques for the treatment of fractures around the knee has become more popular over the last decades. Nevertheless, limited types of fractures are amenable to arthroscopy (some tibial plateau fractures, tibial spine avulsions, and osteochondral lesions) and open surgery still remains the gold standard in several cases (i.e., patellar, femoral condyles, and complex tibial plateau fractures). The treatment of osteochondral lesions has been previously described, and this chapter will be mainly focused on arthroscopic treatment of tibial plateau fractures and tibial spine avulsions.

TIBIAL PLATEAU FRACTURES

Clinical Evaluation

Tibial plateau fractures represent only 1% of all fractures (1). They commonly result from varus/valgus stresses across the knee joint, direct traumas, or excessive axial loads to the extended lower limb. They mainly occur in motor vehicle accidents (i.e., bumper trauma and motorcycle accidents), in sports (i.e., skiing and high-contact sports) and falls from height.

A correct classification of the fracture is mandatory for the decision-making and to assess the prognosis. We commonly use Schatzker's classification. Its advantages compared with other classification systems (i.e., Hohl, Moore, Honkonen and Jarvinen, AO, etc.) include handiness as well as a good correlation with severity, treatment, and prognosis of the fracture (2). Type I is a wedge fracture of the lateral hemiplateau, without articular depression. Type II is a wedge fracture of the lateral hemiplateau associated with articular depression. Type III is an isolated articular depression fracture involving the lateral plateau. Type IV is a medial tibial plateau fracture, most likely associated with tibial eminence fracture. Type V is a bicondylar tibial fracture, without metaphyseal involvement. Type VI is an unicondilar or bicondilar tibial fracture, with metaphyseal involvement.

Clinically, the traumatic mechanism should be investigated, a dislocation excluded and the physical examination

should be mainly focused on the neurovascular evaluation and assessment of possible associated lesions. The knee is usually swollen as well as painful and stability maneuvers must be carried out under anesthesia, before surgery.

For a correct assessment of the fracture type, the workup must include anteroposterior (AP) and lateral X-ray views as well as a CT scan of the involved knee. MRI is not routinely required, but may be useful when associated ligamentous injuries are suspected, even though ligaments reconstruction is usually delayed untill after fracture healing.

Treatment

The management of the fracture depends on several factors and these include (1) fracture configuration (2); concomitant soft-tissue injury (3); patient's age and activity level; and (4) bone quality. Arthroscopic reduction and internal fixation (ARIF) is indicated in Schatzker type I to III (Fig. 84.1), when the displacement is more than 5 mm, in compliant patients and in nonarthritic knees (Table 84.1). Nevertheless, in some Schatzker type II fractures, if the bone quality is poor or the wedge fragment is comminuted, open reduction and internal fixation (ORIF) with plating is recommended.

Arthroscopic-assisted techniques have been described for Schatzker type IV fractures (wedge medial plateau fragment, with an additional fragment involving the tibial eminences). These fractures usually result from high-energy traumas, with soft-tissue injuries (skin, ligaments, and capsule) and are more difficult to reduce by external maneuvers. Therefore, we recommend ORIF in these cases to avoid as well possible arthroscopic fluid leakage in the soft tissues.

Many open and arthroscopic-assisted techniques have been proposed. All of them allow a direct visualization of fracture reduction and a precise evaluation and treatment of associated intraarticular lesions, with a minimally invasive procedure. They generally have in common the indirect reduction through an en masse elevation of the depressed fragment (Schatzker type II to IV) from below the involved hemiplateau, using a bone punch. Nevertheless, they differ in the type of fixation and in the way of

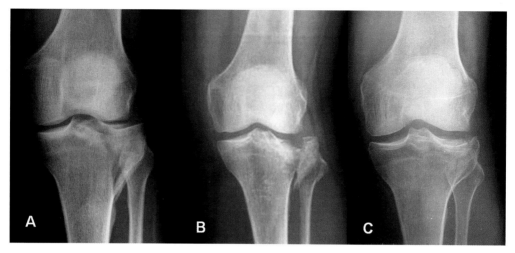

FIGURE 84.1. Tibial plateau fractures amenable to ARIF include Schatzker **A:** type I, **B:** type II, and **C:** type III fractures.

Table 84.1

Indications for proximal tibial fractures

Fracture Type (Schatzker Classification)	Treatment
Type I (lateral plateau wedge fracture, without articular depression)	ARIF and percutaneous lag screw fixation
Type II (lateral plateau wedge fracture with articular depression)	ARIF and percutaneous lag screw fixation vs ORIF and plating (if poor bone quality or high comminution of the wedge fragment)
Type III (lateral plateau articular depression only)	ARIF and percutaneous lag screw fixation
Type IV (medial tibial plateau fracture with tibial eminence fracture)	ORIF and plating vs ARIF and percutaneous lag screw fixation (if low energy trauma and isolated involvement of the medial plateau, either wedge or depressed fragment)
Type V (bicondylar tibial fracture, without metaphyseal involvement)	ORIF and double plating vs external fixation
Type VI (unicondilar or bicondilar tibial fracture, with metaphyseal involvement)	ORIF and double plating vs external fixation

filling the metaphyseal void under the fracture. Recent studies advocate the use of PMMA (polymethylmethacrylate) or bone substitutes such as carbonate apatite or calciumphosphate cement, instead of autologous iliac crest graft, to reduce donor site morbidity and permit early weight-bearing. Nevertheless, with bone substitutes, the disadvantages are high cost as well as less osteoinductive and osteoconductive properties, and with acrylic cement, the risk of thermal osteonecrosis should be considered.

Authors' Preferred Technique

To overcome the necessity of using bone graft or substitutes, we proposed an alternative arthroscopic-assisted technique (1, 3) for Schatzker types II and III fractures.

The patient is positioned supine in general or spinal anesthesia, with the tourniquet placed on the proximal thigh. The knee stability is then evaluated under anesthesia. Arthroscopic examination is performed using gravity inflow, through classical anteromedial and anterolateral portals. The heamarthrosis is drained and any osteochondral fragments removed. The degree of fracture depression and soft-tissues injury is assessed. A longitudinal 3-cm skin incision is made on the medial aspect of the tibia, starting 10 cm from the articular surface and extended distally. A cortical window (10 × 20 mm) is opened on the medial tibia and a hollow trephine cutter (diameter 10 mm), with a sawtoothed tip, is introduced in the tibia itself (Figs. 84.2 to 84.4).

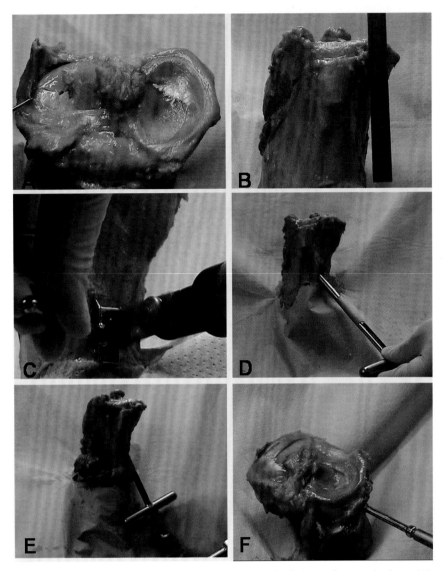

FIGURE 84.2. In this human specimen, ARIF for lateral tibial plateau fractures is shown (**A**). On the anteromedial tibia, 10 cm below the articular surface (**B**), a cortical window is opened (**C**). A cannulated cutter is inserted in the cortical window (**D**) and positioned 2 cm below the lateral plateau. A bone tamp is inserted in the cutter and the fracture reduced (**E**). Two or three cannulated screws are inserted percutaneously from lateral to medial (**F**).

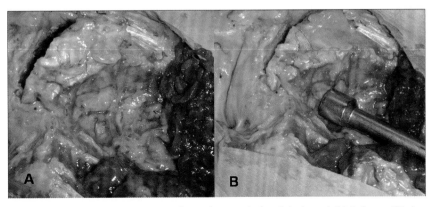

FIGURE 84.3. This human specimen shows the vascularity of the lateral tibial plateau (**A**) that can be damaged by inserting the bone tamp (**B**) in the lateral column and not in the medial one.

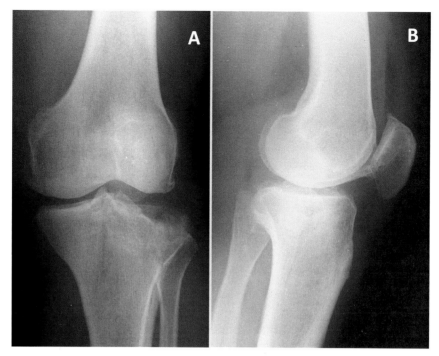

FIGURE 84.4. Schatzker type II fracture in AP **(A)** and lateral view **(B)**.

Under fluoroscopic control (AP and lateral views), the edge of the cutter is placed 2 cm below the lateral plateau fracture (Fig. 84.5). A bone punch (diameter 9 mm) is then inserted into the cutter and, with a hammer, the cancellous bone block (base 9 mm diameter, height about 100 mm) is impacted under the fracture to obtain an indirect reduction (Fig. 84.2). If the articular surface is severely compacted, this procedure could be repeated placing the cutter in another direction, through the same window. The anatomical reconstruction of the articular surface is assessed arthroscopically (Fig. 84.6). Once the optimal reduction is achieved, the fracture is then fixed with two or three cancellous cannulated screws (6.5 mm), inserted percutaneously from lateral to medial and 1 cm under the articular surface (Fig. 84.2). The cutter and the punch are then removed and the tibial cortex replaced in situ (1). Neither iliac crest graft nor bone substitutes are used with this technique.

In Schatzker type I fractures (wedge fractures, without articular surface depression), the en masse elevation is not required and, under arthroscopic control, the wedge fragment is usually reduced by external maneuvers. These include a digital compression on the wedge fragment that is usually distally displaced, a varus stress on the knee (playing on the ligamentotaxis by the articular capsule) and the use of a K wire as a *joystick*. Once the fracture is reduced and the articular surface restored, a percutaneous fixation with screws is performed, as previously described.

Complications, Controversies, and Special Considerations

The advantages of this technique include (1) preserving the fractured lateral tibial column from further surgical damages (i.e., cortical window opening and cancellous

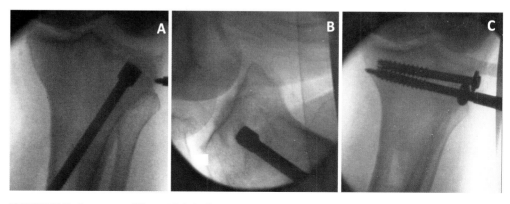

FIGURE 84.5. Same case of Figure 84.4. **A:** Fluoroscopy in AP **(A)** and lateral **(B)** view of fracture reduction using the bone tamp from medial to lateral. **C:** Fluoroscopy of synthesis with cannulated screws.

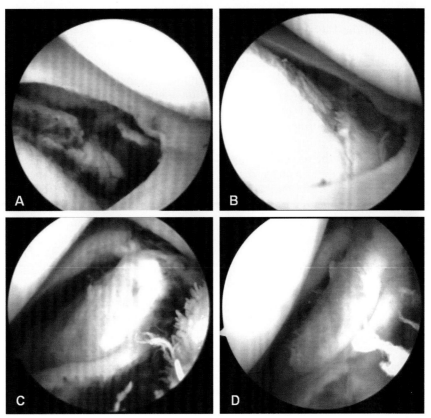

FIGURE 84.6. Arthroscopic evaluation before (**A**) and after (**B**) reduction of the same fracture described in Figures 84.4 and 84.5. Arthroscopic evaluation before (**C**) and after (**D**) reduction of another case.

bone mobilization) (2); preserving the lateral plateau blood supply (Fig. 84.3) (3); playing on the inclined plane effect of the tunnel (that is oblique from medial to lateral and not vertical right below the depressed plateau); and, therefore (4), avoiding bone or bone substitutes augmentation.

The short- and midterm results reported in literature for any ARIF techniques are comparable to ORIF (1). Nevertheless, as previously mentioned, ARIF allows direct visualization of fracture reduction as well as precise evaluation and treatment of associated intraarticular lesions, with a minimally invasive procedure.

Cassard et al. (4) treated 26 patients with ARIF and reported a mean KSS score of 94.1 for pain and 94.7 for function. In their series, Schatzker type I to IV fractures were included and no bone graft was used. Gill et al. (5) treated arthroscopically a 29-patient series, reporting a mean postoperative Rasmussen score of 27.5. Schatzker type I to IV fractures were included in the study and coral hydroxyapatite was used as bone substitute. Hung et al. (6) arthroscopically operated 31 patients and report HSS scores excellent in 81%, good in 13%, fair in 6%. Iliac crest autograft was used for bone augmentation in all the patients. Roche et al. (7) in a 10-patient series described the use of surgical cement to allow immediate weight-bearing. In their study, 9 out of 10 patients had no secondary displacement.

In our 46-patient case series (1), at 5 years follow-up evaluation knee score was excellent in 37 patients (80%), good in 6 (13%), fair in 3 (7%). Function score was excellent in 38 patients (83%), good in 5 (11%), fair in 3 (6%). HSS score was excellent in 41 patients (89%), good in 5 (11%). Schatzker type II and III fractures were included in this study and no bone or bone-substitute augmentation was used.

The most common complications related to tibial plateau fractures, regardless of the surgical management decided, include (1) nonunion (2); loss of correction and malunion, with consequent knee malalignment (3); posttraumatic knee arthritis (4); infection (5); thromboembolism (6); joint stiffness; and (7) compartment syndrome.

The use of arthroscopy in these fractures may raise some concerns about possible compartment syndrome. There is no evidence in literature supporting an increased risk of compartment syndrome with arthroscopy. Nevertheless, we recommend the use of gravity inflow during the arthroscopic phase and, if the procedure is prolonged, we suggest to open the cortical window, in order to allow the saline to leak out of the knee.

Pearls and Pitfalls

As previously mentioned, we recommend to use a gravity inflow arthroscope, in order to reduce the risk of compartment syndrome and to perform an anterome-dial cortical window to elevate the lateral tibial plateau depressed fragment with a bone punch. If, arthroscopically, the articular surface is not reduced, the reduction procedure can be repeated placing the cutter and the bone punch in another direction, through the same window.

If an intraarticular overcorrection is verified under ar-throscopic control, a gentle knee flexion more than 90° also associated with a valgus stress is performed, in order to allow the femoral condyles to push the prominent fragment back into the tibia and to restore the articular surface.

Rehabilitation

Immediate active motion 0° to 90° is allowed in a hinged knee brace. The brace is removed after 4 weeks and partial weight-bearing allowed after 8 weeks. Full weight is permitted after 3 months. CPM (continuous passive motion) is not required.

TIBIAL SPINE AVULSIONS

Clinical Evaluation

Fractures of the anterior tibial spine are uncommon injuries in children, with a reported incidence of 3/100,000 per year (8) and are even rarer in adults. The traumatic mechanism is comparable to anterior cruciate ligament (ACL) ruptures (mainly valgus stress and external tibial rotation or hyperextension). These fractures are mostly related to motor vehicle accidents, falls from bicycle and sports injuries.

Meyers and McKeever (9) classified tibial spine avulsion into three types. In type-I fracture, the intercondylar eminence is slightly elevated anteriorly. In type II, the fracture is hinged posteriorly, elevated anteriorly, and shows a beak-like pattern. The fragment in the type-III fracture is completely separated from its bone bed (Figs. 84.7 and 84.8). Zaricznyj (10) added type IV in which the fragment is comminuted.

Clinically, the traumatic mechanism should be investigated and the physical examination should be mainly focused on assessing knee stability (Lachman, Pivot Shift, anterior drawer, varus and valgus stress tests) and possible associated lesions.

In the work-up plain AP, lateral and tunnel X rays views are usually sufficient to assess the fracture type. A CT scan may be indicated if the degree of displacement is not clear on plain radiographs and to evaluate the integrity of the medial spine posterior hinge. MRI is indicated if associated lesions are suspected or if inadequate reduction is achieved after closed reduction maneuvers. In this case, MRI may show the interposition of the transverse meniscal ligament or the meniscal anterior horn.

Treatment

Type I injuries do not require reduction and can be immobilized in a cylinder cast for 4 to 6 weeks. We recommend cast

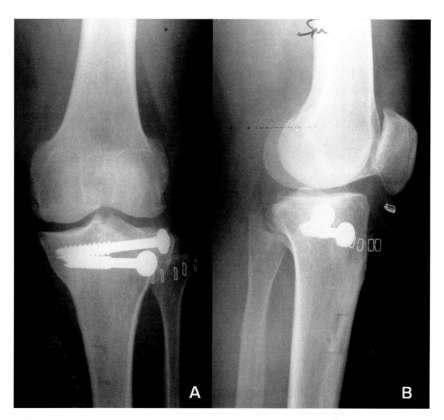

FIGURE 84.7. Postoperative AP **(A)** and lateral view **(B)** of the same case described in Figures 84.4 to 84.6.

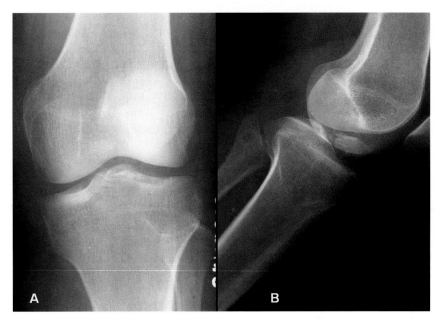

FIGURE 84.8. AP **(A)** and lateral **(B)** views of a tibial spine avulsion (Meyers and McKeever type III).

in full extension (not in hyperextension), in order to reduce the risk of extension deficit (high in this kind of fractures). Nevertheless, some authors suggest the use of a cast at 20° to 30° of knee flexion, in order to reduce ACL tension.

The treatment of type II fractures is controversial. Both conservative and surgical treatments (ARIF and ORIF) have been proposed. Our management include (1) heamarthrosis drainage (2); combined intraarticular injection of local anesthetic (3); closed reduction, bringing the knee to full extension; and (4) cast immobilization in full extension (not in hyperextension). If postimmobilization radiographs show insufficient reduction, MRI is requested to assess any soft-tissue interpositions between the fragments and ARIF is performed.

Surgical treatment is always indicated in type III and IV fractures as well as in nonunions. Either ARIF or ORIF can be performed (Table 84.2).

Eilert (11) first described arthroscopic reduction on tibial spine fracture in 1978. Since then, it has become a common practice to treat tibial spine fracture arthroscopically and many techniques have been proposed. All of them have in common the accurate debridement of the fracture site, the ACL integrity evaluation, and the careful reduction. The differences are basically about the fixation devices adopted and these include (1) cannulated screws (12) (2); suture anchors (13) (3); metallic tension band wiring (14) (4); K-wires (15); and (5) pullout suturing (16).

Authors' Preferred Technique

We commonly use a rigid fixation with cannulated screws when the avulsed fragment is voluminous. When the fragment is small or comminuted (type IV fractures), we use a pullout technique (with braided sutures). In children, we

---

Table 84.2

Indications for tibial spine avulsions

Fracture Type (Meyers and McKeever Classification)	Treatment
Type I: Slight elevation of the anterior margin of the fragment	Cast immobilization for 4–6 wk
Type II: Beak-like fracture, hinged posteriorly	Reduction and cast immobilization for 4–6 wk vs ARIF or ORIF (if inadequate reduction)
Type III: Complete avulsion from bone bed	ARIF (all techniques possible) or ORIF
Type IV (Zaricznyj): Complete avulsion with comminution of the fragment	ARIF (pullout suture technique) or ORIF

prefer an intra-epiphyseal fixation either with screws or with pullout sutures. Transphyseal techniques (obviously not with screws) have been described in children without any growth disturbances because of the minimal physeal drilling. Nevertheless, we recommend an intra-epiphyseal fixation to avoid the necessity of hardware removal.

The patient is positioned supine in general or spinal anesthesia, with the tourniquet placed on the proximal thigh. The knee stability is then evaluated under anesthesia. Arthroscopic examination is performed using a water pump, through classical anteromedial and anterolateral portals. The heamarthrosis is drained and any osteochondral fragments removed. A complete diagnostic examination is performed to assess for any associate lesions. The fracture site is carefully debrided to clear any fibrous or soft-tissue interpositions. The tibial spine is carefully reduced and the integrity of the ACL fibers is probed. The dimensions and the integrity of the avulsed fragment are evaluated. If the fragment is wide enough and not comminuted, screw fixation is performed. Two 1.1 mm guide wires are inserted into the fragment and the proximal tibia from the anteromedial portal. In this phase, a lateral mid-patellar portal may improve the arthroscopic visualization. The reduction achieved and the guide wires positioning is then evaluated fluoroscopically with AP and lateral views. In children, the physis sparing should be verified as well. A 2-mm hole is drilled with a cannulated tip on the guide wires, and two 3.0 mm partially threaded cancellous lag screws are inserted (Fig. 84.9). Once fixation is achieved, the knee laxity is evaluated.

If the avulsed fragment is too small or comminuted for a screw fixation, a pullout suturing is performed (Fig. 84.10). A hook suture passer is used to load the ACL fibers with two strands of no. 2 braided suture (Ethibond, Ethicon, Somerville, NJ). Absorbable monofilament sutures (PDS, Ethicon, Somerville, NJ) can be used as well. The ends of the sutures are then pulled outside the joint through the anterolateral portal. A 2-cm longitudinal skin incision is performed on the anteromedial tibia. A tip-to-tip ACL guide is inserted in the knee through the anteromedial portal, and two 2.5-mm guide K-wires are drilled lateral and medial to the tibial bed of the fracture. The 2.5-mm tunnels should be positioned more anterior than posterior, in order to avoid secondary anterior displacement of the tibial spine with consequent impingement and extension deficit. In children, the tunnels should be drilled more proximal and horizontal, in order to spare the growth plate, and the K-wires position must be verified under fluoroscopy. A Hewson suture passer in then inserted in the tunnels, and the sutures pulled out from the anterior tibia. Keeping the sutures in tension, the reduction is arthroscopically evaluated, and the knee stability is assessed with the Lachman test. The sutures are then tied together on the anteromedial tibia.

Complications, Controversies, and Special Considerations

In the literature, there are no conclusive data regarding the treatment of such a rare pathology. Nevertheless, there seems to be no difference between the open and the

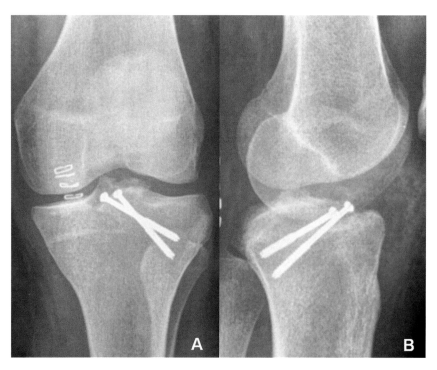

FIGURE 84.9. AP **(A)** and lateral **(B)** postoperative views of a tibial spine fracture, treated with ARIF and cannulated screws synthesis.

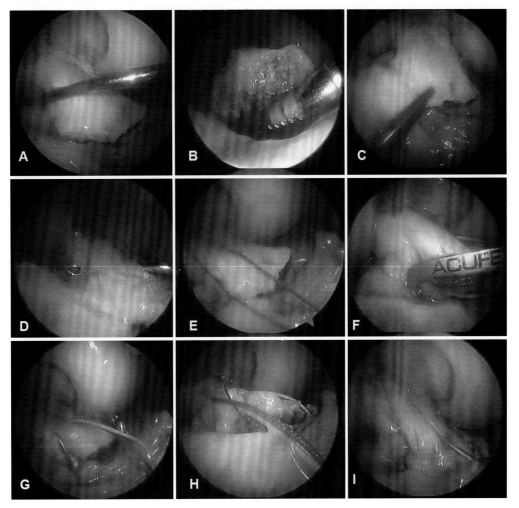

FIGURE 84.10. Arthroscopic pullout suturing technique for tibial spine avulsions. **A:** ACL integrity evaluation. **B:** Debridement of fracture site. **C:** Evaluation of the reduction. **D:** Insertion of the first-braided suture with a hook suture passer (**E**) in the distal fibers of the ACL. **F:** Use of the ACL reconstruction guide to drill two tunnels (**G**), medial and lateral to the fracture bed. **H:** Use of a Hewson suture passer to pull the sutures out of the anterior tibia. The sutures are then tied together on the anteromedial tibia, if (**I**) the reduction is satisfactory.

arthroscopic techniques described (17). Even though the results reported are good, in this pathology, there is a high rate of complications, regardless of the treatment methods.

Several authors have reported varying amounts of ligamentous laxity after these fractures. Baxter and Wiley (18) reported that 51% of their patients had a positive anterior drawer test at last follow-up and that all patients had a loss of extension, ranging from 4° to 15°; 64% of the patients were aware of the difference between their knees. Grönkvist et al. (19) stated that younger children compensate somewhat for any anterior instability as the skeleton grows and recommended operative repair, especially in older children, if satisfactory closed reduction is not achieved.

In their report of 50 patients with tibial eminence fractures, Willis et al. (20) noted that, although most children (64% at clinical examination and 74% at KT-1000 arthrometer) have objective evidence of ACL laxity at long-term follow-up, only 10% of patients complained

of pain and none complained of instability at follow-up. No correlation was found between long-term stability and method of treatment (open or closed). They concluded that most anterior tibial eminence fractures should be treated conservatively, with surgery reserved for irreducible fractures. They also stated that arthroscopy may be useful to ensure adequate reduction of the fragment.

Pearls and Pitfalls

We recommend to perform a vertical anteromedial portal, in order to eventually convert the arthroscopic procedure in mini-open, if inadequate reduction or synthesis are achieved arthroscopically. This will allow to include the anteromedial portal in a 4-cm medial parapatellar arthrotomy.

A lateral midpatellar portal can be useful for better visualization either in screw fixation or in pullout suturing.

When performing a pullout suturing technique, we recommend to position the tibial tunnels more anterior than posterior, in order to avoid secondary anterior displacement of the tibial spine, with consequent impingement and extension deficit.

Rehabilitation

For 30 days from surgery, partial weight-bearing is allowed and a hinged knee brace (locked in extension) is used. At 30 days from surgery, full weight-bearing is allowed and the knee brace is unlocked. At 60 days from surgery, the brace is discontinued.

CONCLUSIONS AND FUTURE DIRECTIONS

Even if technically more difficult, the arthroscopic treatment of tibial plateau fractures and tibial spine avulsions has become more popular over the last two decades. The results of ARIF seem to be comparable to ORIF in both pathologies. Nevertheless, arthroscopy allows direct visualization of fracture reduction as well as assessment and treatment of associated intraarticular lesions, with a minimally invasive procedure.

REFERENCES

1. Rossi R, Bonasia DE, Blonna D, et al. Prospective follow-up of a simple arthroscopic-assisted technique for lateral tibial plateau fractures: results at 5 years. *Knee.* 2008;15:378–383.
2. Bonasia DE, Rossi R, Bardelli A. Tibial plateau fractures. A review of classifications. *Minerva Ortopedica e Traumatologica.* 2005;56:457–463.
3. Rossi R, Castoldi F, Blonna D, et al. Arthroscopic treatment of lateral tibial plateau fractures: a simple technique. *Arthroscopy.* 2006;22:678.e1–678.e6.
4. Cassard X, Beaufils P, Blin JL, et al. Osteosynthesis under arthroscopic control of separated tibial plateau fractures. 26 case reports. *Rev Chir Orthop Reparatrice Appar Mot.* 1999;85:257–266.
5. Gill TJ, Moezzi DM, Oates KM, et al. Arthroscopic reduction and internal fixation of tibial plateau fractures in skiing. *Clin Orthop Relat Res.* 2001;383:243–249.
6. Hung SS, Chao E, Chan Y, et al. Arthroscopically assisted osteosynthesis for tibial plateau fractures. *J Trauma.* 2003;54:356–363.
7. Roche O, Aubrion JH, Sirveaux F, et al. Use of surgical cement in tibial plateau fractures in the elderly. *J Bone Joint Surg Br.* 2001;83-B(suppl 2):242.
8. Skak SV, Jenson TT, Paulsen TD, et al. Epidemiology of knee injuries in children. *Acta Orthop Scand.* 1987;58:78–81.
9. Meyers MH, McKeever FM. Fracture of the intercondylar eminence of the tibia. *J Bone Joint Surg Am.* 1959;41:209–222.
10. Zaricznyj B. Avulsion fracture of the tibial eminence: treatment by open reduction and pinning. *J Bone Joint Surg Am.* 1977;59:1111–1114.
11. Eilert RE. Arthroscopy and arthrography in children and adolescent. In: *AAOS Symposium on Arthroscopy and Arthrography of the Knee.* St Louis, MO: Mosby; 1978:12.
12. Van Loon T, Marti RK. A fracture of the intercondylar eminence of the tibia treated by arthroscopic fixation. *Arthroscopy.* 1991;7:385–388.
13. Vega JR, Irribarra LA, Baar AK, et al. Arthroscopic fixation of displaced tibial eminence fractures: a new growth plate-sparing method. *Arthroscopy.* 2008;24:1239–1243.
14. Osti L, Merlo F, Liu SH, et al. A simple modified arthroscopic procedure for fixation of displaced tibial eminence fractures. *Arthroscopy.* 2000;16:379–382.
15. Medler RG, Jansson KA. Arthroscopic treatment of the fractures of the tibial spine. *Arthroscopy.* 1994;10:292–295.
16. Kogan MG, Marks P, Amendola A. Technique for arthroscopic suture fixation of displaced tibial intercondylar eminence fractures. *Arthroscopy.* 1997;13:301–306.
17. Rademakers MV, Kerkhoffs GM, Kager J, et al. Tibial spine fractures: a long-term follow-up study of open reduction and internal fixation. *J Orthop Trauma.* 2009;23:203–207.
18. Baxter MP, Wiley JJ. Fractures of the tibial spine in children. An evaluation of knee stability. *J Bone Joint Surg Br.* 1988;70:228–230.
19. Grönkvist H, Hirsch G, Johansson L. Fracture of the anterior tibial spine in children. *J Pediatr Orthop.* 1984;4:465–468.
20. Willis RB, Blokker C, Stoll TM, et al. Long-term follow-up of anterior tibial eminence fractures. *J Pediatr Orthop.* 1993;13:361–364.

Foot and Ankle

Topographic and Arthroscopic Anatomy of the Ankle

Sami Abdulmassih • Fernando Pena • Annunziato Amendola

The first efforts at arthroscopic intervention, dating back to 1918, were made by Dr. K. Takagi at the University of Japan. Considering the technologic limitations at that time, the knee joint was the focus of interest. Burman, in 1931, in New York, reported on arthroscopy of 100 knees, 25 shoulders, 20 hips, 15 elbows, 6 wrists, and 3 ankles (1). He stated that the ankle "is not suitable for arthroscopy." The congruency of the ankle joint and the diameter of the cannula (4 mm) seemed to be the most limiting factors. Later, M. Watanabe, a protégé of Dr. K. Takagi, developed new arthroscopes and expanded arthroscopy to joints other than the knee. In 1977, Dr. Hiroshi Ikeuchi, a student of Dr. Watanabe, presented one of the first series on ankle arthroscopy with clear examples of intra-articular pathology (2). As described in Guhl's book (2), this presentation inspired Guhl and others to pursue further interest in this field of arthroscopy. More recently, several authors, among them Ewing, Ferkel, and Guhl, have popularized arthroscopy of the ankle joint (2–5). Although it is still an evolving area of arthroscopic surgery, ankle arthroscopy has demonstrated high rates of success and minimal complications with proper technique and indications.

Complications associated with ankle arthroscopy can be avoided or significantly decreased by a solid knowledge and familiarity with the anatomy of the ankle joint and the structures crossing along this joint. Feiwell and Frey (6), as well as Sitler et al. (5), described in detail the relationship of structures at risk with placement of standard ankle portals. These and other reports added to the improved visualization and access to the ankle joint, allowing an expansion in indications for ankle arthroscopy.

This chapter reviews the normal topographic anatomy, vital structures, and arthroscopic anatomy of the ankle joint.

TOPOGRAPHIC ANATOMY

The ankle joint consists of the distal tibia, the fibula, and the talus. The configuration of bony anatomy makes the ankle joint a very congruent joint with limited access if the soft tissue and bony structures are respected. Therefore, ankle arthroscopy represents a challenge to achieve full visualization and working access to the joint, without creating any iatrogenic injury.

The medial malleolus extends approximately 1 cm distal to the joint line. The posterior tibialis tendon lies on the posterior half of the malleolus; posterior to it, the tibial nerve, the tibial artery, and the flexor hallucis longus (FHL) tendon are found and protected. Anterior to the medial malleolus lie the most distal and fine branches of the saphenous nerve, which are posterior and medial to the great saphenous vein. These branches may extend as far distally as the first metatarsophalangeal joint, where they anastomose with the most medial branches of the superficial peroneal nerve. The "soft spot" of the ankle joint is located between the anterior tibialis tendon and the medial malleolus. This represents a safe area to place an anteromedial portal; however, the portal should be placed as close as possible to the medial aspect of the anterior tibialis tendon, in order to avoid the saphenous nerve and vein as well as the medial malleolus (3) (Fig. 85.1).

Anteriorly, the thin subcutaneous tissue allows easy palpation of the anterior compartment structures. From medial to lateral, there are the anterior tibialis tendon, the extensor hallucis longus tendon, the anterior tibial artery and vein, the deep peroneal nerve, and the extensor digitorum longus tendon. Previous publications described the anterocentral portal, which provides a broad anterior visualization of the ankle joint (4, 7, 8). More recent reports (6, 9) have pointed out the risk of injuring the anterior structures with the use of this portal. In addition, adequate access through anteromedial and anterolateral portals has made the anterocentral portal unnecessary for full visualization (Fig. 85.2).

The superficial peroneal nerve may be found along the lateral half of the anterior aspect of the ankle. Plantar flexing and inverting the foot facilitate visualization of this nerve under the skin in many cases. Because injury to this nerve is the most common complication when using the anterolateral

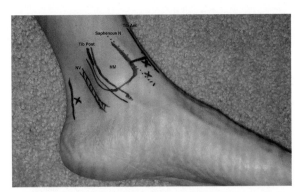

FIGURE 85.1. Medial aspect of the ankle with location of the anteromedial, accessory me dial, and posteromedial portals. MM, medial malleolus; NV, neurovascular bundle; N, nerve.

portal, it is important to discuss the anatomy in detail (2, 4). Although multiple anatomic variations have been described, the nerve becomes subcutaneous approximately 10.5 cm proximal to the tip of the fibula in 91% of specimens (10). At this level, it is most likely to be found along the anterior margin of the fibula. From that point, it branches into the medial terminal branch and the intermediate dorsal cutaneous branch. In 92% of specimens, this division occurs 6.5 cm proximal to the tip of the fibula (11). The medial terminal branch crosses the ankle joint line along the anterior middle third, adjacent to the extensor hallucis longus tendon. More distally, it trifurcates into three final branches to innervate the dorsal aspect of the medial half of the foot. The most lateral branch, the intermediate dorsal cutaneous

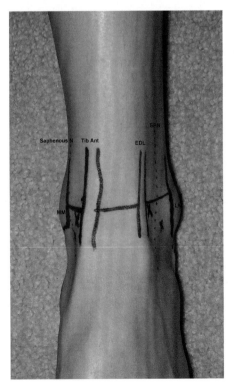

FIGURE 85.2. Anterior aspect of the ankle with location of the accessory medial, anteromedial, anterolateral, and accessory lateral portals. SPN, superficial peroneal nerve; MM, medial malleolus; LM, lateral malleolus; N, nerve; EDL, extonsor digitorum longus.

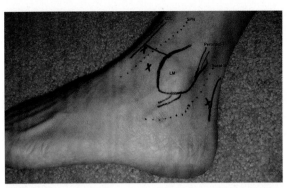

FIGURE 85.3. Lateral aspect of the ankle with location of the anterolateral, accessory lateral, and posterolateral portals. EDL, extensor digitorum longus; SPN, superficial peroneal nerve; LM, lateral malleolus; T, tendon; N, nerve.

branch, crosses the ankle joint subcutaneously at the level of the fourth and fifth extensor digitorum longus tendons, and from there it aims for the third intermetatarsal space (Fig. 85.3). This is the branch at risk when an anterolateral portal is created. More distally, it may have some anastomosis with the most dorsal branches of the sural nerve. The medial and the intermediate branches provide sensation to most of the dorsal skin of the foot. The deep peroneal nerve innervates the dorsal aspect of the first web space.

The lateral malleolus extends more posteriorly and distally than its medial counterpart. The tip of the malleolus is, on average, 2 cm distal to the joint line and 1 cm posterior to the medial malleolus. Posterior to the fibula, the peroneal tendons curve inferiorly, and the sural nerve may be found more posteriorly. The sural nerve is located an average of 1 to 1.5 cm distal and 1.5 to 2 cm posterior to the tip of the fibula. It travels anteriorly and laterally to the lesser saphenous vein, which may be found in the immediate vicinity of the nerve. As mentioned previously, at the level of the tuberosity of the fifth metatarsal, it divides into its terminal medial and lateral branches to anastomose with the intermediate dorsal cutaneous branch of the superficial peroneal nerve (Fig. 85.3).

The posterior topographic anatomy of the ankle is better assessed with the patient in the prone position. At the level of the ankle joint, the Achilles tendon is slightly lateral to the midline. The joint line can be palpated and identified medial, lateral, and anterior to the tendon. The superior border of the calcaneus is used as a reference, and dorsiflexion of the ankle joint helps in feeling the posterior process of the talus. Both medial and lateral portals are placed at the level of the tibiotalar joint (Fig. 85.4). The posterolateral portal is placed adjacent to the lateral border of the Achilles tendon (Fig. 85.5), and the sural nerve remains anterior to it by an average of 3.2 mm (5). On the medial side, the portal is again placed adjacent to the margin of the tendon (Fig. 85.6), and the neurovascular bundle remains at a safe distance (on average, 9.7 mm) anterior to it (5) (Fig. 85.7).

We recommend identifying and delineating the structures described here with a marking pen before beginning the procedure, in order to have a better appreciation of their

VI. Foot and Ankle

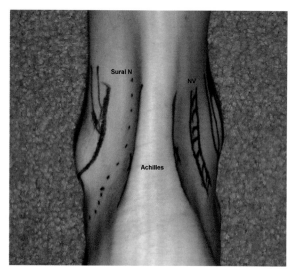

FIGURE 85.4. Posterior aspect of the ankle with location of the posteromedial and posterolateral portals in relation to the nearby at risk structures. NV, neurovascular bundle; N, nerve.

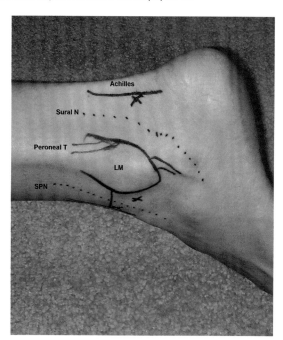

FIGURE 85.5. Lateral aspect of the ankle in the prone position and the setting for hindfoot arthroscopy with location of the posterolateral, accessory lateral, and anterolateral portals. N, nerve; T, tendon; LM, lateral malleolus; SPN, superficial peroneal nerve.

location and thus decrease the chances for injury. In addition, the use of blunt dissection and minimal number of reentries through the same portal decrease the risk of injury.

The technique and instrumentation required for ankle arthroscopy are discussed in Chapter 61.

INTRA-ARTICULAR ANATOMY

Ferkel (4) described a 21-point inspection for the intra-articular anatomy of the ankle. This method represents one of many ways to explore the ankle joint. Regardless of the methodology used by the surgeon, we recommend, as

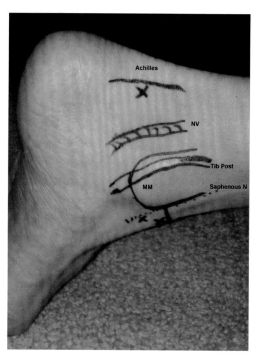

FIGURE 85.6. Medial aspect of the ankle in the prone position and the setting for hindfoot arthroscopy with location of the posteromedial, accessory medial, and anteromedial portals. NV, neurovascular bundle; MM, medial malleolus; N, nerve.

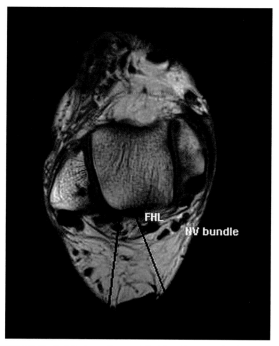

FIGURE 85.7. Axial view of an ankle MRI showing the location and direction of the posterior portals in hindfoot arthroscopy in relation to the Achilles tendon and the neurovascular structures. FHL, flexor hallucis longus; NV, neurovascular.

with any joint arthroscopy, a systematic way of examination in order to avoid missing any portions or pathology of the ankle joint. The dome of the talus presents a convexity in the anterior–posterior plane and a concavity in the medial–lateral plane. This particular morphology, as well as the inherent stability of the ankle joint, makes access to it more challenging than for some other joints.

The methodology and technique described in this chapter are performed with a 2.7-mm arthroscope and noninvasive ankle distraction (Fig. 85.8). Invasive ankle distraction through the use of calcaneal pin might also be utilized if needed (Figs. 85.9 and 85.10). Once the pathology has been identified and located, a change to the 4.0-mm arthroscope and release of the distraction may take

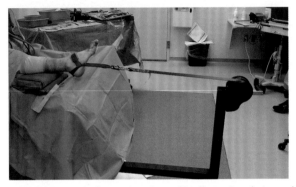

FIGURE 85.8. Setup for noninvasive ankle distraction during ankle arthroscopy using an ankle strap.

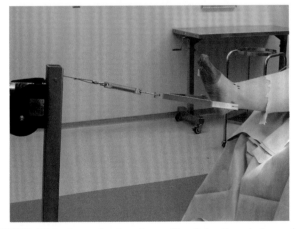

FIGURE 85.9. Setup for invasive ankle distraction during ankle arthroscopy.

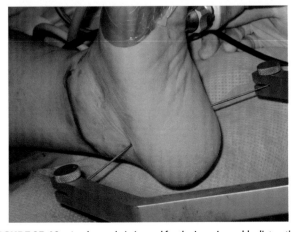

FIGURE 85.10. A calcaneal pin is used for the invasive ankle distraction.

place, particularly to relax the capsule anteriorly. Dowdy and colleagues (12) concluded that noninvasive distraction of 30 lb (13.6 kg) for less than 60 minutes is a safe setup to avoid injury to the nerves crossing the ankle joint.

Our preference is to begin with an anteromedial and anterolateral portals, with subsequent portals being created depending on the location of the pathology. As previously recommended by other authors (7, 13), the medial and lateral portals provide better visualization of the medial and lateral structures, respectively. In general, the arthroscope is inserted through the portal opposite to the pathology, and the working instruments are inserted through the portal on the same side of the pathology.

Anteromedial Portal

Through the anteromedial portal, the anterolateral part of the ankle joint is initially visualized. The junction of the anterior portion of the talus with the tibia superiorly and with the fibula laterally is inspected (Fig. 85.11). In this area, the intra-articular portion of the anterior inferior tibiofibular ligament (AITFL) is seen (Fig. 85.12). These fibers run obliquely at 45 degrees from above the articular portion of the distal tibia. An acute or chronic tear in the AITFL might be evaluated (Figs. 85.13 and 85.14). More anteriorly, the capsule inserts into the neck of the talus (Fig. 85.15). This area is difficult to assess if proper intra-articular pressure is not maintained, because the soft tissues collapse on themselves from lack of distention. More medially, the neck of the talus is inspected. Here can be visualized any anterior impingement between the neck of the talus and the anterior distal tibia (Fig. 85.16). Some erosion of the dorsal aspect of the neck of the talus created by the anterior margin of the distal tibia may be noticed. Osteophytes might be found over the anterior aspect of the tibia, with the anteromedial portion the most common location (Fig. 85.17). The capsule is reflected on intimate contact with the most superior portion of the osteophytes. This portion of the capsule must be peeled off before osteophyte removal.

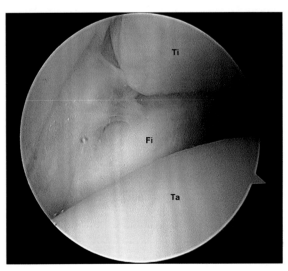

FIGURE 85.11. From anteromedial portal, view of tibiotalofibular junction.

VI. Foot and Ankle

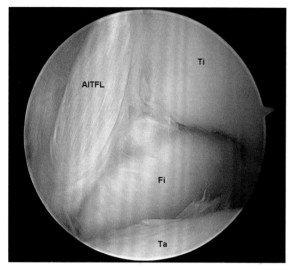

FIGURE 85.12. From anteromedial portal, view of AITFL.

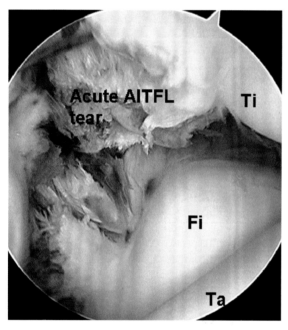

FIGURE 85.13. From anteromedial portal, view of acutely torn AITFL. Ti, tibia; Ta, talus; Fi, fibula.

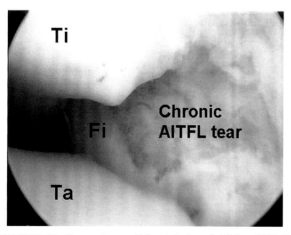

FIGURE 85.14. From anteromedial portal, view of deficient AITFL due to chronic tear.

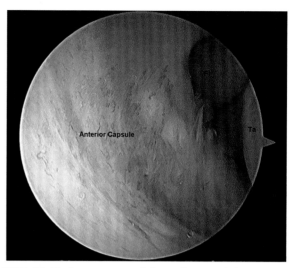

FIGURE 85.15. From anteromedial portal, view of the insertion of anterior capsule into the talus.

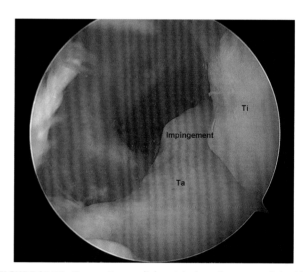

FIGURE 85.16. From anteromedial portal, view of anteromedial ankle impingement between the distal tibia and the talar neck.

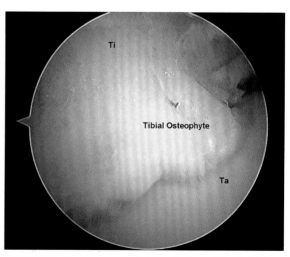

FIGURE 85.17. From anteromedial portal, view of distal tibial spiked osteophyte.

Next, the surgeon may proceed posteriorly to assess the syndesmosis and the relationship between the tibia and the fibula. A probe can be inserted between the tibia and the fibula to assess the widening of the syndesmosis (Figs. 85.18 and 85.19). In posttraumatic cases, some impingement of soft tissues at the most superior aspect of the syndesmosis may be seen. Wolin et al.(14) described this as the meniscoid lesion of the ankle. Posterior to this level, the intra-articular portion of the posterior inferior tibiofibular ligament is also seen (Fig. 85.20). The most posterior aspect of the talus, the distal tibia, and the posterior capsule are visualized (Fig. 85.21). Continuing from lateral to medial, the medial half of the posterior aspect of the tibiotalar joint is also inspected, and osteochondral

injuries are ruled out (Fig. 85.22). Most of the posttraumatic osteochondral lesions are found between the middle and the posterior thirds of the medial aspect of the dome of the talus (Fig. 85.23). The integrity of the medial wall of the body of the talus can be inspected, as can, more distally, the medial gutter (Fig. 85.24). Over the most distal portion of the gutter, the presence of loose bodies is ruled out, and the status of the deepest fibers of the deltoid ligament is evaluated (Fig. 85.25). Finally, moving anteriorly, the most anterior aspect of the medial malleolus may be seen (Fig. 85.26). On some occasions, an anterior spur is seen in intimate relationship with the anteromedial aspect of the capsule (Fig. 85.27). As described for the anterior impingement, some kissing lesions between the talus and

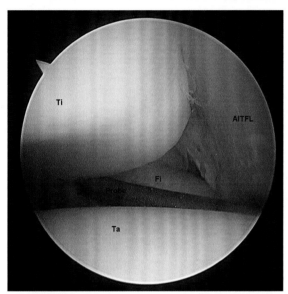

FIGURE 85.18. From anteromedial portal, assessment of the syndesmosis using a probe.

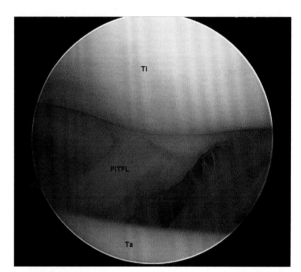

FIGURE 85.20. From anteromedial portal, view of posterior inferior tibiofibular ligament (PITFL).

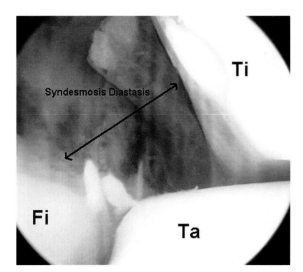

FIGURE 85.19. From anteromedial portal, view of syndesmosis diastasis.

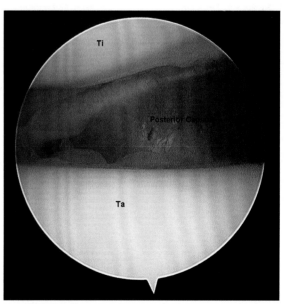

FIGURE 85.21. From anteromedial portal, view of the posterior aspect of the ankle joint with the posterior capsule.

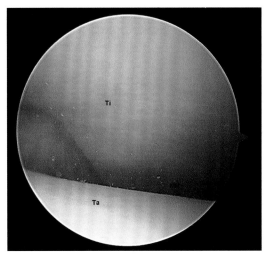

FIGURE 85.22. From anteromedial portal, view of the medial half of the posterior aspect of the tibiotalar joint.

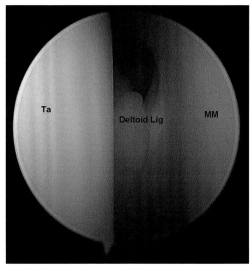

FIGURE 85.25. From anteromedial portal, view of the most distal portion of the medial gutter with intact deep deltoid ligament.

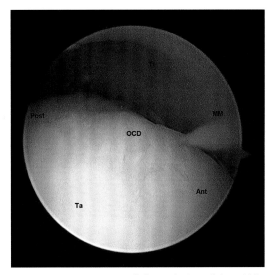

FIGURE 85.23. From anteromedial portal, view of the middle aspect of the medial talus with an OCD lesion.

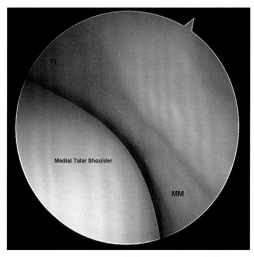

FIGURE 85.26. From anteromedial portal, view of the most anterior aspect of the medial malleolus and the medial talar shoulder.

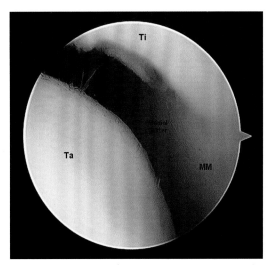

FIGURE 85.24. From anteromedial portal, view of the medial wall of the talus and the middle aspect of medial gutter.

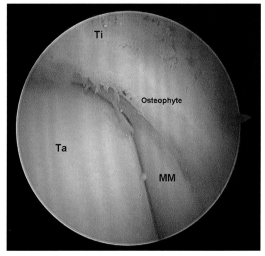

FIGURE 85.27. From anteromedial portal, view of impinging medial malleloar anterior osteophyte.

the medial malleolus may be seen during forced ankle dorsiflexion.

Anterolateral Portal

With the arthroscope in the anterolateral portal, the first area of inspection is the anteromedial aspect of the tibiotalar joint (Fig. 85.28) and the most dorsal aspect of the talus and its capsular insertion (Fig. 85.29). Talar osteophytes (Fig. 85.30) as well as Cam lesion of the talus is best seen and evaluated from this portal, and debridement is usually performed through the anteromedial portal (Figs. 85.31–85.34). A better visualization of the anterior aspect of the medial malleolus can also be achieved through this portal. It is usually easier to identify the presence of spurs along the medial malleolus and the medial distal tibia, as well as the amount

that must be removed for adequate debridement, using the anterior cortex of the medial malleolus as a reference point (Figs. 85.35 and 85.36).

From there, evaluation of the posterior half of the articular surface of the ankle joint is possible (Fig. 85.37). An Oste chondritis dessicans (OCD) lesion of the medial talar dome is usually visualized through this portal while the anteromedial portal is used as the working portal (Fig. 85.38). Once the most posterior portion of the lateral aspect of the ankle is reached, the posterior inferior tibiofibular ligament can be identified. This ligament may be clearly visualized with distinct fibers running obliquely from anterior to posterior. A synovial fold may be seen, which represents the intra-articular imprint of the transverse tibiofibular ligament (Fig. 85.39). Still moving

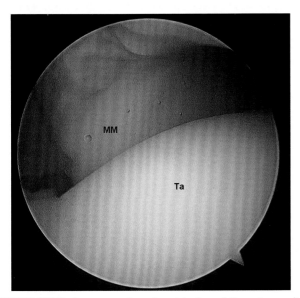

FIGURE 85.28. From anterolateral portal, view of the anteromedial aspect of the ankle joint.

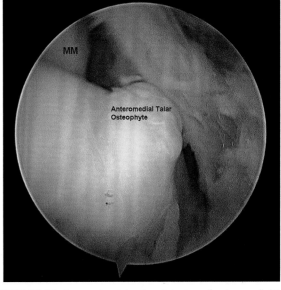

FIGURE 85.30. From anterolateral portal, view of anteromedial talar osteophyte.

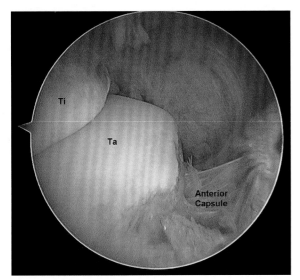

FIGURE 85.29. From anterolateral portal, view of the insertion of the anterior capsule into the talus.

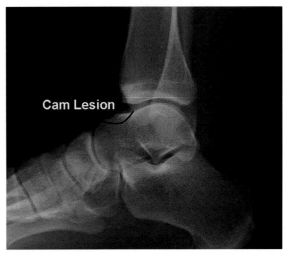

FIGURE 85.31. Lateral XR of the ankle showing Cam lesion of the talus.

VI. Foot and Ankle

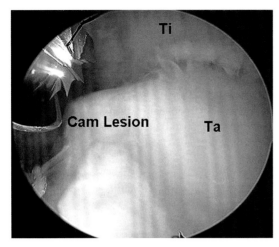

FIGURE 85.32. From anterolateral portal, view of Cam lesion of the talus.

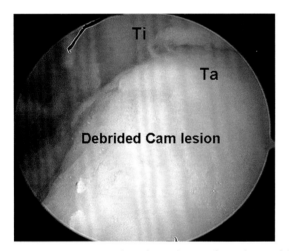

FIGURE 85.33. From anterolateral portal, view of Cam lesion of the talus after debridement.

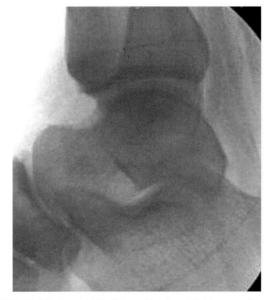

FIGURE 85.34. Lateral XR of the ankle after debridement of the Cam lesion of the talus.

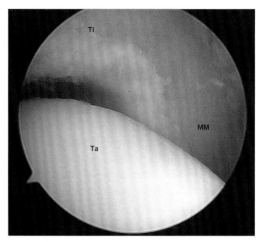

FIGURE 85.35. From anterolateral portal, view of the anterior aspect of the talus and the medial malleolus after osteophytes debridement.

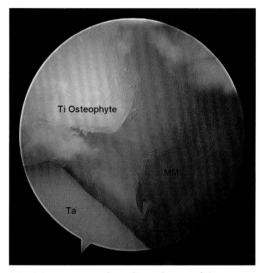

FIGURE 85.36. From anterolateral portal, view of the anterior cortex of the medial malleolus as a reference point for adequate debridement of the distal tibial impinging osteophytes.

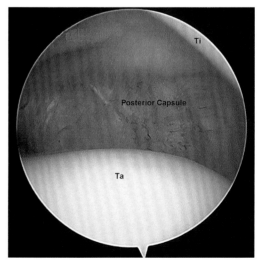

FIGURE 85.37. From anterolateral portal, view of the posterior aspect of the ankle joint.

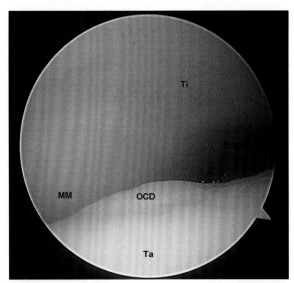

FIGURE 85.38. From anterolateral portal, view of the middle aspect of the medial talus with OCD lesion.

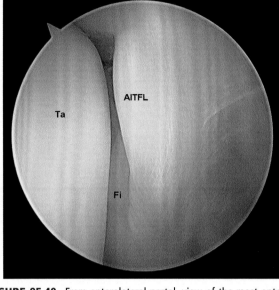

FIGURE 85.40. From anterolateral portal, view of the most anterior aspect of the lateral malleolus with intact AITFL fibers.

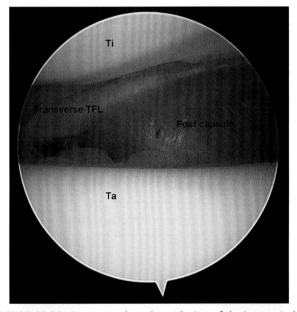

FIGURE 85.39. From anterolateral portal, view of the intra-articular imprint of the transverse tibiofibular ligament.

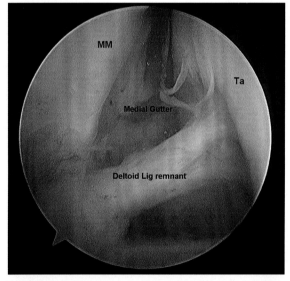

FIGURE 85.41. From accessory anteromedial portal, view of the most distal portion of medial gutter with deep deltoid ligament injury. Only attenuated remnant fibers of the ligament are left.

anteriorly, the syndesmosis is visualized and, specifically, the most distal portion of the lateral gutter, where the presence of loose bodies or soft tissue impingement from previous trauma must be ruled out as a source of pathology. Finally, the most inferior fibers of the AITFL are visualized as the inspection from this portal is concluded (Fig. 85.40).

Accessory Anterior Portals

In certain cases, it is necessary to create accessory portals for better access to the most distal portion of the respective gutters.

The accessory anteromedial portal provides exposure to the most distal fibers of the deltoid ligament (Fig. 85.41). Its placement is approximately 1 cm anterior and distal to the medial malleolus, and still medial to the tibialis anterior tendon. As mentioned earlier, loose bodies embedded in the synovial tissue or ossicles from previous trauma may be found and removed from this portal.

The accessory anterolateral portal allows better access with instruments to the lateral gutter (Fig. 85.42). It is located at the level of the tip of the distal malleolus

VI. Foot and Ankle

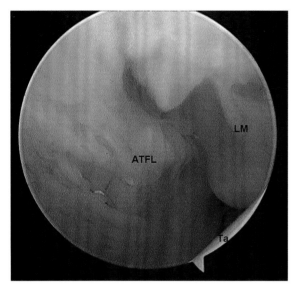

FIGURE 85.42. Anterolateral accessory portal gives better working access to the distal lateral gutter. ATFL, anterior talofibular ligament.

and 1 cm anterior to it. In addition, the anterior and posterior talofibular ligaments may be visualized from this portal although their integrity should be evaluated from a dynamic perspective rather than during arthroscopy.

Posterolateral Portal

Via a posterolateral portal, the posterior aspect of the lateral gutter is examined (Fig. 85.43) then the FHL tendon should be visualized medially and used as a medial boundary to protect the posteromedial neurovascular bundle

(Fig. 85.44). It is usually easier to enter the ankle joint below the transverse tibiofibular ligament after debriding part of the posterior capsule (Fig. 85.45). The fibers of the transverse tibiofibular ligament are intra-articular but extrasynovial and represent the most inferior portion of the posterior inferior tibiofibular ligament. The posterior lateral and posterior medial aspects of the tibiotalar joint are visualized and treated from this portal (Figs. 85.46 and 85.47).

Posteromedial Portal

Several authors (6, 9, 15) have discouraged the use of a posteromedial portal because of an increased risk of injury

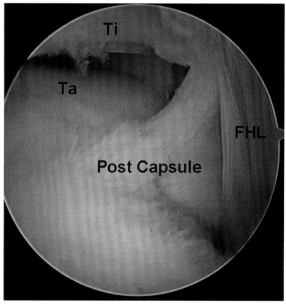

FIGURE 85.44. From posterolateral portal, view of the posterior aspect of the tibiotalar joint after debriding part of the posterior capsule to allow access to the joint. FHL, flexor hallucis longus.

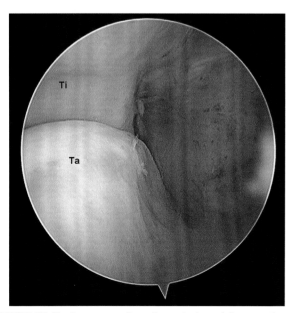

FIGURE 85.43. From posterolateral portal, view of the posterior aspect of the lateral gutter.

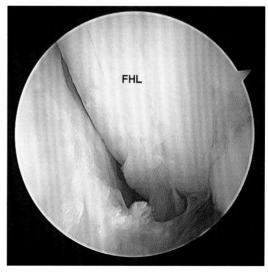

FIGURE 85.45. From posterolateral portal, view of the FHL tendon.

to the calcaneal nerve, a branch of the tibial nerve. Sitler et al. (3) concluded that the tibial nerve and calcaneal nerve branches remain safe if this portal is approached with the patient in a prone position, and adjacent to the medial border of the Achilles tendon. We believe that a postero-medial portal may be safely used to address posterior pathology. Before getting into the ankle joint, a virtual space can be created between the posterior capsule anteriorly and the pre-Achilles bursa posteriorly. In this space, the tendon sheath for the FHL may be appreciated medially, as may the presence of an os trigonum (Figs. 85.48). From this approach, this ossicle may be removed, although the posterior capsule must be violated during the resection, considering its intra-articular location (Fig. 85.49). This portal allows evaluation of the most medial and posterior aspect of the talus and distal tibia, and finally, the most posterior aspect of the medial gutter to rule out the presence of loose bodies (Fig. 85.50).

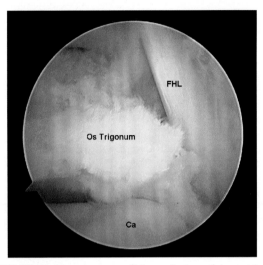

FIGURE 85.48. From posteromedial portal, view of an os trigonum abutting the FHL tendon.

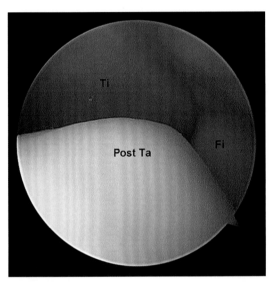

FIGURE 85.46. From posterolateral portal, view of the posterior lateral aspect of the tibiotalar joint.

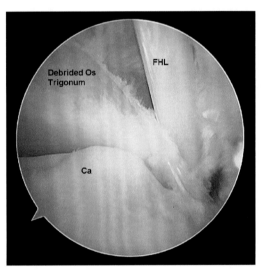

FIGURE 85.49. From posteromedial portal, view of the FHL tendon after debriding the OS trigonum.

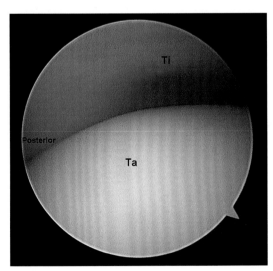

FIGURE 85.47. From posterolateral portal, view of the posterior medial aspect of the tibiotalar joint.

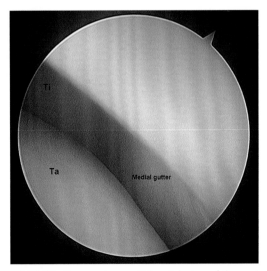

FIGURE 85.50. From posteromedial portal, view of the posterior aspect of the medial gutter.

VI. Foot and Ankle

REFERENCES

1. Burman MS. Arthroscopy or the direct visualization of joints. *J Bone Joint Surg Am.* 1931;13:669–695.

2. Guhl JF. *Ankle Arthroscopy.* Thorofare, NJ: SLACK Inc; 1988:1–6.

3. Ewing JW, Tasto JA, Tippett JW. Arthroscopic surgery of the ankle. *Instr Course Lect.* 1995;44:325–340.

4. Ferkel RD. *Arthroscopic Surgery: The Foot and Ankle.* Philadelphia, PA: Lippincott-Raven; 1996:85–103.

5. Sitler DF, Amendola A, Bailey CS, et al. *Posterior Ankle Arthroscopy: An Anatomic Study.* Presented at: 68th American Academy of Orthopaedic Surgery; March 4, 2001; San Francisco, CA. *J Bone Joint Surg Am.* May 2000.

6. Feiwell LA, Frey C. Anatomic study of arthroscopic portal sites of the ankle. *Foot Ankle.* 1993;14:142–147.

7. Drez D Jr, Guhl JF, Gollehon DL. Ankle arthroscopy: technique and indications. *Clin Sports Med.* 1982;1:35–45.

8. Ferkel RD, Heath DD, Guhl JF. Neurological complications of ankle arthroscopy. *Arthroscopy.* 1996;12:200–208.

9. Voto SJ, Ewing JW, Fleissner PR Jr, et al. Ankle arthroscopy: neurovascular and arthroscopic anatomy of standard and trans-Achilles tendon portal placement. *Arthroscopy.* 1989;5:41–46.

10. Sarrafian SK. Anatomy of the foot and ankle: descriptive, topographic, functional. Philadelphia, PA: Lippincott; 1993:356–374.

11. Horwitz MT. Normal anatomy and variations of the peripheral nerves of the leg and foot. *Arch Surg.* 1938;36:626.

12. Dowdy PA, Watson BV, Amendola A, et al. Noninvasive ankle distraction: relationship between force, magnitude of distraction, and nerve conduction abnormalities. *Arthroscopy.* 1996;12:64–69.

13. Carson WG, Andrews JR. Arthroscopy of the ankle. *Arthroscopy.* 1987;6:503–512.

14. Wolin I, Glassman F, Sideman S. Internal derangement of talofibular components of the ankle. *Surg Gynecol Obstet.* 1950;91:193–200.

15. Stetson WB, Ferkel RD. Ankle arthroscopy: I. Technique and complications. *J Am Acad Orthop Surg.* 1996;4:17–23.

Ankle Arthroscopy: Setup and Complications

James P. Tasto • Amar Arora • John H. Brady

The indications for ankle arthroscopy have broadened considerably over the past few decades as technologic advances have made the surgery safer and the results more predictable. Many ankle procedures that once required an extensive open approach followed by a prolonged recovery can now be effectively done arthroscopically. In many cases, this has resulted in decreased morbidity, preservation of soft-tissue structures, and generally a quicker return to function. However, ankle arthroscopy can still be fraught with minor as well as major complications. This chapter is dedicated to the proper setup for anterior ankle arthroscopy and the potential complications related to it. Hopefully, by thoroughly understanding the potential pitfalls, one can learn to avoid them.

ANTERIOR ARTHROSCOPY SETUP

Anterior ankle arthroscopy is considered the workhorse for most arthroscopic procedures of the foot and ankle. It is certainly the most common and many consider it the most routine. Still, the success of this procedure relies on careful preoperative planning, patient positioning, portal placement, and equipment management. The most common indications for anterior ankle arthroscopy include osteochondral lesions of the talus, soft-tissue impingement lesions, bony anterior impinging osteophytes, loose body removal, and arthroscopic ankle fusion. Specific details of these conditions and their treatments are not discussed in this chapter but are covered elsewhere.

Ankle arthroscopy is frequently performed under general anesthesia. This is both for patient comfort, as well for the added benefit of soft-tissue relaxation during distraction of the ankle. The patient is placed supine, and a thigh or calf tourniquet is placed onto the operative extremity. It should be noted that the use of a tourniquet is optional. The operative leg is then placed in a well-leg holder or on a bolster. The thigh should be secured in a slightly flexed position, with the end of the table flexed and the knee extended distally enough to prevent the table from interfering with possible posterior instrumentation if necessary (Fig. 86.1). The opposite leg must also be well padded and flexed at the hip to prevent femoral nerve injury. Next, the distraction device is secured according to the manufacture's specifications. Currently, there are

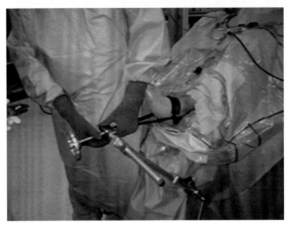

FIGURE 86.1. Demonstration of the correct patient position for anterior ankle arthroscopy. Note that both the hip and knee are placed in slight flexion.

multiple noninvasive ankle joint distraction devices available that securely attach to the foot of the operating table and use a foot strap and lever arm to provide gentle ankle distraction. This also affords the surgeon greater access to the ankle with minimal obstruction (Fig. 86.2). Noninvasive traction of up to 25 lb (11.3 kg) can be safely applied.

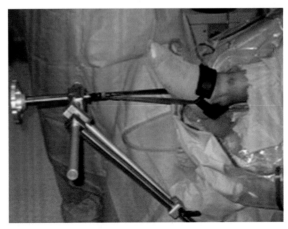

FIGURE 86.2. A distraction device secured to the end of the table will improve joint visibility during anterior ankle arthroscopy.

Special attention to inflow pressure and flow is also a crucial aspect of the ankle arthroscopy setup. Modern flow-regulated arthroscopic pumps enable the surgeon to carefully monitor soft-tissue fluctuations clinically, correlate this with pump pressure settings, and adjust them accordingly. Outflow can be managed through judicious use of a shaver and suction, or the use of a cannula. In addition, some authors routinely use the posterolateral portal to manage their outflow. Whichever technique the surgeon chooses, he or she must closely monitor flow dynamics and adjust them based on clinical observation to ensure safe soft-tissue management during ankle arthroscopy.

Planning ahead with the proper arthroscopic instruments will also help to make this procedure more routine. A 30°, 2.7-mm scope with the accompanying set of hand instruments including graspers, curettes, and baskets is necessary (Fig. 86.3). Smaller 2.0 mm scope sets are often too small and delicate for use in the ankle joint. They may bend or brake, and often do not provide the necessary inflow. However, they should be available for backup use in case the joint is excessively tight. Conversely, larger instruments often reserved for the shoulder or knee may be too large and may inadvertently cause iatrogenic damage to the articular surfaces. Either 3.5 or 2.0 mm arthroscopic shavers can be used according to surgeon preference, and joint tightness.

Prior to starting surgery, the extremity should be carefully examined. Outline the bony landmarks including the medial and lateral malleolar tips and the joint line. Next, carefully outline the neurovascular and tendinous structures anteriorly and posteriorly. Finally, mark the anticipated portals, anteromedial, anterolateral, and posterolateral if needed (Fig. 86.4).

The anteromedial portal is established just medial to the anterior tibialis tendon at the level of the joint line. An 18G spinal needle is introduced and directed toward the center of the joint and 10 mL of normal saline is injected. Proper placement of the spinal needle in the joint is confirmed by distention of the joint capsule medially and laterally and by return of fluid through the spinal needle (Fig. 86.5). Although this area is free from major neurovascular structures, this portal must be placed as medial to the tendon as possible. Placement of this portal too medial will limit access and visualization of the medial gutter. Once the appropriate location is identified, use a no. 11 blade scalpel to make a vertical 5-mm incision through the skin only. Use a hemostat to spread soft tissues down to the joint capsule using the "nick and spread" technique. This is followed by placement of the blunt trochar and cannula, thus establishing the anteromedial portal through which the scope is introduced.

The anterolateral portal is established after inserting the scope medially. Injury to the superficial peroneal nerve or its branches is one of the primary risks of anterior ankle arthroscopy (Fig. 86.6). This risk can be reduced by marking the path of the nerve preoperatively, and by

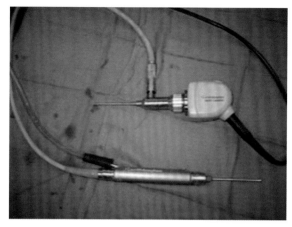

FIGURE 86.3. A 2.7-mm arthroscope accompanied by a 2.0-mm shaver will help decrease the risk of iatrogenic injury to the articular surface during ankle arthroscopy.

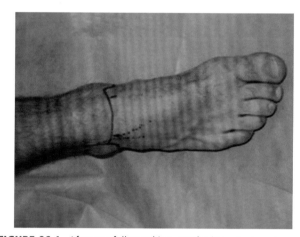

FIGURE 86.4. After carefully marking out the important anatomy of the ankle, the medial portal is placed just medial to the Tibialis anterior tendon, and the lateral portal is adjacent to the Peroneus tertius tendon.

transilluminating the joint through the medial portal to attempt to visualize the nerve and its branches. With the foot slightly plantarflexed and adducted, the nerve can often be located coursing toward the fourth toe. The portal is then established lateral to the peroneus tertius carefully using a similar "nick and spread" technique.

POSTERIOR ARTHROSCOPY SETUP

Posterior ankle arthroscopy is a useful tool for evaluating and treating pathologic conditions of the posterior ankle joint and its related structures. The most common indications include posterior impingement often associated with the os trigonum and the flexor hallucis, Haguland deformity correction and subtalar arthrodesis. It is best preformed with the patient in the prone position, with a bump under the distal tibia to elevate the foot. Distraction may or may not be necessary depending on how

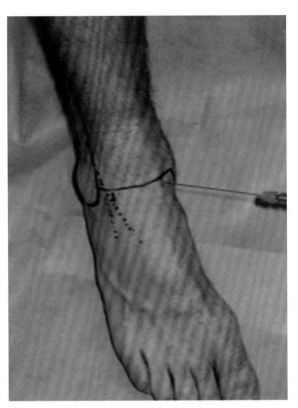

FIGURE 86.5. After identifying the appropriate landmarks, an 18G spinal needle is introduced through the medial portal site and the ankle joint is distended.

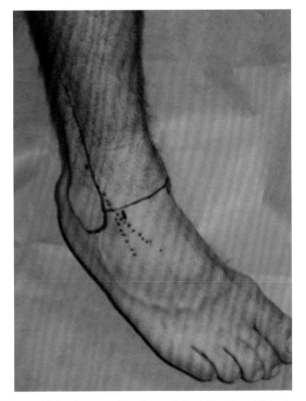

FIGURE 86.6. The anterolateral portal should be placed 2 to 4 mm lateral to the peroneus tertious tendon. This will decrease the risk of iatrogenic injury to the superficial peroneal nerve.

much visualization is needed. When working outside the joint capsule, a large bore arthroscope is helpful because it provides the flow necessary for using a larger 4.5 mm shaver. As with anterior ankle arthroscopy, pump pressures should be kept as low as clinically possible (40 to 50 mm Hg) to prevent excessive extravasation.

The medial and lateral borders of Achilles tendon are the primary landmarks for portal placement during posterior ankle arthroscopy. The portals are usually placed approximately 1 cm proximal to the level of the distal tip of the fibula, immediately adjacent to the Achilles tendon using the "nick and spread" technique. Anatomic studies have demonstrated that precise portal placement will be 6 to 7 mm from the tibial nerve and 3 to 4 mm from the sural nerve (1). Great care, therefore, should always be used when considering posterior ankle arthroscopy.

ANKLE ARTHROSCOPY COMPLICATIONS

A thorough understanding of the surface anatomy of the foot and ankle is mandatory for the prevention of the myriad of potential complications associated with ankle arthroscopy. The overall complication rate with ankle arthroscopy has been reported to be anywhere between 9% and 17% (2–6, 15). Broadly, complications of ankle arthroscopy can be divided into surgical and postoperative complications (Table 86.1). One of the most preventable complications is an improper diagnosis prior to undertaking ankle arthroscopy. If ankle arthroscopy is being considered one must understand that there are both intraarticular as well as extraarticular causes. Isolated lateral ankle pain without instability, subtalar pathology, occult talar process fractures, tendinopathies, and tendon tears may be playing a role in the patient's symptoms. Isolated ankle arthroscopy in these settings may not be the best treatment option. A careful physical examination, appropriate imaging studies, differential injections, and a detailed history will help differentiate between diagnoses that may be helped with ankle arthroscopy. Arthroscopy should not supercede the role of a careful history and physical examination.

Neurologic complications account for the large majority of reported arthroscopic complications. The superficial peroneal nerve is most commonly at risk for injury, especially during the establishment of the anterolateral portal. This nerve and its branches lie superficially around the anterolateral ankle and should be identified prior to portal placement. The superficial peroneal nerve divides into the medial dorsal cutaneous nerve and the intermediate dorsal cutaneous nerve proximal to the fibula. As the intermediate dorsal cutaneous nerve crosses the ankle, it runs anterior to the common extensor tendons toward the area between the third and fourth metatarsals. At that point, this nerve divides into its terminal dorsal digital branches. The medial dorsal cutaneous nerve runs anterior to the common extensor tendons at the ankle before it runs lateral to the extensor hallucis longus tendon and eventually

Table 86.1

Complications of ankle arthroscopy

Surgical complications

Inappropriate diagnosis

Neurovascular injuries

Tendon injuries

Ligament injuries

Articular cartilage injuries

Radiofrequency related injuries

Instrument breakage

Compartment ischemia/syndrome

Fluid-management complications

Distraction-related complications

Intraoperative fractures

Inadequate resection of osteophytes

Excessive soft-tissue resection

Inadequate debridement of OCD lesions

Arthroscopic ankle fusion technical errors

Postoperative complications

Tourniquet complications

Wound complications/incisional pain/fistula formation

Infection—superficial and deep

Hemarthrosis

Postoperative effusion

Regional pain syndrome

Postoperative fracture/stress fracture

Joint stiffness/arthrofibrosis

Deep vein thrombosis

divides into its terminal dorsal digital nerves. Ferkel et al. (3) reported complications involving the superficial peroneal nerve accounting for 56% of all neurologic complications. The sural nerve, greater saphenous nerve, and the deep peroneal nerve are all at risk and proper technique for portal establishment is necessary to avoid neurologic complications. The use of the "nick and spread" technique for portal placement can help avoid potential neurologic complications. In most reported cases, issues with neurologic complications resolved within 6 months (3).

Proper placement of portals is also necessary to avoid potential vascular complications. Although rare,

pseudoaneurysm of the anterior tibial artery after ankle arthroscopy has been reported in five cases in the literature (3, 7, 9, 10, 12, 14). Anatomic variations of the artery can lead to increased incidence of injury when creating standard portals. The incidence of anatomic variations has been reported to run between 1.5% and 12% in the literature. In general, the nick and spread technique for the establishment of arthroscopic ankle portals can safely reduce neurovascular complications. With this technique, a vertical incision is made over the portal site only through the most superficial layers of the skin and dermis. Deeper layers are penetrated safely with the use of a mosquito clamp, and the joint is accessed with the use of a blunt trocar. Injecting the ankle with 8 to 10 mL of saline prior to portal establishment may help identify relative anatomy and help reduce iatrogenic injury to neurovascular structures. In addition, avoidance of the anterocentral and posteromedial portals, except in the most necessary cases, can reduce the possibility of vascular injuries. If there are any questions about anomalous arterial anatomy, the use of preoperative vascular studies or intraoperative Doppler studies may be helpful. One should also be careful when using noninvasive distraction techniques with ankle arthroscopy. Incorrect placement of anterior strap may cause unwanted compression of the anterior tibial artery as well as branches of the superficial peroneal nerve. This may increase possibility of iatrogenic injury of the anterior tibial artery during ankle arthroscopy especially when performing a synovectomy of the ankle (10). In addition, while performing anterior synovectomy of the ankle, one must be cognizant of the position of the foot. With plantar flexion of the ankle, the anterior structures become tight and care must be taken when the performing anterior ankle procedures. Dorsiflexing the ankle or releasing traction during these procedures will help prevent iatrogenic injury to the anterior neurovascular structures.

Infection is a potentially devastating complication that can be reduced by adhering to established arthroscopic surgical techniques. Ferkel et al. reported infection accounting for 18% (n = 10) of all types of complications. Barber et al. (2) reported an overall 17% complication rate with ankle arthroscopy with infection accounting for 33% (n = 3) of all types of complications. Deep infections have been reported in the literature to be anywhere between 0.1% and 10%. Various risk factors have been postulated to contribute to superficial and deep infections. Damage to the thin subcutaneous tissue with repetitive instrument use, prolonged arthroscopy times, and comorbid risk factors can all be potential causative factors. In addition, fistula formation has been reported in the literature as a potential complication of ankle arthroscopy (Fig. 86.7). Many theories have been proposed for the cause of this complications including excessive soft-tissue resection during ankle arthroscopy, possible use of tape for portal closure instead of sutures, limited distance between portal sites, and early mobilization following ankle arthroscopy.

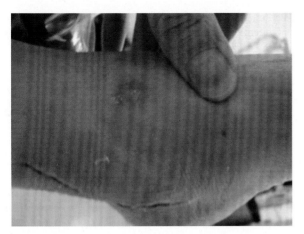

FIGURE 86.7. Fistula formation following ankle arthroscopy.

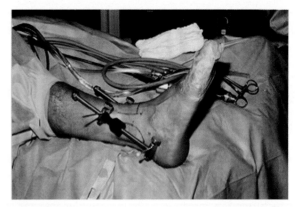

FIGURE 86.8. Invasive distraction of the ankle during ankle arthroscopy.

The use of prophylactic preoperative antibiotics may help reduce the incidence of deep or superficial infections though the literature has yet to show definitive evidence.

Fluid management is an extremely important part of ankle arthroscopy. One can use both gravity assisted or pump-based systems to help with fluid delivery. We prefer to use a pump-based system so that we can monitor the pressure and flow to the ankle. Fluid-based complications can range from prolonged ankle swelling following ankle arthroscopy to compartment syndrome of the foot or lower extremity. Compartment syndrome has rarely been reported in the literature following ankle arthroscopy. Imade et al. (8) reported one case of compartment syndrome following ankle arthroscopy in the treatment of an acute Maisonneuve fracture. Excessive extravasation of fluid during ankle arthroscopy may be a potential risk factor for the development of compartment syndrome. In addition, perioperative position of the lower extremity may be a contributing factor to the development of compartment syndrome (11, 13). In addition to the potential risk of compartment syndrome, one should be cognizant of the development of deep vein thrombosis in the lower extremity following ankle arthroscopy. This complication has been reported and its development must be watched in the perioperative period. Close monitoring of the lower extremity following ankle arthroscopy is merited. Postoperative swelling of the ankle is common for ankle arthroscopy and initial management with elevation, compression, and the use of ice may help reduce immediate postoperative swelling (15).

The use of distraction can also increase the chances of complications (Fig. 86.8). Invasive distraction has been associated with the incidence of intraoperative fractures secondary to pin placement or secondary postoperative stress fractures of the tibia and fibula (15). Ferkel has reported transient pin-tract pain that resolved uneventfully when using invasive techniques (15). Noninvasive distraction can theoretically increase the chance of neurovascular compression especially with the use of the anterior ankle strap. Newer techniques have been introduced that avoid the use of invasive and noninvasive distraction techniques. Instead, these techniques rely on dorsiflexion and plantar flexion of the ankle to gain access to different compartments (16). It is possible that the use of nondistraction techniques in certain situations may reduce the potential complications associate with distraction while still allowing for successful arthroscopic ankle surgery.

Various radiofrequency devices are available for use in arthroscopy. Radiofrequency devices can be used to treat many disorders specific in ankle arthroscopy including synovitis, chondral lesions, arthofibrosis, and instability. Although few complications have been reported with the use of radiofrequency in the ankle, long-term studies are still needed to verify its safety and efficacy. Potential complications have been reported including articular cartilage damage, persistent pain, and possible burns (Fig. 86.9).

Technical errors during surgery may lead to poor results following ankle arthroscopy. Inappropriate screw placement or inadequate cartilage resection during arthroscopically aided ankle arthrodesis may lead to lower fusion rates. Inadequate resection of OsteoChondritis

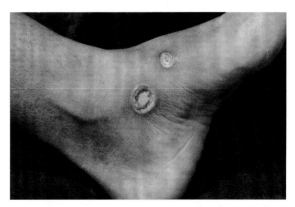

FIGURE 86.9. Remote thermal burn on the contralateral ankle following ankle arthroscopy and the use of a radiofrequency device.

Dessicans (OCD) lesions can occur. This may occur when treating posteromedial-based lesions. Taking extratime, using various instruments to be certain that a stable resection has been created and possibly changing portals for both instruments and for the arthroscope can help minimize this problem. Inadequate resection of osteophytes, especially from the anterior tibiotalar joint, may lead to persistent pain following ankle arthroscopy. Direct visualization of the osteophyte or assistance from the use of fluoroscopy may help reassure the surgeon that the entire symptomatic osteophyte has been removed. Other reported complications include instrument failure, ligament/tendon injury, iatrogenic articular damage, incisional pain, and postoperative regional pain syndrome. Careful preoperative planning, knowledge of proper techniques, and experience of the surgeon can limit technical complications of ankle arthroscopy.

REFERENCES

1. Amendola A, Lee KB, Saltzman CL, et al. Technique and early experience with posterior arthroscopic subtalar arthrodesis. *Foot Ankle Int.* 2007;28:298–302.
2. Barber FA, Click J, Britt BT. Complications of ankle arthroscopy. *Foot Ankle.* 1990;10:263.
3. Darwish A, Ehsan O, Marynissen H, et al. Pseudoaneurysm of the anterior tibial artery after ankle arthroscopy. *Arthroscopy.* 2004;20(6):63–64.
4. Ferkel RD, Heath DD, Guhl JF. Neurological complications of ankle arthroscopy. *Arthroscopy.* 1996;12(2):200–208.
5. Ferkel RD, Scranton PE. Current concepts review: arthroscopy of the ankle and foot. *J Bone Joint Surg Am.* 1993;75:1233.
6. Ferkel RD, Karzel RP, Del Pizzo W. Arthroscopic treatment of anterolateral impingement of the ankle. *Am J Sports Med.* 1991;19:440–446.
7. Jang EC, Kwak BK, Song KW, et al. Pseudoaneurysm of the anterior tibial artery after ankle arthroscopy treated with ultrasound-guided compression therapy: a case report. *J Bone Joint Surg Am.* 2008;90:2235–2239.
8. Imade S, Takao M, Miyamoto W, et al. Leg anterior compartment syndrome following ankle arthroscopy after Maisonneuve fracture. *Arthroscopy.* 2009;25(2):215–218.
9. Kotwal RS, Acharya A, O-Doherty D. Anterior tibial artery pseudoaneurysm in a patient with hemophilia: a complication of ankle arthroscopy. *J Foot Ankle Surg.* 2007;46:314–316.
10. Mariani PP, Mancini L, Giorgini TL. Pseudoaneurysm as a complication of ankle arthroscopy. *Arthroscopy.* 2001;17:400–402.
11. Meyer RS, White KK, Smith JM, et al. Intramuscular and blood pressures in legs positioned in the hemilithotomy position: clarification of risk factors for well-leg acute compartment syndrome. *J Bone Joint Surg Am.* 2002;84-A:1829–1835.
12. O'Farrell D, Dudeney S, McNally S, et al. Pseudoaneurysm formation after ankle arthroscopy. *Foot Ankle Int.* 1997;18:578–579.
13. Olson SA, Glasgow RR. Acute compartment syndrome in lower extremity musculoskeletal trauma. *J Am Acad Orthop Surg.* 2005;13(7):436–444.
14. Salgado CJ, Mukherjee D, Quist MA, et al. Anterior tibial artery pseudoaneurysm after ankle arthroscopy. *Cardiovasc Surg.* 1998;6:604–606.
15. Stetson WB, Ferkel RD. Ankle arthroscopy: I. Technique and complications. *J Am Acad Orthop Surg.* 1996;4:17–23.
16. Van Dijk CN, van Bergen CJ. Advancements in ankle arthroscopy. *J Am Acad Orthop Surg.* 2008;16(11):635–646.

Subtalar Arthroscopy

John E. Femino

CLINICAL EVALUATION

History

Patients with subtalar joint pain commonly complain of the lateral hindfoot or posterior ankle pain, since most pathologies involve the posterior facet. Infrequently, medial hindfoot pain may be related to the subtalar joint. Two examples would be medial subtalar coalition and ganglion cysts from the subtalar joint causing impingement on the posteromedial soft tissue structures such as the tarsal tunnel or flexor hallucis longus (FHL).

Pain is typically worse with walking and running on uneven surfaces such as grass. Cutting sports are likely to aggravate lateral pain in the foot that is planted, since this when the subtalar joint is maximally everted, a position of subtalar joint impingement of the anterior and lateral posterior facet. Some sports, such as soccer, gymnastics, and dance, may have non weight-bearing motions that can aggravate subtalar joint problems. Pain may also be made worse with climbing stairs as this involves the extremes of ankle and subtalar motion.

A history of trauma or inversion injury is common in athletes presenting with subtalar joint problems. Inversion injury mechanisms place the subtalar joint in a position where joint congruence contributes the least to joint stability and therefore most of the joint stabilization is provided by ligamentous constraints. Under these conditions, ligamentous stabilizers can yield to excessive tensile load and result in tearing of intra-articular ligaments, which can lead to soft tissue impingement lesions.

Physical Examination

Diagnosis of pathologies around the ankle and subtalar joint can be difficult since very many structures are close together. Successful arthroscopic treatments depend on precise diagnosis of a patient's cause of pain. Physical examination of the leg, ankle, and foot should always be performed together since many of the major soft tissue structures around the ankle and hindfoot pass longitudinally from the leg and are redirected by the retinacula and bony gliding surfaces as these structures terminate in the foot. Superficial examination of the skin, sensation, and palpation for pulses can be done by inspection and light palpation without exacerbating painful intra-articular conditions. Neurogenic causes of pain such as neuropraxia of the superficial peroneal nerve or complex regional pain syndrome, which can occur after ankle injuries, should be ruled out.

Examination of muscle strength testing the extrinsic muscles that move the ankle, hindfoot, and toes should be performed. Aggravation of symptoms with resisted active motions can help to further localize pain and reveal adjacent problems such as tendonitis or peroneal tendon instability at the superior peroneal retinaculum.

Evaluation of passive motions of the ankle, subtalar joint, and transverse tarsal joints can reveal any limitation of motion such as with a subtalar coalition.

Palpation of the ankle and foot is the key to pinpointing painful structures. Thorough knowledge of the musculoskeletal anatomy will help the examiner to identify specific painful structures beneath the skin. The ability to decipher the anterolateral ankle recess, lateral ankle gutter, and the anterior and lateral joint lines of the posterior subtalar facet is essential, yet all of these periarticular locations are within a few centimeters of each other. Impingement is a common pathology of the subtalar joint and ankle, and a positive impingement test is very helpful in localizing pain. Each joint has a unique motion that ranges from an open to a closed position. Pressure over a joint in the open position is held while the joint is moved to a closed position recreating the impingement event. Locations of soft tissue impingement include the posteromedial ankle, posterior ankle, lateral aspect of the posterior facet of the subtalar joint, anterior joint line of the posterior facet (sinus tarsi), the anterolateral ankle recess and lateral gutter, and the anteromedial ankle recess and gutter.

The impingement tests for the anterior and lateral subtalar joint posterior facet are distinct in location. The anterior subtalar impingement test is performed by placing the subtalar joint in the open position of plantarflexion and inversion. Mild to moderate digital pressure over the sinus tarsi displaces redundant soft tissue into the joint line. With digital pressure held at a constant pressure, the hindfoot is everted while the ankle is dorsiflexed, thus closing the subtalar joint. If the patient's stated pain is reproduced, it is typically a clear diagnosis. Occasionally, the impingement may be more subtle, and repeated gentle impingement maneuvers may recreate the pain more gradually. Crepitus can be felt at the moment of impingement and coincides with reproduction of the patient's pain.

Flexor hallucis longus (FHL) stenosis is a condition that occurs at the level of the posteromedial subtalar joint where the posterior tibiotalar ligament attaches onto the trigonal process of the talus. This fibro-osseous tunnel can be an area of stenosis of a low-lying FHL muscle belly that occurs near the distal limit of FHL excursion in dorsiflexion of the ankle and first metatarsophalangeal (MTP) joints. Other possible causes of pain at this level include posttraumatic bony irregularity from a posteromedial tubercle fracture of the talus, an unstable or irregular os trigonum or a medial subtalar coalition. The test FHL stenosis is performed with the ankle in neutral and the first metatarsal head supported to simulate standing in foot flat stance. The first MTP joint is isolated and dorsiflexed. In cases of stenosis, this motion is severely limited to 10° or less. The limitation of dorsiflexion is resolved with ankle plantarflexion unlike hallux rigidus where there is a bony block to dorsiflexion. Palpation of FHL under tension and without tension will elicit greater pain with the tendon under tension. Posteromedial ankle soft tissue impingement can be differentiated from FHL symptoms because tension on the tendon will shield the posteromedial ankle gutter and ankle neutral open the posterior ankle joint.

Evaluation for instability of ankle and subtalar joint is performed with the patient seated and relaxed. Stability testing should be done moderately, not suddenly. The patient should be informed of the purpose of the maneuvers to avoid surprise. Sudden forceful maneuvers will often alarm patients and may elicit unnecessary pain and apprehension. The resulting splinting by the patients muscles will confound any further diagnostic examination efforts. Lateral ankle instability and subtalar joint instability can be difficult to differentiate by physical examination. Subtalar instability can be diagnosed when the ankle is stable, but is not reliably diagnosed with an unstable ankle since gross motion of an unstable ankle is much greater than the gross motion of an unstable subtalar joint. Also, the stresses for testing the two joints are similar and therefore the ankle joint instability masks instability of the subtalar joint. Testing for lateral ankle instability traditionally has been described by using two tests, anterior drawer and talar tilt. Instability, however, is actually elicited best by a combination of these forces that recreates the mechanism of injury with inversion ankle injuries. This is done by placing the stabilizing hand on the distal tibia in such a way that the long finger can be used to palpate lateral gutter of the ankle between the fibula and the talus. Anterolateral rotatory stress with inversion stress is performed with the ankle in plantarflexion. As the stress is applied, and if instability exists, the gap

of the lateral gutter will be felt to widen. Comparison with the unaffected side will also make it apparent that the depth of palpation into the lateral gutter is greater than normal, indicating deficiency of the anterior talofibular ligament (ATFL). Often this stress will elicit pain and/or apprehension. Tilting of the talus with inversion stress will be pronounced with combined deficiency of the calcaneofibular ligament (CFL). Subtalar instability is identified when talar tilt alone elicits gross increase of inversion in the setting of a stable ankle. In such cases where the lateral subtalar joint opens, there is likely combined deficiency of the CFL and the interosseous talocalcaneal ligament (ITCL).

Imaging

Radiographs of foot and ankle are important for assessing the normal shape and alignment of the talus and calcaneus. Alignment of the hindfoot can demonstrate deformity such as lateral subluxation of the subtalar joint in a flat foot. Radiographs or CT scan can also demonstrate degenerative joint changes, peritalar fractures, bony irregularities such as a symptomatic trigonal process or os trigonum, subtalar coalitions, and bony variations such as an accessory facet of the lateral talar process, which can contribute to subtalar impingement in the sinus tarsi (Fig. 87.1).

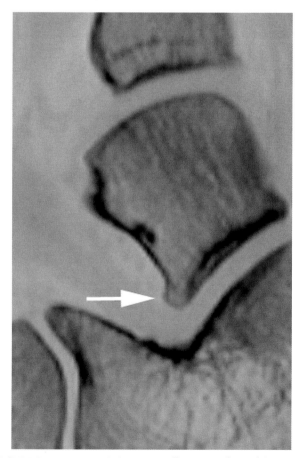

FIGURE 87.1. Arrow pointing to a small accessory facet of the lateral talar process that contributes to anterior impingement in the sinus tarsi.

MRI is helpful for demonstrating an effusion of the subtalar joint, which is not easily seen on plain radiographs. Bone marrow edema can be seen as an indicator of bony impingement as with an accessory facet, an unstable os trigonum, or medial subtalar coalition. FHL tenosynovitis can be evidenced by increased peritendinous fluid signal behind the talus (Fig. 87.2). Peroneal tendon pathology can be assessed as well and may be included in any operative planning. MRI can also help to identify occult masses such as ganglion cysts or other tumors. Subchondral cysts or osteochondral lesions may be identified.

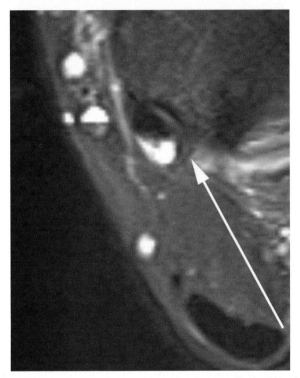

FIGURE 87.2. Axial T2-weighted MRI demonstrates fluid within the sheath of the FHL. The *arrow* points to the fibrous bands attaching to the trigonal process of the talus, which create the entrance to the FHL tunnel. The *arrow* indicates also the direct line from the posterolateral portal through which a shaver can be placed to release this from the talus.

Dynamic ultrasound can be useful for evaluating causes of periarticular pain such as peroneal tendon pathology or instability.

CT scanning can be helpful in both diagnosis and preoperative planning can detect osseous abnormalities such as occult peritalar fractures and other periarticular bony irregularities, which can be amenable to arthroscopic debridement. Improving software can provide three-dimensional surface rendered CT scans to add to the precision of preoperative planning (Fig. 87.3).

Finally, intra-articular contrast can add to the level of diagnostic accuracy for some pathologies such as loose bodies. However, extravasation of dye can also hinder evaluation of some periarticular soft tissue pathologies such as FHL tenosynovitis.

TREATMENT

Nonoperative treatment of subtalar joint pain includes short-term immobilization, ice and anti-inflammatory modalities such as nonsteroidal anti-inflammatory drugs (NSAIDs) and steroid injections, all of which may calm synovitis of the subtalar joint. However, most pathologies that are amenable to subtalar arthroscopy are mechanical in nature and, therefore, are not likely to be resolved in the long term by these nonoperative means. Malalignment due to flat foot should always be considered as a possible underlying cause. Correction with custom medial forefoot posted orthoses or surgical realignment may be necessary to correct overpronation.

OPERATIVE INDICATIONS

Most patients with symptoms suggestive of subtalar joint pathology have a history of injury such as inversion injuries or fractures of the ankle, talus, or calcaneus. Therefore, many of these patients have had either operative or nonoperative treatment for their injuries, and present in a delayed fashion after reasonable efforts of nonoperative treatment. Persistent pain referable to the subtalar joint should lead to an appropriate examination and diagnostic workup. Operative indications can include synovitis,

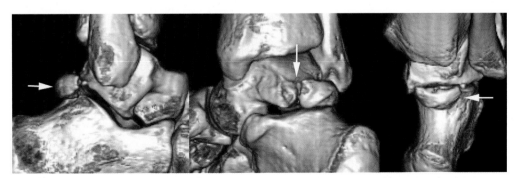

FIGURE 87.3. A sequence of three-dimensional CT reconstructions showing in detail the anatomy of an os trigonum. This is helpful in preoperative planning for prone arthroscopic excision.

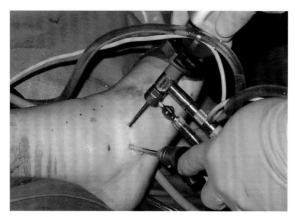

FIGURE 87.4. Supine subtalar arthroscopy is performed through the anterolateral and lateral portals providing good access to pathology in the anterior and lateral regions of the posterior subtalar facet. The lateral portal can also be used to visualize the peroneal tendons.

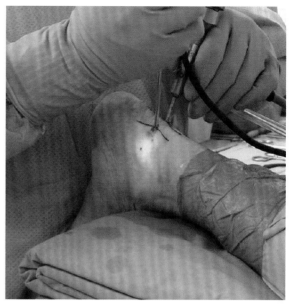

FIGURE 87.5. Prone arthroscopy is performed through paramedian portals placed on either side of the Achilles tendon providing direct access to the posterior ankle and subtalar joints.

arthrofibrosis, cartilagenous lesions, and bony impingement in the sinus tarsi, subfibular region, or posterior talar region (1–15). In addition, cases of early degenerative joint disease may not be apparent by radiographic techniques (4, 16, 15). The role of diagnostic subtalar arthroscopy should be a consideration, especially in the presence of combined ankle symptoms, such as instability and impingement (3, 4, 5, 11, 15). In most reports, the focus of treatment has centered on the sinus tarsi or anterior joint space of the posterior facet of the subtalar joint, which is the most common site of pain referable to the subtalar joint. Soft tissue impingement due to torn ligaments and/or synovitis in this area is a common diagnosis. Underlying anatomic variation of the anterior aspect of the lateral talar process may contribute to impingement due to an accessory facet in this location (17). The supine semilateral approach to the subtalar joint is the most expeditious, and consists mainly of the anterolateral and lateral portals (Fig. 87.4). In the posterior talar region there is, by nature of the anatomy of the talus, confluence of the ankle and subtalar joints. Posterior periarticular causes of pain such as an os trigonum, FHL stenosis/tenosynovitis, and different types of posterior soft tissue impingement can be approached by using a posterolateral and lateral portal (14) but are more directly seen and treated by the prone posterior arthroscopic approach, which allows more direct evaluation and treatment of posterior pathologies of the ankle and subtalar joints (Fig. 87.5) (13, 15). The immediate use of subtalar arthroscopy for fractures, such as those of the calcaneus, is an evolving and promising technique (18–20).

Loose bodies are a well-accepted indication for arthroscopic surgery in a number of joints including the shoulder, elbow, knee, and ankle. They are, however, relatively uncommon in the subtalar joint. The normal subtalar joint, in the absence of external distraction forces, has such tightly apposed articular surfaces that there is essentially no room for a loose body to become interposed. A grossly unstable subtalar joint could have a loose body

interposed in the joint. Periarticular bony fragments or prominences are more likely causes of subtalar symptoms by impingement. There are relatively few reported cases of loose body excision with subtalar arthroscopy (4, 5, 15). Two of these series reported one case each out of a combined 41 patients who underwent operative subtalar arthroscopy. Neither of these reports described the location of the loose body. The third report had three cases of loose bodies out of 18 patients. This study specified that the loose bodies were located in the posterior recess of the subtalar joint, along the margin of the posterior joint. None of these studies report patient histories of catching or locking suggesting that this diagnosis is more of a periarticular problem.

A painful os trigonum is a well-established pathology in ballet dancers, athletes, and nonathletes that involves the subtalar joint, the ankle joint, and the FHL tendon at the entrance to the fibro-osseous tunnel at the posteromedial ankle and subtalar joint (21–23). The association with FHL stenosis in diagnosis can in practical terms be assumed and clinically both are treated with excision of the os trigonum, which effectively releases the posterior tibiotalar fibers of the superficial Deltoid ligament that create the proximal FHL tunnel at the posteromedial subtalar joint (12). Endoscopic excision of the os trigonum and release of the proximal FHL tunnel have been described with the lateral subtalar arthroscopic technique; but more recently, the prone endoscopic technique using posteromedial and posterolateral portals has been reported to be very effective and safe (1, 12, 15). The efficacy of this approach for improved visualization and direct access to posterior pathologies has also been demonstrated anatomically (24). While this technique has been shown to be safe and effective by surgeons well experienced with this technique, the proximity of the posteromedial neurovascular bundle warrants that the arthroscopist has circumspect knowledge of the local anatomy and the technique (Fig. 87.2). However, the same degree of anatomic knowledge and caution is needed if approaching these posterior pathologies from the lateral arthroscopic approach as well.

TIMING

After most inversion injuries, usual nonoperative treatment and rehabilitation should be pursued for at least 3 to 4 months. Progress in recovery usually continues up to 6 months or more. In many cases, there is a more chronic presentation and patients will have already undergone extensive therapy or even surgery. For ongoing pain, a clear anatomic cause is pursued through physical examination, imaging, and diagnostic injections. When a clear anatomic diagnosis is made, then subtalar arthroscopy should be considered. Without a clear anatomic diagnosis, diagnostic subtalar arthroscopy can be considered too. However, patients should be counseled that results in cases with degenerative joint disease are much less favorable (3, 14).

TECHNIQUES

Supine Semilateral Position

The supine semilateral technique of subtalar arthroscopy is best performed with a bump beneath the ipsilateral hip and a sterile bump beneath the ankle that allow the foot to fall passively into inversion, thus opening the sinus tarsi and subtalar joint (Fig. 87.6). The joint can be insufflated

with saline by medially directed injection into the sinus tarsi. In cases of large sinus tarsi fat pads, this can aid in prospecting for the ideal portal placement. The anterolateral portal is made over the sinus tarsi beginning just distal to the midpoint between the lateral talar process and the anterior process of the calcaneus, the "soft spot" of the sinus tarsi is actually just below the fat pad. This allows for entrance into the joint space just anterior to the posterior facet and should allow easy access to the tarsal canal medially. Deep to the skin, this passes through the inferior sinus tarsi fat pad and punctures the intermediary root of the inferior extensor retinaculum that inserts at the base of the anterior calcaneal process. The "nick and spread" technique should be employed for all portals, and a fine straight hemostat is effective for creating a straight track. The portal should not puncture the inferior extensor retinaculum too medially as this will constrain use of the arthroscope to visualize the lateral aspect of the joint line. The arthroscope can be placed and the anterior joint assessed.

The direct lateral portal is placed at the anterior margin of the lateral talar facet, and dorsal to the peroneal tendons, which course just plantar to the level of the calcaneal side of the sinus tarsi (Fig. 87.7). Incidentally, this allows for a convenient portal for inspecting the peroneal tendons as well. From this lateral position the arthroscope can visualize the anterior joint space and the posterolateral recess. In cases of subtalar instability it offers a good view of the articular surface. Anterior pathologies such as soft tissue impingement and bony impingement due to the lateral talar process can be treated using these two portals (Fig. 87.8). Placement of the arthroscope through the lateral portal allows good visualization of a shaver for debridement of anteromedial soft tissue impingement lateral to the ITCL (Fig. 87.9). Also, a burr can be used to remove a prominent accessory facet from the lateral process of the talus (Fig. 87.10). Integrity of the ITCL can be assessed by direct inspection and an anterior drawer test of the

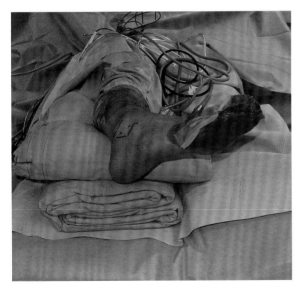

FIGURE 87.6. Positioning for supine subtalar arthroscopy is performed with a bump beneath the ipsilateral hip and another beneath the ankle that allows the foot to passively invert, opening the subtalar joint anteriorly. This same position can be used for anterior ankle arthroscopy and can allow a direct posterior portal as in prone ankle/subtalar arthroscopy.

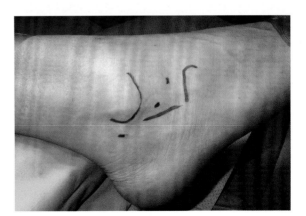

FIGURE 87.7. The placement of the anterolateral and lateral portals is not in proximity to the sural or superficial peroneal nerves, but the posterolateral portal is very close to being over the sural nerve in some patients, even when placed directly behind the peroneal tendons.

VI. Foot and Ankle

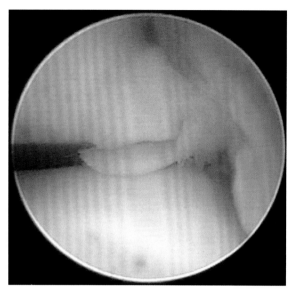

FIGURE 87.8. Soft tissue impingement, at the anteromedial aspect of the posterior facet, which is overlying the ITCL. The inflamed soft tissues become entrapped in the joint when eversion occurs.

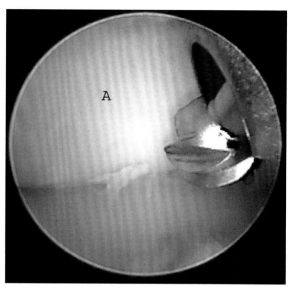

FIGURE 87.10. A burr placed through the anterolateral portal is used to remove the prominence of the accessory facet.

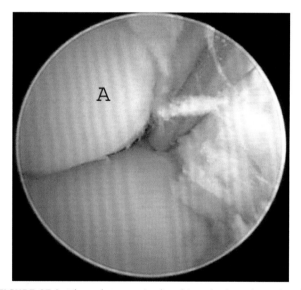

FIGURE 87.9. The arthroscope is placed into the lateral portal and the shaver through the anterolateral portal to debride the impingement lesion. An accessory facet of the lateral talus (A) also contributes to impingement in this location.

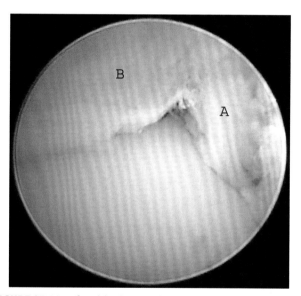

FIGURE 87.11. After debridement of the soft tissue impingement and accessory facet (B), the ITCL (A) is clearly seen with intact fibers. The middle facet of the subtalar joint lies medial to the ligament.

calcaneus will show deficiency (Fig. 87.11). If the middle subtalar facet is visualized it is an indication of loss of the ITCL, which should cover this facet on its lateral side. Relief of anterior impingement can be demonstrated when full eversion is performed and the anterior joint space can still be visualized, which indicates enough room for the arthroscope in this position. For this reason the impingement lesion due to a large bony prominence cannot often be photographed until debridement has occurred.

Placement of the arthroscope into the anterolateral portal affords good visualization of lateral impingement

lesions and the CFL and can visualize the lateral gutter to the posterolateral recess while the lateral portal is used for the shaver or bur (Fig. 87.12). Lateral impingement can demonstrated as with physical examination by placing digital pressure over the sinus tarsi and visualizing the tongue of tissue extending into the joint, even in the inverted position (Figs. 87.13 and 87.14). This can be debrided by placing the arthroscope into the anterolateral portal and the shaver or bur into the lateral portal (Fig. 87.15). Debridement begins at the anterolateral margin of the posterior facet and continues in a posterior direction medial to the CFL, which can be tested by using a probe. The CFL is the lateral boundary of the debridement

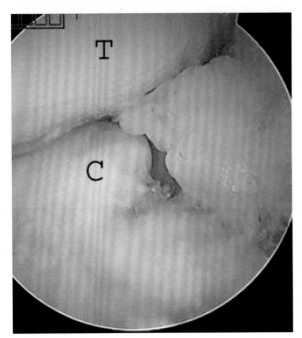

FIGURE 87.12. An example of a lateral impingement lesion, which bears the fibrotic appearance of chronic impingement, as viewed from the anterolateral portal. The tongue like tissue can become entrapped between the talus *(T)* and the calcaneus *(C)* causing pain with eversion.

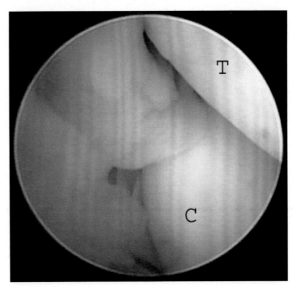

FIGURE 87.14. The same joint in Figure 87.13 is seen with mild digital pressure over the impingement lesion. The extension of the tongue-like soft tissue lesion into the joint is evident even in this distended and inverted joint.

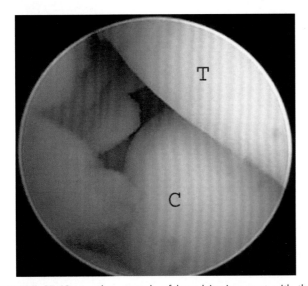

FIGURE 87.13. Another example of lateral impingement with the joint opened in inversion, viewed from the anterolateral portal.

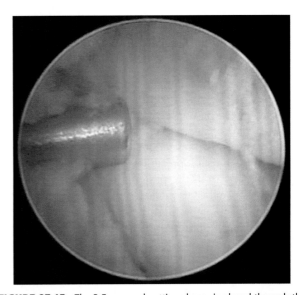

FIGURE 87.15. The 3.5 mm end-cutting shaver is placed through the lateral portal to remove the impingement lesion.

(Fig. 87.16). Combined loss of ITCL and CFL function will allow inversion stress to open the joint laterally. Traction in this condition will allow good visualization of the posterior facet.

The posterior recess and posterior talus can be visualized by using the lateral and a posterolateral portal. The posterolateral portal has been described by various authors and all agree that the sural nerve and lesser saphenous vein are at risk. Placing the portal midway between the Achilles tendon and the fibula is the most likely location to injure the nerve. Placing the portal closer to the posterior margin of the peroneal tendons decreases, but does not eliminate this risk, as the anatomic course of the nerve and vein varies (Fig. 87.7). The posterolateral portal described for prone posterior arthroscopic technique is safer and can be easily used in the semilateral position by creating a portal along the lateral margin of the Achilles tendon and directing it anteriorly to the posterior subtalar joint line. Both the posterolateral portal behind the peroneal tendons and the posterolateral portal adjacent to the Achilles can be used in this position for procedures such as removal of an os trigonum or loose body.

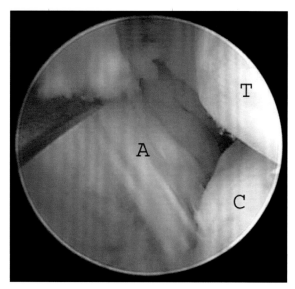

FIGURE 87.16. After debridement, the CFL *(A)* is clearly demonstrated and the lateral aspect of the posterior facet between the talus *(T)* and the calcaneus *(C)* is now clear of impingement.

Prone Position

Prone posterior ankle and subtalar arthroscopy provides the best view and access to posterior pathologies. The portals are paramedian to the Achilles tendon and are made with respect to the fascia of the superficial and deep posterior compartments. The posterolateral and posteromedial portals are begun adjacent to the Achilles tendon and hemostat spreading is directed centrally and posterior the Achilles tendon. The fascia of the deep posterior compartment is entered in the midline through a common hole created by hemostat spreading. The arthroscope can be placed initially from the posteromedial or posterolateral portal, but in either case, the scope is directed into the posterolateral recess behind the ankle and subtalar joint once the deep posterior compartment has been entered (Fig. 87.17). By maintaining this protocol, the posteromedial neurovascular structures are easily protected. Some initial soft tissue debridement can be performed to clarify the ankle and subtalar joints and the trigonal process or os trigonum. Debridement proceeds from lateral to medial and anterior to posterior. Once the posterolateral aspect of the ankle joint, subtalar joint, and os trigonum/trigonal process are visualized, the shaver can work toward the medial side staying close to the posterior ankle joint line. Once the FHL is identified, aided by passively dorsiflexing the hallux, then release of the ligamentous attachment on the medial side of the os trigonum or trigonal process can be safely performed (Fig. 87.18). Once the soft tissue attachments are released, the os can be mobilized by using blunt elevators, shavers, and biters. Once free, it can be removed by enlarging the posterolateral portal. In cases of FHL stenosis, an irregular or large trigonal process can be removed or trimmed using an arthroscopic bur. Careful consideration should be exercised in using

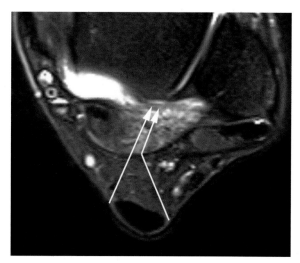

FIGURE 87.17. An axial MRI with arrows demonstrating the direction of instrument placement for prone arthroscopy. Both portals begin anterior the Achilles tendon and pass into the deep posterior compartment in the midline. The instruments are then directed to the posterolateral recess of the ankle where inspection and debridement can begin, moving medially with the FHL as a medial boundary.

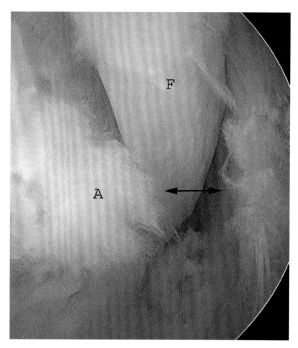

FIGURE 87.18. An example of an FHL retinacular release from the trigonal process of the talus *(A)*. The *arrow* indicates the former location of the proximal edge of the fibrous tunnel. The FHL *(F)* can be seen to pass freely beyond the posterior talus, with ample room for the distal muscle to move without further stenosis.

osteotomes, even curved ones, to remove a trigonal process or even an os trigonum. The optimum angle necessary to avoid violating the talar body and the subtalar joint is nearly impossible to achieve even with maximal ankle dorsiflexion, due to the oblique slope of the subtalar joint, which mirrors the angle achieved with an osteotome used from posteriorly (Fig. 87.19). A lateral fluoroscopy image should be used and will often dissuade the use of an osteotome. An arthroscopic bur is effective and avoids this potential complication.

AUTHOR'S PREFERRED TREATMENT

The prone technique is used for any posterior pathology of the ankle and subtalar joint. The supine semilateral technique is advantageous in cases where concomitant anterior ankle arthroscopy or other anterior procedures are planned, including anterior subtalar problems and lateral subtalar joint impingement. Both 30° and 70° 2.7-mm arthroscopes should be available (Fig. 87.20). The author's preferred instruments are pictured (Fig. 87.21). Distraction can be applied for both ankle and subtalar arthroscopy, but other than for arthrodesis or osteochondral lesions, the nature of the pathologies most commonly treated do not make this necessary and may impede the manipulation of the joint, which is helpful in evaluating impingement lesions. The anterior joint space is most effectively opened

by allowing passive inversion rather than distraction in a plantarflexed position. Peroneal tendoscopy can be added to the procedure in cases where exploration or treatment of peroneal pathology is being considered. In cases where both anterior and posterior pathology requires treatment, it is reasonable to turn a patient from the prone position to the supine position to allow for the optimal treatment of both locations. It is possible to place an arthroscope down the lateral aspect of the subtalar joint from the posterolateral portal in the prone position and place an anterolateral portal for debridement of anterior impingement. A 70° scope makes this relatively easy.

With the prone technique, the larger 4.0-mm scope can be used, but the 2.7-mm scope works well in most circumstances. Debridement and burring with the anterior technique joint is best accomplished with a 3.5-mm end-cutting shaver. Some cases may require a shaver as small as 2.0 mm, particularly in the lateral subtalar region where damage to the soft calcaneal subchondral bone can occur, and space is limited with an intact CFL ligament.

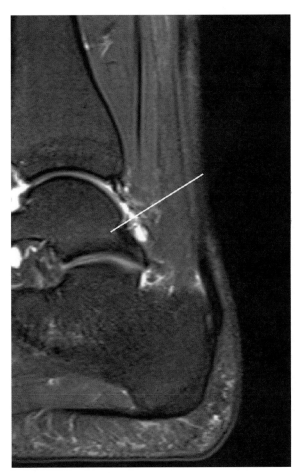

FIGURE 87.19. A sagittal MRI demonstrates the difficulty with using an osteotomy to remove an os trigonum or large trigonal process. The line indicates the direction of an instrument placed through a posterior portal. Even with maximal dorsiflexion, this line would not improve sufficiently to avoid cutting into the subtalar joint excessively.

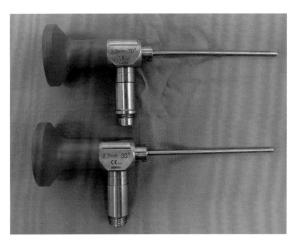

FIGURE 87.20. 30° and 70° 2.7-mm arthroscopes are sufficient for most subtalar arthroscopy. Smaller scopes may be needed in small adolescent patients. A 4.0-mm scope can be used in prone arthroscopy if preferred.

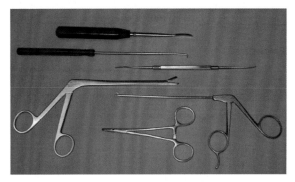

FIGURE 87.21. The author's preferred instruments for supine and prone subtalar arthroscopy. Curved elevators, probe, pituitary rongeur, straight biter, and a straight hemostat usually all that is required beyond the powered shaver and burr.

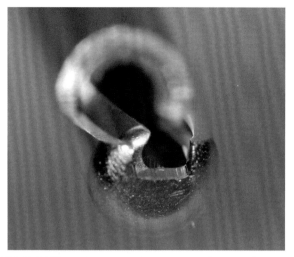

FIGURE 87.22. A close-up of the 3.5-mm end-cutting shaver preferred by the author. The cutout at the end allows for debridement of soft tissues when the shaver is pointing directly ahead. This circumstance is common in both supine and prone subtalar arthroscopy. The overall length of the opening is short. This allows for precise debridement and limits risk of shaving adjacent soft tissues that are not intended to be removed. The 3.5-mm shaver fits on a standard large shaver handpiece, but does not suction too much water so that the 2.7-mm scope can still be used for inflow.

Shavers that are too large will suction the fluid out of a joint when using smaller scopes, and therefore, the shaver size must be matched to the inflow capacity of the scope. An end-cutting shaver is particularly helpful as much of the debridement in subtalar and ankle arthroscopy is done with the shaver directed at the lesion, and the cutting area is shorter and therefore more precise (Fig. 87.22). Burs of various sizes can be used with any scope since suction is not applied continuously but intermittently to clear the visual field.

COMPLICATIONS, CONTROVERSIES, AND SPECIAL CONSIDERATIONS

Reported complications after supine and prone subtalar arthroscopy are rare, but the proximity of neurovascular structures should always be considered. Neurovascular injuries are the most concerning with subtalar arthroscopy.

Supine Semilateral Technique

One case of a lesser saphenous vein injury has been reported with the use of a posterolateral portal placed behind the peroneal tendons. Bleeding was controlled with a skin's suture and compression (5). One case of tarsal tunnel syndrome after removal of an os trigonum was treated with delayed tarsal tunnel release (14). One reported series had three cases of transient neuritis and one sinus tract with superficial infection, which was successfully treated with nonoperative care and antibiotics (3).

Prone Technique

One case of transient medial hindfoot numbness was treated by observation alone (12). Temporary numbness around the portals in five patients and temporary stiffness in one were all treated by observation in another study (15).

Controversy continues regarding the use of prone ankle/subtalar arthroscopy and the use of the posteromedial portal despite a lack of reported complications. Certainly, a posteromedial portal should never be attempted with a patient in the supine semilateral position, but in the prone position, this has proven to be safe and reliable in reports from two centers with extensive experience with this technique. As with all new techniques, surgeons should gain experience after self-study through observation of others experienced with the technique and by skills training on anatomic specimens.

REHABILITATION

Rehabilitation after subtalar arthroscopy can begin very soon after surgery. This has sped the progress to weight-bearing activities, motion, and physical therapy compared with traditional open operative techniques since the concern for wound healing is minimal with small arthroscopic portal incisions. Depending on the extent of internal dissection and the amount of bony work that may increase postoperative bleeding, progression to active motion and unrestricted weight bearing may vary, but usually begins within a few days to a week from the time of surgery. For example, in some cases of removal of a large os trigonum, a portal incision may have to be extended and a short delay in motion may be appropriate. Motion after operative treatment of fractures may also begin motion earlier for the same reason, although weight-bearing restrictions will apply due to the necessity for fracture healing. Even though skin healing occurs reliably and early compared with open techniques, patients should be counseled that there will still be a period of several months of postoperative swelling and loss of proprioception in many cases that warrants a progressive return to sports.

CONCLUSIONS AND FUTURE DIRECTIONS

The knowledge and experience gained from performing subtalar joint arthroscopy has improved our diagnostic accuracy in evaluating and treating subtalar joint pathologies. The previous common default diagnosis of "sinus tarsi syndrome" has now been replaced by specific anatomic diagnoses as was predicted by Parisien in his original proposal of arthroscopy of the anterolateral subtalar joint (3–5, 11, 14, 25). Likewise, posterior and posteromedial pathologies of the ankle and subtalar joints are now being treated and more fully understood with the advent of prone posterior ankle and subtalar arthroscopy (13, 14). In general, the intimate relationship of the ankle and subtalar joints, both in normal function and in the injured state, warrants a new comprehensive approach that would include evaluating these joints as a single complex rather than as two completely separate anatomic sites.

In the future, broader application of subtalar joint arthroscopy for assisting in the acute treatment of fractures will continue to develop (18, 19, 20). The previously exclusive realms of arthroscopy and trauma surgery of the foot and ankle will continue to meld. Subtalar arthroscopy may also extend into earlier treatment of some inversion injuries in order to decrease the length of disability for those injuries that go on to have chronic pain due to problems such as soft tissue impingement. This depends on developing circumspect studies to find reliable ways of determining which injuries are most likely to go on to chronically painful conditions. Arthroscopic-assisted treatment of ankle and subtalar joint instability has been described, and may become a more common technique in the future (26).

PEARLS AND PITFALLS

Pearls

1. Use dynamic examination techniques to evaluate impingement and instability.
2. Repeat impingement test to assess debridement.
3. Consider not using traction or using intermittent traction in cases of impingement.
4. Use end-cutting shaver to facilitate debridement of "end-on" pathology.
5. Position the ankle in prone arthroscopy so that the ankle and hallux can be fully dorsiflexed.

Pitfalls

1. Avoid posterolateral portals near sural nerve due to variable anatomy.
2. Avoid placing anterolateral portal too medially that hinders lateral visualization.
3. Consider anatomic variant of lateral talus with accessory facet in cases of impingement, which may warrant bony debridement.
4. Posterior arthroscopy portals in the prone position should always enter the deep posterior compartment in the midline.
5. Prone arthroscopy should always begin at the posterolateral ankle and proceed medially with the FHL as a medial marker.

REFERENCES

1. Amendola A, Lee KB, Saltzman CL, et al. Technique and early experience with posterior arthroscopic subtalar arthrodesis. *Foot Ankle Int.* 2007;28(3):298–302.
2. Elgafy H, Ebraheim NA. Subtalar arthroscopy for persistent subfibular pain after calcaneal fractures. *Foot Ankle Int.* 1999;20(7):422–427.
3. Frey C, Feder KS, Di Giovanni C. Arthroscopic evaluation of the subtalar joint: does sinus tarsi syndrome exist? *Foot Ankle Int.* 1999;20(3):185–191.
4. Goldberger MI, Conti SF. Clinical outcome after subtalar arthroscopy. *Foot Ankle Int.* 1998;19(7):462–465.
5. Jerosch J. Subtalar arthroscopy—indications and surgical technique. *Knee Surg Sports Traumatol Arthrosc.* 1998;6(2):122–128.
6. Lee KB, Bai LB, Song EK, et al. Subtalar arthroscopy for sinus Tarsi syndrome: arthroscopic findings and clinical outcomes of 33 consecutive cases. *Arthroscopy.* 2008;24(10):1130–1134.
7. Lee KB, Chung JY, Song EK, et al. Arthroscopic release for painful subtalar stiffness after intra-articular fractures of the calcaneum. *J Bone Joint Surg Br.* 2008;90(11):1457–1461.
8. Lui TH. Arthroscopic subtalar release of post-traumatic subtalar stiffness. *Arthroscopy.* 2006;22(12):1364.e1–1364.e4.
9. Niek van Dijk C. Anterior and posterior ankle impingement. *Foot Ankle Clin.* 2006;11(3):663–683.
10. Oloff LM, Schulhofer SD, Bocko AP. Subtalar joint arthroscopy for sinus tarsi syndrome: a review of 29 cases. *J Foot Ankle Surg.* 2001;40(3):152–157.
11. Parisien JS. Arthroscopy of the posterior subtalar joint: a preliminary report. *Foot Ankle.* 1986;6(5):219–224.
12. Scholten PE, Sierevelt IN, van Dijk CN. Hindfoot endoscopy for posterior ankle impingement. *J Bone Joint Surg Am.* 2008;90(12):2665–2672.
13. van Dijk CN, Scholten PE, Krips R. A 2-portal endoscopic approach for diagnosis and treatment of posterior ankle pathology. *Arthroscopy.* 2000;16(8):871–876.
14. Williams MM, Ferkel RD. Subtalar arthroscopy: indications, technique, and results. *Arthroscopy.* 1998;14(4):373–381.
15. Willits K, Sonneveld H, Amendola A, et al. Outcome of posterior ankle arthroscopy for hindfoot impingement. *Arthroscopy.* 2008;24(2):196–202.
16. Lee KB, Bai LB, Park JG, et al. Efficacy of MRI versus arthroscopy for evaluation of sinus tarsi syndrome. *Foot Ankle Int.* 2008;29(11):1111–1116.
17. Martus JE, Femino JE, Caird MS, et al. Accessory anterolateral facet of the pediatric talus. An anatomic study. *J Bone Joint Surg Am.* 2008;90(11):2452–2459.
18. Gavlik JM, Rammelt S, Zwipp H. Percutaneous, arthroscopically-assisted osteosynthesis of calcaneus fractures. *Arch Orthop Trauma Surg.* 2002;122(8):424–428.
19. Gavlik JM, Rammelt S, Zwipp H. The use of subtalar arthroscopy in open reduction and internal fixation of intra-articular calcaneal fractures. *Injury.* 2002;33(1):63–71.
20. Rammelt S, Gavlik JM, Barthel S, et al. The value of subtalar arthroscopy in the management of intra-articular calcaneus fractures. *Foot Ankle Int.* 2002;23(10):906–916.
21. Hamilton WG. Stenosing tenosynovitis of the flexor hallucis longus tendon and posterior impingement upon the os trigonum in ballet dancers. *Foot Ankle.* 1982;3(2):74–80.
22. Kolettis GJ, Micheli LJ, Klein JD. Release of the flexor hallucis longus tendon in ballet dancers. *J Bone Joint Surg Am.* 1996;78(9):1386–1390.
23. Sammarco GJ, Cooper PS. Flexor hallucis longus tendon injury in dancers and nondancers. *Foot Ankle Int.* 1998;19(6):356–362.
24. Phisitkul P, Tochigi Y, Saltzman CL, et al. Arthroscopic visualization of the posterior subtalar joint in the prone position: a cadaver study. *Arthroscopy.* 2006;22(5):511–515.
25. Parisien JS, Vangsness T. Arthroscopy of the subtalar joint: an experimental approach. *Arthroscopy.* 1985;1(1):53–57.
26. Lui TH. Arthroscopic-assisted lateral ligamentous reconstruction in combined ankle and subtalar instability. *Arthroscopy.* 2007;23(5):554.e1–554.e5.

VI. Foot and Ankle

Periarticular Endoscopy

C. Niek van Dijk • Gino M. M. J. Kerkhoffs • Peter A. J. de Leeuw
• Maayke N. van Sterkenburg

In 1931, Burman (1) found the ankle joint unsuitable for arthroscopy because of its typical anatomy. Tagaki and later Watanabe (2) made considerable contributions to arthroscopic surgery, and the latter published a series of 28 ankle arthroscopies in 1972. Since the late 70s, numerous publications have followed. Over the last 30 years, arthroscopy of the ankle joint has become an important procedure with numerous indications for both anterior as well as posterior pathology and pathology of tendons. Endoscopic surgery offers the possible advantages of direct visualization of structures, improved assessment of articular cartilage, less postoperative morbidity, faster and functional rehabilitation, earlier resumption of sports, and outpatient treatment (3–5). The value of diagnostic arthroscopy nowadays is considered limited (6,7). Posterior ankle problems pose a diagnostic and therapeutic challenge, because of their nature and the deep location of hindfoot structures. This makes direct access more difficult. Historically, the hindfoot was approached by a three-portal technique, that is, the anteromedial, anterolateral, and posterolateral portals, with the patient in the supine position (8–10). The traditional posteromedial portal is associated with potential damage to the tibial nerve, the posterior tibial artery, and local tendons (11). A two-portal endoscopic approach with the patient in the prone position was introduced in 2000 (12). This technique has shown to give excellent access to the posterior ankle compartment, the subtalar joint, and extra-articular structures (12–15). This chapter provides up-to-date information on posterior ankle arthroscopy and tendoscopy with a wide variety of indications highlighted.

STANDARD TWO-PORTAL HINDFOOT APPROACH

Introduction

Posterior ankle pathology can be treated by means of a standard two-portal hindfoot approach. The posteromedial and lateral hindfoot portals have proved to be anatomically safe and reliable (16,17) and clinically provide excellent access to the posterior aspect of the ankle and subtalar joint, including extra-articular hindfoot structures (12). Hindfoot arthroscopy compares favorably to open surgery with regard to an overall lesser morbidity and quicker recovery. Since the introduction of the technique in 2000 (12), an increasing number of pathologic conditions can be treated. These will be discussed in the upcoming paragraphs. First, the standard technique for hindfoot endoscopy, including its pearls and pitfalls, will be discussed (12, 18). The individual pearls and pitfalls for each indication will be mentioned in the corresponding subchapters.

Technique

Hindfoot endoscopy can be carried out in an outpatient setting under general, spinal, or regional anesthesia. The affected side is marked preoperatively, and the patient is placed in prone position. Prophylactic antibiotics are not routinely administered. A tourniquet is applied above the knee and pressured at 300 mm Hg prior to instrument insertion. The ankle is positioned slightly over the distal edge of the operating table with a small triangular support under the lower leg, allowing free movement of the ankle. Normal saline or Ringer solution by gravity flow is used for irrigation. A 4.0-mm 30° arthroscope is routinely used and distraction is not persistently applied; however, a soft-tissue distractor may be used when indicated (19).

For correct portal placement, several anatomical landmarks must be taken into account; these include the sole of the foot, the lateral malleolus, and the medial and lateral borders of the Achilles tendon. The authors prefer to mark each of the anatomical references on the skin. The ankle is subsequently brought in the neutral position (90°), and a straight line, parallel to the sole of the foot, is then drawn from the tip of the lateral malleolus to the Achilles tendon, and is extended over the Achilles tendon to the medial side.

The posterolateral portal is located just proximal to, and 5 mm anterior to, the intersection of the straight line with the lateral border of the Achilles tendon. The posteromedial portal is located at the same level as the posterolateral portal, but on the medial side of the Achilles tendon (Fig. 88.1).

First, the posterolateral portal is made as a vertical stab incision, and a mosquito clamp is used to spread the subcutaneous layer. The foot is now in a slightly plantarflexed position. The clamp is directed anteriorly, toward the first interdigital webspace. When the tip of the clamp touches bone, it is exchanged for a 4.5-mm arthroscopic cannula with the blunt trocar pointing in the same direction. The trocar is situated extra-articularly at the level of the posterior talar process and is exchanged for the 4.0-mm 30° arthroscope, pointing laterally. At this time, the scope is still outside the joint in the fatty tissue overlying the capsule.

Second, the posteromedial portal is made with a vertical stab incision, and a mosquito clamp is introduced through the posteromedial portal and directed toward the arthroscope shaft at a 90° angle until the clamp contacts the arthroscope. The ankle is still in a slightly plantarflexed position, and the arthroscope has remained in position through the posterolateral portal, still directing toward the first interdigital webspace. The arthroscope shaft is used as a guide for the mosquito clamp to travel anteriorly. While in contact with the arthroscope shaft, the clamp glides over the shaft toward the ankle joint until bone is reached. Once the arthroscope and clamp are both touching bone, the mosquito clamp is left in position and the arthroscope is pulled slightly backward and tilted until the tip of the clamp comes into view. The soft tissue layer covering the joints consists of fatty tissue and the deep crural fascia. At the lateral side, a specialized part of the crural fascia can be recognized, which is called the Rouvière ligament.

The clamp is now directed to the lateral side in an anterior and slightly plantar direction. This movement creates an opening in the crural fascia just lateral to the posterior talar process. The fatty tissue and subtalar joint capsule are subsequently opened. The mosquito clamp is exchanged for a 5-mm full radius shaver (Fig. 88.2). With a few turns of the shaver, the subtalar joint capsule and soft tissue are gently removed. The opening of the shaver

blade is facing bone. This part of the procedure is carried out in a blind fashion. The shaver is then retracted, and the scope is brought anteriorly through the opening in the crural fascia to visualize the posterolateral aspect of the subtalar joint. Once the joint is recognized, the opening in the crural fascia is enlarged to create more working area. At the level of the ankle joint, the posterolateral talar prominence and the posterior talofibular ligament (PTFL) are recognized. Just proximal to the PTFL, the intermalleolar ligament or tibial slip is recognized and more proximal and deep part of the tibiofibular ligament, also named transverse ligament, can be assessed.

The cranial part of the posterior talar process is freed from the Rouvière ligament and crural fascia to identify the flexor hallucis longus (FHL) tendon. The FHL tendon is an important safety landmark. Since the neurovascular bundle runs just medial to this tendon, the area lateral to the FHL tendon is regarded as being safe (Fig. 88.3).

Once the safe working area is defined, pathology can be addressed. Applying manual distraction to the calcaneus opens up the posterior compartment of the ankle and instruments can be introduced. We prefer to apply a soft-tissue distractor at this point (19). When indicated, a synovectomy and/or capsulectomy can be performed. The talar dome can be inspected over almost its entire surface as well as the complete tibial plafond. Possible osteochondral defects (OCDs) can be debrided, drilled, and microfractured.

In the following sections, each of the different indications is explained in detail.

Pearls and Pitfalls

- Create the posterolateral portal just proximal and lateral to the imaginary intersection of the horizontal line, perpendicular to the foot sole, from the tip of the lateral malleolus to the Achilles tendon with the ankle in the neutral position.
- The posteromedial portal is located at the same level as the posterolateral portal, just medial to the Achilles tendon.

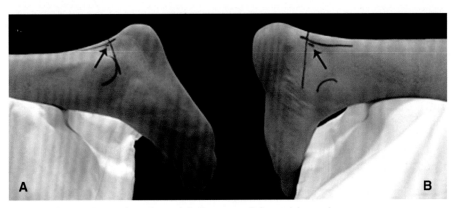

FIGURE 88.1. A: Posterolateral portal. **B:** Posteromedial portal *(arrows).*

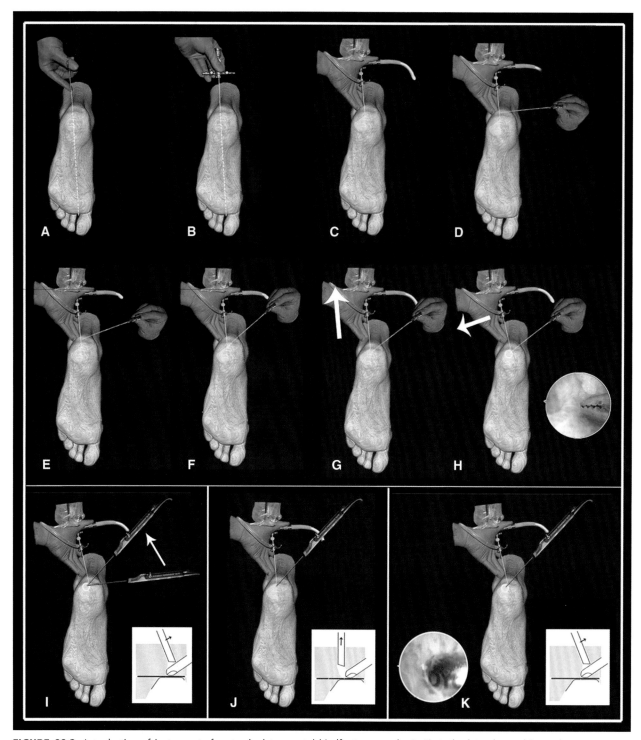

FIGURE 88.2. Introduction of instruments for standard two-portal hindfoot approach. **A:** First, the lateral portal is made. **B:** Instruments are introduced in the lateral portal pointing toward the first webspace. **C:** Direction of view is always to the lateral side. **D:** Through the medial portal the instrument is introduced horizontally, until it touches the shaft of the scope. **E, F:** The scope is used as a guide for the instrument in the medial portal to travel anteriorly. When the instrument touches bone, the scope is slightly lifted (**G**) and tilted laterally, until the instrument comes into view (**H**). **I, J, K:** The same maneuvre is performed each time an instrument is introduced into the medial portal.

- Use the arthroscopic shaft, inserted through the posterolateral portal and directed toward the interdigital webspace in between the first and the second toe, as a guide to travel anteriorly with the instruments inserted through the posteromedial portal.

- Exchanging instruments through the posteromedial portal requires a careful step-by-step procedure to prevent iatrogenic damage to the neurovascular structures. The direction of the arthroscope is hereby essential. At the start, the instruments must always be directed

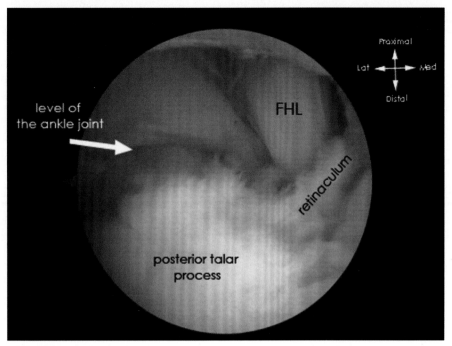

FIGURE 88.3. Overview after standard two-portal hindfoot approach. Safe working area.

toward the first webspace with the ankle in slight plantarflexion. Subsequent instrument insertions through the posteromedial portal must be perpendicular to the arthroscope until they are in contact. The arthroscopic shaft should routinely be used to guide the instruments inserted through the posteromedial portal up to the level of the bone. For accurate orientation, the arthroscopic view (30° angulation) should always be directed to the lateral side.

- Proximal and lateral to the posterior talar process the crural fascia can be quite thick; this local thickening is called the ligament of Rouvière. This ligament should at least be partially excised of sectioned, using arthroscopic punch or scissors, to reach the level of the subtalar joint and/or ankle joint.
- Always operate lateral from the FHL tendon to prevent damage to the neurovascular bundle, which is located just medially from the FHL tendon.
- Posterior ankle arthroscopy is an advanced endoscopic procedure; surgeons not familiar with endoscopic surgery are advised to practice in a cadaveric setting (20).

POSTERIOR ANKLE IMPINGEMENT

Introduction

The pathophysiological mechanism to produce this syndrome can be divided into an *overuse* and a *trauma group.*

The *overuse* group mainly consists of ballet dancers, downhill runners, and soccer players (21–23)." In these different sports, hyperplantarflexion is common, resulting in compression of the anatomical structures between the calcaneus and the posterior part of the tibia.

A hyperplantarflexion *trauma* and supination *trauma* can cause damage to these structures and can finally lead to a chronic posterior ankle impingement syndrome. A differentiation must be made between the two groups, since overuse trauma seems to have a better prognosis (24) and patients are more satisfied after arthroscopic treatment (25). Congenital anatomic anomalies such as a prominent posterior talar process, an os trigonum, or a bipartite talus (26) can facilitate the occurrence of the syndrome. An os trigonum is estimated to be present in 1.7% to 7% and occurs bilateral in 1.4% people (27–29). These congenital anomalies in combination with a traumatic or overuse injury facilitate the occurrence of symptoms (23, 30–32).

In the presence of a congenital bony anomaly, the soft tissue structures in the hindfoot are more prone to injury. With plantarflexion, bony anomalies impinge between the posterior part of the distal tibia and the calcaneus. The posterior ankle ligaments, such as the intermalleolar ligament, transverse ligament, and/or the PTFL, can become damaged during these ankle movements in the presence of bony anomalies. The posterior ankle impingement syndrome is, therefore, most frequently a combination of soft and bony impingement. Nevertheless also pure soft tissue ankle impingement can be present, as for instance, an isolated injury to the intermalleolar ligament (33), and pure bony impingement such as loose bodies can be present.

History and Physical Examination

Posterior ankle impingement syndrome is by definition a pain syndrome. The pain is mainly present in the hindfoot during forced plantarflexion. A specific test to detect posterior ankle impingement is the forced passive hyper-plantarflexion test. The forced hyperplantarflexion test is performed with the patient in a sitting position with the knee flexed to 90°. The test must be performed with repetitive quick passive hyperplantarflexion movements. The test can be repeated in slight external rotation or slight internal rotation of the foot relative to the tibia. The test is considered positive when the patient complains of recognizable pain during the test. A negative test rules out the posterior ankle impingement syndrome. A positive test is followed by a diagnostic infiltration with Xylocaine. Disappearance of pain following infiltration confirms the diagnosis.

Diagnostic Imaging

In patients with a posterior ankle impingement, the anteroposterior (AP) ankle view typically does not show abnormalities. Osteophytes, calcifications, loose bodies, chondromatosis as well as hypertrophy of the posterosuperior calcaneal border can often be detected by the lateral ankle radiograph. In case of doubt for the differentiation between hypertrophy of the posterior talar process or an os trigonum, we recommend a lateral radiograph view with the foot in 25° of exorotation (Fig. 88.4). Especially in posttraumatic cases, a spiral CT scan can be important to ascertain the extent of the injury and the exact location of calcifications or fragments. Soft tissue pathology and the posterior ankle ligaments can be visualized best using an MRI scan (34, 35).

Treatment Options

The deep location of hindfoot structures makes direct access difficult. Historically, the hindfoot was approached by a three-portal technique (i.e., anteromedial,

anterolateral, posterolateral), with the patient in the supine position (36). The traditional posteromedial portal is associated with potential damage to the tibial nerve, the posterior tibial artery, and local tendons (37). We describe the treatment of the most common posterior ankle impingement etiologies through the two-portal hindfoot approach with the patient in the prone position, as is discussed in detail previously.

During the standard endoscopic hindfoot approach, first the FHL tendon must be localized, as this is the safety landmark during the entire procedure that determines the medial border of the working area. Now the hindfoot can be inspected for specific pathologies.

Loose bodies can be localized and removed according to the preoperative planning based on the CT scan. Routinely inspect the posterior ankle ligaments, that is, the intermalleolar, transverse, and PTFL. From distal to proximal, the PTFL, intermalleolar ligament, and transverse ligament can subsequently be recognized. Distinguishing the intermalleolar ligament from the transverse ligament can be difficult. Ankle dorsiflexion tensions both ligaments, creating a gap mainly at the lateral side. In case the ligaments are swollen, partially ruptured or in case of fibrosis, the ligaments can be (partly) removed or debrided.

Specific soft tissue impingement such as synovitis, chondromatosis, and/or excessive scar tissue can be removed using a shaver.

Removal of a symptomatic os trigonum (Fig. 88.5), a nonunion of a fracture of the posterior talar process or a symptomatic large posterior talar prominence, involves partial detachment of the PTFL and release of the flexor retinaculum and a release of the talocalcaneal ligament, which all attach to the posterior talar prominence. Detachment is achieved using an endoscopic punch.

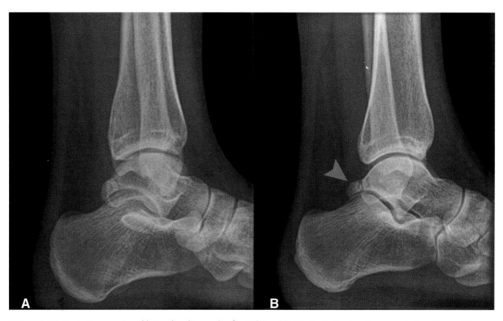

FIGURE 88.4. A: Conventional lateral radiograph of a right ankle. **B:** Posterior impingement view. An os trigonum is now visible.

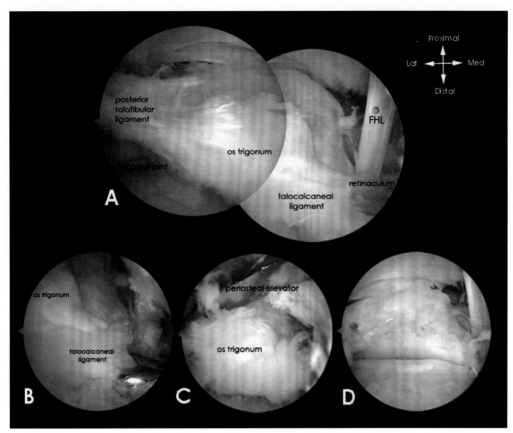

FIGURE 88.5. A: Endoscopic overview of the hindfoot after identification of the FHL tendon. An os trigonum is visible. **B:** With a punch, the posterior talofibular and talocalcaneal ligaments are released. **C:** With a periosteal elevator, the os trigonum is released and removed thereafter with a grasper. **D:** View after removal of the os trigonum.

In case of a symptomatic large posterior talar prominence, the bony prominence should additionally be detached from the talus using a chisel to allow removal with a grasper.

Rehabilitation Protocol

The patient can be discharged the same day of surgery and weight bearing is allowed as tolerated. The patient is instructed to elevate the foot when not walking to prevent edema. The dressing is removed 3 days postoperatively, and the patient is permitted to shower. Performing active range of motion exercises for at least three times a day for 10 minutes each is encouraged. With satisfaction of the surgeon and patient, no further outpatient department contact is necessary. Patients with limited range of motion are directed to a physiotherapist.

Pearls and Pitfalls

- Ankle dorsiflexion creates a gap in between the intermalleolar and the transverse ligament at the lateral side, allowing a clear distinction between both ligaments on inspection.
- If a hypertrophic posterior talar process is removed by using a chisel, care must be taken not to place

the chisel too far anteriorly. Only the inferoposterior part of the process should be removed with the chisel. The remnant of the process can be taken away with a bonecutter shaver. If initially the chisel is placed too much anteriorly, it is hard to avoid taking away too much bone at the level of the subtalar joint.

OSTEOCHONDRAL DEFECT POSTERIOR COMPARTMENT ANKLE JOINT

Introduction

An OCD is a lesion involving both the articular cartilage and the subchondral bone. The incidence of OCDs of the talar dome in patients with acute lateral ankle ligament ruptures is 4% to 7% (6, 38). OCDs are usually located on the posteromedial (58%) or anterolateral (42%) side of the talus (39). Medial lesions are typically deep and cup-shaped; lateral lesions are shallow and wafer-shaped (40). Inappropriate treatment of OCDs may eventually result in osteoarthritis of the ankle (40).

The etiology of OCD is a previous trauma to the ankle joint, which is reported in 93% of lateral lesions and

61% of medial lesions (39). In lateral lesions, the trauma mechanism is usually a combination of inversion and dorsiflexion; in medial lesions, the combination is inversion, plantar flexion, and rotation (41). In nontraumatic OCDs, possible causes are genetic, metabolic, vascular, endocrine, or degenerative as well as morphologic abnormalities (41, 42).

History and Physical Examination

Patients with a chronic lesion typically experience persistent or intermittent deep ankle pain during or after activity, sometimes accompanied by swelling and limited range of motion. Often, on examination, few abnormalities are found. Affected ankles may have a normal range of motion with the absence of swelling and no recognizable tenderness on palpation.

Diagnostic Imaging

Routine radiographs consist of weight-bearing anteroposterior and lateral views of both ankles. The radiographs may show an area of detached bone surrounded by radiolucency.

Initially, the damage may be too small to be visualized on a routine radiograph. A heel rise mortise view may reveal the posterior OCD (43). For further diagnostic evaluation, CT and MRI have demonstrated similar accuracy (43). A multislice helical CT scan is preferred because it is more helpful for preoperative planning.

Treatment Options

For asymptomatic of low symptomatic lesions, conservative therapy must be tried prior to any surgical intervention for at least 6 months. Conservative measures for these lesions may consist of rest and/or restriction of (sporting) activities with or without treatment with nonsteroidal anti-inflammatory drugs (NSAIDs). Also, a cast to immobilize the ankle is a possibility (42, 44). The aim is to unload the damaged cartilage, so edema can resolve and necrosis is prevented. Another objective of the conservative treatment could be healing of a (partly) detached fragment to the surrounding bone.

A surgical intervention must be considered for symptomatic OCDs interfering with daily activity. Symptomatic lesions are treated primarily by debridement and bone marrow stimulation, consisting of removal of all the unstable cartilage, including the underlying necrotic bone (39). Any cysts underlying the defect are opened and curetted. The sclerotic-calcified zone that is most commonly present is perforated by means of microfracturing into the vascularized subchondral bone. The underlying intraosseous blood vessels are disrupted and growth factors are released, leading to the formation of a fibrin clot in the created defect. The formation of local new blood vessels is stimulated, marrow cells are introduced into the OCD,

and fibrocartilaginous tissue is formed (45). In case of a cystic defect ≥15 mm in size, we consider placing a cancellous bone graft in the defect (46).

Retrograde drilling, combined with cancellous bone grafting when necessary, may be performed for primary OCDs when there is intact cartilage with a large subchondral cyst (47). When primary treatment fails, osteochondral autograft transfer system (OATS) or autologous chondrocyte implantation (ACI) are options for talar defects (48, 49). With OATS, one or more osteochondral plugs are harvested from a lesser weight-bearing area of the knee and transplanted into the defect (49). Although most reports show excellent results, the technique is associated with donor site morbidity, and a medial malleolar osteotomy is often required (50–52). ACI is the implantation of in vitro-cultured autologous chondrocytes, using a periosteal tissue cover after expansion of isolated chondrocytes. Despite excellent results reported by some investigators (48, 53), disadvantages include the two-stage surgery, high cost, and reported donor site morbidity (51, 53). Talar fragment fixation with one or two lag screws is preferred in acute or semiacute situations in which the fragment is ≥15 mm. In adolescents, fixation of an OCD always should be considered following failure of a 6-month period of conservative treatment.

Surgical Technique

Most OCDs will not exceed 15 mm. These lesions are treated with debridement and drilling. Depending on the location of the lesion, which must be mapped preoperatively, ideally with a CT scan, a noninvasive soft-tissue distraction device can be very helpful (19). Lesions located in the tibia plafond are difficult to assess without such a device.

After having determined the posterior working area, which is lateral to the FHL tendon, the intermalleolar ligament must be tilted using a hook to enter the talocrural joint. The lesion can now be addressed and its extent can be determined with a probe or hook. Debridement is performed by means of the bonecutter shaver or a small closed cup curette. It is important to remove all necrotic bone and overlying unstable cartilage (54). After full debridement, the sclerotic zone is perforated several times at intervals of approximately 3 mm. Perforation can be achieved by using a 2-mm drill, a microfracture awl or a 1.4-mm K-wire. A K-wire has the advantage of flexibility, whereas a drill may break more easily if the position of the ankle is changed during drilling. Microfracturing by means of a microfracture awl offers the possibility to work "around the corner" and results in microfractures of the trabeculae rather than destruction of the bone (55), but any created small bony particles should be carefully removed (56). Sufficient hemorrhage can be checked by loosening the tourniquet (Fig. 88.6).

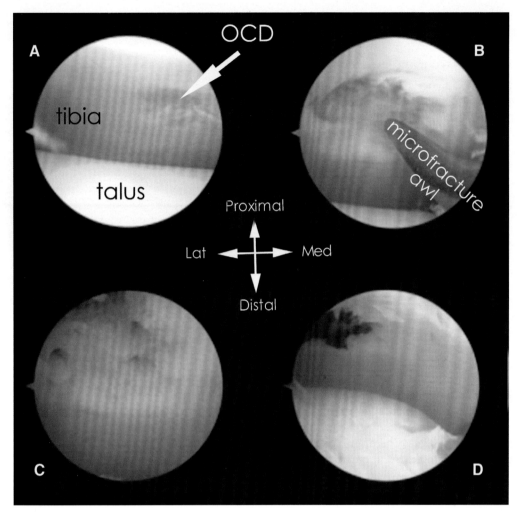

FIGURE 88.6. Debridement and microfracturing of an OCD of the posterior tibial plafond. **A:** OCD. **B:** After debridement with a curette, a microfracture probe is introduced. **C:** OCD after microfracturing. **D:** On release of the tourniquet, bleeding of subchondral bone is visible.

Rehabilitation Protocol

Active plantarflexion and dorsiflexion are encouraged. Partial weight bearing (eggshell) is allowed as tolerated. It is the senior author's practice to allow progress to full weight bearing within 2 to 4 weeks in patients with central or posterior lesions of up to 1 cm. Larger lesions require partial weight bearing up to 6 weeks. Running on even ground is permitted after 12 weeks (42). Sport is resumed after an average of 15.1 weeks (57). Full return to normal and sporting activities is usually possible 4 to 6 months after surgery (58).

Pearls and Pitfalls

- Loose bony particles can easily be created with the microfracture awl in case of puncturing the subchondral plate in OCDs. They can become detached upon withdrawal of the awl. If the particles are not removed properly, they may act as loose bodies (56).

- A noninvasive soft-tissue distraction device is advised mainly in case of osteochondral lesions located in the tibia plafond.

RETROCALCANEAL BURSITIS

Introduction

A symptomatic inflammation of the retrocalcaneal bursa is caused by repetitive impingement of the bursa between the anterior aspect of the Achilles tendon and a bony posterosuperior calcaneal prominence. In 1928, the Swedish orthopedic surgeon Haglund (59) described a patient with a painful hindfoot caused by a prominent posterosuperior aspect of the calcaneus in conjunction with a sharp rigid heel counter.

Often, Haglund syndrome, Haglund disease, Haglund deformity, pump-bump, and retrocalcaneal bursitis are used interchangeably although they are different entities (60–66). To avoid confusion, we use the term "retrocalcaneal bursitis," which is the source of pain and the main reason for treatment.

History and Physical Examination

Patients complain of pain after a day of strenuous activity or when starting to walk after a period of rest. Wearing shoes with rigid heel counters is often avoided. Physical examination reveals swelling on both sides of the Achilles tendon at the level of the posterosuperior calcaneal prominence. Pain is aggravated by palpating this area just medial and lateral to the Achilles tendon.

Retrocalcaneal bursitis can be accompanied by insertional tendinopathy. In case of insertional tendinopathy, there is pain at the bone–tendon junction, which gets worse after exercise. The area of maximal tenderness is often located in the central part of the insertion.

Diagnostic Imaging

Close consultation between orthopedic surgeon and radiologist is necessary to decide upon optimal radiographic diagnostics (67).

Always start with routine weight-bearing radiographs in an AP and lateral direction. In general, soft tissue pathology consequently can be visualized best using an MRI scan. However, obliteration of the normally radiolucent retrocalcaneal recess on a lateral weight-bearing radiograph has shown to be of great diagnostic value in patients with a retrocalcaneal bursitis, resulting in a higher cost-effectiveness and quicker treatment (68). When uncertainty remains, MRI or ultrasonography can still be used.

Treatment Options

Multiple conservative treatment options have been described to manage chronic retrocalcaneal bursitis, including avoidance of tight shoe heel counters, cast immobilization, NSAIDs, activity modification, padding, shockwave treatment, physical therapy, and a single injection of corticosteroids into the retrocalcaneal space. When these measures fail, endoscopic calcaneoplasty can be performed. Surgery is performed with the patient in prone position under general or regional anesthesia. The involved leg is marked with an arrow by the patient to avoid wrong side surgery. The feet are positioned just over the edge of the operation table. The involved leg is slightly elevated by placing a bolster under the lower leg. The position of the foot is in plantarflexion through gravity. Prior to surgery, important anatomical structures are marked. These include the medial and lateral border of the Achilles tendon and the calcaneus (Fig. 88.7).

The lateral portal is made first, just lateral of the Achilles tendon at the level of the superior aspect of the calcaneus. This portal is produced as a small vertical incision through the skin only. The retrocalcaneal space

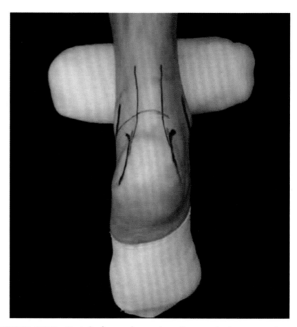

FIGURE 88.7. Portals for endoscopic calcaneoplasty are made precisely above the posterosuperior calcaneus and just lateral and medial from the Achilles tendon.

is penetrated with a blunt trocar. A 4.0-mm arthroscope with an inclination angle of 30° is introduced through a 4.5-mm shaft.

Irrigation is performed by gravity flow. A 70° arthroscope can also be used, but is seldom necessary. Under direct vision, a spinal needle is introduced just medial to the Achilles tendon, again at the level of the superior aspect of the calcaneus, to locate the medial portal. After having prepared the medial portal by a vertical stab incision, a 5.5-mm bonecutter shaver is introduced and visualized by the arthroscope. The inflamed retrocalcaneal bursa is removed first to provide a better view. Now the superior surface of the calcaneus is visualized and its fibrous layer and periosteum are stripped off. During resection of the bursa and the fibrous layer and periosteum of the superior aspect of the calcaneus, shaver is facing the bone to avoid damage to the Achilles tendon (Fig. 88.8).

When the foot is brought into full dorsiflexion, impingement between the posterosuperior calcaneal edge and the Achilles tendon can be perceived. The foot is subsequently brought into plantarflexion and now the posterosuperior calcaneal rim is removed. This bone is quite soft and can be removed by an aggressive full radius resector. The portals are used interchangeably for both the arthroscope and the shaver, so as to remove the entire bony prominence. It is important to remove a sufficient amount of bone at the posteromedial and lateral corner. These edges have to be rounded off by moving the shaver beyond the posterior edge onto the lateral respectively medial wall of the calcaneus.

The Achilles tendon is protected throughout the entire procedure by keeping the closed end of the shaver

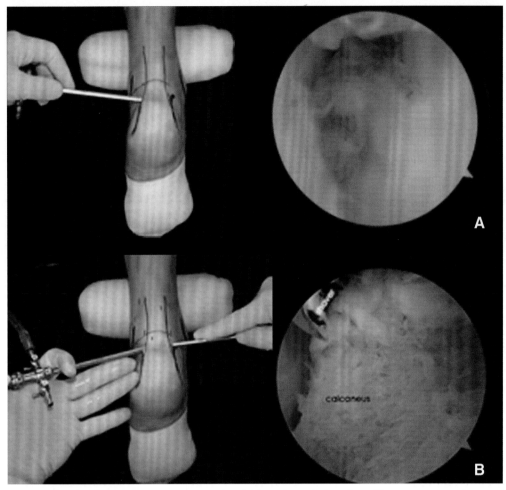

FIGURE 88.8. A: When the scope is introduced in the lateral portal, the inflamed bursa comes into view. **B:** Shaving off the posterosuperior side of the calcaneus through the medial portal.

against the tendon. With the foot in full plantarflexion, the insertion of the Achilles tendon can be visualized. The shaver is placed on the insertion against the calcaneus to smoothen this part of the calcaneus. Finally, debris is removed and possible rough edges are smoothened. Fluoroscopic control can be used to ascertain whether sufficient bone has been resected. With some experience, this will not be necessary. Also when confident with the anatomy and the procedure, the retrocalcaneal space can be freed blindly with a 4.5-mm arthroscopic shaft at the start of the procedure.

To prevent sinus formation, at the end of the procedure, the skin incisions are closed with 3.0 Ethilon sutures. The incisions and surrounding skin are injected with 10 mL of a 0.5% bupivacaine/morphine solution. A sterile compressive dressing is applied.

Rehabilitation Protocol

Postoperatively, the patient is allowed weight bearing as tolerated and is instructed to elevate the foot when not walking. The dressing is removed 3 days postoperatively, after which the patient is allowed to shower. Patients are encouraged to perform active range of motion exercises at least three times a day for 10 minutes each. The patient is allowed to return to wearing regular shoes as soon as tolerated. The sutures are removed after 2 weeks. A conventional lateral radiograph is made to ensure that sufficient bone has been excised (see Fig. 88.10). With satisfaction of the surgeon and patient, no further outpatient department contact is necessary. Patients with limited range of motion are directed to a physiotherapist.

Pearls and Pitfalls

- During resection of the bursa and the fibrous layer and periosteum of the superior aspect of the calcaneus, the full radius resector should routinely face the bone to prevent damage to the Achilles tendon.
- Routinely change portals during the procedure to ascertain that sufficient bone is released, also use fluoroscopy when inexperienced in this matter.

ENDOSCOPY OF TENDONS AROUND THE ANKLE (TENDOSCOPY)

In the last three decades, arthroscopy has become the preferred technique to treat intra-articular ankle pathology. However, extra-articular problems of the ankle have traditionally demanded open surgery. Open ankle surgery has been associated with some serious complications. The percentage of complications reported with open surgery for posterior ankle impingement varies between 15% and 24%. The incidence of these complications has stimulated the development of extra-articular endoscopic techniques. Endoscopic surgery offers the advantages related to any minimally invasive procedure, such as fewer wound infections, less blood loss, smaller wounds, and less morbidity. Aftertreatment is functional, and surgery is performed on an outpatient basis. In order to become familiar to the different endoscopic techniques in foot and ankle surgery, international courses are yearly organized in which surgeons can train themselves in a cadaveric setting (69, 70). Van Dijk et al. were the first to describe endoscopic access to the tendons by tendoscopy. Tendoscopy can be performed for the treatment and diagnosis of various pathologic conditions of the Achilles tendon, the posterior tibial tendon (PTT), the peroneal tendons, and the FHL tendon. These endoscopic procedures and their indications are discussed in detail in this second part of our chapter.

ACHILLES TENDOSCOPY

Introduction

The combination of tendon pain, swelling, and impaired performance should be given the clinical label of tendinopathy, and includes the histopathologic entities peritendinitis and tendinosis (71). The most common clinical diagnosis of Achilles overuse injuries is paratendinopathy and/or tendinopathy (55% to 65%), followed by insertional problems such as retrocalcaneal bursitis and insertional tendinopathy (20% to 25%).

The anatomy of the Achilles tendon is different from that of other tendons inserting into the foot. It lacks a true synovial sheath, but rather has a peritendineum. The peritendineum functions as an elastic sleeve and permits free movement of the tendon within the surrounding tissues. The peritendineum is richly vascularized, and provides blood supply to the Achilles tendon itself. The midportion of the tendon is minimally vascularized and, therefore, has a low metabolic rate. This is where noninsertional complaints are invariably situated. Neural supply to the Achilles tendon and the surrounding paratenon is provided by nerves from the attaching muscles and by the sural nerve.

Differentiation between tendinopathy of the main body of the Achilles tendon and paratendinopathy may be confusing, and frequently these entities coexist in the chronic phase. Currently, there is no consensus on what causes the pain, the peritendineum, the tendon proper, or a combination of both. Several studies described degenerative changes of the Achilles tendon in as many as 34% of subjects with no complaints (72–75). It is questionable whether degeneration of the tendon itself is the main cause of the pain. Therefore, the authors focus on endoscopic management of chronic paratendinopathy, leaving the (possibly pathologic) tendon proper untouched.

History and Physical Examination

General symptoms include painful swelling typically 2 to 6 cm proximal to the insertion, and stiffness especially when getting up after a period of rest. Pain is often most prominent on the medial side of the tendon (76).

Patients with tendinopathy of the main body can present with three patterns: diffuse thickening of the tendon, local degeneration of the tendon, which is mechanically intact, or insufficiency of the tendon with a partial tear. In paratendinopathy, there is local thickening of the paratenon. Clinically, a differentiation between tendinopathy and paratendinopathy can be made, but often these entities coexist. Maffulli and coworkers (77,78) describe the Royal London Hospital test, which is positive in patients with isolated tendinopathy of the main body of the tendon: The portion of the tendon originally found to be tender on palpation shows little or no pain with the ankle in maximum dorsiflexion. Paratendinopathy can be acute or chronic. *Acute* isolated paratendinopathy manifests itself as peritendinous crepitus as the tendon tries to glide within the inflamed covering. Areas of increased erythema, local heat, and palpable tendon nodules or defects may also be present at clinical examination. In *chronic* Achilles paratendinopathy, exercise-induced pain is still the cardinal symptom whereas crepitation and swelling diminish. The area of swelling does not move with dorsiflexion and plantarflexion of the ankle, where it does in tendinopathy (77, 79, 80). In addition, ankle instabilities and malalignment of the lower extremity, especially in the foot, should be looked for in patients with Achilles complaints.

Differential diagnoses are partial rupture, an insertional disorder, anomalous soleus muscle, and complete rupture. All these show a marked overlapping of the findings in history and physical examination. In clinical practice, overuse injuries often do have features of more than one pathophysiologic entity; however, in most cases, thorough history taking and physical examination should provide with the correct diagnosis.

Diagnostic Imaging

In the acute phase of Achilles tendinopathy, ultrasonography reveals fluid surrounding the tendon. In its more chronic form, peritendinous adhesions can be seen as thickening of the hypoechoic paratenon with poorly defined borders. Discontinuity of tendon fibers, focal hypoechoic intratendinous areas, and localized tendon swelling and thickening are the most characteristic ultrasonographic findings in patients with surgically verified intratendinous lesion of the Achilles tendon. Ultrasound imaging is known as a cost-effective and accurate measure to evaluate disorders of the Achilles tendon.

Although MRI is expensive and time-consuming, its ability to acquire images from multiple planes is a clear advance, and is especially important for preoperative planning. The tendon proper may show fusiform expansion on T1-weighted images and central enhancement of the signal within the tendon. In the acute phase of Achilles paratendinopathy, MRI shows high signal around the Achilles tendon on short tau inversion recovery (STIR) and T2. In the chronic phase, the peritendineum is thickened.

Treatment Options

Conservative measures should be tried for at least 6 to 12 months before considering surgery. The first step may be to remove the precipitating factors by resting or modifying training regimes. Foot and ankle malalignments may be addressed by orthotics, and decreased flexibility and muscle weakness may be treated by appropriate physiotherapists. Shoe modifications and inlays can be given. An eccentric exercise program should be recommended as the first treatment of choice, which can be combined with icing and NSAIDs (81–85). Shockwave treatment, a night splint, and cast immobilization are alternative conservative methods.

The percentage of patients requiring surgery is around 25% (77, 86, 87). The goal of Achilles tendoscopy is to release adhesions of the peritendineum, remove pathologic peritendinous tissue, and to release the plantaris tendon at the level of complaints.

This procedure can be performed on an outpatient basis. Local, epidural, spinal, and general anesthesia can be applied. The patient is in prone position. A tourniquet is placed around the thigh of the affected leg, and a bolster is placed under the foot. Because the surgeon needs to be able to obtain full plantar and dorsiflexion, the foot is placed right over the end of the table.

The authors mostly use a 2.7-mm arthroscope with a 30° angle. This small-diameter short arthroscope yields an excellent picture comparable to the standard 4-mm arthroscope; however, it cannot deliver the same amount of irrigation fluid per time as the 4-mm sheath. This is important in procedures in which a large diameter shaver is used (e.g., in endoscopic calcaneoplasty). When a 4-mm arthroscope is used, gravity inflow of irrigation fluid is usually sufficient. A pressurized bag or pump device sometimes is used with the 2.7-mm arthroscope.

The distal portal is located on the lateral border of the Achilles tendon, 2 to 3 cm distal to the pathologic nodule. The proximal portal is located medial to the border of the Achilles tendon, 2 to 4 cm above the nodule. In this situation, it is possible to visualize and work around the complete surface of the tendon, over a length of approximately 10 cm.

The distal portal is made first. After making the skin incision, the mosquito clamp is introduced, followed by the blunt 2.7-mm trocar in a craniomedial direction. With this blunt trocar, the paratenon is approached, and is blindly released from the tendon by moving around it. Subsequently, the arthroscope is introduced (Fig. 88.9). To minimize the risk of iatrogenic damage, it should be kept on the tendon. At this moment, it can be confirmed whether the surgeon is in the right layer between the peritendineum and the Achilles tendon. If not, now it can be identified and release can be repeated.

The proximal portal is made by introducing a spinal needle under direct vision, followed by a mosquito clamp and probe. In a typical case of local paratendinopathy, the plantaris tendon, the Achilles tendon, and the paratenon are tight together in the process. The plantaris tendon can be identified at the anteromedial border of the Achilles

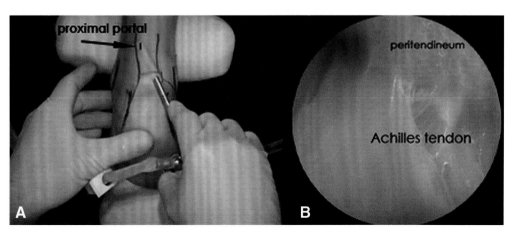

FIGURE 88.9. A: Blind release of the peritendineum from the Achilles tendon. **B:** Endoscopic view when in the correct layer.

tendon. It is cut at the level of the nodule. With a 2.7-mm full radius resector, neovessels and residual pathologic tissue can be removed. Changing portals can be helpful. At the end of the procedure, it must be possible to move the arthroscope over the entire symptomatic area of the Achilles tendon.

After the procedure, the portals are sutured with 3.0 Ethilon, and a compression bandage is applied.

Rehabilitation Protocol

Aftercare consists of leaving the compressive dressing on for 2 to 3 days. Patients are encouraged to actively perform range-of-motion exercises. Full weight bearing is allowed as tolerated. Initially, the foot must be elevated when not walking.

Pearls and Pitfalls

- The incisions should be made vertically, to prevent iatrogenic (partial) ruptures when accidentally placing them into the Achilles tendon.
- To prevent iatrogenic damage, keep the trocar onto the tendon when blindly releasing the peritendineum from the Achilles tendon.
- Make sure you stay away from the sural nerve, which runs dorsolaterally slightly proximal to the midportion of the tendon.

POSTERIOR TIBIAL TENDOSCOPY

Introduction

In the absence of intra-articular ankle pathology, postero-medial ankle pain is most often caused by disorders of the PTT.

Inactivity of the PTT gives midtarsal instability and is the most common cause of adult onset flatfoot deformity. The relative strength of this tendon is more than twice that of its primary antagonist, the peroneus brevis tendon. Without the activity of the PTT, there is no stability at the midtarsal joint, and the forward propulsive force of the gastrocnemius–soleus complex acts at the midfoot instead of at the midtarsal heads. Total dysfunction eventually leads to a flatfoot deformity.

These disorders can be divided into two groups: The younger group of patients with dysfunction of the tendon, caused by some form of systemic inflammatory disease (e.g., rheumatoid arthritis); and an older group of patients whose tendon dysfunction is mostly caused by chronic overuse (88).

Following trauma, surgery, and fractures, adhesions and irregularity of the posterior aspect of the tibia can be responsible for symptoms in this region.

Mostly, a dysfunctioning PTT evolves in a painful teno-synovitis. Tenosynovitis is also a common extra-articular manifestation of rheumatoid arthritis, where hindfoot problems are a significant cause of disability. Tenosynovitis in rheumatoid patients eventually leads to a ruptured tendon (89).

Although the precise etiology is unknown, the condition is classified on the basis of clinical and radiographic findings.

History and Physical Examination

In the early stage of dysfunction, patients complain of per-sisting ankle pain medially along the course of the tendon, in addition to fatigue and aching on the plantar medial aspect of the ankle. When a tenosynovitis is present, swelling is common (90, 91). A typical observation is abnormal wear of the medial sides of the shoes. Pain increases on walking and participation in sports activities becomes difficult.

Careful clinical examination is important and both feet should be examined. Valgus angulation of the hind-foot is frequently seen with accompanying abduction of the forefoot, the "too-many-toes" sign (91). This sign is positive when inspecting the patient's foot from behind: In case of significant forefoot abduction, three or more toes are visible lateral to the calcaneus, where normally only one or two toes are seen.

With the patient seated, the strength of the tendon and location of pain are evaluated by asking the patient to invert the foot against resistance.

Intra-articular lesions such as a posteromedial im-pingement syndrome, subtalar pathology, calcifications in the dorsal capsule of the ankle joint, loose bodies or OCDs should be excluded. Entrapment of the posterior tibial nerve in the tarsal canal is commonly known as a tarsal tunnel syndrome. Clinical examination is normally sufficient to adequately differentiate these disorders from an isolated PTT disorder.

Diagnostic Imaging

After initial history taking and physical examination, di-agnosis can be confirmed or rejected using radiography. Conventional radiographs may show abnormal alignment like flattening of the plantar arch or bony changes such as bony irregularity and hypertrophic change at the navicular attachment, providing an important clue to the presence of longstanding problems with the PTT (92). However, pathology to this soft tissue structure is easier to identify using ultrasound or MRI. Ultrasound imaging is known as a cost-effective and accurate to evaluate disorders of the PTT (93). Thickening of the tendon and/or periten-dinous soft tissue, hypoechoic texture, ill-definition of the fibrillar pattern, associated hypervascularity on color Doppler, thinning, splitting, or rupture may be useful clues (92). In our practice, MRI is the method of choice since the images can be interpreted by the orthopedist in contrast to ultrasound images and therefore are more helpful for preoperative planning. It is also considered the gold standard of assessing tibialis posterior dysfunction and related soft tissue injuries (92). A major advantage is the ability to detect bony edema. Findings can be fluid or synovitis around the tendon, hypertrophy of the tendon, intrasubstance tears showing increased signal, longitudinal tears, and complete tendon tears (92).

Treatment Options

Initially, conservative management is indicated, with rest, combined with NSAIDS, and immobilization using a plaster cast or tape. There is no consensus whether to use corticosteroid injections; cases of tendon rupture following corticosteroid injections have been described (94).

Surgery is indicated if conservative management for 3 to 6 months does not resolve complaints (95). This can be done open or endoscopically. An open synovectomy is performed by sharp dissection of the inflamed synovium, while preserving blood supply to the tendon. Postoperative management consists of plaster cast immobilization for 3 weeks, with the possible disadvantage of new formation of adhesions, followed by wearing a functional brace with controlled ankle movement for another 3 weeks and physical therapy.

Endoscopic synovectomy is indicated when access allows radical removal of inflamed synovium (96). Several studies have been published in which endoscopic synovectomy was successfully performed, offering the advantages that are related to minimally invasive surgery (97–99).

The procedure can be performed on an outpatient basis under local, regional, or general anesthesia. The patient is placed in the supine position. A tourniquet is placed around the upper leg. Before anesthesia, the patient is asked to actively invert the foot, so that the PTT can be palpated and the portals can be marked. Access to the tendon can be obtained anywhere along its course.

We prefer to make the two main portals directly over the tendon 2 to 3 cm distal and 2 to 3 cm proximal to the posterior edge of the medial malleolus. The distal portal is made first: The incision is made through the skin, and the tendon sheath is penetrated by the arthroscopic shaft with a blunt trocar. A 2.7-mm 30° arthroscope is introduced, and the tendon sheath is filled with saline. Irrigation is performed using gravity flow.

Under direct vision, the proximal portal is made by introducing a spinal needle, and subsequently, an incision is made into the tendon sheath. Instruments as a retrograde knife, a shaver system, blunt probes, and scissors can be used. For synovectomy in patients with rheumatoid arthritis, a 3.5-mm shaver can be used. The complete tendon sheath can be inspected by rotating the arthroscope around the tendon.

Synovectomy can be performed with a complete overview of the tendon from the distal portal, over the insertion of the navicular bone to approximately 6 cm above the tip of the medial malleolus.

Special attention should be given while inspecting the tendon sheath, the posterior aspect of the medial malleolar surface, and the posterior ankle joint capsule. The tendon sheath between the PTT and the flexor digitorum longus is relatively thin: Assessment of the correct tendon should always be checked. This can be accomplished by passively flexing and extending the toes; if the tendon sheath of the flexor digitorum longus tendon is entered, the tendon will move up and down.

When remaining in the PTT sheath, the neurovascular bundle is not in danger.

When a rupture of the PTT is seen (Fig. 88.10), endoscopic synovectomy is performed, and the rupture is repaired through a mini-open approach. Magnifying the tendon endoscopically pronounces the localization and extent of the rupture, thereby minimizing the incision for repair. At the end of the procedure, the portals are sutured to prevent sinus formation.

Rehabilitation Protocol

Postoperative management consists of a pressure bandage and partial weight bearing for 2 to 3 days. Active range of motion exercises are encouraged from the first day.

Pearls and Pitfalls

- It is important to identify the location of the PTT before creating the portals. Ask the patient to actively invert the foot, identify the tendon, and mark the location of the portals on the skin.
- In cases where you have entered the tendon sheath of the flexor digitorum longus, you can easily see tendons move up and down when you passively flex and extend the toes.
- The tendon sheath between the PTT and the flexor digitorum longus is quite thin. Always check to ensure that you are inspecting the correct tendon.
- Remaining in the tendon sheath of the PTT keeps the neurovascular bundle out of danger.
- Surgeons not familiar with endoscopic surgery are advised to train themselves in a cadaveric setting (69, 70).

PERONEAL TENDON PATHOLOGY

Introduction

The peroneal muscles are located in the lateral compartment of the leg, also known as the peroneal compartment. Both muscles are innervated by the superficial peroneal nerve, and the peroneal and medial tarsal arteries supply the muscles with blood through separate vinculae (99, 100). The peroneus brevis tendon is situated dorsomedially to the peroneus longus tendon from its proximal aspect up to the fibular tip, where it is relatively flat. Just distal to this tip, the peroneus brevis tendon becomes rounder, and crosses the round peroneus longus tendon. The distal

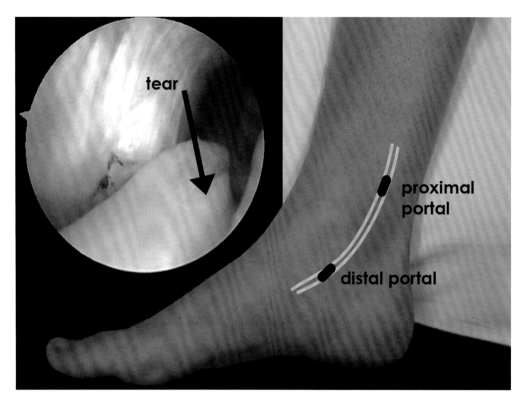

FIGURE 88.10. The scope is introduced through the distal portal. A probe slides into a longitudinal tear.

posterolateral part of the fibula forms a sliding channel for the two peroneal tendons. This malleolar groove is formed by a periosteal cushion of fibrocartilage that covers the bony groove (101). Posterolaterally, the tendons are held into position by the superior peroneal retinaculum (102, 103).

Because the peroneal tendons act as lateral ankle stabilizers, in chronic ankle instability, more strain is put on these tendons, resulting in hypertrophic tendinopathy, tenosynovitis, and ultimately in tendon tears (103).

In 1803, Montegggi(104) was the first to describe peroneal tendon dislocation in a female ballet dancer. These tendons dislocate if the superior peroneal retinaculum ruptures, frequently due to an inversion/dorsiflexion trauma of the foot with the tendons contracted, or is congenitally absent or weak (102). A nonconcave fibular groove predisposes the dislocation to occur. Another cause is explained through the cartilaginous rim, located laterally from the fibular groove that adds to the overall depth of the groove (105). In case this rim is absent or flat, the tendons are more likely to dislocate (106).

History and Physical Examination

Tendinopathy of the peroneal tendons often coexists with a lateral ankle sprain. The diagnosis of peroneal tendon pathology can therefore be difficult in a patient with lateral ankle pain (107). The anterior drawer test and varus stress test are applied routinely to detect laxity of the ankle ligaments. In acute cases, the detailed history should include

reconstruction of the trauma mechanism. The presence of associated conditions such as rheumatoid arthritis, psoriasis, hyperparathyroidism, diabetic neuropathy, calcaneal fracture, fluoroquinolone use, and local steroid injections is important since these can all increase the prevalence of peroneal tendon dysfunction (108). A diagnostic differentiation must be made with fatigue fractures or fractures of the fibula, posterior impingement of the ankle, and lesions of the lateral ligament complex. Posttraumatic or postsurgical adhesions and irregularities of the posterior aspect of the fibula (peroneal groove) can also be responsible for symptoms in this region.

In case of tendinopathy, there is crepitus and recognizable tenderness over the tendons on palpation. Swelling, tendon dislocation, and signs of tenosynovitis can be found at the lateral aspect of the posterior ankle.

In case of peroneal tendon dislocation, patients typically complain of lateral instability, giving way and sometimes a popping or snapping sensation over the lateral aspect of their ankle. On physical examination, the tendons can be subluxated by active dorsiflexion and eversion, which provokes the pain (109) (Fig. 88.11).

Diagnostic Imaging

If the Ottawa ankle rules do not show abnormalities, it should be questioned whether to apply diagnostics in the acute phase following an inversion trauma. However, when there is suspicion of peroneal tendon pathology, additional

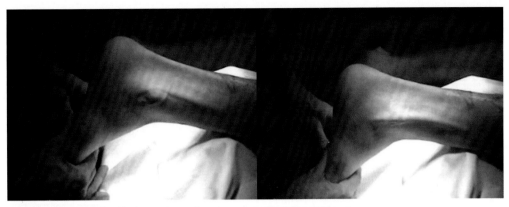

FIGURE 88.11. On dorsiflexion and eversion, the peroneal tendons subluxate.

diagnostics should be applied. Also, if posterolateral ankle pain persists after the initial trauma, diagnostic imaging should be considered. Routine weight-bearing radiographs in the anteroposterior and lateral direction are advised in these cases to rule out (avulsion) fractures, spurs, calcifications, or ossicles.

Peroneal tendon dislocation is a clinical diagnosis; nevertheless, it is frequently accompanied by a tendon rupture. Additional investigations such as MRI and ultrasonography may be helpful in diagnosing (partial) tears of the tendon of peroneus brevis or longus (110). Both are considerably accurate and precise; nevertheless, ultrasonography cost-effectively is preferable (111).

Treatment Options

Conservative management should be attempted first. This includes activity modification, footwear changes, temporary immobilization, and corticosteroid injections. Also, lateral heel wedges can take the strain off the peroneal tendons, which may allow healing (108).

In case conservative treatment fails, surgery can be indicated. For the tendoscopic treatment of peroneal tendon pathology, the patient is placed in the lateral decubitus position. Alternatively, the patient can also be placed in the supine position with the foot in exorotation. A support can be placed under the leg, being able to move the ankle freely. Before anesthesia is administered, the patient is asked to evert the foot, hereby the peroneal tendons can usually be visualized clearly. Its course is drawn on the skin, and the location of the portals is marked. The surgery can be performed under local, regional, epidural, or general anesthesia. After exsanguination, a tourniquet is inflated around the thigh of the affected leg.

A distal portal is made first, 2 to 2.5 cm distal to the posterior edge of the lateral malleolus. An incision is made through the skin, and the tendon sheath is penetrated with an arthroscopic shaft with a blunt trocar. After this, a 2.7-mm 30° arthroscope is introduced.

The inspection starts approximately 6 cm proximal to the posterior tip of the fibula, where a thin membrane splits the tendon compartment into two separate tendon chambers. More distally, the tendons lie in one compartment. A second portal is made 2 to 2.5 cm proximal to the posterior edge of the lateral malleolus under direct vision by placing a spinal needle, producing a portal directly over the tendons. Through the distal portal, a complete overview of both tendons can be obtained (Fig. 88.12).

By rotating the arthroscope over and in between both tendons, the whole compartment can be inspected. When a total synovectomy of the tendon sheath has to be performed, it is advisable to make a third portal more distal or more proximal than the portals described previously.

When a rupture of one of the tendons is seen, endoscopic synovectomy is performed, and the rupture is repaired through a mini-open approach.

In patients with recurrent dislocation of the peroneal tendon, endoscopic fibular groove deepening can be performed through this approach. It is, however, a time consuming procedure, because of the limited working area. Groove deepening is performed from within the tendon sheath with the risk of iatrogenic damage to the tendons.

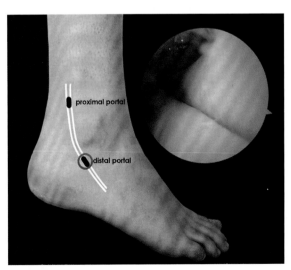

FIGURE 88.12. View on the peroneal tendons when the scope is introduced in the distal portal.

VI. Foot and Ankle

We, therefore, prefer an approach, based on the two-portal hindfoot technique, with an additional portal located 4 cm proximal to the posterolateral portal (112).

Rehabilitation Protocol

Postoperative management consists of a pressure bandage and partial weight bearing for 2 to 3 days. Full weight bearing is allowed as tolerated and active range of motion exercises are advised starting immediately postsurgery.

Pearls and Pitfalls

- It is important to identify the location of the peroneal tendons before creating the portals. Ask the patient to actively evert the foot, identify the tendon, and mark the location of the portals on the skin.
- Place a support under the affected ankle prior to surgery, so that the ankle can be moved freely.
- Patients with chronic lateral ankle instability and lateral retromalleolar ankle pain should be suspected for tendon ruptures. Specifically, pay attention to this pathology during the tendoscopy.

FLEXOR HALLUCIS LONGUS TENDOSCOPY

Introduction

FHL tenosynovitis is a well-recognized cause of posteromedial ankle pain. In ballet dancers, this entity has been described as "dancer's tendinitis" (113). Athletes performing repetitive forceful push-offs are at risk to develop an FHL tendinitis (114).

FHL tendinitis and posterior ankle impingement based on the os trigonum syndrome are distinct entities; nevertheless frequently coexist because of their close anatomical orientation (22, 115, 116). If conservative treatment fails, surgical intervention involves removal of the os trigonum, tendon debridement, and a release of the flexor retinaculum and tendon sheath at the level of the posterior talar process. Also, extra-articular structures of the hindfoot such as the os trigonum and FHL can be assessed (12).

History and Physical Examination

Patients typically complain of pain located at the posteromedial aspect of the ankle, which exacerbates with ankle motion and hallux dorsiflexion and diminishes at rest. The tendon can be palpated behind the medial malleolus at the level of the subtalar joint. Asking the patient to repetitively flex the big toe with the ankle in 10° to 20° of plantarflexion will increase the ability to palpate the tendon in its gliding channel. This maneuver will also differentiate between FHL and PTT pathology. The FHL tendon glides up and down under the palpating finger of the examiner. In case of stenosing tendinitis or chronic inflammation, crepitus and recognizable tenderness can be provoked. In some patients, a nodule can be palpated moving up and down with active movement of the great toe.

In patients with associated posterolateral ankle pain, a posterior impingement syndrome must be ruled out by means of a hyperplantarflexion test. The forced passive hyperplantarflexion test is positive when the patient experiences recognizable posterior ankle pain. A negative test rules out a posterior ankle impingement syndrome. A positive test is followed by a diagnostic infiltration with Xylocaine (AstraZeneca, Zoetermeer, The Netherlands) in the posterior ankle compartment. Disappearance of pain following infiltration confirms diagnosis.

Diagnostic Imaging

After history taking and physical examination, diagnosis can be confirmed or rejected based on different available imaging techniques. In case history taking and physical examination do not reveal abnormalities, additional diagnostics can be used to search for a clue or to rule out pathology, or for medicolegal reasons.

In patients without a history of trauma but with isolated recognizable posteromedial ankle pain during flexion of the great toe while palpating the tendon at the level of the gliding channel, no additional diagnostics are needed. In case conservative treatment options fail, the intervention will be a release regardless of the pathology. An MRI scan can be valuable to rule out tendon ruptures.

Treatment Options

Nonoperative treatment options include rest, activity modification, ice therapy, NSAIDs, and physical therapy modalities, as for instance stretching exercises (22, 115). An infiltration with corticosteroids around the tendon at the level of the tunnel can be performed as a next step. Be cautious for iatrogenic neurovascular bundle and tendon lesions. Frequently, conservative treatment options do not completely resolve the complaints. Also, a highly active professional ballet dancer with a competitive attitude will not permit himself to be inactive for several months. In these cases, release of the tendon and resection of posterior located bony or soft tissue impediment is indicated.

The authors decided to describe the hindfoot endoscopic approach, as was previously described. The procedure is carried out as outpatient surgery under general anesthesia or spinal anesthesia. The standard two-portal hindfoot approach is performed (see above) and the safe working area is reached. After resection of the soft tissue overlying the posterior talar process, the FHL comes into view. In case of isolated tendinitis of the FHL tendon, the flexor retinaculum can be released by detaching it from the posterior talar process or os trigonum with an arthroscopic punch. Subsequently, the tendon sheath can be opened distally up to the level of the sustentaculum tali. The tendon sheath can now be entered with the scope, allowing accurate tendon inspection and if necessary a further release can be performed (Fig. 88.13).

Possible length ruptures are debrided. The proximal part of the tendon and the distal part of the muscle belly are inspected and debrided if inflamed, thickened or if nodules are present. Adhesions and excessive scar tissue are removed.

Bleeding is controlled by electrocautery at the end of the procedure. To prevent sinus formation, the skin incisions are sutured with 3.0 Ethilon. The incisions and surrounding skin are injected with 10 mL of a 0.5% bupivacaine/morphine solution. A sterile compressive dressing is applied. Prophylactic antibiotics are not routinely given.

Postoperative Rehabilitation Protocol

The patient can be discharged the same day of surgery and weight bearing is allowed as tolerated. The patient is instructed to elevate the foot when not walking to prevent edema. The dressing is removed 3 days postoperatively after which the patient is permitted to shower.

Performing active range of motion exercises for at least three times a day for 10 minutes each is encouraged. Patients with limited range of motion are directed to a physiotherapist.

Pearls and Pitfalls

- Use an arthroscopic punch to detach the flexor retinaculum from the posterior talar process and to release the tendon sheath in case of tendinopathy of the FHL.
- Sufficiently release the tendon sheath all the way down toward the sustentaculum tali in case of isolated tendinopathy of the FHL.
- Be cautious while removing a hypertrophic posterior talar process with a chisel.
- Only remove the inferoposterior part and remove the remnant with the bonecutter shaver in order to prevent removing too much bone at the level of the subtalar joint.
- Surgeons not familiar with endoscopic surgery are advised to train themselves in a cadaveric setting (69, 70).

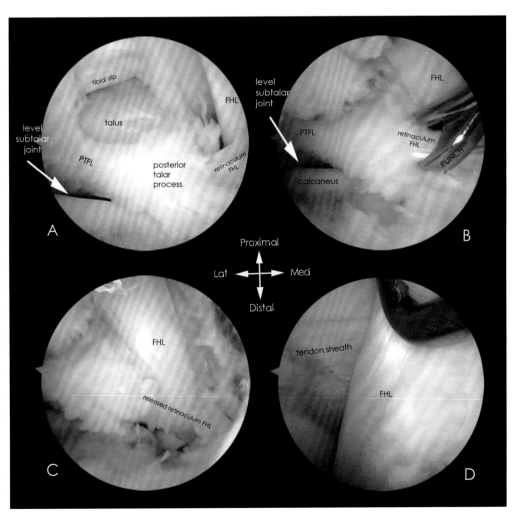

FIGURE 88.13. Release of the FHL tendon. **A:** Overview of the working area. **B:** The flexor retinaculum is cut. **C:** Cut retinaculum. **D:** Scope has entered the tendon sheath for inspection.

FUTURE DIRECTIONS

Future directions include the refinement of arthroscopic arthrodesis techniques. Indications include the subtalar, talonavicular, and calcaneocuboid joints; double arthrodesis and triple arthrodesis will be performed arthroscopically. Subtalar prostheses will be developed, and placement under arthroscopic control will be a possibility.

REFERENCES

1. Burman MS. Arthroscopy of direct visualization of joints: an experimental cadaver study. *J Bone Joint Surg Am.* 1931;13:669–695.
2. Watanabe M. *Selfoc-Arthroscope (Watanabe No. 24 Arthroscope). Monograph.* Tokyo, Japan: Teishin Hospital; 1972.
3. Guhl JF. Operative arthroscopy. *Am J Sports Med.* 1979;7:328–335.
4. Myerson MS, Quill G. Ankle arthrodesis. A comparison of an arthroscopic and an open method of treatment. *Clin Orthop Relat Res.* 1991;268:84–95.
5. Scranton PE Jr, McDermott JE. Anterior tibiotalar spurs: a comparison of open versus arthroscopic debridement. *Foot Ankle.* 1992;13:125–129.
6. van Dijk CN, Scholte D. Arthroscopy of the ankle joint. *Arthroscopy.* 1997;13:90–96.
7. van Dijk CN, Verhagen RA, Tol JL. Arthroscopy for problems after ankle fracture. *J Bone Joint Surg Br.* 1997;79:280–284.
8. Andrews JR, Previte WJ, Carson WG. Arthroscopy of the ankle: technique and normal anatomy. *Foot Ankle.* 1985;6:29–33.
9. Ferkel RD, Scranton PE Jr. Arthroscopy of the ankle and foot. *J Bone Joint Surg Am.* 1993;75:1233–1242.
10. Guhl JF. *Foot and Ankle Arthroscopy.* New York, NY: Slack; 1993.
11. Ferkel RD, Small HN, Gittins JE. Complications in foot and ankle arthroscopy. *Clin Orthop Relat Res.* 2001;381:89–104.
12. van Dijk CN, Scholten PE, Krips R. A 2-portal endoscopic approach for diagnosis and treatment of posterior ankle pathology. *Arthroscopy.* 2000;16:871–876.
13. Beimers L, de Leeuw PA, van Dijk CN. A 3-portal approach for arthroscopic subtalar arthrodesis. *Knee Surg Sports Traumatol Arthrosc.* 2009;17(7):830–834.
14. Scholten PE, Sierevelt IN, van Dijk CN. Hindfoot endoscopy for posterior ankle impingement. *J Bone Joint Surg Am.* 2008;90:2665–2672.
15. van Dijk CN. Hindfoot endoscopy. *Foot Ankle Clin.* 2006;11:391–414, vii.
16. Lijoi F, Lughi M, Baccarani G. Posterior arthroscopic approach to the ankle: an anatomic study. *Arthroscopy.* 2003;19:62–67.
17. Sitler DF, Amendola A, Bailey CS, et al. Posterior ankle arthroscopy: an anatomic study. *J Bone Joint Surg Am.* 2002;84-A:763–769.
18. van Dijk CN, de Leeuw PA, Scholten PE. Hindfoot endoscopy for posterior ankle impingement. Surgical technique. *J Bone Joint Surg Am.* 2009;91(suppl 2):287–298.
19. van Dijk CN, Verhagen RA, Tol HJ. Technical note: resterilizable noninvasive ankle distraction device. *Arthroscopy.* 2001;17:E12.
20. Amsterdam Foot & Ankle Platform. http://www.ankleplatform.com/page.php?id=97. 2009.
21. Hamilton WG, Geppert MJ, Thompson FM. Pain in the posterior aspect of the ankle in dancers. Differential diagnosis and operative treatment. *J Bone Joint Surg Am.* 1996;78:1491–1500.
22. Hedrick MR, McBryde AM. Posterior ankle impingement. *Foot Ankle Int.* 1994;15:2–8.
23. van Dijk CN, Lim LS, Poortman A, et al. Degenerative joint disease in female ballet dancers. *Am J Sports Med.* 1995;23:295–300.
24. Stibbe AB, van Dijk CN, Marti RK. The os trigonum syndrome. *Acta Orthop Scand.* 1994;(suppl 262):59–60.
25. Scholten PE, Sierevelt IN, van Dijk CN. Hindfoot endoscopy for posterior ankle impingement. *J Bone Joint Surg Am.* 2008;90:2665–2672.
26. Weinstein SL, Bonfiglio M. Unusual accessory (bipartite) talus simulating fracture. A case report. *J Bone Joint Surg Am.* 1975;57:1161–1163.
27. Bizarro AH. On sesamoid and supernumerary bones of the limbs. *J Anat.* 1921;55(pt 4):256–268.
28. Lapidus PW. A note on the fracture of os trigonum. Report of a case. *Bull Hosp Joint Dis.* 1972;33:150–154.
29. Sarrafian SK. *Anatomy of the Foot and Ankle: Descriptive, Topographic, Functional.* Philadelphia, PA: Lippincott; 1983.
30. Brodsky AE, Khalil MA. Talar compression syndrome. *Am J Sports Med.* 1986;14:472–476.
31. Hamilton WG. Stenosing tenosynovitis of the flexor hallucis longus tendon and posterior impingement upon the os trigonum in ballet dancers. *Foot Ankle.* 1982;3:74–80.
32. Howse AJ. Posterior block of the ankle joint in dancers. *Foot Ankle.* 1982;3:81–84.
33. Golano P, Mariani PP, Rodriguez-Niedenfuhr M, et al. Arthroscopic anatomy of the posterior ankle ligaments. *Arthroscopy.* 2002;18:353–358.
34. Boonthathip M, Chen L, Trudell DJ, et al. Tibiofibular syndesmotic ligaments: MR arthrography in cadavers with anatomic correlation. *Radiology.* 2010;254:827–836.
35. Oh CS, Won HS, Hur MS, et al. Anatomic variations and MRI of the intermalleolar ligament. *AJR Am J Roentgenol.* 2006;186:943–947.
36. Ferkel RD, Heath DD, Guhl JF. Neurological complications of ankle arthroscopy. *Arthroscopy.* 1996;12:200–208.
37. Ferkel RD, Fischer SP. Progress in ankle arthroscopy. *Clin Orthop Relat Res.* 1989;240:210–220.
38. Bosien WR, Staples OS, Russell SW. Residual disability following acute ankle sprainsuy. *J Bone Joint Surg Am.* 1955;37-A:1237–1243.
39. Verhagen RA, Struijs PA, Bossuyt PM, et al. Systematic review of treatment strategies for osteochondral defects of the talar dome. *Foot Ankle Clin.* 2003;8:233–239.
40. Canale ST, Belding RH. Osteochondral lesions of the talus. *J Bone Joint Surg Am.* 1980;62:97–102.
41. Berndt AL, Harty M. Transchondral fractures (osteochondritis dissecans) of the talus. *J Bone Joint Surg Am.* 1959;41-A:988–1020.
42. Zengerink M, Szerb I, Hangody L, et al. Current concepts: treatment of osteochondral ankle defects. *Foot Ankle Clin.* 2006;11:331–359, vi.
43. Verhagen RA, Maas M, Dijkgraaf MG, et al. Prospective study on diagnostic strategies in osteochondral lesions of the

talus. Is MRI superior to helical CT? *J Bone Joint Surg Br.* 2005;87:41–46.

44. Schuman L, Struijs PA, van Dijk CN. Arthroscopic treatment for osteochondral defects of the talus. Results at follow-up at 2 to 11 years. *J Bone Joint Surg Br.* 2002;84:364–368.

45. O'Driscoll SW. The healing and regeneration of articular cartilage. *J Bone Joint Surg Am.* 1998;80:1795–1812.

46. Giannini S, Buda R, Faldini C, et al. Surgical treatment of osteochondral lesions of the talus in young active patients. *J Bone Joint Surg Am.* 2005;87(suppl 2):28–41.

47. Taranow WS, Bisignani GA, Towers JD, et al. Retrograde drilling of osteochondral lesions of the medial talar dome. *Foot Ankle Int.* 1999;20:474–480.

48. Baums MH, Heidrich G, Schultz W, et al. Autologous chondrocyte transplantation for treating cartilage defects of the talus. *J Bone Joint Surg Am.* 2006;88:303–308.

49. Hangody L, Fules P. Autologous osteochondral mosaicplasty for the treatment of full-thickness defects of weight-bearing joints: ten years of experimental and clinical experience. *J Bone Joint Surg Am.* 2003;85-A(suppl 2):25–32.

50. Baltzer AW, Arnold JP. Bone-cartilage transplantation from the ipsilateral knee for chondral lesions of the talus. *Arthroscopy.* 2005;21:159–166.

51. Giannini S, Vannini F. Operative treatment of osteochondral lesions of the talar dome: current concepts review. *Foot Ankle Int.* 2004;25:168–175.

52. Reddy S, Pedowitz DI, Parekh SG, et al. The morbidity associated with osteochondral harvest from asymptomatic knees for the treatment of osteochondral lesions of the talus. *Am J Sports Med.* 2007;35:80–85.

53. Whittaker JP, Smith G, Makwana N, et al. Early results of autologous chondrocyte implantation in the talus. *J Bone Joint Surg Br.* 2005;87:179–183.

54. Takao M, Ochi M, Naito K, et al. Arthroscopic drilling for chondral, subchondral, and combined chondral-subchondral lesions of the talar dome. *Arthroscopy.* 2003;19:524–530.

55. Steadman JR, Rodkey WG, Rodrigo JJ. Microfracture: surgical technique and rehabilitation to treat chondral defects. *Clin Orthop Relat Res.* 2001;391S:S362–S369.

56. van Bergen CJ, de Leeuw PA, van Dijk CN. Potential pitfall in the microfracturing technique during the arthroscopic treatment of an osteochondral lesion. *Knee Surg Sports Traumatol Arthrosc.* 2008;17(2):184–187.

57. Saxena A, Eakin C. Articular talar injuries in athletes: results of microfracture and autogenous bone graft. *Am J Sports Med.* 2007;35:1680–1687.

58. Chuckpaiwong B, Berkson EM, Theodore GH. Microfracture for osteochondral lesions of the ankle: outcome analysis and outcome predictors of 105 cases. *Arthroscopy.* 2008;24:106–112.

59. Haglund P. Beitrag zur Klinik der Achillessehne. *Zeitschr Orthop Chir.* 1928;49:49–58.

60. Brunner J, Anderson J, O'Malley M, et al. Physician and patient based outcomes following surgical resection of Haglund's deformity. *Acta Orthop Belg.* 2005;71:718–723.

61. Harris CA, Peduto AJ. Achilles tendon imaging. *Australas Radiol.* 2006;50:513–525.

62. Jerosch J, Schunck J, Sokkar SH. Endoscopic calcaneoplasty (ECP) as a surgical treatment of Haglund's syndrome. *Knee Surg Sports Traumatol Arthrosc.* 2007;15:927–934.

63. Leitze Z, Sella EJ, Aversa JM. Endoscopic decompression of the retrocalcaneal space. *J Bone Joint Surg Am.* 2003;85-A:1488–1496.

64. Lohrer H, Nauck T, Dorn NV, et al. Comparison of endoscopic and open resection for Haglund tuberosity in a cadaver study. *Foot Ankle Int.* 2006;27:445–450.

65. Ly JQ, Bui-Mansfield LT. Anatomy of and abnormalities associated with Kager's fat Pad. *AJR Am J Roentgenol.* 2004;182:147–154.

66. Ortmann FW, McBryde AM. Endoscopic bony and soft-tissue decompression of the retrocalcaneal space for the treatment of Haglund deformity and retrocalcaneal bursitis. *Foot Ankle Int.* 2007;28:149–153.

67. van Dijk CN, de Leeuw PA. Imaging from an orthopaedic point of view. What the orthopaedic surgeon expects from the radiologist? *Eur J Radiol.* 2007;62:2–5.

68. van Sterkenburg MN, Muller B, Maas M, et al. Appearance of the weight-bearing lateral radiograph in retrocalcaneal bursitis. *Acta Orthop.* 2010; 81:387-390.

69. Arthroscopy Association of North America. Master courses: Foot/Ankle. http://www.aana.org/cme/MastersCourses/descriptions.aspx#Foot/Ankle. Accessed March 9, 2009.

70. Amsterdam Foot & Ankle Platform. http://www.ankleplatform.com/page.php?id=854. Accessed March 9, 2009.

71. Maffulli N, Khan KM, Puddu G. Overuse tendon conditions: time to change a confusing terminology. *Arthroscopy.* 1998;14:840–843.

72. Emerson C, Morrissey D, Perry M, et al. Ultrasonographically detected changes in Achilles tendons and self reported symptoms in elite gymnasts compared with controls—An observational study. *Man Ther.* 2009;15(1):37–42.

73. Haims AH, Schweitzer ME, Patel RS, et al. MR imaging of the Achilles tendon: overlap of findings in symptomatic and asymptomatic individuals. *Skeletal Radiol.* 2000;29:640–645.

74. Kannus P, Jozsa L. Histopathological changes preceding spontaneous rupture of a tendon. A controlled study of 891 patients. *J Bone Joint Surg Am.* 1991;73:1507–1525.

75. Khan KM, Forster BB, Robinson J, et al. Are ultrasound and magnetic resonance imaging of value in assessment of Achilles tendon disorders? A two year prospective study. *Br J Sports Med.* 2003;37:149–153.

76. Segesser B, Goesele A, Renggli P. The Achilles tendon in sports. *Orthopade.* 1995;24:252–267.

77. Maffulli N, Walley G, Sayana MK, et al. Eccentric calf muscle training in athletic patients with Achilles tendinopathy. *Disabil Rehabil.* 2008;30(20–22):1677–1684.

78. Maffulli N, Kenward MG, Testa V, et al. Clinical diagnosis of Achilles tendinopathy with tendinosis. *Clin J Sport Med.* 2003;13:11–15.

79. Steenstra F, van Dijk CN. Achilles tendoscopy. *Foot Ankle Clin.* 2006;11:429–438, viii.

80. Williams JG. Achilles tendon lesions in sport. *Sports Med.* 1993;16:216–220.

81. Magnussen RA, Dunn WR, Thomson AB. Nonoperative treatment of midportion Achilles tendinopathy: a systematic review. *Clin J Sport Med.* 2009;19:54–64.

82. Mafi N, Lorentzon R, Alfredson H. Superior short-term results with eccentric calf muscle training compared to concentric training in a randomized prospective multicenter

VI. Foot and Ankle

study on patients with chronic Achilles tendinosis. *Knee Surg Sports Traumatol Arthrosc.* 2001;9:42–47.

83. Norregaard J, Larsen CC, Bieler T, et al. Eccentric exercise in treatment of Achilles tendinopathy. *Scand J Med Sci Sports.* 2007;17:133–138.

84. Ohberg L, Lorentzon R, Alfredson H. Eccentric training in patients with chronic Achilles tendinosis: normalised tendon structure and decreased thickness at follow up. *Br J Sports Med.* 2004;38:8–11.

85. Silbernagel KG, Thomee R, Thomee P, et al. Eccentric overload training for patients with chronic Achilles tendon pain—a randomised controlled study with reliability testing of the evaluation methods. *Scand J Med Sci Sports.* 2001;11:197–206.

86. Kvist M. Achilles tendon injuries in athletes. *Ann Chir Gynaecol.* 1991;80:188–201.

87. Maffulli N. Augmented repair of acute Achilles tendon ruptures using gastrocnemius-soleus fascia. *Int Orthop.* 2005;29:134.

88. Myerson MS. Adult acquired flatfoot deformity: treatment of dysfunction of the posterior tibial tendon. *Instr Course Lect.* 1997;46:393–405.

89. Michelson J, Easley M, Wigley FM, et al. Posterior tibial tendon dysfunction in rheumatoid arthritis. *Foot Ankle Int.* 1995;16:156–161.

90. Bulstra GH, Olsthoorn PG, van Dijk CN. Tendoscopy of the posterior tibial tendon. *Foot Ankle Clin.* 2006;11:421–427, viii.

91. Trnka HJ. Dysfunction of the tendon of tibialis posterior. *J Bone Joint Surg Br.* 2004;86:939–946.

92. Kong A, Van Der Vliet A. Imaging of tibialis posterior dysfunction. *Br J Radiol.* 2008;81:826–836.

93. Miller SD, Van HM, Boruta PM, et al. Ultrasound in the diagnosis of posterior tibial tendon pathology. *Foot Ankle Int.* 1996;17:555–558.

94. Porter DA, Baxter DE, Clanton TO, et al. Posterior tibial tendon tears in young competitive athletes: two case reports. *Foot Ankle Int.* 1998;19:627–630.

95. Lui TH. Endoscopic assisted posterior tibial tendon reconstruction for stage 2 posterior tibial tendon insufficiency. *Knee Surg Sports Traumatol Arthrosc.* 2007;15:1228–1234.

96. Paus AC. Arthroscopic synovectomy. When, which diseases and which joints. *Z Rheumatol.* 1996;55:394–400.

97. van Dijk CN, Kort N, Scholten PE. Tendoscopy of the posterior tibial tendon. *Arthroscopy.* 1997;13:692–698.

98. van Dijk CN, Scholten PE, Kort N. Tendoscopy (tendon sheath endoscopy) for overuse tendon injuries. *Oper Techn Sports Med.* 1997;5:170–178.

99. van Dijk CN, Kort N. Tendoscopy of the peroneal tendons. *Arthroscopy.* 1998;14:471–478.

100. Sobel M, Geppert MJ, Hannafin JA, et al. Microvascular anatomy of the peroneal tendons. *Foot Ankle.* 1992;13:469–472.

101. Benjamin M, Qin S, Ralphs JR. Fibrocartilage associated with human tendons and their pulleys. *J Anat.* 1995;187(pt 3):625–633.

102. Kumai T, Benjamin M. The histological structure of the malleolar groove of the fibula in man: its direct bearing on the displacement of peroneal tendons and their surgical repair. *J Anat.* 2003;203:257–262.

103. Scholten PE, van Dijk CN. Tendoscopy of the peroneal tendons. *Foot Ankle Clin.* 2006;11:415–420, vii.

104. Monteggi GB. *Instituzini Chirurgiche.* Italy: Milan; 1803.

105. Edwards ME. The relations of the peroneal tendons to the fibula, calcaneus and cuboideum. *Am J Anat.* 1928;42:213–253.

106. Eckert WR, Davis EA Jr. Acute rupture of the peroneal retinaculum. *J Bone Joint Surg Am.* 1976;58:670–672.

107. Molloy R, Tisdel C. Failed treatment of peroneal tendon injuries. *Foot Ankle Clin.* 2003;8:115–129, ix.

108. Heckman DS, Reddy S, Pedowitz D, et al. Operative treatment for peroneal tendon disorders. *J Bone Joint Surg Am.* 2008;90:404–418.

109. Safran MR, O'Malley D Jr, Fu FH. Peroneal tendon subluxation in athletes: new exam technique, case reports, and review. *Med Sci Sports Exerc.* 1999;31:S487–S492.

110. Rosenberg ZS, Bencardino J, Astion D, et al. MRI features of chronic injuries of the superior peroneal retinaculum. *AJR Am J Roentgenol.* 2003;181:1551–1557.

111. Rockett MS, Waitches G, Sudakoff G, et al. Use of ultrasonography versus magnetic resonance imaging for tendon abnormalities around the ankle. *Foot Ankle Int.* 1998;19:604–612.

112. de Leeuw PAJ, Golano P, van Dijk CN. A 3-portal endoscopic groove deepening technique for recurrent peroneal tendon dislocation. *Tech Foot Ankle Surg.* 2008;7:250–256.

113. Hamilton WG. Tendonitis about the ankle joint in classical ballet dancers. *Am J Sports Med.* 1977;5:84–88.

114. Leach RE, DiIorio E, Harney RA. Pathologic hindfoot conditions in the athlete. *Clin Orthop Relat Res.* 1983;177:116–121.

115. Sammarco GJ, Cooper PS. Flexor hallucis longus tendon injury in dancers and nondancers. *Foot Ankle Int.* 1998;19:356–362.

116. van Dijk CN. Hindfoot endoscopy for posterior ankle pain. *Instr Course Lect.* 2006;55:545–554.

Soft Tissue and Bony Impingement

James Stone

SOFT TISSUE ANKLE IMPINGEMENT

Until 1950 the concept that abnormal soft tissue within the ankle joint could be responsible for pain and mechanical symptoms was not the subject of orthopedic investigation. In 1950, Wolin and associates published a paper on soft tissue impingement lesions of the ankle joint, which they termed "meniscoid" lesions because of their tactile resemblance to knee meniscus tissue (1). They reported on nine patients with chronic ankle pain after inversion ankle sprains, who were found at open surgery to have impingement lesions in the lateral gutter and improved after removal of the abnormal soft tissue. Although patients often complained of instability, they did not demonstrate objective signs of joint laxity, and their instability symptoms resolved after excision of the synovial-based lesion. The authors proposed that the inciting factor was the inversion injury that caused tissue disruption and bleeding. Although most patients gradually resolve such injuries, the ones who develop synovial impingement lesions develop a chronic synovitis with gradual thickening and fibrosis of the material in the anterolateral gutter of the ankle joint. Japanese investigators performed some of the earliest arthroscopic evaluations of the ankle joint and may have been the first to describe similar lesions on arthroscopic examination.

In 1987, McCarroll et al. (2) reported on four soccer players who developed chronic ankle symptoms after recurrent ankle sprains and did not improve with nonoperative treatment. Arthroscopic examination revealed abnormal fibrous tissue bands in each patient, and after resection of the lesions and appropriate rehabilitation, each patient returned to competitive soccer. Martin et al. (3) reported on 16 patients undergoing ankle arthroscopy for chronic ankle pain mainly after inversion sprains and found that all patients demonstrated hypertrophic synovial tissue at arthroscopy, and good or excellent results were noted in 75% of the patients after excision. Ferkel and Fischer (4) reported on 100 ankle patients who underwent ankle arthroscopy, 24 of whom had chronic anterolateral impingement symptoms. Pain and instability

were common symptoms, but stress radiographs failed to document objective ligament laxity. Plain radiographs were not helpful in predicting these synovial lesions, but the authors suggested that MRI could be useful in delineating abnormal anterolateral soft tissues. In a follow-up study, Ferkel et al. (5) reported on 31 patients with chronic anterolateral ankle joint pain following inversion ankle sprain. None had objective evidence of joint laxity and the preoperative MRI scan was found to reliably show abnormal soft tissue synovial thickening in the anterolateral gutter. At the time of arthroscopy these patients were noted to have "proliferative synovitis and fibrotic scar tissue," sometimes associated with adjacent chondromalacia of the talar articular cartilage. There were good or excellent results in 26 of the patients after arthroscopic excision of the abnormal tissue. Numerous other studies in the orthopedic literature support the utility of arthroscopy for resection of soft tissue impingement lesions of the ankle joint with good results in patients who do not have associated degenerative changes in the joint (6–11).

Bassett (12) has delineated a specific type of anterior ankle soft tissue impingement caused by mechanical impingement of the distal fascicle of the anterior inferior tibio fibular ligament on the adjacent talus. The anatomy and clinical relevance of the syndrome have been explored by others (13)

We generally refer to these problems as posttraumatic synovial impingement lesions rather than meniscoid lesions because there is a wide range of lesions varying in organization or "hyalinization" from a localized inflammatory synovitis to a well-organized mass of firm tissue. In addition, we have recognized that impingement lesions can occur in any part of the ankle including the lateral gutter, medial gutter, anterior joint, or posterior joint.

History

Patients with soft tissue ankle impingement present to the physician with persistent ankle symptoms after ankle ligament injury that fail to resolve with standard treatment of the ankle sprain. When evaluated soon after an ankle sprain, conservative measures including rest, ice, elevation, compression, nonsteroidal anti-inflammatory medications, and a limited period of nonweight bearing immobilization in a removable orthosis may be instituted. Most patients will recover with a physician-directed rehabilitation protocol emphasizing range of motion exercises, strengthening exercises, and gradual return to weight-bearing functional activities. However, other patients with more severe injuries or those who participate in high demand work or sports activities may benefit from a supervised exercise and rehabilitation program under the direction of a physical therapist.

A small group of these patients may present to the orthopedic surgeon with persistent symptoms of pain, catching, or giving way of the ankle despite a reasonable period of rehabilitation of up to 12 weeks. In general the pain symptoms are well localized either medially or laterally but may be more diffuse anteriorly and on occasion may occur posteriorly. Persistent or intermittent swelling associated with attempts to resume activities may occur.

Physical Examination

The physical examination of the patient with soft tissue impingement of the ankle joint is not specific. The clinician should first observe the ankle for signs of localized or generalized swelling or ecchymosis, which may direct the examination to a specific anatomic location. The range of motion of the ankle and the subtalar joints should be assessed and compared with the opposite ankle to detect subtle or obvious limitations. It is very important to assess the hindfoot alignment for fixed valgus or varus deformities as the presence of alignment abnormality may predispose the patient to recurrent injury and may influence the nature of the nonoperative intervention, for example using orthotic devices, or of the surgical procedures to be considered should nonoperative treatment fail to alleviate symptoms.

The examiner then assesses for specific areas of tenderness and correlates those areas with the area where the patient complains of pain. Specific examination must attempt to determine whether the tenderness is, for example, over the joint line and therefore potentially associated with soft tissue impingement versus tenderness localized to the bony structures of the ankle or possibly abnormal bony structures such as osteophytes. Soft tissue impingement lesions may be associated with palpable soft tissue prominence and perhaps palpable clipping or snapping beneath the examining finger with passive or active motion of the joint.

Much of the physical examination is dedicated to other structures to exclude other diagnoses from the differential diagnosis list. In particular, the examiner should assess the tendons about the anterior ankle to be certain that there is no evidence of chronic tendinitis or tendon tearing. For patients complaining of posterior ankle pain, the examiner must carefully palpate and assess the strength of the posterior tibial tendon, flexor digitorum

tendon, flexor hallucis longus tendon, the peroneal tendons, along with the Achilles tendon. The examination of these tendons should include palpation to assess tenderness and palpation during active and passive motion of the isolated tendons to assess for crepitus, snapping, or weakness.

The neurovascular structures must also be assessed carefully. Pulses should be assessed along with a careful sensory and motor examination of the ankle and foot.

Radiographic Studies

Patients presenting to the orthopedic surgeon with ankle pain should have routine anteroposterior (AP), lateral, and mortise views of the ankle. In addition, patients with potential foot complaints should have weight-bearing AP, lateral, and oblique radiographs of the foot. Standing radiographs of the ankle may assist in assessing the degree of degenerative changes in the ankle joint and in assessing the alignment of the hindfoot joints.

A CT of the ankle and subtalar joints can be useful for assessing the bony characteristics of osteochondral lesions of the talar dome or bony osteophytes. However, this study will not contribute to the workup of soft tissue abnormalities.

Early studies of the use of MRI to assess for soft tissue impingement lesions of the ankle gave equivocal or contradictory results regarding sensitivity, specificity, and diagnostic accuracy (14, 15). The more recent orthopedic and radiologic literature has suggested that with improved equipment and image quality along with increased awareness of these lesions, the MRI is able to diagnose these lesions with a high level of accuracy (16–18). It is also the most appropriate study to assess other soft tissue causes of ankle pain such as tendinitis or tendon tearing. In addition, the MRI visualizes bone to assess for chondral or osteochondral abnormalities in the bones comprising the ankle and subtalar joints, and the presence of bone edema in an area of the talus or tibia may be the only radiographic manifestation of injury, for example, owing to posterior impingement.

Treatment of Soft Tissue Impingement Lesions

Most patients with an acute ankle sprain will recover uneventfully from their injury with standard nonoperative treatment. In some patients there may be a propensity to develop excessive scar tissue after injury, or in the case of recurrent injury the ankle is never given adequate opportunity to complete the healing sequence with gradual resorption of inflammatory tissue associated with the healing ligament injury.

An adequate period of nonoperative treatment of up to 12 weeks should be pursued. During this time, the conservative measures mentioned above will usually decrease pain and swelling and allow the gradual resumption of weight bearing, range of motion, and strengthening.

In patients with persistent discomfort an intra-articular corticosteroid injection may be useful for both diagnostic and therapeutic purposes. When combined with a local anesthetic and injected into the ankle joint, the patient with a soft tissue impingement lesion should have at least temporary relief of their symptoms. The corticosteroid may control inflammation in the joint and allow further healing without need for surgery. If the patient denies even temporary relief during the period of anesthetic effectiveness, the evaluating physician should entertain the possibility that the patient's problem does not emanate from the ankle joint. At this point another injection into the subtalar joint may be indicated to assess the possibility that the symptoms are arising from that joint rather than the ankle joint. Some patients may have communication between the two joints that may make interpretation of the diagnostic injection difficult. If neither injection affords symptom relief, the evaluating physician must consider other causes of persistent ankle pain arising from the soft tissue structures in the vicinity of the ankle or ankle pain secondary to a completely different source such as neurologically mediated ankle pain.

Surgical treatment is reserved for those patients with symptoms and signs consistent with soft tissue impingement of the ankle joint who fail to respond to nonoperative measures. Ankle arthroscopy is performed with the patient positioned supine on the operating table with the hip and knee of the affected side flexed and supported by a well-padded leg holder (Fig. 89.1). The leg holder should have a long thigh support segment and a short portion extending past the posterior knee crease so that when traction is applied to the joint, the force is placed against a broad area of the thigh rather than being concentrated over a short area in the popliteal fossa, which might contribute to increased venous obstruction and increase the chance of deep vein thrombosis.

After routine skin preparation and sterile draping, a noninvasive commercially available ankle distraction apparatus is placed and gentle traction is applied to the ankle joint (Fig. 89.2). The author recommends routine

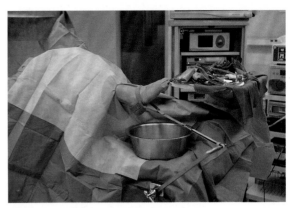

FIGURE 89.2. After routine skin preparation and sterile draping, the commercially available noninvasive joint distraction apparatus is attached. The distractor is completely sterile and allows the leg to hang in a plantigrade position, with good access to both anterior and posterior portals and with free intraoperative joint motion possible.

placement of anteromedial, anterolateral, and posterolateral portals on every patient (Fig. 89.3). The inflow is placed posteriorly, the arthroscope is initially placed anteromedially, and instruments are introduced through the anterolateral portal. Every ankle should be surveyed in an organized and reproducible manner by the operating surgeon. The author begins the evaluation from the anteromedial portal at the tip of the medial malleolus visualizing the deltoid ligament and then proceeds up the anteromedial gutter to the dome of the talus. The arthroscope is then directed in a posterolateral direction so that the entire talar dome and tibial plafond are visualized and palpated. The posterior joint is evaluated at this point and gentle manual pumping of the posterior soft tissues may help to visualize any hidden posterior loose bodies. The arthroscope is then turned laterally to visualize the "trifurcation" where the distal tibia, distal fibula, and the lateral talar dome are seen. The inferior bundle of the anterior inferior tibiofibular ligament is visualized as a vertically oriented structure at the anterior margin of the trifurcation. Bassett has suggested that hypertrophy of this structure may cause anterolateral impingement and may be associated with adjacent chondromalacia of the talar dome. The arthroscope is then directed into the anterolateral gutter to visualize the anterior talofibular ligament and the tip of the lateral malleolus. As the arthroscope is withdrawn across the anterior joint, the distal tibia and the talar neck can be evaluated. This exposure may be improved by diminishing the traction applied to the joint in combination with ankle dorsiflexion, which relaxes the anterior capsule to create increased space anteriorly.

The instruments are then switched so that the arthroscope is in the anterolateral portal and the probe or other instruments in the anteromedial portal, and a similar complete evaluation in reverse is performed. As a final view, the arthroscope may be placed in the posterolateral portal to enhance visualization of the posterior ankle compartment.

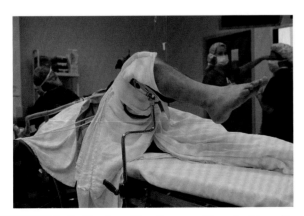

FIGURE 89.1. Position for ankle arthroscopy: The patient is supine on the operating table with the hip and knee flexed and supported by a well-padded leg holder with a long thigh support and minimal extension past the popliteal fossa.

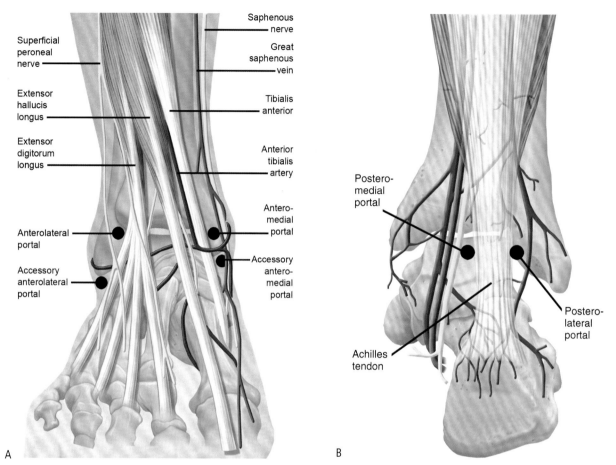

A

B

FIGURE 89.3. **A:** Anterior anatomy pertinent to ankle arthroscopy. The anteromedial portal is placed immediately adjacent to the medial border of the tibialis anterior tendon at the level of the joint line. Good position for this portal is determined by introducing a needle into the joint to confirm that it can be passed across the joint without injuring the tibial or talar articular surfaces. Position is adjusted superior or inferior as needed to allow safe passage of the needle and then the instruments. An accessory medial portal may be placed 1 cm or more from the anteromedial portal, as guided intraoperatively by placement of a hypodermic needle. **B:** Posterior anatomy pertinent to ankle arthroscopy. The posterolateral portal is placed immediately adjacent to the lateral border of the Achilles tendon 1 to 2 cm distal to the level of the anterior portals. This more distal location allows for a needle to pass into the joint smoothly, accommodating the curved surface of the talar dome.

The most common location for impingement lesions is in the anterolateral gutter and in the distal tibiofibular joint (Fig. 89.4). The abnormal tissue may be removed using a shaver if the lesion is soft. Firmer tissue may be removed using basket forceps or a radiofrequency device that achieves both tissue ablation and hemostasis (Fig. 89.5). Anterolateral impingement may be on account of the inferior fascicle of the anterior inferior tibiofibular ligament. The lesion was originally identified by Bassett who noted that the hypertrophic ligament may physically impinge upon the talus during ankle dorsiflexion. A popping sensation may be noted by the patient, and physical examination may show local tenderness over the anterolateral talar dome made worse with dorsiflexion and eversion of the ankle joint. In the presence of ligament hypertrophy, the diagnosis is supported by the presence of adjacent chondromalacia of the talus. Resection of

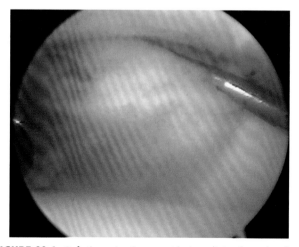

FIGURE 89.4. Soft tissue impingement lesion arising from the distal tibiofibular joint.

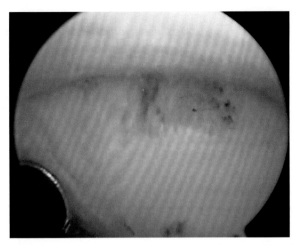

FIGURE 89.5. Arthroscopic view after resection of the soft tissue impingement lesion of the distal tibiofibular joint.

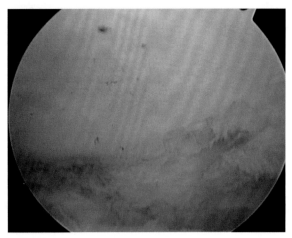

FIGURE 89.7. Medial soft tissue impingement lesion after resection.

the visible intra-articular portion of the ligament does not destabilize the syndesmosis and represents the definitive surgical treatment of this lesion.

Soft tissue impingement may also be noted medially (Fig. 89.6). Synovial hypertrophy with increased rigidity of the soft tissue in the area of the medial gutter is diagnostic of medial synovial impingement. This lesion is also removed using shaver, basket forceps, and/or radiofrequency probe (Fig. 89.7).

The patient is placed into a posterior plaster splint or immobilizing short leg walker for 1 week before the-sutures are removed. The immobilizing device is discontinued as the patient is allowed to increase weight bearing as tolerated. The patient may be instructed on exercises to increase the range of motion and strength on his/her own or the patient may be referred to a physical therapist to supervise the rehabilitation process. Rehabilitation after soft tissue impingement surgery should allow return to full activity including sports in 6 to 8 weeks.

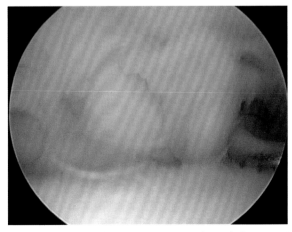

FIGURE 89.6. Medial soft tissue impingement lesion before resection.

BONY ANKLE IMPINGEMENT

Osteophytes are bony excrescences that originate from the joint margins in response to articular cartilage damage as seen in degenerative arthritis or owing to joint injuries not associated with articular cartilage damage as seen in bony impingement lesions. In the ankle these bony impingement lesions arise most commonly from the anterior tibia and may be associated with adjacent bony lesions on the talar neck. Impingement occurs with forced ankle dorsiflexion. Osteophytes may also arise posteriorly on the tibial margin and be associated with posterior bony impingement in ankle plantar flexion. Most often they are associated with overuse or repetitive joint injury, but the etiology of these lesions has not been well defined. Early studies suggested that repetitive traction injury, in the case of the anterior ankle repetitive plantar flexion injury, stimulated formation of anterior tibial osteophytes. (19, 20). This mechanism would imply traction of the capsule itself on the bone to be the inciting mechanism. However, it has been noted that the osteophytes actually form distal to the capsular insertion on the tibia (21). This finding would suggest that the osteophytes form in response to repetitive trauma rather than the capsular traction injury. In another study, 28 talus specimens were examined regarding the location of bony outgrowths in comparison with the talar head. The authors found that on the medial aspect of the anterior talus, bone spur formation occurred in an intra-articular location suggesting a true osteophyte. In contrast, on the more lateral aspect of the anterior talus the outgrowths occurred in an extra-articular location and appeared to occur in response to capsular traction injury (22). More recently it has been noted by van Dijk that tibial osteophytes most commonly form over the medial side of the tibia and often include the anterior surface of the medial malleolus. He postulated that recurrent inversion of the ankle resulting in contact of these surfaces was the initiating factor. 23 This mechanism might also imply that ankle instability with recurrent inversion sprains increases the incidence of anterior tibial osteophytes.

Anterior tibial osteophytes have been classified by Scranton and McDermott (24) into four categories (Fig. 89.8). Type I bony impingement includes bone spurs up to 3 mm. Type II lesions include bony spurs greater than 3 mm without talar spurring. Type III lesions include both anterior tibial spurs and talar spurs. Type IV lesions include those patients with both bony spurs and concomitant degenerative changes on plain radiographs. These authors have found that resection of bony osteophytes generally results in diminished symptoms of ankle pain especially when the osteophytes are not present with significant degenerative arthritis of the joint. Tol et al (21, 23, 25). came to a similar conclusion in a prospective study of 57 patients treated for anterior ankle impingement. They found that at an average follow-up of 6.5 years in all patients without evidence of osteoarthritis had good or excellent results. Those patients who exhibited joint space narrowing along with osteophyte impingement had a 53% incidence of good or excellent results.

Van Dijk has pointed out that despite the fact that anterior tibial osteophytes appear in some patients to abut talar neck osteophytes, when lateral radiographs are obtained in ankle dorsiflexion, these osteophytes actually seldom make contact. He found that the osteophytes occur more commonly over the medial aspect of the anterior

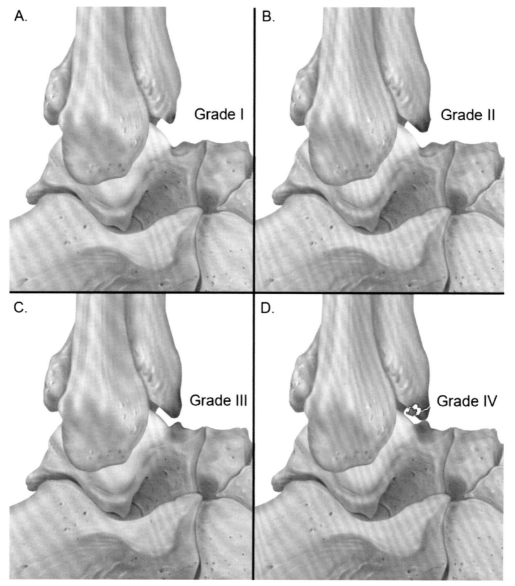

FIGURE 89.8. Classification of anterior ankle osteophytes by Scranton and McDermott: **A:** Grade I: Anterior tibial spur 3 mm or less. **B:** Grade II: Anterior tibial spur greater than 3 mm. No talar neck osteophyte. **C:** Grade III: Anterior tibial spur associated with talar neck osteophyte. **D:** Grade IV: Anterior tibial and talar spurs associated with generalized ankle arthritic changes.

tibia, sometimes being contiguous with osteophyte all the way along the medial malleolus into the medial gutter (25). In addition, he noted that routine lateral radiographs may underestimate the size or fail to identify these osteophytes. Therefore, van Dijk (26) suggested an easily obtained oblique lateral ankle radiograph that identifies these osteophytes more accurately (Fig. 89.9). It is easily performed in the office setting and is a valuable adjunct to the routine AP, lateral, and mortise radiographs obtained to evaluate ankle pain.

Osteophytes may also occur in the posterior ankle joint, associated with bony impingement of a prominent posterior talar process or os trigonum against the posterior tibia with forced plantar flexion maneuvers. Certain types of athletes including soccer players and ballet dancers appear to be more prone to posterior ankle impingement, although it may occur in other sports or be related to workplace exposure (27).

History

The main complaint of patients with ankle osteophytes is pain but may be limitation of range of motion of the joint. Pain is usually localized to the specific area where the osteophyte is located. However, coexisting degenerative arthritis may cause the patient to have more nonspecific pain complaint localization. Osteophytes may grow over time causing increasing symptoms, and they ultimately may break off, creating a loose body within the joint. In this case, a patient may complain of locking of the ankle joint or the sensation of instability as the loose body intermittently impinges within the joint. However, these patients do not display objective signs of joint laxity.

Physical Examination

As with any other ankle physical examination, the entire lower extremity should be examined including the

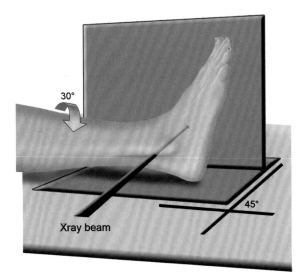

FIGURE 89.9. Technique of van Dijk for oblique lateral radiograph to visualize extension of anterior tibial osteophyte to the medial malleolus.

condition of the skin, overall extremity alignment, and the range of motion, stability, and alignment of the hip, knee, and ankle joints. Specifically, the ankle should be examined and the range of dorsi and plantar flexion along with subtalar mobility noted. Every ankle should be examined to determine whether a fixed varus or valgus hindfoot alignment is present. Stability of the ankle joint, especially to inversion and anterior stress, should be assessed. When osteophytes are suspected, specific palpation over the area of osteophytes should be performed. Osteophytes of the medial malleolus are often palpable beneath the skin. Discomfort with forced dorsiflexion of the joint is an evocative maneuver for anterior ankle osteophytes as is the forced plantar flexion test for posterior osteophytes.

Radiographic Studies

As noted earlier, each patient should have AP, lateral, and mortise radiographs. Patients with suspected anterior osteophytes should have an oblique lateral radiograph as described by van Dijk (26). Although a CT scan will accurately depict the location and extent of bony osteophytes, the examination is seldom necessary and exposes the patient to significant radiation . MRI also has the ability to visualize osteophytes, but its main advantage over plain radiographs and CT scanning is the ability of this study to visualize the soft tissues. The MRI can be useful in ruling out other potential causes of ankle pain to pare down the list of potential diagnoses of the various entities on the differential diagnosis (28–31).

SURGICAL TECHNIQUE

The surgical technique is performed as described earlier, with the patient placed supine on the operating table and with the flexed hip and knee supported by a well-padded leg holder. Noninvasive ankle distraction is applied to the joint and routine anteromedial, anterolateral, and posterolateral portals are made. The entire joint is examined in an organized and reproducible fashion. If an anterior tibial osteophyte possibly associated with a talar neck osteophyte is the pathology found during the arthroscopic examination, it may be useful to diminish the amount of traction force applied to the joint and to dorsiflex the ankle to relax the anterior capsule and allow easier exposure of the distal tibia and talar neck.

The presence of a large anterior tibial osteophyte, possibly associated with a talar neck osteophyte, may make initial visualization of the joint difficult especially when associated with significant anterior joint synovitis. The joint space may be difficult to delineate. The best approach is to insert the arthroscope through the anteromedial portal and then establish fluid flow with the inflow in the posterolateral portal. The shaver is then introduced from the anterolateral portal in such a way that the shaver blade contacts the arthroscope shaft. The shaver is "walked" down the arthroscope shaft in the next step until it becomes visible at the tip. The hypertrophic synovium is then carefully debrided. It is especially important during this initial attempt at visualization that the shaver blade is directed toward the joint space rather than anteriorly so that the anterior capsule is not inadvertently penetrated risking iatrogenic injury to the anterior neurovascular structures. Once the joint is exposed, it is also important to expose the osteophyte properly. The anterior capsule must be stripped from the anterior surface of the osteophyte. This may be done using the shaver, again being careful to direct the shaver blade against the osteophyte itself rather than the anterior capsule. Alternatively, a bipolar or monopolar radiofrequency wand may be used for this process (Fig. 89.10). This method has the advantage of accomplishing simultaneous tissue ablation and hemostasis. The entire osteophyte must be exposed from its most lateral to its most medial extent. As noted above, the medial extent may go all the way to the medial malleolus toward its tip. It is not uncommon to observe wearing of the articular cartilage of the talus appearing as a grooving of the surface owing to erosion of the surface during dorsi and plantar flexion of the joint.

Once the osteophyte is exposed, excision may be performed using two techniques. First, a power burr may be used to gradually resect the osteophyte (Fig. 89.11). A 4-mm round abrader is ideally suited for this procedure. Second, a small osteotome may be introduced into the joint, and the osteophyte may be separated from the anterior tibia and then removed using a loose body forceps.

The amount of resection should approximate the normal contour of the anterior tibia and eliminate any contact of the anterior tibia with the talus during full range of motion of the ankle as observed arthroscopically. In general, resection should proceed until normal thickness of the

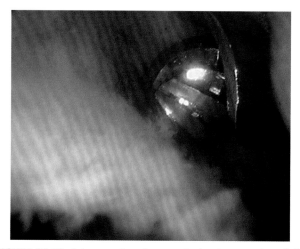

FIGURE 89.11. Intraoperative photograph showing resection of the anterior tibial osteophyte using a 4 mm round burr.

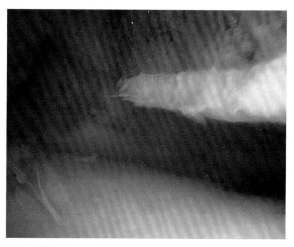

FIGURE 89.12. Intraoperative photograph showing the anterior tibia after resection of the bony osteophyte.

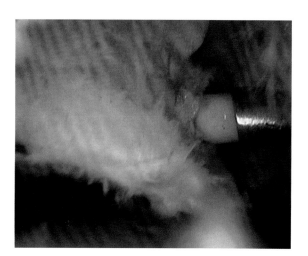

FIGURE 89.10. Intraoperative photograph showing the method of exposure of the anterior tibial osteophyte by stripping the anterior capsule off the superior surface using a radiofrequency wand.

remaining articular cartilage is noted along the anterior tibia (Fig. 89.12). If there is any question regarding the adequacy of resection, an intraoperative radiograph may be obtained.

The talar neck must be exposed to be certain that any talar neck osteophyte is removed. This is performed using a round abrader or an osteotome as above.

Posterior ankle joint osteophytes are more challenging to resect. There are three techniques for approaching these osteophytes. First, in a joint that displays adequate laxity, the arthroscope can be advanced from one of the anterior portals to the back of the joint, adequately visualizing the posterior tibial osteophyte. Then, a motorized abrader may be introduced from the posterolateral portal and the osteophyte removed while visualizing from anterior.

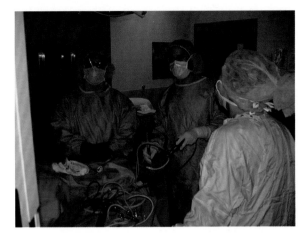

FIGURE 89.13. Positioning for posterior ankle arthroscopy.

The second technique is the direct posterior approach to the joint (32, 33). This approach was pioneered by van Dijk and is performed with the patient positioned prone on the operating table utilizing two portals, one placed at the medial and the other at the lateral border of the Achilles tendon approximately at the level of the tip of the fibula (Fig. 89.13). The arthroscope is introduced through the posterolateral portal and directed toward the first web space. The shaver is introduced through the posteromedial portal perpendicular to the arthroscope until contact is made between the shaver tip and the arthroscope (Fig. 89.14). The shaver is then advanced to the tip of the arthroscope until it is visualized and a space is created lateral to the flexor hallucis longus tendon (Fig. 89.15). The capsule of the posterior ankle joint is resected to evaluate the joint (Fig. 89.16).

This approach is excellent for approaching posterior tibial osteophytes, a prominent posterior talar process, or os trigonum causing posterior impingement. Resection of the osteophyte or posterior talar process may be performed under direct visualization using a 4-mm round burr.

An inconvenience of this approach is the requirement for the patient to be positioned prone on the operating table. If anterior surgery is required first, then switching to prone position with redo skin preparation and draping is required. Another alternative has been proposed by Allegra with posterior visualization utilizing double posteromedial portals (34). The first portal

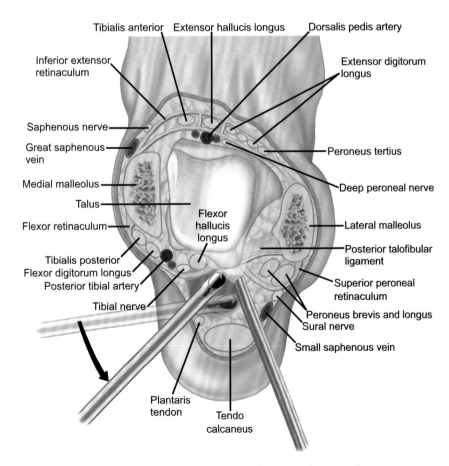

FIGURE 89.14. Technique for placement of arthroscope for posterior ankle arthroscopy, after van Dijk.

VI. Foot and Ankle

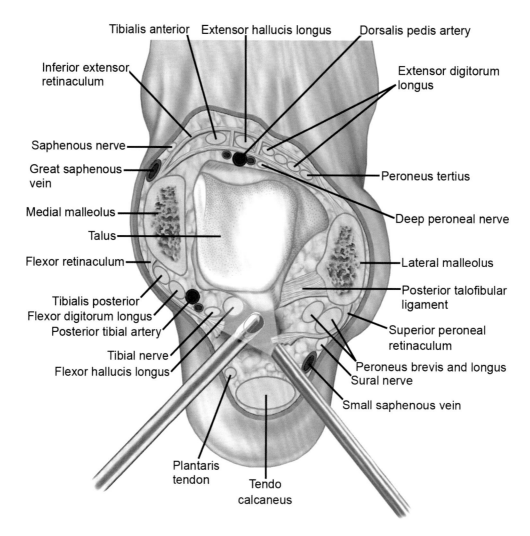

Tibialis anterior Extensor hallucis longus Dorsalis pedis artery

Inferior extensor retinaculum

Extensor digitorum longus

Saphenous nerve

Great saphenous vein

Peroneus tertius

Medial malleolus

Deep peroneal nerve

Talus

Flexor retinaculum

Lateral malleolus

Tibialis posterior
Flexor digitorum longus
Posterior tibial artery

Posterior talofibular ligament

Tibial nerve
Flexor hallucis longus

Superior peroneal retinaculum

Peroneus brevis and longus
Sural nerve

Small saphenous vein

Plantaris tendon

Tendo calcaneus

FIGURE 89.15. Technique for safely creating the posterior space for posterior ankle and subtalar arthroscopy, after van Dijk.

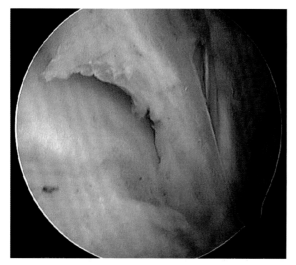

FIGURE 89.16. Intraoperative photograph of posterior ankle arthroscopy showing the ankle joint after resection of the posterior capsule to expose the joint, with the flexor hallucis longus tendon visible at the right side of the photograph.

is placed similar to that advocated by van Dijk, and the second approximately 3 cm proximal to the first. This approach has the advantage of being possible with the patient supine on the operating table and thus possible to be performed without need for repositioning after anterior ankle arthroscopy.

POSTOPERATIVE CARE

A short leg posterior splint is applied in the operating room after closing each portal with a simple suture. The splint is removed from 7 to 10 days postoperative and then weight-bearing is advanced as tolerated and an exercise program is instituted to regain range of motion and to strengthen the ankle. The assistance of a licensed physical therapist may help the patient to return to work and sports activity more quickly. Return to sports activities is expected at approximately 6 weeks postoperative.

REFERENCES

1. Wolin I, Glassman F, Sideman S, et al. Internal derangement of the talofibular component of the ankle. *Surg Gynecol Obstet.* 1950;91:193–200.
2. McCarroll JR, Schrader JW, Shelbourne KD, et al. Meniscoid lesions of the ankle in soccer players. *Am J Sports Med.* 1987;15:255–257.
3. Martin DF, Curl WW, Baker CL. Arthroscopic treatment of chronic synovitis of the ankle. *Arthroscopy.* 1989;5:110–114.
4. Ferkel RD, Fischer SP. Progress in ankle arthroscopy. *Clin Orthop Relat Res.* 1989;240:210–220.
5. Ferkel RD, Karzel RP, Del Pizzo W, et al. Arthroscopic treatment of anterolateral impingement of the ankle. *Am J Sports Med.* 1991;19:440–446.
6. Meislin RJ, Rose DJ, Parisien JS, et al. Arthroscopic treatment of synovial impingement of the ankle. *Am J Sports Med.* 1993;21:186–189.
7. DeBerardino TM, Arciero RA, Taylor DC. Arthroscopic treatment of soft tissue impingement of the ankle in athletes. *Arthroscopy.* 1997;13:492–498.
8. Kim SH, Ha KI. Arthroscopic treatment of impingement of the anterolateral soft tissues of the ankle. *J Bone Joint Surg Br.* 2000;82-B:1019–1021.
9. Gulish HA, Sullivan RJ, Aronow M. Arthroscopic treatment of soft tissue impingement lesions of the ankle in adolescents. *Foot Ankle Int.* 2005;26:204–207.
10. Urguden M, Soyuncu Y, Ozdemir H, et al. Arthroscopic treatment of anterolateral soft tissue impingement of the ankle: evaluation of factors affecting outcome. *Arthroscopy.* 2005;21:317–322.
11. Koczy B, Pyda M, Stoltny T, et al. Arthroscopy for anterolateral soft tissue impingement of the ankle joint. *Ortop Traumatol Rehabil.* 2009;11:339–345.
12. Basset FH III, Gates HS III, Billys BJ, et al. Talar impingement by the anteroinferior tibiofibular ligament. A cause of chronic pain in the ankle after inversion sprain. *J Bone Joint Surg Am.* 1990;72A:55–59.
13. Van den Bekerom MP, Raven EE. The distal fascicle of the anterior inferior tibiofibular ligament as a cause of tibiotalar impingement syndrome: a current concepts review. *Knee Surg Sports Traumatol Arthrosc.* 2007;15:465–471.
14. Rubin DA, Tishkoff NW, Britton CA, et al. Anterolateral soft tissue impingement in the ankle: diagnosis using MR imaging. *AJR Am J Roentgenol.* 1997;169:829–835.
15. Liu SH, Nuccion SL, Finerman G. Diagnosis of anterolateral ankle impingement: comparison between magnetic resonance imaging and clinical examination. *Am J Sports Med.* 1997;25:389–393.
16. Robinson P, White LM, Salonen D, et al. Anteromedial impingement of the ankle. Using MR arthrography to assess the anteromedial recess. *AJR Am J Roentgenol.* 2002;178:601–604.
17. Lee JW, Suh JS, Huh YM, et al. Soft tissue impingement syndrome of the ankle: diagnostic efficacy of MRI and clinical results after arthroscopic treatment. *Foot Ankle Int.* 2004;25:896–902.
18. Ferkel RD, Tyorkin M, Applegate GR, et al. MRI evaluation of anterolateral soft tissue impingement of the ankle. *Foot Ankle Int.* 2010;31:655–661.
19. Morris LH. Athlete's ankle. *J Bone Joint Surg Am.* 1943;25:220.
20. McMurray TP. Footballer's ankle. *J Bone Joint Surg Br.* 1950;32B:68–69.
21. Tol JL, van Dijk CN. Etiology of the anterior ankle impingement syndrome: a descriptive anatomical study. *Foot Ankle Int.* 2004;25:382–386.
22. Hayeri MR, Trudell DJ, Resnick D. Anterior ankle impingement and talar bony outgrowths: osteophyte or enthesophyte? Paleopathologic and cadaveric study with imaging correlation. *AJR Am J Roentgenol.* 2009;193:W334–W338.
23. Tol JL, Slim E, van Soest AJ, et al. The relationship of the kicking action in soccer and anterior ankle impingement syndrome. A biomechanical analysis. *Am J Sports Med.* 2002;30:45–50.
24. Scranton PE Jr, McDermott JE. Anterior tibiotalar spurs. A comparison of open versus arthroscopic debridement. *Foot Ankle.* 1992;13:125–129.
25. Tol JL, Verhagen RA, Krips R, et al. The anterior ankle impingement syndrome. Diagnostic value of oblique radiographs. *Foot Ankle Int.* 2004;25:63–68.
26. van Dijk CN, Wessel RN, Tol JL, et al. Oblique radiograph for the detection of bone spurs in anterior ankle impingement. *Skeletal Radiol.* 2002;31:214–221.
27. Maquirriain J. Posterior ankle impingement syndrome. *J Am Acad Orthop Surg.* 2005;13:365–371.
28. Karasick D, Schweitzer ME. The os trigonum syndrome. Imaging features. *AJR Am J Roentgenol.* 1996;166:125–129.
29. Bureau NJ, Cardinal E, Hobden R, et al. Posterior ankle impingement syndrome. MR imaging findings in seven patients. *Radiology.* 2000;215:497–503.
30. Peace KA, Hillier C, Hulme A, et al. MRI features of posterior ankle impingement syndrome in ballet dancers. A review of 25 cases. *Clin Radiol.* 2004;59:1025–1033.
31. Willits K, Sonneveld H, Amendola A, et al. Outcome of posterior ankle arthroscopy for hindfoot impingement. *Arthroscopy.* 2008;24:196–202.
32. Van Dijk CN. Anterior and posterior ankle impingement. *Foot Ankle Clin.* 2006;11:663–683.
33. van Dijk CN, Scholten PE, Krips R. A 2-portal endoscopic approach for diagnosis and treatment of posterior ankle pathology. *Arthroscopy.* 2000;16:871–876.
34. Allegra F, Maffulli N. Double posteromedial portals for posterior ankle arthroscopy in supine position. *Clin Orthop Relat Res.* 2010;468:996–1001.

Osteochondral Lesions of the Talar Dome: Autologous Chondrocyte Implantation

Terence Y.P. Chin • Steve Mussett • Richard Ferkel • Mark Glazebrook • Johnny Tak-Choy Lau

Osteochondral lesions of the talus (OLT) are defects of the cartilaginous surface and underlying subchondral bone of the talar dome. In some instances, an associated subchondral cyst(s) forms subjacent to the OLT. The etiology of this condition remains uncertain although many follow a twisting injury to the ankle. In the absence of preceding trauma, a primary vascular insult is thought to be the cause. Patients with OLT report ankle pain, swelling, and mechanical symptoms of clicking or locking (1, 2).

OLT commonly occur on the anterolateral or posteromedial aspects on the talar dome. Trauma precedes up to 90% of anterolateral and 70% of posteromedial talar OLT (3). Loren and Ferkel (4) found a 61% incidence of traumatic talar articular surface lesions with acute ankle fractures. In addition, Hintermann et al (5) found an incidence of 79% cartilage lesions in 288 acute ankle fractures treated. Stufkens, Hintermann, and associates recently performed a long-term follow-up study of their consecutive prospective cohort of 288 ankle fractures, previously described above. One hundred and nine patients (47%) were available for follow-up at a mean of 12.9 years. Their findings showed that the initial cartilage damage seen arthroscopically following an ankle fracture was an independent predictor of the development of posttraumatic or osteoarthritis. They found lesions on the anterior and lateral aspects of the talus and on the medial malleolus correlated the highest with an unfavorable clinical outcome (6). OLT occur bilaterally 10% of the time (7).

Berndt and Harty's (8) X-ray classification of OLT is still widely used. However, CT or MRI is essential to staging the lesion and guiding treatment (9, 10). The radiologic staging of OLTs is discussed in detail in the preceding chapters.

TREATMENT

Treatment of OLT depends on whether the lesion is acute or chronic, the radiologic stage and size of the lesion as well as the severity of the patient's symptoms. This chapter will focus on the treatment of chronic OLT. Symptomatic high-grade lesions with significant detachment or

displacement require surgery. Overall, nonoperative treatment has been shown to be ineffective in 25% to 45% of patients with symptomatic OLT (1, 11).

The aims of treatment are to reduce pain, restore ankle function, and protect the ankle joint from degenerative change. Ideally, this is achieved by restoring normal hyaline articular cartilage to cover the subchondral plate. If lower limb malalignment or ankle instability is present, these need to be addressed as well, particularly if any cartilage restoration procedure is contemplated.

Surgical options available for chronic OLT include the following:

- *Marrow stimulation*: abrasion, drilling, or microfracture.
- *Cartilage restoration*: osteochondral autologous transplantation system (OATS), osteochondral allograft transplantation, or chondrocyte implantation (e.g., autologous chondrocyte implantation [ACI]).

Loose and irreparable OLT must be removed. Marrow stimulation techniques produce nonhyaline fibrocartilage (predominantly type I collagen) with mechanical properties inferior to and likely less durable than native hyaline cartilage (12). Current treatment modalities that aim to restore hyaline or hyaline-like cartilage (consisting of mainly type II collagen) include OATS, osteochondral allograft transplantation, and ACI. OATS utilizes small hyaline cartilage covered bone plugs, harvested from the nonweight bearing areas of the knee joint to fill the OLT. Although good intermediate term results have been reported with OATS, concerns persist with regard to significant donor site morbidity, technical difficulties with the procedure, insufficient graft volume for larger lesions, chondrocyte death from plug impaction, difficulty with grafting "shoulder" lesions, mismatches of knee to ankle articular cartilage, and incomplete defect coverage (13–16). Osteochondral allografts have been used to treat mainly large OLTs, and acceptable results have been reported in several case series (level 4) (17–19). Compared with autologous osteochondral grafts (harvested usually from nonweight bearing areas of the knee), talar allografts have the advantage of harvesting not only larger donor grafts, but also grafts that are more anatomically congruent. With preoperative CT scans, the allograft can also be matched exactly to fit the recipient defect. The disadvantages of allografts, however, include the potential for disease transmission, fresh allograft availability, and longer healing times.

OVERVIEW OF ACI

ACI technologies and techniques is a rapidly evolving field. A comprehensive review of this topic is beyond the scope of this chapter and the reader is referred to the references for further information (20, 21). Presently there are three generations of chondrocyte implantation techniques for osteochondral defects:

- *First-generation chondrocyte implantation* involves the implantation of autologous chondrocytes under an autologous periosteal flap (classic ACI).
- *Second-generation chondrocyte implantation* involves the implantation of autologous chondrocytes under a tissue-engineered collagen covering (e.g., Chondro-Gide and Bio-Gide, Geistlich Biomaterials, Wolhusen, Switzerland) or, more commonly, the implantation of a tissue-engineered scaffold seeded with autologous chondrocytes. The latter includes matrix-induced autologous chondrocyte implantation (MACI; Genzyme, Cambridge, MA) and Hyalograft C scaffold (Fida Advanced Biopolymers, Abano Terma, Italy).
- *Third-generation chondrocyte implantation* essentially involves the creation ex vivo and implantation of a three-dimensional chondral grafts (21). Features of generation III techniques include the use allogeneic juvenile chondrocytes, novel chondroinductive and chondroconductive scaffolds, and specialized techniques to mechanically condition the developing chondral tissue ex vivo to enhance their material properties prior to implantation (22). Examples of these include the "Denovo" Engineered Tissue (ET) Graft (Zimmer, Warsaw, MO) and Neocart (Histogenics, Waltham, MA) (22).

Currently, only first-generation ACI techniques are in use in the United States for OLTs (23). Second-generation ACI is widely used in Europe and Australia, but are not currently approved by the FDA (24, 25). Third-generation chondrocyte implantation methods are in the early phases of human clinical trials in the United States. Others are not yet approved by the FDA for marketing (22).

FIRST-GENERATION ACI

First-generation ACI involves the implantation of previously harvested autologous chondrocytes that have been cultured and expanded in vitro. The implanted chondrocytes are secured to the defect by an overlying periosteal flap. Good results for the treatment of knee osteochondral lesions have been reported at 9- to 11-year follow-up (26).

ACI's success in the knee joint has led to its increasing use in the ankle as well as other joints.

ACI for OLT is performed in two stages. The first stage involves arthroscopically harvesting 200 to 300 mg of cartilage from nonweight bearing areas of the ipsilateral knee (edges of femoral condyles or intercondylar notch) or ankle. In the ankle joint, cartilage harvest has been described from the anterior edge of talar dome or tibial plafond, from the edges of the OLT during debridement or from removed loose fragment of OLT (27–29). These cartilage specimens are then sent to the laboratory for chondrocyte isolation and proliferation (Genzyme, Cambridge, MA). A formal ankle arthroscopy is also performed to assess the size and depth of the OLT and whether bone grafting is required for large subchondral bony defects. In addition, associated pathology not accessible by future osteotomy is treated at the same time.

Details of chondrocyte isolation and culture are beyond the scope of this chapter and the reader is directed to the suggested reading list for more information (13, 30, 31). Briefly, the harvested cartilage is minced, washed with antibiotic solution, enzymatically digested, filtered, and centrifuged to obtain the chondrocytes. The chondrocytes are cultured to achieve a suspension consisting of 5×10^6 cells. The entire process requires 3 to 4 weeks.

The second stage is performed once the cultured chondrocytes are ready for implantation. In most cases, a lateral malleolar or medial malleolar osteotomy is required to access lateral and medial OLT, respectively (27, 29, 32, 33). The OLT is debrided to stable native cartilage at the rim of the lesion and to subchondral bone at the base. A flap of periosteum equal or slightly larger to the size of the defect is harvested from the distal tibial metaphysis and sutured to the defect with the cambium layer facing the subchondral bone using interrupted 5/0 Vicryl sutures. Fibrin glue is then used to seal the periphery of the flap, leaving a gap for the introduction of the chondrocytes. Normal saline is initially injected through this gap to confirm a water-tight seal and then removed. The cultured cells are then injected under the periosteal flap and the gap sealed with fibrin glue. The malleolar osteotomies are then internally fixed in the standard fashion (27, 29, 30, 32–34).

In some cases, a large cystic cavity underlies the OLT. This cavity has to be filled with cancellous bone graft and the level of the subchondral bone reconstituted prior to ACI. Some authors have implanted the autologous chondrocytes directly over the bone graft and sutured the periosteum over the defect (29, 30). Most, however, use the "sandwich technique" aimed at isolating the implanted chondrocytes from the underlying raw cancellous bone graft, thereby protecting the chondrocytes from unwanted bleeding and pluripotential cell contamination (27, 32–34) (Fig. 90.1). After debridement and drilling of the base of the cyst, it is then filled with autogenous cancellous bone graft to the level of the subchondral plate.

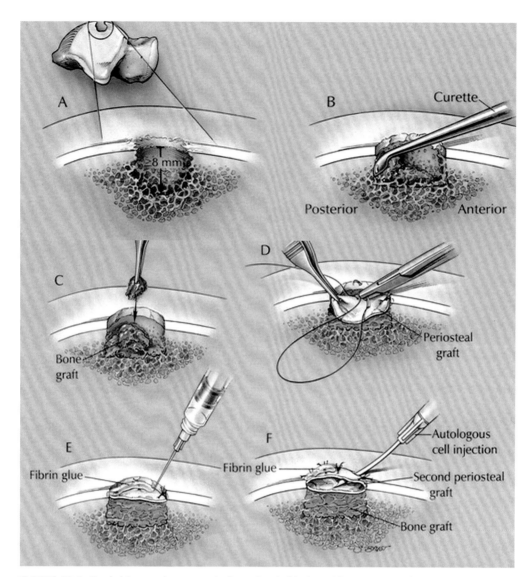

FIGURE 90.1. Sandwich procedure steps. **A:** Osteochondral lesion with cyst greater than or equal to 8 mm. **B:** Curette is used to remove the osteochondral lesion and the underlying cyst. **C:** Bone graft is obtained from the iliac crest or tibia and is impacted to just below the subchondral bone plate. **D:** A periosteal flap is inserted to cover the bony defect at the level of the subchondral bone plate, with the cambium layer facing the joint. The flap is anchored with horizontal suture into the cartilage. **E:** Fibrin glue is injected between the flap and the bone graft to seal off the marrow cavity from the joint, and the tourniquet is released to check for any bleeding that may penetrate the periosteal cover. **F:** A second periosteal flap is sutured to the cartilage edges with the cambium layer facing the defect, and fibrin glue is used to seal off the intervals between the sutures. After a water test is done, the chondrocytes are injected between the two layers of periosteum. (Copyright, Richard D. Ferkel, MD.)

A periosteal flap with the cambium layer facing away from the bone graft is secured to the OLT with sutures and fibrin glue. A second periosteal flap with the cambium layer facing into the initial periosteal flap (i.e., away from the joint surface) is then secured over the first with sutures and fibrin glue. The space between the two periosteal flaps represents an isolated chamber into which the chondrocytes are injected. The implanted chondrocytes are therefore "sandwiched" between the two periosteal flaps. The osteotomy is anatomically reduced with internal fixation.

EVIDENCE FOR FIRST-GENERATION ACI

A search of the English literature from 1994 (first report on ACI in humans by Brittberg et al. (13)) to August 2009 was performed in PubMed. Search terms included a combination of the following: "ankle," "talar," "osteochondral," "osteochondritis dissecans," and "chondrocyte implantation." This revealed six studies on ACI for talar OLT (27, 29, 30, 32–34). All were level 4 prospective case series with small numbers (largest study *n* = 14) and short to medium follow-up (2 to 5 years). Over 80% of patients reported improvement in symptoms and high patient satisfaction. The vast majority of first ACIs was performed in patients who had failed previous marrow stimulation procedures.

Peterson et al. (34) were the first investigators to perform ACI for osteochondral lesions of the knee and they have since published their early experience with OLT. They reported on 14 patients with ACI ± sandwich procedure (34). The average OLT size was 1.7 cm^2 (range 0.3 to 3.5 cm^2). Four had concomitant lateral ligament reconstruction. The results of this study are reported in more detail by Peterson in a separate publication (35). At an average follow-up of 32.4 months, 80% of patients reported improvement. Seven patients required repeat arthroscopy for periosteal hypertrophy and there was one patient with graft delamination.

In a level 4 prospective study, Whittaker et al. (33) utilized ACI in 10 patients with OLT. Two had the "sandwich" bone grafting procedure. The OLT had a mean area of 1.95 cm^2 (1 to 4 cm^2). Six of these had previous arthroscopic or open surgery. At an average follow-up of 23 months (range 12 to 54 months), the mean Mazur ankle score had improved from 51 pre-op to 71 post-op ($P < .0005$). Nine of 10 patients were pleased or extremely pleased with the result. Second-look arthroscopies were performed in nine patients at a mean of 13 months post-ACI. All OLTs had filled with macroscopically stable, but slightly softer and more irregular cartilage compared with the surrounding native cartilage. A full-thickness biopsies were performed in five patients showing hyaline-like cartilage in some regions in two patients and predominantly fibrocartilage in three patients.

Giannini et al. (30) reported similarly good results in a level 4 case series of eight patients treated with ACI as the primary procedure. The average OLT size was 3.3 cm^2 (range 2.2 to 4.3 cm^2) with average 26 months follow-up. One patient required bone grafting for a subchondral cyst, with the chondrocytes implanted directly over the cancellous bone graft and then covered with the periosteal flap (nonsandwich technique). One required a tibial osteotomy to correct malalignment. All patients were satisfied with the procedure, with AOFAS hindfoot scores improving from 32.1 to 91. Repeat arthroscopies in all eight patients showed complete filling of the defect with hyaline-type cartilage containing type II collagen.

Koulalis et al. (29) performed ACI in a level 4 series of eight patients with a mean lesion size of 1.84 cm^2 (1 to 6.25 cm^2). Cartilage was harvested from the nonarticular anterior rim of the talar dome of the same ankle joint. Subchondral bony defects were filled with autogenous cancellous bone, using the "nonsandwich" technique. At an average of 17.6 months follow-up (range 8 to 26), the Finsen ankle score improved from an average of 3.4 pre-op to 0.6 post-op, with all patients achieving good or excellent results. Repeat arthroscopy was performed in three patients for division of capsular adhesions. Inspection of the graft site during the repeat arthroscopy showed coverage of

the OLT with "cartilage-like" tissue. Biopsy performed in one of the three repeat arthroscopy patients showed mainly fibrocartilage and cartilaginous metaplasia. Type I collagen was seen, however, with immunohistochemical staining. With the addition of four more patients, this cohort of patients was later included in a longer follow-up by Baums et al. (27) They reported statistically significant improvements in AOFAS (43.5 to 88.4) and Hanover ankle rating score (40.4 to 85.5) at an average of 63-month follow-up (range 48 to 84 months). Eleven of the 12 patients reported good or excellent results. MRI scans were performed at the most recent follow-up, which demonstrated nearly congruent joint surface, with integration of the graft with adjacent native cartilage and subchondral bone in seven patients. The remaining patients had graft irregularity with some fissuring.

In 2009, Nam et al. (32) (prospective level 4 study) reported their experience in 11 patients. All had failed previous surgical treatment. In this series of 11 patients, 6 had the "sandwich" procedure for subchondral cysts (mean depth 11.5 mm, range 9 to 15 mm). The average OLT size was 2.7 cm^2 (range 1.8 to 4.2 cm^2). At an average follow-up of 38 months (range 24 to 60 months), statistically significant improvements were recorded in AOFAS (47.4 to 84.3), Tegner activity scores (1.3 to 4.0), and Finsen score in all categories. Nine of 11 patients were classified as good or excellent. Follow-up MRI in nine patients showed varying degrees of articular surface incongruity, but good to moderate fill of the defect (Fig. 90.2). All patients had restoration of subchondral bone albeit with some depression and focal defects. Bone marrow edema resolved in all but one patient. Second-look arthroscopy was performed in 10 patients at a mean postoperative time of 14.2 months. All OLTs were completely filled with smooth cartilage-like repair tissue, with a line of demarcation between the graft and the surrounding native cartilage (Fig. 90.3). Periosteal overgrowth was noted in two patients at repeat arthroscopy.

Recently, Ferkel and associates (personal communication) have completed a study of the first 32 ACI patients with long-term follow-up. There were 16 male and 16 female patients, with a mean age of 34. Twenty-four patients had medial lesions and eight had lateral, with an average size of 198 mm^2. Twenty-three patients underwent ACI of the talus alone, whereas nine had ACI with a sandwich procedure. Mean follow-up was 66 months. Preoperatively, 25 patients rated their ankle as poor and 3 as fair, using the simplified symptomatology evaluation. At last follow-up, 8 were classified as excellent, 12 as good, 5 as fair, and 1 as poor. The poor patient had an ankle fusion 4 years after the ACI procedure because of degenerative arthritis, which existed prior to the ACI procedure. Patients' overall Tegner activity level improved from 1.6 to 4.4, and the Finsen score showed significant improvement in the total score. AOFAS score improved from 50.2 to 86.4 and correlated well with the Finsen score. Nine of the 11 previously reported patients continued to make some

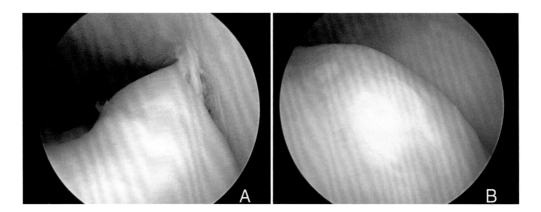

FIGURE 90.2. Arthroscopic views of a 23-year-old female figure skating instructor who underwent ACI after a failed drilling procedure in the right ankle. **A:** Loose osteochondral flap before ACI insertion. **B:** Second-look arthroscopy 9 months after ACI. (Reprinted with permission from Nam EK, Ferkel RD, Applegate GR: Autologous chondrocyte implantation of the ankle. A 2 to 5 Year Follow-up. Am J Sports Med 2009;37:274–284)

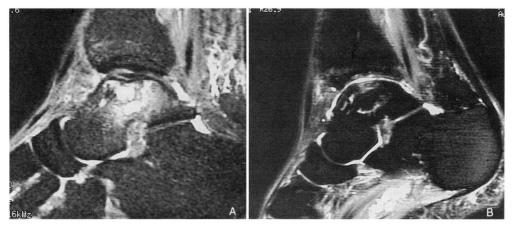

FIGURE 90.3. An MRI evaluation of the ACI patient. **A:** Preoperative sagittal T2-weighted MRI of the left ankle, with subchondral collapse and cyst formation. Significant bone marrow edema is present. **B:** Sagittal T2-weighted MRI of the left ankle performed 28 months after sandwich procedure demonstrates "good fill" at the articular surface and bone replacing the subchondral cysts. (Reprinted with permission from Nam EK, Ferkel RD, Applegate GR: Autologous chondrocyte implantation of the ankle. A 2 to 5 Year Follow-up. Am J Sports Med 2009;37:274–284)

improvement in Tegner, Finsen, and AOFAS scores (personal communication).

SECOND-GENERATION ACI

Traditional first-generation ACI consists of the direct injection of chondrocytes into a water-tight chamber formed by a periosteal flap and the subchondral bone. On a basic science level, many questions regarding the biology of chondrocyte metabolism and differentiation in such a biomechanical environment remain unanswered. Implanted chondrocytes have not been demonstrated to produce the proper chondrocyte to extracellular matrix ratio as native hyaline cartilage (25). The hyaline-like cartilage produced consists of disorganized collagen fibers, which do not yet replicate the well-ordered layered anatomy of hyaline cartilage. Furthermore, concerns remain with regard to the difficulty of achieving a watertight seal with the periosteal flap, with potential cellular leakage leading to suboptimal

cartilage production. In an effort to address some of these concerns, much attention has been paid to the development of biologic membrane scaffolds in which to seed, proliferate, orient, and finally to deliver chondrocytes into the OLT (25, 36).

Matrix-induced autologous chondrocyte implantation (MACI; Genzyme, Cambridge, Mass) is widely used in Europe, South America, Australia, and New Zealand (25). It has yet to be approved for use in the United States or Canada. In the MACI technique, harvested chondrocytes are first embedded into a bilayer membrane consisting of porcine type I/III collagen. This collage scaffold has a smooth external layer (higher density of collagen fibers), which serves as a barrier. The inner layer (where the chondrocytes are seeded) is porous and allows for seeding of the chondrocytes. This membrane is then directly implanted into the OLT and sealed with fibrin glue (36).

The Hyalograft C (Fidia Advanced Polymers, Abano Terme, Italy) scaffold is another system being used in

Europe (37). It uses a hyaluronic acid-based scaffold instead of porcine collagen. Similar to MACI, chondrocytes are expanded in vitro and seeded onto the membrane prior to implantation. Hyalograft C has self-adhesive properties, which do not require fibrin glue to secure the graft. A fully arthroscopic technique using specially designed instruments has been described for this technique for OLT (see below) (38).

Second-generation ACI is performed in two stages. As for first-generation ACI, the first stage involves chondrocyte harvesting and initial debridement of the OLT. The harvested cartilage is then sent to the laboratory for processing and the chondrocytes obtained are embedded into the biomembrane scaffold. At the second-stage procedure, the chondrocyte-rich membrane is cut to fit the OLT, applied to the subchondral bone and sealed with fibrin glue. Depending on the location of the OLT, the delivery and sealing of the membrane can be performed arthroscopically, without the need for a malleolar osteotomy (38).

EVIDENCE FOR SECOND-GENERATION ACI

As with traditional ACI, much of the current published data on the use of scaffolds are in the treatment of osteochondral lesions in the knee (25, 39). The short-term results (2- to 3-year follow-up) for MACI and Hyalograft C demonstrate equivalent histologic and functional knee outcome results to first-generation ACI, but without the need for harvesting and meticulous suturing of periosteal flaps. Second-generation ACI can potentially be performed with significantly reduced surgical time and complexity compared with traditional ACI.

Cherubino et al. (40) reported their preliminary experience with MACI on 11 patients (nine osteochondral lesions were in the knee and two in the talus). The mean defect size was 3.5 cm^2 (2.0 to 4.5 cm^2). They reported no complications at an average follow-up of 6.5 months. Improvements in knee scores were reported in six patients with a minimum 6-month follow-up. No ankle scores were mentioned. Postoperative MRI showed filling of the defect with cartilage with a signal pattern similar to hyaline cartilage. Two years later, the same authors reported on six patients with OLT treated with MACI (41) In this prospective case series, the average lesion size was 3.4 cm^2 (2.5 to 4.0 cm^2). Malleolar osteotomies were performed for access. At a mean follow-up of 33.8 months (25 to 43 months), five patients reported clinically significant improvements in their AOFAS scores (raw data not provided). Repeat arthroscopy in these patients showed complete filling of lesion with stable hyaline-like cartilage, which was macroscopically similar to surrounding native cartilage. Biopsies were not performed. Follow-up MRIs showed good filling and integration of the repair cartilage. The remaining patient had a kissing lesion, which failed to fill with repair tissue.

In a large level 4 study, Giannini et al. (38) used Hyalograft C in 46 patients with talar dome OLT. Twenty-three of these patients had failed prior surgery, and one had failed mosaicplasty. The average age was 31.4 years (20 to 47 years) and follow-up was up to 36 months for all patients. All procedures were done arthroscopically, with the delivery of the membrane to the defect being done with specially designed introducers. Mean lesion size was 1.6 cm^2 (0.5 to 2.5 cm^2). At 36 months follow-up, mean AOFAS scores improved from 57.2 to 89.5 ($P < .0005$). Thirty-eight patients had good or excellent results. Previous surgery ($P < .0005$) and increasing age ($P = .05$) were associated with poorer outcomes. Second-look arthroscopy was performed in three patients showing good defect fill and integration to the surrounding cartilage. Biopsies showed remodeling hyaline-like cartilage with type II collagen. This is the first study to describe a fully arthroscopic ACI procedure for OLT.

SUMMARY OF EVIDENCE AND RECOMMENDATIONS

The short- to medium-term results (2 to 5 years) of first-generation ACI for OLT show good/excellent results in 80% to 90% of patients. These results are reported mainly in patients with failed prior surgery. Experience with second-generation ACI (MACI and Hyalograft C) suggests that it is comparable with first-generation ACI. Only two studies in the English literature could be found on second-generation ACI for OLT, both of which were level 4 studies showing encouraging short-term (36 months) results. One of these reported on a completely arthroscopic approach (38). Using the criteria proposed by Wright et al. (42), the current levels of evidence warrant a grade C recommendation for first- and second-generation ACI for the treatment of OLT. At this juncture, the histology of the repair tissue produced from ACI is, at best, hyaline-type cartilage containing type II collagen. Nevertheless, studies performed in the knee show that this hyaline-type cartilage is biomechanically superior to fibrocartilage, and comparable with native hyaline cartilage (43). Currently, marrow stimulation procedures (drilling and microfracture) have reported good outcomes in 50% to 80% of patients with medium- to long-term follow-up (1, 23, 44). However, most are level 4 studies, with no or limited description of the size of the OLT treated (23, 44). There is evidence to suggest the results of marrow stimulation for OLT are poorer for lesions greater than 1.5 cm^2 (level 3) (45), and results may deteriorate over time (level 4) (23). Further investigation is required to determine if this hyaline-like cartilage produced by ACI translates to better and more durable clinical outcomes in the longer term.

Clearly, randomized trials with greater patient numbers and longer follow-up are required to further elucidate ACI's efficacy and, in particular, to establish its place in relation to marrow stimulation techniques. However, as

VI. Foot and Ankle

marrow stimulation procedures are substantially simpler and cheaper to perform, with less morbidity to the patient compared with ACI, it is the authors' opinion that they should be considered first-line treatment for OLT, with chondrocyte implantation reserved for patients who have failed marrow stimulation (16, 32, 35, 45). Caveats to this may be the larger (>1.5 cm²) OLT, or the presence of a significant subchondral cyst (>8 mm) where ACI with "sandwich" bone grafting is more likely to restore the congruity of the articular surface and underlying bone (16, 32, 34, 35) Prospective randomized studies with long-term follow-up are needed to assess the efficacy of ACI in comparison with marrow stimulation.

AUTHORS' RECOMMENDED TECHNIQUE FOR TREATING OLT

The authors currently perform first-generation ACI with a periosteal flap for OLT. This is performed in two stages. The first stage involves performing an ankle arthroscopy to confirm the procedure is appropriately indicated by thoroughly assessing the OLT and debriding the areas of the ankle that would not be accessible from the subsequent osteotomy. The actual OLT should be left alone to serve as a map of the exact lesion for definitive debridement at the second-stage small joint (2.7 mm) arthroscopes and associated instruments are normally used during ankle arthroscopy, although 4.0-mm 30° arthroscopes can also be utilized. A routine arthroscopic examination of the ankle joint is performed followed by a thorough assessment and initial debridement of the OLT (10). In the presence of a subchondral cystic defect greater than or equal to 8 mm, the bone grafting "sandwich" procedure is planned for the second stage. A biopsy harvest of 200 to 300 mg of cartilage is then obtained to provide donor chondrocytes for culture. This can be obtained from the ankle (the periphery of the OLT, from removed unstable fragments of cartilage or from the nonweight bearing anterior talar dome or tibial plafond) or the ipsilateral knee (edges of femoral condyles or trochlear notch). The authors prefer the latter as there is some laboratory evidence that chondrocytes harvested from damaged cartilage of the OLT have decreased cartilage-forming capacity (46). With completion of the first stage, the ankle is irrigated and the portals are closed with interrupted 4.0 nylon vertical mattress suture. A sterile dressing is applied followed by compression bandaging or posterior splint. Weight bearing and range of movement should be restricted for a week to allow the wounds to heal and then the sutures and splint are removed at 1 week.

The second stage follows no earlier than 4 to 6 weeks later and consists of excision of the OLT and implantation of the cultured chondrocytes. The preoperative routine, preparation, and draping are as for the first-stage procedure. The use of a tourniquet is recommended to ensure a bloodless field to prevent bleeding into the implanted chondrocytes. A malleolar osteotomy is usually required

to provide adequate access to the OLT (Fig. 90.4). The use of fluoroscopy is strongly recommended to ensure an appropriate level of the osteotomy. On the medial side, an oblique osteotomy of the malleolus is performed after it is predrilled and pretapped to accommodate two 4.0 cancellous lag screws (Fig. 90.5). It is critical that the osteotomy is made lateral to the osteochondral lesion, so as to allow access for suturing the periosteum over the defect. Maintaining its distal soft tissue attachments, the osteotomized fragment is hinged open to provide access to the ankle joint. If the osteochondral lesion is on the lateral talar dome, an oblique fibular osteotomy is performed. Prior to making the cuts, two interfragmentary oblique screw holes are drilled to facilitate easier reduction at the end of the

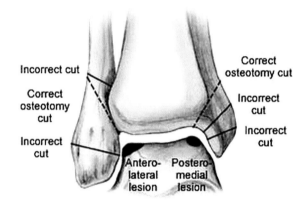

FIGURE 90.4. Positioning of the malleolar osteotomy is critical to providing adequate exposure of the entire osteochondral lesion and performing the ACI procedure. In addition, application of appropriate hardware for stabilization of the osteotomy is facilitated by the appropriate osteotomy. (Reprinted with permission from Bazaz R, Ferkel RD: Treatment of osteochondral lesions of the talus with autologous chondrocyte implantation. Tech Foot Ankle Surg 2004;3:45–52.)

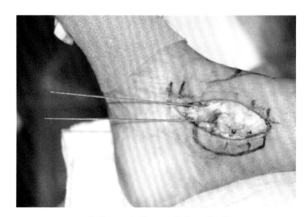

FIGURE 90.5. Predrilling of the medial malleolar osteotomy. Two cannulated screws from the 4.0 AO cannulated screw set are inserted parallel to each other and then a cannulated drill is passed just across the proposed osteotomy site. Guide pins are then removed from the osteotomy and the oblique medial malleolar osteotomy is performed in a right ankle.

procedure. A low-profile 3.5-mm semitubular plate can then be contoured after the interfragmentary screws are inserted. Following the osteotomy, the capsule and anterior talofibular ligament are released, leaving a cuff of tissue on the fibula, and the osteotomized fibula can then be hinged open to provide access to the lateral ankle joint (47).

With adequate exposure, the OLT is carefully debrided sharply back to a stable circular or oval rim of native cartilage and down to subchondral bone at the base of the lesion (Fig. 90.6). Care must be taken not to penetrate the subchondral bone in order to prevent unwanted bleeding and contamination of the implanted chondrocytes. If necessary, thrombin-soaked pledgets may be applied to the bed of the OLT. The OLT is measured, and a flap of periosteum 2 to 3 mm larger than the size of the defect is harvested from the distal tibial metaphysis. This allows for some shrinkage of the flap after harvest. Sterile tracing paper (sterile glove packaging) can be used to template the size of the defect. The periosteal patch is harvested from the distal tibia through the same medial malleolar osteotomy incision, or a separate incision is made when the lateral malleolar osteotomy is performed. The edges of the periosteal patch are incised on three sides and then elevated with a periosteal elevator prior to incision of the remaining fourth side. The flap is sutured to the defect with the cambium layer facing the subchondral bone using interrupted 6.0 Vicryl suture. The flap is assessed for water tightness using a saline-filled syringe and an 18G catheter. Additional sutures are placed in areas of leakage. The water is removed, the cartilage is dried, and the periphery is sealed with Tisseel fibrin glue, leaving a gap for the introduction of the chondrocytes. A second water tightness test is then performed to ensure an adequate seal. If a good seal is obtained, the water is removed and the cultured cells are then drawn up and injected into the far end of the defect, slowly withdrawing the catheter using a side-to-side motion for even dispersal of cells. Careful technique should be used when handling the chondrocyte transport vials and drawing up the

cultured cells to avoid a break in sterile technique, which may contaminate the procedure. Avoidance of priming the application needle will prevent unwanted premature clogging of the needle. Once the cells are injected, the opening is sutured closed and sealed with fibrin glue.

In the presence of a subchondral defect greater than or equal to 8 mm in depth, the authors recommend the "sandwich technique" (Fig. 90.1). The base of the cyst is debrided and drilled under direct visualization and then packed with harvested autogenous tibial, iliac crest, or calcaneal cancellous bone graft to the level of the subchondral plate (Fig. 90.7). The bone is then covered with fibrin glue. The base of the defect is measured and a periosteal flap is harvested and placed in position with the cambium layer facing *away* from the bone graft. It is secured with interrupted sutures and fibrin glue. A second periosteal flap with the cambium layer facing *into* the initial periosteal flap (i.e., away from the joint surface) is then secured over the first with sutures and fibrin glue as previously described. Water tightness is once again confirmed prior to injection of the cultured chondrocytes and final closure of the periosteal flap with suture and fibrin glue (Fig. 90.8).

The medial osteotomy is reduced with screws and the lateral malleolar osteotomy is reduced with screws and a plate to give secure fixation and allow early motion of the ankle (Fig. 90.9).

REHABILITATION

The goals of rehabilitation after chondrocyte implantation for OLT are first to aid graft healing, incorporation, and remodeling and second to return to function. In basic terms, the rehabilitation process following chondrocyte implantation should be guided by the "timeline" of graft healing, incorporation, and maturation (48, 49). Our understanding, however, of this "timeline" is still in its infancy and largely based on canine studies (48). The evidence base therefore for any specific rehabilitation protocol in clinical

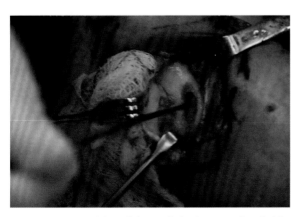

FIGURE 90.6. Excision of the medial talus osteochondral lesion. The medial malleolus is retracted and the OLT is excised and then measured. This picture shows a probe palpating the lesion in a right ankle.

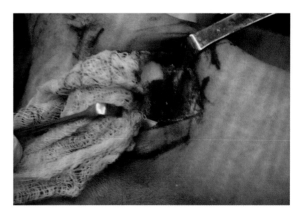

FIGURE 90.7. Bone grafting of a cystic lesion of the medial malleolus in a right ankle. Bone graft is obtained from the proximal tibia and inserted just below the subchondral plate. Note excellent exposure with the medial malleolus retracted inferiorly hinged on the deltoid ligament.

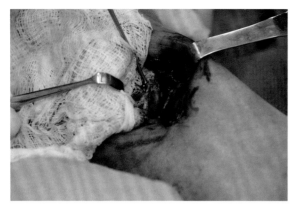

FIGURE 90.8. Final picture after the sandwich procedure. The cells have been injected between the two periosteal layers and the hole closed and then sealed with fibrin glue.

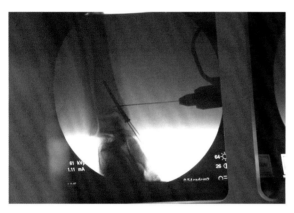

FIGURE 90.9. Internal fixation of the medial malleolar osteotomy with three 4.0 cannulated screws. After the two oblique screws are inserted, a third transverse screw is placed between the two oblique screws to prevent proximal migration of the osteotomy.

practice is level 5. Although rehabilitation protocols vary between studies (e.g., weight bearing, use of CPM), most authors agree that strict patient compliance to a prescribed rehabilitation regime under the supervision of a knowledgeable physiotherapist is crucial to optimal outcomes (27, 30, 32, 35).

A summary of the authors' recommended rehabilitation protocol is outlined in Table 90.1 (32). Postoperatively, patients are casted for 2 weeks and then placed into a removable CAM boot. Partial weight bearing (30 lb [13.6 kg]) and range of motion exercises are initiated at 2 weeks (phase I healing). Gentle range of movement and protected load bearing provide important stimuli for chondrocyte development while avoiding high-shear stresses, which could dislodge/damage the immature graft (35, 50). Gradual advancement to full weight bearing is indicated by radiographic healing of the osteotomies. At 6 weeks (phase II transitional), patients are prescribed a lace-up figure-of-eight brace and pool therapy is initiated. Nonresistance stationary bike exercises are commenced at 4 to 6 weeks, aiming to achieve full range of ankle movement by

6 to 8 weeks. During this phase, proprioceptive exercises, isometric and eccentric muscle strengthening, and closed chain exercises are also started. At 12 to 32 weeks (phase III remodeling), duration and intensity of activities (cycling, walking, jogging, etc.) are progressively increased as tolerated. In the final phase (maturation phase) approximately 32 weeks postsurgery, sport-specific training can be carefully initiated. Patients are allowed to return to nonimpact sports at 6 months and impact sports at 9 months (32).

EVIDENCE FOR THIRD-GENERATION ACI

Presently there is not good third-generation data published for either short-term or long-term studies, but research is underway in the United States and abroad.

PEARLS AND PITFALLS

1. It is important to address instability and limb malalignment prior to considering ACI. Patients undergoing corrective osteotomy for malalignment should be given 4 to 6 months to adequately consolidate the osteotomy site. Lateral ligament reconstruction can be performed at the second stage in conjunction with chondrocyte implantation.
2. Fluoroscopy should be used to guide the placement of malleolar osteotomies to ensure adequate access to the OLT. Predrilling and pretapping allow for an anatomic repair once the procedure is complete.
3. Compliance with a progressive structured rehabilitation program should be stressed to the patient and progress should be monitored vigilantly.
4. Avoid utilizing too small a piece of periosteum, since it always shrinks somewhat leading to inadequate coverage is of the defect.
5. Suture periosteum passing the needle from the normal cartilage to the periosteal graft. Gently tie the knots to avoid pulling the sutures out of either side using "micro" instruments.
6. Leave a large enough gap between sutures to allow insertion of the autologous chondrocytes. However, put the suture through the gap prior to inserting the chondrocytes to make it easier to close this gap more quickly.
7. Use a third transverse screw for medial malleolar osteotomies to prevent translation of the proximal medial malleolar fragment proximally.
8. Use fluoroscopy to assess the osteotomy reduction.
9. Reassure the patient that it takes time (6 to 12 months) for appropriate healing.

COMPLICATIONS

Complications specific to ACI in OLT include periosteal hypertrophy, capsular adhesion/arthrofibrosis, and prominent metal ware from osteotomy fixation.

Periosteal hypertrophy, confirmed at second-look arthroscopy, was noted by Nam et al. (32) (2 of 11) and

Table 90.1				
Rehabilitation After Autologous Chondrocyte Implantation for Talus Osteochondral Lesions *(Reprinted from Am J Sports Med vol. 37, p. 278, 2009, with permission)*				
Phase	**Weightbearing**	**Range of Motion**	**Muscle Strength**	**Functional Training**
Phase I: healing, weeks 0–6	30 lb PWB	CPM × 2 weeks (optional); cycle > 4 weeks	Isometric ADF/ APF	Water training; cycle ↓ resist
Phase 2: transitional, weeks 6–12	Advance to FWB	Achieve FROM DF/PF	Eccentric training	Cycle ↑ resist; proprio-cetive training
Phase 3: remodeling, weeks 12–32	FWB	Start Pro/Sup range of motion	↑ load training	Cycling; skate; cross-training; light jogging
Phase 4: maturation, weeks 32–52	FWB; impact WB	Maintain FROM	↑ load and repetition	Sport-specific training

ADF/APF = active dorsiflexion/active plantar flexion; CPM = continuous passive motion; DF/PF = dorsiflexion/plantar flexion; FROM = full range of motion; FWB = full weightbearing; Pro/Sup = pronation/supination; PWB = partial weightbearing.

Peterson et al. (7 of 14) (34, 35). These were successfully treated with arthroscopic debridement and physiotherapy. One case of graft delamination was also described by Peterson et al. (34) Koulalis et al. (29) performed repeat arthroscopies for capsular adhesions in 3 of 10 patients following ACI.

Donor site morbidity after knee harvest of cartilage has also been reported by Whittaker et al. (33), with 7 of 10 patients with 15% reduction in Lysholm scores at 1 year. This has not been seen by other authors (27, 32).

CONCLUSIONS

There is level 4 evidence to support the use of first- and second-generation ACI for the treatment of OLT. This permits a grade C recommendation for these procedures based on the criteria set out by Wright et al. (42) Given the greater morbidity and the higher cost and complexity of ACI, it is the authors' opinion that ACI be reserved for patients who have failed marrow stimulation procedures. The exception to this may be the larger (size >1.5 to 2.0 cm^2) OLT or those associated with a significant sub-chondral cyst (depth >5 to 8 mm) (44). Since there is level 3 evidence indicating poorer results in marrow stimulation procedures for OLT ≥ 1.5 cm^2, ACI may be considered an appropriate first-line intervention in these circumstances (45). ACI may be considered an appropriate first-line intervention in these circumstances. However, there are to date no reports published to substantiate this.

The field of cartilage restoration is rapidly advancing with new products and biotechnologies (21). Continued advances in tissue engineering will undoubtedly lead to the greater use of second- and third-generation chondrocyte implantation techniques as well as other novel methods of cartilage restoration (e.g., use of minced allogeneic cartilage, chondrocyte optimization, use of growth factors, injection of autogenous stem cells) for the treatment of OLT (21, 22, 24).

REFERENCES

1. Tol JL, Struijs PA, Bossuyt PM, et al. Treatment strategies in osteochondral defects of the talar dome: a systematic review. *Foot Ankle Int.* 2000;21(2):119–126.
2. Zengerink M, Szerb I, Hangody L, et al. Current concepts: treatment of osteochondral ankle defects. *Foot Ankle Clin.* 2006;11(2):331–359, vi.
3. Flick AB, Gould N. Osteochondritis dissecans of the talus (transchondral fractures of the talus): review of the literature and new surgical approach for medial dome lesions. *Foot Ankle.* 1985;5(4):165–185.
4. Loren GJ, Ferkel RD. Arthroscopic assessment of occult intra-articular injury in ankle fractures. *Arthroscopy.* 2002;18:412–421.
5. Hintermann B, Regazzoni P, Lampert C, et al. Arthroscopic findings in acute fractures of the ankle. *J Bone Joint Surg Br.* 2000;82:345–351.
6. Stufkens SA, Knupp M, Horisberger M, et al. Cartilage lesions and the development of osteoarthritis after internal fixation of ankle fractures. *J Bone Joint Surg Am.* 2010;92:279–286.
7. Hermanson E, Ferkel RD. Bilateral osteochondral lesions of the talus. *Foot Ankle Int.* 2009;30(8):723–727.
8. Berndt AL, Harty M. Transchondral fractures (osteochondritis dissecans) of the talus. *J Bone Joint Surg Am.* 1959;41-A:988–1020.
9. Anderson IF, Crichton KJ, Grattan-Smith T, et al. Osteochondral fractures of the dome of the talus. *J Bone Joint Surg Am.* 1989;71(8):1143–1152.
10. Ferkel RD. *Arthroscopic Surgery: The Foot and Ankle.* Philadelphia, PA: JB Lippincott; 1996.
11. Verhagen RA, Struijs PA, Bossuyt PM, et al. Systematic review of treatment strategies for osteochondral defects of the talar dome. *Foot Ankle Clin.* 2003;8(2):233–242, viii–ix.
12. Alford JW, Cole BJ. Cartilage restoration, part 2: techniques, outcomes, and future directions. *Am J Sports Med.* 2005;33(3):443–460.
13. Brittberg M, Lindahl A, Nilsson A, et al. Treatment of deep cartilage defects in the knee with autologous chondrocyte transplantation. *N Engl J Med.* 1994;331(14):889–895.

14. Getgood A, Brooks R, Fortier L, et al. Articular cartilage tissue engineering: today's research, tomorrow's practice? *J Bone Joint Surg Br*. 2009;91(5):565–576.
15. Hangody L, Fules P. Autologous osteochondral mosaicplasty for the treatment of full-thickness defects of weight-bearing joints: ten years of experimental and clinical experience. *J Bone Joint Surg Am*. 2003;85-A(suppl 2):25–32.
16. Mitchell ME, Giza E, Sullivan MR. Cartilage transplantation techniques for talar cartilage lesions. *J Am Acad Orthop Surg*. 2009;17(7):407–414.
17. Gortz S, DeYoung AJ, Bugbee WD. Fresh osteochondral allografting for osteochondral lesions of the talus. *Foot Ankle Int*. 2010;31:283–290.
18. Gross AE, Agnidis Z, Hutchison CR. Osteochondral defects of the talus treated with fresh osteochondral allograft transplantation. *Foot Ankle Int*. 2001;22(5):385–391.
19. Hahn DB, Aanstoos ME, Wilkins RM. Osteochondral lesions of the talus treated with fresh talar allografts. *Foot Ankle Int*. 2010;31:277–282.
20. Kerker JT, Leo AJ, Sgaglione NA. Cartilage repair: synthetics and scaffolds: basic science, surgical techniques, and clinical outcomes. *Sports Med Arthrosc*. 2008;16(4):208–216.
21. McNickle AG, Provencher MT, Cole BJ. Overview of existing cartilage repair technology. *Sports Med Arthrosc*. 2008;16(4):196–201.
22. Hettrich CM, Crawford D, Rodeo SA. Cartilage repair: third-generation cell-based technologies—basic science, surgical techniques, clinical outcomes. *Sports Med Arthrosc*. 2008;16(4):230–235.
23. Ferkel RD, Zanotti RM, Komenda GA, et al. Arthroscopic treatment of chronic osteochondral lesions of the talus: long-term results. *Am J Sports Med*. 2008;36(9):1750–1762.
24. Kon E, Delcogliano M, Filardo G, et al. Second generation issues in cartilage repair. *Sports Med Arthrosc*. 2008;16(4):221–229.
25. Safran MR, Kim H, Zaffagnini S. The use of scaffolds in the management of articular cartilage injury. *J Am Acad Orthop Surg*. 2008;16(6):306–311.
26. Peterson L, Minas T, Brittberg M, et al. Two- to 9-year outcome after autologous chondrocyte transplantation of the knee. *Clin Orthop Relat Res*. 2000;(374):212–234.
27. Baums MH, Heidrich G, Schultz W, et al. Autologous chondrocyte transplantation for treating cartilage defects of the talus. *J Bone Joint Surg Am*. 2006;88(2):303–308.
28. Giannini S, Buda R, Grigolo B, et al. The detached osteochondral fragment as a source of cells for autologous chondrocyte implantation (ACI) in the ankle joint. *Osteoarthritis Cartilage*. 2005;13(7):601–607.
29. Koulalis D, Schultz W, Heyden M. Autologous chondrocyte transplantation for osteochondritis dissecans of the talus. *Clin Orthop Relat Res*. 2002;(395):186–192.
30. Giannini S, Buda R, Grigolo B, et al. Autologous chondrocyte transplantation in osteochondral lesions of the ankle joint. *Foot Ankle Int*. 2001;22(6):513–517.
31. Peterson L, Brittberg M, Kiviranta I, et al. Autologous chondrocyte transplantation. Biomechanics and long-term durability. *Am J Sports Med*. 2002;30(1):2–12.
32. Nam EK, Ferkel RD, Applegate GR. Autologous chondrocyte implantation of the ankle: a 2- to 5-year follow-up. *Am J Sports Med*. 2009;37(2):274–284.
33. Whittaker JP, Smith G, Makwana N, et al. Early results of autologous chondrocyte implantation in the talus. *J Bone Joint Surg Br*. 2005;87(2):179–183.
34. Peterson L, Brittberg M, Lindahl A. Autologous chondrocyte transplantation of the ankle. *Foot Ankle Clin*. 2003;8(2):291–303.
35. Mandelbaum BR, Gerhardt MB, Peterson L. Autologous chondrocyte implantation of the talus. *Arthroscopy*. 2003;19(suppl 1):129–137.
36. Levine D. Tissue-engineered cartilage products. In: Lanza R, Langer R, Vacanti J, ed. *Principles of Tissue Engineering*. New York, NY: Elsevier; 2007:1215–1223.
37. Aigner J, Tegeler J, Hutzler P, et al. Cartilage tissue engineering with novel nonwoven structured biomaterial based on hyaluronic acid benzyl ester. *J Biomed Mater Res*. 1998;42(2):172–181.
38. Giannini S, Buda R, Vannini F, et al. Arthroscopic autologous chondrocyte implantation in osteochondral lesions of the talus: surgical technique and results. *Am J Sports Med*. 2008;36(5):873–880.
39. Bartlett W, Skinner JA, Gooding CR, et al. Autologous chondrocyte implantation versus matrix-induced autologous chondrocyte implantation for osteochondral defects of the knee: a prospective, randomised study. *J Bone Joint Surg Br*. 2005;87(5):640–645.
40. Cherubino P, Grassi FA, Bulgheroni P, et al. Autologous chondrocyte implantation using a bilayer collagen membrane: a preliminary report. *J Orthop Surg (Hong Kong)*. 2003;11(1):10–15.
41. Ronga M, Grassi FA, Montoli C, et al. Treatment of deep cartilage defects of the ankle with the matrix-induced autologous chondrocyte implantation (MACI). *Foot Ankle Surg*. 2005;11:29–33.
42. Wright JG, Einhorn TA, Heckman JD. Grades of recommendation. *J Bone Joint Surg Am*. 2005;87(9):1909–1910.
43. Henderson I, Lavigne P, Valenzuela H, et al. Autologous chondrocyte implantation: superior biologic properties of hyaline cartilage repairs. *Clin Orthop Relat Res*. 2007;455:253–261.
44. Robinson DE, Winson IG, Harries WJ, et al. Arthroscopic treatment of osteochondral lesions of the talus. *J Bone Joint Surg Br*. 2003;85(7):989–993.
45. Choi WJ, Park KK, Kim BS, et al. Osteochondral lesion of the talus: is there a critical defect size for poor outcome? *Am J Sports Med*. 2009;37(10):1974–1980.
46. Candrian C, Miot S, Wolf F, et al. Are ankle chondrocytes from damaged osteochondral fragments a suitable source for cartilage repair? In: 8th World Congress of the International Cartilage Repair Society; 2009; Miami, FL.
47. Ferkel RD, Chams RN. Chronic lateral instability: arthroscopic findings and long-term results. *Foot Ankle Int*. 2007;28:24–31.
48. Breinan HA, Minas T, Hsu HP, et al. Effect of cultured autologous chondrocytes on repair of chondral defects in a canine model. *J Bone Joint Surg Am*. 1997;79(10):1439–1451.
49. Hambly K, Bobic V, Wondrasch B, et al. Autologous chondrocyte implantation postoperative care and rehabilitation: science and practice. *Am J Sports Med*. 2006;34(6):1020–1038.
50. Buckwalter JA. Articular cartilage: injuries and potential for healing. *J Orthop Sports Phys Ther*. 1998;28(4):192–202.

Arthroscopy and Management of Ankle Fractures

Beat Hintemann

Despite having adequate open reduction and internal fixation, ankle fractures may still be associated with poor clinical outcomes (1–4). Residual problems such as chronic pain, arthrofibrosis, recurrent swelling, and perceived instability continue to occur unpredictably after ankle fractures. The cause of such poor outcomes is unclear, yet may be related to occult articular trauma (5–8). The use of arthroscopy allowed comprehensive evaluation of the pattern and extent of articular injury associated with acute ankle fractures (9–12).

SURGICAL TECHNIQUE

The operative procedure is performed under general, spinal, or epidural anesthesia. The patient is positioned supine with a padded bolster placed under the ipsilateral pelvis. The knee is flexed to about 70° using the knee holder, which allows the foot to hang free. No distraction device is used for the ankle. Following sterile preparation, surface anatomy is carefully outlined. In the swollen ankle, more care is necessary to delineate the important structures. To avoid iatrogenic lesions of the soft tissues and articular cartilage, the joint is first inflated with saline, and the portals are created by blunt dissection. The anterior approach at the lateral border of the anterior tibial tendon is used to insert the 4.5- or 2.7-mm, 30° arthroscope. If necessary, accessory anteromedial or anterolateral portals are used for the insertion of instruments. After having copiously irrigated the joint, the joint is inspected systematically (13).

Arthroscopic Assessment

Chondral lesions are carefully assessed with regard to extent and severity, and graded as described by Outerbridge (14). Unstable chondral flaps are debrided, and free osteochondral fragments are removed. Articular surface lesions and intra-articular ligament integrity and syndesmosis stability are evaluated (Fig. 91.1).

Arthroscopic Reduction and Internal Fixation

The use of arthroscopic reduction and internal fixation (ARIF) is surgeon dependent. Reported indications for ARIF include transchondral talar dome fracture, talar fracture, low-grade fracture of the distal tibia, syndesmotic disruption, malleolar fracture, and chronic pain following definitive management of fracture about the ankle. Among the potential benefits are less extensive exposure, preservation of blood supply, and improved visualization of the pathology.

Percutaneous manipulation of fracture fragments under direct visualization is performed using fluoroscopy as needed. If arthroscopically assisted reduction of the medial malleolus or distal tibia fracture is successful, cannulated screw fixation under fluoroscopy control is undertaken without open exposure of the fracture site. If the fracture morphology precludes arthroscopic reduction, open reduction and fixation (ORIF) are then performed. This is typically the case for a fracture of the fibula.

Postoperative Care

Postoperatively, the ankle is routinely immobilized in a posterior splint until swelling-down and safe wound-healing. Thereafter, the patients are kept in a cast or a walker for a minimum of 6 weeks following surgery with a period of 4 to 6 weeks of partial weight-bearing immobilization, and additional 2 or more weeks of weight-bearing immobilization.

RESULTS

With the studies available, arthroscopy was found to be a valuable tool in acute ankle fractures in identifying and managing intra-articular damage that otherwise remain unrecognized (Fig. 91.2) (9–13). Arthroscopy also provides prognostic information regarding the outcome (4). A relative contraindication to arthroscopy is important soft-tissue damage associated with fracture-dislocation because of the risk related to fluid extravasation.

Chondral Lesions

In general, chondral lesions (Fig. 91.3) were found more often than expected (Table 91.1).

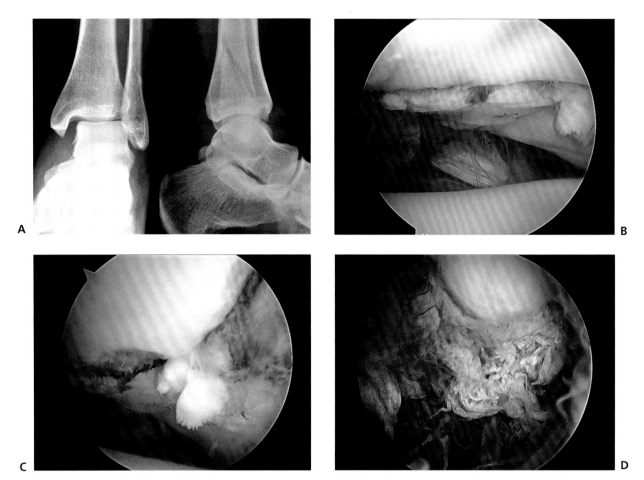

FIGURE 91.1. In this 36-year-old female patient who sustained a PER injury (**A**), arthroscopy evidenced a bony avulsion of posterior tibiofibular ligament with extended involvement of posterior tibial plafond and preserved intermalleolar ligament (**B**) with some intermediate osteoarticular debris (**C**). It also showed a complete avulsion of deltoid ligament from medial malleolus (**D**).

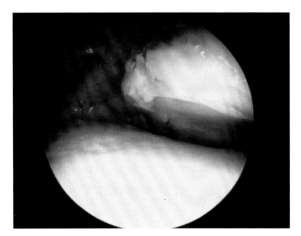

FIGURE 91.2. In this 32-year-old soccer player with a type-A fracture, arthroscopy evidenced an impaction fracture at medial tibial plafond, indicating the severity of sustained injury. This lesion would not have been detected otherwise.

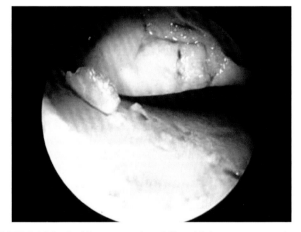

FIGURE 91.3. Besides osseous instability with incongruency, arthroscopy reveals extended lesions to articular surface (a 48-year-old female patient after PER injury).

Hintermann et al., (11) in a prospective study on 288 patients, first reported on arthroscopic findings in acute ankle fractures. They found a 79% rate of articular lesions. The frequency and severity of chondral lesions increased from type-B to type-C ankle fractures ($P < .05$), as classified with use of the AO-Danis-Weber criteria, but there was no difference between type-A and type-B fractures with regard to the frequency and severity of chondral lesions. There were more lesions in men than in women, and

Table 91.1

Amount and localization of chondral lesions

	Year	n (%)	Total (%)	Talar Dome (%)	Tibial Plafond (%)	Lateral Malleolus	Medial Malleolus	Loose Bodies
Hintermann et al. (11)	2000	288	79	69	46	45	41	14
Thordarson et al. (12)	2001	9	89	89	n.i.	n.i.	n.i.	11
Loren and Ferkel (13)	2002	48	63[a]	40	23	n.i.	n.i	28
Ono et al. (15)	2004	105	20	6	5	7	3	n.i.
Takao et al. (16)	2004	41[b]	–	73	n.i.	n.i.	n.i.	n.i.
Yoshimura et al. (17)	2008	4	100	100	0	0	0	100
Leontaritis et al. (9)	2009	84	73	61	6	5	5	15

[a]Osteochondral lesions of >5 mm of diameter.
[b]All 41 cases, type B-fractures (Danis-Weber) fractures.
n.i., not indicated.

in general, they were more severe in men ($P < .05$). They also tended to be worse in patients under 30 years and in those older than 60 years. Within each type of fracture, the lesions increased from subgroups 1 to 3 ($P < .05$).

Loren and Ferkel (10) conducted a prospective study of 48 fractures classified with use of the Lauge-Hansen and AO-Danis-Weber criteria, with the inclusion of plafond-variant fractures, and found chondral lesions in 63% of the ankles; they determined that patients with an ankle fracture have a high prevalence of concomitant intra-articular pathology. However, they did not further subclassify or stage the fractures with use of the Lauge-Hansen criteria; as a result, no correlation could be made between the severity of the fracture pattern and the severity of intra-articular injury.

Ono et al. (15) prospectively reviewed the arthroscopic findings and surgical outcomes for 105 malleolar fractures that had been classified with use of the Lauge-Hansen system. Chondral lesions were found in 21 patients (20%), and the authors concluded that these lesions could occur regardless of the fracture stage or type. No correlation was found between the fracture type and the site of the chondral lesion or between the mechanism of injury and the severity of the chondral damage.

Leontaritis et al. (9) retrospectively reviewed the medical charts of 84 ankle fractures. Chondral lesions were found in 61 patients (73%). Of 17 fractures graded as pronation-external rotation (PER) or supination-external rotation (SER) type I according to the Lauge-Hansen classification, 15 were associated with one or no chondral lesion and two, with two or more chondral lesions. Of 10 fractures graded as PER or SER type II, 9 were associated with one or no chondral lesion and one, with two or more chondral lesions. Of 56 fractures graded as PER or SER type IV, 27 were associated with one or no chondral lesion

and 29, with two or more chondral lesions. Type-IV PER and SER ankle fractures were more likely to be associated with two or more chondral lesions than type-I fractures or type-II fractures.

Thordarson et al. (12) assessed the role of arthroscopy on the surgical management of ankle fractures in a prospective, randomized study. They found in eight of the original nine patients (89%) who underwent arthroscopic evaluation of the joint to have articular damage to the talar dome.

Ligamentous Injuries

A fewer studies have focused on arthroscopic assessment of ligamentous injuries in acute ankle fractures (Table 91.2).

Hintermann et al. (11) found injuries to the lateral ligament more often in type-B than in type-C fractures, but there was no difference in the frequency of injuries of the deltoid ligament (Fig. 91.4) with the exception of type-B1 fractures. Damage to the anterior tibiofibular (syndesmosis) ligament was noted with increasing frequency from type-B1 to type-C3 fractures (Fig. 91.5), although it was not ruptured in all cases.

Loren and Ferkel (10) found in 10 of 24 SER fractures at least partial interstitial disruption or incomplete articular avulsion of the syndesmosis ligaments. Only one SER injury had an unstable syndesmosis necessitating fixation, whereas, a disrupted and unstable syndesmosis ligament complex was found in all PER fractures and in the sole pronation-abduction (PAB) injuries. They also found that syndesmosis disruption portended a particularly high risk of articular surface injury to the talar dome.

Analogously, Yoshimura et al., (17) in their series of four Maisonneuve fractures, all ankles evidenced a complete disruption of syndesmosis ligament (Fig. 91.6) and also extended cartilage lesions to talar dome.

Table 91.2

Amount and localization of ligament injuries

	Year	n (%)	Total (%)	ATiF (%)	Deltoid Ligament (%)	ATF Ligament (%)
Hintermann et al. (11)	2000	288	79	70	40	45
Loren and Ferkel (10)	2002	48	63	48	41	4
Ono et al. (15)	2004	105	51	52	5	3
Takao et al. (16)	2004	38[a]	87	80	29	n.i.
Yoshimura et al. (17)	2008	4[b]	100	100	75[c]	100

[a]All 41 cases, type B-fractures (Danis-Weber) fractures.
[b]All four cases, Maisonneuve fractures.
[c]Fourth case, fracture of medial malleolus.
ATiF, anterior tibiofibular ligament (syndesmosis).
n.i., not indicated.

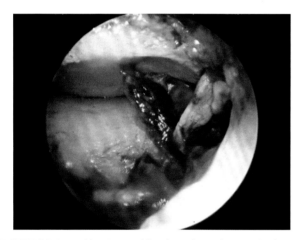

FIGURE 91.4. In this 56-year-old male patient who sustained a PER trauma, arthroscopy revealed a highly unstable ankle joint with syndesmotic disruption. There are also extended lesions to articular surfaces.

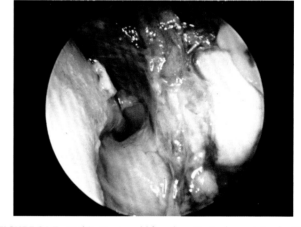

FIGURE 91.5. In this 41-year-old female patient who sustained a PER injury arthroscopy evidenced interposition of ruptured anterior deltoid ligament into the medial gutter, the deep deltoid ligament being partially ruptured. In this case, the interpositioned part of deltoid ligament was arthroscopically repositioned, and ORIF was done for the fracture of fibula.

ARIF

In their consecutive series of 288 acute ankle fractures, Hintermann et al. (11) used arthroscopy successfully to assist in the removal of debris and frayed cartilage and bone in 41 patients (14.2%), in the reduction of interposed stumps of ruptured ligaments in 9 (3.2%), in the reduction of interposed periosteum in 4 (1.4%), in pinning back a loose osteochondral fragment into place in 6 (2.1%), and in closed reduction of a fracture and fixation in 21 (7.3%) (11). Ono et al.,(15) who considered arthroscopic osteosynthesis in those patients in whom fractures could be reduced manually or arthroscopically, were able to perform this procedure successfully in 16 of 105 patients (16%). In 9 of these patients, the lesions were located at the medial malleolus and in 7 at the lateral malleolus.

The main advantages of ARIF include limited exposure, preservation of blood supply, and improved visualization of the pathology (18). However, ARIF requires increased surgical time, is technically more challenging than ORIF, and may result in soft-tissue swelling. Although ARIF may cost more initially, it may result in reduced long-term costs associated with chronic conditions.

Given the lack of evidence-based literature, it is not possible to definitively recommend the use of ARIF or arthroscopically assisted ORIF for the management of ankle fractures. However, there seems to be general agreement regarding the high incidence of intra-articular pathology associated with ankle fractures. In ankle fractures managed

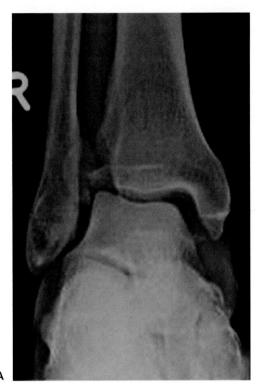

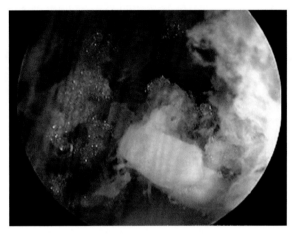

FIGURE 91.6. In this 39-year-old tennis player who sustained a Maisonneuve fracture with two bony fragments suggesting a bony avulsion of both the anterior and the posterior tibiofibular ligament (**A**), arthroscopy showed that the anterior bony fragment was an isolated fragment (**B**).

with ORIF, some of these conditions may be missed, resulting in chronic complaints.

Although arthroscopy is increasingly used in the setting of trauma, the effectiveness of ARIF compared with ORIF for the management of ankle fractures has yet to be determined. Most of these fractures are effectively managed with open procedures.

Arthroscopy for Chronic Pain Following Ankle Fracture

Several studies of adults with ankle fractures have shown poor results in some patients despite anatomic realignment and even after removal of hardware (1, 8, 9). Brown et al. (1) assessed late pain associated with hardware and found that, despite improvement after hardware removal, nearly half of the patients continued to experience pain. Such ongoing pain may result from intra-articular injury sustained at the time of the fracture.

van Dijk et al. (8) arthroscopically assessed 34 consecutive patients with residual complaints following fracture. They compared prospectively two groups: Group I comprised 18 patients with complaints that could be clinically attributed to anterior bony or soft-tissue impingement. In group II, the complaints of the 16 patients were more diffuse and despite extensive investigation, the definitive diagnosis was unclear before arthroscopy. Arthroscopic treatment consisted of removal of the anteriorly located osteophytes and/or scar tissue. After 2 years,

group I showed a significantly better score for patient satisfaction. There were good or excellent results in group I in 76% and group II in 43%. The authors concluded that patients with residual complaints after an ankle fracture and clinical signs of anterior impingement may benefit from arthroscopic surgery.

Amendola et al., (19) in a series comparing the outcomes of arthroscopy to manage various diagnoses in 79 ankles, concluded that arthroscopic debridement of well-reduced ankle fracture with chronic pain was helpful. Thomas et al. (6) performed arthroscopy in 50 patients who presented with chronic pain following the management of an acute ankle fracture. They found synovitis in 46 ankles, transchondral fractures in 45, arthrofibrosis in 20, spurs in 15, and loose bodies or debris in 9. Utsugi et al. (7) performed arthroscopy at the time of hardware removal in 33 patients and found arthrofibrosis in 24 patients. Debridement of fibrous tissue resulted in improved function in 29 patients who presented with functional limitation before arthroscopy.

SUMMARY AND CONCLUSIONS

The use of arthroscopy has brought more insight to type and extent of intra-articular damage in an acute ankle fracture. Chondral lesions are commonly found after an acute ankle fracture. There is evidence that the number of intra-articular chondral lesions associated with the more severe ankle fracture patterns (PER and SER type-IV fractures) is greater than the number associated with the less severe ankle fracture patterns. Among the ligament injuries, a disruption of syndesmosis ligament is obviously associated with a high risk of articular surface injury to the talar dome. Analogously, ankles with injuries to the deltoid ligament seem to evidence chondral lesions more frequently than those with intact deltoid ligament. Despite of advanced arthroscopic techniques, fracture fixation under fluoroscopic control may remain limited to fixation of fractures of medial malleolus and tibia. Finally, patients with residual complaints after an ankle fracture and clinical signs of anterior impingement may benefit from arthroscopic surgery.

To determine if early arthroscopic intervention will minimize poor outcomes after malleolar fractures, a prospective randomized comparative study is necessary. Thordarson et al. (12) performed a prospective randomized comparative study for surgical treatment of malleolar fractures with or without ankle arthroscopy. They reported no significant difference between arthroscopic techniques and standard open techniques. Their study consisted of a small group of patients (19 patients), and the average follow-up time was short (21 months). However, a larger group of patients and long-term follow-up times may be necessary to show the usefulness of arthroscopic intervention. Nevertheless, as arthroscopy was found to provide reliable information about the present intra-articular lesions that may often not be detected, it enables the surgeon to understand the injury pattern and to optimize the treatment modalities. This, in turn, may result in a better outcome at long term.

REFERENCES

1. Brown OL, Dirschl DR, Obremskey WT. Incidence of hardware-related pain and its effect on functional outcomes after open reduction and internal fixation of ankle fractures. *J Orthop Trauma.* 2001;15(4):271–274.
2. Beris AE, Kabbani KT, Xenakis TA, et al. Surgical treatment of malleolar fractures. A review of 144 patients. *Clin Orthop Relat Res.* 1997;341:90–98.
3. Day GA, Swanson CE, Hulcombe BG. Operative treatment of ankle fractures: a minimum ten-year follow-up. *Foot Ankle Int.* 2001;22(2):102–106.
4. Stufkens SA, Knupp M, Horisberger M, et al. Cartilage lesions and the development of osteoarthritis after internal fixation of ankle fractures: a prospective study. *J Bone Joint Surg Am.* 2010;92(2):279–286.
5. Pritsch M, Lokiec F, Sali M, et al. Adhesions of distal tibiofibular syndesmosis. A cause of chronic ankle pain after fracture. *Clin Orthop Relat Res.* 1993;(289):220–222.
6. Thomas B, Yeo JM, Slater GL. Chronic pain after ankle fracture: an arthroscopic assessment case series. *Foot Ankle Int.* 2005;26(12):1012–1016.
7. Utsugi K, Sakai H, Hiraoka H, et al. Intra-articular fibrous tissue formation following ankle fracture: the significance of arthroscopic debridement of fibrous tissue. *Arthroscopy.* 2007;23(1):89–99.
8. van Dijk CN, Verhagen RA, Tol JL. Arthroscopy for problems after ankle fracture. *J Bone Joint Surg Br.* 1997;79(2):280–284.
9. Leontaritis N, Hinojosa L, Panchbhavi VK. Arthroscopically detected intra-articular lesions associated with acute ankle fractures. *J Bone Joint Surg Am.* 2009;91(2):333–339.
10. Loren GJ, Ferkel RD. Arthroscopic assessment of occult intra-articular injury in acute ankle fractures. *Arthroscopy.* 2002;18(4):412–421.
11. Hintermann B, Regazzoni P, Lampert C, et al. Arthroscopic findings in acute fractures of the ankle. *J Bone Joint Surg Br.* 2002;82(3):345–351.
12. Thordarson DB, Bains R, Shepherd LE. The role of ankle arthroscopy on the surgical management of ankle fractures. *Foot Ankle Int.* 2001;22(2):123–125.
13. Ferkel RD, Fasulo GJ. Arthroscopic treatment of ankle injuries. *Orthop Clin North Am.* 1994;25(1):17–32.
14. Outerbridge RE. The etiology of chondromalacia patellae. *J Bone Joint Surg Br.* 1961;43-B:752–757.
15. Ono A, Nishikawa S, Nagao A, et al. Arthroscopically assisted treatment of ankle fractures: arthroscopic findings and surgical outcomes. *Arthroscopy.* 2004;20(6):627–631.
16. Takao M, Ochi M, Naito K, et al. Arthroscopic diagnosis of tibiofibular syndesmosis disruption. *Arthroscopy.* 2001;17(8):836–843.
17. Yoshimura I, Naito M, Kanazawa K, et al. Arthroscopic findings in Maisonneuve fractures. *J Orthop Sci.* 2008;13(1):3–6. Epub 2008 Feb 16.
18. Bonasia DE, Rossi R, Saltzman CL, et al. The role of arthroscopy in the management of fractures about the ankle [review]. *J Am Acad Orthop Surg.* 2011;19(4):226–235.
19. Amendola A, Petrik J, Webster-Bogaert S. Ankle arthroscopy: outcome in 79 consecutive patients. *Arthroscopy.* 1996;12(5):565–573.

The Role of Arthroscopy in the Treatment of Chronic Ankle Instability

Annunziato Amendola • Davide Edoardo Bonasia

Ankle sprains are among the most common injuries encountered in work and sport with well over two million individuals experiencing ankle ligament trauma each year in the United States (1). Although most of these respond well to conservative management, acute ankle sprains are frequently associated with pathology resulting in chronic symptoms including pain and instability that persist beyond the expected recovery period (1). The incidence of chronic symptoms after ankle sprains has been reported as high as 50% (1). The obvious question is what causes residual dysfunction following sprains? There are many causes that have been described that may be responsible for chronic pain following ankle sprains, including (1) intra-articular pathologies (chondral lesions, loose bodies, ossicles, synovitis, and arthrosis); (2) impingements (anterior and anterolateral); and (3) instabilities (lateral, syndesmotic, and medial). The incidence of the most common disorders associated with chronic ankle instability is reported in Table 92.1.

After optimal nonoperative conservative treatment, surgery may be indicated. The open lateral reconstruction still remains the gold standard, but the combined arthroscopic evaluation of the ankle has evolved considerably over the past two decades. It is now possible to directly examine intra-articular structures that were only partially accessible via traditional approaches while avoiding much of the morbidity associated with open arthrotomy. Indeed, advances in technology and expertise have resulted in an expanded role of arthroscopy in many surgical procedures around the foot and ankle. Yet while it is generally accepted that arthroscopy can be very helpful in the diagnosis and treatment of many ankle injuries, there is still some controversy regarding specific indications and effectiveness for its use. The purpose of this chapter was to review the use and indications of arthroscopy or periarticular endoscopy in adjunct to treating ankle instability at the time of open ligamentous stabilization.

CLINICAL EVALUATION

The history of patients with chronic ankle pain should be thoroughly investigated. The patient may report (1) isolated or recurrent ankle sprains; (2) pain during normal or sustained activities; (3) giving way of the ankle; and (4) locking or catching. Associated swelling, stiffness, and weakness about the ankle are also common. Symptoms are typically exacerbated by prolonged weight-bearing or high-impact activities such as running or jumping sports.

Physical examination to evaluate medial and lateral instability should include (1) inversion stress test; (2) eversion stress test; and (3) the anteroposterior stress test (anterior drawer sign). Special tests for the evaluation of syndesmosis injuries include (1) the squeeze test; (2) the external rotation stress test; (3) the fibula translation test; (4) the Cotton test; (5) the crossedleg test; and (6) the stabilization test. The stabilization test is performed by tightly applying several layers of 5 cm athletic tape just above the ankle joint to stabilize the distal syndesmosis. The patient is then asked to stand, walk, and perform a toe raise and jump. The test result is positive if these maneuvers are less painful after taping. This test is particularly useful to confirm diagnosis during the subacute or chronic phase of injury, once acute swelling and pain have subsided. All of the stress tests cited must clearly demonstrate a significant difference between the affected and normal ankles before they can be considered diagnostic.

The flexion-extension range of motion must be evaluated as well, in order to exclude anterior or posterior impingement. Joint effusion and localized tenderness over the joint line may indicate intrarticular disorders (ossicles, loose bodies, osteochondral lesions [OCLs], arthritis, etc.). The foot alignment evaluation is mandatory and some deformities (i.e., hindfoot varus, first ray plantar flexion, and midfoot cavus) may predispose to recurrent sprains.

A correct work-up must include plain radiographs with weight-bearing anteroposterior, lateral, and mortise views of both ankles. Stress radiographs may be useful to confirm the diagnosis, but are not mandatory. MRI evaluation is essential in demonstrating ligament injury signs (ligament swelling, discontinuity, a lax or wavy ligament, and nonvisualization) and associated causes of ankle pain (chondral injury, bone bruising, radiographically occult fractures, sinus tarsi injury, periarticular tendon tears, and impingement syndrome) (Fig. 92.1).

Table 92.1

Literature review regarding disorders associated with chronic lateral ankle instability

References	No. of Cases	Syndesmotic Lesions (%)	Deltoid Lesions (%)	Chondral Lesions (%)	Ossicles (%)	Loose Bodies (%)	Synovitis (%)	Arthrosis (%)	Bony and Soft Tissue Impingement (%)
Taga et al. (2)	31	—	—	89–95	—	—	—	—	—
Schäfer and Hintermann (3)	110	7	6	71	—	—	38	—	—
Ogilvie-Harris et al. (4)	100	9	—	51	—	5	3	2	28
Komenda and Ferkel (5)	55	—	—	25	25	21	69	11	—
Hintermann et al. (6)	148	9	40	66	—	—	32	—	—
Okuda et al. (7)	30	—	—	63	—	—	—	—	—
Ferkel and Chams (8)	21	—	—	52	29	24	76	19	48
Choi et al. (9)	65	29	—	23	38	—	—	11	81
		7–29	6–40	23–95	25–38	21–24	3–76	2–19	28–81

Intra-articular pathology is a common finding in chronic ankle instability (Table 92.1), and the main role of arthroscopy is found here in diagnosing and treating these conditions.

The accuracy of arthroscopy in diagnosing ankle pathologies associated with lateral instability has been reported by many authors. A recent investigation by Hintermann et al. (6) demonstrated the sensitivity of arthroscopy in diagnosing abnormalities in the chronically unstable ankle. In their study, 148 patients with chronic ankle instability (>6 months) underwent arthroscopic evaluation. All structural changes were noted and compared with the original diagnosis as assessed by standardized physical exam and imaging. Arthroscopy demonstrated that over 50% of the cases had cartilage lesions of the talus, whereas the preoperative diagnosis was made in only

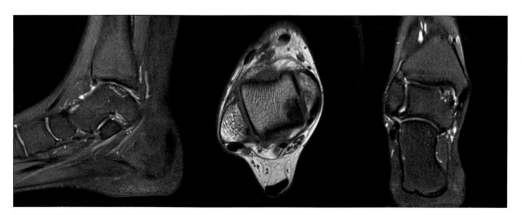

FIGURE 92.1. MRI showing a chondral lesion of the posteromedial aspect of the talar dome in a patient with associated lateral ankle instability.

4% of the patients. Arthroscopic examination also revealed cartilage lesions of the tibial pilon (8%), medial malleolus (11%), and lateral malleolus (2.5%) that were not identified preoperatively. Furthermore, arthroscopic examination provided a more sensitive means to diagnose medial and rotational instability as well as visualize synovitis. Similar findings were seen in Kibler's (10) study of 44 patients (46 ankles) who underwent a modified Broström procedure to repair the anterior talofibular ligament (ATFL) and the calcaneofibular ligament (CFL) in chronically symptomatic ankles. Arthroscopy identified intra-articular pathology in 38 (83%) of the 46 ankles. Preoperative diagnosis of intra-articular pathologies based on physical exam was made in only 28 (60%) cases.

Takao et al. (11) reported the results of 14 patients with apparent functional ankle instability. All subjects had no clinically demonstrable lateral instability and underwent standard stress radiography, MRI, ankle arthroscopy, and anatomical reconstruction of ATFL. Arthroscopic assessment revealed three cases with scar tissue and no ligamentous structure, nine cases with partial ligament tears and scar tissue on the disrupted ATFL fiber, and two cases of abnormal course of the ligament at the fibular or talar attachment. MRI revealed the following: five cases of discontinuity of the ATFL; two cases of narrowing of the ATFL; four cases of high-intensity lesion in the ATFL; and three normal cases. The authors concluded that both MRI and arthroscopy are excellent tools in the diagnosis of ankle disorders, with arthroscopy being more accurate in detecting small lesions.

Taga et al. (2) performed an arthroscopic investigation of ankles prior to lateral ligament reconstruction to look for associated cartilage lesions. Of the 22 patients with chronic ankle instability, chondral lesions were detected in 21 (95%). The articular surface of the medial tibial plafond was noted to be the most frequently and severely involved site with 7 (33%) of the ankles exhibiting grade 3 or 4 lesions at this location. Furthermore, given that the higher grade injuries were not noted radiographically, only arthroscopic evaluation could accurately diagnose the presence of associated chondral lesions. They suggested that arthroscopic evaluation should be performed to evaluate ankles with lateral ligament damage to aid patient counseling and direct further intervention.

Choi et al. (9) described, out of 65 cases of lateral ankle instability, 63 (96.9%) intra-articular lesions, of which 53 (81.5%) showed soft tissue impingement as the most common associated lesion. Other associated intra-articular lesions included ossicles at the lateral malleolus (38.5%), syndesmosis widening (29.2%), and OCL of the talus (23.1%).

Komenda and Ferkel (5) in their series of 55 patients with lateral instability demonstrated intra-articular abnormalities in 93% of ankles prior to lateral ankle stabilization. However, the incidence of chondral injuries in this study was only 25% compared with 95% reported by

Taga et al. (2) Additional abnormalities including loose bodies (22%), synovitis (69%), adhesions (15%), and osteophytes (11%) were discovered.

Ankle arthroscopy seems to be essential even when an open surgery is planned, like in lateral stabilization, for example. Ferkel and Chams (8) in their series of 21 patients with lateral ankle instability reported that arthroscopy showed 95% of intra-articular lesions, and only the 20% of them could be noted during the following open procedure. On the other hand, Ogilvie-Harris et al. (4) stated that in the ankles treated with lateral ligament reconstruction, the chondral lesions detected arthroscopically (23 out of 27 patients) could all have been treated during open surgery. Nevertheless, the authors concluded that arthroscopy was useful to confirm the abnormal talar tilt when the diagnosis of lateral instability was not certain.

In review of the literature, high rate of associated intra-articular lesions (Table 92.1) is evident along with the essential role that arthroscopy has in detecting them. Nevertheless, the types of lesions differ somewhat across studies, which may reflect the variety of anatomic lesions likely to produce chronic symptoms.

TREATMENT

The first step in the management of patients with chronic ankle instability is a functional and prophylactic rehabilitation program, which may be supplemented with external splinting.

Surgery is indicated after failure of an adequate conservative treatment.

The open surgical techniques described for the treatment of chronic ankle instability can be divided in two main categories: anatomic and nonanatomic. The aim of anatomic techniques (i.e., Broström, Broström-Gould) is to restore normal anatomy as well as joint mechanics and to maintain ankle and subtalar motion. The Broström technique involves midsubstance imbrications and suture of the ruptured ligament ends. Gould et al. (19) augmented the Broström repair with the mobilized lateral portion of the extensor retinaculum, which was attached to the fibula. Nevertheless, the outcome of these techniques is highly dependent on the quality of ligament remnants. Nonanatomic techniques (i.e., Watson-Jones, Evans, and Chrisman-Snook) are mainly tenodesis stabilizations and restrict ankle motion without repair of the injured ligaments.

A few arthroscopic lateral stabilization techniques have been described, including the arthroscopic stapling of the anterolateral capsule and the thermal-assisted capsular shift. Despite the promising results, a high success rate (85% to 100%) was reported for nearly all open ankle reconstructions, regardless of whether they were augmented or nonaugmented, anatomic or nonanatomic. For this reason, the open procedures still remain the gold standard treatment in chronic ankle instability.

VI. Foot and Ankle

As previously mentioned, the main role of arthroscopy in chronic medial instability is assessing and treating associate disorders. These can be summarized in (1) OCLs; (2) impingements; (3) loose bodies and avulsion fractures; (4) peroneal tendon pathology; (5) syndesmotic instability; and (6) medial instability.

Osteochondral Lesions

The incidence of OCLs associated with lateral ankle instability is 23% to 95%. The treatment of OCLs depends on the age and BMI of the patient, the size of the lesion, the quality of the articular surface, the quality of the subchondral bone, and the chronicity.

OCLs of the talus that are asymptomatic or discovered incidentally can be treated nonoperatively. Low-grade OCLs, particularly osteochondritis dissecans lesions in the pediatric population, may resolve completely with variable need for immobilization or protected weight-bearing. However, it is rarer to observe spontaneous healing in adult patients, most of all if chronic lateral instability is associated.

Traumatic osteochondral fragments that have not detached from the underlying bone may be suitable for fixation. Whenever possible, large unstable OCLs with a viable bony component are preferentially treated with stabilization rather than debridement alone. The synthesis may be achieved with both metallic or bioabsorbable pins. With associated lateral instability, it is rare to encounter this condition and OCLs usually show chronic patterns.

Retrograde drilling is indicated for subchondral bone lesions over which the overlying cartilage remains intact, with the clear advantage of protecting the integrity of the articular cartilage, compared with anterograde drilling. Bone or bone substitutes augmentation as well as platelet rich plasma (PRP) injection may be used respectively to avoid articular collapse and to promote healing. Once again, it is rare to find this type of OCLs associated with lateral instability. They are more likely encountered in early stages of osteochondritis dissecans.

The goal of microfractures and abrasion debridement procedures is to stimulate fibrocartilage development by breaching the subchondral plate and achieving a bone marrow stimulation (Fig. 92.2). Although the efficacy of microfracture in ankle OCLs is somewhat controversial compared with abrasion alone, most series have demonstrated that it provides symptomatic relief. In the presence of young and light patients, with small (<6 mm) and shear-type lesions, characterized primarily by chondral damage, these techniques may be optimal.

Impingements

Bony or soft tissue impingements are associated with lateral ankle instabilities in 28% to 81% of the cases (Table 92.1). Of bony impingements, anterior impingement is more common (Fig. 92.3). Although anterior impingement (spurs on the anterior tibia and anterior neck of the talus) indicates a long-standing disorder of the ankle, sprains usually exacerbate the symptoms that may require surgery in previously asymptomatic patients. Ogilvie-Harris et al. (4) treated 11 patients with anterior impingement, become symptomatic after multiple sprains. The patients complained of pain, stiffness, limp, and limitation of activities and not of substantial instability. The spurs were arthroscopically removed without any other combined procedure. The range of motion in dorsiflexion was significantly improved from an average of 0° dorsiflexion preoperatively to 10° postoperatively. Nine of the patients were completely satisfied and two were only partially satisfied.

Another condition associated with ankle sprains and instability is the anterolateral impingement syndrome, which is a synovial thickening consistent with impingement in the anterolateral ankle gutter (4). In these patients, the pain is characteristically increased by plantar flexion of the ankle and a talar dome chondral lesion is often associated. Arthroscopy reported good results in treating this condition. Ferkel et al. (12) evaluated 31 patients with anterolateral impingements. Arthroscopic synovectomy and debridement of scar tissue from the lateral gutter were performed in all patients. The outcomes of more than a 2-year follow-up were excellent in 15 cases, good in 11, fair in 4, and poor in 1. Ogilvie-Harris et al. (4) treated arthroscopically 17 cases with anterolateral impingement. Thirteen patients were completely satisfied, three partially satisfied, and only one was dissatisfied with the results.

Loose Bodies and Avulsion Fractures

With recurrent sprains, often avulsion injuries occur around the ankle (med malleolus, fibular malleolus, medial and lateral wall of the talus, posteromedial talus). At the time of ankle stabilization, arthroscopic removal of the loose bodies (Fig. 92.4) and unstable avulsions (Fig. 92.5) may be of benefit to prevent any discomfort when returning to play after stabilization.

Peroneal Tendon Pathology

Another condition that may be associated with chronic ankle instability is peroneal tendons pathology, even though the real incidence of this association is unknown. As the peroneal muscles act as lateral ankle stabilizers, more strain is placed on these tendons in chronic lateral instability resulting in hypertrophic tendinopathy, tenosynovitis, and, ultimately, in (partial) tendon tears (13).

These conditions, along with adhesions, tendon ruptures, and exostosis, can be easily treated with tendoscopy (Fig. 92.6), when a proper conservative treatment fails. Endoscopic release in combination with synovectomy has several advantages: outpatient procedure, diminished pain, quick work, and sports resumption, and no need for a plaster (13). Grade 1 and 2 injuries of the superior peroneal retinaculum accounts for more than 80% of peroneal instabilities (14). In these cases, the anatomical reattachment of the retinaculum is indicated (14). Lui (14) described

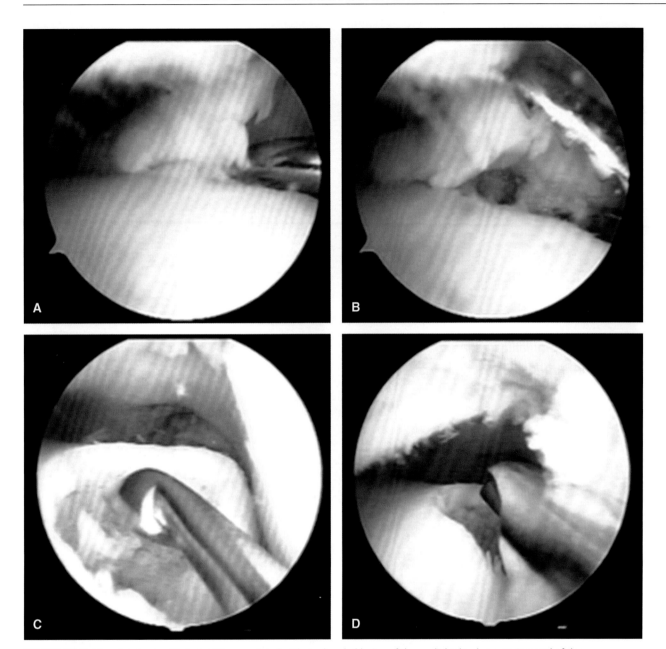

FIGURE 92.2. Chronic lateral ankle instability, associated with **A:** chondral lesion of the medial talar dome. **B:** Removal of the cartilage fragment. Debridement of the lesion with **C:** curette and **D:** shaver.

the endoscopic technique for superior retinaculum repair, using three anchor sutures inserted in the fibula. This procedure seems to have the advantages of minimal invasive surgery, better cosmesis results and less subjective tightness at peroneal tendons (14). An endoscopic approach can allow better assessment of retinaculum integrity, grading of the injury, detection of other pathology (e.g., exostosis of the retromalleolar sulcus), (14) and can also be easily converted to an open procedure.

In the patients with peroneal snap without a clinically evident dislocation over the lateral malleolus, the peroneal tendons are likely to snap over each other at the level of the tip of the lateral malleolus. The treatment of this condition is still debated. Both resection of the peroneal brevis

vincula and tenodesis have been proposed, but the results are still controversial (13).

Syndesmotic Instability

A disruption of the distal tibiofibular syndesmosis is a common finding in chronic lateral instabilities with an incidence ranging from 7% to 29%. The treatment of syndesmotic instability regardless of the involvement of lateral ligaments is still controversial. Current indications for surgical treatment of acute syndesmosis injuries include frank diastasis of the syndesmosis or diastasis on stress radiographs (15). In these cases, surgical treatment should include reduction and trans-syndesmotic fixation with one or two metallic screws (15). Arthroscopic

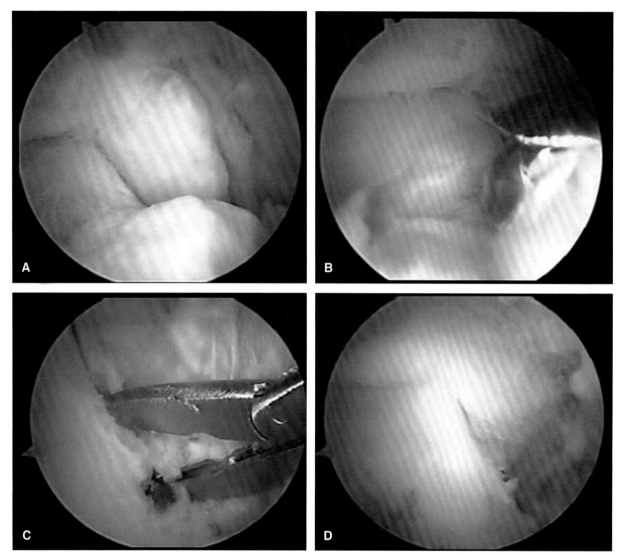

FIGURE 92.3. Chronic lateral ankle instability associated with **A:** anterior impingement. **B:** Removal of the bumps with a bur. **C:** Debridement of the ankle medial gutter. **D:** Tibiotalar joint after osteoplasty.

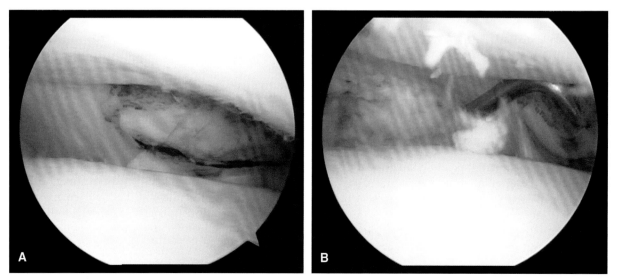

FIGURE 92.4. chronic lateral instability associated with **A:** loose body. **B:** Probing of the lateral ligaments tension and confirmation of the instability, after the loose body removal.

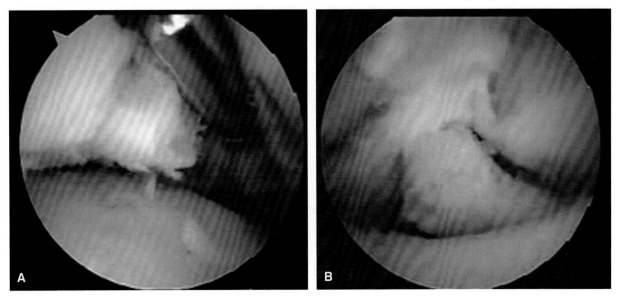

FIGURE 92.5. Chronic lateral ankle instability associated with **A:** anterior impingement and **B:** medial malleolus avulsion (which may be indicative of medial instability).

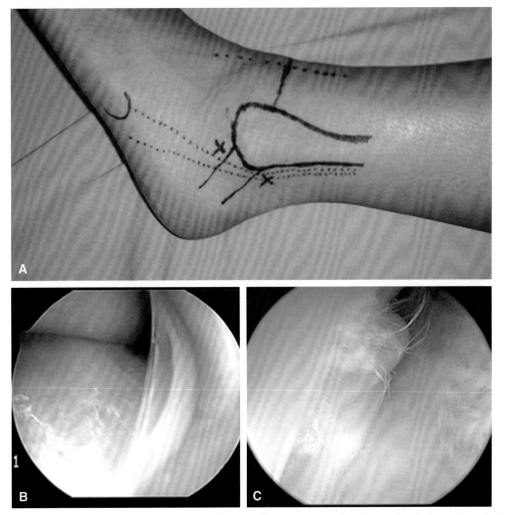

FIGURE 92.6. A: Portals' positioning for tendoscopy. If Broström procedure is associated, the incision should be posterior paramalleolar, including the two portals. **B** and **C:** Endoscopic images of the peroneals, with tendon degeneration.

evidence of syndesmotic instability is another indication for operative treatment. Nevertheless, when there are no radiographic signs of syndesmotic diastasis, the treatment of choice is controversial. Ogilvie-Harris et al. (4) treated nine patients with syndesmotic instability and normal radiographs. The diagnosis was made clinically and confirmed arthroscopically. The treatment involved an arthroscopic removal of the torn portions of the interosseous ligament and posterior-inferior tibiofibular ligament along with a debridement of the chondral damage if present. No screw fixation was performed. Seven patients were completely satisfied with the result and only two were partially satisfied. The authors concluded that the pain was caused by the intra-articular disruption, not by

biomechanical laxity, and that arthroscopic debridement was sufficient in these patients.

On the other hand, Wolf and Amendola (16) advocate the use of percutaneous fixation (Fig. 92.7). Fourteen athletically active patients underwent arthroscopic debridement at the level of the anterior-inferior tibiofibular ligament (to allow adequate visualization of the syndesmosis) and percutaneous trans-syndesmotic fixation with arthroscopic demonstration of syndesmotic instability. Three patients required additional lateral ligament reconstruction (Broström). Two of 14 patients (14%) had an excellent result, 10 of 14 (71%) had a good result, and 2 of 14 (14%) had a fair result (according to Edwards and DeLee scale).

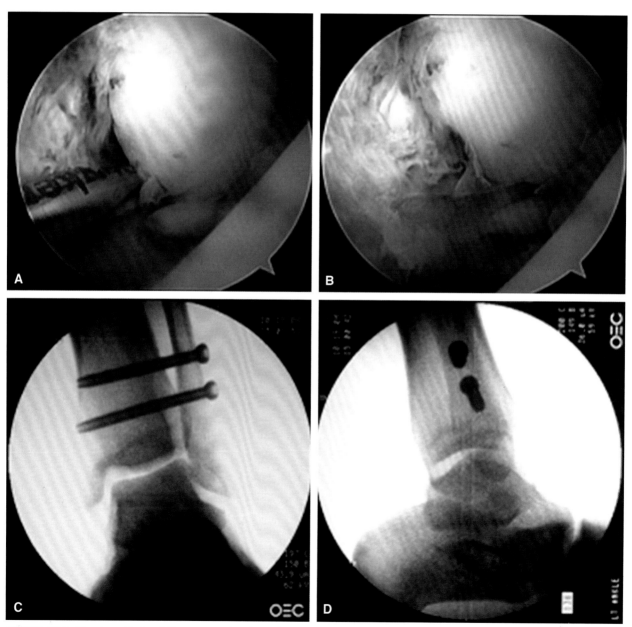

FIGURE 92.7. Chronic ankle instability associated with syndesmotic instability. **A** and **B**: Debridement of the syndesmosis. **C** and **D**: Intraoperative fluoroscopy to assess screws positioning and adequate mortise reduction.

Medial Instability

Although limited data are available in the literature regarding medial ankle instability, in patients with lateral ankle instability, it is common to observe an associated lesion of the deltoid ligament (6% to 40%). Similarly, a high incidence of lateral ligaments lesions (77%)(17) is detectable in chronic medial instability. Hintermann et al. (17) stated that this phenomenon is probably due to repetitive rotatory shift of the talus within the medial ankle mortise, provoking overuse and attenuation of the lateral ankle ligaments. Nevertheless, the authors raised the doubt that the "primum movens" of combined medial and lateral instability can be the lateral insufficiency. Another interesting datum regarding medial ankle instability is the high association with chondral lesions (100%).

Although once again arthroscopy has the important role in confirming the diagnosis often underestimated, the clinical relevance of medial ligament insufficiency is not exactly known, and the wide tendency is to not treat it surgically, as in deltoid disruptions associated to ankle fractures. The only study reporting results on medial ankle stabilization is the one by Hintermann et al (17). The authors treated 52 consecutive ankles with medial ankle instability. The surgical technique involved an arthroscopic diagnostic procedure before an open medial repair with anchors and with augmentation (plantaris tendon graft), if the tissue quality was poor. Additional lateral ligaments shortening and reinsertion were performed if an associated lateral instability was detected. At average 4.43 years after surgery, the clinical result was considered to be good/excellent in 46 cases (90%), fair in 4 cases (8%), and poor in 1 case (2%).

AUTHORS' PREFERRED TREATMENT

Presently, once the decision to stabilize an ankle has been made, my preferred method is a modified Broström with a Gould modification. In patients with excessive laxity or failed Broström, augmentation with an allograft semitendinosus or Achilles, or autograft hamstring tendon may be used. In addition, an arthroscopic evaluation is conducted prior to the incision to confirm the status of the joint, remove and synovial impingement, any bony impingement, loose bodies, and if necessary confirm the syndesmosis is intact. Anteromedial and anterolateral portals are used. The anterolateral portal is incorporated into the Broström incision anteriorly (Fig. 92.8). Swelling from fluid extravasation is present but usually of no impediment to identifying anatomy and carrying out the procedure.

In general, if there is any pain associated with the choric instability, arthroscopy is recommended at the time of stabilization to deal with any of the associated pathologies as noted above.

Most commonly a modified Broström is performed as the procedure of choice, but a lateral reconstruction with autograft or allograft transplantation can be used.

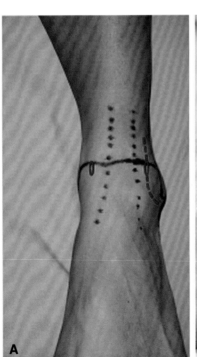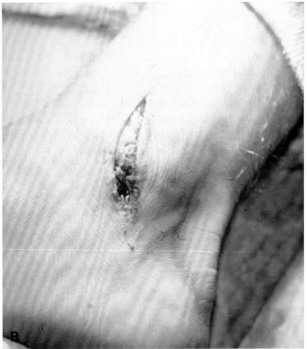

FIGURE 92.8. Ankle arthroscopy associated with Broström procedure. **A:** Positioning of the AM and AL portals *(red ovals)* and approach to the lateral compartment, including the AL portal *(red dashed line)*. **B:** Anterolateral approach for Broström procedure. AM, anteromedial; AL, anterolateral.

COMPLICATIONS, CONTROVERSIES, AND SPECIAL CONSIDERATIONS

There are still some debated issues mainly about osteochondral defects. Although other intra-articular disorders reported good results with arthroscopic treatment and seem to not affect the outcome of lateral reconstruction, it is still controversial whether chondral lesions correlate with poor results. Komenda and Ferkel (5) in the previously cited study reported good or excellent results in 96% of cases, further suggesting a benefit for the use of arthroscopy in diagnosing and treating all intra-articular lesions at the time of ligament repair. Okuda et al. (7) reported in a 30-patient series a 63% rate of focal chondral lesion diagnosed arthroscopically. The lesions were located on the medial side of the tibial plafond in 13 ankles (43%), on the lateral side in 2 ankles (7%), on the lateral side of the talar dome in 3 ankles (10%), and on the medial side in 9 ankles (30%). The authors noticed no significant differences in the clinical and radiologic results between patients with and without chondral damages. Hence, they concluded that lateral stabilization can be successful regardless of the presence of focal chondral lesions in patients with chronic lateral ankle instability when preoperative weight-bearing radiographs of the ankle do not show any joint space narrowing. Nevertheless, long-term results of patients with chondral lesion are not yet known.

On the other hand, Takao et al. (18) described the results of 16 lateral ankle instabilities with moderate arthrosis (7 cases with stage 2 and 9 cases with stage 3 degeneration, according to Takakura classification). All patients underwent lateral stabilization and arthroscopic drilling of the cartilage lesions. The authors recommended the combined procedures only for stage 2 arthrosis. Similar results were reported by Taga et al. (2) in the previously described paper, which stated that all the patients included in the study had sustained functional stability and mobility at 1-year follow-up. However, four of the patients with grade 3 or 4 lesions continued to experience medial ankle pain with activity. Physical examination of these patients revealed point tenderness at the anteromedial joint line corresponding to the location of the chondral lesions. The authors concluded that these symptomatic lesions may affect the final outcome of ankle stabilization procedures. Choi et al. (9) in a 65-case series evaluated the effect of associated lesions on the outcome of lateral ankle stabilization and concluded that arthroscopic diagnosis and treatment of intra-articular lesions is a safe and effective method. Nevertheless, the presence of any combination of associated intra-articular lesions resulted in a poor outcome. The strongest risk indicators for patients' dissatisfaction were syndesmosis widening, OCLs of the talus, and ossicles.

Another controversy in the literature is whether chondral lesions are correlated to the degree and the duration of ankle instability. In the study by Taga et al., (2) the severity and extent of cartilage lesions increased with the duration of symptoms, but did not correlate with the number of ligaments involved. The authors concluded that even single ligament lesions should be treated to prevent further cartilage damage. On the contrary, Hintermann et al. (6) showed no correlation between the severity and extent of cartilage lesions and the duration of ankle instability, but found an increased incidence of cartilage lesions in the presence of deltoid ligament rupture.

PEARLS AND PITFALLS

We recommend the use of a 30° 5.5-mm arthroscope and a fluid pump for ankle arthroscopy, in order to obtain a wider joint opening. No traction is required during the procedure.

We recommend for Broström procedure an anterolateral paramalleolar approach, if ankle arthroscopy is associated, and a posterolateral paramalleolar approach, if peroneal tendoscopy is planned. This will allow the surgeon to incorporate the arthroscopic portals in the Broström incision.

REHABILITATION

If a modified Broström procedure is performed, crutches are used for the first 7 days, until swelling subsides, and then a short leg walking cast is applied with the ankle in neutral, and weight-bearing is allowed as tolerated. The cast is removed at 4 weeks, and an air splint is worn 4 more weeks for protection. At 4 weeks after surgery, gentle range-of-motion exercises and isometric peroneal strengthening are begun. Return to sports is usually at 8 to 12 weeks after surgery. Complete rehabilitation of the peroneals is essential.

If retrograde drilling, microfractures, or abrasions are associated to lateral repair, weight-bearing is not allowed for 4 weeks.

If syndesmosis fixation is associated, nonweight-bearing is continued for a total of 8 weeks, and the syndesmosis screw is removed at 8 to 10 weeks.

CONCLUSIONS AND FUTURE DIRECTIONS

Chronic dysfunction following an ankle sprain or recurrent sprains is common occurrence. Despite surgical restoration of objective stability, many of these ankles are likely to continue to be problematic. In addition, traditional approaches to repair damaged ligaments offer limited exposure to intra-articular structures. As the use of arthroscopy expands, previously undiagnosed articular lesions suggest etiologies for unsatisfactory outcomes. Ankle arthroscopy has progressed immensely over the past several decades as previous limitations give way to improved technology, experiences, and techniques. Its use prior to ankle ligament reconstruction will aid the surgeon in assessing for additional damage while conferring minimal additional time or morbidity. Surgically amenable lesions can then be addressed and the patients can be more accurately counseled regarding the condition of their ankle. Although it is likely that preoperative arthroscopy will improve outcomes in surgically stabilized ankles, controlled prospective studies are lacking to truly assess its efficacy.

REFERENCES

1. Amendola A, Bonasia DE. When is ankle arthroscopy indicated in ankle instability? *Oper Tech Sports Med.* 2010;18:2–10.
2. Taga I, Shino K, Inoue M, et al. Articular cartilage lesions in ankles with lateral ligament injury. An arthroscopic study. *Am J Sports Med.* 1993;21(1):120–127.
3. Schäfer D, Hintermann B. Arthroscopic assessment of the chronic unstable ankle joint. *Knee Surg Sports Traumatol Arthrosc.* 1996;4(1):48–52.
4. Ogilvie-Harris DJ, Gilbart MK, Chorney K. Chronic pain following ankle sprains in athletes: the role of arthroscopic surgery. *Arthroscopy.* 1997;13(5):564–574.
5. Komenda GA, Ferkel RD. Arthroscopic findings associated with the unstable ankle. *Foot Ankle Int.* 1999;20(11):708–713.
6. Hintermann B, Boss A, Schafer D. Arthroscopic findings in patients with chronic ankle instability. *Am J Sports Med.* 2002;30(3):402–409.
7. Okuda R, Kinoshita M, Morikawa J, et al. Arthroscopic findings in chronic lateral ankle instability: do focal chondral lesions influence the results of ligament reconstruction? *Am J Sports Med.* 2005;33(1):35–42.
8. Ferkel RD, Chams RN. Chronic lateral instability: arthroscopic findings and long term results. *Foot Ankle Int.* 2007;28(1):24–31.
9. Choi WJ, Lee JW, Han SH, et al. Chronic lateral ankle instability: the effect of intra-articular lesions on clinical outcome. *Am J Sports Med.* 2008;36(11):2167–2172.
10. Kibler WB. Arthroscopic findings in ankle ligament reconstruction. *Clin Sport Med.* 1996;15(4):799–803.
11. Takao M, Innami K, Matsushita T, et al. Arthroscopic and magnetic resonance image appearance and reconstruction of the anterior talofibular ligament in cases of apparent functional ankle instability. *Am J Sports Med.* 2008;36(8):1542–1547.
12. Ferkel RD, Karzel RP, Del Pizzo W, et al. Arthroscopic treatment of anterolateral impingement of the ankle. *Am J Sports Med.* 1991;19(5):440–446.
13. Van Dijk CN, Kort N. Tendoscopy of the peroneal tendons. *Arthroscopy.* 1998;14(5):471–478.
14. Lui TH. Endoscopic peroneal retinaculum reconstruction. *Knee Surg Sports Traumatol Arthrosc.* 2006;14(5):478–481.
15. Williams GN, Jones MH, Amendola A. Syndesmotic ankle sprains in athletes. *Am J Sports Med.* 2007;35(7):1197–1207.
16. Wolf BR, Amendola A. Syndesmosis injuries in the athlete: when and how to operate. *Curr Opin Orthop.* 2002;13:151–154.
17. Hintermann B, Valderrabano V, Boss A, et al. Medial ankle instability: an exploratory, prospective study of fifty-two cases. *Am J Sports Med.* 2004;32(1):183–190.
18. Takao M, Komatsu F, Naito K, et al. Reconstruction of lateral ligament with arthroscopic drilling for treatment of early-stage osteoarthritis in unstable ankles. *Arthroscopy.* 2006;22(10):1119–1125.
19. Gould N, Seligson D, Gassman J. Early and late repair of lateral ligament of the ankle; Foot and Ankle, 1980 Sep;1(2):84–9.

Arthroscopic Ankle Arthrodesis

Brad D. Blankenhorn • Troy M. Gorman • Florian Nickisch
• Timothy C. Beals • Charles L. Saltzman

Arthroscopic ankle arthrodesis was first developed in the mid 1980s, and the technique has been refined over the past 20 years. In the appropriate patient, arthroscopic joint preparation combined with percutaneous joint stabilization allows for a minimally invasive approach to ankle arthrodesis that can decrease a patient's perioperative risks. The main advantage of arthroscopic arthrodesis over open arthrodesis is that it can be utilized in patients who have a compromised soft tissue envelope from trauma, previous surgeries, rheumatoid arthritis, or diabetes.

Over the past two decades, arthroscopic ankle arthrodesis has become a viable alternative to the open procedure and has shown consistently encouraging results (1–4). Proposed advantages of arthroscopic techniques are less postoperative pain and morbidity, decreased blood loss, and a shorter hospital stay.

ANATOMY AND PATHOGENESIS

The ankle joint is formed by the interaction of the tibia, talus, and fibula. The distal tibia along with the medial and lateral malleoli forms the ankle mortise. The talar dome is contained within this mortise. The ankle mortise confers inherent bony stability due to its congruency, but is also further stabilized by soft tissue structures. These structures include the ligaments of the syndesmosis, the ankle capsule, the anterior and posterior talofibular ligament, the calcaneofibular ligament (CFL), the intermalleolar ligament, and the deltoid ligament complex.

Ankle arthritis differs from hip and knee arthritis in that the principle cause of end-stage ankle arthritis is posttraumatic degeneration. The relative resistance of the ankle joint to primary osteoarthritis is likely due to a combination of its congruency, which results in inherent stability and restrained motion, and the cartilage's unique tensile properties and distinct metabolic characteristics. Unfortunately, the ankle seems quite susceptible to posttraumatic arthritis, and this may be related to its thinner and stiffer articular cartilage not being able to accommodate articular step-offs or the stresses of improperly constrained motion.

Step-offs lead to increased local contact stresses that the thin cartilage of the ankle may not be able to accommodate as well as the thicker cartilage in the hip and knee (5, 6). These increased localized contact stresses likely contribute to the degeneration in articular cartilage that is seen following trauma. Other disease processes such as Charcot arthropathy or osteochondritis with large osteochondral defects can lead to step-offs or incongruity in the articular surface resulting in increased contact stresses.

Secondary osteoarthritis of the ankle can develop after fracture or ligamentous injury. Rotational ankle fractures and ligamentous injury with recurrent instability are the most common causes (7–11). In the senior authors' practice over a 13-year time period, 445/639 (70%) patients with Kellgren-Lawrence grade 3 and 4 ankle arthritis were posttraumatic, and only 46 (7.2%) had primary osteoarthritis (9). Other recorded etiologies in this study for ankle arthritis include neuropathic disease (Charcot neuroarthropathy), inflammatory arthropathies (RA), crystalline arthropathies (pseudogout), osteochondritis, osseous necrosis, and postinfectious arthropathy.

INDICATIONS

General indications for ankle arthrodesis include degenerative arthritis with significant pain unresponsive to nonoperative interventions, large OsteChondritis Dessicans (OCD) not amendable to other interventions, osseous necrosis of the talus, failed total ankle replacement, and malalignment or instability from a paralytic deformity.

Indications for arthroscopic ankle arthrodesis remain the same with the exception of failed total ankle replacement. Well-aligned ankles and those that are easily realigned are excellent candidates for arthroscopic fusion (Fig. 93.1). Patients with soft tissue compromise (previous trauma, burn victims, patients with muscle flaps or skin grafts) or vasculopathy are strongly considered for an arthroscopic approach. Previously, it was felt that ankle varus or valgus greater than 5° was an absolute contraindication to arthroscopic arthrodesis. However, recent reports have

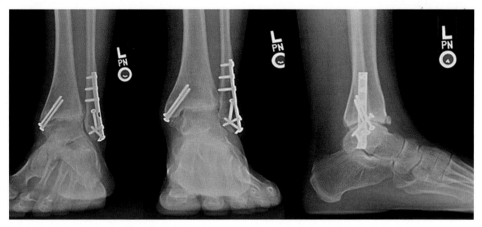

FIGURE 93.1. Anteroposterior, mortise, and lateral radiographs of a 29-year-old female with end-stage posttraumatic tibiotalar arthritis. There is minimal coronal or sagittal plane deformity with minmal disease in the distal tibiofibular joint and lateral gutter. This patient is an ideal candidate for arthroscopic tibiotalar arthrodesis.

suggested substantial ankle varus or valgus is a relative contraindication rather than an absolute one (12–14). The authors consider any ankle that can be realigned properly after arthroscopic debridement appropriate, but acknowledge that patients should be counseled that conversion to an open approach is prudent if an extensive capsulotomy or bony resection is required to achieve correct alignment. Additional contraindications for the arthroscopic procedure are significant focal bone loss and deformity and extremely rigid ankles. In general, the desired position of the arthrodesis is neutral dorsiflexion, 0° to 5° of ankle valgus, equal or slightly greater external rotation compared with the contralateral leg, and placement of the anterior aspect of the talar dome at or posterior to the level of the anterior aspect of the tibia.

CONTRAINDICATIONS

Absolute contraindications include active infection and active Charcot arthropathy. However, after appropriate treatment of an infection and resolution of the metabolic issues associated with Charcot arthropathy, arthrodesis is an acceptable treatment for these problems. Some surgeons may consider active smoking by the patient a relative contraindication.

CLINICAL EVALUATION

Physical Exam

Examination begins with observation, especially when you have the opportunity to watch the patient walk into the exam room. Having the patient walk as part of the exam is informative, and observing overall lower extremity alignment and gait pattern is critical. Restricted ankle motion leads to early heel rise and a bent knee gait. The posture of the forefoot when it strikes the ground should

be noted, as excessive forefoot varus or valgus is important to consider in surgical planning. Upon standing, the position of the hindfoot should be recorded as well. External rotation of the lower extremity is a common feature of patients with ankle arthritis.

The seated exam includes evaluation of range of motion in the ankle, hindfoot, midfoot, and forefoot. Ankle stability should be assessed by drawer testing, with the foot in both plantarflexion and neutral position. This investigates the competence of the anterior talofibular ligament (ATFL) and CFL, respectively. Talar tilt should also be assessed. Foot alignment is important as deformity in the foot may cause secondary ankle disease. For example, pes planus with medial column instability may be associated with secondary ankle valgus and eventual degenerative change. Conversely, realignment of a deformed ankle can alter the foot position and adversely or positively affect function of other joints, particularly the subtalar joint. If compensatory foot deformities are noted on exam, their passive correctability has to be assessed. Tendons should be palpated to identify potential confounding sources of pain. Furthermore, finding the point of maximal tenderness during the exam may help in diagnosis if there are multiple degenerative joints. A vascular exam should be performed with palpation of pulses and assessment of the distal capillary refill. The exam is completed with a neurologic assessment looking for motor or sensory deficits.

Imaging

Weight-bearing radiographs will better elicit deformity or soft tissue instability and should be obtained if possible. The four radiographic views we use in our clinic to evaluate ankle pain include the anteroposterior, lateral, mortise, and hindfoot alignment view. Radiographs of the degenerative ankle will show joint space narrowing, osteophyte formation, subchondral sclerosis, and subchondral cysts. When considering arthroscopic tibiotalar arthrodesis,

VI. Foot and Ankle

increased scrutiny should be applied to evaluating these standard radiographs. Anterior subluxation of the talus should be noted. Significant anterior subluxation will be difficult to correct with the limited capsular releases afforded during an arthroscopic approach. Special attention should be directed toward assessing degeneration of the distal tibiofibular joint and the formation of osteophytes in the medial and lateral gutters of the ankle. Failure to identify bony impingement in these areas can result in the inability to correct deformity or result in persistent pain postoperatively. If there is concern that these areas cannot be dealt with adequately through an arthroscopic approach, then open tibiotalar arthrodesis should be pursued.

The hindfoot alignment view is important in the evaluation hindfoot varus/valgus and ankle coronal plane deformity (Fig. 93.2) (15). It is taken with the patient standing on a platform facing a collector that angles away from the platform at 20°. The X-ray tube is posterior to the ankle with the beam perpendicular to the plane of the film at the level of the ankle. On average, the most inferior aspect of the calcaneus is centered along the longitudinal mid-axis of the tibia.

CT is an excellent adjunct to standard radiographs to better delineate the three-dimensional bony anatomy. Arthroscopic tibiotalar arthrodesis may be difficult in the setting of significant bone loss or collapse, and CT allows for better evaluation of the bony structures. In addition, due to the high prevalence of posttraumatic tibiotalar arthritis, there is often orthopedic hardware from previous interventions present, and unlike MRI, cCTallows for visualization near hardware. Noninvasive joint distraction plus air-contrast arthrography enhances visualization of the ankle articular features, and can be used if there is a need to delineate between focal and global ankle arthritis (16). MRI has limited use unless one suspects an osteochondral lesion of the talus, osseous necrosis or ligamentous abnormality that will alter patient care. In such cases, MRI arthrography may be advantageous.

Selective fluoroscopically guided injections can also be helpful in patients who have clinical or radiographic findings that suggest more than one source of pain. It is reasonable to expect 75% pain relief in an area that is injected (17). It is important to identify the patients' ankle pain as global (affecting a majority of the joint) or focal (specific region), as this distinction may guide the treatment options. It is particularly important to identify patients with coexisting subtalar pain as that population needs to be counseled more intensely about the risks of residual pain and progression of adjacent joint arthritis.

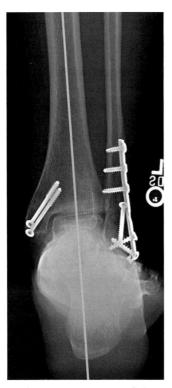

FIGURE 93.2. Hindfoot alignment view of the same 29-year-old patient. A line is drawn from the center of the intramedullary canal through the center of the tibiotalar joint and extended distally. If there is no malalignment of the hindfoot, this line should pass through the most plantar portion of the calcaneus. This patient shows normal hindfoot alignment.

TREATMENT

Both nonoperative and operative treatments can help reduce symptoms and improve function of painful ankle arthritis. Nonoperative interventions primarily focus on treating symptoms through either medications or mechanical unloading and immobilization. The authors' experience with nonsteroidal anti-inflammatory drugs (NSAID)s is that they seem to have variable efficacy in addressing the pain of ankle arthritis, but are still a mainstay of nonoperative treatment of ankle arthritis. The judicious use of corticosteroid or hyaluronate-based injections may provide temporary relief and be beneficial in acute exacerbations in someone who has tolerable steady state pain. Mechanical unloading or immobilization typically is conducted with a rigid ankle foot orthosis (AFO) or a leather ankle lacer with an imbedded polypropylene shell (18). If tolerated, bracing can be an effective means of controlling the pain associated with ankle arthritis. Adding a rocker bottom sole to a shoe or the use of a solid ankle cushioned heel (SACH) may also provide relief by reducing ankle excursion with gait.

Operative intervention should be considered only after failure of nonoperative treatment methods. When planning surgical interventions, it is critical to remember that recreating normal foot alignment will encourage improved foot function regardless of the chosen surgical technique. Surgical options for end-stage degenerative ankle arthritis include osteotomies about the ankle, debridement, distraction arthroplasty, total ankle arthroplasty, and ankle arthrodesis. Ankle arthrodesis currently has the most predictable and consistent results for the treatment of end-stage ankle arthritis, and can be performed in a variety of ways including open, mini-open, and arthroscopic techniques.

If arthrodesis is the surgical treatment of choice, the next step is ensuring appropriate alignment at the fusion site. This requires taking the alignment of the entire limb into account. Malalignment or angulation of the tibia may require special consideration. In addition, adjustment may need to be made in the position of the fusion to ensure a plantigrade foot if the foot has significant forefoot varus or valgus or other foot malalignment. For example, if a patient has significant fixed forefoot varus, the ankle joint needs to be positioned in a little more valgus so a plantigrade foot can be created. Concomitant knee and ankle arthritis and deformity should be fully assessed and realignment at the knee is a priority prior to ankle arthrodesis. If there is significant deformity, arthroscopic ankle arthrodesis should be abandoned in favor of an open approach.

Careful scrutiny of the patient's physical and radiographic exam are essential during the process of deciding which approach to take toward an ankle arthrodesis. If there is minimal or correctable coronal or sagittal plane deformity coupled with minimal degeneration of the distal tibiofibular joint and medial and lateral gutters, the patient is a good candidate for arthroscopic tibiotalar arthrodesis. A description of the technique follows.

ANTERIOR ARTHROSCOPIC SURGICAL TECHNIQUE

We recommend a general anesthetic to relax the gastrocnemius–soleus complex augmented with a regional block to aid in post-op pain control. At our center, a popliteal level indwelling catheter and a single injection saphenous block are placed with ultrasound imaging.

Patient Positioning

An arthroscopic ankle arthrodesis can be completed through either anterior or posterior arthroscopic portals. The anterior approach is favored for most cases, unless a subtalar fusion is also considered or there are soft tissue reasons (e.g., free flap, severe burns) not to do an anterior approach. In this situation, prone positioning and posterior portals would allow for arthroscopic preparation of both the tibiotalar and subtalar joints. For an anterior arthroscopic approach, the patient is placed in a supine position on the operating table with the operative leg in either a well leg holder (Fig. 93.3) or flat on the operative table depending on the type of external distractor used. When the leg is left out of the well leg holder, the bed can be adjusted (combination of reflex, Trendelenberg, and leg lowering) to create countertraction. Invasive distraction with a calcaneal or talar "skinny" wire or noninvasive distraction with an ankle strap can be used to facilitate joint

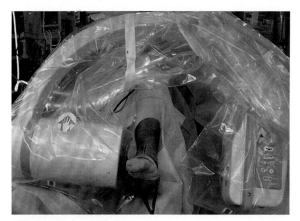

FIGURE 93.3. Positioning for arthroscopic tibiotalar arthrodesis using a well leg holder. The external distraction strap is placed around the ankle to aid in visualization. A mini C-arm is brought above the ankle to allow for fluoroscopic evaluation without interfering with access to the ankle for the arthroscopic procedure.

visualization. If external strapping techniques are used to distract the joint, the force (generally <25 lb [11.3 kg]) should be decreased during preparation of the anterior talar dome, as this takes tension off the anterior capsule, allowing for easier access to talar dome. Use of thigh tourniquet is optional; we always place a tourniquet in case needed, and rarely inflate it. Prepping above the knee allows for assessment of rotational alignment. Prior to portal creation, we mark out landmarks including malleoli, palpable branches of the superficial peroneal nerve, and the expected level of the tibiotalar joint space.

Portal Creation

For anterior arthroscopy, standard anteromedial and anterolateral portals are created. The joint is insufflated by injecting approximately 20 cc (20 mL) of normal saline using an 18G needle placed anteromedially into the joint. The anterolateral portal is created after needle localization under direct arthroscopic visualization (Fig. 93.4). Both portals are created using the "nick and spread" technique to minimize the risk of injury to branches of the superficial peroneal nerve. For arthroscopic arthrodesis, the portals should be made larger than would normally be done for standard arthroscopy. The larger portals aid in the introduction of larger instruments that will facilitate a timely arthroscopic debridement. To enhance visualization and fluid flow, a 4.0-mm scope is routinely used for arthroscopic visualization. An arthroscopic pump is typically used to distend the joint; the pump is set at the lowest pressure needed to achieve visualization, and is generally adjusted several times in the operation to reduce tissue edema. It is not uncommon to have a significant amount of anterior capsular scarring and synovitis, which can make access to the joint difficult. This synovitis and scarring should be removed to facilitate visualization (Fig. 93.4).

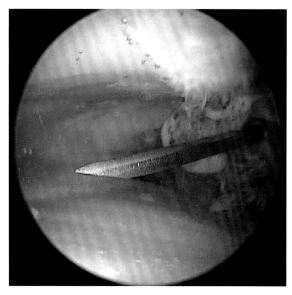

FIGURE 93.4. View of the tibiotalar joint in a left ankle from the anteromedial portal. The 18G needle is used to localize the lateral portal. There is a significant amount of synovitis seen in the anterior joint. This will need to be excised in order to visualize the anterior talus for joint preparation.

Joint Preparation

Once the joint is accessed and adequate visualization obtained, the tibiotalar joint surfaces are denuded of cartilage and prepared for arthrodesis. Cartilage debridement is conducted with a combination of curettes, elevators, and arthroscopic instruments (Fig. 93.5). It is advantageous to have a wide array of curettes and elevators available to facilitate access to as much of the joint as possible. Cartilage debridement within the medial and lateral gutters can be difficult to visualize, and may need to be done by palpation with minimal visual assistance. When the lateral gutter has little or no degeneration, we do not include it in the preparation or fusion—focusing solely on the tibiotalar joint. Once the remaining cartilage is removed, the joint surface is prepared for arthrodesis by perforating the subchondral bone with a 4.0-mm burr (Fig. 93.6). This creates a viable bed of bleeding bone. Adequacy of debridement is then inspected by deflating the tourniquet if it has been inflated, turning off the pump, and inspecting the joint for adequate bony bleeding (Fig. 93.7). If desired, dimineralized bone matrix can be injected into the joint using a 1-cc (1 mL) syringe through either portal. Attempted incorporation of the distal fibula into the fusion construct is determined by preexisting disease within this joint and the lateral gutter of the ankle.

Alignment

Aligning the foot correctly under the tibia is the critical step. As most arthroscopic patients have mild deformity, the goal is getting the foot plantigrade and neutral in the sagittal plane. This can sometimes still be very challenging.

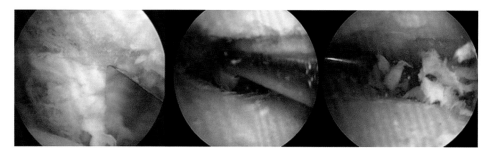

FIGURE 93.5. Arthroscopic views of the tibiotalar joint during removal of the remaining articular cartilage. Various instruments including a periosteal elevator and curettes are used to remove any residual articular cartilage.

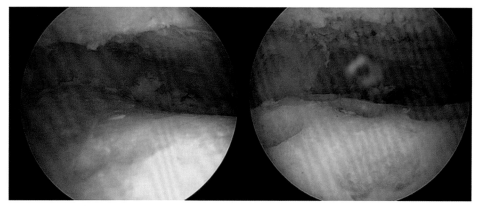

FIGURE 93.6. Arthroscopic views of the tibiotalar joint after cartilage removal and then after decortication with an arthroscopic burr. Decortication is a crucial step to allow facilitate fusion across the joint.

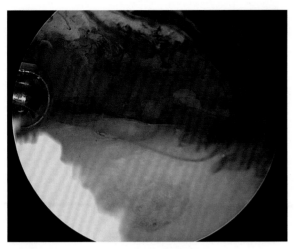

FIGURE 93.7. Arthroscopic view of bleeding bone after the subchondral bone has been decorticated with an arthroscopic burr.

We recommend placing the ankle in what you feel is the best position clinically and temporarily fixing it with two large K-wires or cannulated pins. Mechanically compressing the bones while the pins are placed can be helpful to achieve proper compression. Next, have your assistant hold the leg without grabbing the foot and go to the side of the patient to assess the sagittal position of the ankle with the foot gently dorsiflexed. Check the alignment of the heel. If it looks to be perfectly straight, it probably will be in a little varus when the patient stands. The position must be perfect before you move onto fixation. In addition, straighten the leg to ensure proper ankle coronal plane and rotational alignment.

Fixation

Fixation of the arthrodesis is done in a percutaneous manner. Two to three partially threaded screws can be placed in multiple configurations. Typically, one to two screws are placed from the anteromedial tibia into the talus (Fig. 93.8). Care must be taken not to injure the posterior tibial tendon when placing these screws. Avoidance of screws crossing at the joint surface facilitates stability of the construct. A screw can also be placed from the lateral tibia to the talus to increase construct rigidity (Fig. 93.9).

We typically use variable pitch headless compression screws for arthroscopic tibiotalar arthrodesis. Due to screw placement along the medial border of the tibia, there has been a documented high rate of screw removal with standard partially threaded compression screws (19). Variable pitch compression screws potentially decrease the rate of symptomatic hardware by burying the head of the screw below the medial cortex (20). A multiplane external fixator can also be employed if there has been a previous infection. If the lateral gutter (fibulotalar articulation) has no significant arthritis, it does not need to be debrided or fixed. However, if the fibulotalar joint is arthritic, a screw is placed from posterolateral in the fibula to infero-central into the talar neck and body. We often downsize the width of that screw to avoid cracking the fibula and add accessory screw(s) directed from the fibula to the talar dome (Fig. 93.10). Another consideration is to perform a transverse osteotomy of the fibula a few centimeters proximal to the joint line to decouple forces from the proximal fibula to the distal fibular fragment. This may enhance fusion of the syndesmotic region, and the distal fibular fragment can be secured with the same screw arrangement described above. Usually, some small gaps exist between the bony surfaces after fixation. If the lateral malleolus is included in the fusion, there will often be a small gap laterally as the medial screw may pull the talus medially.

POSTOPERATIVE CARE

Postoperative care for an arthroscopic tibiotalar arthrodesis is similar to postoperative protocol for an open arthrodesis. The ankle is placed in a well-padded posterior splint. The splint and sutures are removed at 10 to 14 days, and a below knee cast is placed. We allow patients 5 to 10 lb (2.2 to 4.5 kg) of heel weight-bearing so they can maintain their balance. Others have reported allowing full weight-bearing (21). Our group has no experience with early full weight-bearing.

At 6 to 8 weeks, radiographs are taken. At this point, we hope to see early bridging, which will have a ground glass appearance in the joint space. If there is doubt about adequacy of fusion, a CT scan can be used to better

VI. Foot and Ankle

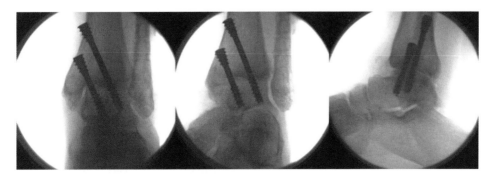

FIGURE 93.8. Intraoperative fluoroscopy showing fixation of an arthroscopic tibiotalar arthrodesis using two screws placed medially without incorporation of the fibula into the construct.

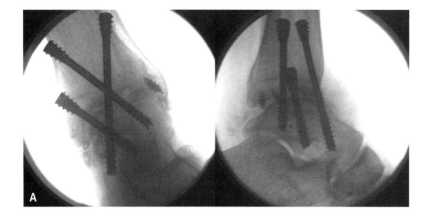

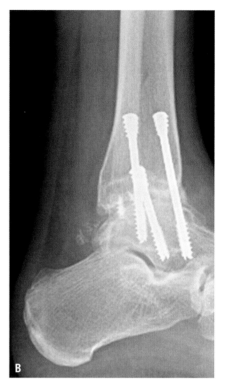

FIGURE 93.9. A: Intraoperative fluoroscopy showing fixation of an arthroscopic tibiotalar arthrodesis using three screws. Two screws were placed medially and a third screw was placed from the anterolateral direction. **B:** The fibula was not included in the construct. The talus appears to be slightly plantarflexed. On standing, in follow-up, the tibia is perpendicular to the floor, suggesting plantigrade sagittal plane alignment has been achieved.

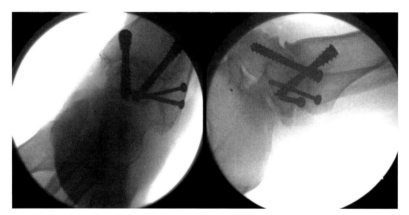

FIGURE 93.10. Intraoperative fluoroscopy showing fixation of an arthroscopic tibiotalar arthrodesis using two screws placed from the posteromedial and anterolateral directions with incorporation of the distal fibula into the construct.

visualize the joint. If fusion is apparent and the patient has minimal pain in the joint, the leg is placed into a removable boot. It should be worn at all times except for sleeping, bathing, and sitting. The patient then begins progressive weight-bearing as tolerated in the boot, as long as there is no significant pain.

At 10 weeks, a second set of radiographs is taken. If the radiographs show increased bridging and the patient has no pain with standing, they are weaned from the boot. Formal physical therapy is not mandated, but a 4- to 8-week course of balance and gait training after removal of the boot seems to speed recovery, particularly in elderly patients.

OUTCOMES

Many clinical series have been published since 1990 reporting on the outcomes of arthroscopic ankle arthrodesis. All the studies are retrospective in nature and only a few have compared the outcomes against an open treatment group. Myerson and Quill (3) published the first comparison study of arthroscopic versus open techniques. They had 17 patients treated with arthroscopic ankle arthrodesis versus 16 patients treated with an open technique consisting of a medial malleolar osteotomy. The authors found that the arthroscopic group had a shorter average time to fusion

(8.7 vs. 14.5 weeks) and a much shorter hospital stay (1.5 vs. 4 days). The arthroscopic group had one pseudoarthrosis for a fusion rate of 94.1% compared with 100% in the open group. However, this study was not controlled and the two groups were dissimilar, with the open group having patients with greater deformity and bone loss. O'Brien and colleagues (4) attempted to devise a better study by having two comparable groups in regard to the amount of deformity. They had 19 patients treated arthroscopically and 17 treated with open arthrodesis with "flat-cuts." The authors reported an 84% fusion rate in the arthroscopic group versus 82% in the open group. They found the arthroscopic group had a shorter surgery time by 12 minutes (166 vs. 184 minutes) and a significantly shorter hospital stay (1.6 vs. 3.4 days). The complication rate was similar between the groups.

The following results are compiled from an additional 15 clinical series in the literature (Table 93.1). Reported fusion rates range from 70% to 100% (1, 2, 12, 13, 21–30).

Five studies report 100% fusion rates, whereas the other 10 studies had rates ranging from 89% to 97%, with only one study reporting a fusion rate below 89% (30). A common definition for fusion in the literature is an ankle that is clinically stable on exam, pain-free on weight-bearing, and also has radiographic signs of bridging trabeculae. Five studies reported mean fusion times under 10.5 weeks, with the fastest mean time to fusion reported at 8.9 weeks (2, 23, 28–30). The other studies reported mean fusion time ranging from 11 to 16 weeks.

Five of the series report on the clinical outcome of patients with good or excellent results in 80% to 95% of patients with follow-up ranging from 14 months to 18 years (1, 2, 13, 27, 30). In the largest of the studies, Winson et al. (13) reported good to excellent results in 83 of 104 (80%) at average follow-up of 5.4 years. In addition, 95% to 100% satisfaction rates have been reported in the literature (28, 29).

Table 93.1

Published series of arthroscopic ankle arthrodesis

Study	No. of Patients	% Posttraumatic	Fusion Rate (%)	Time to Fusion	Complication Rate (%)
Myerson and Quill(3)	17 Arthroscopic	59	94	8.7 wk	11.70
	16 Open	75	100	14.5 wk	18.70
O'brien et al. (4)	19 Arthroscopic	63	84	Not reported	16
	17 Open	82	82		18
Olgivie-Harris et al. (27)	19	74	89	12 wk	26
Dent et al. (26)	8	60	100	Not reported	0
De Vriese et al. (25)	10	—	70	4 mo	30
Turan et al. (29)	8 (10 ankles)	0 (All rheumatoid)	100	10 wk	0
Corso and Zimmer(23)	16	75	100	9.5 wk	12.50
Glick and Morgan(2)	34	—	97	9 wk	5.80
Crosby et al. (24)	42	90	93	5.5 mo	55
Cameron and Ullrich(22)	15	33	100	11.5 wk	40
Zvijac et al. (30)	21	90	95	8.9 wk	4
Cannon et al. (21)	36	55	100	77% fused at 8 wk 100% at 16 wk	33
Saragas(28)	26	92	96	10.5 wk	34
Ferkel et al. (1)	35	77	97	11.8 wk	23
Winson et al. (13)	116 (118 ankles)	57	92	12 wk	32
Gougoulias et al. (12)	74 (78 ankles)	49	97	12.5 wk	31
Nielsen et al. (19)	58 Arthroscopic	64	95	1 y	33
	48 Open	67	84	1 y	40
Odutola et al. (20)	32	31	88	14 wk	12
Totals	594 ankle	52	90	—	22

COMPLICATIONS

In general, complications with the arthroscopic procedure compare favorably with those reported with open techniques. Complications rates in the literature range from 0% to 55%. However, prominent or painful hardware are responsible for much of the reported complications that result in eventual additional procedures. In an early study that focused on complications in arthroscopic ankle fusion, Crosby et al. reported an overall complication rate of 55% in a series consisting of 42 patients. There were three (7%) nonunions, two (5.1%) delayed unions, two stress fractures at the tibial pin sites used for distraction, five infections (four superficial infections at the sites pins were used and one deep infection), and six (14%) cases of painful hardware (four elected to have screws removed), and four patients went on to have painful subtalar arthritis (24). The amount of subsequent subtalar arthritis is similar to that reported in other studies (12, 13, 22). Other reported complications include cutaneous nerve injury, deep peroneal nerve palsy, malunion, dorsalis pedis pseudoaneurysm, and deep venous thrombosis with nonfatal pulmonary embolism (2, 13, 21, 23, 27).

SUMMARY

Reported series of arthroscopic ankle arthrodesis generally have comparable or improved rates of fusion, patient satisfaction, and adverse outcomes compared with traditional open fusion techniques. Arthroscopic tibiotalar arthrodesis is an excellent option for patients with minimal deformity in the coronal plane and those with a compromised soft tissue envelope. Postoperative morbidity is less than with an open approach and patients spend less time in the hospital following treatment. In addition, patient satisfaction is high. Thus, for surgeons with arthroscopy skills, arthroscopic ankle arthrodesis is an attractive and viable option for treating patients with end-stage ankle degenerative disease.

REFERENCES

1. Ferkel RD, Hewitt M. Long-term results of arthroscopic ankle arthrodesis. *Foot Ankle Int.* 2005;26(4):275–280.
2. Glick JM, Morgan CD, Myerson MS, et al. Ankle arthrodesis using an arthroscopic method: long-term follow-up of 34 cases. *Arthroscopy.* 1996;12(4):428–434.
3. Myerson MS, Quill G. Ankle arthrodesis. A comparison of an arthroscopic and an open method of treatment. *Clin Orthop Relat Res.* 1991;268:84–95.
4. O'Brien TS, Hart TS, Shereff MJ, et al. Open versus arthroscopic ankle arthrodesis: a comparative study. *Foot Ankle Int.* 1999;20(6):368–374.
5. Ateshian GA, Soslowsky LJ, Mow VC. Quantitation of articular surface topography and cartilage thickness in knee joints using stereophotogrammetry. *J Biomech.* 1991;24(8):761–776.
6. Athanasiou KA, Niederauer GG, Schenck RC Jr. Biomechanical topography of human ankle cartilage. *Ann Biomed Eng.* 1995;23(5):697–704.
7. Demetriades L, Strauss E, Gallina J. Osteoarthritis of the ankle. *Clin Orthop Relat Res.* 1998;349:28–42.
8. Harrington KD. Degenerative arthritis of the ankle secondary to long-standing lateral ligament instability. *J Bone Joint Surg Am.* 1979;61(3):354–361.
9. Saltzman CL, Salamon ML, Blanchard GM, et al. Epidemiology of ankle arthritis: report of a consecutive series of 639 patients from a tertiary orthopaedic center. *Iowa Orthop J.* 2005;25:44–46.
10. Schafer D, Hintermann B. Arthroscopic assessment of the chronic unstable ankle joint. *Knee Surg Sports Traumatol Arthrosc.* 1996;4(1):48–52.
11. Wyss C, Zollinger H. The causes of subsequent arthrodesis of the ankle joint. *Acta Orthop Belg.* 1991;57(suppl 1):22–27.
12. Gougoulias NE, Agathangelidis FG, Parsons SW. Arthroscopic ankle arthrodesis. *Foot Ankle Int.* 2007;28(6):695–706.
13. Winson IG, Robinson DE, Allen PE. Arthroscopic ankle arthrodesis. *J Bone Joint Surg Br.* 2005;87(3):343–347.
14. Dannawi Z, Nawabi DH, Patel A, et al. Arthroscopic ankle arthrodesis: are results reproducible irrespective of pre-operative deformity? *Foot Ankle Surg.* 2011;17:294–299.
15. Saltzman CL, el-Khoury GY. The hindfoot alignment view. *Foot Ankle Int.* 1995;16(9):572–576.
16. El-Khoury GY, Alliman KJ, Lundberg HJ, et al. Cartilage thickness in cadaveric ankles: measurement with double-contrast multi-detector row CT arthrography versus MR imaging. *Radiology.* 2004;233(3):768–773.
17. Khoury NJ, el-Khoury GY, Saltzman CL, et al. Intraarticular foot and ankle injections to identify source of pain before arthrodesis. *AJR Am J Roentgenol.* 1996;167(3):669–673.
18. Saltzman CL, Shurr D, Kamp J, et al. The leather ankle lacer. *Iowa Orthop J.* 1995;15:204–208.
19. Nielsen KK, Linde F, Jensen NC. The outcome of arthroscopic and open surgery ankle arthrodesis a comparative retrospective study of 107 patients. *Foot Ankle Surg.* 2008;14:153–157.
20. Odutola AA, Sheridan BD, Kelly AJ. Headless compression screw fixation prevents symptomatic metalwork in arthroscopic ankle arthrodesis. *Foot Ankle Surg.* 2012;18:111–113.
21. Cannon L. Early weight bearing is safe following arthroscopic ankle arthrodesis. *Foot Ankle Surg.* 2004;10:135–139.
22. Cameron SE, Ullrich P. Arthroscopic arthrodesis of the ankle joint. *Arthroscopy.* 2000;16(1):21–26.
23. Corso SJ, Zimmer TJ. Technique and clinical evaluation of arthroscopic ankle arthrodesis. *Arthroscopy.* 1995;11(5):585–590.
24. Crosby LA, Yee TC, Formanek TS, et al. Complications following arthroscopic ankle arthrodesis. *Foot Ankle Int.* 1996;17(6):340–342.
25. De Vriese L, Dereymaeker G, Fabry G. Arthroscopic ankle arthrodesis. Preliminary report. *Acta Orthop Belg.* 1994;60(4):389–392.
26. Dent CM, Patil M, Fairclough JA. Arthroscopic ankle arthrodesis. *J Bone Joint Surg Br.* 1993;75(5):830–832.
27. Ogilvie-Harris DJ, Lieberman I, Fitsialos D. Arthroscopically assisted arthrodesis for osteoarthrotic ankles. *J Bone Joint Surg Am.* 1993;75(8):1167–1174.
28. Saragas N. Results of arthroscopic arthrodesis of the ankle. *Foot Ankle Surg.* 2004;10:141–143.
29. Turan I, Wredmark T, Fellander-Tsai L. Arthroscopic ankle arthrodesis in rheumatoid arthritis. *Clin Orthop Relat Res.* 1995;(320):110–114.
30. Zvijac JE, Lemak L, Schurhoff MR, et al. Analysis of arthroscopically assisted ankle arthrodesis. *Arthroscopy.* 2002;18(1):70–75.

Arthroscopic Subtalar Arthrodesis

Phinit Phisitkul • Tanawat Vaseenon

Subtalar arthrodesis has been successfully used for the treatment of subtalar arthritis, subtalar instability, tibialis posterior tendon dysfunction, and talocalcaneal coalition. Advances in foot and ankle arthroscopy and instruments allowed the arthroscopic arthrodesis of the posterior subtalar joint to be technically feasible in select cases. Tasto (1) described the technique with the patient in a lateral position using a combination of portals placed laterally. Amendola et al. (2) described posterior arthroscopic subtalar arthrodesis (PASTA) using the posterior hindfoot endoscopy portals, with the patient in a prone position. The efficacy and safety of the technique was supported by anatomical studies and a number of case series. The advantages of this technique include minimal pain, less scarring, fewer wound complications, high fusion rate, and that it is performed as outpatient surgery. With proper patient selection and familiarity with the technique, the arthroscopic subtalar arthrodesis may be found to be a useful addition to the surgeon's armamentarium.

CLINICAL EVALUATION OF SUBTALAR PAIN

History and Physical Examination

Patients with subtalar joint problems usually present with activity-related pain and swelling in the hindfoot aggravated by walking on uneven grounds. Common pathologies of the subtalar joint include primary arthritis, inflammatory arthritis, posttraumatic arthritis, and talocalcaneal (T-C) coalition. History of underlying systemic arthropathy or previous injuries should be obtained. Patients with T-C coalition have the onset of pain in the second decade but some presents in their 30s, often after an injury.

Physical examination should include screening for the involvement of the hips, the knees, and the back. Thorough examination of the foot and ankle is the cornerstone of the clinical evaluation. Gait and limb alignment should be observed with the patient both standing and walking

(Fig. 94.1A, B). Swelling of the subtalar joint is located around the subfibular area. Disappearance of the subfibular concavity is sometimes observed. Any surgical scar seen should be documented. Patients with T-C coalition involving the middle facet may have a bony prominence in the posteromedial ankle (Fig. 94.2). This structure may compress the tibial nerve simulating symptoms and signs of a tarsal tunnel syndrome in up to one-third of the cases. Tenderness on palpation of the subtalar joint is the most useful test in the evaluation of subtalar problems. Maximum tenderness is usually triggered by palpation along the subtalar joint laterally just distal to the tip of the fibula. Attention should be paid to rule out pain from the peroneal tendons, which are located superficial to the subtalar joint. Direct palpation over the peroneal tendons while the patient holds the foot in dorsiflexion and eversion can help differentiate the source of tenderness. The sinus tarsi area is sensitive to direct pressure, therefore a comparative evaluation of the contralateral side is recommended. Crepitus can be felt at the joint line while the foot is passively everted and inverted. Patient with a T-C coalition may have tenderness on palpation over the middle facet just dorsal to the sustentaculum tali. Range of motion of the subtalar joint is evaluated with the knee in 90° of flexion in prone or sitting position. In patients with a T-C coalition, the range of subtalar motion can be deceptively normal due to the compensatory motion through the transverse tarsal joint. Peroneal spastic flatfoot, if present, is suggestive of the presence of T-C coalition. The peroneal muscle spasms can be demonstrated by passive forced plantarflexion or inversion. Flexibility of the coronal plane malalignment, varus or valgus, can be evaluated using Coleman's blocks. When the alignment is improved with the blocks, medial or lateral forefoot postings can be applicable as a mean of nonoperative treatment.

Imaging

Radiographic evaluation is essential for the evaluation of subtalar joint. We recommend weight-bearing, orthogonal views of the foot and ankle, oblique views of the foot, and a hindfoot alignment view. Ankle joint should be carefully

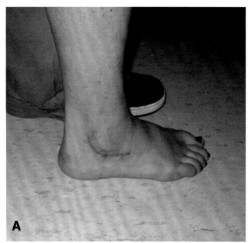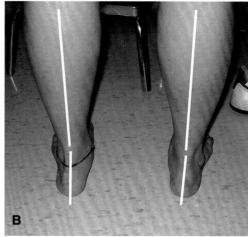

FIGURE 94.1. The patient is observed from the lateral **(A)** and the posterior **(B)** aspects. The surgical incision and a mild degree of subfibular swelling over the subtalar joint are documented. The hindfoot alignment of the right side is in slight varus compared with the normal valgus alignment of the contralateral limb.

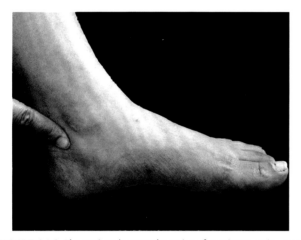

FIGURE 94.2. The patient locates the point of maximum pain corresponding to a bony prominence due to a T-C coalition.

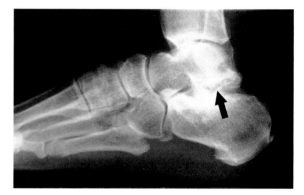

FIGURE 94.3. A weight-bearing lateral view of the left foot in a patient with posttraumatic arthritis of the subtalar joint is demonstrated. Subchondral sclerosis and obliteration of the joint space is observed in the posterior facet *(arrow).*

evaluated because of the high incidence of overlapping symptoms. The subtalar joint is best visualized on the lateral view. Subchondral sclerosis, subchondral cysts, osteophytes, and joint space narrowing are common findings in arthritis (Fig. 94.3). Articular incongruities and surgical implants often present in posttraumatic arthritis after a calcaneus fracture. Evidence of T-C coalition includes nonvisualization of the middle facet, dysmorphic sustentaculum tali, shortening of the talar neck, and the C-sign (3,4) (Fig. 94.4). Talar beaking is most commonly seen in T-C coalition (39%) but can be associated with calcaneonavicular coalition (19%) as well (5). A Harris view of the calcaneus can sometimes demonstrate a coalition in the middle facet as well as medial osteophytes. A hindfoot alignment view can give objective evidence of coronal plane deformity of the hindfoot, which may be helpful in surgical planning.

Image-guided injection of local anesthetic agent is particularly useful as a part of making a therapeutic diagnosis

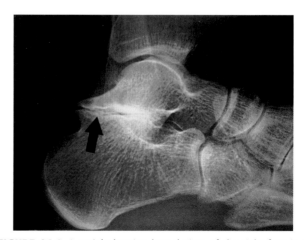

FIGURE 94.4. A weight-bearing lateral view of the right foot in a 25-year-old patient with T-C coalition is demonstrated. Large bone spurs are evident on the posterior aspect of the posterior facet *(arrow).* The sustentaculum tali is poorly visualized.

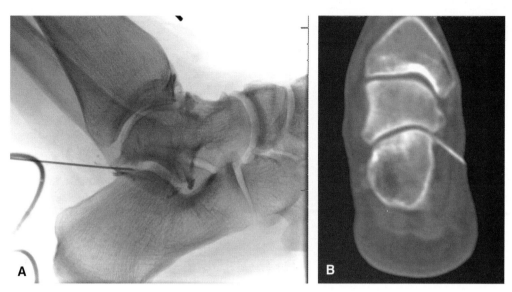

FIGURE 94.5. Flouroscopic-guided injection of the posterior subtalar joint is demonstrated **(A)**. In this case, contrast media is seen in the anterolateral, posterior, and medial aspects of the posterior subtalar joint. Expansion of the contrast media in to the ankle joint is also observed. CT-guided injection of the posterior subtalar joint in a postoperative case with a painful stiffness of the subtalar joint is shown **(B)**.

(Fig. 94.5A, B). Injections under fluoroscopic guidance have been shown to be helpful in differentiating pain from the ankle and/or the subtalar joint prior to an arthrodesis. However, the communication between the ankle and the posterior subtalar joint is present in about 10% of patients. Cortisone can be added if the anti-inflammatory effects are desired after risks and benefits have been explained to the patient. Pain relief can be more predictable after a subtalar arthrodesis when all or most of the pain is eliminated immediately after the injection.

A CT scan can best demonstrate the osseous anatomy of the subtalar joint. It is considered the gold standard for diagnosing a T-C coalition (6). The degree of arthritis can be clearly shown together with periarticular osteophytes and loose bodies (Fig. 94.6A, B). MRI has not been commonly used for the evaluation of the subtalar joint due to availability and cost. However, it has a definitive role in the evaluation of bone edema, stress fracture, and nonosseous coalition (Fig. 94.7).

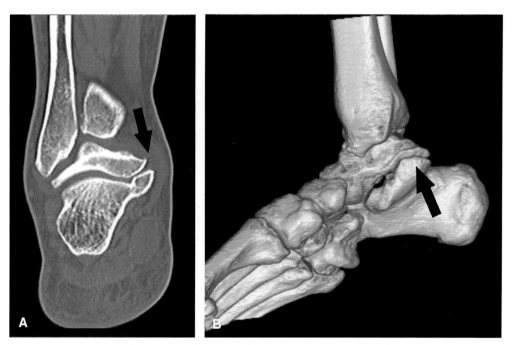

FIGURE 94.6. A and **B:** The CT coronal image and the 3D-reconstruction view of the right foot in a patient with T-C coalition are shown. The extent and shape of the involved part of the posterior subtalar joint is well illustrated *(arrow)*.

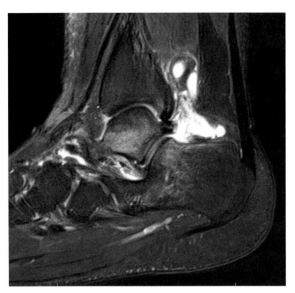

FIGURE 94.7. The sagittal T2 MRI image of a patient with pain from an overuse injury of the subtalar joint is demonstrated. The marrow edema and joint effusion around the posterior subtalar joint is seen.

Decision-Making Algorithms

We have not seen a classification of the subtalar arthritis reported in English literature. Most clinicians rely on the presence of symptoms and the response to nonoperative management to guide further treatments. The subtalar joint is mechanically delicate and can cause substantial pain in spite of minimal radiographic changes (1). On the other hand, severe arthrosis of the subtalar joint may allow little motion and can be asymptomatic. Subtalar arthrodesis is usually the only available option after a failure of nonoperative treatment.

The pathology of the tarsal coalition can be classified into osseous, fibrous, or cartilaginous. The amount of articular involvement can be determined with a CT scan, as the degree of posterior facet involvement has shown association with success after a resection (7). There is no universally accepted protocol in the treatment of T-C coalition. From the available evidence, the resection of coalition is suitable for adolescents with posterior facet involvement of less than 50%; while an arthrodesis is indicated in adolescents with posterior facet involvement greater than 50%, or in patients of any age with arthritis. The treatment in adults with symptomatic coalition without arthritis is inconclusive. We reserve the resection of the T-C coalition for only select cases with minimal involvement of the posterior facet, normal posterior facet joint space, relatively preserved subtalar motion, and absence of tenderness of the lateral subtalar joint. The decision-making algorithms are shown in Figure 94.8.

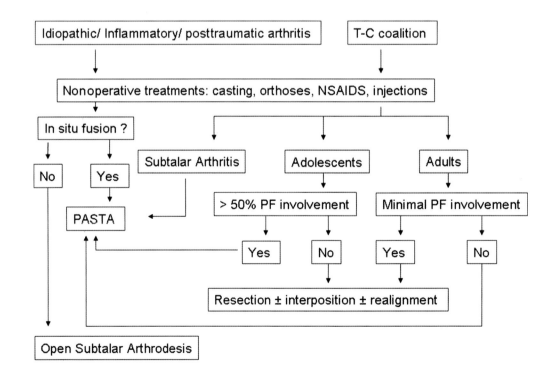

PF = posterior facet of the subtalar joint

FIGURE 94.8. Decision-making algorithms for subtalar arthritis and T-C coalition.

TREATMENT

Nonoperative Treatment

Nonoperative methods are effective and should be used routinely as first-line treatment, especially for symptomatic T-C coalitions; they have a success rate up to 80%. The goal is to decrease inflammation and mechanical overload of the joint. Anti-inflammatory medication and acetaminophen can be helpful additions. Intra-articular cortisone injections are effective in cases with inflammatory arthropathy such as rheumatoid arthritis, seronegative spondyloarthropathy, systemic lupus erythematosus, and gout. Repetitive injections may accelerate cartilage degradation and increase risk of joint infection. Orthoses are the mainstays of nonoperative treatment (Fig. 94.9). Various types of orthoses with different degree of corrective and accommodative characteristics have been used with the goal of decreasing subtalar motion and normalizing tibial rotation. An optimal amount of medial or lateral forefoot

posting can be applied to the orthosis if the deformity is supple. Shoe inserts are generally helpful in shock absorption and mild alignment control. The University of California Biomechanics Laboratory (UCBL) shoe inserts have improved hindfoot control due to their higher trim-lines. Ankle-foot-orthoses and Arizona braces are reserved for cases with severe deformity necessitating a control proximal in the calf. Below-the-knee walking casts or boots are useful as short-term treatment when the pain is severe.

Operative Indications, Timing, and Technique

The most common operative indication for subtalar arthrodesis is intractable pain due to an arthritis or a T-C coalition. Patient should have failed nonoperative treatment for at least 3 to 6 months before considering operative treatment. The surgery can be performed with either an open or an arthroscopic approach. Isolated subtalar arthrodesis by an open approach has been widely used, with a fusion rate of 84% to 100% in primary cases

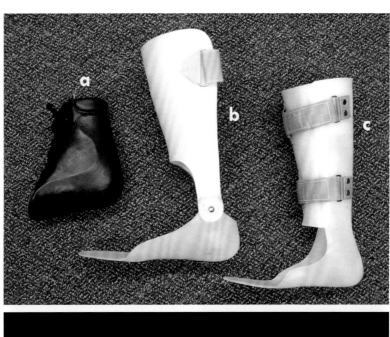
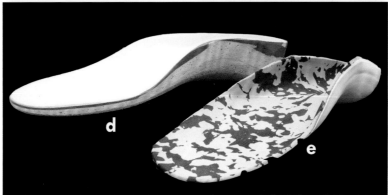

FIGURE 94.9. Commonly used orthoses for subtalar joint pain are demonstrated. (**A:** Arizona brace; **B:** hinged AFO; **C:** rigid AFO; **D:** composite custom insert; **E:** UCBL insert.) (Courtesy of Donald G Shurr, C.P.O., P.T.)

VI. Foot and Ankle

(8–10). The open technique is recommended in a postoperative situation when extensive scar formation prevents arthroscopic access. Lateral extensile exposure also allows surgeons to remove hardware or osseous mass on the lateral side of the calcaneus as well as an opportunity for the realignment calcaneus osteotomy and structural bone grafting to be done (Fig. 94.10). The overall favorable outcome of the open subtalar arthrodesis was mixed with relatively high complication in some series (11–13). Arthroscopic approach is advantageous in preserving blood supply to the bone, minimizing soft tissue injury, and decreasing postoperative pain and scarring. The fusion time of the arthroscopic approach is generally shorter than the open technique (9, 14). Although arthroscopic approach has been used mainly for an in situ fusion, a considerable amount of hindfoot alignment can be changed through arthroscopic release and joint debridement. Arthroscopic-assisted arthrodesis, however, requires greater arthroscopic understanding of the anatomy of the hindfoot and some laboratory cadaver training. The posterior facet is the only joint to be fused for most subtalar arthrodeses. It can be approached from either the lateral or the posterior aspect. The lateral approach uses a combination of anterior, middle, and posterior portals for the cartilage debridement in lateral decubitus position (1, 15). We have found it quite difficult to debride the cartilage in the posteromedial aspect of the subtalar joint because of the contour and the tightness of the joint. The posterior approach to the subtalar joint using three posterior portals allows a more direct approach to the entire posterior facet (Fig. 94.11). Access to the posteromedial aspect of the joint is possible due to the release of the posterior T-C ligaments and flexor retinaculum overlying the flexor hallucis longus (FHL) tendon. The addition of posteromedial portal increases the working area in the posterior aspect of the subtalar joint by 45% (16). The alignment of the hindfoot is better controlled in this position and allows

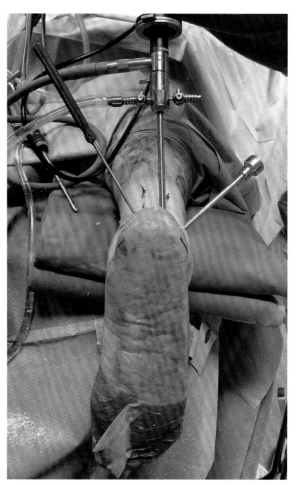

FIGURE 94.11. The PASTA is performed through three hindfoot portals with the patient in prone position.

straight posterior observation. Indications and contraindications of the arthroscopic subtalar arthrodesis are listed in Table 94.1.

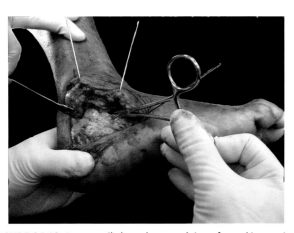

FIGURE 94.10. An extensile lateral approach is performed in a patient with neglected calcaneal fracture. It allows exostectomy of the lateral calcaneal wall as well as distraction arthrodesis of the subtalar joint.

Table 94.1

Indications and contraindications of arthroscopic subtalar arthrodesis

Indications

Idiopathic/ inflammatory/posttraumatic arthritis of the subtalar joint
Most talocalcaneal coalitions in adults
Talocalcaneal coalitions involving 50% or more in adolescents

Contraindications

Overlying soft tissue infection
Severe postoperative scarring or joint ankylosis

AUTHORS' PREFERRED TREATMENT

Posterior Arthroscopic Subtalar Arthrodesis

Patient Positioning

The procedure is performed with the patient under general anesthesia combined with a regional block. Preoperative intravenous antibiotics are routinely administered. A thigh tourniquet is placed while the patient is in the supine position. Padding is properly placed on the operating table. The patient is then turned into prone position with the feet hung free, allowing full dorsiflexion. The operated foot is observed from the end of the bed to make sure the long axis of the foot is in a vertical line. External rotation of the foot can make orientation difficult and pose risks of the neurovascular injuries. The bed can be tilted toward the operated side, with a post placed next to the ipsilateral iliac crest to prevent the patient from falling (Fig. 94.12).

Room Setup

The arthroscopic monitor is placed at the head of bed on the contralateral side. The operating room nurse and the instrument table are toward the middle of the bed on the ipsilateral side. The area around the end of the bed is kept free for the surgeon, assistants, and the fluoroscopic machine (Fig. 94.13).

Instruments

The required instruments for PASTA are shown in Figure 94.14. We generally use 4.0-mm arthroscope because it provides a wide visual field (115°) and stable pictures. This big arthroscope also tolerates stiff joints and aggressive instrumentation better than small ones. The scope does not need to be inserted between joint surfaces as much as it needs to directly observe them from behind. We have found 4-mm shavers to be appropriate for cartilage removal.

Portals

Three portals are required for visualization and instrumentation (Fig. 94.15). The posterolateral and the

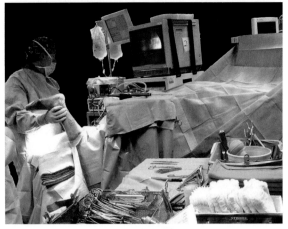

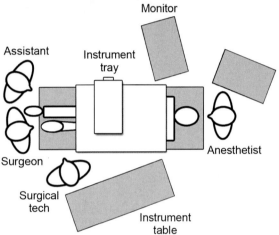

FIGURE 94.13. The diagram demonstrates the room setup for PASTA. (**A:** surgeon; **B:** assistant; **C:** scrub nurse; **D:** instrument table; **E:** arthroscopic instrument tray; **F:** arthroscopic tower and monitor; **G:** anesthesiologist's area.)

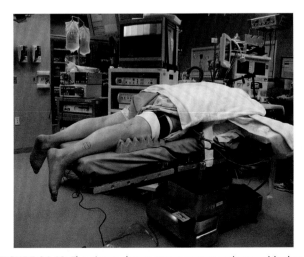

FIGURE 94.12. The picture demonstrates proper patient positioning.

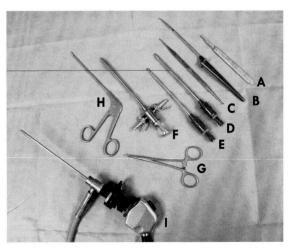

FIGURE 94.14. Required instruments for PASTA. (**A:** scapel; **B:** small joint probe; **C:** Small curette; **D:** 4.0 mm round burr; **E:** 4.0 mm bone cutting shaver; **F:** arthroscopic cannula; **G:** curved hemostat; **H:** arthroscopic scissors; **I:** 4.0 mm 30° arthroscope and camera.)

VI. Foot and Ankle

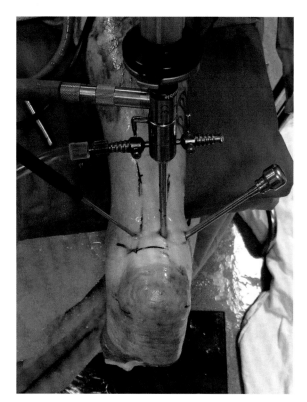

FIGURE 94.15. The intraoperative picture of PASTA on the right leg with the patient in prone position is demonstrated. The arthroscope is inserted through the posterolateral portal while a probe is placed through the posteromedial portal. An arthroscopic trocar is inserted through the accessory posterolateral portal for joint distraction.

posteromedial portals, as described by van Dijk, are created at the beginning of the procedure. They are located just next to the Achilles tendon on either side at about 1.5 to 2 cm proximal to the proximal aspect of the calcaneal tuberosity. The accessory posterolateral portal is usually created under direct visualization at approximately 1 cm proximal and 1 cm posterior to the tip of the lateral malleolus. It is located just posterior to the peroneal tendon sheath at an angle parallel to the joint surface.

Surgical Technique

The step-by-step pictures of PASTA are shown in Figure 94.16A–O. The surgery is performed under tourniquet to maximize visualization. The posterolateral portal is first established using a scalpel. A curved hemostat is used to carefully dissect through the subcutaneous tissue toward the second toe. Often, the trigonal process or the os trigonum is palpable as a small bony prominence. The blunt arthroscopic trocar and cannula is inserted at the same direction until a bony stop is felt. The posteromedial portal is made and a curved hemostat is used to create a soft tissue tunnel directly toward the arthroscopic cannula in the plane just anterior to the Achilles tendon. The tip of the hemostat is then advanced anteriorly along the shaft of the cannula toward the tip while keeping both instruments in direct contact. In essence, the cannula in the posterolateral portal is used as a guide so that

the risk of neurovascular injury from the posteromedial portal placement is minimized. The tip of the hemostat is visualized with the arthroscope. A 4-mm shaver is inserted through the posteromedial portal into the same soft tissue tunnel after the hemostat is removed. The shaver tip is visualized and advanced toward the lateral aspect of the subtalar joint. The shaver tip should be palpable just distal to the fibula and anterior to the peroneal tendons. Capsulectomy and partial synovectomy of the subtalar joint is made until the subtalar joint is visualized. Thick transverse fibers of the posterior talofibular ligament (PTFL) are observed proximal to the shaver. The shaver is then placed directly on the proximal aspect of the PTFL. While the face is turned laterally, the posterior capsule of the ankle joint is partially debrided toward the medial aspect. The FHL is identified on the posteromedial aspect of the ankle joint by passively moving the big toe. At this stage, the posterior ankle joint can be examined if needed. The FHL is used as a landmark to avoid the neurovascular structures just medial to it. The FHL tendon sheath is partially released with arthroscopic scissors until the posteromedial aspect of the subtalar joint is visualized. The soft tissue in the posterior aspect of the subtalar joint can be thoroughly debrided with a shaver. The accessory posterolateral portal is localized using a no. 18 needle as described earlier. A curved hemostat is used to bluntly dissect down to the joint while avoiding the adjacent sural nerve. A trocar or a narrow osteotome is inserted through the accessory posterolateral portal into the most lateral aspect of the posterior subtalar joint. The instrument is wedged into the joint and holds the joint open. The cartilage is debrided through the posterolateral and the posteromedial portal. The most lateral aspect of the joint is debrided through the posterolateral portals whereas the trocar is inserted through the posteromedial portal into the medial aspect of the joint. The entire articular cartilage of the posterior facet is removed with a shaver, a burr, and multiangled curettes. Care is taken to avoid altering the joint geometry. A 4-mm round bur can be helpful to create spot-welds for vascular ingrowth in the subchondral bone. Alternatively, a narrow osteotome is inserted through the posterolateral portal to make shingles on both facets. The joint is positioned into inversion or eversion through the manipulation of the midfoot and forefoot. In cases with significant bone loss, injectable demineralized bone matrix (DBX; Synthes; Oberdorf, Switzerland) is used to fill into the gap. Two 6.5- or 7.3-mm cannulated screws are used to stabilize the construct. They are inserted under fluoroscopic monitoring to make sure that all the threads are with the talus, and there is no penetration into the ankle joint. The screw heads should be countersunk to avoid heel pad irritation on weight-bearing.

COMPLICATIONS, CONTROVERSIES, AND SPECIAL CONSIDERATIONS

Although high level of evidence is lacking, the overall results of PASTA are encouraging. Amendola et al. (2)

reported early experience of PASTA performed at the University of Iowa in 11 ft. The preoperative diagnoses were posttraumatic arthritis after a fracture of the calcaneus (2 ft), a fracture of the talus (one patient), primary subtalar arthritis (three patients, one bilateral), residual T-C coalition (three patients), and inflammatory arthritis after Crohn's disease (one patient). Ten of them fused by 10 weeks and one became a nonunion. Carro et al. (17) performed PASTA in 4 ft with posttraumatic arthritis after intra-articular calcaneal fractures. The authors used posteromedial and posterolateral portals without joint distraction. Radiographic union was evident in all at a mean of 8 weeks. Beimers et al. (14) reported PASTA in three patients with T-C coalition. The authors distracted the joint by introducing a blunt trocar through a sinus tarsi portal.

The bony union was evident by radiographs at 6 weeks following surgery in all three patients.

Tasto (1) reported arthroscopic subtalar arthrodesis through a lateral approach in 25 patients. The diagnoses were posttraumatic arthritis (10 patients), osteoarthritis (8 patients), posterior tibial tendon dysfunction (4 patients), rheumatoid arthritis (2 patients), and T-C coalition (1 patient). The subtalar joint of all the patients completely fused clinically and radiographically at the mean of 8.9 weeks. Glanzmann et al. (15) successfully fused 41 primary and posttraumatic subtalar joints arthroscopically through the lateral approach. The authors advocate a resection of the interosseous ligament and extension of the joint debridement into the middle and anterior facets. Proximal tibia autograft was used routinely

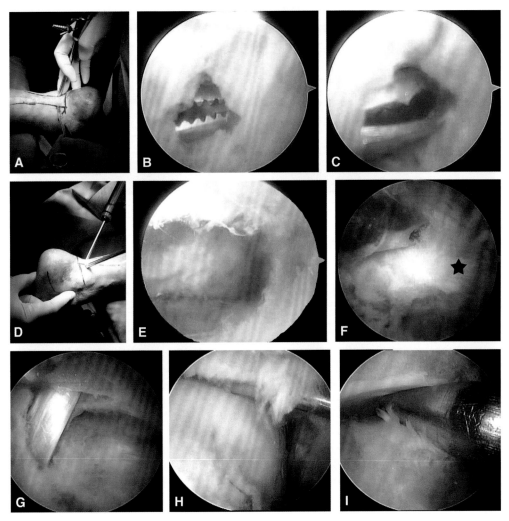

FIGURE 94.16. The surgical steps of PASTA in a patient with posttraumatic arthritis of the right subtalar joint are demonstrated. **A:** A curved hemostat is inserted from the posteromedial portal toward the arthroscopic cannula. **B:** The tip of the hemostat is visualized in the deep soft tissue plane. **C:** The hemostat is replaced by an arthroscopic shaver. **D:** The shaver is advanced toward the lateral aspect of the posterior subtalar joint. The shaver tip is palpable just distal to the fibula. **E:** A partial capsulotomy of the subtalar joint is performed by gentle shaving. The posterior subtalar joint is visualized through the debrided capsule. **F:** The posterior ankle capsule is debrided with shaver tip just proximal to the PTFL (*star*). **G:** The FHL tendon is visualized in the posteromedial aspect of the ankle joint. **H:** The accessory posterolateral portal is located using a no. 19 needle. **I:** A blunt trocar is inserted through the accessory posterolateral portal to distract the joint.

VI. Foot and Ankle

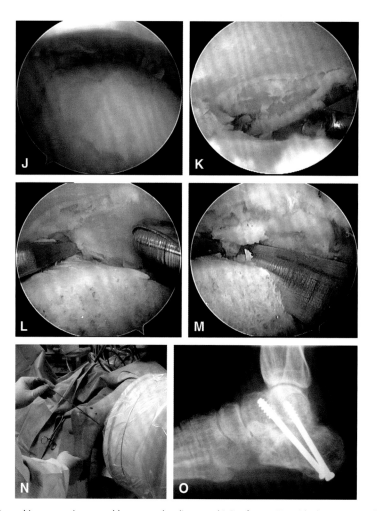

FIGURE 94.16. *(continued)* **J:** A working space is created between the distracted joint facets. **K:** With the trocar in the lateral aspect of the joint, the cartilage is debrided using a shaver and curettes. **L:** The joint is distracted with a narrow osteotome from the posteromedial portal while the cartilage on the lateral aspect of the joint is debrided. **M:** Shingles are made on both sides of the joint using a narrow osteotome. **N:** The trajectory of the screws is determined under fluoroscopic guidance. **O:** The postoperative lateral radiograph of PASTA with two 6.5-mm cannulated screws.

to promote fusion. Scranton (18) successfully performed arthroscopic subtalar arthrodesis in 5 patients with degenerative or posttraumatic arthritis through the lateral approach. An AO distractor was used for joint distraction.

Complications

The complication rate from arthroscopic subtalar arthrodesis has been shown to be very low in the published case series. Apart from three cases with a delay union in Glanzmann's series (15) and a case of nonunion in Amendola's series (2), there has been no other complication reported in English literature. This may reflect the fact that the technique is performed only by a limited group of experienced surgeons. However, other potential complications are possible in this technique and should be prevented including neurovascular injuries, hindfoot malalignment, and hardware-related problems.

Controversies

There are variations of the joint distraction methods used in the arthroscopic subtalar arthrodesis. Joint preparation

can be performed without distraction by removing a block of cartilage and subchondral bone at the same thickness of a shaver or a bur while observing through the scope posteriorly. (17). Distraction of the joint will allow the surgeons to selectively remove the cartilage and preserve the subchondral bone. As described previously, we generally use a blunt trocar or a narrow osteotome to wedge the joint opened from an accessory posterolateral portal. The trocar can also be inserted from the sinus tarsi, in line with the joint, and wedged in the joint to serve the same purpose (14). Additional techniques have been described for joint distraction through the lateral approach including using a small laminar spreader inserted through the sinus tarsi or using an AO distractor.

There is no evidence to support or to discourage the use of morselized cancellous allograft or autograft in arthroscopic subtalar arthrodesis. Most of the authors achieved a very high fusion rate without using any bone graft (1, 14, 17). The use of bone graft is not indicated in a simple case where well vascularized subchondral surfaces are obtained. Bone graft may be helpful, if available, in cases with significant bone loss or a persistent gap after the osteosynthesis.

There is no consensus in the postoperative weight-bearing status after the subtalar fusion. Tasto (1) allowed patient to bear full weight in an AFO right after the surgery. Carro et al. immobilized the patient in a short leg cast but allowed weight-bearing at 3 weeks. Similar to Amendola et al. (2) and Beimers et al. (14), we have been generally conservative: 6 weeks of non–weight-bearing in a cast or a boot.

Special Considerations

Heel pad irritation due to prominent screw heads can be troublesome. Following an open subtalar fusion, screw removal was required in 20% to 39% of cases (11, 15, 19). Using headless screws, there was no need of screw removal in Carro's series. It has been our experience as well those headless screws are particularly useful in this location. Alternatively, for the headed screws, we pay attention to the location of the screw head on the calcaneus, which should be just proximal to the heel pad. The thick cortical bone should be countersunk to allow the screw head to be less prominent.

Posterior hindfoot endoscopies are not without risk. Surgeons should be aware of anatomical variations that can lead to complications, especially neurovascular injuries. Variations of the arteries in the hindfoot may allow an arterial injury even in the area lateral to the FHL tendon, especially those whose posterior tibial artery is thin or absent (0% to 2%) with dominant peroneal artery at risk traversing across the posterolateral ankle toward the tarsal tunnel. Preoperative evaluation of the pedal pulses is essential. The peroneocalcaneus internus muscle, "The False FHL," can imitate the FHL, causing the surgeon to direct the shaver toward the neurovascular bundles. This muscle has much less excursion than the real FHL when the big toe is passively moved and can be identified using preoperative MRI. Variations in the cutaneous nerve of the foot are very common. Surgeon should take care of the arthroscopic portal as if there is a nerve directly underneath. The accessory posterolateral is particularly close to the sural nerve and gentle soft tissue manipulation is required.

PEARLS AND PITFALLS

1. Ensure proper patient selection. Local anesthetic injection may help differentiating pain between the ankle and the subtalar joint.
2. Arthroscopic subtalar arthrodesis is recommended for surgeons familiarized with small joint endoscopy techniques and hindfoot anatomy. Laboratory cadaver training can be helpful.
3. For PASTA, patients should be positioned so that the foot is in a vertical plane to ensure proper orientation of the surgeons.
4. To avoiding neurovascular injuries, all portals should be established and handled with care. Always be vigilant for anatomical variations.

5. The joint should be sufficiently distracted using a trocar or a narrow osteotome inserted from an accessory portal.
6. The subcondral bone should be preserved but subsequently stimulated by making multiple spot welds or shingles.
7. Two large cannulated screws are preferred for the fixation of posterior facet of the subtalar joint. Headless screws may help avoid heel pad irritation.

REHABILITATION

The patient is usually placed in a postoperative plaster splint for 10 to 14 days followed by a boot or a cast for 4 more weeks. At 6 weeks, the radiographs are taken to verify a union. The patient is then allowed to bear weight as tolerated and wean off from the boot. If the union is uncertain, the patient is allowed to walk in a boot and radiographic studies are repeated 4 weeks later. The cannulated screws do not require a routine removal. However, they can be removed after a successful arthrodesis if needed due to heel pad irritation.

CONCLUSIONS AND FUTURE DIRECTIONS

Arthroscopic subtalar arthrodesis is a minimally invasive technique, and it is one that shows the advantages of endoscopic surgery. It has a high fusion rate and low complications. The techniques are simple, but there is a learning curve that requires laboratory skill practice. Currently, it is indicated for in situ arthrodesis or in cases with mild deformity. Because of its versatility, more advances in the technique will allow arthroscopic subtalar arthrodesis to be applicable to more complicated cases, for example, revision arthrodesis or moderate to severe hindfoot malalignment in conjunction with open or percutaneous osteotomies. Computer navigation may assist in alignment correction and hardware placement. Other invasive or noninvasive means of subtalar joint distraction may improve the access to the joint. Biologic manipulation and the use of growth factors or bone grafting may be found applicable in very high-risk patients.

REFERENCES

1. Tasto JP. Arthroscopy of the subtalar joint and arthroscopic subtalar arthrodesis. *Instr Course Lect.* 2006;55:555–564.
2. Amendola A, Lee KB, Saltzman CL, et al. Technique and early experience with posterior arthroscopic subtalar arthrodesis. *Foot Ankle Int.* 2007;28(3):298–302.
3. Lateur LM, Van Hoe LR, Van Ghillewe KV, et al. Subtalar coalition: diagnosis with the C sign on lateral radiographs of the ankle. *Radiology.* 1994;193(3):847–851.
4. Crim JR, Kjeldsberg KM. Radiographic diagnosis of tarsal coalition. *AJR Am J Roentgenol.* 2004;182(2):323–328.
5. Nalaboff KM, Schweitzer ME. MRI of tarsal coalition: frequency, distribution, and innovative signs. *Bull NYU Hosp Jt Dis.* 2008;66(1):14–21.
6. Herzenberg JE, Goldner JL, Martinez S, et al. Computerized tomography of talocalcaneal tarsal coalition: a clinical and anatomic study. *Foot Ankle.* 1986;6(6):273–288.

7. Wilde PH, Torode IP, Dickens DR, et al. Resection for symptomatic talocalcaneal coalition. *J Bone Joint Surg Br.* 1994;76(5):797–801.

8. Dahm DL, Kitaoka HB. Subtalar arthrodesis with internal compression for post-traumatic arthritis. *J Bone Joint Surg Br.* 1998;80(1):134–138.

9. Mann RA, Baumgarten M. Subtalar fusion for isolated subtalar disorders. Preliminary report. *Clin Orthop Relat Res.* 1988;(226):260–265.

10. Mann RA, Beaman DN, Horton GA. Isolated subtalar arthrodesis. *Foot Ankle Int.* 1998;19(8):511–519.

11. Easley ME, Trnka HJ, Schon LC, et al. Isolated subtalar arthrodesis. *J Bone Joint Surg Am.* 2000;82(5):613–624.

12. Carr JB, Hansen ST, Benirschke SK. Subtalar distraction bone block fusion for late complications of os calcis fractures. *Foot Ankle.* 1988;9(2):81–86.

13. Flemister AS Jr, Infante AF, Sanders RW, et al. Subtalar arthrodesis for complications of intra-articular calcaneal fractures. *Foot Ankle Int.* 2000;21(5):392–399.

14. Beimers L, de Leeuw PA, van Dijk CN. A 3-portal approach for arthroscopic subtalar arthrodesis. *Knee Surg Sports Traumatol Arthrosc.* 2009;17(7):830–834.

15. Glanzmann MC, Sanhueza-Hernandez R. Arthroscopic subtalar arthrodesis for symptomatic osteoarthritis of the hindfoot: a prospective study of 41 cases. *Foot Ankle Int.* 2007;28(1):2–7.

16. Phisitkul P, Tochigi Y, Saltzman CL, et al. Arthroscopic visualization of the posterior subtalar joint in the prone position: a cadaver study. *Arthroscopy.* 2006;22(5):511–515.

17. Carro LP, Golano P, Vega J. Arthroscopic subtalar arthrodesis: the posterior approach in the prone position. *Arthroscopy.* 2007;23(4):445.e1–445.e4.

18. Scranton PE Jr. Comparison of open isolated subtalar arthrodesis with autogenous bone graft versus outpatient arthroscopic subtalar arthrodesis using injectable bone morphogenic protein-enhanced graft. *Foot Ankle Int.* 1999;20(3):162–165.

19. Radnay CS, Clare MP, Sanders RW. Subtalar fusion after displaced intra-articular calcaneal fractures: does initial operative treatment matter? *J Bone Joint Surg Am.* 2009;91(3):541–546.

Index

Note: Page numbers followed by *f* indicate figures; those followed by *t* indicate tables.